PASS CCRN®!

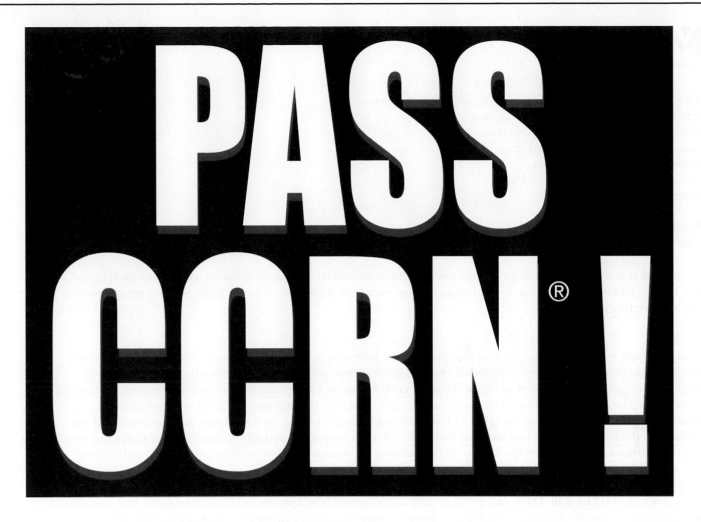

Second edition

ROBIN DONOHOE DENNISON
RN, MSN, CCRN, CS
Critical Care Consultant
Lexington, KY

With 241 illustrations

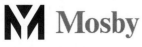 Mosby

An Affiliate of Elsevier

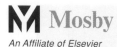

Mosby
An Affiliate of Elsevier

Vice President and Nursing Editorial Director: Sally Schrefer
Executive Editor: Barbara Nelson Cullen
Developmental Editor: Cindi Anderson
Associate Developmental Editor: Eric Ham
Project Manager: John Rogers
Senior Production Editor: Beth Hayes
Designer: Kathi Gosche

SECOND EDITION
Copyright © 2000 by Mosby, Inc.

NOTICE

Pharmacology is an ever-changing field. Standard safety precautions must be followed, but as new research and clinical experience broaden our knowledge, changes in treatment and drug therapy may become necessary or appropriate. Readers are advised to check the most current product information provided by the manufacturer of each drug to be administered to verify the recommended dose, the method and duration of administration, and contraindications. It is the responsibility of the treating physician, relying on experience and knowledge of the patient, to determine dosages and the best treatment for each individual patient. Neither the publisher nor the editor assumes any liability for any injury and/or damage to persons or property arising from this publication.

Permissions may be sought directly from Elsevier's Health Sciences Rights Department in Philadelphia, USA: phone: (+1)215-238-7869, fax: (+1)215-238-2239, email: healthpermissions@elsevier.com. You may also complete your request on-line via the Elsevier Science homepage (http://www.elsevier.com), by selecting 'Customer Support' and then 'Obtaining Permissions'.

Mosby, Inc.
An Affiliate of Elsevier
11830 Westline Industrial Drive
St. Louis, Missouri 63146

Printed in China

Library of Congress Cataloging-in-Publication Data

Dennison, Robin.
    Pass CCRN®!/Robin Donohoe Dennison.—2nd ed.
        p. ; cm.
    Includes bibliographical references and index.
    ISBN 0-323-00999-9
        1. Intensive care nursing—Examinations, questions, etc. I. Title: Pass Certified Critical-Care Registered Nurse!. II. Title.
        [DNLM: 1. Critical Care—Examination Questions. 2. Critical Care—Outlines.
    3. Critical Illness—nursing—Examination Questions. 4. Critical Illness—nursing—Outlines.
    5. Nursing Assessment—Examination Questions. 6. Nursing Assessment—Outlines. WY 18.2 D411p 2000]
    RT120.I5 D46 2000
    610.73'61'076—dc21
                                                                                    99-051958

04   CL/MV   9   8   7   6

*This second edition is dedicated to my husband, my family,
my friends, my church, and my God. Thank you for loving
me and supporting me when I really need it.*

CONTRIBUTORS

Contributors to First Edition

Betty Nash Blevins, RN, MSN, CCRN, CS
Susan Carver, RN, BSN
Frank Hicks, RN, MSN, CCRN
Wendy M. Johnson, RN, CCRN
Paul Langlois, RN, PhD, CCRN

Julie Mueller, RN, MS, CCRN
Paulette Rollant, RN, PhD, CCRN
Gail Tagney, RN, MSN, CCRN, CEN, CFRN
Ann M. Walthall, Illustrator

Contributors to This Edition

Janice Dobbins Andrews, RN, MSN
JAMARDA Resources, Inc.
Winston-Salem, North Carolina

Chapter 13: Response to Diversity

Betty Nash Blevins, RN, MSN, CCRN, CS
Associate Professor of Nursing
Bluefield State College
Bluefield, West Virginia

Test questions: Neurologic, Gastrointestinal

Kimberly A. Litton, RN, MS, CS, CCRN
Clinical Education Coordinator
Harris Methodist Fort Worth
Fort Worth, Texas

Test questions: Cardiovascular, Pulmonary

Leanna R. Miller, RN, MN, CCRN, CEN, APRN
Education Specialist—Burn, Flight, Trauma
Vanderbilt University
Nashville, Tennessee

Chapter 13: Systems Thinking, Advocacy/Moral Agency, and Clinical Inquiry

Julie Gottemoller Mueller, RN, MS, CCRN
Clinical Nurse Specialist
Health Care Centers of Illinois
Blue Island, Illinois

Test questions: Cardiovascular, Gastrointestinal, Pulmonary, Renal

Connie O'Daniel, RN, MSN, CCRN
Clinical Education Specialist
Harris Methodist Fort Worth
Fort Worth, Texas

Test questions: Cardiovascular

Toni E. Simpson, RN
Staff Nurse, ICU
Veteran's Administration Medical Center
Lexington, Kentucky

Chapter 13: Response to Diversity

Linda Weld, MSN, CCRN
Director, Quality Management
Doctors Hospital
Dallas, Texas

Test questions: Cardiovascular, Pulmonary

REVIEWERS

Jeanette K. Chambers, PhD, RN, CS, CNN
The Ohio State University
Grant/Riverside Methodist Hospitals
Columbus, Ohio

Kendra Ellis, RN, MS, CCRN
Medical Education Seminars Education
  Consultant
Grandview, Texas

**Leanna R. Miller, RN, MN, CCRN, CEN,
  APRN**
Vanderbilt University
Nashville, Tennessee

Gail Tagney, RN, MSN, CCRN, CEN, CFRN
St. Xavier University
Chicago, Illinois

Linda Weld, RN, MSN, CCRN
Director, Quality Management
Doctors Hospital
Dallas, Texas

PREFACE

This book provides a selective but comprehensive review of critical care nursing. It is intended for registered nurses planning to take the CCRN® examination for certified critical care practice offered by the American Association of Critical-Care Nurses (AACN) Certification Corporation. Information is organized according to the current CCRN® examination blueprint. The blueprint is issued by the AACN Certification Corporation to identify the content areas to be tested and the percentage of the examination devoted to the content areas. Only content included in the test blueprint is included in this book, eliminating extraneous information that is not likely to be tested. This book reviews critical content and provides learning activities to assist in learning key concepts. Multiple-choice questions are provided on CD-ROM so that test-taking skills can be practiced in the same method as testing occurs.

The intent of this book is to provide various study ad preparation opportunities for nurses preparing to take the CCRN® examination offered by the AACN Certification Corporation. Teaching seminars to prepare nurses for this examination for the last 15 years has helped me learn what nurses need in order to prepare for this test and the strengths and weaknesses of current books on the market for CCRN® examination preparation.

My goal in writing this book is to help nurses prepare for the CCRN® examination by providing a pertinent content review, fun but challenging learning activities, realistic practice questions, and comprehensive practice examinations that reflect the content and complexity of the CCRN® examination.

Content Review

A succinct outline format is used, and information is written so that it is easy to read, understand, and remember. Illustrations and tables further explain and clarify content. Figures and diagrams are used to illustrate key concepts and add to verbal explanations. Numerous tables organize information in a helpful manner.

An anatomy and physiology review is included for each core body system. Although anatomy and physiology questions are unlikely to be on the examination, knowledge of anatomy and physiology is often helpful, if not essential, in correctly answering questions about assessment, intervention, or evaluation.

Assessment includes health history, physical assessment, diagnostic studies, and system-specific assessment such as hemodynamic monitoring and electrocardiography in the cardiovascular chapter, arterial blood gas interpretation in the pulmonary chapter, and intracranial pressure monitoring in the neurology chapter.

Pathologic conditions listed on the CCRN® blueprint are included in the content review. Headings in this area are Definition, Etiology, Pathophysiology, Nursing Diagnoses, Clinical Presentation, and Collaborative Management. Collaborative Management includes medical and

nursing management specific to the disease entity. Also included in this second edition is a review of key content areas found in the new component of the test referred to as Professional Caring and Ethical Practice.

Learning Activities

Learning activities test recall, organize information in a new manner, and ask questions in a different way. In his book, *A Whack on the Side of the Head,* Roger von Oeck advocates changing the question to come up with the right answer or right answers. This is the basis for the learning activities. You will not see matching questions, essays, table completion exercises, or crossword puzzles on the CCRN® examination. They are used here to encourage you to look at the information in a different way. I hope you will find the crossword puzzles and other activities an enjoyable way to review terminology, anatomy and physiology, and pharmacology.

Review Questions

The review questions are written in the same format as the CCRN® examination. There are questions for each component of the blueprint. If you want to work on cardiovascular questions, choose "cardiovascular" from the menu. Two 200-item final examinations are also included on the CD-ROM. Again, these tests are in the same format as the examination, and the content distribution matches that identified on the CCRN® blueprint.

Answers, rationale, and test-taking strategies are given for all practice questions. Rationale explains why the correct answer is the best answer, while test-taking strategies show how to think through questions if you do not know the content. Both of these will make you a better test-taker on the important day of the CCRN® examination. Analysis of your performance on the practice examination will help you to focus your final preparation on your weak areas.

Appendix A is a table with the nursing diagnoses commonly used in critical care. The table includes Nursing Diagnoses, Defining Characteristics, Nursing Interventions, and Expected Outcomes. Appendix B is a list of abbreviations used in this book and common in critical care. The term is always written out in the text the first time it is mentioned, but if you see it later, you may not remember what the letters stand for. This abbreviation list is to help you at that time. Appendix C lists laboratory studies that are important in the care of critically ill adults and the normal range of laboratory values for each. I recommend that you study this just before you go to take the exam, because you are expected to know the normal range of common laboratory tests. Appendix D is a listing of formulae commonly used in the evaluation of the critically ill patient. Appendix E is a table describing common critical care drugs. Knowledge of these drugs is very important in your preparation for the CCRN® examination.

This book is not a comprehensive critical care text. The focus is what is likely to be on the CCRN® examination. I believe this book is the only one you will need to help you prepare for the examination, but if you would like an additional text in which to do more reading on your weak areas, I recommend *Critical Care Nursing Diagnosis and Management,* third edition, by Thelan et al., published by Mosby, Inc.

Critical care nursing has never been more exciting and challenging. For those of us who thrive on this excitement and challenge, keeping up with new developments, research, and clinical changes provides yet another challenge. This book provides a review of selected areas of critical care and is a ready resource for succinct summary of important content.

CCRN® certification is a prestigious and important credential to hold for those of us who specialize in critical care nursing. If you study the content of this book and practice your test-taking skills, you will pass the examination. I would love to hear from you regarding your success with the test and your comments on how this book helped you or how you feel it could be more helpful. E-mail me at rddennison@aol.com or write to me at: Nursing Editorial Department, Mosby, Inc., 11830 Westline Industrial Drive, St. Louis, MO 63146.

I believe that this book will prove to be your most valuable resource in preparing for the CCRN® examination. Good luck!

Robin Donohoe Dennison

ACKNOWLEDGMENTS

First and foremost, I thank the critical care nurses who have attended CCRN® review courses that I have taught over the last 15 years. You have taught me what works and what does not, what you want and what you do not want, and how you learn and remember content. I have heard from so many critical care nurses over the last 4 years regarding how helpful this book has been. Thank you so much for that feedback.

I thank all the reviewers and item writers for this text. Objective reviews are so valuable, and writing good test questions is a special talent. I really appreciate your efforts.

I thank my wonderful editor and friend, Cindi Anderson. Flexibility is such a wonderful quality, and I have appreciated your flexibility, your encouragement, and your friendship.

And finally, I thank my physician husband, R. Russell Dennison, Jr., M.D., for listening, thinking, discussing, finding references, and encouraging me through this second edition.

CONTENTS

Contents

PASS CCRN®!

The Critical Care Certification Examination

Why Take This Examination?

- **Self-Satisfaction: Validation of Your Knowledge of Nursing Critically Ill Patients**
- **Career Mobility: A National Credential That Is as Prestigious in One State as Another**
- **Clinical Promotion**

I. This is a *clinical* credential; you must maintain a clinical practice (144 hours per year) to maintain your certification

II. Certification is often required or recommended for promotion up a clinical career ladder

Money

I. Some hospitals offer a bonus for CCRN® certification

II. Some hospitals offer an hourly differential for CCRN® certification

III. Some hospitals prefer certified nurses for clinical or administrative promotion

IV. Most hospitals reimburse the nurse for the expense of taking the test if a passing score is attained

Requirements to Take the Examination

- **Current Unrestricted RN License in the U.S. or in Any of Its Territories That Use the NCLEX for RN Licensure**
- **Clinical Practice in Critical Care**

I. Clinical hours in critical care nursing: 1750 hours within the previous 2-year period with 875 of the hours accrued in the most recent year preceding application to take the examination

II. Recommended critical experiences: these experiences are no longer required to sit for the examination but experience with these types of patients may be helpful in answering examination questions

A. Hemodynamic instability that required any of the following:
   1. Arterial pressure monitoring
   2. Central venous pressure monitoring
   3. Pulmonary artery pressure monitoring
   4. Invasive cardiac output/index determination
   5. Direct RA/LA/PA pressure monitoring
   6. Intravenous vasoactive agents
   7. Fluid resuscitation

B. Life-threatening conditions that required emergency drug administration (e.g., epinephrine, atropine)

C. Compromised air exchange that required any of the following:
   1. Continuous respiratory monitors
   2. Endotracheal intubation
   3. Newly inserted tracheostomy
   4. Nasal/facial continuous positive airway pressure (CPAP)
   5. Conventional mechanical ventilation
   6. High-frequency ventilation

D. Cardiac dysfunction that required any of the following:
   1. Continuous ECG monitoring
   2. Temporary pacemaker
   3. Elective cardioversion
   4. 12-lead ECG interpretation
   5. Transcutaneous (external) pacemaker
   6. Newly inserted permanent pacemaker
   7. Intravenous antidysrhythmic agents
   8. Intravenous thrombolytic agents
   9. Defibrillation
   10. Intravenous phosphodiesterase (PDE) inhibitors (e.g., amrinone)
   11. Mediastinal chest tube(s)
   12. Automatic implantable cardioverter defibrillator (AICD)

E. Neurologic dysfunction that required intracranial pressure monitoring devices

F. Physiologic alterations that required administration of any of the following:
   1. Intravenous paralytic agents
   2. Continuous intravenous insulin infusion
   3. Intravenous push anticonvulsant agents

BSN Not a Requirement
I. Although the American Nurses' Certification Corporation (ANCC) does require a BSN to sit for its certification examinations, the AACN is not a member of this Corporation and does not require a BSN to sit for the CCRN® examination

Maintaining Your Certification
I. Certification is for a three-year period
II. Recertification is achieved by retaking the examination or submitting the appropriate information about your continuing education and professional activities

To Obtain Application: Call AACN at (800) 899-2226

The CCRN® Examination
Basic Information About the Test
I. The test is computerized and consists of 200 multiple-choice questions to be completed within 4 hours
II. The test is administered by Professional Examination Services (PES) and is offered nationwide at Sylvan Prometric Testing Centers; these centers are open 6 days a week from 9 AM to 6 PM
   A. Instructions are given at the beginning of the examination; do take the time to read the instructions carefully
   B. You will not need a pencil; calipers and calculators are not permitted
   C. The test is designed to evaluate your command of the common body of knowledge needed to function effectively in a critical care setting

Blueprint for the CCRN® Examination
(Table 1-1)
I. The blueprint identifies the categories tested and the percentage of questions in each category
II. The blueprint is based on a Role Delineation/CCRN® Validation Study conducted by the AACN in 1998; in essence, this study identified tasks, knowledge, and experiences required of a registered nurse practicing in a critical care setting and what should be on the examination
III. The blueprint identifies what percentage of questions is in each area as well as what disease entities are on the examination
   A. Note: This book includes only content and disease entities that are on the blueprint and the examination; although it may be important to understand myxedema coma, it is not on the blueprint, not on the examination, and not in this book; focus on what is on the blueprint and the examination

Table 1-1	Blueprint for the CCRN® Examination Indicating the Distribution of Questions on Each System	
Clinical Judgment		**80%**
Cardiovascular		29%
Pulmonary		17%
Multisystem		10%
Neurology		7%
Gastrointestinal		6%
Renal		5%
Endocrine		3%
Hematology/immunology		3%
Professional Caring and Ethical Practice		**20%**
Advocacy/moral agency		4%
Caring practices		4%
Collaboration		4%
Systems thinking		2%
Response to diversity		2%
Clinical inquiry		2%
Facilitator of learning		2%

IV. The Synergy Model serves as the organizing framework (AACN, 1999)
   A. Core concept: the needs or characteristics of patients and families influence and drive the characteristics or competencies of nurses
   B. Assumptions
      1. Patients are biologic, psychologic, social, and spiritual entities who present at a particular developmental stage
      2. The patient, family, and community all contribute to providing a context for the nurse-patient relationship
      3. Patients can be described by a number of characteristics
      4. Nurses can be described in a number of dimensions
      5. A goal of nursing is to restore a patient to an optimal level of wellness as defined by the patient
   C. Patient characteristics
      1. Resiliency: the capacity to return to a restorative level of functioning using compensatory coping mechanisms; the ability to bounce back quickly after an insult
      2. Vulnerability: susceptibility to actual or potential stressors that may adversely affect patient outcomes
      3. Stability: the ability to maintain a steady-state equilibrium
      4. Complexity: the intricate entanglement of two or more systems (e.g., body, family, therapies)
      5. Resource availability: extent of resources (e.g., technical, fiscal, personal, psychologic, social)
      6. Participation in care: extent to which the patient and family engage in aspects of care

7. Participation in decision making: extent to which the patient and family engage in decision making
8. Predictability: a summative characteristic that allows one to expect a certain trajectory of illness

D. Nurse characteristics
1. Clinical judgment: clinical reasoning, which includes clinical decision making, critical thinking, and a global grasp of the situation, coupled with nursing skills acquired through a process of integrating formal and experiential knowledge
2. Advocacy/moral agency: working on another's behalf and representing the concerns of the patient, family, and community; serving as a moral agent in identifying and helping to resolve ethical and clinical concerns within the clinical setting
3. Caring practices: the constellation of nursing activities that are responsive to the uniqueness of the patient and family and that create a compassionate and therapeutic environment, with the aim of promoting comfort and preventing suffering
4. Collaboration: working with others in a way that promotes and encourages each person's contributions toward achieving optimal and realistic patient goals; collaboration involves intradisciplinary and interdisciplinary work with all colleagues
5. Systems thinking: the body of knowledge and tools that allow the nurse to appreciate the care environment from a perspective that recognizes the holistic interrelationship that exists within and across healthcare systems
6. Response to diversity: the sensitivity to recognize, appreciate, and incorporate differences into the provision of care
7. Clinical inquiry or innovator/evaluator: the ongoing process of questioning and evaluating practice, providing informed practice, and innovating through research and experiential learning
8. Facilitator of learning of patient/family educator: the ability to facilitate patient and family learning

Cognitive Levels of Questions
I. Knowledge questions require you to remember previously learned information
II. Comprehension questions require you to understand the information
III. Application questions require you to use information
IV. Analysis questions require you to break down information into its component parts and recognize commonalities, differences, and interrelationships
V. Synthesis questions require you to put parts of information together to form a new conclusion

Table 1-2   Cognitive Level Distribution of Questions on the CCRN® Examination

Level 1	Knowledge/comprehension	36%
Level 2	Application/analysis	39%
Level 3	Synthesis/evaluation	25%

Table 1-3   Nursing Process Breakdown of Questions on the CCRN® Examination

Assessment	32%
Planning	15%
Intervention/implementation	40%
Evaluation	13%

VI. Evaluation questions require you to judge the value of information
VII. Table 1-2 shows the cognitive level distribution of questions on the CCRN® examination

Nursing Process Distribution of Questions
I. All phases of nursing process are included on the examination
II. Table 1-3 shows the nursing process distribution of questions on the CCRN® examination

Passing Scaled Score: 130 of 200
I. The difficulty of the examination determines the actual number of questions that must be answered correctly to earn a scaled score of 130
II. If you receive a slightly more difficult version, you will need to correctly answer fewer questions than if you receive a less difficult version
III. Scaled scores are reported for each category so that you can evaluate how well you performed in each area and identify your weaknesses; no minimal score is required for each category, cognitive level, or nursing process component
IV. Since July 1989, the passing rate has been between 66% and 68% for nurses taking the test for the first time; nurses retaking the test for recertification have a higher passing rate

Preparation to Improve Performance
Be Positive!
I. Remember that this test is strictly for you
II. Avoid negative self-talk; "I'll never pass this exam" can be a self-fulfilling prophecy because you begin to believe it
III. Practice positive self-talk
   A. Write affirmations (positive statements); suggested affirmations are listed in Box 1-1
   B. Say these and other affirmations that you have written over and over again throughout your

1-1 Affirmations

I am a knowledgeable critical care nurse.
I understand the information important for this
examination.
I am an excellent test-taker.
I feel prepared for this examination.
I will pass this examination.

preparation time; say them like you believe them
and you will!

C. Record your affirmations on audiotape and play
them over and over; play them in the car or
while you walk or do dishes, or any other time
when you can listen

Prepare for the Test

I. Establish a realistic schedule for your preparation;
one- to two-hour time slots are probably the most
helpful
A. Study examination content: plan to review a
system per evening, day, or weekend, depending on how much time you have left before
the examination
1. Priority setting
a) Study your weak areas first
b) Study the large percentage content areas
even if you feel confident about them: you
should feel especially confident about
cardiac, pulmonary, and multisystem
content since these three areas constitute
56% of the examination
B. Practice using your test-taking skills by doing
practice questions
1. In addition to looking at the answer, read the
rationale; remember that the question may
not be written exactly the same as the practice question, but the concept may be on the
examination
2. If you still do not understand why you
missed the question, refer back to the
section in this book or a critical care text to
understand why the correct answer is
better than your answer
3. In addition to looking at the answer and the
rationale, read the test-taking strategy; this information will help you identify how to approach a question to which you do not know
the answer
4. Analyze why you missed a question; consider:
a) Did you not know the content? Study this
content again
b) Did you misread the question? Slow down
and read the question thoroughly
c) Did you misread the options? Slow down
and read all of the options and select the
best one
d) Did you miss an important element such
as age, diagnosis, or parameter? Again,
slow down and read the question care-

fully; mentally highlight those critical
points in the case study that you feel are
important
e) Did you read into the question? Do not
assume information that is not given; take
the question at face value
II. If you like study groups, organize a study group
with nurses who are also preparing for the examination and who will actually work for the group
A. Choose your members carefully: You do not
want to choose a member who will not prepare
to present information to the group or who
will not collect resources that the group needs
B. Establish guidelines for the group
1. When will you meet?
2. What will you do at the meetings?
3. What are the group members' expectations?
III. Create memory joggers
A. Almost everyone knows "On Old Olympus' Tow-
ering Tops A Fin And German Viewed Some
Hops" to remember the 12 cranial nerves; establish others that help you identify things that
you have trouble remembering
B. Remember case study links: For example, you
remember a patient with a triglyceride level
over 2000 mg/dl who developed acute pancreatitis, and then ARDS helps you remember
that a major risk factor for acute pancreatitis is
hypertriglyceridemia and that a major complication of acute pancreatitis is ARDS
IV. Take a practice test 1 week before the examination; use this test to identify weak areas for final
study time
A. Analyze which categories (systems) are your
weakest and strongest
B. Analyze which cognitive level question is the
most difficult for you
C. Analyze which component of the nursing
process is most difficult for you

Schedule the Examination

I. Complete the application and send it to the AACN
II. AACN will send you an authorization letter indicating that you meet the requirements to take the examination, along with instructions on how to
schedule the examination at a Sylvan Prometric
Testing Center
III. Call Sylvan to schedule your examination date and
time
A. This flexibility in scheduling allows you to avoid
scheduling conflicts between the examination
and major life events such as a family wedding,
graduation, or birth
B. Schedule the time of the examination according
to when you do your best thinking or are most
productive: Schedule early in the morning if
you are a lark or late in the afternoon if you are
an owl
IV. DO SCHEDULE THE EXAM so that you have a
target date; you can reschedule up to 2 days prior
to the scheduled test day if something comes up

that interferes with your ability to complete the examination on the scheduled day; you must reschedule the examination within 90 days of the date printed on your authorization letter

Final Preparations

I. Don't cram the night before the examination; cramming usually just decreases your self-confidence and increases your anxiety
II. Go to bed at your usual time; if you go to bed early, you probably won't go to sleep anyway and will just worry about the test
III. Do not consume alcohol or other sedating drugs the night before or the day of the examination
IV. Take a watch and a sweater; don't forget your glasses, if you wear them
V. Eat a healthy but light meal before the examination; avoid simple carbohydrates such as doughnuts or Danishes
VI. Be sure to take a government-issued photo identification that contains a signature
VII. You must arrive 15 minutes before your scheduled appointment; thumbprints will be taken prior to the examination

Performance During the Examination

Control of Anxiety

I. Remember that some anxiety increases your performance; panic does not
II. Feeling adequately prepared decreases anxiety; take the time to prepare for this examination, including practicing your test-taking strategies
III. Use visualization: See yourself receiving your passing score
IV. Use deep breathing and/or progressive muscle relaxation
    A. Progressive muscle relaxation is performed by contracting a group of muscles and then relaxing it: leg, leg, arm, arm, back, face
        1. Use this technique in the car before you go in to take the examination and at anytime during the examination that you feel tense
    B. Deep breathing is performed by putting your hand below your costal margin and breathing deeply enough to raise your hand; focus on your breathing instead of anything else
        1. Use this method at anytime during the examination when you feel frustrated or stressed
        2. Use meditation or prayer depending on your religious beliefs: These techniques are also helpful in verbalizing your goals and desires

Test-taking Skills

I. Read questions thoroughly
    A. Look for key words such as: except, least, most, never, always, initially, first, last, early, late, indicated, contraindicated, priority, best
    B. Read all options as well as the stem
    C. After you read the stem, answer the question without looking at the options; if your answer is there, it's probably right; however, still go ahead and read all options—there may be one better than your answer
II. Do not assume information that is not given; the only assumption is an ideal situation
    A. All important information is included
        1. Do not read into the question such as "maybe she's a diabetic;" if she were and it were important to the question, that information would be included
    B. Included information is probably important
        1. Extraneous information is not usually included, so if the case study or question gives you a point of information, ask yourself why this information was given and how it is important to this situation
III. Don't leave any question blank; unanswered questions are counted as incorrect
    A. Answer easy questions first
    B. Mark questions that you feel unsure of and want to go back to; at the end of the test, the computer allows you to go back to these marked items and review them before unmarking them and continuing to the end of the examination
IV. Priority questions
    A. Priority one is always whatever must be done to prevent death; always follow the ABC order: airway, then breathing, and finally circulation
    B. Priority two is whatever must be done to prevent disability or serious complication; consider this D for disability
    C. Priority three is pain or discomfort; if nothing in the case study or question could cause death or disability, pain should be considered the priority
    D. Actual problems always take precedence over potential problems; for example, actual hypoxemia takes precedence over potential oxygen toxicity
V. Answers with multiple answers (also referred to as multiple multiples)
    A. If the option has more than one answer (such as x and y), both (or all) of the answers must be correct for the option to be correct
VI. Guessing
    A. Guessing should be used only as a last resort
    B. First eliminate any choices that you can; it is better to guess between two choices than to guess among four
    C. If you still do not know the answer, then look for the option that is different from the others; for example, if there are 3 beta-blockers and 1 calcium channel blocker, then choose the calcium channel blocker; among 3 very specific and 1 very general, choose the general, etc.
VII. Changing answers
    A. If you tend to miss questions because you don't read them thoroughly and you realize

that you misread this question, then by all means change your answer

B. If you tend to miss questions even though you read them thoroughly, don't change your initial answer since first impressions are probably best

VIII. Math questions

A. Math questions on the CCRN® examination are usually a drug calculation such as dopamine in micrograms per kilogram per minute

B. Recheck your math if you have time

IX. Budget your time

A. You will have 4 hours to answer 200 questions, but if you are a slow test-taker, you may run short on time

B. You should be at least halfway (#100) through the examination in 90 to 100 minutes

1. This halfway point will leave you some time to recheck your math and go back to the marked items

C. Do not be distressed by people finishing before you; we all take examinations at different speeds, and they are probably not even taking the CCRN® exam; several exams are given at the same place and same time

D. It may be helpful to read the question (at end of case study) and then go back and read the case study; this technique saves you time by knowing what you are looking for in the case study

X. Water or restroom breaks

A. You may ask permission to get a drink of water or go to the restroom

B. You may need minor analgesics for headache, antihistamines for allergies, etc.; avoid drugs that may sedate you

Congratulations for Having the Initiative to Take This Exam!

Use this book to review the content for the examination, complete the learning activities, practice your test-taking skills with practice questions at the end of each chapter, take a practice examination 1 week before the examination and use your final study time to study your weak areas, and then use your test-taking skills during the exam.

You will receive a preliminary result of pass or fail before you leave the testing center; your final score with category breakdown will arrive within weeks.

Good luck! I would love to hear from you regarding how well you felt that this book prepared you for the exam; E-mail me at: rddennison@aol.com or write to me at Mosby.

LEARNING ACTIVITIES

1. Why do you want to take this examination?
_____
_____
_____
_____
_____

2. List your top five life priorities for the next year. Is CCRN® certification on this list? What is the ranking for CCRN® certification?

1st_____
2nd_____
3rd_____
4th_____
5th_____

3. Prioritize this list from 1 (least comfortable) to 9 (most comfortable). Use this list to schedule your preparation with 1 being first and 9 being last.

Knowledge Area	Comfort Level
Cardiovascular	
Pulmonary	
Multisystem	
Neurology	
Gastrointestinal	
Renal	
Endocrine	
Hematology/immunology	
Professional caring and ethical practice	

4. Describe your plan to prepare for the CCRN® examination.

a. _____
b. _____
c. _____
d. _____
e. _____

5. List three new test-taking strategies that you have learned and will use while taking the CCRN® examination.

a. _____
b. _____
c. _____

Bibliography and Selected References

Biel M et al: Evolving trends in critical care nursing practice: results of a certification role delineation study, *Am J Crit Care* 8 (5):285, 1999.

Caterinicchio M: Redefining nursing according to patients' and families' needs: an evolving concept, *AACN Clinical Issues,* 6 (1):153, 1995.

Curley MAQ: Patient nurse synergy: optimizing patient outcomes, *Am J Crit Care* 7 (1):64, 1998.

Czerwinski S, Blastic L, Rice B: The synergy model: building a clinical advancement program, *Critical Care Nurse* 19 (4):72, 1999.

Edwards D: The synergy model: linking patient needs to nurse competencies, *Critical Care Nurse* 19:98, 1999.

Moloney-Harmon P: The synergy model: contemporary practice of the clinical nurse specialist, *Critical Care Nurse* 19 (2):101, 1999.

Nuggent P, Vitale B: *Test success,* ed 2, Philadelphia, 1993, FA Davis.

Rollant P: *Soar to success: Do your best on nursing tests,* St Louis, 1999, Mosby.

Sides M, Korchek N: *Nurses' guide to successful test-taking,* Philadelphia, 1994, JB Lippincott.

Villaire M: The synergy model of certified practice: creating safe passage for patients, *Critical Care Nurse* 16:95, 1996.

Cardiovascular System: Physiology and Assessment

CHAPTER 2

Selected Concepts in Anatomy and Physiology

General Information About the Cardiovascular System

I. The cardiovascular system is a continuous, fluid-filled elastic circuit with a pump

II. The cardiovascular system provides communication among all body parts through transportation of oxygen, nutrients, hormones, water, enzymes, vitamins, minerals, buffers, leukocytes, antibodies, buffers, and wastes; these functions maintain dynamic equilibrium to maintain homeostasis

III. The cardiovascular system consists of the heart and vascular system

The Heart

I. Bioelectrically driven, muscular, four-chamber organ that provides forward propulsion of blood into the vascular system

II. Size of a closed fist: usually approximately 9 cm wide and 12 cm long; weighs approximately 4 g/kg of ideal body weight

III. Lies in the mediastinum between the sternum (anterior) and the spine (posterior) with two thirds of the heart to the left of the midline and one third of the heart to the right of the midline (Fig. 2-1)

IV. Shaped like a blunt cone
  A. Apex
    1. Inferior, anterior, and to the left
    2. Normally at fifth left intercostal space (LICS) at the midclavicular line (MCL)
    3. On the upper surface of the diaphragm
  B. Base
    1. Superior, posterior, and to the right
    2. Normally at level of second intercostal space

V. Cardiac walls (Fig. 2-2)
  A. Pericardium: maintains the heart in a stationary position

1. Fibrous
  a) Loose-fitting, white fibrous layer
  b) Acts as a barrier against infection and neoplastic invasion
2. Serous
  a) Parietal layer: lines inner surface of fibrous pericardium
  b) Visceral layer: lines the surface of the heart; synonymous with epicardium
3. Pericardial space
  a) Located between the parietal and visceral layers of the serous pericardium
  b) Contains 10 to 30 ml of lubricating fluid
    (1) Protects the heart against friction and erosion
    (2) Provides a well-lubricated sac in which the heart moves during contraction
  B. Epicardium: synonymous with visceral layer of serous pericardium
  C. Myocardium
    1. Largest portion of the cardiac wall
    2. Consists of the following:
      a) Specialized conduction fibers
      b) Interlacing cardiac muscle fibers
  D. Endocardium
    1. Consists of the following:
      a) Connective tissue
      b) Elastic fibers
      c) Endothelial cells
        (1) Form a smooth surface for blood contact
        (2) Deter clot formation
    2. Contiguous with the lining of the great vessels
    3. Lines heart chambers and valves

VI. Cardiac skeleton
  A. Composed of continuous dense connective tissue
  B. Located at base of heart and in interventricular septum

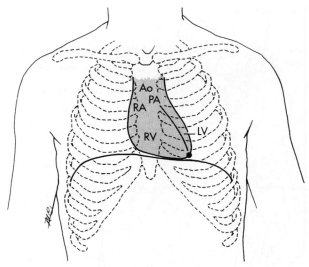

Figure 2-1 Location and orientation of the heart within the thorax. (From Price SA, Wilson LM: *Pathophysiology—clinical concepts of disease processes,* ed 5, St Louis, 1996, Mosby.)

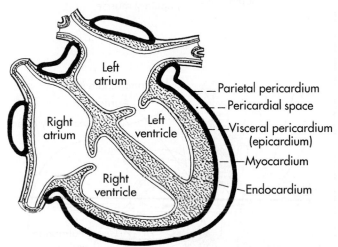

Figure 2-2 Layers of the cardiac wall. (From Copstead L: *Perspectives on pathophysiology,* Philadelphia, 1995, WB Saunders.)

C. Serves as point of origin and insertion for cardiac muscle fibers
D. Supports the heart valves; includes the four valve rings (annuli)

VII. Cardiac chambers (Fig. 2-3)
  A. Atria
    1. Located posterior, superior, and to the right of the corresponding ventricles
    2. Contain interatrial septum to divide left and right atria
    3. Contain trabeculae to divide atria and ventricles
    4. Thin-walled, low-pressure chambers
      a) Right: 2 mm thick, 2 to 6 mm Hg pressure
      b) Left: 3 mm thick, 6 to 12 mm Hg pressure

    5. Act as reservoirs and booster pumps for the ventricles
      a) Passive ventricular filling: 70% to 75% of ventricular filling is passive because blood falls straight through atrium into ventricle
      b) Active ventricular filling: 25% to 30% of ventricular filling is active because the atrium contracts at the end of ventricular diastole
    6. Right atrium
      a) Inflow tracts
        (1) Superior vena cava
        (2) Inferior vena cava
        (3) Coronary sinus
        (4) Thebesian veins
      b) Outflow tract: through tricuspid valve to right ventricle
    7. Left atrium
      a) Inflow tracts: four pulmonary veins (only case of veins carrying oxygenated blood)
      b) Outflow tract: through mitral valve to left ventricle
  B. Ventricles
    1. Located anterior, inferior, and to the left of the corresponding atria
    2. Contain interventricular septum to divide left and right ventricles
    3. Contain trabeculae to divide atria and ventricles
    4. Act as pumps receiving blood from the atria and pumping blood into the great vessels
    5. Right ventricle
      a) Thin-walled: 3 to 5 mm
      b) Low-pressure pump: 25/5 mm Hg
      c) Inflow tract
        (1) Right atria via tricuspid valve
        (2) Thebesian veins
      d) Outflow tract: pulmonary artery (only case of artery carrying deoxygenated blood)
    6. Left ventricle
      a) Thick-walled: 8 to 15 mm
      b) High-pressure: 120/5 mm Hg
      c) Inflow tract
        (1) Left atria via mitral valve
        (2) Thebesian veins
      a) Outflow tract: aorta

VIII. Cardiac valves (Fig. 2-4)
  A. Purposes
    1. Permit antegrade flow
    2. Prevent retrograde flow
  B. Atrioventricular (AV) valves: tricuspid and mitral valves
    1. Located between atria and ventricles
      a) Tricuspid valve is between right atria and right ventricle
      b) Mitral valve is between left atria and left ventricle
    2. Consist of annulus (fibrous supporting ring), cusps (two for mitral, three for tricuspid),

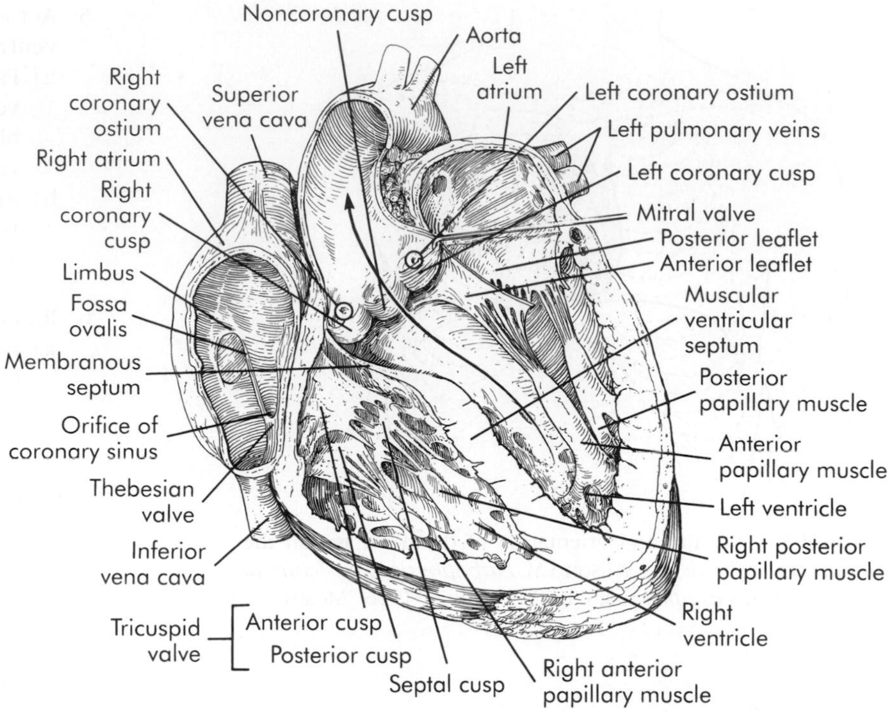

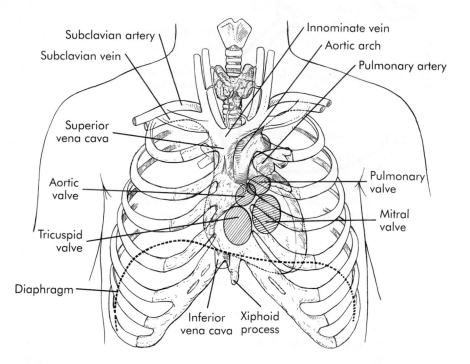

Figure 2-3 Interior of the heart showing cardiac chambers (pulmonary artery removed for visualization). (From Seifert PC: *Mosby's perioperative nursing series: cardiac surgery,* St Louis, 1994, Mosby.)

Figure 2-4 Position of the cardiac valves. (From Seifert PC: *Mosby's perioperative nursing series: cardiac surgery,* St Louis, 1994, Mosby.)

and papillary muscles, which attach to valve cusps by chordae tendineae (Fig. 2-5); the cusps are joined for 0.5 to 1.0 cm at the annulus (referred to as a *commissure*)

3. Open passively during diastole
4. Close when papillary muscles contract
5. Cause the first heart sound, S_1, when they close; two components of S_1: M_1 and T_1

C. Semilunar valves: aortic and pulmonic valves
  1. Located between ventricles and great vessels
    a) Pulmonic valve is located between the right ventricle and the pulmonary artery
    b) Aortic valve is located between the left ventricle and the aorta
  2. Consist of annulus and three cusps

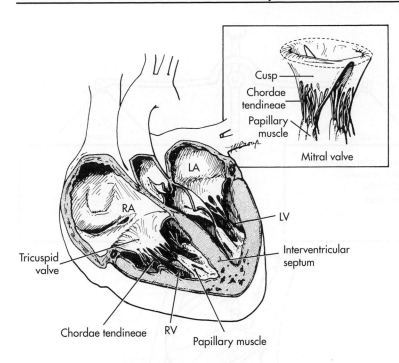

Cusp

Chordae
tendineae

Papillary
muscle

Mitral valve

LA

RA

LV

Interventricular
septum

Tricuspid
valve

Chordae tendineae   RV   Papillary muscle

Figure 2-5   Atrioventricular valve. (From Price SA, Wilson LM: *Pathophysiology: clinical concepts of disease processes,* ed 5, St Louis, 1996, Mosby.)

3. Function by pressure gradients
4. Cause the second heart sound, S_2, when they close; two components of S_2: A_2 and P_2

IX. Coronary vasculature
  A. Coronary arteries are the first branch off the aorta, immediately outside the aortic valve
  B. Coronary arteries lie on the epicardium, but branches penetrate through to the myocardium and subendocardium
  C. The myocardium receives 5% of cardiac output and extracts 65% to 80% of oxygen in the blood even at basal rate
    1. Blood flow through the coronary arteries is determined almost entirely by local autoregulation in response to the metabolic needs of the myocardium
    2. Myocardial blood flow is increased by dilation of the coronary arteries
  D. Coronary artery perfusion
    1. Effect of cardiac cycle
      a) The left ventricle is perfused primarily during diastole because of compression of musculature around intramuscular vessels during systole
      b) The right ventricle is perfused throughout the cardiac cycle but more during diastole
    2. Effect of aortic pressure
      a) The pressure in the aorta immediately outside the aortic valve (referred to as *aortic root pressure*) is significant in coronary artery filling pressure
      b) Coronary artery perfusion pressure (CAPP) is equal to the diastolic BP minus the pulmonary artery occlusive pressure (PAOP) (previously known as *pulmonary artery wedge pressure*

or *pulmonary capillary wedge pressure*); normal CAPP is 60 to 80 mm Hg
  3. Myocardial oxygen consumption (Fig. 2-6)
    a) Determinants of myocardial oxygen demand include the following:
      (1) Heart rate
      (2) Preload
      (3) Afterload
      (4) Contractility
    b) Determinants of myocardial oxygen supply include the following:
      (1) Patent arteries
      (2) Diastolic pressure
      (3) Diastolic time
      (4) Oxygen extraction
        (a) Hgb
        (b) Sao_2
    c) Imbalances between supply and demand cause ischemia; prolonged imbalance causes infarction
  E. Coronary arteries and distribution (Fig. 2-7)
    1. Left coronary artery (LCA) before bifurcation is referred to as the *left main coronary artery;* the LCA then divides into left anterior descending and left circumflex arteries
      a) Left anterior descending (LAD) coronary artery supplies the following:
        (1) Anterior left ventricle
        (2) Anterior two thirds of the interventricular septum
        (3) Apex of left ventricle
        (4) Bundle of His and bundle branches
      b) Left circumflex coronary artery supplies the following:
        (1) Left atrium
        (2) SA node in 45% of hearts

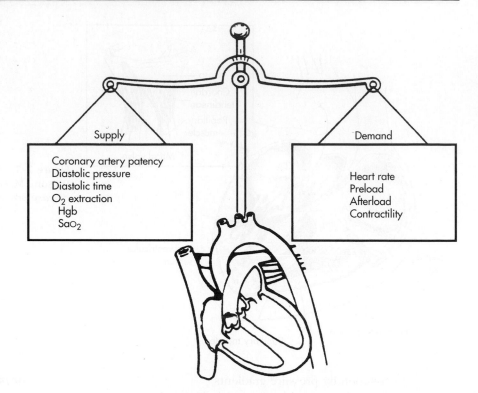

Figure 2-6 Factors influencing myocardial oxygen supply and demand. (Courtesy of Baxter Healthcare Corporation, Irvine, Calif.)

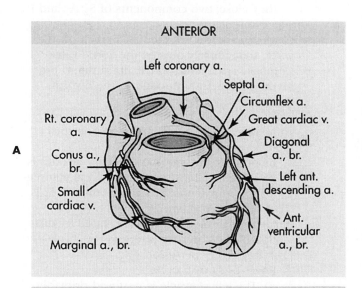

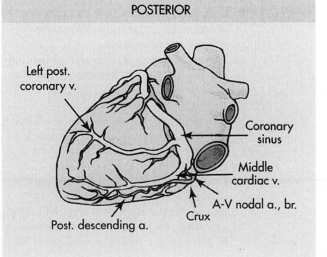

Figure 2-7 The coronary circulation. **A,** Anterior surface. **B,** Posterior surface. (*a.,* artery, *v.,* vein, *br.,* branch, *ant.,* anterior, *post.,* posterior) (From Kinney M et al: *AACN clinical reference for critical care nursing,* St Louis, 1998, Mosby.)

(3) AV node in 10% of hearts

(4) Obtuse marginal branch supplies the following:

    (a) Lateral left ventricle

    (b) Posterior left ventricle

2. Right coronary artery (RCA) supplies the following:

  a) Right atrium

  b) SA node in 55% of hearts

  c) Left posterior hemibundle (dual blood supply: LAD and RCA)

  d) AV node in 90% of hearts

  e) Marginal branch supplies:

    (1) Lateral right ventricle

    (2) Inferior right ventricle

  f) In RCA-dominant hearts (approximately 80% of hearts), a branch of RCA referred to as the *posterior descending artery* supplies the following:

    (1) Anterior right ventricle

    (2) Inferior wall of left ventricle

    (3) Posterior left ventricle

    (4) Posterior one third of septum

3. Collateral circulation

  a) Consists of interarterial vessels that connect, or anastomose, with each other

  b) Factors that foster development of collateral flow include anemia, hypoxemia, and arteriosclerosis (gradual occlusion)

F. Coronary veins

1. Most coronary veins empty into the coronary sinus, which empties into the right atrium

2. The thebesian veins drain some venous blood from the myocardium directly into the right atrium, right ventricle, and left ventricle rather than through the coronary sinus; this venous blood emptying directly into the left ventricle accounts for normal physiologic shunt because it slightly decreases oxygen saturation

G. Lymph vessels

1. Main cardiac channel empties into the pretracheal node and then into the right lymphatic duct

2. Drainage system facilitated by cardiac contraction

X. Electrophysiology and the conduction system

A. Properties of cardiac cells

1. Automaticity: ability of certain cardiac cells to initiate impulses regularly and spontaneously

2. Excitability: ability of the cardiac cells to respond to a stimulus by initiating a cardiac impulse

3. Conductivity: ability of cardiac cells to respond to a cardiac impulse by transmitting the impulse along cell membranes

4. Contractility: ability of the cardiac cells to respond to an impulse by muscle contraction

B. Action potential of myocardial cells (Fig. 2-8)

1. Phase 4: resting membrane potential

  a) This phase coincides with isoelectric line between T and QRS

  b) Electrical charge within the cell is −80 to −95 mV

  c) Negativity is maintained by the sodium-potassium pump

    (1) When cellular energy (ATP) supplies are low, such as during shock, this resting membrane potential cannot be maintained and irritability occurs

    (2) An active transport system requires energy to pump sodium out of the cell and potassium into the cell

2. Phase 0: rapid depolarization of the cell

  a) This phase coincides with QRS

  b) It occurs when a stimulus is applied to the cell

  c) Cell membrane permeability to sodium increases significantly so that sodium rushes into the cell (influx) and potassium begins to move out (efflux)

  d) If the stimulus is strong enough to reach a critical level known as the *threshold potential* (approximately −60 to −70 mV), then the cell responds entirely and depolarization occurs

  e) This phase is referred to as the *sodium* (or *fast*) channel

  f) Class I antidysrhythmic agents (e.g., procainamide, lidocaine) block the influx of sodium into the cell, thereby

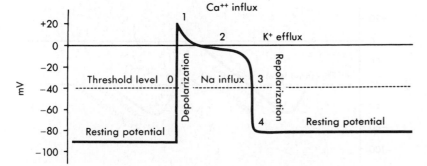

Figure 2-8 Action potential of a myocardial cell. (From Thelan LA et al: *Critical care nursing: diagnosis and management,* ed 3, St Louis, 1998, Mosby.)

preventing the achievement of threshold potential and depolarization

3. Phase 1: brief, rapid initiation of repolarization
   a) Sodium channels close
   b) Chloride influx occurs
4. Phase 2: slowing of the repolarization causing a plateau
   a) This phase coincides with ST segment
   b) It allows the cardiac muscle a more sustained contraction
   c) This phase is referred to as *calcium* (or *slow*) channel
   d) Class IV antidysrhythmics (calcium channel blockers such as verapamil) block the movement of calcium and prolong repolarization and refractoriness
5. Phase 3: sudden acceleration in the rate of repolarization
   a) Potassium movement accelerates during this phase; movement out of the cell occurs at the beginning of phase 3 and back into the cell at the end of phase 3
   b) Class III antidysrhythmics (e.g., bretylium, amiodarone) block the movement of potassium during this phase and prolong refractoriness
6. Phase 4: resting membrane potential

C. Action potential of pacemaker cells (Fig. 2-9)
1. Pacemaker cells have the property of self-excitation
2. They demonstrate slow diastolic depolarization because of a time-dependent leak of sodium into the cell
3. When enough sodium has entered the cell that threshold potential is reached, spontaneous depolarization occurs
4. Rate of diastolic depolarization determines intrinsic rate of pacemakers
   a) Sinoatrial (SA) node: 60 to 100/min
   b) Atrioventricular (AV) junction: 40 to 60/min
   c) Purkinje fibers: 20 to 40/min

D. Refractoriness (Fig. 2-10)
1. Absolute refractory period
   a) No matter how strong the impulse is, the cell cannot be depolarized again during this period

b) This period correlates with the period from phase 0 through mid-phase 3 on the action potential and from the QRS to the peak of the T-wave on the ECG

2. Relative refractory period
   a) If the impulse is strong enough, the cell may respond but may respond abnormally (e.g., R on T may cause ventricular tachycardia or ventricular fibrillation)
   b) This period correlates with late phase 3 of the action potential and the descending limb of the T-wave on the ECG
3. Effective refractory period: the absolute refractory period plus the relative refractory period

E. Conduction system (Fig. 2-11)
1. Sinoatrial (SA) node
   a) Functions as the natural pacemaker of the heart because it has the fastest intrinsic rate (60-100/min)
   b) Located in right atrial wall near opening of superior vena cava
2. Internodal pathways
   a) Three pathways between SA node and AV node
      (1) Anterior tract (Bachmann's)
      (2) Middle tract (Wenckebach's)
      (3) Posterior tract (Thorel's)
3. Bachmann's bundle (interatrial pathway): pathway that takes impulse from right atrium to left atrium
4. Atrioventricular (AV) node
   a) Located at base of right atrium at top of interventricular septum
   b) Accounts for physiologic delay of 0.08 to 0.12 seconds to allow the atria to completely depolarize, contract, and finish filling the ventricles before the ventricles are stimulated
   c) Contains no pacemaker cells; primary function is to slow the impulse down
5. Atrioventricular (AV) junction
   a) Tissue surrounding AV node and Bundle of His that contains pacemaker cells
   b) Functions as a secondary pacemaker with intrinsic rate of 40 to 60/min

Figure 2-9   Action potential of a pacemaker cell. (From Thelan LA et al: *Critical care nursing: diagnosis and management,* ed 3, St Louis, 1998, Mosby.)

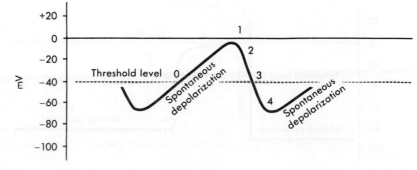

6. Bundle of His
   a) First portion of interventricular conduction system
7. Bundle branches
   a) Right bundle branch (RBB) takes the impulse to the right ventricular myocardium

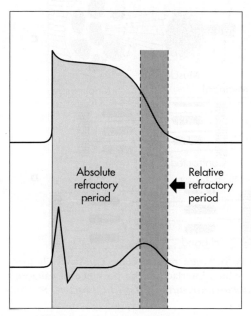

Figure 2-10 Absolute and relative refractory periods correlated with the myocardial cell action potential and with ECG tracing. (From Thelan LA et al: *Critical care nursing: diagnosis and management,* ed 2, St Louis, 1994, Mosby.)

   b) Left bundle branch (LBB) divides into two hemibundles
      (1) Left anterior hemibundle (LAH) to anterior and superior left ventricle
      (2) Left posterior hemibundle (LPH) to posterior and inferior left ventricle
   c) These three branches (RBB, LAH, LPH) are referred to as *fascicles* as in unifascicular, bifascicular, trifascicular block
8. Purkinje fiber system
   a) Takes the impulse from the bundle branches through the wall of the ventricles to subendocardial layers
   b) Acts as a final tertiary pacemaker if upper pacemakers fail at the inherent rate of 20 to 40/min
   F. Depolarization of cardiac chambers occurs from endocardium to epicardium
   G. Repolarization of cardiac chambers occurs from epicardium to endocardium
XI. Muscle mechanics
   A. Cardiac muscle is similar to skeletal muscle except for the following:
      1. Cardiac muscle has more mitochondria than skeletal muscle; cardiac muscle has greater ATP requirements because of the high energy requirements of the repetitive muscular action of the heart
      2. Cardiac muscle remains contracted 150 to 300 times longer than skeletal muscle
      3. Cardiac muscle forms a functional syncytium
         a) Intercalated disks lie between myocardial cells; they offer low electrical im-

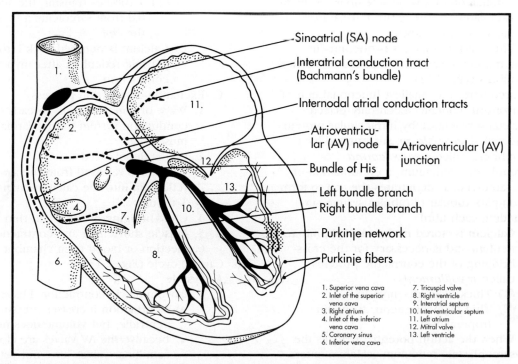

1. Superior vena cava
2. Inlet of the superior vena cava
3. Right atrium
4. Inlet of the inferior vena cava
5. Coronary sinus
6. Inferior vena cava
7. Tricuspid valve
8. Right ventricle
9. Interatrial septum
10. Interventricular septum
11. Left atrium
12. Mitral valve
13. Left ventricle

Figure 2-11 The conduction system. (From Huszar RJ: *Basic dysrhythmias: interpretation and management,* ed 2, St Louis, 1994, Mosby.)

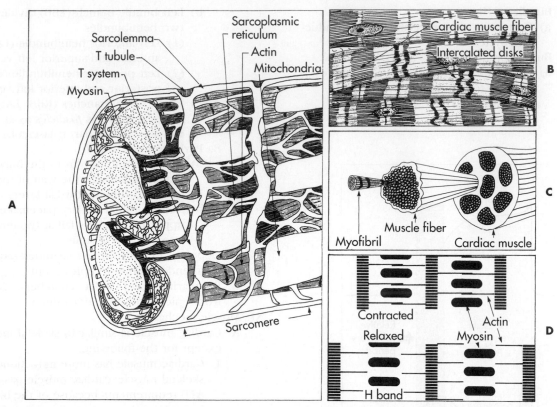

Figure 2-12 Cardiac muscle. **A,** The ultrastructure. **B,** Intercalated disks lie between muscle cells. **C,** Myofibrils form muscle fibers, which form cardiac muscle. **D,** Actin and myosin are myofilaments, which interlace in the presence of calcium to cause muscle contraction and shortening. (From Guzzetta CE, Dossey BM: *Cardiovascular nursing: holistic practice,* St Louis, 1992, Mosby.)

pedance, allowing electrical stimuli to pass with ease from cell to cell
   b) Stimulation of any muscle fiber results in stimulation of the entire muscle mass (all-or-none response)
   c) The heart acts as if it is one muscle
B. Cardiac muscle fibers are composed of bundles of myofibrils (Fig. 2-12)
   1. A sarcomere, the smallest functional unit of a myofibril, contains a centrally placed nucleus surrounded by intracellular protein fluid called *sarcoplasm;* surrounded by a membrane called a *sarcolemma*
   2. Sarcoplasmic reticulum, a continuation of the sarcolemma, penetrates the cell to form a complex tubular (T-tubule) system surrounding each fibril
      a) Calcium is stored in the sarcoplasmic reticulum and is necessary for the cross-bridging of the contractile proteins called *myofilaments*
         (1) Thick filaments: myosin
         (2) Thin filaments: actin, troponin, tropomyosin
      b) When the action potential reaches the sarcoplasmic reticulum, calcium enters the cell through calcium channels in the

sarcolemma and in the invaginations of the sarcolemma, the T-tubules
         (1) T tubules transmit the action potential from sarcolemma to interior of the cell
      c) Calcium is pumped back into the sarcoplasmic reticulum after myocardial contraction
   C. Excitation-contraction process
      1. Wave of depolarization spreads through conduction system to myocardial muscle cell
      2. Cell is depolarized
      3. Calcium is released from the sarcoplasmic reticulum into the calcium channels and T tubules
      4. Cross-bridging of thick and thin filaments
      5. Muscle shortening and contraction
      6. Ejection of blood from chamber
XII. Cardiac cycle (Fig. 2-13)
   A. Systole
      1. Isovolumetric contraction: Phase 1
         a) Contraction increases pressure in the ventricle, but volume does not change because the AV valves are closed and the semilunar valves have not yet opened
         b) Ventricular pressure must exceed the

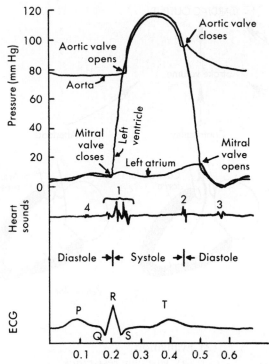

Figure 2-13 Wenger diagram: demonstrates cardiac cycle showing ECG events, heart sounds, and pressure curves. (From Wenger N et al: *Cardiology for nurses,* St Louis, 1980, McGraw-Hill.)

pressure in the great vessel to open the semilunar valve

     c) This subphase accounts for two thirds of oxygen consumption of the ventricle

     d) This subphase follows the QRS

   2. Maximal ejection: Phase 2

     a) When the pressure in the ventricle exceeds the pressure in the great vessel, the semilunar valve opens and blood is rapidly ejected into the great vessel

     b) Aortic and pulmonary artery pressures increase rapidly and ventricular volume decreases sharply

     c) This subphase occurs during the ST-segment

   3. Reduced ejection (also referred to as *proto-diastole*): Phase 3

     a) Blood is slowly ejected from the ventricle to the great vessel

     b) Ventricular pressure and volume decrease

     c) When the pressure in the great vessel is greater than the pressure in the ventricle, the semilunar valve closes and systole ends

     d) This subphase occurs during the T-wave

B. Diastole

   1. Isovolumetric relaxation: Phase 1

     a) Relaxation occurs and ventricular pressure decreases, but volume does not change because the semilunar valves

have closed and the AV valves have not yet opened

     b) This subphase occurs after the T-wave

   2. Rapid filling: Phase 2

     a) During this phase, the AV valves open and blood rushes into the ventricles

     b) Atrial and ventricular pressure decreases and ventricular volume increases

     c) Ventricular pressure is less than atrial pressure

     d) This subphase occurs during the TP interval

   3. Reduced filling (also referred to as *diastasis*): Phase 3

     a) Atrial and ventricular pressures slowly increase and ventricular volumes increase with slow filling of ventricles

     b) Coronary artery blood flow is optimal

     c) This subphase occurs during the TP interval

   4. Atrial contraction: Phase 4

     a) This subphase is also referred to as the *atrial kick*

     b) Atrial contraction accounts for 15% to 30% of diastolic filling volume; may be up to 50% when left ventricular filling is impeded (e.g., mitral stenosis)

     c) Atrial pressure decreases and ventricular volume and pressure increase

     d) This subphase occurs after P-wave

XIII. Regulation of cardiac function

A. Intrinsic control of the heart

   1. Determinants of cardiac output (Fig. 2-14 and Table 2-1)

     a) Heart rate

       (1) Definition: number of times per minute that the ventricles contract

       (2) Evaluation

         (a) Count rate at apex with stethoscope

         (b) Note HR on ECG monitor (confirm that a pulse is present with each QRS)

       (3) Effect of heart rate on cardiac output

         (a) If HR is less than 50 or greater than 150, cardiac output often falls and the tendency to dysrhythmias increases

       (4) Effect of heart rate on myocardial oxygen consumption

         (a) Although an increase in heart rate may increase cardiac output in patients with coronary artery disease, an increase in heart rate greater than 120/minute tends to increase myocardial oxygen demand more than coronary blood flow, causing ischemia

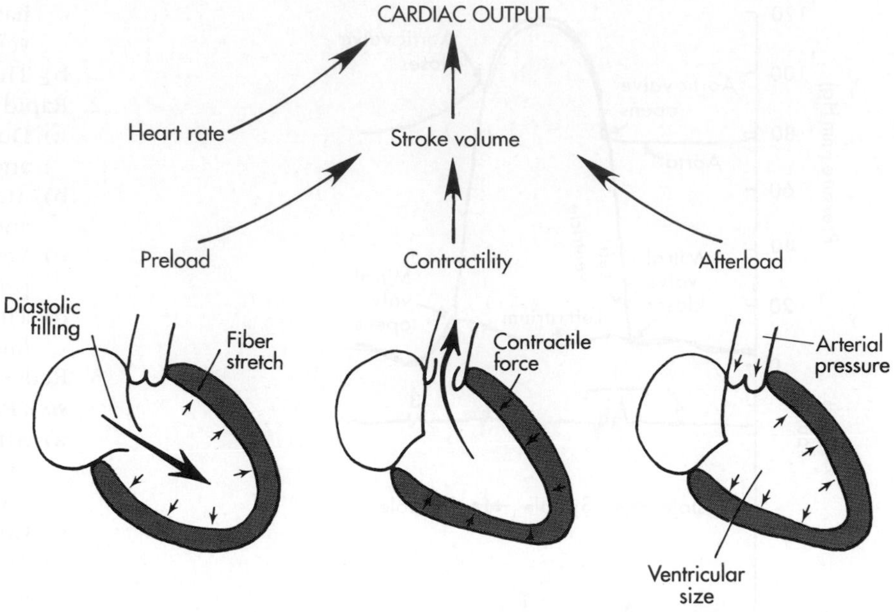

Figure 2-14 Determinants of cardiac output. (From Price SA, Wilson LM: *Pathophysiology: clinical concepts of disease processes,* ed 5, St Louis, 1996, Mosby.)

(5) Table 2-1 describes factors affecting heart rate

b) Preload
   (1) Definition: the stretch on the myofibrils at the end of diastole; determined by the pressure in the ventricle at the end of diastole
   (2) Evaluation: atrial pressure correlates to end-diastolic pressure for the respective ventricle
      (a) RV preload = central venous pressure (CVP) or right atrial pressure (RAP)
      (b) LV preload = pulmonary artery occlusive pressure (PAOP) or left atrial pressure (LAP)
   (3) Effect of preload on stroke volume and cardiac output
      (a) Starling's law of the heart and the Frank-Starling mechanism: Within physiologic limits, the greater the stretch on the myofibrils, the greater the force of the subsequent contraction (Fig. 2-15)
         (i) Both understretching and overstretching of the myofibrils results in a less than optimal contraction
   (4) Effect of preload on myocardial oxygen consumption: as preload increases, myocardial oxygen consumption increases
   (5) Table 2-1 describes factors affecting preload

c) Afterload
   (1) Definition: the pressure against which the ventricle must pump to open the semilunar valve

   (2) Evaluation
      (a) Vascular resistance
         (i) RV afterload = pulmonary vascular resistance (PVR) and pulmonary vascular resistance index (PVRI)
         (ii) LV afterload = systemic vascular resistance (SVR) and systemic vascular resistance index (SVRI)
      (b) Ventricular diameter
      (c) Mass and viscosity of blood
   (3) Effect of afterload on stroke volume and cardiac output (Fig. 2-16)
   (4) Effect of afterload on myocardial oxygen consumption: as afterload increases, myocardial oxygen consumption increases
   (5) Table 2-1 describes factors affecting afterload

d) Contractility
   (1) Definition: contractile force of the heart independent of preload and afterload
   (2) Evaluation: calculated parameter
      (a) RV contractility = right ventricular stroke work index (RVSWI)
      (b) LV contractility = left ventricular stroke work index (LVSWI)
   (3) Effect of contractility on stroke volume and cardiac output (Fig. 2-17)
   (4) Effect of contractility on myocardial oxygen consumption: as contractility increases, myocardial oxygen consumption increases
   (5) Table 2-1 describes factors affecting contractility

Table 2-1

Determinants of Cardiac Output

Parameter	Conditions		Treatments	
	Increased	**Decreased**	**To Increase**	**To Decrease**
Heart rate: evaluated by apical rate and/or ECG monitor	• SNS stimulation (e.g., exercise, fever, infection, pain, anxiety, hypovolemia or hypervolemia, most physiologic or psychologic stressors)	• PNS (vagal) stimulation (e.g., Valsalva maneuver, coughing, suctioning, vomiting, carotid stimulation) • Conduction abnormalities (e.g., sinus blocks, second- or third-degree AV blocks) • Drug effects (e.g., beta-blockers)	• Sympathomimetic drugs (e.g., epinephrine, isoproterenol) • Parasympatholytic drugs (e.g., atropine) • Pacemaker	• Cardiac glycosides (e.g., digoxin) • Beta-blockers (e.g., propranolol, esmolol) • Calcium channel blockers (e.g., verapamil, diltiazem) • Other antidysrhythmic drugs dependent on rhythm • Vagal maneuvers • Overdrive pacemaker • Cardioversion or defibrillation

Afterload: evaluated by calculation of SVR and SVRI (LV) and PVR and PVRI (RV)	• Vasoconstriction as from sympathetic nervous system (SNS) stimulation or vasopressors
	 • Hypertension
	 • Aortic valve disease
	 • Hypercoagulability
	 • Pulmonary hypertension (RV)
		• Hypotension
		 • Vasodilation (e.g., vasogenic shock, septic shock, neurogenic shock, anaphylactic shock)
			• Vasopressors (e.g., dopamine, norepinephrine)	• Arterial vasodilators
				   • Nitroprusside (NTP)
				   • Hydralazine
				   • Calcium channel blockers (e.g., nifedipine)
				   • Alpha blockers (e.g., phentolamine, labetalol)
				   • Angiotensin converting enzyme (ACE) inhibitors (e.g., captopril, enalapril)
				 • PDE inhibitors (e.g., amrinone, milrinone)
				 • Intraaortic balloon pump
				 Right ventricle specifically
				 • Oxygen
				 • Pulmonary vasodilators (e.g., aminophylline)

Preload: evaluated by PAOP (LV) and RAP (RV)	• HF
	 • Hypervolemia
	 • Brady-dysrhythmias
		• Hypovolemia
		 • Excessive vasodilation (e.g., vasogenic shock)
		 • Increased intrathoracic pressure
		 • Cardiac tamponade
		 • Right ventricular failure or infarction (LV)
		 • Tachydysrhythmias
		 • Loss of atrial contraction (e.g., atrial fibrillation)
			• Isotonic crystalloids (e.g., normal [0.9%] saline, lactated Ringer's)
			 • Colloids (e.g., albumin, plasma protein fraction (PPF), dextran, hetastarch)
			 • Blood and/or blood products
			 • Adjustment of vasodilator dosage
				• Diuretics (e.g., furosemide)
				 • Venous vasodilators
				   • Nitroglycerin (NTG)
				   • Morphine sulfate
				   • Nitroprusside
				   • Calcium channel blockers (e.g., nifedipine)
				 • ACE inhibitors (e.g., captopril, enalapril)

Contractility: evaluated by calculation of stroke volume and LVSWI (LV) and RVSWI (RV)	• SNS stimulation (see heart rate for selected factors that stimulate SNS) • Sympathomimetic drugs (e.g., epinephrine, isoproterenol)	• Myocardial ischemia or infarction • Cardiomyopathy • Hypoxemia • Acidosis • Drug adverse effects (e.g., barbiturates, anesthetics, beta-blockers, calcium channel blockers, most antidysrhythmics)	• Cardiac glycosides (e.g., digoxin) • Sympathomimetics (e.g., dobutamine, dopamine at medium [~5 µg/kg/min] dose) • Phospho-diesterase (PDE) inhibitors (e.g., amrinone, milrinone) • Calcium • Glucagon	• Beta-blockers (e.g., propranolol, metoprolol) • Calcium channel blockers (e.g., diltiazem, verapamil)

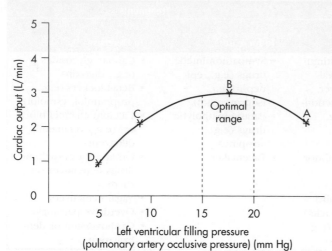

Figure 2-15 Relationship between PAOP and cardiac output. *A,* Overstretched myofibrils resulting in decreased contractility and cardiac output; *B,* Optimally stretched myofibrils resulting in optimally stretched myofibrils and optimal cardiac output; *C,* Normal stretched myofibrils resulting in normal (but suboptimal) cardiac output; *D,* Understretched myofibrils resulting in decreased contractility and cardiac output.

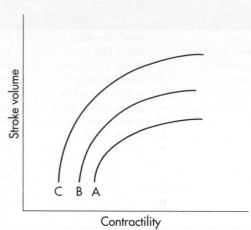

Figure 2-17 Relationship between contractility and stroke volume. *A,* Decreased contractility; *B,* normal contractility; *C,* enhanced contractility.

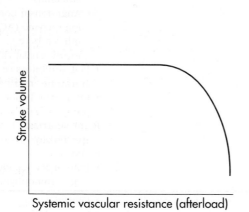

Figure 2-16 Relationship between afterload and stroke volume.

B. Extrinsic control of the heart
   1. Neurologic control of the heart
      a) Autonomic nervous system
         (1) Cardiac effects
            (a) Chronotropic: effect on heart rate
            (b) Inotropic: effect on contractility
            (c) Dromotropic: effect on conductivity
         (2) Sympathetic nervous system (SNS)
            (a) This branch is referred to as *fight or flight*
            (b) SNS is innervated by physiologic or psychologic stress
            (c) It causes positive chronotropic, inotropic, and dromotropic effects
            (d) SNS receptors and effects are listed in Table 2-2

Table 2-2 Sympathetic Nervous System (Adrenergic) Receptors and Effects

Receptor	Location of Receptors	Effects
Alpha	Vessels	Vasoconstriction of most vessels, especially the arterioles
Beta$_1$	Heart	Increased heart rate (chronotropic effect), contractility (inotropic effect), and conductivity (dromotropic effect)
Beta$_2$	Bronchial and vascular smooth muscle	Bronchodilation, vasodilation
Dopaminergic	Renal and mesenteric artery bed	Dilation of renal and mesenteric arteries

            (e) Sympathomimetic drugs are frequently used in critical care to augment these effects, especially after the patient's endogenous supplies are depleted; these drugs vary in their receptor stimulation and the potency of the stimulation (Table 2-3)
         (3) Parasympathetic (vagal) nervous system (PNS)
            (a) This branch maintains steady state
            (b) PNS causes negative chrono-

Table 2-3	Sympathomimetic Agents and Receptor Stimulation		
Drug	Alpha	Beta$_1$	Beta$_2$
Phenylephrine	++++	0	0
Norepinephrine	++++	++	0
Epinephrine	++++	++++	++
Dopamine	++>5 µg/ kg/min; +++>10 µg/ kg/min	++++ <10 µg/ kg/min	+
Dobutamine	+	++++	++
Isoproterenol	0	++++	++++

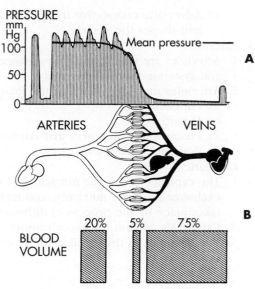

Figure 2-18 The vascular system. **A,** Mean pressure in components of vascular system. **B,** Volume in components of vascular system. (Reprinted with permission from Rushmer R: *Cardiovascular dynamics,* ed 4, Philadelphia, WB Saunders.)

tropic, inotropic, and dromotropic effects; the cardiovascular effects of the PNS are generally undesirable in critical care
  (c) Parasympatholytic (or vagolytic) agents (e.g., atropine) block these effects
    b) Chemoreceptors
      (1) Chemoreceptors are located in carotid and aortic bodies
      (2) They are sensitive to changes in Pao$_2$, Paco$_2$, and pH
      (3) Hypoxia, hypercapnia, and acidosis cause changes in heart rate and respiratory rate
    c) Baroreceptor reflex
      (1) Baroreceptors are located in the carotid sinus and aortic arch
      (2) They are sensitive to arterial pressure
      (3) Increased BP causes vagal stimulation, resulting in decreased heart rate and contractility
    d) Bainbridge reflex
      (1) Accelerator receptors are located in the right atrium
      (2) These receptors are sensitive to right atrial pressure
      (3) Increased right atrial pressure causes increased heart rate
    e) Respiratory reflex
      (1) Inspiration decreases intrathoracic pressure, which increases venous return to the right side of the heart, which causes the Bainbridge reflex; when the increased venous return reaches the left side of the heart, left ventricular cardiac output increases, which increases arterial BP and decreases the heart rate through stimulation of baroreceptors
      (2) This process is at least partly responsible for sinus dysrhythmia; an inter-

action between the respiratory and cardiac centers in the medulla also contributes
XIV. The endocrine function of the heart: atrial natriuretic factor (ANF)
  A. A hormonelike substance that is synthesized and stored by specialized atrial muscle cells
  B. ANF is secreted in response to increased atrial stretch
  C. ANF is an important regulator of blood volume and BP

Vascular System

  I. Function: to supply blood, nutrients, and hormones to the tissues and to remove metabolic wastes from the tissues
 II. Resistance to flow depends on the following:
  A. Diameter of vessels
  B. Viscosity of blood
  C. Elastic recoil of vessels
III. Components (Fig. 2-18)
  A. Arteries
    1. The delivery system that distributes and regulates the amount of oxygenated blood flow to various tissue beds
    2. Arteries are able to stretch during systole and recoil during diastole
    3. The arterial system is a high-pressure circuit
    4. The layers of the artery consist of the following (Fig. 2-19):
      a) Intima: thin lining of endothelium and a small amount of elastic tissue; decreases resistance to flow and minimizes the chance of platelet aggregation
      b) Media: smooth muscle and elastic tissue; changes the lumen diameter as needed

c) Adventitia: connective tissue; strengthens and shapes the vessels

B. Arterioles
   1. Arterioles are vital to the maintenance of BP and systemic vascular resistance
   2. Arterioles may lead to any of the following:
      a) Capillaries
      b) Metarterioles
      c) Precapillary sphincters that control blood flow into capillary bed

C. Capillaries
   1. The capillary bed is the nutrient bed where exchange of gases, nutrients, and metabolites takes place by the process of diffusion
   2. Capillaries contain no smooth muscle
   3. The diameter of the capillary depends

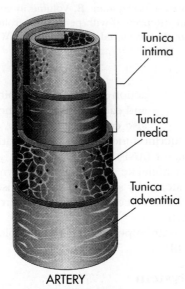

ARTERY

Figure 2-19 Layers of the arterial wall. (From Copstead L: *Perspectives on pathophysiology*, Philadelphia, 1995, WB Saunders.)

on changes in precapillary and postcapillary tone

   4. Capillary dynamics are influenced by four pressures (Fig. 2-20)
      a) Hydrostatic pressures push
         (1) Capillary hydrostatic pressure pushes fluid out of the capillary and into the interstitium
         (2) Interstitial hydrostatic pressure pushes fluid out of the interstitium and into the capillary
      b) Colloidal oncotic pressures pull
         (1) Capillary colloidal oncotic pressure pulls and holds fluid in the capillary
         (2) Interstitial colloidal oncotic pressure pulls and holds fluid in the interstitium
      c) Pressures pushing fluid out of the capillary dominate at the arterial end; pressures pushing fluid back into the capillary dominate at the venous end
      d) Edema is caused by an imbalance in these pressures or an increase in capillary permeability; *third spacing* is a term used to describe fluid accumulation in any space that is not intravascular or intracellular (e.g., interstitial edema, ascites, pleural effusion, pericardial effusion, into the lumen of the intestine)
         (1) Heart failure: Peripheral edema is caused by venous congestion and excessive hydrostatic pressure at the venous end
         (2) Malnutrition: Decrease in plasma proteins decreases capillary colloidal oncotic pressure and allows excessive fluid to leak out of the capillary

D. Veins
   1. The venous sytem is the return system that brings deoxygenated blood back to the heart and lungs

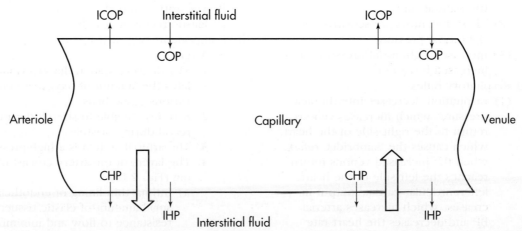

Figure 2-20 Capillary dynamics. Forces out of the capillary dominate at the arteriole end while forces back into the capillary dominate at the venule end. *CHP,* Capillary hydrostatic pressure; *IHP,* Interstitial hydrostatic pressure; *COP,* Capillary oncotic pressure; *ICOP,* Interstitial colloidal oncotic pressure.

2. Veins act as a reservoir; the venous system holds 65% to 70% of total blood volume
3. The venous pump sends blood back to the right side of the heart; the skeletal muscles contract, compress veins, and propel blood toward the heart
4. Valves in the veins prevent retrograde blood flow

IV. Blood pressure
   A. Regulation
     1. Autonomic nervous system
     2. Renin-angiotensin-aldosterone system (Fig. 2-21)
       a) Renin secreted by the kidney in response to:
         (1) Decreased BP stimulating stretch receptors in juxtaglomerular cells
         (2) Sympathetic nervous system stimulation
         (3) Hyponatremia
       b) Renin stimulates the conversion of angiotensinogen to angiotensin I
       c) Angiotensin I is converted to angiotensin II by angiotensin-converting enzyme (occurs in the lung)
       d) Angiotensin II causes vasoconstriction and secretion of aldosterone; vasoconstriction and sodium and water retention increase blood pressure and decrease renin secretion
     3. Capillary fluid shifts: especially from interstitial to intravascular
     4. Local control mechanisms
   B. Factors affecting arterial BP
     1. BP = Cardiac output × systemic vascular resistance (Fig. 2-22)
       a) Heart rate
       b) Arterial elasticity
       c) Blood viscosity
       d) Blood volume
       e) Sympathetic nervous system stimulation
       f) Drug effects
     2. Age
     3. Body size (body surface area)
     4. Electrolyte levels: sodium; potassium
   C. Pulse pressure (Fig. 2-23)
     1. The difference between systolic and diastolic pressures
     2. Affected by stroke volume and arterial elastance
   D. Mean arterial pressure (Fig. 2-23)
     1. The average pressure in the aorta and its major branches during cardiac cycle
     2. Calculated:
       a) [BP systolic + (BP diastolic × 2)] ÷ 3 OR
       b) BP diastolic + ⅓ pulse pressure
     3. Normal: 70 to 105 mm Hg
     4. Affected by cardiac output and systemic vascular resistance

V. Control and regulation of peripheral blood flow
   A. Local control mechanisms
     1. Autoregulation is the ability of the tissues to control blood flow; vasodilation is caused by hypoxia, hypercapnia, and acidosis
     2. Precapillary sphincters that precede every

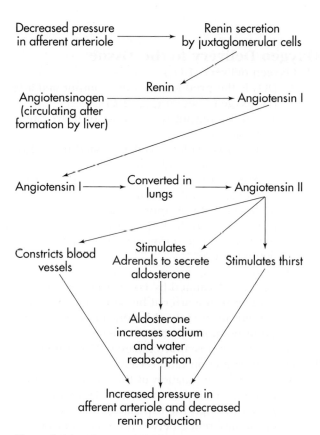

Figure 2-21   The renin-angiotensin-aldosterone system.

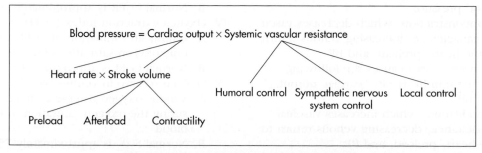

Figure 2-22   Determinants of blood pressure.

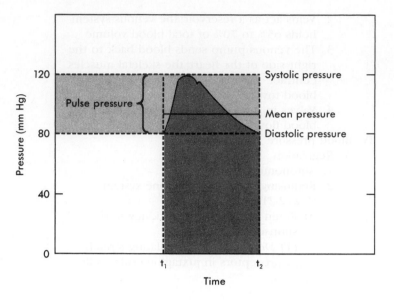

Figure 2-23 Blood pressure, pulse pressure (difference between systolic and diastolic pressures), and mean arterial pressure (calculated or measured average pressure). (Modified from Berne RM, Levy MN: *Cardiovascular physiology,* ed 7, St Louis, 1997, Mosby.)

capillary bed relax and permit more blood flow when oxygen tension falls; they constrict and restrict blood flow when oxygen tension rises

B. Autonomic nervous system
  1. Increased sympathetic nervous system stimulation: vasoconstriction
    a) Maintains arterial pressure
    b) Decreases vascular capacitance, increasing venous return to the heart and preload
  2. Decreased sympathetic nervous system stimulation: vasodilation

C. Baroreceptors
  1. Increase in BP or blood volume results in the following:
    a) Decreased heart rate and contractility
    b) Peripheral vasodilation
    c) Decrease in systemic vascular resistance and blood pressure
  2. Decrease in BP or blood volume results in the following:
    a) Increased heart rate and contractility
    b) Peripheral vasoconstriction
    c) Increase in systemic vascular resistance and blood pressure

D. Vasomotor center in medulla
  1. Vasoconstrictor area causes the following:
    a) Increase in heart rate, cardiac output, and blood pressure
    b) Venoconstriction, which decreases vascular capacitance, increasing venous return to the heart, preload, and BP
  2. Vasodepressor area causes the following:
    a) Decrease in heart rate, cardiac output, and BP
    b) Venodilation, which increases vascular capacitance, decreasing venous return to the heart, preload, and BP

Oxygen Delivery to the Tissue

I. Oxygen delivery (DO_2)
  A. DO_2 is the product of cardiac output and arterial oxygen content (Fig. 2-24)
    1. Cardiac output is a product of heart rate and stroke volume
      a) Stroke volume is determined by preload, afterload, and contractility
    2. Arterial oxygen content is a product of hemoglobin and arterial saturation
    3. Normal DO_2 is approximately 1000 ml/min
  B. DO_2I is the product of cardiac index and arterial oxygen content; normal DO_2I is approximately 600 ml/min/m^2

II. Oxygen consumption or extraction (VO_2)
  A. VO_2 is determined by comparing the oxygen content in the arterial blood to the oxygen content in the mixed venous blood (e.g., distal tip of pulmonary artery catheter)
  B. Normal VO_2 is approximately 250 ml/min

III. Oxygen extraction ratio (O_2ER)
  A. O_2ER is an evaluation of the amount of oxygen that is extracted from the arterial blood as it passes through the capillaries; it is the ratio of the difference between the content of oxygen in the arterial blood and the content of oxygen in venous blood to the content of oxygen in the arterial blood
  B. Normal O_2ER is approximately 25%

IV. Oxygen extraction index (O_2EI)
  A. O_2EI is an estimation of O_2EI calculated using only oxygen saturations (SaO_2 and SvO_2)
  B. Normal O_2EI is approximately 25%

V. Oxygen reserve in venous blood
  A. Venous oxygen reserve is determined by measuring the oxygen saturation in mixed venous blood
  B. Normal SvO_2 is approximately 75%

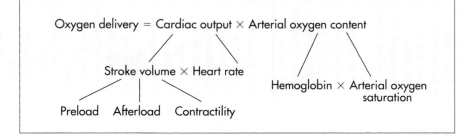

Oxygen delivery = Cardiac output × Arterial oxygen content

Stroke volume × Heart rate

Preload   Afterload   Contractility

Hemoglobin × Arterial oxygen saturation

Figure 2-24   Determinants of oxygen delivery. (From Daily EK, Schroeder JS: *Techniques in bedside hemodynamic monitoring,* St Louis, 1994, Mosby.)

Cardiovascular Assessment
Interview

I. Chief complaint: Identifies why the patient is seeking help and the duration of the problem

II. Symptoms related to cardiac disorders
   A. Chest pain
      1. May also be identified as indigestion, burning, discomfort, tightness, or pressure in midchest, epigastrium, or left arm (Table 2-4 describes differentiation of chest pain)
      2. PQRST format for describing complaint
         a) P
            (1) Provocation: What provokes or worsens the pain?
            (2) Palliation: What relieves the pain? (also include what was used but did not relieve the pain)
         b) Q
            (1) Quality: What does the pain feel like?
         c) R
            (1) Region: Where is the pain?
            (2) Radiation: If the pain radiates, to what area does the pain radiate?
         d) S
            (1) Severity: How severe is the pain? A 0 to 10 scale with 0 being no pain and 10 being the most severe pain
         e) T
            (1) Timing: Is the pain intermittent or continuous? What is the relationship to other events or activities?
   B. Dyspnea
      1. Shortness of breath or "breathlessness"
      2. Exertional dyspnea
      3. Orthopnea: Patient is unable to lie flat because of dyspnea
      4. Paroxysmal nocturnal dyspnea (PND): Patient awakens with a feeling of suffocation 1 to 2 hours after going to sleep; if accompanied by wheezing, may be called *cardiac asthma*
   C. Cough: Cardiac cough usually occurs at night and is precipitated by supine position, exertion, or by turning to one side
   D. Headache: may be related to hypertension
   E. Ascites: may be related to right ventricular failure (RVF)
   F. Abdominal pain: may be related to RVF
   G. Edema or weight gain: frequently related to RVF; also described as bloated feeling, swelling, tightening of clothing, tightening of shoes, marks left from constricting garments
   H. Fatigue or weakness: may be related to RVF
   I. Syncope
      1. Effort syncope: transient loss of consciousness that occurs shortly after heavy activity is started; may be associated with aortic or subaortic stenosis
      2. Stokes-Adams attack: dramatic loss of consciousness; related to heart block or rhythm disturbances
      3. Pacemaker syncope: syncope caused by malfunction or failure of an artificial pacemaker
      4. Hypersensitive carotid sinus syncope: syncope caused by pressure applied on a carotid sinus body of a patient with atherosclerotic and hypersensitive carotid arteries
   J. Palpitations: unpleasant awareness of the heartbeat when at rest; may be described as skipping, pounding, thumping sensation; associated with premature beats or other rhythm disturbances
   K. Hemoptysis: may be related to mitral stenosis or pulmonary edema
   L. Intermittent claudication: hip, thigh, or calf pain that occurs with exercise and ceases with rest; indicative of peripheral arterial disease
   M. Nocturia: may be related to HF
   N. Diaphoresis: may be related to sympathetic nervous system stimulation or infection
   O. Unexplained joint pain: may be related to rheumatic fever
   P. Calf tenderness: may be related to thrombophlebitis; may be accompanied by red, warm skin over vein
   Q. Varicose veins: dilated, sometimes painful, veins

III. History of present illness: use PQRST format
   A. Provocation, palliation
   B. Quality, quantity
   C. Region, radiation
   D. Severity
   E. Timing
   F. Associated symptoms

Text continued on p. 30

Table 2-4	Differentiation of Chest Pain						
Cause	**Provocation**	**Palliation**	**Quality**	**Region/Radiation**	**Severity**	**Timing**	**Associated Signs/ Symptoms**
ANGINA PECTORIS	• Exercise • Exertion • Exposure to cold • Emotional stress • Eating • Smoking	• Rest • Oxygen • Nitroglycerin • Calcium channel blocker (e.g., nifedipine)	• Heaviness or pressure • Tightness • Squeezing • Dull ache • Burning • Not always described as pain but as discomfort	• Substernal • May be diffuse and vague • May radiate to arms, neck, jaw, back, and upper abdomen	• Mild to severe	• Gradual or sudden onset • Duration: usually 1-4 minutes but may be 5-15 minutes	• Tachycardia, tachypnea • Dyspnea • Nausea, vomiting • Diaphoresis • Weakness • Anxiety • May have ST-T-wave changes with pain
ACUTE MYOCARDIAL INFARCTION	• No specific precipitator • Lifestyle change and stress • Usually occurs within 3 hours of awakening	• Narcotics • Reperfusion by thrombolytics or interventional cardiology procedure • No relief with rest and/or NTG	• As for angina • Heaviness or pressure • May show Levine's sign (clenched fist over sternum)	• As for angina	• No symptoms to severe • Absence of pain is common in patients with diabetes mellitus and in older adults	• Sudden onset • Duration: >30 minutes; usually 1-2 hours	• As for angina • Tachycardia, tachypnea • Dyspnea • Feeling of impending doom • S_4 • ECG changes: T-wave inversion, ST segment elevation, eventually Q-waves
DISSECTING AORTIC ANEURYSM	• Peripheral vascular disease • Marfan syndrome • Aortitis • Hypertension and/or hypertensive crisis • Chest trauma	• Narcotics • Surgery • No relief with rest and/or NTG	• Tearing • Ripping	• Anterior chest • Radiation to shoulders, neck, back, and abdomen	• Severe	• Sudden onset • Worse at onset • Duration: hours to days	• Tachycardia, tachypnea • Dysphagia • Confusion • Diaphoresis • Syncope • Dyspnea • Diaphoresis • Anxiety • Unilateral absence of pulse; BP differences between sides • Motor/sensory changes • Murmur of aortic regurgitation

PERICARDITIS	• Myocardial infarction • Cardiac surgery • Trauma • Infections • Uremia • Lupus erythematosus	• Nonsteroidal antiinflammatory agents (e.g., ibuprofen; indomethacin) • Sitting up and leaning forward	• Sharp • Stabbing • Knifelike • Worsened by inspiration, coughing, movement, recumbent position	• Precordial • Substernal • Radiation to neck, shoulders, arms, and back	• Mild to severe	• Sudden onset • Duration: days	• Tachycardia, tachypnea • Fever • Dyspnea • Pericardial friction rub • Leukocytosis • Diffuse ST segment elevation across the precordial leads
PULMONARY EMBOLISM	• Venous stasis (e.g., immobility, pelvic surgery, atrial fibrillation) • Hypercoagulability (e.g., oral contraceptives, malignancy, polycythemia) • Injury to vessel wall (e.g., IVs, vascular surgery) • Long-bone fracture (fat embolus)	• Narcotics • High Fowler's position • Splinting of chest	• Sharp • Knifelike • Shooting • Deep ache • Pressure • Increased by deep inspiration or coughing	• Substernal or lateral chest • Radiation to shoulder or neck	• Mild to severe	• Sudden onset • Duration: minutes to hours	• Tachycardia, tachypnea • Dyspnea • Pallor or cyanosis • Cough • Anxiety, feeling of impending doom • Sinus tachycardia or atrial dysrhythmias • Accentuated P_2 • Right-sided S_4, possible right-sided S_3 • If RVF: JVD • If pulmonary infarction: pleural friction rub; hemoptysis, fever

Continued

Table 2-4 **Differentiation of Chest Pain—cont'd**

Cause	Provocation	Palliation	Quality	Region/Radiation	Severity	Timing	Associated Signs/Symptoms
PNEUMOTHORAX	• Congenital bleb • Emphysematous bullous • Large tidal volumes or positive end-expiratory pressure (PEEP) on mechanical ventilator • Chest trauma • Exacerbated by coughing, exertion, or Valsalva maneuver	• Narcotics • Insertion of chest tube	• Tearing • Sharp • Increased with breathing	• Lateral chest • May radiate to shoulder, back, and arms	• Mild to severe	• Sudden onset • Duration: hours to days	• Tachypnea • Tachycardia • Dyspnea • Anxiety • JVD • Hyperresonance on percussion of affected side • Diminished breath sounds on affected side • Subcutaneous emphysema may be seen • Tracheal deviation may be seen, especially with tension pneumothorax
PLEUROPULMONARY (E.G., PLEURISY)	• Respiratory infection • Aspiration	• Narcotics • Relief with sitting up	• Sharp • Increased by coughing, inspiration, or movement	• Lateral chest • May radiate to shoulder, neck	• Moderate	• Gradual onset • Duration: days to weeks	• Tachypnea • Tachycardia • Dyspnea • Fever • Productive cough • Pleural friction rub

Type	Precipitating Factors	Relieving Factors	Character	Location	Severity	Onset/Duration	Associated Symptoms
GASTROINTESTINAL CHEST PAIN	• Cold liquids • Food intake, especially spicy foods, acidic foods, or foods high in fat • Alcohol • Caffeine • Stress • Smoking • Exercise	• Sitting up • Antacids • Esophageal spasm may be relieved by nitroglycerin	• "Heartburn" • Dull, burning • Squeezing • Increased by eating or supine position	• Retrosternal or lower substernal • Upper abdomen • Midline • May radiate to left arm, neck, jaw, upper abdomen, back, and shoulder	• Mild to moderate	• Gradual or sudden onset • Duration: minutes to days	• Dyspnea • Diaphoresis • Anxiety • Dysphagia • Eructation • Vomiting
MUSCULOSKELETAL CHEST PAIN	• Neck or arm strain • Movement • Coughing • Deep breathing • CPR	• Rest • Heat • Antiinflammatory agents (e.g., aspirin, ibuprofen)	• Soreness • Stabbing or sticking sensation • Tenderness • Increased with inspiration and movement	• Localized to one side of chest	• Mild to moderate	• Gradual or sudden onset • Duration: weeks	• Tachypnea • Splinting respirations • Localized tenderness over site of pain
PSYCHOSOMATIC CHEST PAIN	• Stress • Fatigue	• Rest • Anxiolytics	• Dull ache • Sharp • Stabbing • Superficial	• Precordium • Localized; frequently on left side • No radiation	• Mild to moderate	• Gradual or sudden onset • Duration: minutes to days	• Hyperpnea • Dyspnea • Palpitations • Dry mouth • Dizziness • Tingling of hands, mouth • Fatigue • Frequent sighing

IV. Past medical history
  A. Past illnesses
    1. Coronary artery disease
       a) Angina
       b) Myocardial infarction
    2. Hypertension
    3. Cerebrovascular disease: transient ischemic attacks or cerebral infarction (stroke)
    4. Peripheral vascular disease
    5. Rheumatic fever or rheumatic heart disease
    6. Murmur or known valvular heart disease
    7. Pulmonary disease (e.g., asthma; COPD)
    8. Connective tissue disorders
    9. Endocrine disorders
    10. Kidney disease
    11. Alcoholism
    12. Anemia
    13. Bleeding disorders
  B. Past chest trauma: history of recent past trauma is important to differentiate myocardial infarction from myocardial contusion; recent chest trauma would serve as a contraindication for thrombolytics
  C. Past surgical procedures
    1. Cardiac surgery: identify whether coronary artery bypass grafting, valve replacement, or other type of cardiac surgery
    2. Percutaneous coronary intervention: angioplasty, atherectomy, stent placement, valvuloplasty
    3. Pacemaker insertion
  D. Allergies and type of reaction
  E. Past diagnostic studies (e.g., stress ECG, cardiac catheterization, echocardiogram)
V. Family history
  A. Coronary artery disease (CAD)
  B. Cerebrovascular disease
  C. Peripheral vascular disease
  D. Hypertension
  E. Diabetes mellitus
  F. Hyperlipidemia
  G. Kidney disease
  H. Bleeding disorders
VI. Social history
  A. Relationship with spouse or significant other; family structure
  B. Occupation
  C. Educational level
  D. Stress level and usual coping mechanisms
  E. Personality type
    1. Type A: sense of time urgency, hostility, aggression, ambition, competitiveness, impatience, frustration
    2. Type B: none of the above qualities
  F. Recreational habits
  G. Exercise habits
  H. Dietary habits
  I. Caffeine intake
  J. Tobacco use: recorded as pack-years (number of packs per day times the number of years he or she has been smoking)
  K. Alcohol use: recorded as alcoholic beverages consumed per month, week, or day
  L. Toxin exposure
  M. Travel
VII. Medication history
  A. Prescribed drug, dosage, frequency, time of last dose
  B. Nonprescribed drugs
    1. Over-the-counter drugs
    2. Substance abuse (e.g., cocaine, amphetamines)
  C. Patient's understanding of drug actions, side effects
  D. Drugs causing potential problems for patients with cardiovascular disease
    1. Sinus or cold remedies: may contain ephedrine and increase BP
    2. Aspirin: prolongs blood clotting
    3. Tricyclic antidepressants: may cause dysrhythmias (e.g., torsades de pointes)
    4. Phenytoin: may cause dysrhythmias
    5. Phenothiazines: may cause dysrhythmias, hypotension
    6. Oral contraceptives: may predispose to embolus, thrombosis
    7. Doxorubicin (Adriamycin): may cause cardiomyopathy
    8. Lithium: may cause dysrhythmias
    9. Corticosteroids: cause sodium and fluid retention and exacerbate heart failure
    10. Theophylline preparations: cause tachycardia and may cause dysrhythmias
    11. Cardiac stimulants (e.g., cocaine): cause tachycardia and may cause dysrhythmias and coronary artery spasm

Landmarks (Fig. 2-25)

I. Anatomic
  A. Clavicle
  B. Sternum
  C. Ribs
  D. Intercostal spaces
  E. Angle of Louis
  F. Xiphoid process
  G. Costal margin
  H. Costal angle
II. Imaginary
  A. Midsternal line (MSL)
  B. Midclavicular line (MCL)
  C. Anterior axillary line (AAL)
  D. Midaxillary line (MAL)
  E. Posterior axillary line (PAL)
  F. Scapular line
  G. Midspinal line
III. Location of heart
  A. Between the sternum and spinal column
  B. Lies between second ICS and fifth ICS
  C. Apex normally at fifth LICS at MCL

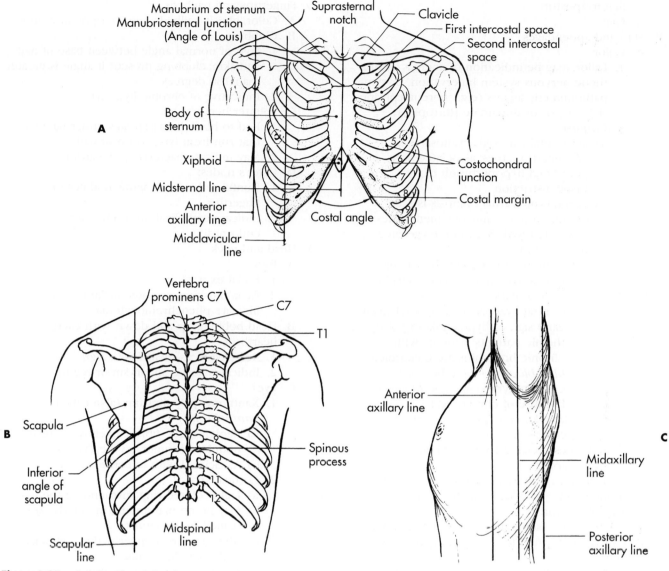

Figure 2-25   Landmarks of the thorax. **A,** anterior. **B,** posterior. **C,** lateral. (From Barkauskas V: *Health and physical assessment,* St Louis, 1994, Mosby.)

Inspection and Palpation

I. Vital signs
  A. BP: sitting, lying, standing
    1. Reduction of up to 15 mm Hg in systolic and 5 mm Hg in diastolic BP when standing is normal; greater reduction indicates orthostatic changes
    2. Variation of up to 15 mm Hg between arms is normal
    3. BP in lower extremities is expected to be 10 mm Hg higher than in upper extremities
    4. Narrowed pulse pressure frequently indicates vasoconstriction as occurs with innervation of sympathetic nervous system (SNS) (e.g., hypovolemic shock); widened pulse pressure frequently indicates excessive vasodilation as occurs with excessive vasodilatory mediator release (e.g., septic shock)

  B. Heart rate
    1. Rhythm is monitored if ECG monitor available
    2. Tachycardia frequently indicates innervation of SNS
  C. Respiratory (ventilatory) rate: Tachypnea frequently indicates innervation of SNS
  D. Temperature: Fever may indicate inflammatory or infectious process (e.g., myocardial infarction, pericarditis, endocarditis)
  E. Height
  F. Weight
II. General survey
  A. Apparent health status: consistency of apparent age and chronologic age
  B. Level of consciousness
  C. Gross deformity
  D. Nutritional status

E. Stature/posture

F. Gait

III. Skin and appendages

  A. Color

    1. Pallor: may be indication of anemia, sympathetic nervous system innervation, or sympathomimetic agents (e.g., norepinephrine [Levophed] or dopamine [Intropin])

    2. Cyanosis

      a) Peripheral (or cold) cyanosis is seen on fingertips, toes; associated with peripheral hypoperfusion or vasoconstriction

      b) Central (or warm) cyanosis is seen on lips, tongue, mucous membranes; associated with 5 g of deoxygenated hemoglobin

        (1) Central cyanosis may be late or impossible sign of hypoxemia in anemic patients

        (2) Central cyanosis may be a relatively early sign of hypoxemia in polycythemic patients; patients with chronic bronchitis are nicknamed *blue bloaters*—*blue* because of chronic hypoxemia and *bloaters* because of chronic RVF

      c) In dark-skinned patients, cyanosis appears as an ashen color

    3. Ruddiness: related to polycythemia or hypercapnia

  B. Moisture: diaphoresis, dryness

  C. Temperature: cold skin may be related to hypoperfusion

  D. Turgor: decrease in skin turgor, also referred to as *tenting,* related to interstitial dehydration

  E. Edema

    1. Edema indicates increase in interstitial fluid of 30% above normal

    2. Note the location of the edema

      a) Facial

        (1) Allergies: profound facial edema in anaphylaxis

        (2) Steroids: exogenous (e.g., prednisone) or endogenous (e.g., Cushing's syndrome)

        (3) Renal disease (e.g., nephrotic syndrome)

      b) Dependent: RVF

      c) Generalized (anasarca): end-stage HF, end-stage renal failure, hypoproteinemia

    3. Degree of pitting

      a) Grade 1+ = 0 to ¼ inch

      b) Grade 2+ = ¼ to ½ inch

      c) Grade 3+ = ½ to 1 inch

      d) Grade 4+ = more than 1 inch

  F. Lesions

    1. Arterial disease may cause ulcers at toes or points of trauma

    2. Venous disease may cause ulcers at sides of ankles

IV. Fingertips and nailbeds

  A. Color: bluish nailbeds with peripheral cyanosis

  B. Clubbing

    1. Loss of normal angle between base of nail and skin; clubbing present if angle is greater than 180 degrees

    2. Indicative of chronic hypoxia

  C. Splinter hemorrhages

    1. Red to black linear streaks under nailbed that run from base to tip of nail

    2. May indicate bacterial endocarditis

  D. Osler's nodes:

    1. Painful red subcutaneous nodules on fingertips

    2. Indicate embolization in infective endocarditis

V. Head and neck

  A. Face

    1. Facial expression

    2. Facial flushing: episodic facial flushing may indicate pheochromocytoma

  B. Head bobbing up and down with each heartbeat

    1. Referred to as *de Musset's sign*

    2. Indicates aortic aneurysm or regurgitation

  C. Eyes

    1. Xanthoma palpebrarum (also called *xanthelasma*)

      a) Benign, fatty, fibrous, yellowish plaque, nodule, or tumor on the eyelids

      b) Associated with hyperlipidemia

    2. Corneal arcus

      a) Light-colored ring surrounding the iris

      b) May be normal finding in elderly patient (called *arcus senilis*)

      c) Abnormal in younger patient; associated with hyperlipidemia

    3. Exophthalmos: may be seen in advanced HF with pulmonary hypertension

  D. Ears

    1. Diagonal bilateral earlobe creases (referred to as *McCarty's sign*): may indicate coronary artery disease if seen in individuals less than 45 years of age

  E. Neck

    1. Jugular vein distention

      a) To evaluate JVD (Fig. 2-26)

        (1) Place patient at a 45-degree angle

        (2) Identify the sternal angle: raised notch that is created where the manubrium and the body of the sternum join; also called *manubriosternal junction* or *angle of Louis*

        (3) Measure height of neck vein distention above the level of the sternal angle

        (4) Normal height of neck vein distention is 1 to 2 cm above the sternal angle

      b) Neck vein distention of greater than 2

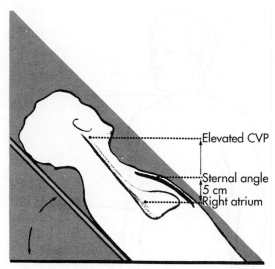

Figure 2-26 Jugular venous distention and estimation of central venous pressure: assess jugular venous distention with patient in 45-degree angle; determine height of jugular venous distention above the sternal angle; add 5 cm to this measurement to estimate central venous pressure. (From Guzzetta CE, Dossey BM: *Cardiovascular nursing: holistic practice,* St Louis, 1992, Mosby.)

cm above the sternal angle is indicative of any of the following:
(1) Right ventricular failure
(2) Hypervolemia
(3) Tension pneumothorax
(4) Cardiac tamponade
c) To estimate central venous pressure (CVP)
(1) Add 5 cm to the height of neck vein distention
(2) Normal CVP (in centimeters of water): 3 to 8
d) To evaluate hepatojugular (or abdomino-jugular) reflux
(1) Apply pressure over right upper quadrant
(2) Evaluate increase in neck vein distention
(3) Increase in neck vein distention greater than 3 cm is indicative of hepatojugular reflux and right ventricular failure
VI. Precordium: inspect and palpate entire precordium
A. Point of maximal impulse (PMI) or apical impulse
1. Frequently visible and usually palpable
2. Location
a) Normal location of the PMI is at the fifth LICS at the MCL
b) Lateral displacement is associated with any of the following:
(1) Left ventricular dilation (e.g., aortic or mitral insufficiency)
(2) Upward displacement of the diaphragm (e.g., pregnancy, ascites)

(3) Right to left mediastinal shift (e.g., right pleural effusion or tension pneumothorax)
(4) Left ventricular hypertrophy or failure
c) Medial displacement may occur with any of the following:
(1) Downward displacement of the diaphragm (e.g., COPD)
(2) Left to right mediastinal shift (e.g., left pleural effusion or tension pneumothorax)
3. Intensity
a) Normal intensity is only a light tap
b) Failure may increase the intensity and cause a heave
4. Size
a) Normal size is approximately 1 to 2 cm
b) The size is more diffuse with ventricular aneurysm
B. Heave
1. Lifting of the chest wall indicative of failure
2. Left ventricular heave felt at or near the apex
3. Right ventricular heave (or lift) felt at or near the sternum
C. Thrill
1. Palpable vibration associated with murmur or bruit
2. Felt where the murmur is heard the loudest or at location of bruit
VII. Abdomen
A. Aortic pulsation
1. Normally visible, especially during expiration
2. Normally palpable at midline or slightly to left of midline; feel for lateral expansion, which might be indicative of aneurysm
VIII. Extremities
A. Arterial versus venous disease (Table 2-5)
B. Temperature
1. Coolness or coldness may indicate decreased blood flow because of hypoperfusion or vasoconstriction
2. Excessive warmth may indicate hyperthyroidism or fever
C. Peripheral pulses
1. Location (Fig. 2-27)
a) Carotid: palpate only lower half and never palpate both carotids simultaneously
b) Brachial
c) Radial
d) Ulnar
e) Femoral
f) Popliteal
g) Posterior tibialis
h) Dorsalis pedis
2. Rate and rhythm
3. Amplitude
a) 0 = not palpable

Table 2-5	Comparison of Clinical Indications of Arterial and Venous Peripheral Vascular Disease	
	Arterial	**Venous**
PAIN	• Excruciating in acute occlusion • Intermittent claudication in chronic occlusion	• Crampy pain • Homan's sign in thrombophlebitis
PULSES	• Diminished or absent	• Normal (but may be difficult to palpate because of edema)
COLOR	• Pale	• Normal or ruddy
TEMPERATURE	• Cool or cold	• Warm
EDEMA	• Absent	• Present; may be severe
SKIN CHANGES	• Thin, shiny, atrophic skin • Loss of hair • Thickened toenails	• Brown pigmentation at ankles
ULCERATIONS	• At toes or points of trauma	• At sides of ankles

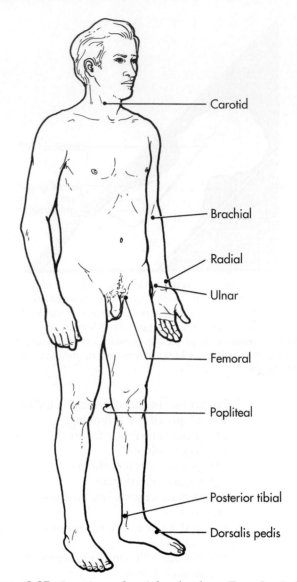

Figure 2-27 Locations of peripheral pulses. (From Lewis SM, Collier IC: *Medical-surgical nursing: assessment and management of clinical problems,* ed 3, St Louis, 1992, Mosby.)

b) 1+ = weak and thready, easily obliterated
c) 2+ = normal, not easily obliterated
d) 3+ = full and bounding, cannot obliterate
4. Doppler pulse
   a) A Doppler stethoscope is used to identify presence of pulse if the pulse is not palpable and may be used to confirm that the pulse palpated is the patient's and not the nurse's
5. Doppler pressure
   a) A Doppler stethoscope is used to measure the blood pressure distal to vascular lesions or surgery
   b) Apply sphygmomanometer on calf or below graft site and inflate to pressure above the patient's systolic brachial pressure; allow pressure to decrease and note pressure when pulse is audible again; note posterior tibial and dorsalis pedis pressure
   c) Use the best pressure (posterior tibial or dorsalis pedis) to calculate the ankle-brachial index (ABI); divide the brachial

pressure by the ankle pressure (ankle-brachial) to calculate the ABI
   (1) Normal: 1.0 or greater
   (2) Mildly abnormal: 0.95 to 0.75
   (3) Claudicant: 0.75 to 0.50
   (4) Ischemic: 0.50 to 0.25
   (5) Severe ischemia: less than 0.25
   (6) Clinically significant: decrease of 0.15 or more
6. Capillary refill rate
   a) Color should return to blanched area within 3 seconds; delay beyond 3 seconds indicates hypoperfusion
7. Apical-radial pulse deficit
   a) Performed by two nurses using one watch
   b) Deficit (radial pulse rate less than apical rate) indicative of dysrhythmia (e.g., atrial fibrillation, ventricular ectopy)

ARTERIAL PULSE ABNORMALITIES

Type	Description
Pulsus magnus	Pulse is readily palpable, not easily obliterated by fingers, and does not fade Pulse is felt as a brisk impact; can occur with or without increased pulse pressure
Pulsus parvus	Pulse is difficult to feel, easily obliterated by the fingers, and may fade out Pulse is slow to rise, has a sustained summit, and falls slowly If both weak and variable in amplitude, pulse is termed "thready"
Pulsus alternans	Pulses have large amplitude beats followed by pulses of small amplitude Rhythm remains normal
Pulsus paradoxus	Pattern is exaggerated (>10 mm Hg) during insipiration, and amplitude is increased during expiration Heart rate and rhythm are unchanged
Pulsus bisferiens (double-peaked)	Best felt by palpating carotid artery Two systolic peaks can occur in disorders that cause rapid left ventricular ejection of large stroke volume with wide pulse pressure
Water-hammer, collapsing	Pulse has greater amplitude than normal pulse Pulse marked by rapid rise to a narrow summit followed by a sudden descent

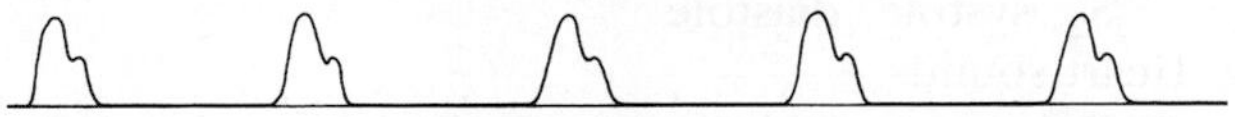

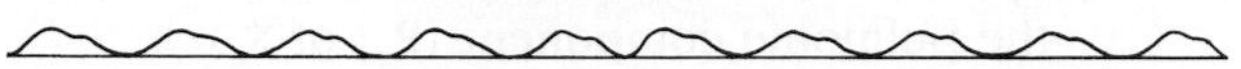

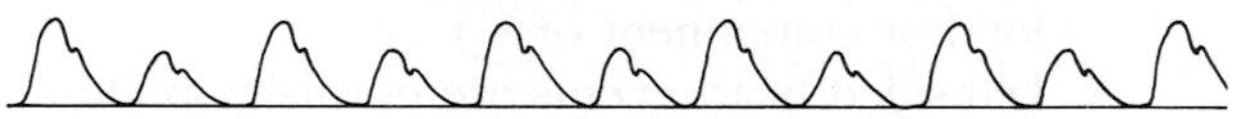

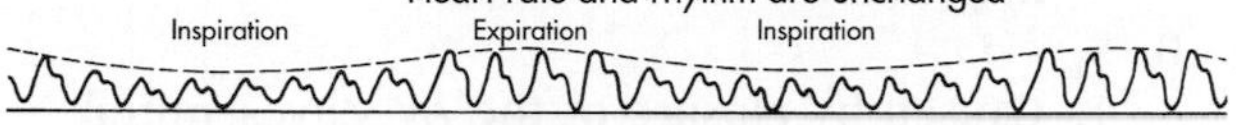

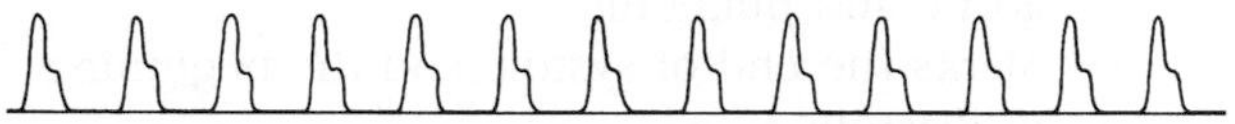

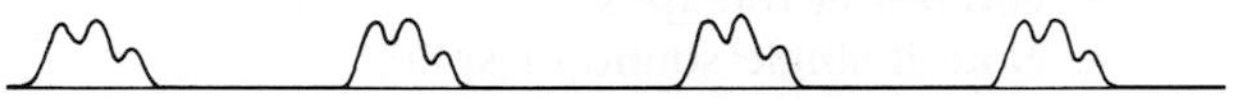

Figure 2-28 Pulse contour. (Modified from Cannobio MM: *Cardiovascular disorders,* St Louis, 1990, Mosby.)

8. Pulse contour (Fig. 2-28)
   a) Pulsus magnus
      (1) Strong, bounding pulses with rapid upstroke and downstroke
      (2) Characteristic of any of the following:
         (a) Hypertension
         (b) Thyrotoxicosis
         (c) Aortic insufficiency
         (d) Patent ductus arteriosus
         (e) Arteriovenous fistula
   b) Pulsus parvus
      (1) Small, weak pulse
      (2) Characteristic of any of the following:
         (a) Aortic stenosis: also tardus (late)
         (b) Mitral stenosis
         (c) Constrictive pericarditis
         (d) Cardiac tamponade
   c) Pulsus alternans
      (1) Alternating pulse waves, every other

beat being weaker than the preceding one
      (2) Characteristic of left ventricular failure
   d) Pulsus paradoxus
      (1) Pulsus paradoxus is an exaggeration of normal physiologic response to inspiration
      (2) The normal decrease in BP during inspiration is 10 mm Hg or less
      (3) BP drop of more than 10 mm Hg during inspiration is pulsus paradoxus
      (4) Characteristic of any of the following:
         (a) Pericardial effusion
         (b) Constrictive pericarditis
         (c) Cardiac tamponade
         (d) Severe lung disease
         (e) Advanced HF
         (f) Hemorrhagic shock
   e) Pulsus bisferiens
      (1) Two pulses palpated during systole with second slightly weaker than the first
      (2) Characteristic of any of the following:
         (a) Hypertrophic cardiomyopathy
         (b) Constrictive cardiomyopathy
         (c) Aortic stenosis or regurgitation
   f) Water-hammer (or *Corrigan's*) pulse
      (1) Increased pulse pressure with a rapid upstroke and downstroke and shortened peak
      (2) Characteristic of aortic regurgitation
D. Homan's sign
   1. Identified by dorsiflexing the foot with the knee slightly bent
   2. Homan's sign is present if the patient has pain in the calf with this action
   3. Suggestive of thrombophlebitis
E. Petechiae or ecchymosis
F. Varicose veins
G. Neurovascular assessment
   1. Assess neurovascular status in all of the following situations:
      a) In patients at risk for mural thrombi (e.g., atrial fibrillation, ventricular aneurysm)
      b) After cardiac catheterization
      c) After percutaneous coronary intervention (e.g., angioplasty, atherectomy, valvuloplasty)
      d) When the patient has intraaortic balloon pump catheter in place
      e) When the patient has an extremity fracture (to monitor for compartment syndrome)
      f) When the patient has a circumferential burn of an extremity
   2. Monitor for clinical indications of acute arterial occlusion: 6 P's (Box 2-1)

H. Clinical indications of hypoperfusion (Table 2-6); because hypoperfusion is progressive, the earlier these changes are identified, the more appropriate the management and the chances for successfully reversing these changes

Auscultation

I. Stethoscope
   A. Qualities of a good stethoscope
      1. Snug-fitting earplugs to eliminate extraneous sounds
      2. Tubing
         a) Two tubings are preferable for high-frequency sounds
         b) Tubing should not be longer than 12 to 15 inches
      3. Chest piece
         a) Diaphragm
            (1) Used for high-pitched sounds (e.g., S_1, S_2, splits of S_1 and S_2, pericardial friction rubs, most murmurs)
            (2) Held firmly against skin
         b) Bell
            (1) Used for low-pitched sounds (e.g., S_3, S_4, murmurs of AV valve stenosis)
            (2) Held only tightly enough against skin to create a seal
II. Auscultatory areas (Fig. 2-29)
   A. Mitral: fifth LICS at MCL
   B. Tricuspid: fifth LICS at LSB
   C. Erb's point: third LICS at LSB
   D. Pulmonic: second LICS at LSB
   E. Aortic: second RICS at RSB

III. Method of cardiac auscultation
   A. Ensure a quiet room by turning off television and radio and asking others to be quiet
   B. Listen to all four auscultatory areas with both bell and diaphragm
   C. Concentrate on one cardiac event at a time: S_1, S_2, systole, diastole
IV. Heart sounds
   A. Rules to consider
      1. Left-sided heart events precede right-sided heart events (i.e., the mitral component (M_1) precedes the tricuspid component [T_1] of S_1 and the aortic component [A_2] precedes the pulmonic component [P_2] of S_2)
      2. Left-sided heart events are normally louder than right-sided heart events (i.e., M_1 is the loudest component of S_1, and A_2 is the loudest component of S_2)
      3. Left-sided heart events are normally loudest during expiration, and right-sided heart events are normally loudest during inspiration
   B. S_1
      1. Caused by closure of the AV valves: mitral and tricuspid
      2. Marks the end of diastole and the beginning of systole
      3. Loudest at the apex
      4. Note if single sound or split
      5. Note any increase in intensity (closing snap)
   C. S_2
      1. Caused by closure of the semilunar valves: aortic and pulmonic
      2. Marks the end of systole and the beginning of diastole
      3. Loudest at the base
      4. Note if single sound or split
      5. Note any increase in intensity
   D. Splits
      1. Split S_1
         a) Both components (M_1 and T_1) of S_1 can be heard
         b) A split S_1 is heard best at the tricuspid area
         c) A narrowly split S_1 may be normal
         d) A split S_1 is more often abnormal than

BOX 2-1 Clinical Manifestations of Acute Arterial Occlusion

Pain
Pallor
Pulselessness
Paresthesia
Paralysis
Polar (cold)

Note: these 6 P's are your format for neurovascular assessment

---

Table 2-6 Clinical Indications of Hypoperfusion

Normal	Subclinical Hypoperfusion	Clinical Hypoperfusion	Shock
CI 2.5-4.0 L/min/m^2	CI 2.2-2.5 L/min/m^2	CI 2.0-2.2 L/min/m^2	CI <2.0 L/min/m^2
• Normal	• No clinical indications of hypoperfusion but "something different"	• Tachycardia • Narrowed pulse pressure • Tachypnea • Cool skin • Oliguria • Diminished bowel sounds • Restlessness to confusion	• Dysrhythmias • Hypotension • Tachypnea • Cold, clammy skin • Anuria • Absent bowel sounds • Lethargy to coma

normal and is associated with any of the following:
(1) RBBB
(2) Left ventricular (epicardial) pacemaker
(3) Left ventricular ectopy
2. Split S_2
   a) Both components (A_2 and P_2) of S_2 can be heard
   b) A split S_2 is heard best at the pulmonic area
   c) Inspiratory only split of S_2 is normal
      (1) Called a *physiologic split of S_2*
      (2) Normal and frequently heard in individuals under 50 years of age
      (3) Split only during inspiration
      (4) Caused by changes in intrathoracic pressure related to ventilation; increased venous return to right ventricle and decreased venous return to left ventricle delay pulmonic valve closure (P_2)
   d) Expiratory split of S_2 is abnormal
      (1) Increased splitting during inspiration (split on expiration but split more during inspiration); associated with any of the following:
         (a) RBBB
         (b) Left ventricular ectopy
         (c) Left ventricular (epicardial) pacemaker
         (d) Severe mitral regurgitation
         (e) Pulmonary stenosis
         (f) Pulmonary hypertension
         (g) Ventricular septal defect
      (2) Fixed splitting (split the same on inspiration and expiration); associated with atrial septal defect

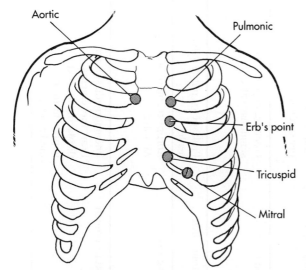

Figure 2-29 Cardiac auscultatory areas. (From Price SA, Wilson LM: *Pathophysiology: clinical concepts of disease processes,* ed 4, St Louis, 1994, Mosby.)

(3) Paradoxical split (split on expiration but not on inspiration); associated with any of the following:
   (a) LBBB
   (b) Right ventricular (endocardial) pacemaker
   (c) Right ventricular ectopy
   (d) Severe aortic stenosis or regurgitation
   (e) Patent ductus arteriosus
E. Extra heart sounds (Table 2-7 is a summary of extra heart sounds)
   1. S_3
      a) Also called a *ventricular gallop*
      b) Dull, low-pitched sound occurring early in diastole after S_2; may sound like "Ken-tuc-ky" with the "ky" being the S_3
      c) Caused by rapid rush of blood into a dilated ventricle; considered abnormal in patients more than 30 years of age
      d) Heard best with bell, with the patient lying on his or her left side
         (1) Left-sided S_3
            (a) Heard best at apex
            (b) Heard best during expiration
         (2) Right-sided S_3
            (a) Heard best at sternum
            (b) Heard best during inspiration
      e) Associated primarily with failure
      f) May also be associated with any of the following:
         (1) Fluid overload
         (2) Cardiomyopathy
         (3) Ventricular septal defect or patent ductus arteriosus
         (4) Mitral or tricuspid regurgitation
   2. S_4
      a) Also called an *atrial gallop*
      b) Dull, low-pitched sound occurring late in diastole before S_1; may sound like "Ten-nes-see" with the "Ten" being the S_4
      c) Caused by atrial contraction and propulsion of blood into a noncompliant ventricle; abnormal in adults
      d) Heard best with bell with patient lying on his or her left side
         (1) Left-sided S_4: heard best at apex
         (2) Right-sided S_4: heard best at sternum
      e) Associated with any of the following:
         (1) Myocardial ischemia or infarction
         (2) Hypertension
            (a) Systemic: left-sided S_4
            (b) Pulmonary: right-sided S_4
         (3) Ventricular hypertrophy
         (4) AV blocks
         (5) Severe aortic or pulmonic stenosis
   3. Quadruple rhythm: all four heart sounds heard
   4. Summation gallop
      a) All four heart sounds plus tachycardia

Table 2-7 Extra Sounds

Sound	Cause	Timing	Location	Pitch	Position	Respiratory Effect
S_3 (also called *ventricular gallop*)	Rapid ventricular filling into dilated ventricle	Early diastole (rapid filling phase of diastole)	Mitral if LV; tricuspid if RV	Low	Heard best in left lateral position	LV S_3 increases with expiration; RV S_3 increases with inspiration
S_4 (also called *atrial gallop*)	Atrial contraction into noncompliant ventricle	Late diastole (atrial contraction phase of diastole)	Mitral area if LV; tricuspid area if RV	Low	Heard best in left lateral position	LV S_4 increased with expiration; RV S_4 increased with inspiration
Quadruple rhythm	All four heart sounds are heard	S_3 heard in early diastole, and S_4 heard in late diastole	Apex	Low	Heard best in left lateral position	As for S_3, S_4
Summation gallop	S_1, S_2 heard along with merged S_3 and S_4; occurs with tachycardia	Middiastole	Apex	Low	Heard best in left lateral position	As for S_3, S_4
Pericardial friction rub	Constriction of the pericardium	Early diastole	Lower left sternal border	High	Heard best with patient leaning forward	Heard best if patient holds his breath after expiration
Pericardial knock	Constriction of the pericardium	Early diastole	Lower left sternal border	Low	Heard best with patient leaning forward or in left lateral position	Heard best if patient holds his breath after expiration
Ejection click	Opening of defective semilunar valve	Early systole	Aortic or pulmonic	High	Heard best with patient leaning forward	Aortic: not affected by respiratory phase Pulmonic: increased with expiration
Midsystolic click	Prolapse of mitral valve leaflet	Mid-systole	Mitral	High	Heard best in left lateral position	Increased with expiration
Opening snap	Abrupt recoil of stenotic AV valve	Early diastole	Mitral	High	Heard best in left lateral position	Mitral: increased with expiration Tricuspid: increased with inspiration
Mediastinal crunch	Pneumomediastinum; heart movements displacing air that is present in the mediastinum	Random	Apex or lower left sternal border	High	Heard best in left lateral position	Increased with inspiration

b) Merging of S_3 and S_4 causes a louder mid-diastolic sound

5. Pericardial friction rub
   a) High-pitched "to-and-fro" scratchy sound; usually triphasic including systolic, early diastolic, and late diastolic components
   b) Heard best at the fourth-fifth intercostal space at lower LSB with patient leaning forward
   c) Differentiate between pericardial and pleural friction rubs: Ask the patient to hold his or her breath; if the rub persists, it is a pericardial friction rub
   d) Caused by inflammation of the pericardium; commonly heard after MI or cardiac surgery

6. Pericardial knock
   a) Loud, early-diastolic sound heard best at lower LSB
   b) Caused by constrictive pericarditis

7. Snaps
   a) Opening snap
      (1) Short, high-pitched sound heard early in diastole at third to fourth LICS at LSB; earlier, sharper, higher pitched than S_3
      (2) Caused by either of the following:
          (a) Opening of stenotic AV valve; usually precedes a diastolic murmur
          (b) Increased flow (e.g., ventricular septal defect, patent ductus arteriosus)
   b) Closing snap
      (1) Really a loud S_1
      (2) Caused by closure of AV valve

8. Clicks: high pitched sounds heard during systole
   a) Aortic ejection click
      (1) High-pitched sound heard early in systole over aortic area to apex; may precede systolic ejection murmur
      (2) Caused by aortic valve disease or dilated aorta (e.g., aortic aneurysm or coarctation)
   b) Pulmonic ejection click
      (1) High-pitched sound heard early in systole over pulmonic area
      (2) Caused by pulmonic valve disease, pulmonary embolism, pulmonary hypertension, hyperthyroidism
   c) Midsystolic click
      (1) High-pitched sound heard best at apex or lower left sternal border
      (2) May occur alone or prior to a late systolic murmur
      (3) Caused by mitral valve prolapse or mitral regurgitation
   d) Prosthetic valve click: metallic click caused by opening and closing of prosthetic valve

9. Mediastinal crunch
   a) Crunching sound heard best at apex or along LSB in left lateral position
   b) Caused by air in mediastinum

F. Murmurs
   1. Causes of turbulence (referred to as a *murmur* if intracardiac or referred to as a *bruit* if extracardiac) (Fig. 2-30)
      a) Increased flow across a normal valve (e.g., flow murmur)
         (1) May also be called *functional* (as opposed to structural); they are always soft (not louder than grade II/VI) and systolic (but never holosystolic)
         (2) Caused by any of the following:
             (a) Hyperthermia
             (b) Anemia
             (c) Pregnancy
             (d) Hyperthyroidism
      b) Forward flow through a stenotic valve
      c) Backward flow through a regurgitant (also called *insufficient* or *incompetent*) valve
      d) Flow through an AV fistula or septal defect
      e) Flow into a dilated chamber or a portion of a vessel
   2. Description
      a) Timing
         (1) Systolic
             (a) Holosystolic: AV regurgitation or ventricular septal defect
             (b) Ejection (midsystolic): semilunar stenosis
             (c) Late: papillary muscle dysfunction, mitral valve prolapse, hypertrophic cardiomyopathy (previously called *idiopathic hypertrophic subaortic stenosis*)
         (2) Diastolic
             (a) Early diastolic: semilunar regurgitation
             (b) Middiastolic or late diastolic: AV stenosis
      b) Location: place at which the murmur is loudest
      c) Radiation: direction in which the murmur radiates
      d) Intensity: Levine scale
         (1) Grade I/VI: barely audible, difficult to detect
         (2) Grade II/VI: clearly audible but quiet
         (3) Grade III/VI: moderately loud, without a thrill
         (4) Grade IV/VI: loud; with or without a thrill
         (5) Grade V/VI: very loud, thrill present, audible with stethoscope partially off the chest

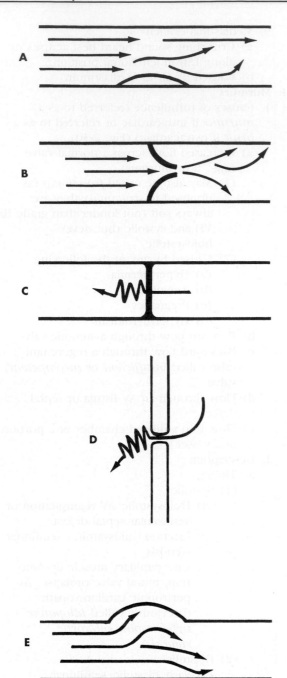

Figure 2-30 Causes of turbulence. **A,** Increased flow across a normal valve. **B,** Forward flow through a stenotic valve. **C,** Backward flow through an incompetent valve. **D,** Flow through a septal defect or an AV fistula. **E,** Flow into a dilated chamber or a portion of a vessel. (From Thompson DA: *Cardiovascular assessment,* St Louis, 1981, Mosby.)

          (6) Grade VI/VI: loudest possible, thrill present, audible with stethoscope off the chest
       e) Configuration
          (1) Crescendo: gets louder
          (2) Decrescendo: gets softer
          (3) Crescendo-decrescendo: louder then softer

          (4) Plateau: even intensity throughout
       f) Pitch
          (1) High-pitched (heard best with diaphragm)
             (a) Mitral and tricuspid regurgitation
             (b) Aortic and pulmonic stenosis
             (c) Aortic and pulmonic regurgitation
          (2) Low-pitched (heard best with bell): mitral and tricuspid stenosis
       g) Quality
          (1) Soft
          (2) Harsh
          (3) Blowing
          (4) Musical
          (5) Rumbling
          (6) Rough
   3. Table 2-8 describes common murmurs
V. Vascular sound: bruit
   A. Turbulent sound
   B. May be heard over carotids, aorta, renals, iliacs, femorals
   C. Associated with plaque or aneurysm

Diagnostic Studies
I. Serum chemistries
   A. Sodium: normal 136 to 145 mEq/L
   B. Potassium: normal 3.5 to 5.0 mEq/L
   C. Chloride: normal 96 to 106 mEq/L
   D. Calcium: normal 8.5 to 10.5 mg/dl
   E. Phosphorus: normal 3.0 to 4.5 mg/dl
   F. Magnesium: normal 1.5 to 2.5 mEq/L or 1.8 to 2.4 mg/dl
   G. Glucose: normal 70 to 110 mg/dl
   H. BUN: normal 5 to 20 mg/dl
   I. Creatinine: normal 0.7 to 1.5 mg/dl
   J. Lactate: 1 to 2 mmol/L
   K. Enzymes
      1. Total CK: normal 55 to 170 U/L for males; 30 to 135 U/L for females
      2. CK-MB: 0% of total CK
      3. LDH: 90 to 200 IU/L
      4. LDH-1: 17% to 25% of total LDH
   L. Muscle proteins
      1. Myoglobin: normal less than 110 ng/ml
      2. Troponin I: normal less than 1.5 ng/ml (although 0.6 to 1.5 ng/ml is considered suspicious)
      3. Troponin T: normal less than 0.1 ng/ml
   M. Lipid profile
      1. Cholesterol: normal 150 to 200 mg/dl
      2. Triglycerides: normal 40 to 150 mg/dl
      3. Lipoprotein-cholesterol fractionation
         a) HDL: normal 29 to 77 mg/dl
         b) LDL: normal 62 to 130 mg/dl
II. Arterial blood gases
   A. pH: normal 7.35 to 7.45
   B. $Paco_2$: normal 35 to 45 mm Hg
   C. HCO_3: normal 22 to 26 mEq/L
   D. Pao_2: normal 80 to 100 mm Hg
   E. Sao_2: more than 95%

Table 2-8	Common Murmurs							
Timing	**Location**	**Radiation**	**Intensity**	**Configuration**	**Pitch**	**Quality**	**Condition**
Holosystolic	Mitral	Toward left axilla	I-VI/VI	Plateau	High	Blowing, harsh, or musical	**Mitral regurgitation**
Holosystolic	Tricuspid	Along right sternal border toward apex if radiates	I-IV/VI	Plateau	High	Blowing, harsh, or musical	**Tricuspid regurgitation**
Holosystolic	3-4 ICS at lower sternal border	Radiates widely throughout precordium	Varies	Plateau	High	Harsh	**Ventricular septal rupture or defect**
Midsystolic (systolic ejection murmur)	Aortic	Toward right side of neck	Varies	Crescendo-decrescendo	Medium to high	Harsh	**Aortic stenosis**
Midsystolic (systolic ejection murmur)	Pulmonic	No radiation or toward left side of neck	III-IV/VI	Crescendo-decrescendo	Medium to high	Harsh	**Pulmonic stenosis**
Early diastole	Aortic or Erb's point	Toward apex	I-VI/VI	Decrescendo	High	Blowing	**Aortic regurgitation**
Early diastole	Pulmonic	Toward apex if radiates	Varies	Decrescendo	High	Blowing	**Pulmonic regurgitation**
Mid to late diastole	Mitral	Usually none	I-II/VI	Crescendo	Low	Rumbling	**Mitral stenosis**
Mid to late diastole	Tricuspid	Usually none; may radiate to apex or xiphoid	Varies	Decrescendo	Low	Rumbling	**Tricuspid stenosis**

III. Hematology
  A. Hematocrit: normal 40% to 52% for males; 35% to 47% for females
  B. Hemoglobin: normal 13 to 18 g/dl for males; 12 to 16 g/dl for females
  C. White blood cells (WBC): normal 3,500 to 11,000 mm^3
  D. Erythrocyte sedimentation rate: normal up to 15 mm/hr for males; up to 20 mm/hr for females

IV. Clotting profile
  A. Prothrombin time (PT): normal 12 to 15 seconds; therapeutic 1.5 to 2.5 times normal
  B. Activated partial thromboplastin time (aPTT): normal 25 to 38 seconds; therapeutic 1.5 to 2.5 times normal
  C. Activated clotting time (ACT): normal 70 to 120 seconds; therapeutic 150 to 190 seconds
  D. Thrombin time: normal 10 to 15 seconds
  E. Bleeding time: normal 1 to 9.5 minutes
  F. International normalized ratio (INR): normal less than 2.0
    1. Therapeutic range for atrial fibrillation: 1.5 to 2.5
    2. Therapeutic range for deep vein thrombosis (DVT) or pulmonary embolus (PE): 2.0 to 3.0
    3. Therapeutic range for prosthetic valves: 2.5 to 3.5
    4. Platelets: normal 150,000 to 400,000/mm^3

V. Urine
  A. Glucose: normal negative
  B. Ketones: normal negative
  C. Specific gravity: 1.005 to 1.030
  D. Osmolality: 50 to 1200 mOsm/L

VI. Other diagnostic studies (Table 2-9)

Electrocardiography
General Information
I. The electrocardiograph measures and records the electrical activity of the heart by measuring electrical potential at the skin surface; the electrocardiogram is a recording of that activity
II. An electrocardiogram is used to detect or demonstrate any of the following:
  A. Rhythm disturbances
  B. Conduction defects
  C. Electrolyte imbalances
  D. Drug toxicity
  E. Chamber enlargement or hypertrophy
  F. Myocardial ischemia, injury, or infarction
III. ECG paper (Fig. 2-31)
  A. Horizontal axis measures time
    1. Each small (1 mm) box is equal to 0.04 seconds
    2. Each large (5 mm) box is equal to 0.20 seconds
    3. Small marks at the top of the paper identify three-second intervals
  B. Vertical axis measures voltage
    1. Useful only if standardized, as on multiple-lead ECG; rhythm strips are not generally standardized because the size (or gain) can be changed
    2. If standardized
      a) Each small (1 mm) box is equal to 0.1 mV
      b) Each large (5 mm) box is equal to 0.5 mV
IV. Rule of electrical flow
  A. Impulses traveling toward the positive pole of a lead cause a positive deflection
  B. Impulses traveling toward the negative (or away from the positive) pole of a lead cause a negative deflection

Rhythm Strip Analysis
I. Monitoring electrode placement (Fig. 2-32)
  A. Lead II: positive at apex; negative under right clavicle; ground usually placed under left clavicle
    1. Advantages
      a) Upright P and QRS-waves
      b) Normal appearance
    2. Disadvantage: ectopy and aberrancy look alike
  B. MCL$_1$: positive at fourth ICS at RSB; negative under left clavicle; ground usually placed under right clavicle
    1. Advantages
      a) Better differentiation of ectopy from aberrancy
      b) Differentiation of LBBB from RBBB
      c) Differentiation of LV ectopy from RV ectopy
    2. Disadvantages
      a) Diphasic P-wave
      b) Negative QRS
  C. MCL$_6$: positive at fifth ICS at left midaxillary line (MAL) has some advantages; may also be used in differentiation of ectopy from aberrancy
II. Components of a single cardiac cycle (Fig. 2-33)
  A. P-wave
    1. Represents atrial depolarization
    2. First deflection from the isoelectric line
    3. Normally less than 2.5 mm tall and less than 0.10 seconds wide (2½ blocks tall and 2½ blocks wide)
  B. PR segment
    1. Represents the delay in AV node
    2. Isoelectric line between P-wave and QRS complex
  C. PR interval
    1. Represents atrial depolarization + delay in AV node
    2. Measured from beginning of P-wave to beginning of QRS complex
    3. Normally 0.12 to 0.20 seconds
  D. Q-wave: the first negative wave after the P-wave but before the R-wave
  E. R-wave: the first positive wave after the P-wave
  F. S-wave: the negative wave after the R-wave

Table 2-9   DIAGNOSTIC STUDIES

Study	Evaluates	Comments
Aortography	• Aortic valve insufficiency • Aneurysms or dissection of ascending aorta • Coarctation of the aorta • Injuries to the aorta and major branches	• Contrast medium used: check for allergy to iodine, shellfish, dye; ensure hydration following procedure • Monitor for clinical indications of anaphylaxis (e.g., flushing, urticaria, stridor) • Monitor puncture site
Cardiac biopsy	• Effect of cardiotoxic drugs • Evidence of cardiac transplant rejection • Inflammatory heart disease • Tumors • Cardiomyopathy	• Observe closely for signs of cardiac perforation and/or cardiac tamponade
Cardiac catheterization and coronary angiography	• Severity of coronary artery stenosis • Cardiac muscle function • Pressures within the heart • Cardiac output and ejection fraction • Blood gas analysis within chambers • Allows angioplasty, atherectomy, intracoronary stents, or lasers to reduce coronary artery obstruction	Prior to test: • Check for allergy to iodine, shellfish, dye (contrast medium used) After the test: • Ensure hydration following procedure (contrast medium used) • Keep extremity in which catheter was placed immobilized in a straight position for 6-12 hours • Monitor arterial puncture point for hemorrhage or hematoma • Monitor neurovascular status of affected limb • Note complaints of back pain and vital sign changes (may indicate retroperitoneal hemorrhage)
Chest X-ray	• Cardiac size and shape • Presence of pulmonary congestion or pleural effusions • Presence of thoracic aneurysm or calcification of the aorta • Position of pulmonary artery and cardiac catheter, pacemaker, wires	• Inquire about possibility of pregnancy
Computed tomography (CT)	• Left ventricular wall motion • Cardiac tumors • Myocardial infarction • Pericardial effusion • Aortic aneurysm • Aortic dissection	• May be done with or without contrast medium • If contrast medium used: check for allergy to iodine, shellfish, dye; ensure hydration following procedure
Digital subtraction angiography	• Vascular disease and degree of occlusion	• Contrast medium used: check for allergy to iodine, shellfish, dye; ensure hydration following procedure • Monitor for clinical indications of anaphylaxis (e.g., flushing, urticaria, stridor) • Monitor puncture site
Doppler ultrasonography	• Vascular disease and degree of occlusion	

Echocardiography
• M-mode: single ultrasound beam
• 2-D: planar ultrasound beam; wider view of heart and structures
• Doppler: addition of Doppler to demonstrate flow of blood through the heart
	• Chamber size and wall thickness
	• Valve functioning
	  • Papillary muscle functioning
	  • Prosthetic valve functioning
	• Ventricular wall motion abnormalities
	• Intracardiac masses
		• Transesophageal echocardiography is especially better if patient is obese, has COPD, chest wall deformity, chest trauma, or thick chest dressings

Continued

Table 2-9 | DIAGNOSTIC STUDIES—cont'd

Study	Evaluates	Comments
• Color flow: Doppler blood flow superimposed on 2-D echocardiogram • Stress echocardiography: images before, during, and after exercise or pharmacologic stress • Transesophageal echocardiography: transducer placed in esophagus	• Presence of pericardial fluid • Intracardiac pressures (Doppler) • Ejection fraction and cardiac output (Doppler) • Valve gradients (Doppler) • Intracardiac shunts (Doppler) • Thoracic aneurysm (transesophageal)	
Electrocardiography (ECG)	• Dysrhythmias • Conduction defects including intraventricular blocks • Electrolyte imbalance • Drug toxicity • Myocardial ischemia, injury, infarction • Chamber hypertrophy	• List what drugs the patient is receiving on ECG request • Be alert to electrical safety hazards
Electrophysiologic studies (EPS)	• Dysrhythmias under controlled circumstances • Best therapy for control of dysrhythmia: drug, required dosage of therapy; pacemaker; catheter ablation	• Patients may have near-death experience during EPS; encourage expression of fears, concerns, anxieties • Monitor puncture site
Holter monitor	• Suspected dysrhythmias over 24-hour period • Pacemaker function • Silent ischemia	• Instruct patient regarding importance of diary-keeping
Intravascular ultrasound (IVUS)	• Coronary artery size and patency • Structure of vessel wall • Coronary artery stent position and patency • Aorta and presence of aneurysm, aneurysm dissections	As for cardiac catheterization
Magnetic resonance imaging (MRI)	• Three-dimensional view of the heart • Anatomy and structure of the heart and great vessels including cardiomyopathy, congenital defect, masses, aneurysm • Changes in chemistry of tissues before structural changes occur	• Does not involve radiation or dyes • Cannot be used in patients with any implanted metallic device, including pacemakers, implantable defibrillators, metallic heart valves, and intracranial aneurysm clips
Multiple-gated acquisition (MUGA) scan (radionuclide angiography)	• Ventricular size and ventricular wall motion • Cardiac output, cardiac index, end-systolic volume, end-diastolic volume, and ejection fraction • Intracardiac shunts	• Assure patient that amount of radioactive material is minimal
Pericardiocentesis and pericardial fluid analysis	• Presence of blood, pus, pathogens, or malignancy • Also used for emergency relief of cardiac tamponade	• Observe closely for signs of cardiac tamponade
Peripheral angiography	• Atherosclerotic plaques, occlusion, aneurysms, or traumatic injury	Prior to test: • Contrast medium used: check for allergy to iodine, shellfish, dye After the test: • Contrast medium used: ensure hydration following procedure • Keep extremity in which catheter was placed immobilized in a straight position for 6-12 hours

Study	Evaluates	Comments
		• Monitor arterial puncture point for hemorrhage or hematoma • Monitor neurovascular status of affected limb • Monitor for indications of systemic emboli
Phonocardiography	• Extra heart sounds and murmurs in relation to the cardiac cycle and ECG	• Rarely used today
Positron emission tomography (cardiac PET scan)	• Severity of coronary artery stenosis • Collateral circulation • Patency of bypass grafts • Size and location of infarcted tissue	• Assure patient that amount of radioactive material is minimal
Stress electrocardiography	• High-risk patients, patients with known CAD, or postsurgical patients for ischemia with exercise or pharmacologic agents (e.g., adenosine, dipyridamole, dobutamine) • Exercise-induced dysrhythmias	• One millimeter or greater transient ST segment depression 80 msec after the J-point is suggestive of CAD • Monitor closely for exercise-induced hypotension or ventricular dysrhythmias
Technetium–99 pyrophosphate scan	• Size, location of acute MI (infarcted areas show increased uptake of radioactivity [hot spots] 1-7 days after MI)	• Assure patient that amount of radioactive material is minimal • Peak accuracy at 12-48 hours after initial symptoms
Thallium stress electrocardiography	• Myocardial ischemia during exercise (ischemic areas show decreased uptake of radioactivity [cold spots])	• Assure patient that amount of radioactive material is minimal
Thallium-201 scan	• Myocardial ischemia (ischemic areas show decreased uptake of radioactivity [cold spots])	• Assure patient that amount of radioactive material is minimal
Vectorcardiography	• Chamber hypertrophy • Bundle branch blocks and hemiblocks • Myocardial ischemia or infarction	
Venography (ascending contrast phlebography)	• Deep leg veins • Presence of deep vein thrombosis (DVT) • Competence of deep vein valves • May be used to locate suitable vein for arterial bypass graft	• Contrast medium used: check for allergy to iodine, shellfish, dye; ensure hydration following procedure • Monitor for clinical indications of anaphylaxis (e.g., flushing, urticaria, stridor) • Monitor puncture site
Ventriculography	• Ventricular wall motion • Wall thickness • Ventricular aneurysm • Mitral valve motion • LV end-diastolic volume, end-systolic volume, stroke volume, ejection fraction • Intracardiac shunt	• Contrast medium used: check for allergy to iodine, shellfish, dye; ensure hydration following procedure • Monitor for clinical indications of anaphylaxis (e.g., flushing, urticaria, stridor) • Monitor puncture site

G. QRS complex
   1. Represents ventricular depolarization
   2. May have one, two, or all three: Q, R, S
   3. Measured from beginning of first wave of complex to end of last wave of complex
   4. QRS interval: normally 0.06 to 0.11

   5. QRS amplitude: normally less than 30 mm in chest leads
H. QT interval
   1. Represents time of ventricular depolarization and repolarization
   2. Measured from first wave of QRS complex to the end of the T-wave

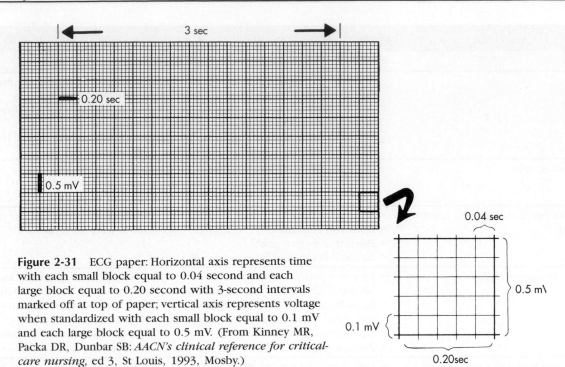

Figure 2-31   ECG paper: Horizontal axis represents time with each small block equal to 0.04 second and each large block equal to 0.20 second with 3-second intervals marked off at top of paper; vertical axis represents voltage when standardized with each small block equal to 0.1 mV and each large block equal to 0.5 mV. (From Kinney MR, Packa DR, Dunbar SB: *AACN's clinical reference for critical-care nursing,* ed 3, St Louis, 1993, Mosby.)

3. Normally not more than one half of preceding RR interval to eliminate the effect of heart rate
4. QTc (QT interval corrected for rate effect)
    a) Calculated by dividing the QT interval by the square root of the RR interval **OR** by dividing the QT interval by the RR interval × ½
    b) QTc is normally 0.32 to 0.44
I. ST segment
    1. Represents the time during which the ventricles have completely depolarized and the beginning of repolarization
    2. Located between the QRS complex and the beginning of the T-wave
    3. Normally isoelectric at baseline
J. J-point
    1. The angle at which the QRS complex ends and the ST segment begins
    2. The J-point deviates from the isoelectric line if the ST segment is elevated or depressed
K. T-wave
    1. Represents ventricular repolarization
    2. Wave after the QRS; may be positive or negative
    3. Normally less than 5 mm in limb leads and less than 10 mm in chest lead
L. U-wave
    1. May represent repolarization of the Purkinje fibers
    2. Small wave after the T-wave; often not seen because of its low voltage
    3. Normally less than or equal to 1 mm
III. Steps in analysis of a rhythm strip (Table 2-10)
IV. Criteria for basic dysrhythmias and blocks (Table 2-11)

A. The pacemaker rule: The fastest rate controls the heart
    1. This is usually the SA node unless an irritable focus (e.g., atrial tissue) is faster; this is called *irritability*
    2. If an upper pacemaker (e.g., SA node) fails, the lower pacemakers (e.g., junctional) assume control: this is called *escape*
V. ECG changes in electrolyte imbalance
    A. Hypokalemia
        1. If 3 mEq/L or less
            a) Flat T with prominent U-wave
            b) T-wave and U-wave of approximately same amplitude
            c) ST segment flattening and/or depression
        2. If 2.0 mEq/L or less
            a) U-wave taller than T-wave
            b) Prolongation of QT interval (this is really QU prolongation since U-waves replace T-waves)
            c) ST segment depression
        3. If 1.0 mEq/L or less: U-wave fuses with T-wave
    B. Hyperkalemia
        1. If greater than 5.5 mEq/L
            a) Tall, narrow, peaked T-waves
            b) QRS complex widens
            c) P-wave widens and becomes shallow
        2. If 6.5 mEq/L or greater: QRS complex widens more
        3. If 8.0 mEq/L or greater
            a) Wide QRS mcrgcd with T-wave
            b) P-wave barely visible
        4. If 12 mEq/L or greater: P-wave disappears
    C. Hypocalcemia
        1. Prolonged QT

2. Prolonged ST segment
D. Hypercalcemia
1. Shortened QT
2. Shortened ST segment
E. Hypomagnesemia
1. Prolonged QT
2. Broad, flattened T-wave
F. Hypermagnesemia
1. PR, QT prolonged
2. Prolonged QRS
VI. Drug effects on the ECG
A. Digitalis
1. Scooping of ST-T-wave (known as *digitalis effect*)
2. Shortened QT
3. PR interval may be prolonged
B. Type IA antidysrhythmics (e.g., procainamide, quinidine, disopyramide)
1. QT prolongation
2. T-wave flattening

Multiple-Lead ECG Analysis

I. ECG leads (Fig. 2-34)
A. Limb leads: frontal plane
1. Lead I: + at LA (left arm); − at RA (right arm)
2. Lead II: + at F (foot); − at RA
3. Lead III: + at F (foot); − at LA
4. Lead aVR: unipolar RA
5. Lead aVL: unipolar LA
6. Lead aVF: unipolar F
B. Chest leads: horizontal plane
1. Lead V_1: 4ICS at right sternal border (RSB)
2. Lead V_2: 4ICS at left sternal border (LSB)
3. Lead V_3: halfway between V_2 and V_4
4. Lead V_4: 5ICS at left midclavicular line (LMCL)
5. Lead V_5: 5ICS at left anterior axillary line (LAAL)
6. Lead V_6: 5ICS at left midaxillary line (LMAL)
7. R-wave gets taller across the precordium from V_1 to V_6 (referred to as *normal progression of the R-wave across the precordium*); the S-wave gets smaller across the precordium (V_1 to V_6)
C. Specialty leads
1. Posterior leads
a) Lead V_7: 5ICS at left posterior axillary line (LPAL)
b) Lead V_8: halfway between V_7 and V_8
c) Lead V_9: 5ICS next to vertebral column
2. Right ventricular leads
a) Lead V_{4R}: 5ICS at RMCL
b) Lead V_{5R}: 5ICS at RAAL
c) Lead V_{6R}: 5ICS at RMAL
d) The standard 12 leads plus V_{4R} to V_{6R} and V_{7-9} make the 18 leads of an 18-lead ECG
e) Right ventricular leads routinely performed on patients with ECG indicators of inferior MI (33% to 50% of patients

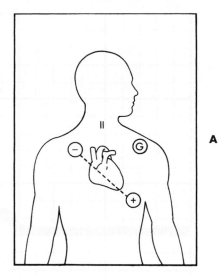

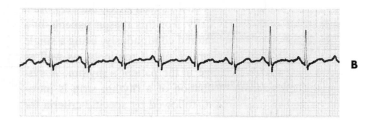

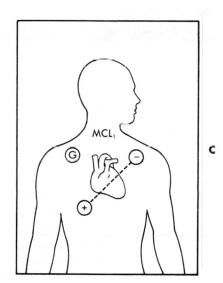

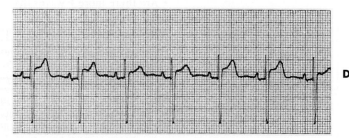

Figure 2-32 Monitoring leads. **A,** Electrode placement for lead II. **B,** Representation of appearance of ECG in lead II. **C,** Electrode placement for MCL_1. **D,** Representation of appearance of ECG in MCL_1. (From Urden LD, Lough ME, Stacy KM: *Priorities in critical care nursing,* St Louis, 1995, Mosby.)

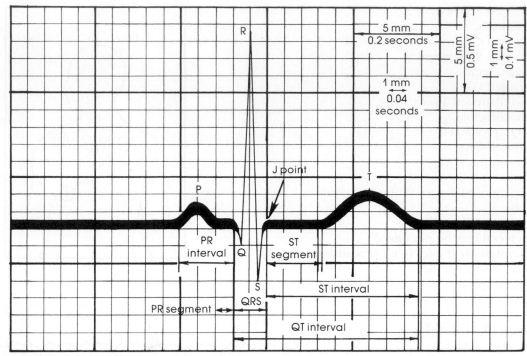

Figure 2-33 Components of a single cardiac cycle. (From Seidel JC: *The Methodist Hospital: Basic electrocardiography: a modular approach,* St Louis, 1986, Mosby.)

Table 2-10	Rhythm Strip Analysis	
Component	**Assessment**
Regularity (rhythm)	• Is it regular? • Is it irregular? • Are there any patterns to the irregularity? • Are there any ectopic beats; if so, are they early or are they late? • Is regularity of P-waves and QRS complexes the same? (If there is only one P-wave for each QRS, only one regularity needs to be recorded)

Rate	• Methods
	  • Count dark lines between P-waves or QRS complexes as 300, 150, 100, 75, 60, 50, 43, 38, 33, 30
	  • Count number of QRS complexes in a six-second strip and multiply by 10
	  • Use a rate ruler
	• Are atrial and ventricular rates the same? (If there is only one P-wave for each QRS, only one rate needs to be recorded)

P-waves	• Are the P-waves regular? • Is there one P-wave for every QRS? • Is there a P-wave in front of the QRS or behind it? • Is the P-wave normal and upright in Lead II? • Are there more P-waves than QRS complexes? • Do all P-waves look alike? • Are irregular P-waves associated with ectopic beats?
PR intervals	• Is PRI measurement within normal range? (normal interval: 0.12-0.20 seconds) • Are all PRIs constant? • If PRI varies, is there a pattern to the changing measurements?
QRS complexes	• Is QRS measurement within normal limits? (normal interval: 0.06-0.11 seconds) • Are all QRS complexes of equal duration? • Do all QRS complexes look alike? • Are unusual QRS complexes associated with ectopic beats? • Are these ectopic beats early or late?
QT interval	• Is the QT measurement within normal limits? (less than one half of RR interval or QTc of 0.32-0.44)
Patient presentation	• Is the patient symptomatic? • Are there clinical indications of hypoperfusion?

Table 2-11 | Criteria for Basic Dysrhythmias and Blocks

Rhythm	Rate	Regularity	P-Waves	PR Interval	QRS Duration
Normal sinus rhythm	60-100/min	Atrial and ventricular rhythms regular	Normal	0.12-0.20 and constant	<0.12
Sinus bradycardia	<60/min	Atrial and ventricular rhythms regular	Normal	0.12-0.20 and constant	<0.12
Sinus tachycardia	>100/min (usually 100-160/min)	Atrial and ventricular rhythms regular	Normal	0.12-0.20 and constant	<0.12
Sinus dysrhythmia	Usually 60-100/min, but may be slower or faster	Atrial and ventricular rhythms regularly irregular; rate increases with inspiration (so RR interval shortens) and decreases with expiration (so RR interval lengthens); difference between shortest and longest RR <0.12	Normal	0.12-0.20 and usually constant; may vary slightly with rate variation	<0.12
Sinus block (sinus exit block)	Dependent on underlying rhythm	Atrial and ventricular rhythms regular with an irregularity; RR interval at block measures an exact multiple of the normal RR interval	One or more entire cardiac cycle is absent; P-wave absent during block	None during block	QRS absent during block
Sinus arrest	Dependent on underlying rhythm	Atrial and ventricular rhythms regular with an irregularity (a pause); RR interval at pause measures more or less than an exact multiple of the normal RR interval	Indefinite period of time without an entire cardiac cycle; P-wave absent during arrest	None during arrest	QRS absent during arrest
Premature atrial contractions	Dependent on underlying rhythm	Dependent on underlying rhythm; PACs interrupt underlying rhythm	P-wave of this early beat differs from sinus P; the ectopic P-wave is early and may be flattened, notched, or lost in preceding T-wave	Usually 0.12-0.20, but may be greater than 0.20	<0.12
Wandering atrial pacemaker	Usually 60-100/min	Atrial and ventricular rhythms usually slightly irregular	P-waves look different beat to beat; at least three different-looking P-waves	0.12-0.20 and may vary	<0.12
Supraventricular tachycardia*	>100/min; usualy 150-250/min	Atrial and ventricular rhythms regular	P-waves are impossible to distinguish; may be lost in QRS or preceding T-wave	Cannot measure	<0.12

*Supraventricular tachycardia refers to any narrow QRS tachycardia whose focus cannot be definitely identified; the term should be used only when a more definitive diagnosis cannot be made.

Continued

Table 2-11	Criteria for Basic Dysrhythmias and Blocks—cont'd				
Rhythm	**Rate**	**Regularity**	**P-Waves**	**PR Interval**	**QRS Duration**
Atrial tachycardia	150- 250/min	Atrial and ventricular rhythms regular	P-wave differs from sinus P; can be lost in preceding T-wave	0.12-0.20	<0.12
Multifocal atrial tachycardia (also called *chaotic atrial rhythm*)	Usually 100-150/min	Atrial and ventricular rhythms usually slightly irregular	P-waves look different beat to beat; at least three different-looking P-waves	0.12-0.20 and may vary	<0.12
Atrial flutter	Atrial rate approximately 300/min; ventricular rate varies with conduction through the AV node; 2:1 atrial flutter has a ventricular rate of approximately 150/min, 4:1 atrial flutter has a ventricular rate of approximately 75/min	Atrial flutter waves regular; ventricular rhythm (response) usually regular	No true P-waves; flutter waves have characteristic sawtooth appearance	No true P-waves	<0.12
Atrial fibrillation	Atrial rate >350/min; ventricular rate varies greatly depending on conduction through AV node	Atrial fibrillatory waves irregular; ventricular rhythm irregularly irregular	No true P-waves; quivering baseline shows fibrillatory waves	No true P-waves	<0.12
Premature junctional contraction	Dependent on underlying rhythm	Dependent on underlying rhythm; PJCs interrupt underlying rhythm	P-wave if visible will be inverted; may be in front of, in, or after the QRS complex	Can be measured only if P-wave is in front of QRS; PR will be <0.12 if measurable	<0.12
Junctional escape rhythm	40-60/min	Atrial and ventricular rhythms regular	If visible, P-wave inverted; may be in front of, in, or after the QRS complex	Can be measured only if P-wave is in front of QRS; PR will be <0.12 if measurable	<0.12
Accelerated junctional rhythm	60-100/min	Atrial and ventricular rhythms regular	If visible, P-wave inverted; may be in front of, in, or after the QRS complex	Can be measured only if P-wave is in front of QRS; PR will be <0.12 if measurable	<0.12

Table 2-11	Criteria for Basic Dysrhythmias and Blocks—cont'd				
Rhythm	**Rate**	**Regularity**	**P-Waves**	**PR Interval**	**QRS Duration**
Junctional tachycardia	>100/min; usually 100-180/min	Atrial and ventricular rhythms regular	If visible, P-wave inverted; may be in front of, in, or after the QRS complex	Can be measured only if P-wave is in front of QRS; PR will be <0.12 if measurable	<0.12
First-degree AV nodal block	Dependent on underlying rhythm	Dependent on underlying rhythm	P-wave normal	>0.20	<0.12
Second-degree AV nodal block Mobitz I* (Wenckebach)	Atrial rate dependent on underlying rhythm; ventricular rate dependent on conduction ratio; atrial rate > ventricular rate	Atrial rhythm regular, ventricular rhythm irregular (PP is regular but RR is irregular); groupings identifiable between P-waves that were not conducted	P-waves normal, but some P-waves not followed by a QRS	Normal PR interval progressively lengthens until a P-wave is not followed by a QRS; entire cycle begins again with normal PR interval	<0.12
Second-degree AV nodal block Mobitz II*	Atrial rate dependent on underlying rhythm; ventricular rate dependent on conduction ratio but usually <60/min; atrial rate > ventricular rate	Atrial rhythm regular, ventricular rhythm regular or irregular depending on whether conduction ratio varies or is constant; PP regular, but some RRs may be twice normal	P-waves normal, but there are P-waves not followed by a QRS without preceding progressive lengthening	Usually 0.12-0.20 of conducted P-waves but may be longer; constant for each conducted QRS	0.12 or >
Third-degree (or complete) AV block	Atrial rate dependent on underlying rhythm; ventricular rate dependent on focus of escape rhythm (40-60/min if escape focus is junctional, 20-40/min if escape focus is ventricular)	Atrial rhythm regular, ventricular rhythm usually regular; PP regular; RR usually regular	Normal but P-waves not followed by (associated with) QRS	No consistent PR interval; no relationship between the P-waves and the QRS complexes	<0.12 if escape focus is junctional; 0.12 or > if escape focus is ventricular
Left bundle branch block (LBBB)	Dependent on underlying rhythm	Dependent on underlying rhythm	P-wave normal	0.12-0.20 as long as no coexisting AV nodal block	0.12 or >; QRS is negative in V_1 or MCL_1
Right bundle branch block (RBBB)	Dependent on underlying rhythm	Dependent on underlying rhythm	P-wave normal	0.12-0.20 as long as no coexisting AV nodal block	0.12 or >; QRS is positive in V_1 or MCL_1

*Note: 2:1 block is a second-degree block but may be either Type I or Type II; the QRS width may be helpful in differentiating between the two; if the QRS is of normal width, it is probably Type I, if the QRS is 0.12 or greater, it is probably Type II

Continued

Table 2-11	Criteria for Basic Dysrhythmias and Blocks—cont'd					
Rhythm	**Rate**	**Regularity**	**P-Waves**	**PR Interval**	**QRS Duration**
Premature ventricular contraction	Dependent on underlying rhythm	Dependent on underlying rhythm; PVCs interrupt underlying rhythm	No associated P-wave	No associated P-waves; cannot measure PR	0.12 or >; QRS of PVC looks different from normal QRSs
Monomorphic ventricular tachycardia	100-250/min *VT is usually ~150/min; VT at 200-250/min may be called ventricular flutter	Ventricular rhythm usually regular; if dissociated P-waves are identifiable, atrial rhythm regular	No associated P-waves but may have dissociated sinus P-waves scattered through the rhythm	No associated P-waves; cannot measure PR	0.12 or >; QRS of VT looks different from normal QRSs
Polymorphic ventricular tachycardia (called Torsades de pointes if preceded by prolongation of the QT interval)	150-250/min	Ventricular rhythm usually regular	None	None	0.12 or > with QRS that seems to twist around a center line; gradual alteration in the amplitude and direction of the QRS
Ventricular fibrillation	None	Irregular; chaotic baseline	None	None	None
Idioventricular rhythm	20-40/min	Ventricular rhythm usually regular; no atrial activity	None	None	0.12 or >
Accelerated idioventricular rhythm	40-100/min	Ventricular rhythm usually regular; no atrial activity	None	None	0.12 or >
Asystole	None	No atrial or ventricular activity	None	None	None

with inferior MI have concurrent right ventricular infarction)

II. Mean QRS axis (Fig. 2-35)
   A. Represents the average direction of ventricular depolarization
   B. Described on a 360-degree circle
   C. Normal axis: downward and to the left (0 to 90 degrees) because of the direction of depolarization from superior to inferior and the larger muscle mass of the left ventricle
   D. Left axis deviation: upward and to the left (0 to 90 degrees); may be caused by any of the following:
      1. Left ventricular hypertrophy
      2. Left anterior hemiblock
      3. Septal infarction
      4. Mechanical shift of heart to more horizontal: ascites, pregnancy, abdominal tumor
   E. Right axis deviation: downward and to the right (+90 to ±180 degrees); may be caused by any of the following:
      1. Right ventricular hypertrophy
      2. Left posterior hemiblock

      3. Lateral infarction
      4. Dextrocardia
   F. Indeterminate axis: upward and to the right (−90 to ±180)
      1. Could be extreme right axis deviation or extreme left axis deviation
      2. May be caused by ventricular tachycardia or multiple infarctions
   G. Two-lead and quadrant method
      1. Lead I
         a) Positive pole is at the left arm and negative pole is at the right arm
         b) If the mean QRS axis is to the left, then a predominantly positive QRS will be in lead I
         c) If the mean QRS axis is to the right, then a predominantly negative QRS will be in lead I
      2. Lead aVF
         a) Positive pole is at the foot
         b) If the mean QRS axis is downward, then a predominantly positive QRS will be in lead aVF

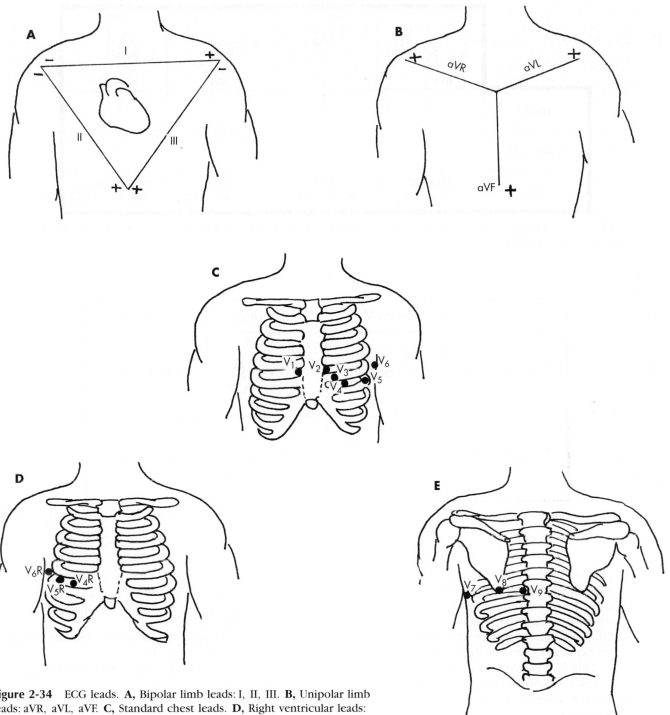

Figure 2-34   ECG leads. **A,** Bipolar limb leads: I, II, III. **B,** Unipolar limb leads: aVR, aVL, aVF. **C,** Standard chest leads. **D,** Right ventricular leads: V_{4R}-V_{6R}. **E,** Posterior leads: V_7-V_9.

c) If the mean QRS axis is upward, then a predominantly negative QRS will be in lead aVF

3. Quadrant determination
   a) If QRS is positive in I and positive in aVF, mean QRS axis is normal (0 to +90)
   b) If QRS is positive in I and negative in aVF, a left axis deviation exists (0 to −90)
   c) If QRS is negative in I and positive in aVF, a right axis deviation exists (+90 to ±180)

d) If QRS is negative in I and negative in aVF, an indeterminate axis deviation exists (−90 to ±180); this axis deviation is sometimes referred to as *extreme right axis deviation* but since it could as easily be an extreme left axis deviation, indeterminant is a better description

III. Bundle branch blocks (Fig. 2-36)
   A. Block of either bundle causes a delay in the conduction through the ventricles and a

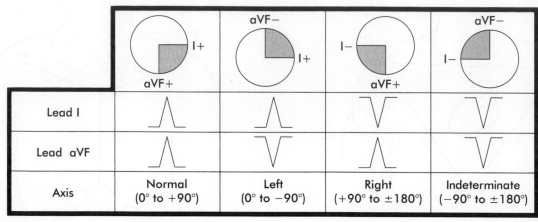

Lead I	⋀	⋀	⋁	⋁
Lead aVF	⋀	⋁	⋀	⋁
Axis	Normal (0° to +90°)	Left (0° to −90°)	Right (+90° to ±180°)	Indeterminate (−90° to ±180°)

Figure 2-35   Two-lead method of axis determination. (Modified from Kinney MR, Packa DR, Dunbar SB: *AACN's clinical reference for critical-care nursing,* ed 4, St Louis, 1998, Mosby.)

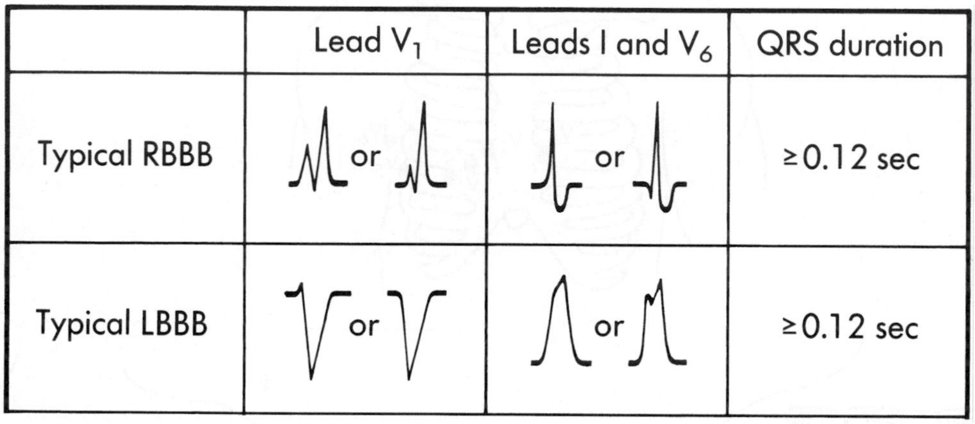

	Lead V₁	Leads I and V₆	QRS duration
Typical RBBB	∿ or ∿	∿ or ∿	≥0.12 sec
Typical LBBB	∨ or ∨	∧ or ∧	≥0.12 sec

Figure 2-36   Bundle branch blocks. (Modified from Grauer K: *Practical guide to ECG interpretation,* St Louis, 1992, Mosby.)

prolongation of the QRS interval; "rabbit ears" or branching of the QRS complex also usually occurs, indicating that the two ventricles are depolarized out of sync

B. LBBB is a bifascicular block (loss of both left hemibundles) and is manifested by:
1. QRS is 0.12 seconds or more
2. QRS is positive in V_6 and negative in V_1
C. RBBB is a unifascicular block and is manifested by:
1. QRS is 0.12 seconds or more
2. QRS is positive in V_1 and negative in V_6

IV. Chamber enlargement and/or hypertrophy
A. Atrial enlargement is manifested by changes in the P-wave; the two best P-wave leads are lead II and lead V_1
1. In lead II: look for tall or wide P-waves
2. In lead V_1 or MCL_1: the first half of the normally diphasic P-wave represents the right atrium, and the second half of the normally diphasic P-wave represents the left atrium; look for a more dominant initial or terminal phase of the diphasic P-wave in V_1 or MCL_1

B. Right atrial enlargement is manifested by the following ECG changes:
1. Tall (greater than 2.5 mm), peaked P-wave in II
2. Larger initial phase of the diphasic P-wave normally seen in V_1
C. Left atrial enlargement is manifested by the following ECG changes:
1. Wide (>.11 seconds), notched P-wave in II
2. Larger terminal phase of the diphasic P-wave normally seen in V_1
D. Ventricular hypertrophy is manifested by changes in the QRS; look at changes in the precordial leads for ventricular hypertrophy
E. Right ventricular hypertrophy causes a change in the usual left ventricular dominance across the precordial leads
1. QRS amplitude: R-wave larger than S-wave in V_1, V_2; S-wave larger than R-wave in V_5, V_6 (indicative of change from the normal dominance of the left ventricle to dominance of right ventricle)
2. Right axis deviation: QRS negative in I; QRS positive in aVF

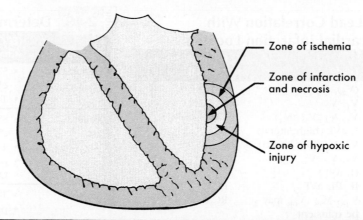

Zone of ischemia

Zone of infarction and necrosis

Zone of hypoxic injury

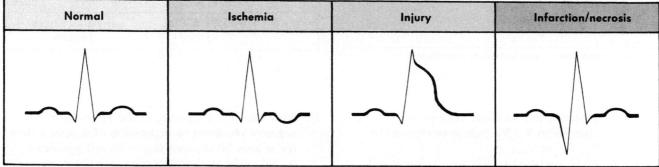

Normal	Ischemia	Injury	Infarction/necrosis

Figure 2-37   ECG indicators of ischemia, injury, infarction. (From McCance KL, Huether SE: *Pathophysiology: the biological basis for disease in adults and children,* ed 2, St Louis, 1994, Mosby.)

3. May have right atrial enlargement
4. ST-T-wave changes in V_1, V_2 indicative of right ventricular strain

F. Left ventricular hypertrophy causes an exaggeration of the usual left ventricular dominance across the precordial leads
   1. QRS amplitude
     a) Deepest S in V_1, V_2 plus tallest R in V_5, V_6 ≥35 mm
     b) R in lead aVL ≥12 mm
   2. Left axis deviation: QRS is positive in I; QRS negative in aVF
   3. May have left atrial enlargement
   4. ST-T-wave changes in V_5, V_6 indicative of left ventricular strain

V. Myocardial ischemia, injury, infarction
  A. ECG indicators (Fig. 2-37)
   1. Ischemia is manifested by T-wave changes; these changes are the earliest in the evolution of myocardial infarction
     a) Indicative change: symmetrically inverted T-waves in leads facing the ischemic area
     b) Reciprocal change: tall T-waves in leads opposite the ischemic area
   2. Injury is manifested by ST segment changes; these changes are intermediate in the evolution of myocardial infarction
     a) Indicative change: ST segment elevation in leads facing the injured area
     b) Reciprocal change: ST segment depression in leads opposite the injured area

3. Necrosis is manifested by Q-wave changes; these changes are the latest in the evolution of myocardial infarction
     a) Indicative change: pathologic Q-waves (0.04 seconds wide and/or one quarter height of R-wave) in leads facing the necrotic area
     b) Reciprocal change: tall R-waves in leads opposite the necrotic area
     c) Q-waves
       (1) Take up to 24 hours to develop
       (2) Related to mass loss of myocardium (e.g., large MI even if subendocardial will cause Q-wave; small MI even if transmural MI will not cause Q-wave)
       (3) To be pathologic must be 0.4 seconds wide and/or one quarter of the height of the R-wave
       (4) Prevented by successful reperfusion therapies (e.g., thrombolytics, angioplasty, atherectomy)

B. Location (Table 2-12)
   1. Anterior left ventricle: indicative changes in V_3, V_4 (possibly V_2)
   2. Septal: indicative changes in V_1, V_2
   3. Lateral left ventricle: indicative changes in I, aVL, and/or V_5, V_6
     a) I, aVL are considered high lateral leads
     b) V_5, V_6 are considered low lateral leads
   4. Inferior left ventricle: indicative changes in II, III, aVF

Table 2-12	ECG Lead Correlation With Myocardial Infarction Locations	
Location	Leads	Coronary Artery Affected
Anterior	(V_2), V_3, V_4	LAD
Septal	V_1, V_2	LAD
Anteroseptal	V_1, V_2, V_3, (V_4)	LAD
Lateral	I, aVL (high lateral), V_5, V_6 (low lateral)	LCA
Anterolateral	V_3, V_4, V_5, V_6, (I, aVL)	LCA
Inferior	II, III, aVF	RCA
RV	V_{4R}, V_{5R}, V_{6R} may be transient	RCA
Posterior	V_7, V_8, V_9 or reciprocal in V_1, V_2, V_3	RCA and/or LCA

Note: changes may also be seen in leads in parentheses

Table 2-13	Determination of Age of MI	
Description	ECG Characteristics	Time From Onset of Pain
Hyperacute	• ST segment elevation • T-wave inversion	• minutes to hours
Acute	• ST segment elevation • T-wave inversion • pathologic Q-waves	• hours to days
Recent	• T-wave inversion • pathologic Q-waves	• weeks to months
Old	• pathologic Q-waves	• after several months

5. Posterior left ventricle: reciprocal changes in V_1, V_2; indicative changes in V_7, V_8, or V_9
6. Right ventricular: indicative changes in V_{4R}, V_{5R}, V_{6R}

C. Determination of age of MI (Table 2-13)

VI. ECG changes in angina

A. Prinzmetal's angina: angina at rest caused by spasm of the coronary artery or arteries; ST segment elevation with pain

B. Wellens syndrome (Fig. 2-38): occlusion of proximal left anterior descending artery
   1. Symmetrical, deeply inverted T-waves with little or no ST segment elevation
   2. Usually seen in V_2, V_3
   3. No Q-wave
   4. Present even when patient is pain free
   5. Little or no enzyme elevation

VII. ECG changes in pericarditis

A. ST segment normal in V_1 and aVR, but all other leads show ST segment elevation

B. Depression of PR interval in limb leads and left chest leads (V_5, V_6)

C. Decrease in QRS voltage if pericardial effusion present

VIII. ECG changes in myocardial trauma (e.g., myocardial contusion)

A. Nonspecific ST and T-wave changes; infarction pattern if necrosis

B. Dysrhythmias and AV nodal blocks

ST Segment Monitoring

I. Definition: Continuous monitoring of ST segment for changes associated with ischemia to allow early indications of ischemia even in the absence of chest pain

II. Choose a lead that best demonstrates ST changes during ischemia or evolving MI; if this information is not available, use lead III or aVF

III. Note significant changes in the ST segment: ST segment elevation or depression of at least 1 mm for at least 60 seconds is considered significant

A. ST segment elevation represents more severe, usually transmural, ischemia

B. ST segment depression represents less severe, usually subendocardial, ischemia or reciprocal changes of ischemia

Hemodynamic Monitoring

Definitions (Table 2-14 lists formulae and normals)

I. Cardiac output (CO): the amount of blood ejected by the ventricle in 1 minute

II. Cardiac index (CI): the cardiac output indexed for differences in body size by dividing by body surface area

III. Stroke volume (SV): the amount of blood ejected by the ventricle with each contraction; also defined as the difference between the end-diastolic volume and the end-systolic volume

IV. Stroke index (SI): the stroke volume indexed for differences in body size by dividing by body surface area

V. Ejection fraction: percentage of blood in the ventricle that is ejected during systole; normal greater than 50%

VI. Afterload: the pressure against which the ventricle must pump; the pressure required to open the semilunar valve

A. RV afterload is evaluated by PVR and PVRI

B. LV afterload is evaluated by SVR and SVRI

VII. Preload: the pressure in the ventricle at the end of diastole (end-diastolic pressure); determines the stretch on the myofibrils and the consequent force of contraction

A. Atrial pressure correlates to the end-diastolic pressure for the respective ventricle and,

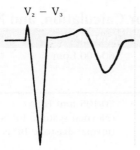

$V_2 - V_3$

Figure 2-38 Wellens syndrome. (From Conover M: *Understanding electrocardiography,* ed 6, St Louis, 1992, Mosby.)

therefore, to the preload for the respective ventricle when ventricular compliance and AV valve function is normal
1. Right ventricular end-diastolic pressure and preload is evaluated by right atrial pressure (RAP)
2. Left ventricular end-diastolic pressure and preload is evaluated indirectly by pulmonary artery occlusive pressure (PAOP) or directly by left atrial pressure (LAP)
VIII. Hemodynamic monitoring: the monitoring of blood flow generally through the use of invasive catheters

General Information Regarding Hemodynamic Monitoring
I. Uses
   A. Measure hemodynamic pressures and record waveforms
      1. Arterial catheter: systemic arterial blood pressure
      2. Central venous pressure catheter: central venous pressure
      3. Pulmonary artery catheter
         a) Right atrial pressure
         b) Pulmonary artery pressure
         c) Pulmonary artery occlusive pressure as an indirect reflection of left atrial pressure
         d) Cardiac output
         e) Specialized catheters also allow the evaluation of:
            (1) Svo_2: oxygen saturation of mixed venous blood
            (2) REF: right ventricular end-diastolic volume, right ventricular stroke volume, and right ventricular ejection fraction
   B. Obtain blood samples
      1. Arterial catheter: arterial (especially helpful for patients being weaned from mechanical ventilation)
      2. Central venous catheter: venous
      3. Pulmonary artery catheter
         a) Right atrial (proximal port): venous
         b) Pulmonary artery (distal port): mixed venous

   C. Provide central venous access for administration of fluids or drugs
      1. Central venous catheter: usually triple-lumen
      2. Pulmonary artery catheter
         a) Right atrial (proximal) port
         b) Pulmonary artery (distal) port: heparinized flush solution only to ensure patency; not to be used for fluid or drug administration
         c) VIP catheters: an extra right atrial port
   D. Perform intracardiac pacing via specialized PA catheter
II. Common indications for hemodynamic monitoring
   A. Shock of any etiology
   B. Myocardial infarction especially with:
      1. Acute left or right ventricular failure
      2. Refractory pain
      3. Significant hypotension or hypertension
   C. Acute right ventricular failure (e.g., after pulmonary embolus)
   D. Pulmonary edema of uncertain etiology: used to differentiate between cardiac and noncardiac pulmonary edema
   E. Postcardiac surgery
   F. Structural defects: severe valvular disease (e.g., papillary muscle rupture); ventricular septal rupture
   G. Cardiac tamponade
   H. Acute respiratory failure (e.g., acute respiratory distress syndrome)
   I. Pulmonary hypertension
   J. Need for evaluation of fluid status and guide fluid resuscitation (e.g., burns, multiple trauma, complex surgical procedures, especially in patients with preexisting cardiopulmonary disease)
   K. Need for evaluation of hemodynamic response to potent pharmacologic agents (e.g., hypertensive crisis treated with nitroprusside)
III. Components of a pressure monitoring system (Fig. 2-39)
   A. Physiologic signal: carried to the transducer by a catheter (inserted into the cardiovascular circuit) and fluid-filled tubing
   B. Transducer: converts the mechanical signal to an electrical signal
   C. Monitor
      1. Amplifier: device that increases the magnitude of the electrical signal and filters out electrical interference
      2. Oscilloscope: device that displays the resultant signal as a pressure waveform and as a numeric value on a digital display
      3. Recorder: device that records the pressure waveform on paper for analysis

Hemodynamic Parameters
I. Arterial and ventricular pressures measured as systolic/diastolic while atrial pressures measured as a mean
II. Systemic arterial blood pressure
   A. Pressure in a systemic artery; reflects systemic arterial blood pressure

Table 2-14 Hemodynamic Parameters, Methods of Measurement or Calculation, and Normals

Parameter	Method of Measurement or Calculation	Normal
Heart rate (HR)	Measured: count rate at apex or number of R-waves by ECG monitor	60-100 bpm
Mean arterial pressure (MAP)	Calculated: [BP systolic + (BP diastolic × 2)] ÷ 3; systolic and diastolic pressures can be obtained directly (arterial line) or indirectly (auscultated using a sphygmomanometer)	70-105 mm Hg (Normal systolic BP is 90-140 mm Hg; normal diastolic BP is 60-90 mm Hg)
Cardiac output (CO)	Measured: usually by thermodilution technique	4-8 L/min
Cardiac index (CI)	Calculated: CO ÷ body surface area (BSA)	2.5-4.0 L/min/m^2
Stroke volume (SV)	Calculated: CO ÷ HR	60-120 ml/beat
Stroke index (SI)	Calculated: SV ÷ BSA	30-65 ml/m^2/beat
Right atrial pressure (RAP)	Measured: at the proximal port of the pulmonary artery catheter; this port is located in the right atrium	2-6 mm Hg 3-8 cm H$_2$O
Pulmonary artery pressure (PAP)	Measured: at the distal port of the pulmonary artery catheter with the balloon deflated; the tip is located in a pulmonary arteriole	Systolic (PAs): 15-30 mm Hg Diastolic (PAd): 5-15 mm Hg Mean (PAm): 10-20 mm Hg
Pulmonary artery occlusive pressure (PAOP)	Measured: at the distal port of the pulmonary artery catheter with the balloon inflated; because right heart pressures are blocked by the inflated balloon, PAOP indirectly reflects left atrial pressure, left ventricular end-diastolic pressure (LVEDP), and left ventricular preload	6-12 mm Hg (Note: Although 6-12 mm Hg is "normal," many patients require a higher pressure [as high as 15-20 mm Hg] to achieve optimal stretch on the myofibrils and optimal preload)
Systemic vascular resistance (SVR)	Calculated: [(MAP − RAP) × 80] ÷ CO	900-1400 dynes/sec/cm^{-5}
Systemic vascular resistance index (SVRI)	Calculated: [(MAP − RAP) × 80] ÷ CI	1700-2600 dynes/sec/cm^{-5}/m^2
Pulmonary vascular resistance (PVR)	Calculated: [(PAm − PAOP) × 80] ÷ CO	100-250 dynes/sec/cm^{-5}
Pulmonary vascular resistance index (PVRI)	Calculated: [(PAm − PAOP) × 80] ÷ CI	225-315 dynes/sec/cm^{-5}/m^2
Left ventricular stroke work index (LVSWI)	Calculated: [SI × (MAP − PAOP)] × 0.0136	45-65 g · m/m^2
Right ventricular stroke work index (RVSWI)	Calculated: [SI × (PAm − RAP)] × 0.0136	5-12 g · m/m^2
Coronary artery perfusion pressure (CAPP)	Calculated: Diastolic BP − PAOP	60-80 mm Hg
Right ventricular end-diastolic volume (RVEDV)	Measured: by thermodilution method with REF pulmonary artery catheter	100-160 ml

Table 2-14	Hemodynamic Parameters, Methods of Measurement or Calculation, and Normals—cont'd	
Parameter	**Method of Measurement or Calculation**	**Normal**
Right ventricular end-diastolic volume index (RVEDVI)	Calculated: RVEDV ÷ BSA	$60\text{-}100 \text{ ml/m}^2$
Right ventricular end-systolic volume (RVESV)	Measured: by thermodilution method with REF pulmonary artery catheter	50-100 ml
Right ventricular end-systolic volume index (RVESVI)	Calculated: RVESV ÷ BSA	$30\text{-}60 \text{ ml/m}^2$
Right ventricular ejection fraction (REF)	Measured: by thermodilution method with REF pulmonary artery catheter	40%-60%
Arterial oxygen saturation (Sao_2)	Measured: by pulse oximetry or by arterial blood gas analysis	95%-100%
Venous oxygen saturation (Svo_2)	Measured: by Svo_2 port of a fiberoptic oximetric PA catheter or by mixed venous blood gas analysis	60%-80%
Arterial oxygen content (Cao_2)	Calculated: $1.34 \times \text{Hgb} \times Sao_2$	18-20 ml/dl
Venous oxygen content (Cvo_2)	Calculated: $1.34 \times \text{Hgb} \times Svo_2$	12-16 ml/dl
Oxygen delivery (DO_2)	Calculated: $CO \times Cao_2 \times 10$	900-1100 ml/min
Oxygen delivery index (DO_2I)	Calculated: $CI \times Cao_2 \times 10$	$550\text{-}650 \text{ ml/min/m}^2$
Oxygen consumption (VO_2)	Calculated: $CO \times \text{Hgb} \times 13.4 \times (Sao_2 - Svo_2)$	200-300 ml/min
Oxygen consumption index (VO_2I)	Calculated: $CI \times \text{Hgb} \times 13.4 \times (Sao_2 - Svo_2)$	$110\text{-}160 \text{ ml/min/m}^2$
Oxygen extraction ratio (O_2ER)	Calculated: $Cao_2 - Cvo_2 \div Cao_2$	22%-30%
Oxygen extraction index (O_2EI)	Calculated: $Sao_2 - Svo_2 \div Sao_2$	20%-27%

B. Blood pressure = CO × SVR; changes in blood pressure are caused by either a change in cardiac output or systemic vascular resistance
C. Measured by a catheter in a peripheral artery or the second lumen of an intraaortic balloon catheter (central aortic arterial line)
   1. Radial artery site is the preferred peripheral site because of collateral circulation provided by ulnar artery
      a) Allen's test must be performed prior to any radial artery puncture to assess patency of radial-ulnar arch; this test is performed by compressing both the radial and ulnar artery to blanch the hand; when the ulnar artery is released, evaluate the time until return of color; if longer than 7 seconds, this radial artery should not be punctured (for arterial blood gases or for radial artery cannulation)
   2. Neurovascular assessment of the limb distal to any arterial line is essential; thrombosis or embolization may cause acute arterial occlusion and loss of limb
D. Systolic arterial pressure: maximal pressure with which the blood is ejected from the left ventricle
E. Diastolic arterial pressure: reflects the rapidity of flow of the ejected blood through the arterial system and the vessel's elasticity
   1. Diastolic pressure is expected to be higher [and pulse pressure narrowed] if endogenous catecholamine release occurs or the patient is receiving sympathomimetic agents (e.g., epinephrine, dopamine [Intropid], or norepinephrine [Levophed])

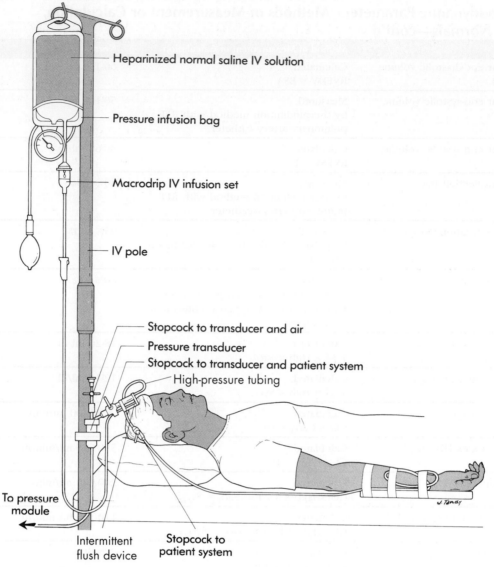

Heparinized normal saline IV solution

Pressure infusion bag

Macrodrip IV infusion set

IV pole

Stopcock to transducer and air
Pressure transducer
Stopcock to transducer and patient system
High-pressure tubing

To pressure module

Intermittent flush device

Stopcock to patient system

Figure 2-39 Components of a pressure monitoring system. (From Flynn JBM, Bruce NP: *Introduction to critical care skills,* St Louis, 1993, Mosby.)

2. Diastolic pressure is expected to be lower [and pulse pressure be widened] if excessive vasodilatory mediators (e.g., septic shock, anaphylactic shock) are present

F. Mean arterial pressure: average pressure occurring in the aorta and its major branches during the cardiac cycle; mean arterial pressure of at least 60 mm Hg is necessary to perfuse the vital organs

G. Normal pressure values
   1. Systolic: 90 to 140 mm Hg
   2. Diastolic: 60 to 90 mm Hg
   3. Mean: 70 to 105 mm Hg

H. Normal waveform (see Fig. 2-23)

I. Causes of abnormal pressures (Table 2-15)

J. Arterial catheter versus cuff pressures
   1. Arterial catheters are a direct measurement and, therefore, are more accurate, espe-

cially in shock states, severe hypertension, vasoconstriction, and obesity
   a) Expect radial artery catheters to show a pressure slightly higher (~10 mm Hg) than brachial cuff measurement
   b) Mean arterial pressures tend to be the same even in these situations and are a more consistent evaluation of perfusion pressure

2. If a significant variation exists between pressure measured by arterial catheter and pressure auscultated using a sphygmomanometer other than in the situations previously listed, do the following:
   a) Check the pressure monitoring system for air bubbles, occlusions, and positioning of catheter against wall of artery

Table 2-15	**Causes of Abnormal Hemodynamic Pressures**	
Parameter	**Increased**	**Decreased**
Systemic arterial BP	• Increase in systemic vascular resistance (e.g., hypertension, sympathetic nervous system innervation) • Increase in cardiac output (e.g., hyperthyroidism)	• Decrease in systemic vascular resistance (e.g., sepsis, anaphylaxis) • Decrease in cardiac output (e.g., myocardial infarction, tachydysrhythmias)

Right atrial pressure (RAP)	• Hypervolemia
	• Tricuspid valve dysfunction: stenosis or regurgitation
	• Right ventricular failure or infarction
	• Ventricular septal defect (VSD) with left-to-right shunt
	• Pulmonic stenosis
	• Pulmonary hypertension
	  • Hypoxemic pulmonary vasoconstriction (Pao_2 <60 mm Hg)
	    • Pulmonary embolism (PE)
	    • Chronic obstructive pulmonary disease (COPD)
	    • Acute respiratory distress syndrome (ARDS)
	  • Mitral valve dysfunction (stenosis or regurgitation)
	• Positive pressure ventilation
	• Constrictive pericarditis
	• Cardiac tamponade
	• Mitral valve dysfunction: stenosis or regurgitation
	• Chronic left ventricular failure (RAP would be a late indication of LVF)
		• Hypovolemia
		• Vasodilation
		  • Venous vasodilators (e.g., nitroglycerin, morphine)
		  • Endogenous systemic vasodilation (e.g., septic shock, anaphylactic shock, neurogenic shock)

Right ventricular pressure	• Right ventricular failure or infarction • Ventricular septal defect (VSD) with left-to-right shunt • Pulmonary hypertension • Mitral valve dysfunction: stenosis or regurgitation • Constrictive pericarditis • Cardiac tamponade • Chronic left ventricular failure	• Hypovolemia • Vasodilation
Pulmonary artery pressure (PAP)	• Hypervolemia • Ventricular septal defect with left-to-right shunt • Pulmonary hypertension • Positive pressure ventilation • Mitral valve dysfunction: stenosis or regurgitation • Constrictive pericarditis • Cardiac tamponade • Left ventricular failure	• Hypovolemia • Vasodilation
Pulmonary artery occlusive pressure (PAOP)	• Positive pressure ventilation, especially with positive end expiratory pressure (PEEP) • Hypervolemia • Mitral valve dysfunction: stenosis or regurgitation • Constrictive pericarditis • Cardiac tamponade • Left ventricular failure • Severe aortic stenosis	• Hypovolemia • Vasodilators

Continued

Table **2-15** **Causes of Abnormal Hemodynamic Pressures—cont'd**

Parameter	Increased	Decreased
Cardiac output	• Sympathetic nervous system (SNS) innervation (endogenous catecholamines) (e.g., stress, exercise) • Exogenous catecholamines (e.g., epinephrine, isoproterenol, dobutamine, dopamine) • Other positive inotropes (e.g., digitalis, amrinone) • Infection, early sepsis • Hyperthyroidism • Anemia	• Decreased contractility (e.g., myocardial infarction [MI], cardiomyopathy, beta-blockers) • Increased afterload (e.g., systemic or pulmonary hypertension, aortic or pulmonic stenosis, polycythemia) • Alteration in preload: excessively increased (e.g., hypervolemia, HF) or decreased (e.g., hypovolemia, cardiac tamponade, mitral or tricuspid valve disease) • Significantly increased or decreased heart rate (e.g., bradydysrhythmias, tachydysrhythmias)

Svo_2	• Increased oxygen supply and delivery
	  • Increased Fio_2, hyperoxemia
	  • Increased cardiac output
	  • Increased hemoglobin
	• Decreased oxygen demand
	  • Anesthesia
	  • Muscle paralysis, sedation
	  • Hypothermia
	  • Sleep
	• Decreased oxygen extraction at tissue level
	  • Early sepsis
	  • Shift of oxyhemoglobin dissociation curve to the left (e.g., alkalosis, hypothermia)
	• Ventricular septal defect with left-to-right intracardiac shunt (e.g., ventricular septal defect)
	• Technical problems
	  • PA catheter in occluded position
	  • Deposits of fibrin on the tip of the catheter
		• Decreased oxygen supply and delivery
		  • Decrease in Sao_2
		  • Decrease in cardiac output
		  • Decrease in Hgb
		• Increased oxygen extraction at tissue level
		  • Increased metabolic needs (e.g., seizures, shivering, restlessness, pain, hyperthermia)
		• Shift of oxyhemoglobin dissociation curve to the right (e.g., acidosis, hyperthermia)

b) Ensure that the transducer is level with the phlebostatic axis

c) Check for overdamping or underdamping using the square wave test (Fig. 2-40)

(1) Fast-flush the system and analyze the waveform after the flush; no peaks should be more than 1 mm apart, and the second peak is less than one third the height of the first peak

(2) If system overdamped, check for occlusion or air in system

(3) If system underdamped:

(a) Add a damping device to absorb unwanted frequency vibration

(b) Turn a stopcock slightly

III. Right atrial pressure (RAP)

A. Pressure in the right atrium

B. Reflects venous return to right heart; also reflects right ventricular end-diastolic pressure and preload as long as right ventricular compliance and tricuspid valve function are normal

C. Measured through catheter in superior vena cava (CVP) or at the proximal port of pulmonary artery catheter (RAP)

1. Insertion of a CVP catheter or pulmonary artery (PA) catheter

a) Preceded by insertion of a venous introducer into the external jugular or subclavian vein; the internal jugular, femoral, or basilic vein can also be used but are less desirable

b) The catheter is then threaded through the introducer into place with the CVP catheter tip in the superior vena cava and the PA catheter tip in a pulmonary arteriole in the dependent area (West zone 3), although the RAP is measured from the proximal port, which is in the right atrium

2. Although these parameters (CVP and RAP) are not actually the same, they are the same in practicality and are frequently used interchangeably

3. Central venous pressure may be measured

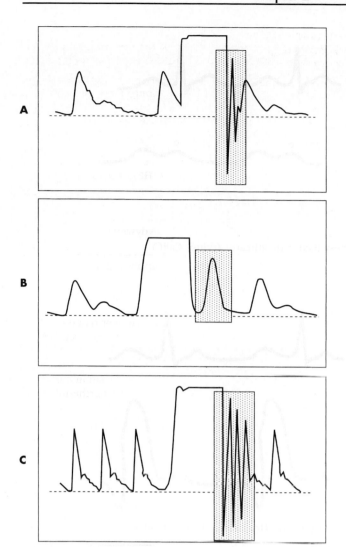

Figure 2-40 Square wave test using the fast-flush valve. **A,** Normal test and accurate waveform. **B,** Overdamped. **C,** Underdamped.

by a water manometer in cm H_2O pressure or by a transducer in mm Hg pressure
4. RAP from the proximal port of the PA catheter is generally measured by a transducer in mm Hg
5. To convert values, remember that 1 mm Hg is equal to 1.36 cm H_2O
D. Normal pressure value: 2 to 6 mm Hg mean (or 3 to 8 cm H_2O)
E. Causes of abnormal pressures (Table 2-15)
F. Normal waveform (Fig. 2-41)
IV. Right ventricular pressure
   A. Pressure in the right ventricle
   B. Measured only during insertion of the PA catheter as the distal tip of the PA catheter is floated through the right ventricle
   C. Normal pressure values
      1. Systolic: 15 to 30 mm Hg
      2. End-diastolic: 0 to 8 mm Hg
   D. Causes of abnormal pressures (Table 2-15)
   E. Normal waveform (Fig. 2-42)

V. Pulmonary artery pressure (PAP)
   A. Pressure in the pulmonary artery with the balloon **deflated**
   B. Measured from the distal tip of the PA catheter with balloon **deflated**
      1. PA systolic pressure (PAs): pressure in the pulmonary artery during RV systole
      2. PA end-diastolic pressure (PAd): pressure in the pulmonary artery at the end of RV diastole; reflects left atrial pressure in the absence of pulmonary disease and LVEDP in the absence of pulmonary disease and mitral valve dysfunction
   C. Normal pressure values
      1. Systolic: 15 to 30 mm Hg
      2. Diastolic: 5 to 15 mm Hg
      3. Mean: 10 to 20 mm Hg
   D. Causes of abnormal pressures (Table 2-15)
   E. Causes for lack of correlation between PAd and PAOP (PAd normally 2 to 5 mm Hg greater than PAOP)
      1. PAd more than 5 mm Hg greater than PAOP caused by any of the following:
         a) Tachycardias greater than 125 beats/min
         b) Pulmonary hypertension
            (1) Hypoxemia with PaO_2 less than 60 mm Hg (e.g., ARDS, COPD, PE)
            (2) Mitral valve dysfunction (stenosis or regurgitation)
      2. PAOP greater than PAd caused by any of the following:
         a) PAd artificially low or PAOP artificially high
         b) Mitral regurgitation with mean of PAOP used rather than the *a*-wave amplitude (since mitral regurgitation causes large *v*-waves on the PAOP-waveform, it increases the PAOP if the mean is used; use the *a*-wave measurement when large *v*-waves are present)
         c) Forceful atrial contraction
   F. Normal waveform (Fig. 2-43)
   G. Changes in waveform (Table 2-16)
      1. Fling (Fig. 2-44)
      2. Damped (Fig. 2-45)
VI. Pulmonary artery occlusive pressure (PAOP) (also referred to as *pulmonary capillary wedge pressure* [PCWP] or *pulmonary artery wedge pressure* [PAWP]
   A. Pressure in the pulmonary artery with the balloon **inflated;** reflects pressure from the left atrium in the absence of pulmonary hypertension
   B. Measured from the distal tip of the PA catheter with the balloon **inflated;** the balloon blocks right heart pressures from the distal tip; left atrial pressure reflects left ventricular end-diastolic pressure and LV preload in the absence of mitral valve disease or left atrial tumor (Box 2-2)
   C. Normal pressure value: 6 to 12 mm Hg (mea-

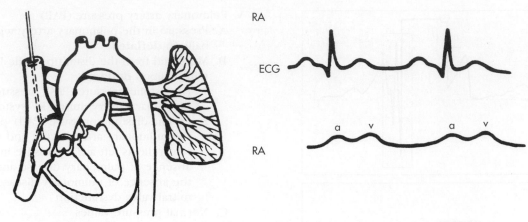

Figure 2-41 Right atrial waveform. (Courtesy Baxter Healthcare, Irvine, Calif.)

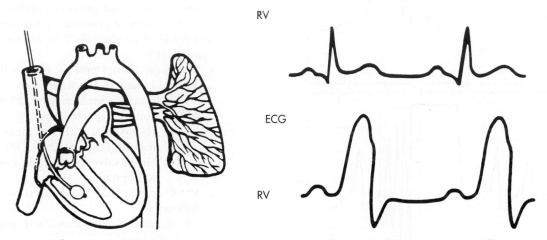

Figure 2-42 Right ventricular waveform. (Courtesy Baxter Healthcare, Irvine, Calif.)

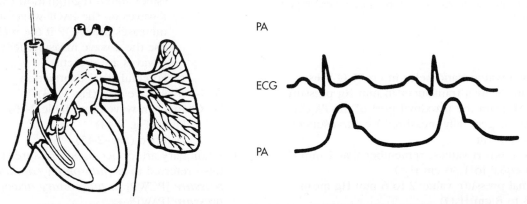

Figure 2-43 Pulmonary artery waveform. (Courtesy Baxter Healthcare, Irvine, Calif.)

sured as a mean); remember that some pa-
tients require a PAOP as high as 15 to 20 mm
Hg for optimal preload
  D. Causes of abnormal pressures (Table 2-15)
  E. Normal waveform (Fig. 2-46)
    1. The *a*-wave correlates with atrial contrac-
    tion: it is the first wave seen after the QRS
    using dual channel recording
    2. The *v*-wave correlates with ventricular con-

traction: it is the first wave after the T-wave
using dual channel recording
  F. Changes in waveform (Table 2-16)
    1. Large *q*-waves
    2. Large *v*-waves
    3. Large *a*-waves and large *v*-waves
VII. Left atrial pressure (LAP)
  A. Pressure in the left atrium; reflects left ventric-
  ular end-diastolic pressure and LV preload in

Table 2-16 Hemodynamic Waveform Abnormalities

Abnormality	Cause	Implications/Treatment
Pulmonary Artery Waveform		

Fling	• Excessive catheter length in RA or RV
	• Catheter tip is located near the pulmonic valve
		• Turn patient to left side to see if catheter will float out into PA
		• Monitor closely for indications that the catheter has flipped back into RV
		  • Loss of dicrotic notch characteristic of an arterial waveform
		  • Decrease in diastolic pressure to close to 0 mm Hg
		  • Ventricular ectopy: PVCs, possible ventricular tachycardia
		• Inflate balloon to increase the chance that it will float distally back into position
		• Catheter needs to be repositioned distally for fling or if catheter is in RV

Damped	• Air bubbles within the pressure monitoring system • Catheter occlusion (e.g., fibrin at the tip of the catheter or catheter tip against the wall of the vessel) • Spontaneous occluded position	• Check the system for bubbles or blood; check that stopcocks are all positioned correctly and that stopcocks are covered with dead-end stopcock port covers (no holes) • Try to aspirate the catheter; DO NOT FLUSH because catheter may be in wedge position; if a clot is aspirated, discard and flush catheter • If still damped, ask patient to take deep breaths, cough, and turn to side; if still in spontaneous occluded position, catheter needs to be repositioned proximally
Pulmonary Artery Occlusive Waveform		
Large *a*-waves	• Mitral stenosis • Severe aortic stenosis • Hypertension • AV block with AV asynchrony	

Large *v*-waves	• Mitral regurgitation
	• Ventricular septal defect
		• Note: in patients with large *v*-waves
		  • The mean PAOP may be higher than PAd; do not use mean as the numeric pressure value for PAOP
		  • Use the measurement of the *a*-wave for the numeric pressure value for PAOP since the mitral valve is open during the *a*-wave (atrial contraction) and this value better evaluates LVEDP

Large *a*- and *v*-waves (looks like M)	• Cardiac tamponade • Constrictive pericarditis • Hypervolemia • Left ventricular failure	

the absence of mitral valve disease or left atrial tumor

B. Measured by a catheter placed directly in the left atrium, usually placed during cardiac surgery

C. A PA catheter is usually used to measure PAOP as an indirect reflection of LAP because of the risk of complications related to direct LA catheter (e.g., air embolus, cardiac tamponade)

D. Normals, waveforms, etc., as for PAOP

VIII. Mixed venous oxygen saturation (Svo$_2$)

A. Oxygen saturation of the blood as it returns to the lung for reoxygenation; reflects how well the body's demand for oxygen is met by the amount of oxygen supplied

B. Measured by a fiberoptic oximetric PA catheter or by blood gas analysis of blood drawn from the distal lumen of the PA catheter

C. Normal Svo$_2$: 60% to 80%

D. Causes of abnormal parameters (Table 2-15)

IX. Cardiac output

A. Amount of blood ejected by the ventricle each minute

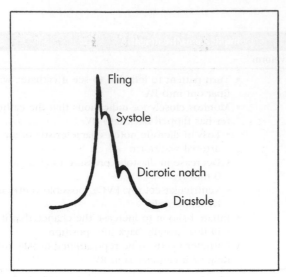

Figure 2-44   Pulmonary artery waveform: catheter fling.

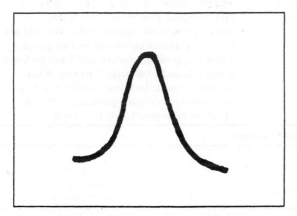

Figure 2-45   Pulmonary artery waveform: damped waveform.

BOX **2-2   Intracardiac Pressures**

RAP = Right heart
PAd = Pulmonary vascular bed
PAOP = Left heart

B. Measured by thermodilution
   1. Intermittent: method
      a) Injection of a known volume of a known temperature solution into an unknown volume of blood at a known temperature
      b) The injectate solution (usually D₅W) is injected into the proximal lumen (RA) of the PA catheter
      c) The injectate is mixed with the blood
      d) The temperature change is sensed downstream at the thermister located 4 cm from the distal tip of the PA catheter
      e) The amount of the unknown volume of blood is deduced from the amount of change in temperature
   2. Continuous (referred to as *continuous cardiac output* [CCO])
      a) Method
         (1) A thermal filament in the right ventricle creates a signal by warming the blood as it flows by
         (2) The thermister at the distal tip measures the temperature of the blood downstream
         (3) The computer produces a thermodilution curve and the cardiac output
         (4) The cardiac output is updated approximately every 5 minutes
      b) Advantages
         (1) May be more accurate in patients with low cardiac output states
         (2) Continuously updated
         (3) Decreases required nursing time
         (4) Reduces risks of contamination and fluid overload
      c) Disadvantages
         (1) Cost: catheter approximately three times the cost of conventional catheter

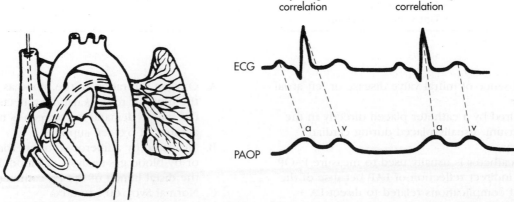

Figure 2-46   Pulmonary artery occlusive pressure waveform. Although the *a* wave correlates physiologically to atrial depolarization and the P wave, and the *v* wave correlates physiologically with the QRS and ventricular depolarization, tubing and catheter cause a time delay. Actually, the first wave seen after the QRS is the *a* wave, and the first wave seen after the T wave is the *v* wave. (adapted from Baxter Healthcare, Irvine, Calif.)

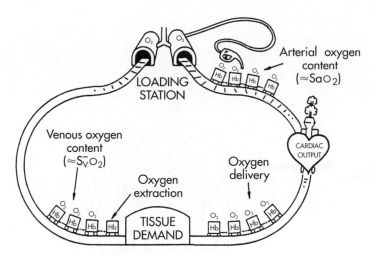

Figure 2-47   Schematic demonstrating DO_2/VO_2 (Understanding continuous mixed venous oxygen saturation monitoring with the Swan Ganz TD System. Baxter Healthcare Corporation, Edwards Critical Care.)

C. Normal value: CO 4 to 8 L/min; CI 2.5 to 4 L/min
D. Causes of abnormal parameter (Table 2-15)

X. Right ventricular parameters
   A. Measured with special REF pulmonary artery catheter
   B. Normal values for right ventricular parameters (Table 2-14)

XI. Oxygenation parameters (Fig. 2-47)
   A. Calculated parameters
   B. Normal values for oxygenation parameters (Table 2-14)

XII. Gastric tonometry: new method to detect regional alterations in tissue perfusion
   A. A vented nasogastric tube with a tonometer balloon located a few inches from the catheter's distal tip is placed into the stomach; a three-way stopcock is placed at the proximal end of the tonometer port
   B. The tonometer balloon is filled with saline and is permeable to carbon dioxide
   C. Samples taken from the balloon are analyzed for CO_2 to reflect the $PICO_2$ (intramucosal carbon dioxide) at the same time that arterial blood is drawn for bicarbonate level
   D. The intramucosal pH (pHi) is then calculated; a low pHi (<7.20) indicates perfusion abnormality
   E. Trends are monitored and interventions evaluated by changes in pHi

Nursing Responsibilities Related to Measurement of Hemodynamic Parameters

I. Maximize accuracy and reproducibility of measured parameters
   A. The transducer must be leveled, balanced to zero, and calibrated with each head of bed position change and/or at least every 12 hours
      1. Leveling
         a) The air-fluid interface (also referred to as the *air reference port*) of the transducer needs to be leveled with the phlebostatic axis to ensure accuracy of measurement; the phlebostatic axis correlates with the right atrium and is at the fourth intercostal space and the midway between the sternum anterior and the spine posterior (Fig. 2-48)
            (1) If transducer too high, reading will be too low
            (2) If transducer too low, reading will be too high
         b) The patient does not need to be flat to take pressure measurements as long as the head of the bed is elevated 60 degrees or less and the air-fluid interface is at the level of the phlebostatic axis (Fig. 2-48); the head of the bed should be elevated no more than 30 degrees for cardiac output determinations
         c) Patients should be supine; lateral positions affect pressure readings as well as cardiac output measurements
      2. Balancing to zero
         a) Zero referencing the transducer requires closing the transducer to the patient, opening the stopcock closest to the transducer to air, and ensuring that the monitor and the recorder read 0 ± 1 mm Hg
         b) This process negates the force exerted by the atmosphere so that only cardiovascular pressures are sensed, measured, and recorded
      3. Calibrating
         a) Some monitors also require calibration
         b) A known pressure is exerted on the transducer to see that the monitor measures and displays it correctly
   B. All pressure readings are done at end-expiration (Fig. 2-49)
      1. Spontaneously breathing patient: expiration is positive (high point of fluctuation)

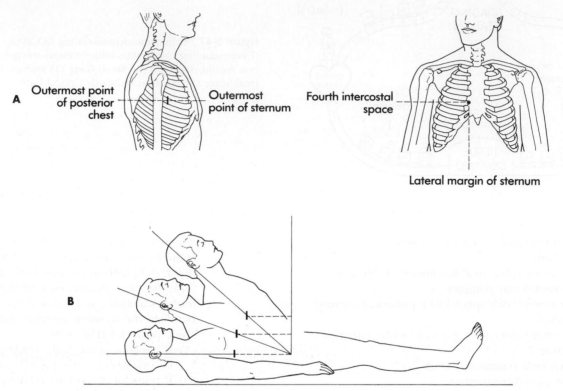

Figure 2-48 Phlebostatic axis. **A,** Location of phlebostatic axis. **B,** Note that the measurements are accurate with head of bed elevated up to 60 degrees as long as the air-fluid interface is level with the phlebostatic axis. (From Flynn JBM, Bruce NP: *Introduction to critical care skills,* St Louis, 1993, Mosby.)

Figure 2-49 Hemodynamic measurements are done at end-expiration. **A,** When a patient is receiving positive pressure mechanical ventilation, inspiration is positive and expiration is neutral. Readings should be done at the valley. Remember: ventilation—valley. **B,** When a patient is spontaneously breathing, inspiration is negative and expiration is positive. Readings should be done at the peak. Remember: patient—peak. (Reprinted with permission from Schermer L: Physiologic and technical variables affecting hemodynamic measurements, *Crit Care Nurse* 8 (2):33, 1988.)

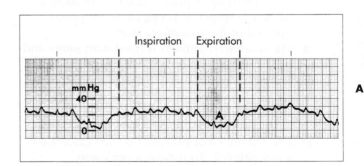

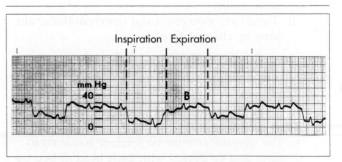

2. Mechanically ventilated patient: expiration is neutral (low point of fluctuation)
3. Remember: ventilator valley, patient peak

C. Room temperature injectates for cardiac output determination by thermodilution are adequate as long as a 12° F difference exists between blood temperature and injectate temperature; keep injectate solution and tubing away from direct sunlight and heat lamps

D. Appropriate computation constant for calculation of cardiac output must be entered into the computer: catheter size and type and volume and temperature of injectate determine the computation constant

E. Cardiac output injectate must be injected within 4 seconds

II. Ensure patency of the catheter by maintaining a heparinized flush system unless contraindicated

A. Usual heparin concentration is 1 U of heparin/ 1 ml of flush solution

1. Heparin is contraindicated in patients with a history of heparin-induced thrombosis and thrombocytopenia (HITT) (also referred to as *heparin-associated thrombosis and thrombocytopenia* [HATT] or *white clot syndrome*)

B. Intermittent flush devices deliver 3 to 5 ml/hr as long as the pressure bag is maintained at 300 mm Hg

III. Correlate numeric value of parameter with the patient's clinical presentation

A. Hemodynamic parameter changes may precede clinical presentation changes (e.g., subclinical hypoperfusion)

B. Hemodynamic parameter changes may reflect inaccurate measurements; care must be taken to be consistent in measuring techniques

IV. Note trends of change of measured parameters over time and in response to therapeutic interventions

V. Notify the physician of significant deviations from patient's normal; a pressure change should be 4 mm Hg or greater before it is considered clinically significant

VI. Utilize hemodynamic parameters in titration of inotropes and vasoactive agents

VII. Prevent and detect complications of hemodynamic monitoring (Table 2-17)

Table 2-17   Complications of Hemodynamic Monitoring

Complications	Prevention/Detection/Treatment
Air emboli	• Utilize Trendelenburg position for insertion of deep vein catheters • Place sterile gloved finger over needle hub with any disconnection during insertion to prevent air emboli • Aspirate air from flush solution bag to avoid air embolus with inadvertent emptying of flush solution bag • Flush all lumens with saline prior to insertion of catheters • Monitor the pressure monitoring system for air bubbles • Use only Luer-Lok connections • Have the patient hold his or her breath during catheter-tubing disconnects (e.g., tubing changes or removal of deep vein catheters) • If air embolus is suspected, turn patient to left side with head down (Durant's maneuver) and administer oxygen
Arterial puncture (during venous cannulation)	• Hold pressure for at least 5-10 minutes; a longer time may be required for patients on anticoagulants or patients who have received thrombolytics
Balloon rupture	• Test the balloon before insertion by inflating the balloon, holding it in a basin of sterile saline, and watching for bubbling • Store catheters away from sunlight and heat • Limit the length of time that catheter is left in (ideally less than 72 hours) • Limit the number of times balloon is inflated to only when indicated (balloons are expected to last about 72 inflations); use PAd as a reflection of LVEDP in patients without pulmonary hypertension • Do not overinflate balloon; stop injecting air as soon as the PAOP waveform is seen • Do not aspirate air from the balloon; allow passive deflation • This complication is particularly dangerous in right-to-left shunt (e.g., neonates [adults shunt left-to-right]) • Indications that the balloon has ruptured include inability to obtain PAOP waveform and absence of resistance during inflation • If balloon rupture has occurred, label balloon lumen accordingly so that others do not continue to try to inflate balloon; use PAd as a reflection of LVEDP in patients without pulmonary hypertension
Clotting and catheter occlusion	• Maintain heparinized normal saline drip with IFD • Monitor for any change in waveform (e.g., damping)

Continued

Table 2-17 | **Complications of Hemodynamic Monitoring—cont'd**

Complications	Prevention/Detection/Treatment
Dysrhythmias: usually ventricular dysrhythmias or RBBB	• Have emergency equipment (including transcutaneous pacemaker) available during insertion • Inflate balloon to capacity when the catheter is in the right atrium during insertion so that the balloon cushions the tip • Monitor the ECG monitor closely during insertion • Have catheter sutured in place to decrease risk of movement • Assess PAP waveform for indication that catheter is flipping back into RV 　• Request catheter repositioning for catheter fling or RV waveform 　• Turn patient to left side to encourage migration of catheter back into pulmonary artery • Remove catheter in a smooth continuous movement with balloon deflated; monitor ECG closely during removal
Emboli	• Aspirate if you suspect small clot rather than flush
Exsanguination	• Use only Luer-Lok connections • Maintain alarms in ON position; pressure alarms are usually set 10-20 mm Hg above and below the patient's normal
Fluid overload	• Limit the number of fast flushes • Use 5 ml instead of 10 ml for cardiac outputs when indicated • Limit frequency of cardiac outputs to every 4 hours unless required more often
Hematoma	• Maintain pressure for 5-10 minutes with single-thickness pressure dressing after catheter removal; a longer time may be required for patients on anticoagulants or patients who have received thrombolytics
Hypothermia	• Use room temperature injectate • Apply blankets and radiant heaters as needed
Infection	• Utilize percutaneous catheter insertion (results in a much lower incidence of infection than does cutdown) • Change flush solution bag every 24 hours • Change tubing every 48-72 hours or according to your hospital protocol • Dress and inspect site using sterile technique every 24-48 hours or according to your hospital protocol • Avoid clear semipermeable dressings in patients with oily skin • Use normal saline rather than D_5W for the heparinized flush solution • Do not allow dried blood to stay in stopcock ports or tubing • Limit the number of stopcocks in the pressure monitoring system • Replace all vented stopcock covers with nonvented "dead-end" caps • Utilize strict sterile technique with blood sampling and cardiac outputs • Encourage use of catheter sleeve over PA catheter to ensure sterility and allow for sterile catheter manipulation • Limit the length of time that catheter is left in place (ideally less than 72-96 hours) • Monitor for clinical indications of catheter sepsis: fever, chills, leukocytosis, positive blood culture and/or catheter culture, redness, swelling, induration, and purulent drainage from catheter insertion site
Microshock	• Recognize that this risk results from elimination of the skin as a protection from microshock in patients with intracardiac catheters • Ensure that all electrical equipment is properly functioning and grounded • Do not touch the patient and a piece of electrical equipment at the same time
Nerve palsy	• Maintain limbs in functional position (e.g., do not keep the wrist hyperextended)
Pneumothorax, hemothorax, chylothorax during insertion	• Have chest x-ray taken after deep vein catheter cannulation • Assist with insertion of chest tube if pneumothorax (air in pleural space), hemothorax (blood in pleural space), or chylothorax (lymph fluid in pleural space) occurs
Pulmonary artery rupture	• Inflate balloon with only enough air to cause PAOP waveform; do not overinflate • Monitor patient for hemoptysis and possible hemorrhage as an indication of pulmonary artery rupture
Pulmonary infarction	• Inflate balloon only long enough to record pressure value and waveform • Continuously monitor PAP so that if catheter advances into PAOP position, it will be noted and catheter repositioned • Request proximal repositioning if it takes less than 1.25 ml to achieve occluded position because this situation indicates that the catheter is positioned too distal and may spontaneously occlude the pulmonary arteriole and cause ischemia and infarction • Monitor for chest pain, dyspnea, and decreased Sao_2 as an indication of pulmonary infarction

| Table | 2-17 | Complications of Hemodynamic Monitoring—cont'd |

Complications	Prevention/Detection/Treatment

Thrombosis	• Maintain heparinized normal saline drip with intermittent flush device (IFD); keep pressure bag at 300 mm Hg
	• Limit length of time that catheter is left in (ideally less than 72 hr)
	• Prevent trauma to the intima by skillful catheter insertion
	• To prevent and detect arterial thrombosis with arterial catheters
	  • Select site with collateral flow (e.g., radial artery for arterial cannulation)
	  • Utilize smallest catheter feasible (e.g., 20-gauge for radial artery cannulation)
	  • Perform neurovascular assessment hourly
	• If arterial occlusion occurs, assist with intraarterial thrombolytic or embolectomy

Table	2-18	Hemodynamic Profiles for Selected Critical Care Conditions

Cardiogenic shock	• CO, CI decreased • RAP, PAP, PAOP increased • SVR, SVRI increased • LVSWI decreased • Svo_2 decreased • DO_2 decreased
Hypovolemic shock	• CO, CI decreased • RAP, PAP, PAOP decreased • SVR, SVRI increased • Svo_2 decreased • DO_2 decreased
Vasogenic shock other than septic (e.g., ana-phylactic shock or neu-rogenic shock)	• CO, CI decreased • RAP, PAP, PAOP decreased • SVR, SVRI decreased • Svo_2 decreased • DO_2 decreased
Septic shock (early) (late as in hypovolemic shock)	• CO, CI increased • RAP, PAP, PAOP decreased • SVR, SVRI decreased • Svo_2 increased • DO_2 increased • VO_2 decreased
Cardiac tamponade	• PAP, PAOP increased • Large a- and v-waves (M) on PAOP waveform • Equalization of intracardiac pressures; RAP, PAd, PAOP will all be increased and within a 5 mm Hg variation • Pulsus paradoxus (drop in BP more than 10 mm Hg during inspiration)

Continued

- **Hemodynamic Profiles for Selected Critical Care Conditions** (Table 2-18)
- **Utilizing hemodynamic parameters in clinical decision-making**
  I. Determination of best PEEP: PEEP that will give the best Pao_2 and Sao_2 without causing a drop in CO and CI
  II. Determination of best PAOP or optimal point on Starling's curve
    A. PAOP that will give the best stroke volume and cardiac output without producing pulmonary edema
    B. Right ventricular end-diastolic volume may be a more valid parameter to monitor in evaluation of best stretch and filling volumes
      1. The main question is *does pressure truly reflect volume?*
      2. Pressure is not a reflection of volume in patients with poor ventricular compliance
      3. Volumetric measurements require a special REF pulmonary artery catheter
  III. Determination of true PAOP with patients on PEEP (especially important if patient is on high levels of PEEP)
    A. Convert cm H_2O measurement of PEEP to mm Hg by dividing by 1.36
    B. Subtract one half of the PEEP (in millimeters of mercury) from the measured PAOP to get a "true" PAOP when evaluating fluid status and filling volumes
    C. This parameter is of questionable clinical value, because trends rather than absolute pressure measurements are of the most clinical significance
  IV. Clinical decision-making
    A. Use indexes to evaluate parameters (e.g., cardiac index versus cardiac output)
    B. Identify why the cardiac index is decreased; physiologic alterations are treated, not just the blood pressure (Fig. 2-50)

Table 2-18	Hemodynamic Profiles for Selected Critical Care Conditions—cont'd
Pulmonary hypertension (COPD, PE, MVD, hypoxia)	• PAd, PVR increased • PAm >20 mm Hg • PAd more than 5 mm Hg >PAOP
Cardiac pulmonary edema	• PAP, PAOP increased • PVR, PVRI increased • Sao_2 decreased • Svo_2 decreased
Noncardiac pulmonary edema (e.g., ARDS)	• PAP elevated, PAOP normal • PVR, PVRI increased • Sao_2 decreased • Svo_2 decreased
Papillary muscle rupture (acute mitral regurgitation)	• PAP, PAOP increased • Large v-waves on PAOP waveform • CO/CI decreased • Svo_2 decreased • DO_2 decreased
Rupture of ventricular septum	• PAP increased • Large v-waves on PAOP waveform may be seen • Svo_2 increased (or mixed venous oxygen saturation) • Increased oxygen gradient (oxygen step-up) between RA and PA • Inaccurate cardiac output measurement: because cardiac output measurement by thermodilution is actually a right ventricular cardiac output, measured cardiac output will be high, but the cardiac output from the left ventricle is actually low
Left ventricular infarction	• RAP, PAP, PAOP may be increased • LVSWI may be decreased • CO/CI may be decreased
Right ventricular infarction	• RAP may be increased • PAP, PAOP may be decreased • RVSWI may be decreased • CO/CI may be decreased

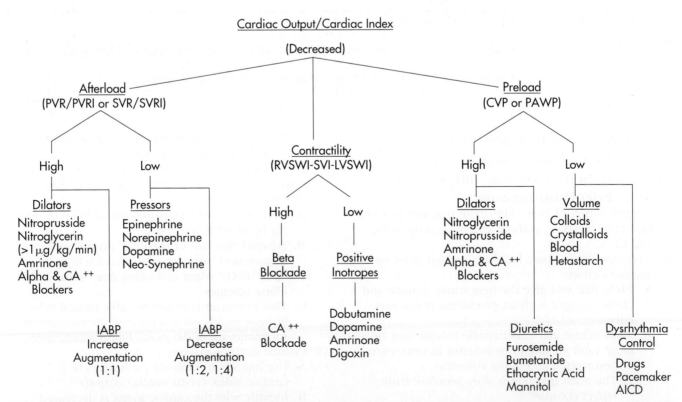

Figure 2-50 Hemodynamic algorithm. (Reprinted with permission from Urban N: Hemodynamic clinical profiles, *AACN Clin Issues Crit Care Nurs* 1:119, 1990.)

LEARNING ACTIVITIES

Note: Remember that you won't see questions like these on the CCRN® examination, but these activities allow you to approach the content from a different perspective to remember it better. Multiple-choice questions similar to those on the CCRN® examination are on the CD-ROM.

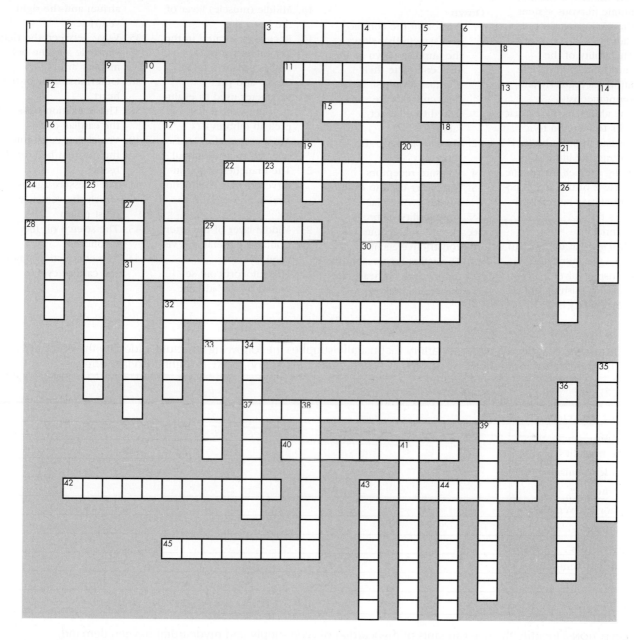

1. DIRECTIONS: Complete the following crossword puzzle dealing with cardiovascular anatomy and physiology.

Across

1. Outermost layer of the artery
3. Cardiac muscle fiber
7. Lower chamber of the heart
11. Vessel leading away from the heart
12. Innermost layer of the heart; contiguous with the heart valves
13. Phase 1 of the action potential may be referred to as the_____ channel
15. Parameter used to evaluate right ventricular afterload (abbrev)
16. The ability of the cardiac cells to respond to a stimulus by muscle contraction
18. Upper chamber of the heart
22. The branch of the autonomic nervous system referred to as the *"fight or flight"* system
24. Parameter used to evaluate left ventricular preload (abbrev)
26. Parameter used to evaluate left ventricular afterload (abbrev)
28. Valve between the left atrium and the left ventricle

29. Innermost layer of the artery
30. Substance secreted by the kidney in response to hypoperfusion
31. Pressure pulling into the capillary
32. The branch of the autonomic nervous system that maintains a steady state
33. The ability of the cardiac cells to initiate impulses regularly and spontaneously
37. The ability of the cardiac cells to respond to a cardiac impulse by transmitting the impulse along the cell membrane
39. Phase 2 of the action potential may be referred to as the_____ channel
40. Muscles that contract to close the mitral and tricuspid valves
42. Pressure pushing out of the capillary

43. Phase 3 of the action potential may be referred to as the_____ channel
45. Fibers that transmit the cardiac impulse throughout the ventricular tissue

Down
1. Portion of the conduction system that slows the impulse down so the atria complete their contraction phase before the ventricles are stimulated to contract (abbrev)
2. Vessel leading to the heart
4. Pressure receptors
5. Parameter used to evaluate left ventricular contractility (abbrev)
6. Potent endogenous vasoconstrictive agent
8. The reflex responsible for the increase in heart rate during inspiration

9. Valve betweeen the left ventricle and the aorta
10. The natural pacemaker of the heart (abbrev)
12. The ability of the cardiac cells to respond to a stimulus by initiating a cardiac impulse
14. Middle (muscle) layer of the heart
17. Receptors located in the carotid and aortic bodies sensitive to Pao_2, $Paco_2$, and pH
19. Parameter used to evaluate right ventricular preload (abbrev)
20. Atrial contraction is also referred to as the atrial___
21. The branches of the interventricular conduction system are referred to as_____
23. Middle layer of the artery
25. Contains parietal and visceral layers
27. Mineralocorticoid secreted by the adrenal

cortex, which causes renal retention of sodium and water
29. Disks that lie between myocardial cells to allow rapid transmission of the cardiac impulse
34. Valve between the right atrium and the right ventricle
35. Valve between the right ventricle and the pulmonary artery
36. Outermost layer of the heart
38. The relaxation phase of the cardiac cycle
39. Vessel that constitutes the nutrient bed for the tissues
41. The pressure against which the ventricle must pump
43. The stretch on the myofibrils
44. The contraction phase of the cardiac cycle

2. **DIRECTIONS:** Identify the coronary artery that usually supplies the following structures. Identify the coronary artery as LAD (left anterior descending artery), LCA (left circumflex artery), or RCA (right coronary artery).

Structure	Coronary Artery
Anterior left ventricle	
AV node	
Bundle branches	
Lateral left ventricle	
Left atrium	
Posterior left ventricle	
Right atrium	
Right ventricle	
Inferior left ventricle	
SA node	
Septum	

3. **DIRECTIONS:** Identify the determinants of myocardial oxygen supply and myocardial oxygen demand.

Myocardial Oxygen Supply	Myocardial Oxygen Demand

4. **DIRECTIONS:** Identify the primary factor or factors affected in each condition and the primary effect or effects of each treatment; indicate increase or decrease of heart rate, preload, afterload, or contractility by appropriate arrows (↑ or ↓).

    Note: sympathetic nervous system responses may be seen in any of these conditions but they are secondary, not primary.

Conditions				
Aortic stenosis	____ Heart Rate	____ Preload	____ Afterload	____ Contractility
Bradydysrhythmias	____ Heart Rate	____ Preload	____ Afterload	____ Contractility
Cardiac tamponade	____ Heart Rate	____ Preload	____ Afterload	____ Contractility
Cardiomyopathy	____ Heart Rate	____ Preload	____ Afterload	____ Contractility
Heart failure	____ Heart Rate	____ Preload	____ Afterload	____ Contractility
Hypertension	____ Heart Rate	____ Preload	____ Afterload	____ Contractility
Hypovolemia	____ Heart Rate	____ Preload	____ Afterload	____ Contractility
Myocardial infarction	____ Heart Rate	____ Preload	____ Afterload	____ Contractility
Pulmonary hypertension	____ Heart Rate	____ Preload	____ Afterload	____ Contractility
Septic shock—early	____ Heart Rate	____ Preload	____ Afterload	____ Contractility
Septic shock—late	____ Heart Rate	____ Preload	____ Afterload	____ Contractility
Tachydysrhythmias	____ Heart Rate	____ Preload	____ Afterload	____ Contractility

Treatments				
Aminophylline	____ Heart Rate	____ Preload	____ Afterload	____ Contractility
Amrinone (Inocor)	____ Heart Rate	____ Preload	____ Afterload	____ Contractility
Digoxin (Lanoxin)	____ Heart Rate	____ Preload	____ Afterload	____ Contractility
Dobutamine (Dobutrex)	____ Heart Rate	____ Preload	____ Afterload	____ Contractility
Dopamine (3-5 µg/kg/min)	____ Heart Rate	____ Preload	____ Afterload	____ Contractility
Dopamine (5-10 µg/kg/min)	____ Heart Rate	____ Preload	____ Afterload	____ Contractility
Dopamine (>10 µg/kg/min)	____ Heart Rate	____ Preload	____ Afterload	____ Contractility
Fluid challenge	____ Heart Rate	____ Preload	____ Afterload	____ Contractility
Furosemide (Lasix)	____ Heart Rate	____ Preload	____ Afterload	____ Contractility
Intraaortic balloon pump	____ Heart Rate	____ Preload	____ Afterload	____ Contractility
Isoproterenol (Isuprel)	____ Heart Rate	____ Preload	____ Afterload	____ Contractility
Nitroglycerin	____ Heart Rate	____ Preload	____ Afterload	____ Contractility
Nitroprusside (Nipride)	____ Heart Rate	____ Preload	____ Afterload	____ Contractility
Phenylephrine (Neo-Synephrine)	____ Heart Rate	____ Preload	____ Afterload	____ Contractility
Propranolol (Inderal)	____ Heart Rate	____ Preload	____ Afterload	____ Contractility

5. **DIRECTIONS:** Match the receptor of the sympathetic nervous system with its physiologic effect.

____ alpha

____ beta$_1$

____ beta$_2$

____ dopaminergic

a. increase in heart rate, contractility, conductivity

b. dilation of the renal and mesenteric arteries

c. vasoconstriction

d. vasodilation, bronchodilation

6. **DIRECTIONS:** Identify which of these sympathomimetic (adrenergic) drugs cause the most powerful stimulation of each of these receptors.

____ alpha

____ beta$_1$

____ beta$_2$

____ dopaminergic

a. isoproterenol

b. dopamine at 2 µg/kg/min

c. phenylephrine

d. dobutamine

7. **DIRECTIONS:** Identify the formula for each of these parameters.

a. Cardiac output	
b. Stroke volume	
c. Blood pressure	
d. Coronary artery perfusion pressure	
e. Cerebral perfusion pressure	

8.   DIRECTIONS: Identify possible causes of the following heart sounds.

Heart Sound	Possible Causes
S$_1$	
S$_2$	
Physiologic split of S$_2$	
Paradoxical split of S$_2$	
Fixed, wide split of S$_2$	
S$_3$	
S$_4$	
Pericardial friction rub	
Midsystolic click	
Holosystolic murmur	
Systolic ejection murmur	
Early diastolic murmur	
Mid- to late-diastolic murmur	

9.   DIRECTIONS: Complete the following table describing common murmurs.

Condition	Timing	Location	Pitch
Mitral regurgitation			
Mitral stenosis			
Aortic regurgitation			
Aortic stenosis			
Mitral valve prolapse			
Papillary muscle dysfunction or rupture			
Ventricular septal defect or rupture			

10.   DIRECTIONS: Match the dysrhythmia to the appropriate characteristic.

_____ 1.   normal sinus rhythm
_____ 2.   sinus bradycardia
_____ 3.   sinus tachycardia
_____ 4.   premature atrial contraction
_____ 5.   atrial fibrillation
_____ 6.   atrial flutter
_____ 7.   supraventricular tachycardia
_____ 8.   premature junctional contraction
_____ 9.   junctional escape rhythm
_____10.   accelerated junctional rhythm
_____11.   junctional tachycardia
_____12.   premature ventricular complex
_____13.   accelerated idioventricular rhythm
_____14.   ventricular tachycardia
_____15.   ventricular fibrillation
_____16.   asystole
_____17.   first-degree AV block
_____18.   second-degree AV block, type I
_____19.   second-degree AV block, type II
_____20.   third-degree AV block

a.   PR interval greater than 0.20 seconds
b.   early P-wave that looks different from other P-waves, followed by normal QRS
c.   sawtooth waves on baseline, no clearly identifiable P-waves, normal QRS
d.   QRS is early, greater than 0.12 seconds, with T-wave in opposite direction of QRS
e.   regular rhythm, normal P-waves, normal QRS complexes, rate less than 60/min
f.   quivering baseline, irregularly occurring QRSs
g.   QRS complex is early with inverted P-wave immediately (less than 0.12 seconds) prior to the QRS, in the QRS, or immediately after the QRS
h.   regular rhythm with rate of 40 to 60/min with narrow QRS and inverted P-wave immediately (less than 0.12 seconds) prior to the QRS, in the QRS, or immediately after the QRS
i.   flat line, no QRS complexes
j.   regular rhythm, normal P-waves, normal QRS complexes, rate more than 100/min
k.   regular rhythm, normal P-waves, normal QRS complexes, rate 60 to 100/min
l.   progressive PR lengthening until a P-wave is not followed by a QRS
m.   regular rhythm with rate of 60 to 100/min with narrow QRS and inverted P-wave immediately (less than 0.12 seconds) prior to the QRS, in the QRS, or immediately after the QRS
n.   wide QRS (more than 0.12 seconds) rhythm with rate of 40 to 100/min

o. regular rhythm with rate of more than 100/min with narrow QRS and inverted P-wave immediately (less than 0.12 seconds) prior to the QRS, in the QRS, or immediately after the QRS

p. regular rhythm with rate of 150 to 250/min without clearly discernible P-waves and narrow QRS

q. P-wave not followed by QRS without preceding progression of PR interval

r. no relationship between P-waves and QRS complexes; escape rhythm established by AV junction or ventricle

s. irregular baseline, absence of QRS complexes

t. wide QRS (more than 0.12 second) rhythm with rate more than 100/minute

11. **DIRECTIONS:** Analyze the following ECG rhythm strips and briefly describe treatment. All strips are 6 seconds.

a.

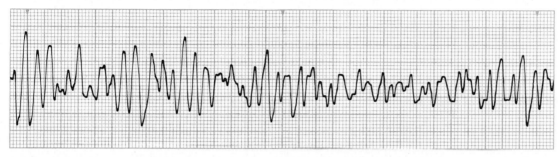

Interpretation:_____

Treatment:_____

b.

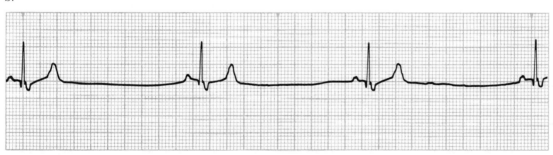

Interpretation:_____

Treatment:_____

c.

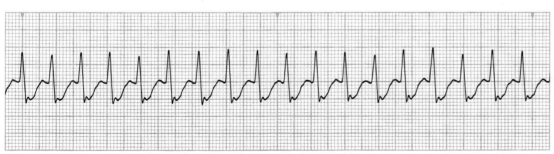

Interpretation:_____

Treatment:_____

d.

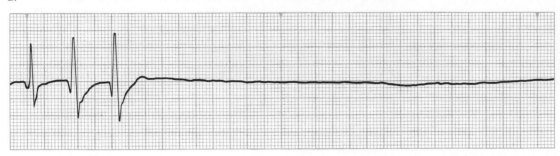

Interpretation:_____

Treatment:_____

e.

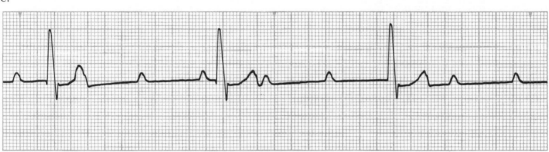

Interpretation:_____

Treatment:_____

f.

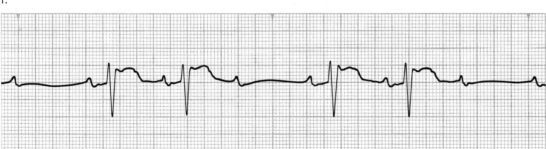

Interpretation:_____

Treatment:_____

g.

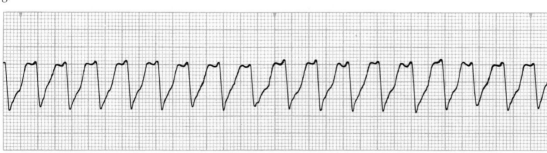

Interpretation:_____

Treatment:_____

h.

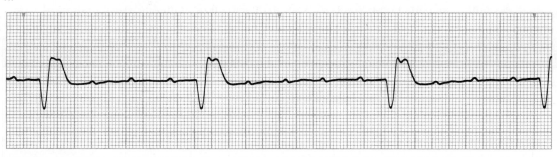

Interpretation:_____

Treatment:_____

i.

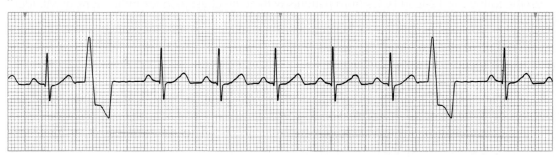

Interpretation:_____

Treatment:_____

12.   DIRECTIONS: Identify the major diagnostic features of the following ECG abnormalities.

Condition	ECG Diagnostic Features
Acute myocardial infarction	
Hypercalcemia	
Hyperkalemia	
Hypocalcemia	
Hypokalemia	
Left atrial enlargement	
Left bundle branch block	
Left ventricular hypertrophy	
Pericarditis	
Prinzmetal's angina	
Right atrial enlargement	
Right bundle branch block	
Right ventricular hypertrophy	
Wellen's syndrome	

13. **DIRECTIONS:** Complete the following table by identifying which cardiac wall the following lead groupings evaluate.

Lead Groupings	Cardiac Wall
II, III, aVF	
V_{4R}	
I, aVL	
V_1, V_2	
V_3, V_4	
V_5, V_6	
V_8, V_9	

14. **DIRECTIONS:** Analyze the following 12-lead ECGs from patients with acute chest pain for indications of MI. Identify location and age of MI if present.

a.

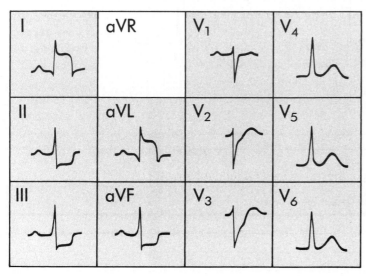

Interpretation:_____

b.

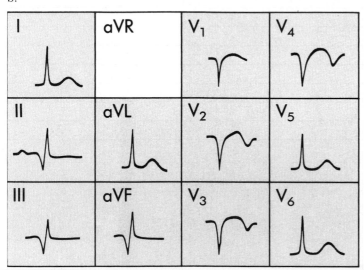

Interpretation:_____

15.   DIRECTIONS: Analyze the following 12-lead ECGs for bundle branch block. Identify if left or right bundle branch block.

a.

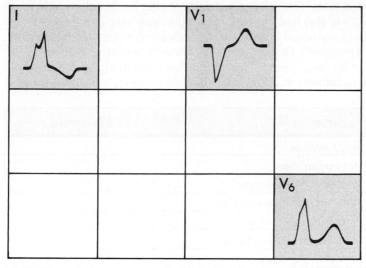

Interpretation:_____

b.

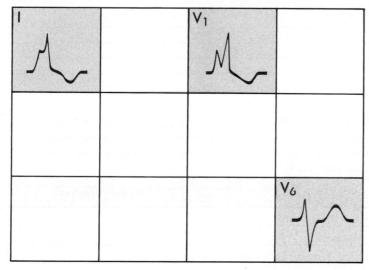

Interpretation:_____

16.   DIRECTIONS: Match the pathologic condition with its hemodynamic profile.

_____cardiac tamponade

_____noncardiac pulmonary edema

_____cardiac pulmonary edema

_____rupture of interventricular septum

_____pulmonary hypertension

_____papillary muscle rupture

_____right ventricular MI

_____cardiogenic shock

_____hypovolemic shock

a.   PAd, PVR, PAm increased; difference between PAd and PAOP greater than 5 mm Hg

b.   RAP, PAd, and PAOP are all elevated and within 5 mm Hg variation; large *a*- and *v*-waves on PAOP waveform

c.   elevated RAP, decreased PAOP, decreased CO/CI

d.   elevated PAP, PAOP, decreased CO/CI, elevated SVR

e.   elevated PAP, normal or decreased PAOP, crackles

f.   elevated PAP and PAOP, crackles

g.   decreased PAP, PAOP, decreased CO/CI, elevated SVR

h.   elevated PAP and PAOP, increased Svo$_2$, falsely elevated CO/CI

i.   elevated PAP and PAOP, large *v*-waves on PAOP waveform

17. **DIRECTIONS:** Identify whether the parameters in these case studies are decreased, normal, or increased. Discuss implications and treatment.

a.

Patient A is a 44-year-old male who was transported to the Emergency Department after having chest pain for 6 hours. He had ST segment elevation from V_2 to V_6. He also has a history of two previous MIs, and the ECG shows a previous inferior MI. The next day, Q-waves are noted from V_2 to V_6 (indicating extensive anterior MI), despite thrombolytic therapy administered in the Emergency Department. He is now hypotensive with an S_3 audible at his cardiac apex and crackles audible in his lung bases. Urine output has been marginal for the last two hours. The physician inserts a pulmonary artery catheter to allow better evaluation of current status as well as response to therapy. BSA 1.7 m^2

Parameter	↑, ↓, or Normal	Parameter	↑, ↓, or Normal
BP: 88/70 mm Hg		SV: 23 ml/beat	
MAP: 76 mm Hg		SI: 14 ml/m^2/beat	
HR: 128 BPM		SVR: 1813 dynes/sec/cm^{-5}	
RA: 8 mm Hg		SVRI: 3022 dynes/sec/cm^{-5}/m^2	
PA: 42/26 mm Hg		PVR: 240 dynes/sec/cm^{-5}	
PAm: 31 mm Hg		PVRI: 400 dynes/sec/cm^{-5}/m^2	
PAOP: 22 mm Hg		LVSWI: 10.3 g • m/m^2	
CO: 3.0 L/min		RVSWI: 2.7 g • m/m^2	
CI: 1.8 L/min/m^2			

Implications and treatment:_____

_____

_____

b.

Patient B is a 65-year-old female admitted with a fractured hip. She had surgery 2 weeks ago. Earlier today she complained about chest pain, shortness of breath, and a feeling of doom. ABGs revealed respiratory alkalosis and hypoxemia. After she was transferred to the critical care unit, the physician inserted a pulmonary artery catheter to aid in diagnosis and evaluation of therapy. BSA 1.6 m^2

Parameter	↑, ↓, or Normal	Parameter	↑, ↓, or Normal
BP: 112/84 mm Hg		SV: 40 ml/beat	
MAP: 93 mm Hg		SI: 25 ml/m^2/beat	
HR: 110 BPM		SVR: 1364 dynes/sec/cm^{-5}	
RA: 18 mm Hg		SVRI: 2182 dynes/sec/cm^{-5}/m^2	
PA: 55/32 mm Hg		PVR: 618 dynes/sec/cm^{-5}	
PAm: 40 mm Hg		PVRI: 989 dynes/sec/cm^{-5}/m^2	
PAOP: 6 mm Hg		LVSWI: 30 g • m/m^2	
CO: 4.4 L/min		RVSWI: 7 g • m/m^2	
CI: 2.75 L/min/m^2			

Implications and treatment:_____

_____

_____

c.

Patient C is a 52-year-old male being admitted to the critical care unit after surgery for repair of hemothorax after a gunshot wound. The Post-Anesthesia Care Unit (PACU) nurse gives you a report of massive blood loss before surgery, and estimated blood loss in the OR was 1 L. He has had 5 L of lactated Ringer's and 2 U of packed red blood cells. Past medical history includes MI 5 years ago and angioplasty 2 years ago for intractable angina. A pulmonary artery catheter was inserted prior to surgery to evaluate fluid status and cardiac function and to aid in fluid resuscitation. BSA 1.9 m²

Parameter	↑, ↓, or Normal	Parameter	↑, ↓, or Normal
BP: 92/70 mm Hg		SV: 24 ml/beat	
MAP: 77 mm Hg		SI: 13 ml/m²/beat	
HR 122 BPM		SVR: 2097 dynes/sec/cm⁻⁵	
RA: 1 mm Hg		SVRI: 4053 dynes/sec/cm⁻⁵	
PA: 20/6 mm Hg		PVR: 221 dynes/sec/cm⁻⁵	
PAm: 11 mm Hg		PVRI: 427 dynes/sec/cm⁻⁵	
PAOP: 3 mm Hg		LVSWI: 13.1 g • m/m²	
CO: 2.9 L/min		RVSWI: 1.8 g • m/m²	
CI: 1.5 L/min/m²			

Implications and treatment:_____

_____

_____

_____

LEARNING ACTIVITIES ANSWERS

1.

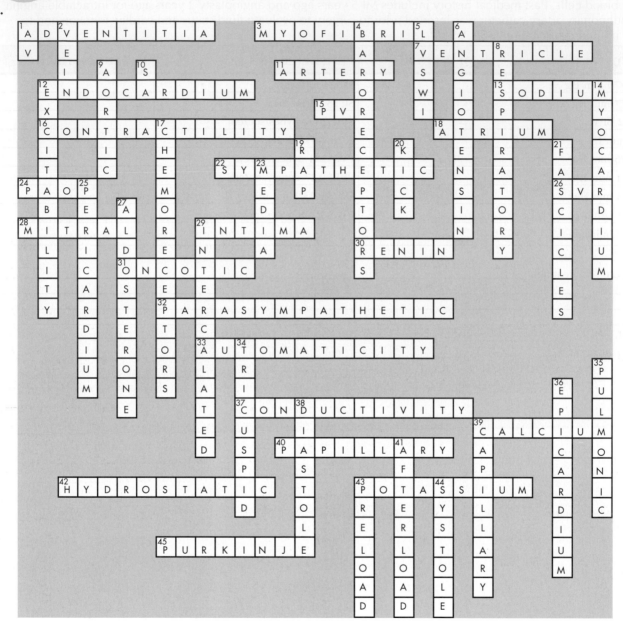

2.

Structure	Coronary Artery
Anterior left ventricle	LAD
AV node	Most commonly RCA; less commonly LCA
Bundle branches	LAD
Lateral left ventricle	LCA
Left atrium	LCA
Posterior left ventricle	Most commonly RCA; less commonly LCA
Right atrium	RCA
Right ventricle	RCA
Inferior left ventricle	RCA
SA node	Most commonly RCA; less commonly LCA
Septum	LAD

3.

Myocardial Oxygen Supply	Myocardial Oxygen Demand
Coronary artery patency	Heart rate
Diastolic pressure	Preload
Diastolic time	Afterload
Oxygen extraction: hemoglobin; Sao_2	Contractility

4.

Conditions							
Aortic stenosis	___ Heart Rate		___ Preload	↑ LV Afterload		___ Contractility	
Bradydysrhythmias	↓ Heart Rate		↑ Preload	___ Afterload		___ Contractility	
Cardiac tamponade	___ Heart Rate		↓ Preload	___ Afterload		___ Contractility	
Cardiomyopathy	___ Heart Rate		___ Preload	___ Afterload		↓ Contractility	
Heart failure	___ Heart Rate		↑ Preload	↑ Afterload		↓ Contractility	
Hypertension	___ Heart Rate		___ Preload	↑ LV Afterload		___ Contractility	
Hypovolemia	___ Heart Rate		↓ Preload	___ Afterload		___ Contractility	
Myocardial infarction	___ Heart Rate		___ Preload	___ Afterload		↓ Contractility	
Pulmonary hypertension	___ Heart Rate		___ Preload	↑ RV Afterload		___ Contractility	
Septic shock—early	___ Heart Rate		↓ Preload	↓ Afterload		___ Contractility	
Septic shock—late	___ Heart Rate		___ Preload	↑ Afterload		___ Contractility	
Tachydysrhythmias	↑ Heart Rate		↓ Preload	___ Afterload		___ Contractility	

Treatments				
Aminophylline	___ Heart Rate	___ Preload	↓ RV Afterload	___ Contractility
Amrinone (Inocor)	___ Heart Rate	↓ Preload	↓ Afterload	↑ Contractility
Digoxin (Lanoxin)	↓ Heart Rate	___ Preload	___ Afterload	↑ Contractility
Dobutamine (Dobutrex)	___ Heart Rate	↓ Preload	↓ Afterload	↑ Contractility
Dopamine (3-5 µg/kg/min)	↑ Heart Rate	___ Preload	___ Afterload	↑ Contractility
Dopamine (5-10 µg/kg/min)	↑ Heart Rate	___ Preload	↑ Afterload	↑ Contractility
Dopamine (>10 µg/kg/min)	↑ Heart Rate	___ Preload	↑ Afterload	___ Contractility
Fluid challenge	___ Heart Rate	↑ Preload	___ Afterload	___ Contractility
Furosemide (Lasix)	___ Heart Rate	↓ Preload	↓ RV Afterload	___ Contractility
Intra-aortic balloon pump	___ Heart Rate	___ Preload	↓ Afterload	___ Contractility
Isoproterenol (Isuprel)	↑ Heart Rate	↓ Preload	↓ Afterload	↑ Contractility
Nitroglycerin	___ Heart Rate	↓ Preload	___ Afterload*	___ Contractility
Nitroprusside (Nipride)	___ Heart Rate	↓ Preload	↓ Afterload	___ Contractility
Phenylephrine (Neo-Synephrine)	___ Heart Rate	___ Preload	↑ Afterload	___ Contractility
Propranolol (Inderal)	↓ Heart Rate	___ Preload	___ Afterload	↓ Contractility

*NTG will decrease afterload if dosage is greater than 1 µg/kg/min or approximately 70 µg/min in a 70-kg patient.

5.

_c_ alpha	a.	increase in heart rate, contractility, conductivity
_a_ beta$_1$	b.	dilation of the renal and mesenteric arteries
_d_ beta$_2$	c.	vasoconstriction
_b_ dopaminergic	d.	vasodilation, bronchodilation

6.

_c_ alpha	a.	isoproterenol
_d_ beta$_1$	b.	dopamine at 2 µg/kg/min
_a_ beta$_2$	c.	phenylephrine
_b_ dopaminergic	d.	dobutamine

7.

a. Cardiac output	heart rate (HR) × stroke volume (SV)
b. Stroke volume	cardiac output (CO) ÷ heart rate (HR)
c. Blood pressure	cardiac output (CO) × systemic vascular resistance (SVR)
d. Coronary artery perfusion pressure	diastolic BP − pulmonary artery occlusive pressure (PAOP)
e. Cerebral perfusion pressure	mean arterial pressure (MAP) − intracranial pressure (ICP)

8.

Heart Sound	Possible Causes
S_1	Closure of mitral and tricuspid valves
S_2	Closure of aortic and pulmonic valves
Physiologic split of S_2	Changes in intrathoracic pressure created by ventilation
Paradoxical split of S_2	LBBB; right ventricular pacemaker or ectopy; severe aortic valve disease; patent ductus arteriosus
Fixed, wide split of S_2	atrial septal defect
S_3	HF; fluid overload; cardiomyopathy; ventricular septal defect; patent ductus arteriosus
S_4	myocardial ischemia or infarction; hypertension; ventricular hypertrophy; AV block; severe aortic or pulmonic stenosis
Pericardial friction rub	pericarditis
Midsystolic click	mitral valve prolapse; mitral regurgitation
Holosystolic murmur	mitral regurgitation; tricuspid regurgitation; ventricular septal defect
Systolic ejection murmur	aortic stenosis; pulmonic stenosis
Early diastolic murmur	aortic regurgitation; pulmonic regurgitation
Mid- to late-diastolic murmur	mitral stenosis; tricuspid stenosis

9.

Condition	Timing	Location	Pitch
Mitral regurgitation	systolic	mitral (apex)	high
Mitral stenosis	diastolic	mitral (apex)	low
Aortic regurgitation	diastolic	aortic (base)	high
Aortic stenosis	systolic	aortic (base)	high
Mitral valve prolapse	systolic	mitral (apex)	high
Papillary muscle dysfunction or rupture	systolic	mitral (apex)	high
Ventricular septal defect or rupture	systolic	LLSB	high

10.

k	1. normal sinus rhythm
e	2. sinus bradycardia
j	3. sinus tachycardia
b	4. premature atrial contraction
f	5. atrial fibrillation
c	6. atrial flutter
p	7. supraventricular tachycardia
g	8. premature junctional contraction
h	9. junctional escape rhythm
m	10. accelerated junctional rhythm
o	11. junctional tachycardia
d	12. premature ventricular complex
n	13. accelerated idioventricular rhythm
t	14. ventricular tachycardia
s	15. ventricular fibrillation
i	16. asystole
a	17. first-degree AV block
l	18. second-degree AV block, type I
q	19. second-degree AV block, type II
r	20. third-degree AV block

11.   a. Interpretation: Ventricular fibrillation
Treatment:
- Confirm pulselessness
- Defibrillate with 200 joules

- If no conversion and still pulseless, defibrillate with 200 to 300 joules
- If no conversion and still pulseless, defibrillate with 360 joules
- While maintaining CPR, establish an IV and airway (intubate when possible)
- Administer 1 mg of epinephrine IV or 2 mg via endotracheal tube if unable to establish IV (repeat epinephrine every 3 to 5 minutes)
- Defibrillate with 360 joules within 30 to 60 seconds
- If no conversion and still pulseless, administer lidocaine at 1.5 mg/kg
- Defibrillate with 360 joules within 30 to 60 seconds
- If no conversion and still pulseless, administer lidocaine at 1.0 mg/kg
- Defibrillate with 360 joules within 30 to 60 seconds
- Consider changing antidysrhythmic to bretylium after lidocaine has been administered to maximum (3 mg/kg) without conversion
- Continue epinephrine 1 mg every 3 to 5 minutes

- Alternate drugs with defibrillation at 360 joules continuing CPR between shocks
- Consider obtaining arterial blood gases to assess pH, oxygenation, and ventilation

b. Interpretation: Sinus bradycardia with wide QRS (BBB should be assessed on 12-lead ECG). Treatment:
  - Considering the rate, this patient is probably symptomatic and atropine 0.5 mg IV should be given
  - Transcutaneous pacing may be considered as a temporary treatment, especially if the patient does not respond to atropine
  - A transvenous pacemaker and eventually a permanent pacemaker may be necessary

c. Interpretation: Supraventricular tachycardia; this is a regular narrow QRS tachycardia with no discernible P-waves; the P-waves could be hidden in the QRS or T-wave, so there is no way to identify where above the ventricle the rhythm originates, but the rate of 180 suggests an atrial origin.
  Treatment:
  - Treatment of cause (e.g., antipyretics for fever; antibiotics for infection, caffeine withdrawal, anxiolytic agents for anxiety)
  - Assess the patient; if patient is symptomatic (e.g., chest pain, hypotension), treatment may include:
    - Valsalva maneuver may be utilized to increase parasympathetic stimulation
    - Adenosine may be utilized
    - Verapamil may be used if the patient is not hypotensive
    - Electrical cardioversion may be needed especially in a hypotensive patient

d. Interpretation: Accelerated idioventricular rhythm progressing to asystole
  Treatment:
  - Confirm asystole with two leads and confirm pulselessness
  - Maintain CPR while establishing IV access and airway (intubate when possible)
  - Epinephrine 1 mg IV
  - Atropine 1 mg IV
  - Transcutaneous pacing should be instituted as soon as possible

e. Interpretation: Underlying sinus rhythm (atrial rate is 90); a third-degree AV block is present with a ventricular escape rhythm (ventricular rate is 35)
  Treatment:
  - Considering the rate, this patient is certainly symptomatic and atropine 0.5 mg IV should be given
  - Transcutaneous pacing may be considered as a temporary treatment, especially if the patient does not respond to atropine
  - A transvenous pacemaker and eventually a permanent pacemaker may be necessary

f. Interpretation: Underlying sinus rhythm (atrial rate is 80); a second-degree Mobitz I (Wenckebach) AV block is present; conduction ratio is 3:2 and ventricular rate is 40 to 50
  Treatment:
  - Considering the rate, this patient may be symptomatic; if hypotension, chest pain, or syncope is present, atropine 0.5 mg IV should be given
  - Mobitz I is usually responsive to atropine, but if symptoms do not abate, transcutaneous pacing may be considered

g. Interpretation: Ventricular tachycardia
  Treatment:
  - Assess the patient
  - If the patient is stable: administer lidocaine 1 mg/kg IV every 5 to 10 minutes to maximum of 3 mg/kg; if lidocaine is unsuccessful in converting the rhythm, bretylium or procainamide may be used
  - If the patient is unstable: electrical cardioversion with 50 joules; if unsuccessful, 100 joules; if unsuccessful, 200 joules; if unsuccessful, 360 joules; start antidysrhythmics after successful conversion
  - If the patient is pulseless: defibrillate at 200 joules and continue as for ventricular fibrillation

h. Interpretation: Underlying rhythm is sinus tachycardia (atrial rate is 145); a second-degree Mobitz II block is present; conduction ratio is variable, but the PR interval of the conducted P-wave is consistent
  Treatment:
  - Considering the rate, this patient is probably symptomatic and atropine 0.5 mg IV should be given initially
  - Mobitz II is rarely responsive to atropine, and transcutaneous pacing should be implemented as a temporary treatment while awaiting transvenous pacemaker insertion
  - Eventually a permanent pacemaker will probably be necessary

i. Interpretation: Sinus rhythm with two unifocal PVCs
  Treatment:
  - If these PVCs continue at the same rate as in this strip, they are occurring at approximately 20/min
  - Consider and treat causes: hypoxia, electrolyte imbalance, acid-base imbalance, ischemia
  - Depending on physician preference and patient situation (e.g., if myocardial ischemia the cause), lidocaine 1 mg/kg may be administered and then an infusion initiated at 2 mg/min

12.

Condition	ECG Diagnostic Features
Acute myocardial infarction	Q-waves at least 0.04 seconds wide and/or one quarter height of R-wave
Hypercalcemia	Shortened QT, shortened ST segment
Hyperkalemia	Tall, peaked T-waves, widening of QRS complex, atrial asystole
Hypocalcemia	Prolonged QT, prolonged ST segment
Hypokalemia	Flat T-waves, prominent U-wave, ST segment depression
Left atrial enlargement	Wide (>0.11 seconds), notched P-wave in lead II, dominant terminal component of P-wave in V_1
Left bundle branch block	Wide (0.12 seconds or >) QRS below the baseline in V_1
Left ventricular hypertrophy	Increased QRS amplitude, left axis deviation, ST-T-wave changes in V_5, V_6
Pericarditis	Diffuse ST segment elevation
Prinzmetal's angina	ST segment elevation with pain
Right atrial enlargement	Tall (>2.5 mm), peaked P-wave in lead II, dominant initial component of P-wave in V_1
Right bundle branch block	Wide (0.12 seconds or >) QRS above the baseline in V_1
Right ventricular hypertrophy	R-wave larger than S-wave in V_1, V_2, S-wave larger than R-wave in V_5, V_6, right axis deviation, ST-T-wave changes in V_1, V_2
Wellen's syndrome	Symmetrically, deeply inverted T-waves in V_2, V_3 with little or no ST segment elevation

13.

Lead Groupings	Cardiac Wall
II, III, aVF	Inferior
V_{4R}	Right ventricular
I, aVL	Lateral (high)
V_1, V_2	Septal
V_3, V_4	Anterior
V_5, V_6	Lateral (low)
V_8, V_9	Posterior

14. a. Interpretation: ST segment elevation in I, aVL indicate acute injury in the lateral wall of the left ventricle. No pathologic Q-waves are in these leads at this time. Reciprocal changes are noted in II, III, aVF. In view of history of acute chest pain, this ECG can be interpreted as hyperacute MI and reperfusion efforts (e.g., thrombolytics or angioplasty) should be initiated.

b. Interpretation: Acute changes are noted in V_1 to V_4. Pathologic Q-waves, ST segment elevation, and inverted T-waves are seen indicative of acute anteroseptal MI. Pathologic Q-waves without acute changes of ST segment elevation or T-wave inversion in II, III, aVF indicate an old MI.

15. a. LBBB: Note indicative changes of BBB in V_6 (LV lead) and the wide QRS is totally below the isoelectric line in V_1.

b. RBBB: Note indicative changes of BBB in V_1 (RV lead) and the wide QRS is totally above the isoelectric line in V_1.

16.

b cardiac tamponade

e noncardiac pulmonary edema

f cardiac pulmonary edema

h rupture of interventricular septum

a pulmonary hypertension

i papillary muscle rupture

c right ventricular MI

d cardiogenic shock

g hypovolemic shock

a. PAd, PVR, PAm increased; difference between PAd and PAOP greater than 5 mm Hg

b. RAP, PAd, and PAOP are all elevated and within 5 PAOP waveform; large *a*- and *v*-waves on PAOP waveform

c. elevated RAP, decreased PAOP, decreased CO/CI

d. elevated PAP, PAOP, decreased CO/CI, elevated SVR

e. elevated PAP, normal or decreased PAOP, crackles

f. elevated PAP and PAOP, crackles

g. decreased PAP, PAOP, decreased CO/CI, elevated SVR

h. elevated PAP and PAOP, increased SvO_2, falsely elevated CO/CI

i. elevated PAP and PAOP, large *v*-waves on PAOP waveform

17.

a.

Parameter	↑, ↓, or Normal	Parameter	↑, ↓, or Normal
BP: 88/70 mm Hg	↓	SV: 23 ml/beat	↓
MAP: 76 mm Hg	↓	SI: 14 ml/m²/beat	↓
HR: 128 BPM	↑	SVR: 1813 dynes/sec/cm⁻⁵	↑
RAP: 8 mm Hg	↑	SVRI: 3022 dynes/sec/cm⁻⁵/m²	↑
PAP: 42/26 mm Hg	↑	PVR: 240 dynes/sec/cm⁻⁵	normal
PAm: 31 mm Hg	↑	PVRI: 400 dynes/sec/cm⁻⁵/m²	normal
PAOP: 22 mm Hg	↑	LVSWI: 10.3 g • m/m²	↓
CO: 3.0 L/min	↓	RVSWI: 2.7 g • m/m²	↓
CI: 1.8 L/min/m²	↓		

Discussion: Patient A is in cardiogenic shock as evidenced by the low cardiac index, increased PAOP and RAP, and the increase in SVR and SVRI. Myocardial oxygen demand is being increased by the increased heart rate, increased preload (note PAOP and RAP), and increased afterload (note SVR). Treatment priorities would include pain management by careful morphine titration (this will decrease preload via venous dilation, decrease heart rate and afterload by decreasing sympathetic nervous system stimulation by obliterating the pain, and decrease anxiety). Titration must be done carefully because of the hypotensive state. Dobutamine would be initiated to increase contractility (note decreased LVSWI and RVSWI). Low-dose dopamine (1 to 2 μg/kg/min) would also be helpful in improving renal perfusion. If preload is not decreased by the morphine and if dobutamine increases the BP, nitroglycerin IV might be administered by careful titration. If afterload is not decreased by pain relief and if dobutamine increases the BP, nitroprusside may be used to decrease afterload. Titration of both of these drugs must be done carefully and cautiously because any further decrease in BP will decrease perfusion pressure including coronary artery perfusion pressure. Diuretics (e.g., furosemide [Lasix]) might be utilized to decrease the preload. Intraaortic balloon pump would be considered to decrease afterload and increase coronary artery perfusion pressure if the patient is not stabilized using a pharmacologic approach. Although beta-blockers are very important for primary and secondary prevention in acute MI patients, beta-blockers would not be utilized in this patient because of the cardiogenic shock.

b.

Parameter	↑, ↓, or Normal	Parameter	↑, ↓, or Normal
BP: 112/84 mm Hg	normal	SV: 40 ml/beat	↓
MAP: 93 mm Hg	normal	SI: 25 ml/m²/beat	↓
HR 110 BPM	↑	SVR: 1364 dynes/sec/cm⁻⁵	normal
RAP: 18 mm Hg	↑	SVRI: 2182 dynes/sec/cm⁻⁵	normal
PAP: 55/32 mm Hg	↑	PVR: 618 dynes/sec/cm⁻⁵	↑
PAm: 40 mm Hg	↑	PVRI: 989 dynes/sec/cm⁻⁵	↑
PAOP: 6 mm Hg	normal	LVSWI: 30 g • m/m²	↓
CO: 4.4 L/min	normal	RVSWI: 7 g • m/m²	normal
CI: 2.75 L/min/m²	normal		

Discussion: Patient B's hemodynamic parameters confirm pulmonary hypertension. Note the increase in PAd with a normal PAOP. Remember that if the PAd is more than 5 mm Hg above the PAOP, pulmonary hypertension exists. The increased PVR is further evidence of pulmonary hypertension. Sympathetic nervous system stimulation has caused the tachycardia and the high normal SVR. Considering the patient's history, you would suspect pulmonary embolism as the cause. V/Q scan would confirm the cause to be a pulmonary embolism. Arterial blood gases should be analyzed for degree of hypoxemia. Treatment of pulmonary embolism in this patient would include oxygen at 5 to 6 L/min. Parenteral anticoagulation with heparin would be initiated. Remember that heparin prevents extension of the clot, but the body must break down the clot. The natural thrombolytic process takes 7 to 10 days. Considering the degree of right ventricular failure (RAP 18 mm Hg), thrombolytics (e.g., tissue plasminogen activate [Activase]) should be considered to accelerate thrombolysis. Although pulmonary embolectomy may be done for mechanical removal of the clot, it is associated with a high mortality rate. Dobutamine may also be used to increase cardiac contractility.

c.

Parameter	↑, ↓, or Normal	Parameter	↑, ↓, or Normal
BP: 92/70 mm Hg	low normal	SV: 24 ml/beat	↓
MAP: 77 mm Hg	normal	SI: 13 ml/m²/beat	↓
HR: 122 BPM	↓	SVR: 2097 dynes/sec/cm⁻⁵	↑
RAP: 1 mm Hg	↓	SVRI: 4053 dynes/sec/cm⁻⁵/m²	↑
PAP: 20/6 mm Hg	↓	PVR: 221 dynes/sec/cm⁻⁵	normal
PAm: 11 mm Hg	↓	PVRI: 427 dynes/sec/cm⁻⁵/m²	normal
PAOP: 3 mm Hg	↓	LVSWI: 13.1 g • m/m²	↓
CO: 2.9 L/min	↓	RVSWI: 1.8 g • m/m²	↓
CI: 1.5 L/min/m²	↓		

Discussion: Patient C is in hypovolemic shock as evidenced by the low cardiac index with low PAOP and RAP. Heart rate and SVR and SVRI are elevated because of sympathetic nervous system stimulation.

Volume replacement will normalize parameters. Considering that the primary fluid loss was blood, blood replacement in the form of either whole blood or packed cells is required along with the normal saline as a primary crystalloid. Hemoglobin is critical for oxygen delivery to the tissues, and the patient's history of coronary artery disease accentuates this need.

BIBLIOGRAPHY AND SELECTED REFERENCES

Adams J, Miracle V: Cardiac biomarkers: past, present, and future, *Am J Crit Care* 7 (6):418, 1998.

Albert N, Spear B, Hammel J: Agreement and clinical utility of 2 techniques for measuring cardiac output in patients with low cardiac output, *Am J Crit Care* 8 (1):464, 1999.

Alspach J, editor: *Core curriculum for critical care nursing*, ed 5, Philadelphia, 1998, WB Saunders.

Barkauskas V: *Health and physical assessment*, St Louis, 1994, Mosby.

Beare P, Myers J: *Adult health nursing*, ed 2, St Louis, 1994, Mosby.

Berne R, Levy M: *Cardiovascular physiology*, St Louis, 1997, Mosby.

Boggs R, Wooldridge-King M: *AACN procedure manual for critical care*, ed 3, Philadelphia, 1993, WB Saunders.

Chang M: Monitoring the critically injured patient, *New Horizons* 7 (1):35, 1999.

Clochesy J et al: *Critical care nursing*, ed 2, Philadelphia, 1996, WB Saunders.

Daily E, Schroeder J: *Techniques in bedside hemodynamic monitoring*, ed 5, St Louis, 1994, Mosby.

Dalton J: An evaluation of facial expression displaced by patients with chest pain, *Heart and Lung* 28 (3):169, 1999.

Drew B et al: 12-lead ST-segment monitoring vs single-lead maximum ST-segment monitoring for detecting ongoing ischemia in patients with unstable coronary syndromes, *Am J Crit Care* 7(5):355, 1998.

Druding M: Integrating hemodynamic monitoring and physical assessment, part I, *Nursing99* 29 (7):32cc1, 1999.

Druding M: Integrating hemodynamic monitoring and physical assessment, part II, *Nursing99* 29 (8):32cc1, 1999.

Ferguson A: Gastric tonometry: evaluating tissue oxygenation, *Crit Care Nurse,* 16 (6):48, 1996.

Gant R, Henkin R, Morton P: The expanding role of signal-averaged electrocardiography, *Critical Care Nurse* 19 (5):61, 1999.

Gawlinski A: Facts and fallacies of patient positioning and hemodynamic measurement, *J Cardiovasc Nurs* 12 (1):1, 1997.

Gawlinski A: Can measurement of mixed venous oxygen saturation replace measurement of cardiac output in patients with advanced heart failure, *Am J Crit Care* 7 (5):374, 1998.

Gawlinski A, Hamwi D: *Acute care nurse practitioner clinical curriculum and certification review,* Philadelphia, 1999, WB Saunders.

Gibbar-Clements T, Shirrell D, Free C: PT and APTT: seeing beyond the numbers, *Nursing97* 27 (7):49, 1997.

Grauer K: *A practical guide to ECG interpretation,* ed 2, St Louis, 1998, Mosby.

Guyton A: *Textbook of medical physiology,* ed 9, Philadelphia, 1996, WB Saunders.

Guzzetta C, Dossey B: *Cardiovascular nursing: holistic practice,* St Louis, 1992, Mosby.

Harrison H: Troponin I, *AJN* 99 (5):24TT, 1999.

Ivanov R et al: Pulmonary artery catheterization: a balanced look at the controversy, *J Crit Illness* 12 (8):469, 1997.

Keen J, Swearingen P: *Mosby's Critical Care Nursing Consultant,* St Louis, 1997, Mosby.

Kiely M et al: Thermodilution measurement of cardiac output in patients with low output: room-temperature versus iced injectate, *Am J Crit Care* 7 (6):436, 1998.

Kinney M et al: *AACN clinical reference for critical care nursing,* ed 4, St Louis, 1998, Mosby.

Kirton C: Assessing S_3 and S_4 heart sounds, *Nursing97* 27 (7):52, 1997.

Lasater M: Noninvasive monitoring with thoracic electrical bioimpedance, *AJN* 99 (8):24JJ, 1999.

Lau K et al: Frequency of ischemia during intracoronary ultrasound in women with and without coronary artery disease, *Crit Care Nurse* 19 (5):48, 1999.

Magdic K, Saul L: ECG interpretation of chamber enlargement, *Critical Care Nurse* 17 (1):13, 1997.

Marino P: *The ICU book,* ed 2, Baltimore, 1998, Williams & Wilkins.

McCloy K et al: Effects of injectate volume on thermodilution measurements of cardiac output in patients with low ventricular ejection fraction, *Am J Crit Care* 8 (2):86, 1999.

Mee C, Possanza C: How to record an accurate 12-lead ECG, *Nursing97* 27 (3):66, 1997.

Mims B et al: *Critical care skills—a clinical handbook,* Philadelphia, 1996, WB Saunders.

Miracle V, Sims J: Making sense of a 12-lead ECG, *Nursing99* 29 (7):35, 1999.

Moccia J: How to use serial and expanded ECGs, *Nursing97* 27 (9):32cc1, 1997.

Moccia J: When an arrhythmia hides a myocardial infarction, *Nursing98* 28 (4):32cc1, 1998.

Montes P: Managing outpatient cardiac catheterization, *AJN* 97 (8):34, 1997.

Morton P: Using the 12-lead ECG to detect ischemia, injury, and infarction, *Critical Care Nurse* 16 (2):85, 1996.

Murphy M: Use of measurements of myoglobin and cardiac troponins in the diagnosis of acute myocardial infarction, *Critical Care Nurse,* 19 (1):58, 1999.

Opie L: *Drugs for the heart,* ed 4, Philadelphia, 1995, WB Saunders Company.

Owen A: Tracking the rise and fall of cardiac enzymes, *Nursing95* 25 (5):35, 1995.

Purdie R, Earnest S: *Pure practice for 12-lead ECGs: a practice workbook,* St Louis, 1997, Mosby.

Ramsey J, Tisdale L: Use of ventricular stroke work index and ventricular function curves in assessing myocardial contractility, *Critical Care Nurse* 15:61, 1995.

Rice K: Measuring thigh BP, *Nursing99* 29 (8):58, 1999.

Rimmer L, Rimmer J: Comparison of 2 methods of measuring the QT interval, *Am J Crit Care* 7 (5):346, 1998.

Sims J, Miracle V: Using the ECG to detect myocardial infarction, *Nursing99* 29 (8):41, 1999.

Stimike C: Understanding intravascular ultrasound, *AJN* 96 (6):40, 1996.

Thelan L et al: *Critical care nursing: diagnosis and management,* ed 3, St Louis, 1998, Mosby.

Varon J, Fromm R: The ICU handbook of facts, formulas, and laboratory values, St Louis, 1997, Mosby.

Vitacco-Grab C, Melzler C: Getting a slant on syncope, *Nursing99* 29 (9):56, 1999.

Waxman A, Sasidhar M: PA catheterization: what it can—and cannot—tell you, *J Resp Dis* 20 (2):106, 1999.

Woods S et al: *Cardiac nursing,* ed 3, Philadelphia, 1995, JB Lippincott.

Wu K, Baker-Carpenter K: ST-T segment changes in a patient with ECG evidence that suggests stenosis of the proximal left anterior descending artery, *Critical Care Nurse* 16 (6):56, 1996.

Zalenski R et al: Assessing the diagnostic value of an ECG containing leads V_{4R}, V_8, V_9: the 15 lead ECG, *Ann Emerg Med* 22 (5):786, 1993.

Cardiovascular System: Pathologic Conditions

Cardiopulmonary Arrest

Definition: A sudden cessation of the cardiac output and effective circulation; cardiac arrest is followed by ventilatory cessation

Etiology

I. Dysrhythmias
II. Electrical shock
III. Drowning
IV. Asphyxiation
V. Trauma
VI. Hypothermia
VII. Terminal phases of a chronic illness (CPR may not be attempted on this patient according to advanced directives and "do not resuscitate" orders)

Pathophysiology

I. Cardiac arrest ceases delivery of oxygen and removal of carbon dioxide, causing tissue hypoxia and metabolic acidosis
II. Ventilatory arrest causes respiratory acidosis and hypoxemia
III. Eventually the cerebral cortex is irreversibly damaged and severe neurologic deficit or biologic death occurs

Clinical Presentation

I. Loss of consciousness: establish unresponsiveness
II. Absence of breathing: look, listen, and feel for air exchange
III. Absence of central pulses: feel for carotid, femoral pulses
IV. Absence of auscultated or palpated BP
V. Anoxic seizures may occur
VI. Urinary and bowel incontinence may occur
VII. ECG
   A. Most commonly ventricular fibrillation
   B. Less commonly ventricular tachycardia
   C. Rarely asystole
D. Cardiopulmonary arrest with a stable electrical rhythm (referred to as *pulseless electrical activity* [PEA])

Collaborative Management

I. Provide cardiopulmonary resuscitation (CPR) and basic life support
   A. Airway and ventilation
      1. Open airway using head tilt–chin lift maneuver; jaw thrust maneuver is used if cervical spine injury is suspected
      2. Provide ventilation by any of the following methods:
         a) Mouth to mask ventilation
         b) Manual resuscitation bag to mask
         c) Manual resuscitation bag to endotracheal (ET) or tracheostomy tube
   B. Compressions
      1. Place heel of one hand over the lower half of sternum; place the other hand over the first hand
      2. Compress the sternum at a depth of 1½ to 2 inches at a rate of 80 to 100/min
   C. Ratio of compressions to ventilation
      1. Maintain a ratio of 15 compressions to 2 ventilations if only one rescuer
      2. Maintain a ratio of 5 compressions to 1 ventilation if two rescuers; allow 1.5- to 2-second pause for ventilation after 5 compressions
   D. Implications
      1. CPR performed expertly provides only 20% of normal cardiac output, but most of this goes to the upper body, including the heart and brain
      2. Mortality rates increase despite prompt CPR if ACLS is delayed beyond 12 minutes
      3. Resistance of ventricular dysrhythmias to defibrillation occurs over time; prompt defibrillation is critical to survival

II. Provide advanced cardiac life support (ACLS)
  A. Use ACLS algorithms to provide assistance with decision making in a cardiopulmonary arrest (Figures 3-1 to 3-5)
  B. Identify and treat the cause of cardiac arrest: especially important in treatment of PEA
  C. Use electrical therapies to change an abnormal cardiac rhythm to a normal one
    1. Principle: by delivering a shock of sufficient strength, a critical mass of myocardium is depolarized simultaneously, allowing emergence of the dominant normal rhythm
    2. Precordial thump
      a) Uses
        (1) For witnessed VF or pulseless ventricular tachycardia only if a defibrillator is not immediately available; do not allow delivery of a precordial thump to delay defibrillation
        (2) For ventricular tachycardia with a pulse only if a defibrillator and pacemaker are readily available because deterioration to VF or asystole may occur
        (3) For use only early for ventricular dysrhythmias; precordial thump delivers minimal voltage (approximately 25 joules), so it is only likely to be effective if the duration of the ventricular dysrhythmia is short
      b) Method: solitary thump with the heel of the hand delivered to the midsternum from a height of 8 to 12 inches
    3. Defibrillation
      a) Uses
        (1) For pulseless ventricular tachycardia and VF
        (2) May also be used in asystole where the rhythm is unclear and could be fine VF
      b) Method
        (1) Check pulse: make sure that VF pattern is not merely artifact caused by loose ECG electrode
        (2) Remove any foil-lined patches from the patient's chest (e.g., nitroglycerin patches) because they may cause arcing and patient burns
        (3) Turn defibrillator on and make sure that the synchronizer switch is off so that charge is delivered as soon as buttons are pushed
        (4) Apply defibrillation pads to chest for paddle placement or apply conductive jelly to paddles
          (a) Anterior: one paddle at the apex and the other just below the right clavicle at the second and third intercostal space
          (b) Anteroposteriorly: one paddle at the second and third right intercostal space and the other at the angle of the left scapula; this paddle placement may be better for obese patients and patients with hyperinflated lungs (e.g., COPD)
          (c) Pacemakers
            (i) In patients with permanent pacemakers, the paddles should not be placed within 5 to 10 cm of the pulse generator
            (ii) Turn temporary pacemaker pulse generator off
        (5) Charge to appropriate voltage for defibrillation: 200 joules initially; 200 to 300 joules for the next shock; then up to 360 joules; all successive shocks are at a voltage of 360 joules
        (6) Apply paddles to defibrillation pads or jellied paddles to chest using firm (~25 lb) pressure
        (7) Say the word *clear* and ensure that no one is touching the patient or the bed
        (8) Press both discharge buttons simultaneously
        (9) Check pulse and monitor
        (10) Administer antidysrhythmic drug therapy after sinus rhythm is restored
      c) Successful defibrillation less likely if any of following present:
        (1) Hypoxia
        (2) Severe acidosis
        (3) Alkalosis
        (4) Local ionic imbalance
        (5) Ischemia
        (6) Long VF duration
      d) Complications
        (1) Dysrhythmias: asystole, bradycardia, AV blocks, VF
        (2) Hypotension
        (3) Myocardial damage
        (4) Pulmonary edema
        (5) Emboli
        (6) Muscle pain
        (7) Skin burns
    4. Temporary pacemaker: for patients who have problem with impulse formation and/or conduction
      a) Transcutaneous pacemaker
        (1) Large surface skin electrodes applied anterior and posterior
          (a) Posterior: positive electrode applied between spine and left scapula at level of heart
          (b) Anterior: negative electrode applied at left fourth ICS at midclavicular line

Text continued on p. 99

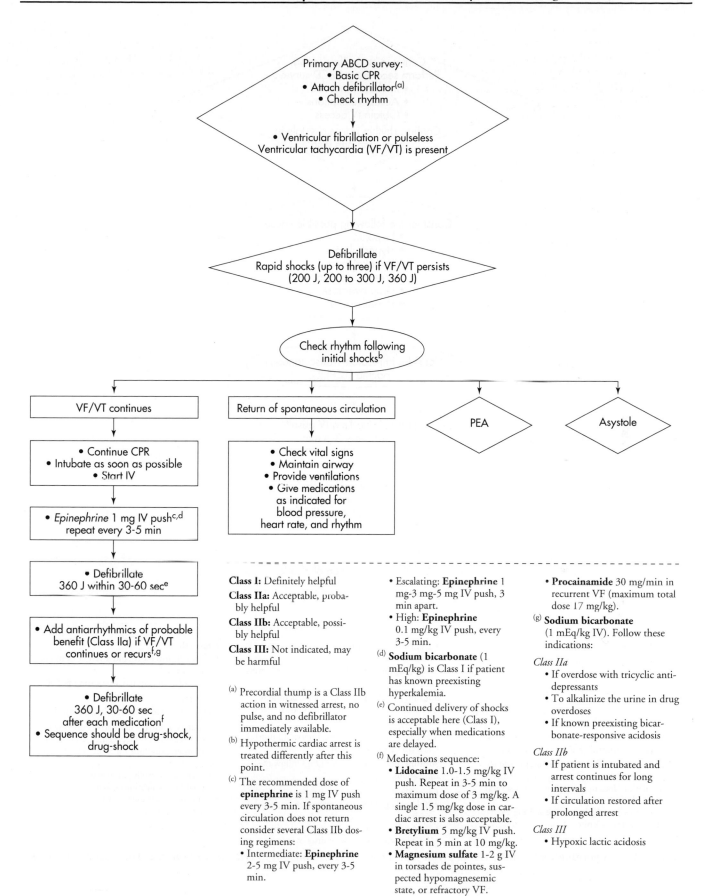

Figure 3-1   Algorithm for ventricular fibrillation or pulseless ventricular tachycardia. (From Flynn JBM, Bruce NP: *Introduction to critical care skills,* St Louis, 1993, Mosby.)

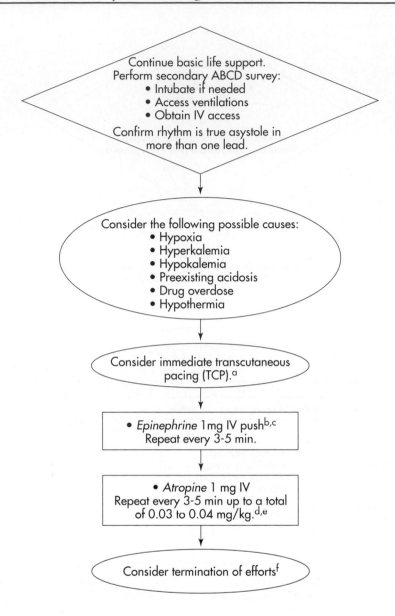

Continue basic life support.
Perform secondary ABCD survey:
- Intubate if needed
- Access ventilations
- Obtain IV access

Confirm rhythm is true asystole in
more than one lead.

Consider the following possible causes:
- Hypoxia
- Hyperkalemia
- Hypokalemia
- Preexisting acidosis
- Drug overdose
- Hypothermia

Consider immediate transcutaneous pacing (TCP).ᵃ

- *Epinephrine* 1mg IV pushᵇ,ᶜ Repeat every 3-5 min.

- *Atropine* 1 mg IV Repeat every 3-5 min up to a total of 0.03 to 0.04 mg/kg.ᵈ,ᵉ

Consider termination of effortsᶠ

Class I: Definitely helpful

Class IIa: Acceptable, probably helpful

Class IIb: Acceptable, possibly helpful

Class III: Not indicated, may be harmful

(a) Pacing is an acceptable intervention (Class IIb). Perform TCP as early as possible, without waiting for the effects of medications. Not recommended as routine treatment for asystole.

(b) The recommended dose of **epinephrine** is 1 mg IV push every 3-5 min. If spontaneous circulation does not return, consider several Class IIb dosing regimens:
- Intermediate: **Epinephrine** 2-5 mg IV push, every 3-5 min

- Escalating: **Epinephrine** 1 mg-3 mg-5 mg IV push, 3 min apart
- High: **Epinephrine** 0.1 mg/kg IV push, every 3-5 min

(c) **Sodium bicarbonate** 1 mEq/kg is definitely indicated (Class I) if patient has known preexisting hyperkalemia.

(d) The shorter **atropine** dosing interval (3 min) is Class IIb in asystolic arrest.

(e) **Sodium bicarbonate** (1 mEq/kg) follow these indications:

Class IIa
- If known preexisting bicarbonate responsive acidosis
- If overdose with tricyclic antidepressants
- To alkalinize the urine in drug overdoses

Class IIb
- If patient intubated and arrest continues for long intervals
- If circulation restored after prolonged arrest

Class III
- Hypoxic acidosis (unventilated patient)

(f) Consider stopping resuscitative efforts when patient remains in documented asystole or other agonal rhythms for more than 10 minutes *after*:
- Patient successfully intubated
- Initial IV medications given
- No reversible causes identified
- Physician concurs

Figure 3-2   Algorithm for asystole. (From Flynn JBM, Bruce NP: *Introduction to critical care skills,* St Louis, 1993, Mosby.)

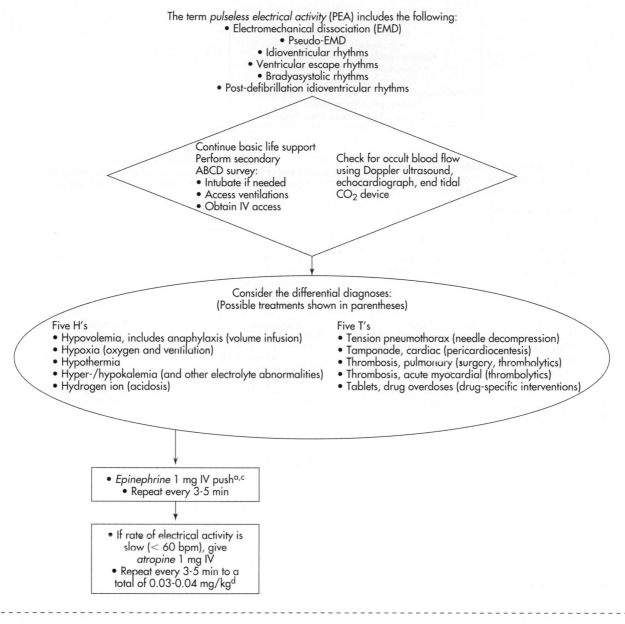

The term *pulseless electrical activity* (PEA) includes the following:
- Electromechanical dissociation (EMD)
- Pseudo-EMD
- Idioventricular rhythms
- Ventricular escape rhythms
- Bradyasystolic rhythms
- Post-defibrillation idioventricular rhythms

Continue basic life support
Perform secondary
ABCD survey:
- Intubate if needed
- Access ventilations
- Obtain IV access

Check for occult blood flow
using Doppler ultrasound,
echocardiograph, end tidal
CO_2 device

Consider the differential diagnoses:
(Possible treatments shown in parentheses)

Five H's
- Hypovolemia, includes anaphylaxis (volume infusion)
- Hypoxia (oxygen and ventilation)
- Hypothermia
- Hyper-/hypokalemia (and other electrolyte abnormalities)
- Hydrogen ion (acidosis)

Five T's
- Tension pneumothorax (needle decompression)
- Tamponade, cardiac (pericardiocentesis)
- Thrombosis, pulmonary (surgery, thrombolytics)
- Thrombosis, acute myocardial (thrombolytics)
- Tablets, drug overdoses (drug-specific interventions)

- *Epinephrine* 1 mg IV push[a,c]
- Repeat every 3-5 min

- If rate of electrical activity is slow (< 60 bpm), give *atropine* 1 mg IV
- Repeat every 3-5 min to a total of 0.03-0.04 mg/kg[d]

Class I: Definitely helpful

Class IIa: Acceptable, probably helpful

Class IIb: Acceptable, possibly helpful

Class III: Not indicated, may be harmful

[a] **Sodium bicarbonate** 1 mEq/kg is Class I if patient has known preexisting hyperkalemia.

[b] **Sodium bicarbonate** (1 mEq/kg) is given as follows:

Class IIa
- If known preexisting bicarbonate-responsive acidosis

- If overdose with tricyclic antidepressants
- To alkalinize the urine in drug overdoses

Class IIb
- If patient is intubated and arrest continues for long intervals
- If circulation is restored after prolonged arrest

Class III
- Hypoxic lactic acidosis (unventilated patient)

[c] The recommended dose of **epinephrine** is 1 mg IV push every 3-5 min. If spontaneous circulation does not return, consider several Class IIb dosing regimens:

- Intermediate: **Epinephrine** 2-5 mg IV push, every 3-5 min.
- Escalating: **Epinephrine** 1 mg-3 mg-5 mg IV push, 3 min apart.
- High: **Epinephrine** 0.1 mg/kg IV push, every 3-5 min.

[d] The shorter atropine dosing interval (3 min) is possibly helpful in cardiac arrest (Class IIb).

Figure 3-3   Algorithm for pulseless electrical activity. (From Flynn JBM, Bruce NP: *Introduction to critical care skills,* St Louis, 1993, Mosby.)

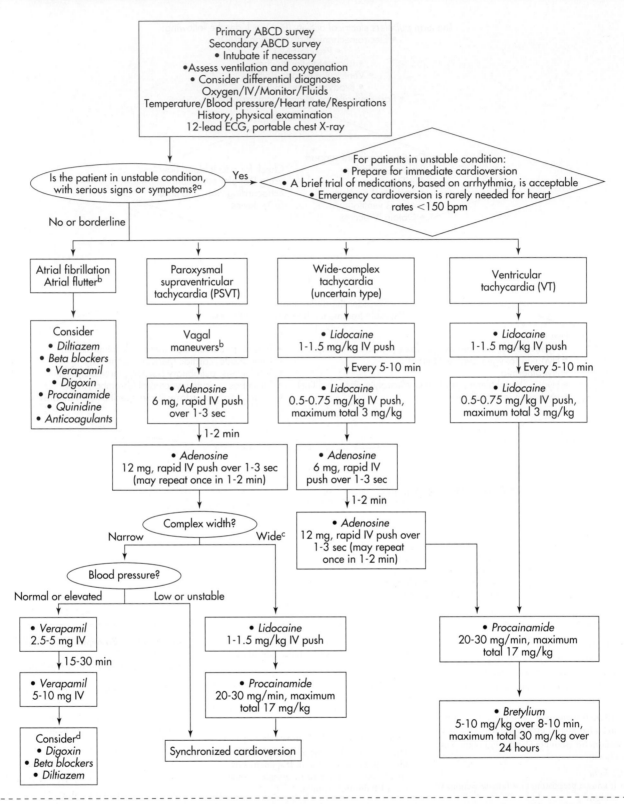

Figure 3-4   Algorithm for tachycardia. (From Flynn JBM, Bruce NP: *Introduction to critical care skills,* St Louis, 1993, Mosby.)

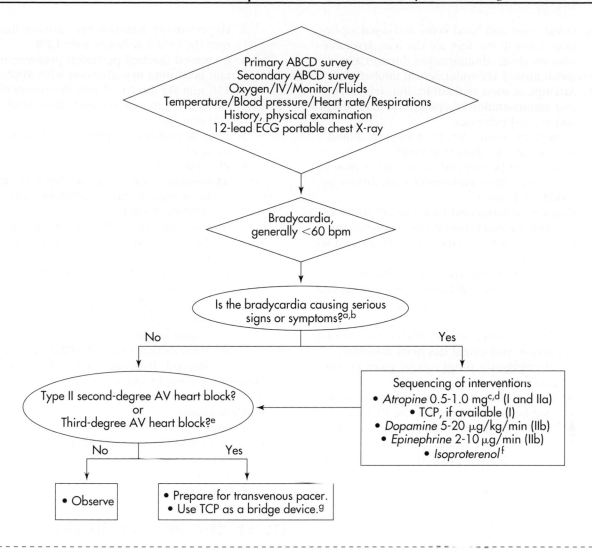

Figure 3-5   Algorithm for bradycardia. (From Flynn JBM, Bruce NP: *Introduction to critical care skills,* St Louis, 1993, Mosby.)

(2) May be painful for patient and should be replaced by transvenous lead as soon as possible

b) Transvenous pacemaker
(1) Lead is threaded into the apex of the right ventricle via subclavian or internal jugular vein

D. Establish/maintain intravenous access
1. Establish patency of existing central or peripheral IV or heparin lock; if a central vein catheter is in place when the arrest occurs, it should be used to administer drugs during the resuscitation
2. Antecubital or external jugular veins are pre-ferred if a venous catheter or additional venous catheters must be established

3. Central vein cannulation may be performed
a) The major disadvantage of central vein cannulation during cardiopulmonary arrest is the need to stop CPR
(1) Internal jugular and subclavian sites do require cessation of CPR
(2) Femoral vein cannulation does not require cessation of CPR
b) Another consideration is that unsuccessful central vein cannulation may contraindi-cate the use of thrombolytics; this point is very important for a patient with acute MI

4. Distal wrist and hand veins and distal saphenous veins in the legs are the least favorable sites for drug administration during CPR

E. Establish airway via endotracheal intubation
1. Attempt as soon as feasible, but defibrillation and administration of epinephrine are first and second priorities
2. Hyperventilation with 100% oxygen should precede any intubation attempt
3. CPR should be stopped for not more than 30 seconds to allow endotracheal intubation by a skilled clinician
4. Confirm endotracheal tube placement by listening for equal bilateral breath sounds initially; chest X-ray is taken after the patient is stabilized
5. Advantages of endotracheal intubation include reduction of the risk of vomiting and aspiration and provision of a relative airway seal
6. If IV route cannot be established but endotracheal tube placement has been achieved, some emergency drugs can be given via the ET tube
   a) Epinephrine, lidocaine, and/or atropine may be administered via the ET tube
   b) ET administration requires adjusting the dose to 2 to 2.5 times the usual dose and diluting the drug to make a total volume of at least 10 ml

F. Provide oxygen therapy
1. Administer 100% oxygen during cardiopulmonary arrest with a bag-valve-mask; a reservoir bag or tubing attached to the bag-valve-mask is required to achieve as high a concentration of oxygen as possible
2. Remember that there is no contraindication to 100% oxygen during cardiopulmonary arrest

G. Administer intravenous fluids: normal saline is used to maintain adequate preload and to mix intravenous drug infusions

H. Administer pharmacologic agents as indicated (Table 3-1)

III. Consider cerebral resuscitation principles
A. Avoid calcium, which has been shown to cause cerebral vessel spasm
B. Avoid dextrose in water: use isotonic normal saline rather than D_5W; the dextrose in D_5W is quickly metabolized to leave only hypotonic water; this hypotonic fluid contributes to hypoosmolality and potentially cerebral edema
C. Utilize other interventions to improve brain outcome as indicated or prescribed
1. Positioning: elevate head of bed 30 degrees; avoid neck flexion or rotation; avoid hip flexion
2. Hyperventilation: maintain $Paco_2$ at 35 mm Hg to cause healthy vessels to constrict, redistributing blood toward unhealthy areas

3. Hyperoxemia: maintain Pao_2 greater than 100 mm Hg for a few hours after CPR
4. Increased cerebral perfusion pressure: maintain brief mild hypertension with MAP 110 to 130 mm Hg for 1 to 5 minutes (contraindicated if neurologic trauma), then MAP 90 to 100 mm Hg
5. Brain hypothermia: apply cooled saline packs to head
6. Pharmacologic agents
   a) Osmotic agents (e.g., mannitol [Osmitrol]) to increase cortical circulation and reduce cerebral edema
   b) Calcium channel blockers (e.g., nimodipine [Nimotop]) to prevent cerebral vasospasm
   c) Anticonvulsants (e.g., phenytoin [Dilantin]) to prevent seizures
   d) Muscle paralytics (e.g., pancuronium [Pavulon]) to decrease cerebral oxygen requirements
   e) Steroids (e.g., methylprednisolone [Solu-Medrol]) to reduce cerebral edema

IV. Monitor for complications of CPR
A. Fracture of sternum, ribs
B. Hemothorax
C. Pneumothorax
D. Laceration of abdominal viscera, especially the liver
E. Myocardial contusion
F. Cardiac rupture

Dysrhythmias and Blocks
Definitions
I. Dysrhythmia: any cardiac rhythm other than sinus rhythm at a normal rate
II. Block: failure of an intrinsic impulse to be conducted through the conduction system

Etiology
I. General
A. Myocardial ischemia or infarction
B. Hypoxemia/hypoxia
C. Electrolyte imbalance
D. Acid-base imbalance
E. Sympathetic nervous system stimulation via endogenous catecholamines or sympathomimetic drugs (e.g., epinephrine, isoproterenol, dopamine)
F. Drug effects or toxicity
II. Table 3-2 describes etiology specific to each dysrhythmia

Pathophysiology: Arrhythmogenic mechanisms
I. Altered automaticity
A. Enhanced automaticity
1. Abnormal condition of latent pacemaker cells in which their firing rate is increased beyond

Table 3-1   Emergency Cardiac Drugs*

Drug	Indications	Dosage (IV injection)	Dosage (IV infusion)	Comments
First-Line Drugs				
Epinephrine (sympathomimetic [alpha, beta])	VF; asystole; PEA	1 mg every 3-5 minutes May be given via ET tube (double dose and dilute to make total volume of 10 ml)	Mix 1 mg in 250 ml (4 µg/ml) and infuse at 2-10 µg/min	• Monitor closely for vital organ hypoperfusion • Monitor closely for infiltration; central vein infusion preferred • Do not administer with alkaline solutions
Atropine (parasympatholytic)	Symptomatic bradycardia; asystole; PEA	0.5-1.0 mg for bradycardia; 1.0 for asystole or PEA; may be repeated in 3-5 minutes Maximum 0.04 mg/kg May be given via ET tube (double dose)	N/A	• Should not be given slowly or in dosages less than 0.5 mg because a paradoxical bradycardia may occur • Use with caution in myocardial ischemia or infarction because myocardial oxygen consumption is increased
Lidocaine (Class IB antidysrhythmic)	Significant PVCs; VF; VT; wide QRS tachycardia of unknown origin	VF: 1.5 mg/kg repeated every 3-5 minutes VT: 1-1.5 mg/kg repeated every 5-10 minutes Max: 3 mg/kg May be given via ET tube (double dose)	Mix 2 g in 500 ml (4 mg/ml) and infuse at 1-4 mg/min	• Monitor for clinical indications of lidocaine toxicity: perioral paresthesia; slurred speech; confusion; muscle twitching; seizures • Use lower dosages in patients with liver disease, hypoperfusion (e.g., HF), shock, or in elderly patients
Adenosine (Adenocard) (nonclassified antidysrhythmic)	SVT	6 mg given within 1-3 seconds using proximal injection site followed by 20 ml normal saline flush; may repeat at 12 mg; 12 mg dose may be repeated once	N/A	• Transient bradycardia or asystole may occur • Dose should be decreased in patients on dipyridamole, increased in patients on theophylline
Second-Line Drugs and Drugs Used to Support the Critically Ill Patient After Cardiopulmonary Arrest				
Bretylium (Bretylol) (Class III antidysrhythmic)	VF; VT	VF: 5 mg/kg repeated every 5 minutes at 10 mg/kg VT: 5-10 mg/kg over 8-10 minutes Max: 30 mg/kg	Mix 2 g in 500 ml (4 mg/ml) and infuse at 1-2 mg/ml	• Contraindicated in digitalis toxicity • Monitor BP closely • Have suction equipment available because this drug frequently causes vomiting
Procainamide (Class IA antidysrhythmic)	Significant PVCs; VF; VT Also used for atrial dysrhythmias	30 mg/min until: dysrhythmia suppressed; QRS widens by 50%; significant hypotension occurs; or maximum given Max: 17 mg/kg	Mix 2 g in 500 ml (4 mg/ml) and infuse at 1-4 mg/min	• Monitor BP closely • Monitor for widening of QRS and prolongation of QT • Consider discontinuance if QT prolongs; this is a forewarning of torsades de pointes

* For more information about these drugs, see Appendix E

Continued

Table 3-1	**Emergency Cardiac Drugs—cont'd**			
Drug	**Indications**	**Dosage (IV injection)**	**Dosage (IV infusion)**	**Comments**
Magnesium sulfate (electrolyte)	Torsades de pointes; refractory VT; VF; acute MI; hypomagnesemia	1-2 g in 10 ml NS given over 1-2 minutes in pulseless VT, VF, or torsades de pointes 1-2 g in 100 ml NS over 1-2 hours in hypomagnesemia, acute MI	Mix 1 g in 100 ml and infuse over 1 hour	• Monitor for signs/symptoms of hypermagnesemia: hyporeflexia; respiratory depression; hypotension • Calcium chloride may be given for hypermagnesemia
Amiodarone (Cordarone) (Class III antidysrhythmic)	VT, VF refractory to lidocaine	150 mg in 100 ml D_5W over 10 minutes followed by infusion	60 mg/hr for next 6 hours, then maintenance of 30 mg/hr for 18 hours	• Hypokalemia, hypomagnesemia should be corrected prior to amiodarone therapy; monitor QTc for prolongation • Use glass bottles • Monitor for hypotension, bradycardia, dysrhythmias, heart failure
Verapamil (Calan) (calcium channel blocker)	SVT	5-10 mg (0.075-0.15 mg/kg) over 2 minutes; may be repeated 5-10 mg q 15-30 minutes Max: 20 mg	N/A	• Do not use if patient is hypotensive; calcium may be given to lessen hypotensive effect of calcium channel blockers • Monitor BP closely • Do not use in patients with AV block, sinus node dysfunction, or HF • Should not be used in Wolff-Parkinson-White syndrome unless antegrade AV nodal conduction with accessory pathway reentry
Diltiazem (Cardizem) (calcium channel blocker)	SVT	0.15-0.25 mg/kg IV over 2 minutes; second dose of 0.35 mg/kg over 2 minutes may be given in 15 minutes	Mix 125 mg in 100 ml for total volume of 125 ml (1 mg/ml) and infuse at 5-15 mg/hr	• Do not use if patient is hypotensive; calcium may be given to lessen hypotension • Monitor BP closely • Do not use in patients with AV block, sinus node dysfunction, or HF • Do not use in Wolff-Parkinson-White syndrome
Esmolol (Brevibloc) (beta-blocker [beta₁])	SVT; VT, especially if caused by excessive catecholamine	500 µg/kg over 1 minute followed by maintenance dose of 50 µg/kg/min for 4 minutes	Mix 5 g in 500 ml (10 mg/ml) and infuse at 50-200 µg/kg/min Max: 300 µg/kg/min	• Monitor for bradycardia, hypotension, AV block • Do not use in HF • Do not administer with alkaline solutions
Propranolol (Inderal) (beta-blocker [beta₁ and beta₂])	SVT; VT, especially if caused by excessive catecholamine MI to decrease myocardial oxygen requirements	0.1 mg/kg in 3 divided doses at rate not to exceed 1 mg/min	N/A	• Monitor for bradycardia, hypotension, AV block • Do not use in HF or obstructive lung disease (e.g., asthma, COPD)

Table 3-1	Emergency Cardiac Drugs—cont'd			
Drug	**Indications**	**Dosage (IV injection)**	**Dosage (IV infusion)**	**Comments**
Dobutamine (Dobutrex) (sympathomimetic [predominantly beta])	Cardiogenic shock; HF	N/A	Mix 250 mg in 250 ml (1000 µg/ml) and infuse at 2-20 µg/kg/min	• Monitor for ventricular ectopy • Beta$_2$ effect (vasodilation) may cause initial hypotension • Do not administer with alkaline solutions
Dopamine (Intropin) (sympathomimetic [alpha, beta, dopaminergic depending on dose])	Hypotension after adequate volume replacement; vasogenic shock	N/A	Mix 400 mg in 250 ml (1600 µg/ml) and infuse at 1-20 µg/kg/min depending on desired effect 1-2 = dopaminergic (renal) 2-5 = beta 5-10 = alpha + beta >10 = alpha	• Monitor for ventricular ectopy • Alpha effect (vasoconstriction) increases afterload and myocardial oxygen consumption • Monitor closely for vital organ hypoperfusion • Monitor closely for infiltration; central vein infusion preferred • Do not administer with alkaline solutions
Digoxin (Lanoxin) (cardiac glycoside)	HF; SVT	0.25-0.5 mg IV to a total digitalizing dose of 1 mg over 24 hours; daily maintenance dose 0.125-0.5 mg	N/A	• Monitor for clinical indications of digitalis toxicity: nausea/vomiting; anorexia; visual changes; dysrhythmias • Ensure adequate potassium, calcium, magnesium levels • Do not give simultaneously with calcium
Amrinone (Inocor) (PDE inhibitor)	Refractory HF	0.75 mg/kg over 2-3 minutes followed by infusion	Mix 500 mg in 500 ml (1000 µg/ml) and infuse at 5-15 µg/kg/min	• Monitor for hepatotoxicity, thrombocytopenia • Monitor for ventricular ectopy
Nitroglycerin (Tridil) (nitrate vasodilator)	Angina; acute MI; HF	N/A	Mix 50 mg in 250 ml (200 µg/ml) and infuse at 10-400 µg/min Max: 400 µg/min	• Monitor BP closely; hypotension may exacerbate myocardial ischemia • May cause reflex tachycardia; this increases myocardial oxygen consumption
Nitroprusside (Nipride)	HF; hypertensive crisis	N/A	Mix 50 mg in 250 ml D$_5$W (200 µg/ml) and infuse at 0.5-10 µg/kg/min Max: 10 µg/min	• Monitor BP closely • Bag or bottle must be wrapped with aluminum foil • Monitor for clinical indications of thiocyanate toxicity: metabolic acidosis; tinnitus; confusion; hyperreflexia; seizures
Norepinephrine (Levophed) (sympathomimetic [predominantly alpha])	Vasogenic shock severe hypotension (<70 systolic) after adequate volume replacement	N/A	Mix 4 mg in 250 ml (16 µg/ml) and infuse at 0.5-30 µg/min Max: 30 µg/min	• Monitor closely for vital organ hypoperfusion • Monitor closely for infiltration; central vein infusion preferred • Do not administer with alkaline solutions

Continued

Table 3-1	Emergency Cardiac Drugs—cont'd			
Drug	Indications	Dosage (IV injection)	Dosage (IV infusion)	Comments
Isoproterenol (Isuprel) (sympathomimetic [beta])	Symptomatic bradycardia that does not respond to atropine; refractory torsades de pointes	N/A	Mix 1 mg in 250 ml (4 µg/ml) and infuse at 2-10 µg/min Max: 30 µg/min	• External pacing is preferred since isoproterenol increases myocardial oxygen consumption • Monitor closely for ventricular ectopy; slow infusion or discontinue • Do not administer with alkaline solutions
Sodium bicarbonate (alkaline buffer)	Severe metabolic acidosis with pH 7.0 or less	1 mEq/kg initially; may be repeated in 10 minutes at 0.5 mg/kg	N/A	• Metabolic acidosis ideally should be reversed by improving perfusion • Worsens acidosis from CO_2 formation and retention and impaired delivery of oxygen to the tissue • Causes electrolyte imbalances: hypernatremia; hypokalemia; hypocalcemia • May contribute to cerebral edema and poor brain outcome • It is more difficult to defibrillate an alkalotic heart
Calcium chloride (electrolyte)	Hypocalcemia; hyperkalemia; hypermagnesemia; calcium channel blocker toxicity; pretreatment of patients with SVT prior to verapamil	500 mg-1 g of 10% calcium chloride administered at rate <50 mg/min	N/A	• Bradycardia may occur if given rapidly • Use with caution in patients on digitalis • Do not give with bicarbonate

their inherent rate (even nonpacemaker cells may spontaneously depolarize)

2. Resting membrane potential is less negative or threshold potential is lower, increasing the chance of depolarization
3. Caused by any of the following:
   a) Hypoxia
   b) Hypercapnia
   c) Ischemia, infarction
   d) Hypokalemia, hypocalcemia
   e) Increased catecholamine levels
   f) Hyperthermia
   g) Digitalis toxicity
   h) Stretching of the heart muscle
4. Cause of most atrial, junctional, and ventricular ectopic beats and most ventricular tachycardia

B. Depressed automaticity
   1. Resting membrane potential is more negative or threshold potential is higher, decreasing the chance of depolarization

2. Caused by any of the following:
   a) Vagal stimulation
   b) Hyperkalemia, hypercalcemia
   c) Decreased catecholamine levels
   d) Hypothermia
   e) Beta-blockers
3. Cause of bradycardia or blocks

II. Triggered activity
   A. Repetitive ectopic firing caused by afterdepolarizations; an afterdepolarization is a transient depolarization occurring during or after repolarization of an action potential
   B. If an afterdepolarization is strong enough to reach threshold, a triggered beat occurs
   C. This activity is not self-generating but is dependent on the preceding beat
   D. They may be early or late
      1. Early: occur when the QT is prolonged
         a) Caused by prolongation of repolarization and effective refractory period
         b) Example: torsades de pointes

Text continued on p. 109

Table 3-2	Basic Dysrhythmias and Blocks: Etiology, Significance, and Treatment		
Rhythm	**Etiology**	**Significance**	**Treatment**
General	• Hypoxia • Ischemia • Electrolyte imbalance • Acid-base imbalance • Drug effect or toxicity	• Dependent on patient's clinical presentation • Monitor for clinical manifestations of hypoperfusion	• Treat cause • Correct ischemia if possible • Correct hypoxemia, hypoxia • Correct electrolyte imbalance • Correct acid-base imbalance • Correct drug toxicity

Sinus bradycardia	• Athletic heart
	• Sleep
	• Vagal stimulation
	• Myocardial ischemia or infarction
	  • Inferior MI
	• Fibrodegenerative changes of the SA node (e.g., sick sinus syndrome)
	• Increased ICP
	• Hypothermia
	• Hypothyroidism
	• Cervical or mediastinal tumor
	• Drug effect: digitalis; beta-blockers; calcium channel blockers; opiates
		• Depends on rate
		• If too slow, cardiac output decreases
		  • Clinical manifestations of hypoperfusion may include hypotension, syncope, chest pain, HF
		• Escape beats (atrial, junctional, or ventricular) may occur
			• None if asymptomatic
			• If clinical manifestations of hypoperfusion occur:
			  • Atropine
			  • Pacemaker

Sinus tachycardia	• Stress, fear, anxiety, pain, anger • Exercise • Hypovolemia or hypervolemia • Shock • Hypoxia • Fever • Anemia • Hyperthyroidism • Inflammatory heart disease • Myocardial ischemic or infarction • Anterior MI • Fibrodegenerative changes (e.g., sick sinus syndrome) • Heart failure • Pulmonary embolism • Drug effect: epinephrine, isoproterenol; dopamine; atropine; caffeine; nicotine; amphetamines; cocaine; alcohol; aminophylline	• Usually not significant except in patients with heart disease—then may cause angina, MI, HF, or shock	• Treat cause • Decrease anxiety, pain, remove stimulants • Usually does not require other treatment, but sedation, beta-blockers, calcium channel blockers, or digitalis may be used
Sinus dysrhythmia	• Normal; variation in sympathetic and parasympathetic stimulation during ventilation • In older patient, may indicate sick sinus syndrome • Digitalis toxicity	• Normal variation • May be seen in digitalis toxicity	• None • Discontinue digitalis if toxicity is cause
Sinus block (sinus exit block)	• Fibrodegenerative changes of the sinus node (e.g., sick sinus syndrome) • Ischemia of SA node (e.g., MI) • Vagal stimulation • Inflammatory heart disease (e.g., myocarditis) • Drug toxicity: digitalis	• Depends on frequency and duration of pauses • If patient loses consciousness (Stokes-Adams attacks), very significant and requires treatment	• Discontinue digitalis if toxicity is cause • Atropine • Pacemaker if frequent pauses, long pauses, or if patient having Stokes-Adams attacks

Continued

Table 3-2	**Basic Dysrhythmias and Blocks: Etiology, Significance, and Treatment—cont'd**		
Rhythm	**Etiology**	**Significance**	**Treatment**
Sinus arrest	• Fibrodegenerative changes (e.g., sick sinus syndrome) • Ischemia of SA node (e.g., MI) • Vagal stimulation • Electrolyte imbalance: potassium, magnesium • Drug toxicity: digitalis	• Depends on frequency and duration of pauses • If patient loses consciousness (Stokes-Adams attacks), very significant and requires treatment	• Discontinue digitalis if toxicity is cause • Atropine • Pacemaker if frequent pauses, long pauses, or if patient having Stokes-Adams attacks
Premature atrial contractions	• Increased sympathetic stimulation: stress, fear, anxiety, pain • Exercise • Inflammatory heart disease (e.g., myocarditis) • Myocardial ischemia • Valvular heart disease (e.g., mitral stenosis; mitral valve prolapse) • Heart failure • Electrolyte imbalance • Hypoxia • Drug effect: caffeine; nicotine; alcohol • Drug toxicity: digitalis	• Usually benign but may precede atrial tachycardia, flutter, or fibrillation • Considered significant if >6/min	• Treatment of cause • Usually no treatment necessary, but if frequent treatment may include digitalis, quinidine, propranolol
Wandering atrial pacemaker	• Vagal stimulation • Sinus bradycardia • Digitalis toxicity	• May represent multiple atrial escape beats	• Usually none needed • Discontinue digitalis if toxicity is suspected • Atropine may be used to increase slow sinus rate
Atrial tachycardia (paroxysmal atrial tachycardia [PAT] refers to the sudden interruption of sinus rhythm by a rapid ectopic focus—starts and ends abruptly)	• Increased sympathetic stimulation: stress, fear, anxiety, pain • Exercise • Inflammatory heart disease (e.g., myocarditis) • Myocardial ischemia or infarction • Hypoxia • Hyperthyroidism • Valvular heart disease (e.g., mitral valve prolapse) • Chronic obstructive pulmonary disease • Wolff-Parkinson-White syndrome • Drug effect: caffeine; nicotine; alcohol • Drug toxicity: digitalis (frequently PAT with block)	• Patient may experience palpitations and clinical manifestations of hypoperfusion (e.g., hypotension, syncope, chest pain, HF) because diastolic filling time and preload is greatly reduced • Myocardial oxygen consumption is increased, and myocardial oxygen supply is decreased	• Depends on patient's tolerance, cause, and history of previous attacks • Rest, sedation • Vagal stimulation • Synchronized cardioversion • Adenosine • Calcium channel blockers (e.g., verapamil, diltiazem) • Beta-blockers (e.g., esmolol) • Digitalis may be used for treatment if not the cause • Discontinue digitalis if toxicity is suspected • Right atrial overdrive pacing
Multifocal atrial tachycardia (may also be called *chaotic atrial rhythm*)	• Pulmonary hypertension (e.g., COPD, pulmonary embolism) • Digitalis toxicity • Valvular heart disease • Congestive heart failure • Electrolyte imbalance: potassium • Drug toxicity: digitalis	• Demonstrates atrial irritability, which may lead to atrial tachycardia, flutter, fibrillation	• Usually none needed • Discontinue digitalis if toxicity is suspected • Digitalis may be used for treatment if not the cause • Calcium channel blockers (e.g., verapamil, diltiazem) • Amiodarone • Potassium, magnesium replacement

Table 3-2	Basic Dysrhythmias and Blocks: Etiology, Significance, and Treatment—cont'd		
Rhythm	**Etiology**	**Significance**	**Treatment**
Atrial flutter	• Heart failure • Myocardial ischemia or infarction • Valvular heart disease • Inflammatory heart disease (e.g., pericarditis) • Hypertension • Postcardiotomy • Pulmonary hypertension (e.g., COPD, pulmonary embolism) • Hyperthyroidism • Drug effect: alcohol • Drug toxicity: digitalis	• No effectiveness of atrial contraction • Significance varies greatly depending on rate • If rate is very rapid may cause clinical manifestations of hypoperfusion (e.g., hypotension, syncope, chest pain, HF) because diastolic filling time and preload is greatly reduced	• Digitalis, beta-blockers, calcium channel blockers, cardioversion, or atrial pacing to control rapid ventricular response rates • Procainamide, quinidine, or amiodarone may also be used • No additional treatment is required if rate is controlled (between 60-100/min)

Atrial fibrillation	• Heart failure
	• Cardiomyopathy
	• Myocardial ischemia or infarction
	  • Especially anterior MI
	• Valvular heart disease (e.g., mitral stenosis, mitral regurgitation)
	• Hyperthyroidism
	• Inflammatory heart disease (e.g., pericarditis)
	• Hypertension
	• Postcardiotomy
	• Pulmonary hypertension (e.g., COPD, pulmonary embolism)
	• Wolff-Parkinson-White syndrome
	• Drug effect: alcohol
		• No effective atrial contraction so loss of atrial kick
		• Mural thrombi formation predisposes to emboli
		• Significance varies greatly on rate: may cause clinical manifestations of hypoperfusion (e.g., hypotension, syncope, chest pain, HF)
			• Digitalis, beta-blockers, calcium channel blockers, or cardioversion to control rapid ventricular response rates
			  • Procainamide, quinidine, or amiodarone may also be used
			• Atropine or pacemaker may be needed for slow ventricular response rates
			  • Digitalis should be considered as cause of slow ventricular response rate; withhold digitalis is cause
			• No additional treatment is required if rate is controlled (between 60-100/min)
			• Anticoagulation is frequently used to prevent mural thrombi and emboli

Premature junctional contraction	• Myocardial ischemia or infarction • Especially inferior MI • Heart failure • Valvular heart disease • Hypoxia • Drug effect: nicotine; caffeine; alcohol • Drug toxicity: digitalis • Also etiology as for PACs	• Usually benign but may predispose to junctional tachycardia if frequent	• Usually none necessary • Discontinue digitalis if toxicity is cause • Sedation • Digitalis if not cause • Beta-blockers
Junctional escape rhythm	• Vagal stimulation • SA block • Complete AV block • Myocardial ischemia or infarction • Valvular heart disease • Hypoxia • Postcardiotomy • Drug toxicity: digitalis	• Protects patient from asystole • Do not suppress	• Treat failure of sinus node • Atropine • Pacemaker may be needed • Discontinue digitalis if digitalis toxicity is cause

Continued

Table 3-2	Basic Dysrhythmias and Blocks: Etiology, Significance, and Treatment—cont'd		
Rhythm	**Etiology**	**Significance**	**Treatment**
Accelerated junctional rhythm	• Vagal stimulation • SA block • Complete AV block • Myocardial ischemia or infarction • Reperfusion of myocardium • Hypoxia • Inflammatory heart disease (e.g., myocarditis) • Postcardiotomy • Drug toxicity: digitalis	• Protects patient from asystole • Do not suppress	• Treat failure of sinus node • Discontinue digitalis if digitalis toxicity is cause
Junctional tachycardia	• Myocardial ischemia or infarction • Reperfusion of myocardium • Inflammatory heart disease • Postcardiotomy • Drug toxicity: digitalis	• Usually stops spontaneously and is usually tolerated well	• Treat cause • Discontinue digitalis if digitalis toxicity is cause • Digitalis may be used if not the cause • Cardioversion
First-degree AV nodal block	• Normal variation • Myocardial ischemia or infarction • Conduction system fibrosis • Inflammatory heart disease (e.g., myocarditis) • Postcardiotomy • Myocardial contusion • Hyperkalemia • Drug toxicity: digitalis; beta-blockers; calcium channel blockers	• Relatively benign but may progress to second- or third-degree block	• Observe closely for progression of block • Discontinue digitalis if digitalis toxicity is cause
Second-degree AV nodal block Mobitz I (Wenckebach)	• Myocardial ischemia or infarction • Inferior MI • Conduction system fibrosis • Inflammatory heart disease • Postcardiotomy • Myocardial contusion • Drug toxicity: digitalis; beta-blockers; calcium channel blockers	• Block is at AV node • Occurs more often in inferior MIs (RCA lesion) • Relatively benign: usually transient and does not usually progress to complete heart block (CHB)	• Does not usually require treatment • Monitor for progression of block • Discontinue digitalis if digitalis toxicity is cause • Atropine may be used if rate slow and patient symptomatic
Second-degree AV nodal block Mobitz II	• Myocardial ischemia or infarction • Anterior MI • Hypertension • Valvular heart disease • Conduction system fibrosis • Inflammatory heart disease (e.g., myocarditis) • Postcardiotomy • Myocardial contusion	• Block is at bundle of His, which accounts for the slight widening of the QRS complex • Occurs more often in anterior MIs (LAD lesion) • Ominous because it often progresses to CHB	• Atropine may be used but is not usually helpful • Prophylactic pacemaker

Third-degree (or complete) AV block	• Myocardial ischemia or infarction
	• Conduction system fibrosis
	• Inflammatory heart disease
	• Postcardiotomy
	• Myocardial contusion
	• Hypoxia
	• Electrolyte imbalance: potassium
	• Drug toxicity: digitalis
		• If no escape rhythm is established, the patient has ventricular asystole	• Observe for clinical manifestations of hypoperfusion if inferior MI with junctional escape rhythm
			• Atropine may be used but is not usually helpful
			• Pacemaker, especially if:
			  • Anterior MI
			  • Inferior MI with ventricular escape rhythm

Table 3-2	Basic Dysrhythmias and Blocks: Etiology, Significance, and Treatment—cont'd		
Rhythm	**Etiology**	**Significance**	**Treatment**
Left bundle branch block (LBBB)	• Myocardial ischemia or infarction • Anterior MI • Fibrodegenerative changes • Postcardiotomy	• Bifascicular block considered more serious than RBBB, especially in presence of acute MI	• New LBBB in acute MI may be treated with prophylactic pacemaker, especially if an AV nodal block is also present • Monitor this patient closely during pulmonary artery catheter insertion because trifascicular block may occur
Right bundle branch block (RBBB)	• Myocardial ischemia or infarction • Anterior or inferior MI • Fibrodegenerative changes • Postcardiotomy • Pulmonary artery catheter insertion • Acute pulmonary embolus	• None; cardiac output is not affected by delayed ventricular depolarization (wide QRS)	• Monitor closely for development of LBBB

Premature ventricular contraction	• Increased sympathetic nervous system stimulation (e.g., endogenous catecholamines or sympathomimetic drugs [e.g., epinephrine, isoproterenol, dopamine])
	• Myocardial ischemia or infarction
	• Reperfusion of myocardium
	• Heart failure
	• Ventricular aneurysm
	• Cardiomyopathy
	• Hypoxia
	• Acidosis
	• Electrolyte imbalance: potassium; calcium; magnesium
	• Drug toxicity: digitalis; aminophylline
		• PVCs of most significance: may predispose to VT or VF
		  • Frequent (>6/min)
		  • Bigeminal
		  • Multifocal
		  • R on T phenomenon
		  • Couplets
		  • Runs of ventricular tachycardia (3 or more PVCs in a row)
		• Pulse amplitude of PVC is reduced due to decreased filling time
			• Treatment of cause (e.g., oxygen, electrolyte replacement, discontinue digitalis)
			• No treatment required if infrequent
			• If frequent: lidocaine, procainamide, bretylium, beta-blockers

Monomorphic ventricular tachycardia	• Myocardial ischemia or infarction • Reperfusion of myocardium • Ventricular aneurysm • Cardiomyopathy • Valvular heart disease • Postcardiotomy • R on T PVC • Hypoxia • Acidosis • Electrolyte imbalance: hypokalemia • Drug toxicity: digitalis	• Ominous because may progress to ventricular fibrillation • Symptoms depend on underlying heart disease, rate, and duration of VT • May cause angina, HF, shock	• If stable: oxygen; lidocaine, procainamide, bretylium; correct electrolyte imbalance, drug toxicity • If having hypotension, chest pain, or pulmonary edema: immediate sedation and cardioversion • If pulseless: treat as VF (e.g., defibrillation, epinephrine, etc.)

Continued

2. Delayed: the result of elevated intracellular calcium
   a) Caused by:
     (1) Electrolyte imbalances
     (2) Increased catecholamine levels
   b) Example: tachycardias of digitalis toxicity
III. Altered conductivity
  A. Reentry (Fig. 3-6): the most common mechanism for tachydysrhythmias
    1. An impulse travels through an area of the myocardium and depolarizes it, but then reenters the same area to depolarize it again
    2. Requirements
     a) An available circuit: Reentry can occur in areas of the heart where conduction velocity is abnormally slow
     b) Unequal responsiveness of two segments of the circuit (delay in one limb of the circuit)

Table 3-2	Basic Dysrhythmias and Blocks: Etiology, Significance, and Treatment—cont'd		
Rhythm	**Etiology**	**Significance**	**Treatment**
Polymorphic ventricular tachycardia (including torsades de pointes)	• Class IA antidysrhythmics (e.g., procainamide, quinidine, disopyramide) • Class III antidysrhythmics (e.g., sotalol, amiodarone) • Tricyclic antidepressants (e.g., amitriptyline [Elavil]) • Phenothiazines (e.g., chlorpromazine [Thorazine]) • Organic insecticides • Electrolyte imbalance (e.g., hypomagnesemia, hypocalcemia, hypokalemia) • Congenital long QT syndrome • Marked bradycardia • Hypothermia • Subarachnoid hemorrhage	• No effective perfusion • May go into and out of this rhythm	• Monitor QT interval closely and discontinue any offending drug when QT prolongs to greater than half of the RR interval • Discontinue any offending drug if characteristic torsades pattern seen • Administer appropriate electrolyte, especially magnesium • Isoproterenol infusion may be given • Atropine may be used to increase intrinsic rate • Overdrive pacing
Ventricular fibrillation	• Myocardial ischemia or infarction • R on T PVC • Electrical shock, including microshock • Near-drowning • Hypothermia • Hypoxia • Drug toxicity: digitalis • Dying heart	• Lethal within 4-6 minutes • No cardiac output • Symptoms include: loss of consciousness, pulse, heart sounds, ventilation, BP, anoxic seizures	• Immediate defibrillation (200 joules, if unsuccessful 200-300 joules, if unsuccessful 360 joules) • CPR • Epinephrine • Intubation • Antidysrhythmics: lidocaine; bretylium; procainamide • Magnesium

Idioventricular rhythm	• Vagal stimulation
	• Failure of higher pacemakers (e.g., ischemia or fibrosis of conduction system)
	• Myocardial ischemia or infarction
	• Third-degree AV block
	• Drug toxicity: digitalis
		• Protects the patient from asystole but very unreliable
		• Do not suppress
			• Accelerate higher pacemakers with atropine
			• Pacemaker
			• If pulseless:
			  • CPR
			  • Epinephrine
			  • Pacemaker

Accelerated idioventricular rhythm	• Failure of higher pacemakers (e.g., ischemia or fibrosis of conduction system) • Myocardial ischemia or infarction • Reperfusion of myocardium • Drug toxicity: digitalis	• Protects the patient from asystole but very unreliable • Do not suppress	• Accelerate higher pacemakers with atropine • Pacemaker
Asystole	• Vagal stimulation • Myocardial ischemia or infarction • Third-degree AV block • Anaphylaxis • Drug overdosage • Hypoxia • Acidosis • Shock • Dying heart	• Lethal within 4-6 minutes • No cardiac output • Symptoms include: loss of consciousness, pulse, heart sounds, ventilation, BP, anoxic seizures	• CPR • Epinephrine • Atropine • Pacemaker

c) An area of slowed conduction or unidirectional block
  (1) Conduction must be slow enough to allow time for the previously stimulated area to recover the ability to conduct

(2) The area of unidirectional block provides a return pathway for the original stimulus to reenter a previously stimulated area in time to repolarize
3. Cause of any of the following:
  a) Some ectopy

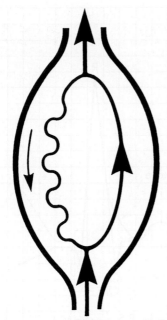

Figure 3-6 Schematic representation of a reentrant circuit depicting two limbs with varying conduction times (straight lines vs. curly line). The tachycardic impulse travels around this circuit, and as it reaches the common end(s), travels to the myocardium, which then depolarizes. A similar reentrant circuit can be located around the sinus node, within the atrial or ventricular myocardium, within the AV node, or between the AV node and an accessory pathway. (From Urban N et al: *Guidelines for critical care nursing,* St Louis, 1995, Mosby.)

    b) Some ventricular tachycardias
    c) Most supraventricular tachycardias
    d) Wolff-Parkinson-White (WPW) tachycardias
  B. Accessory pathways
    1. Lown-Ganong-Levine syndrome
      a) Caused by:
        (1) AV nodal bypass tract
        (2) AV node smaller than normal
        (3) Fibers running through AV node that do not have the built-in delay feature that nodal fibers have
      b) Causes of:
        (1) Short PR, normal QRS
        (2) Tachydysrhythmias
    2. Wolff-Parkinson-White syndrome
      a) Caused by Kent bundle, which bypasses the AV node
        (1) Type A: Kent bundle on left; R-wave in V_1 with inverted T-wave and depressed ST
        (2) Type B: Kent bundle on right; QS in V_1 with upright T-wave and elevated ST
      b) Cause of:
        (1) Short PR, wide QRS with slurring of first portion of QRS (referred to as a *delta wave*) (Fig. 3-7)

    (2) Tachydysrhythmias
      (a) Sinus impulse may take accessory pathway around the AV node (referred to as *preexcitation*), causing elimination of the mandatory delay in the AV node and severe supraventricular tachycardias with a wide QRS
      (b) Impulse may also take AV node but reenter via accessory pathway; narrow QRS
    3. Mahaim fibers
      a) Caused by nodoventricular or fasciculoventricular fibers
      b) Cause of:
        (1) Short PR, wide QRS
        (2) Tachydysrhythmias
  C. Aberrant conduction
    1. Aberrant conduction occurs most often when:
      a) Rate is rapid
      b) Very premature atrial contractions
      c) Changes in cycle length (e.g., atrial fibrillation [QRS that ends a short cycle length after a long cycle length is likely to be conducted aberrantly is referred to as *Ashman's phenomenon*])
    2. Since one of the bundle branches (usually the right) is still refractory when a supraventricular impulse reaches it, the impulse must travel down the nonrefractory bundle and across to the other ventricle; this process causes a wide QRS, which is frequently mistaken for a PVC if a single complex or ventricular tachycardia if several complexes in a row
    3. Unlike ectopy, aberrancy is no more serious than the supraventricular mechanism that caused it (e.g., atrial fibrillation with aberrancy is no more clinically significant than atrial fibrillation)
    4. QRS morphology is the most important criterion in the differentiation between ectopy and aberrancy, but other criteria may also be helpful (Table 3-3); multiple-lead ECG is often helpful to identify P-waves and in looking at the morphology of the QRS
    5. Ectopy is more common than aberrancy; if in doubt, always assume ectopy and treat accordingly

Clinical Presentation

   I. Anxiety, restlessness
  II. Vertigo, syncope
 III. Weakness, fatigue, activity intolerance
 IV. Palpitations
  V. Chest pain
 VI. Clinical indications of LVF: dyspnea, S_3, crackles
VII. Clinical indications of hypoperfusion (see Table 2-6)

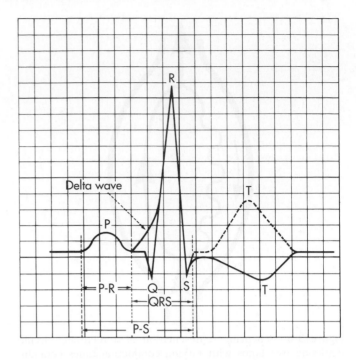

Figure 3-7 Wolff-Parkinson-White syndrome. Note the short PR interval, the delta wave, widened QRS, and T-wave inversion characteristic of preexcitation. (From Kinney MR, Packa DR, Dunbar SB: *AACN's clinical reference for critical-care nursing,* ed 4, St Louis, 1998, Mosby.)

| Table | 3-3 | **Differentiation Between Ventricular Ectopy and Aberrancy** |

Features	Favoring Ventricular Ectopy	Favoring Supraventricular Origin with Aberrancy
Rate	130-150/min	>150/min
Regularity	Regular	Irregular (since most likely to be atrial fibrillation)
P-wave	None or dissociated	Premature
QRS width	>0.14 seconds	0.12-0.14 seconds
QRS morphology in V₁ Note: uppercase letters indicate large waves, lowercase letters indicate small waves	Monophasic R Rr′ with left peak taller Biphasic qR Biphasic Rs or rS	Monophasic QS Biphasic rS Triphasic rSR′ or rR′
QRS morphology in V₆ Note: uppercase letters indicate large waves, lowercase letters indicate small waves	Monophasic QS Biphasic qR Biphasic rS Initial vector opposite normal beats Precordial concordance (all QRSs V₁-V₆ positive or all QRSs V₁-V₆ negative)	Monophasic R Triphasic qRs Initial vector same as normal beats
Fusion beats	Yes	No
Compensatory pause after single beat or at end of run	Yes	No
Axis	Indeterminate or LAD of –30 or greater	Normal or RAD
Patient history	History of PVCs	History of PACs, atrial fibrillation
Response to carotid massage	No effect on ventricular rate	Often causes at least temporary slowing of ventricular rate
BP	Usually very low or absent (but may be normal)	Moderately low or normal
Consciousness	Frequently unconscious (but may be conscious)	May complain of lightheadedness
Seizures	Frequently present (but may be absent)	Absent

VIII. Diagnostic studies
   A. Electrocardiography: multiple-lead ECG
   B. Serum electrolyte levels
   C. Drug levels
   D. Arterial blood gases

Nursing Diagnoses

I. Decreased Cardiac Output related to changes in heart rate, rhythm, or conduction
II. Alteration in Myocardial Tissue Perfusion related to decrease in diastolic time and/or pressure
III. Alteration in Cerebral Tissue Perfusion related to changes in heart rate, rhythm, or conduction
IV. Activity Intolerance related to changes in heart rate, rhythm, or conduction and inability to increase cardiac output in response to exercise
V. Risk for Injury related to use of an electrical device (e.g., defibrillator, pacemaker)
VI. Anxiety related to acute change in health status, emergent procedures
VII. Knowledge Deficit related to antidysrhythmic therapies and drugs

Collaborative Management

I. Assess for clinical manifestations of hypoperfusion (Table 2-6): follow ACLS algorithms for lethal dysrhythmias (see Cardiopulmonary Arrest)
II. Treat etiology of dysrhythmia
III. Correct ischemia if possible
   A. Coronary artery vasodilators and/or antispasmodics: nitrates, calcium channel blockers
   B. Thrombolytics
   C. Percutaneous coronary intervention (PCI): percutaneous transluminal coronary angioplasty (PTCA), atherectomy
   D. Coronary artery bypass graft
IV. Correct hypoxemia/hypoxia
   A. Improve Sao_2 (e.g., oxygen, endotracheal intubation, mechanical ventilation, positive end-expiratory pressure [PEEP])
   B. Improve cardiac output (e.g., inotropes, vasodilators, intraaortic balloon pump)
   C. Improve hemoglobin (e.g., blood)
V. Correct electrolyte imbalances
   A. Replace deficient electrolytes
   B. Decrease excessive electrolyte levels (e.g., electrolyte restriction, diuretics, ion exchange resins, dialysis)
VI. Correct acidosis
   A. Improve perfusion to correct metabolic acidosis caused by lactic acid
   B. Initiate dialysis for patients with renal failure
   C. Provide hydration and insulin therapy for patients in diabetic ketoacidosis
   D. Improve ventilation to correct respiratory acidosis
VII. Eliminate cause of excessive catecholamine release or block effects
   A. Treat pain
   B. Decrease anxiety with relaxation techniques and anxiolytics
   C. Administer beta-blockers for cardioprotection as prescribed
VIII. Initiate standing orders (e.g., IV, oxygen, multiple-lead ECG)
IX. Initiate antidysrhythmic therapy as indicated by standing orders or prescribed
   A. Vaughan-Williams classification system (Table 3-4)
   B. Drugs and treatments of choice for each dysrhythmia (see Table 3-2)
   C. Additional information about antidysrhythmic agents located in Appendix E
X. Utilize electrical therapies as indicated; electrical therapies use the application of electrical energy to the myocardium to change an abnormal cardiac rhythm to a normal one
   A. Principle: By delivering a shock of sufficient strength, a critical mass of myocardium is depolarized simultaneously, allowing emergence of the dominant normal rhythm
   B. Cardioversion
      1. Uses
         a) Urgent cardioversion is used for tachydysrhythmias (other than sinus) that are rapid enough to cause hemodynamic compromise or that have not responded to antidysrhythmic drug therapy
         b) Elective cardioversion is performed for tachydysrhythmias that are reasonably well tolerated hemodynamically but that have not responded to antidysrhythmic drug therapy
      2. Contraindications
         a) Tachydysrhythmias that result from digitalis toxicity
         b) Nonsustained tachydysrhythmias
         c) Long-standing atrial fibrillation
         d) Atrial fibrillation with normal or slow ventricular rate in the absence of AV nodal blocking drugs
         e) Multifocal atrial tachycardia
      3. Method: as for defibrillation except the following:
         a) Conscious patients should be sedated with diazepam (Valium), lorazepam (Ativan), or midazolam (Versed)
         b) Elective procedures should be preceded by at least a 6-hour fast
         c) Emergency equipment and drugs must be available
         d) Synchronizer switch is on so that charge is delivered only during QRS, avoiding the descending limb of the T-wave
         e) Voltage is from 25 to 200 joules
         f) Antidysrhythmic drug therapy is used after sinus rhythm is restored
      4. Complications: as for defibrillation
   C. Defibrillation: see Cardiopulmonary Arrest Section
XI. Utilize pacemaker therapies for patients who have

Table 3-4 Vaughan-Williams Antidysrhythmic Classification System

Class	Effect	Examples
IA	• Blocks sodium influx, which depresses the rate of depolarization • Prolongs repolarization and action potential duration • Decreases contractility (negative inotrope) • Prolongs QT (torsades de pointes potential) and QRS duration	• Quinidine • Procainamide (Pronestyl) • Disopyramide (Norpace)
IB	• Blocks sodium influx during phase 0, which depresses the rate of depolarization • Shortens repolarization and action potential duration • Suppresses ventricular automaticity in ischemic tissue	• Lidocaine (Xylocaine) • Tocainide (Tonocard) • Mexiletine (Mexitil) • Phenytoin (Dilantin)
IC	• Blocks sodium influx, which depresses the rate of depolarization • Does not change repolarization and action potential duration • Has proarrhythmogenic potential	• Flecainide (Tambocor) • Propafenone (Rythmol)
II	• Depresses SA node automaticity • Increases refractory period of atrial and AV junctional tissue to slow conduction • Shortens action potential duration • Inhibits sympathetic activity	Beta-blockers • Propranolol (Inderal) • Esmolol (Brevibloc) • Acebutolol (Sectral) • Sotalol (Betapace) (both II and III)
III	• Blocks potassium movement during phase III • Increases action potential duration • Prolongs effective refractory period	• Bretylium (Bretylol) • Amiodarone (Cordarone) • Sotalol (Betapace) (both II and III) • Ibutilide (Corvert)
IV	• Blocks calcium movement during phase II • Depresses automaticity in the SA and AV nodes • Prolongs conduction time in the AV junction and increases the refractory period at the AV junction • Decreases contractility (negative inotrope)	Calcium channel blockers • Verapamil (Calan) • Diltiazem (Cardizem)
Misc.	• Blocks reentry mechanism • Shortens action potential of atrial tissue with little or no effect on action potential of ventricle • Prolongs AV nodal refractory period • Decreases SA node automaticity and slows sinus rate	• Adenosine (Adenocard)
Misc.	• Blocks parasympathetic nervous system effects to increase SA node firing rate and improve AV nodal conduction	• Atropine
Misc.	• Slows conduction through AV node • Prolongs AV nodal refractory period • Decreases SA node automaticity and slows sinus rate	• Digitalis

problem with impulse formation and/or conduction

A. Definition: An electronic device that delivers an electrical stimulus to the heart to depolarize the myocardium and increase or decrease the heart rate

B. Indications for pacemaker
   1. Sick sinus syndrome with syncope
      a) Symptomatic bradydysrhythmias
      b) Sinus block or sinus arrest with ventricular asystole
      c) Alternating tachycardia and bradycardia (called *tachy-brady syndrome*)
   2. Hypersensitive carotid sinus syndrome
   3. AV blocks (see Table 3-5 for Indications in Acute MI)
      a) Second-degree AV block, Mobitz type II
      b) Third-degree AV block
   4. Bifascicular block with acute MI

   5. Trifascicular block (e.g., bilateral bundle branch block)
   6. Refractory tachydysrhythmias unresponsive to drug therapy or cardioversion (referred to as *tachycardia overdrive*); an important treatment modality for torsades de pointes

C. Components (Fig. 3-8)
   1. Pulse generator
      a) Battery
      b) Circuitry
   2. Lead(s)
      a) Atrial
      b) Ventricular
   3. Electrode(s)
      a) Unipolar
         (1) Negative only
         (2) Metal of pulse generator acts as positive

Table 3-5	Indications for Temporary Transvenous Pacemaker in Presence of Acute MI		
Degree of Block		Inferior MI	Anterior MI
First-degree AV Block		No	No
Second-degree AV Block, Type I		No	NA
Second-degree AV Block, Type II		NA	Yes
Third-degree AV Block with junctional escape rhythm		No if asymptomatic Yes if symptomatic	NA
Third-degree AV Block with ventricular escape rhythm		Yes	Yes

KEY: NA = not applicable because patients with inferior MI do not develop Type II second-degree block, and patients with anterior MI do not develop Type I second-degree block or have junctional escape rhythms.

Adapted from: Grauer K, Cavallaro D: *ACLS: certification preparation and a comprehensive review*, ed 3, St Louis, 1993, Mosby Lifeline.

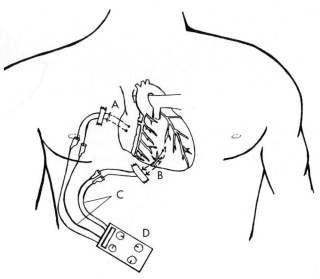

Figure 3-9 Temporary transthoracic epicardial pacing. *A,* Atrial electrodes; *B,* ventricular electrodes; *C,* leads; *D,* external pulse generator. (Drawing by Ann M. Walthall.)

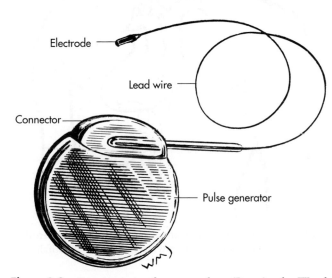

Figure 3-8 Components of a pacemaker. (Drawing by Wendy M. Johnson.)

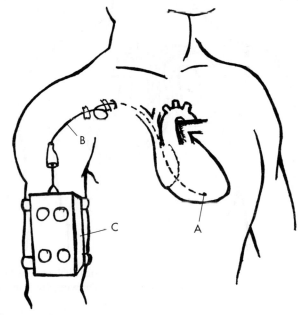

Figure 3-10 Temporary transvenous endocardial pacing. *A,* Electrode; *B,* lead; *C,* external pulse generator. (Drawing by Ann M. Walthall.)

b) Bipolar
   (1) Positive: proximal, sensing
   (2) Negative: distal, pacing
D. Types of pacemakers
   1. Temporary or permanent
      a) Temporary (external pulse generator): hours to weeks
         (1) Transthoracic epicardial (Fig. 3-9)
            (a) Electrodes attached to epicardium of atrium, ventricle, or both during cardiac surgery and brought through the chest wall

         (2) Transvenous endocardial (Fig. 3-10)
            (a) Pacing lead(s) inserted percutaneously via internal jugular or subclavian vein and advanced into RA or RV or both
         (3) Transcutaneous (Fig. 3-11)
            (a) Percutaneous leads applied to chest and back; used during cardiac arrests until transvenous pacer can be inserted
      b) Permanent (internal pulse generator): months to years
         (1) Transvenous endocardial (Fig. 3-12):

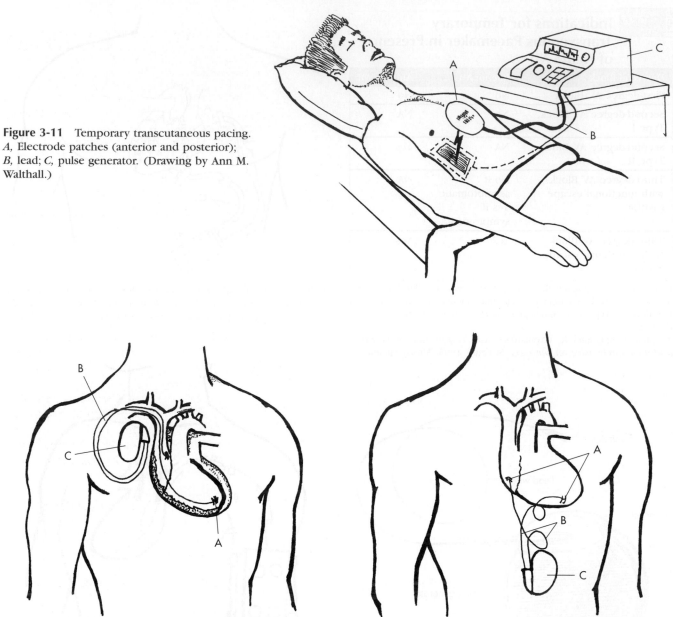

Figure 3-11 Temporary transcutaneous pacing. *A*, Electrode patches (anterior and posterior); *B*, lead; *C*, pulse generator. (Drawing by Ann M. Walthall.)

Figure 3-12 Permanent transvenous endocardial pacemaker. *A*, Electrode; *B*, lead; *C*, pulse generator. (Drawing by Ann M. Walthall.)

Figure 3-13 Permanent epicardial pacemaker. *A*, Electrodes; *B*, leads; *C*, pulse generator. (Drawing by Ann M. Walthall.)

lead inserted into cephalic vein and advanced into RA or RV; pulse generator implanted in subcutaneous fat under clavicle
  (2) Epicardial (Fig. 3-13): electrodes sewn onto epicardium (thoracotomy required); pulse generator implanted in subcutaneous fat of abdomen
2. Asynchronous versus synchronous
  a) Asynchronous
    (1) Also called *fixed rate*
    (2) The pacemaker delivers a pacing stimulus at a fixed rate regardless of the heart's intrinsic activity

    (3) Will cause competition with the heart's intrinsic activity, and the pacing stimulus may land during the descending limb of the T-wave
    (4) Rarely seen today
  b) Synchronous
    (1) Also called *demand*
    (2) The pacemaker delivers a pacing stimulus only when the heart's intrinsic pacemaker fails to function at a predetermined rate
    (3) The pacing stimulus is either inhibited or triggered when the intrinsic activity is seen
E. North American Society of Pacing and Electro-

Table 3-6	The NASPE/BPEG Generic (NBG) Pacemaker Code				
Position	**I**	**II**	**III**	**IV**	**V**
Category	Chamber(s) paced	Chamber(s) sensed	Response to sensing	Programmability, rate modulation	Antitachyarrhythmia function(s)
	O = None	O = None	O = None	O = None	O = None
	A = Atrium	A = Atrium	T = Triggered	P = Simple programmable	P = Pacing (antitachyarrhythmia)
	V = Ventricle	V = Ventricle	I = Inhibited	M = Multiprogrammable	S = Shock
	D = Dual (A + V)	D = Dual (A + V)	D = Dual (T + I)	C = Communicating	D = Dual (P + S)
				R = Rate modulation	
Manufacturers' designation only	S = single (A or V)	S = single (A or V)			

Note: Positions I through III are used exclusively for antibradyarrhythmia function.

physiology (NASPE) generic code (Table 3-6) and types of pacemakers (Table 3-7)
1. Chamber of stimulation
   a) Atrial: AOO, AAI
      (1) Pacing stimulus occurs before the P-wave
      (2) Requires an intact AV node
   b) Ventricular: VOO, VAT, VVI, VVT, VDD
      (1) Pacing stimulus occurs before the QRS complex
   c) Atrioventricular (AV) sequential: DOO, DVI, DDD
      (1) Maintains AV synchrony and the hemodynamic benefit of the atrial kick
      (2) Pacing stimulus before both or either P-wave or QRS complex
      (3) Sufficient AV delay set to allow atrial depolarization and contraction to complete ventricular filling
2. Rate-responsive: The heart rate is adjusted according to demands for cardiac output
   a) Heart rate changes are stimulated by changes in muscle activity, minute ventilation, or blood changes in temperature or pH
   b) Rate-responsive modes: AAIR, VVIR, DDDR
F. ECG evidence of pacing (Fig. 3-14)
   1. Spike before paced event
   2. Wide QRS if ventricular pacer
   3. Presence of T-wave confirms ventricular depolarization
   4. Presence of fusion beats (Fig. 3-15)
G. Complications
   1. Infection
   2. Pneumothorax
   3. Myocardial perforation
   4. Hematoma
   5. Frozen shoulder
   6. Dysrhythmias
   7. Electrical malfunction (Table 3-8)
H. Collaborative management
   1. Temporary

   a) Maintain electrical safety
      (1) Ensure proper grounding of equipment
      (2) Touch siderails before touching patient to discharge static electricity
      (3) Wear rubber gloves when making adjustments
      (4) Avoid sources of electromagnetic interference (EMI) (e.g., electrocautery, defibrillation, MRI, transcutaneous electrical nerve stimulation [TENS] units, radiation therapy, lithotripsy)
   b) Prevent complications
      (1) Cover dial to prevent accidental changes in settings
      (2) Limit mobility of affected extremity to prevent accidental catheter dislodgement
      (3) Observe catheter site for signs of infection
      (4) Observe cardiac monitor for pacemaker malfunction
   2. Permanent
   a) Prevent complications
      (1) Limit mobility for affected upper extremity for 48 hours to prevent lead dislodgement
      (2) Encourage arm exercise after 48 hours to prevent frozen shoulder (ankylosis)
      (3) Observe incision for signs of infection
      (4) Observe cardiac monitor for pacemaker malfunction
   b) Provide patient and family instruction
      (1) Teach patient how to take pulse, symptoms to report
      (2) Teach patient sources of electromagnetic interference (EMI) to avoid (e.g., MRI, metal detectors, radio transmitters, electrical generating plants)

Table 3-7	Types of Pacemakers			
Code	**Description**	**Indications**	**Advantages**	**Disadvantages**
AOO	• Fixed-rate atrial pacer	• Consistently slow sinus rate with intact AV nodal conduction	• Single lead • Maintains AV synchrony	• Atrial competition • No protection in case of AV nodal block
AAI	• Demand atrial pacer	• Sick sinus syndrome • Sinus arrest • Sinus bradycardia • Must have intact AV nodal conduction	• Single lead • Maintains AV synchrony	• No protection in case of AV nodal block
VOO	• Fixed-rate ventricular pacer	• Complete heart block with slow idioventricular rhythm • Rarely used today	• Single lead • Protection from ventricular asystole	• Ventricular competition with possible stimulation of ventricular dysrhythmias
VAT	• Atrial-triggered ventricular pacer	• Complete heart block with intact sinus node	• Synchronized AV conduction with atrial "kick" optimizes cardiac output • Ventricular rate increases with atrial rate so more exercise responsive	• Two leads • May cause pacemaker-mediated tachycardia: rapid ventricular response in sinus or atrial dysrhythmias
VVI	• Demand ventricular pacer	• Sick sinus syndrome • Sinus bradycardia • Sinus arrest • Complete heart block	• Single lead • Simple and reliable • Inexpensive • Protection from ventricular asystole • Little chance of competitive rhythms	• Loss of synchronized AV conduction and atrial "kick" may reduce cardiac output • Not rate responsive (**Note:** VVIR is a VVI with rate-responsiveness)
VVT	• Pacing stimulus delivered if needed or not; stimulus depolarizes ventricle if no intrinsic depolarization; stimulus lands harmlessly in QRS if intrinsic depolarization	• Sick sinus syndrome • Sinus bradycardia • Sinus arrest • Complete heart block	• Single lead • Can evaluate pacer function even if intrinsic activity faster than pacer rate	• Loss of synchronized AV conduction and atrial "kick" may reduce cardiac output • Not rate responsive • Difficult to evaluate QRS morphology
VDD	• Ventricular pacer that can be atrial triggered or inhibited by intrinsic ventricular depolarization	• Sick sinus syndrome • Sinus bradycardia • Sinus arrest • Complete heart block	• Maintains AV synchrony • If atrial activity is present as pacer functions in atrial triggered mode; if no atrial activity, paces the ventricle in demand mode with inhibition to intrinsic ventricular depolarization	• Two leads • May cause pacemaker-mediated tachycardia • Does not pace the atria, so loss of atrial contraction if no intrinsic atrial activity
DOO	• Fixed-rate AV sequential pacer	• Consistently slow atrial and ventricular rate	• Synchronized AV conduction with atrial "kick" optimizes cardiac output	• Two leads • Not rate responsive • Atrial and ventricular competition

XII. Prepare and care for the patient with an automatic, implantable cardioverter defibrillator (AICD)
   A. Definition: implantable device to provide for immediate termination of VT or VF in patients in whom these dysrhythmias cannot be pharmacologically or surgically controlled

B. Tiered therapy (also called *third-generation*) devices have all of the following:
   1. Antitachycardia pacing
   2. Low-energy cardioversion
   3. High-energy defibrillation
   4. Bradycardia backup pacing

Table 3-7	Types of Pacemakers—cont'd			
Code	**Description**	**Indications**	**Advantages**	**Disadvantages**
DVI	• Fixed-rate atrial pacer with demand ventricular pacer	• Sick sinus syndrome • Sinus bradycardia • Sinus arrest • Complete heart block	• Synchronized AV conduction with atrial "kick" optimizes cardiac output	• Two leads • Not rate responsive • Blind to intrinsic atrial activity so atrial competition and even atrial fibrillation may occur
DDD	• Demand atrial and ventricular pacer; ventricular pacing may be atrial triggered or ventricular inhibited	• Sick sinus syndrome • Sinus bradycardia • Sinus arrest • Complete heart block	• Synchronized AV conduction with atrial "kick" optimizes cardiac output • Near normal physiologic function	• Two leads • Most expensive • May cause pacemaker-mediated tachycardia • Difficult troubleshooting • Is not used in atrial fibrillation

PACED HEART ACTIVITY

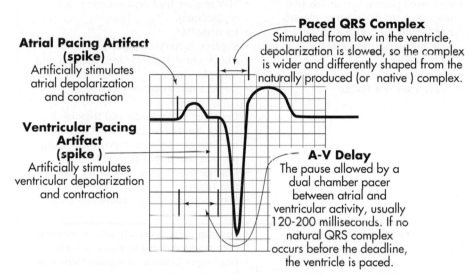

Atrial Pacing Artifact (spike)
Artificially stimulates atrial depolarization and contraction

Ventricular Pacing Artifact (spike)
Artificially stimulates ventricular depolarization and contraction

Paced QRS Complex
Stimulated from low in the ventricle, depolarization is slowed, so the complex is wider and differently shaped from the naturally produced (or native) complex.

A-V Delay
The pause allowed by a dual chamber pacer between atrial and ventricular activity, usually 120-200 milliseconds. If no natural QRS complex occurs before the deadline, the ventricle is paced.

Figure 3-14 ECG evidence of pacing (From Witherell C: Questions nurses ask about pacemakers, *AJN* 90 (12):20, 1990.

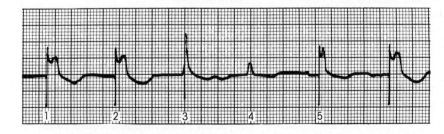

Figure 3-15 Fusion beat. Complexes 1 and 2 are paced complexes; complex 3 is a fusion beat with both the paced impulse and an intrinsic impulse merging to cause this ventricular depolarization; complex 4 is an intrinsic complex; complex 5 is a paced complex. (From Guzzetta CE, Dossey BM: *Cardiovascular nursing: holistic practice,* St Louis, 1992, Mosby.)

C. Indications
   1. Patients with VT or VF that is inducible during EPS studies despite antidysrhythmic therapies
   2. Survivors of non–MI-related cardiac arrest that cannot be induced during EPS studies
D. Contraindications
   1. Frequent episodes of VT or VF (more than 2 events per month)
   2. Uncontrolled HF

   3. Less than 6 to 12 months of productive life expectancy
   4. History of noncompliance
   5. Extreme psychologic barriers to use of the device
E. Components (Fig. 3-16)
   1. Generator
     a) Processes information from the lead system and delivers the electrical impulses

Table 3-8   **Pacemaker Electrical Malfunctions**

Malfunction	Causes	Interventions
Failure to fire (pace) • Pacemaker does not fire when physiologically indicated • Recognized by pauses longer than the automatic interval and absence of pacer spike at end of escape interval	• Loose connections • Battery depletion • Lead displacement • Lead fracture • Sensing malfunction	• Check connections if temporary • Replace battery or pulse generator • Lead repositioning or replacement may be needed • Evaluate patient's own rhythm and patient's response; if inadequate, administer atropine, CPR, and/or apply external transcutaneous pacemaker • May be caused by sensing malfunction; to identify a sensing malfunction, convert pacemaker to asynchronous by placing a magnet over an implanted pacemaker or switching to asynchronous on an external pacemaker • If pacer spikes seen in asynchronous mode, sensing malfunction exists
Failure to capture • Pacemaker fires but depolarization does not occur • Recognized by spike not followed by depolarization (e.g., P-wave if atrial pacer or QRS if ventricular pacer)	• Displacement of lead • Lead fracture • Increased pacing thresholds (e.g., fibrosis at tip of catheter, electrolyte imbalance, drug toxicity, acid-base imbalance, ischemia) • Battery failure • Chamber perforation • Complexes not visible	• Position patient on left side or to whatever position capture was last seen • May require lead repositioning, lead replacement • Increase MA • Replace battery or pulse generator • Check chest X-ray for lead fracture and lead placement • Correct metabolic or electrolyte imbalance • Consider drugs levels and toxicity • Check for diaphragmatic pacing and monitor or cardiac tamponade if catheter perforation is suspected • Change monitoring lead or increase ECG size (gain) • May require external transcutaneous pacing or CPR
Failure to sense • Pacemaker fails to recognize intrinsic activity (e.g., P-wave or QRS) • Recognized by pacer spikes falling closer to the intrinsic beats than the escape interval; spikes land indiscriminately throughout the cardiac cycle, including potentially on the descending limb of the T-wave	• Displacement of lead • Lead fracture • Sensitivity set too low or set on asynchronous • Disconnection of sensing circuit • Inadequate signal (e.g., PVCs) • Battery failure	• Position patient on left side or to whatever position sensing was last seen • Lead repositioning or replacement may be necessary • Make sure that pacer is not set on asynchronous • Increase sensitivity • Check connections on temporary pacemaker • Administer lidocaine if nonsensed QRSs are PVCs • Check chest X-ray for lead placement or lead fracture • Replace battery or pulse generator • If patient's own rhythm adequate, turn pacer off or heart rate down to minimum • If patient's own rhythm inadequate, increase pacer rate to override patient's own rhythm
Oversensing • Pacemaker recognizes extraneous electrical activity or the wrong intrinsic electrical activity as the inhibiting event • Recognized by absence of pacer spikes and failure to fire	• Sensitivity set too high • Electromagnetic interference (EMI) • Oversensing of P-waves or T-waves • Myopotentials • Crosstalk (no ventricular pacing)	• Decrease sensitivity • Remove from EMI • Ensure that all equipment is properly grounded • Decrease atrial output, decrease ventricular sensitivity, increase ventricular blanking period • May require external transcutaneous pacing or CPR

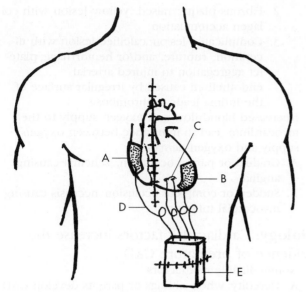

Figure 3-16 Automatic implantable cardioverter defibrillator. *A,* Right atrial defibrillator patch; *B,* left ventricular defibrillator patch; *C,* two unipolar right ventricular electrodes; *D,* leads; *E,* pulse generator. (Drawing by Ann M. Walthall.)

    b) Stores information about the patient's heart rhythm and therapy delivered
    c) Placed in the left upper quadrant of abdomen or under the clavicle
    d) Usually lasts about 3 to 5 years before replacement required
  2. Multi-lead system
    a) Two ventricular patches
      (1) Sewn to the epicardium or placed outside the pericardial sac
      (2) Some models include an additional subcutaneous patch
    b) Two leads that sense cardiac events
F. Method
  1. System evaluates heart rate and probability density function (PDF)
    a) PDF diagnoses the amount of time the ECG spends away from the isoelectric baseline
  2. System is turned on and off by using a donut-shaped magnet
    a) Device is not usually turned on during early postoperative period due to frequent occurrence of sinus tachycardia during this period
  3. When VT is sensed, the AICD will first initiate antitachycardia pacing
  4. If the VT is not successfully pace-terminated, the AICD will cardiovert the rhythm with low-energy synchronized shocks
  5. If the rhythm deteriorates to VF or if VF is the initial rhythm, the AICD will defibrillate at a higher energy level
  6. Once a shock is delivered, the device senses the rhythm

  7. If sinus rhythm is not restored, up to five shocks of 25 to 35 joules are delivered
  8. If the electrical rhythm deteriorates to bradycardia or asystole, the bradycardia backup pacing function is activated
G. Complications
  1. Atelectasis
  2. Pneumonia
  3. Pneumothorax
  4. Lead migration
  5. Lead fracture
H. Collaborative management
  1. Provide postoperative management as for medial sternotomy, lateral thoracotomy, subxiphoid thoracotomy if either of those approaches used; may also be inserted through a small upper anterior thoracic incision or transvenously
  2. Monitor for dysrhythmias and evaluate effectiveness of AICD if firing occurs
    a) Administer antidysrhythmic agents as prescribed
    b) If cardiac arrest occurs, do the following:
      (1) Obtain emergency equipment and prepare to cardiovert or defibrillate if the device fails to resuscitate the patient
      (2) If device is functioning, let it deliver the full series of shocks (usually 3-6 shocks)
      (3) Initiate ACLS protocol if the AICD did not successfully convert the dysrhythmia
      (4) Do not place defibrillator paddles within 5 to 10 cm of the generator
  3. Monitor for complications
    a) Observe incision for signs of infection
    b) Observe for clinical indications of cardiac tamponade
  4. Encourage the patient to express fears and concerns about being shocked
  5. Provide resuscitation efforts in a patient with AICD
XIII. Prepare and care for the patient having ablation therapy
A. Use: To eradicate dysrhythmia in patients who experience frequent, disabling, or life-threatening dysrhythmias that are not suppressed with pharmacologic therapy or in whom pharmacologic therapy is not well tolerated
B. Types
  1. Radio-frequency catheter ablation
    a) A catheter is placed in the heart via cardiac catheterization
    b) Radio-frequency energy is applied to the area in which the dysrhythmia originates or an accessory pathway (e.g., WPW)
    c) Controlled, localized necrosis occurs

d) Postprocedure care is as for cardiac catheterization or angioplasty; monitor closely for dysrhythmias

2. Surgical ablation: The area in which the dysrhythmia originates is either excised or eliminated by cryosurgery or laser

XIV. Prepare for and care for the patient having maze procedure
   A. Cardiothoracic surgery for atrial fibrillation
   B. A maze of carefully planned sutures create an electrical conduction route through atrial myocardium, corralling and herding chaotic atrial impulses from the SA node to the AV node
   C. Provide postoperative management as for cardiothoracic surgery

Coronary Artery Disease

Definition: A progressive disease of the coronary arteries that results in their narrowing or obstruction

Pathophysiology

I. Arteriosclerosis: a group of diseases characterized by thickening and loss of elasticity (calcification) of arterial walls

II. Atherosclerosis: the most common form of arteriosclerosis
   A. A chronic disease process characterized by the build-up of fatty plaque along the subintimal layer of arteries leading to a decrease in arterial lumen
   B. Demand angina caused by 75% occlusion of the coronary artery lumen; angina at rest caused by 99% occlusion
   C. Progression (Fig. 3-17)
      1. Fatty streak: yellow, smooth lesion of lipid

2. Fibrous plaque: raised, yellow lesion with collagen accumulation

3. Complicated lesion: calcified lesion with ulceration, rupture, and/or hemorrhage; platelet aggregation to injured arterial endothelium caused by irregular surface of the intima leads to thrombosis

III. Decreased blood flow and oxygen supply to the myocardium lead to imbalance between oxygen supply and oxygen demand
   A. Gradual or partial occlusion: ischemia causing angina
   B. Sudden or complete occlusion: necrosis causing myocardial infarction

Etiology: Cardiac risk factors increase the incidence of premature CAD

I. Nonmodifiable risk factors
   A. Heredity: when siblings or parents develop CAD before 55 years of age
      1. Maternal history of CAD before 65 years conveys greater risk than paternal history in women
      2. Several risk factors have genetic predisposition (e.g., hypertension, hyperlipidemia, diabetes mellitus)
   B. Advancing age: when age for males is greater than 45 years and for females greater than 55 years
   C. Gender: males have twice the risk of premenopausal females; risk increases in women after menopause but risk is reduced by hormone replacement therapy (HRT)

II. Modifiable risk factors
   A. Hypertension: BP greater than 160/95 mm Hg; desirable BP level is less than or equal to 140/90 mm Hg

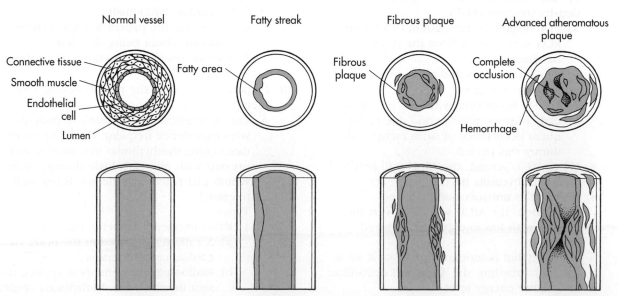

Normal vessel   Fatty streak   Fibrous plaque   Advanced atheromatous plaque

Connective tissue
Smooth muscle
Endothelial cell
Lumen

Fatty area

Fibrous plaque

Complete occlusion

Hemorrhage

Figure 3-17 Progression of atherosclerosis. (From Thelan LA et al: *Critical care nursing: diagnosis and management,* ed 3, St Louis, 1998, Mosby.)

B. Hyperlipidemia: elevated levels of cholesterol, triglycerides, or low-density lipoproteins (LDL) and/or decreased levels of high-density lipoproteins (HDL); desirable levels of lipids are the following:
1. Cholesterol level less than 200 mg/dl
2. LDL level less than 130 mg/dl
3. HDL level more than 35 mg/dl
4. Triglyceride level less than 200 mg/dl

C. Smoking: smoking increases platelet aggregation, fibrinogen levels, and may cause vasospasm; elevated carbon monoxide levels decrease the oxygen-carrying capacity of hemoglobin; complete smoking cessation is desired

D. Diabetes mellitus or glucose intolerance: control of blood glucose in patients with diabetes mellitus is advocated to control risk of sequelae including CAD; desirable fasting glucose level is less than 150 mg/dl

E. Hyperhomocystinemia: homocysteine level more than 15 μmol/L
1. Homocysteine is an essential sulfur-containing amino acid formed during the processing of dietary protein; elevated levels are toxic to the vascular endothelium and increase coagulability
2. Deficiencies of folate, vitamin B_{12}, and vitamin B_6 have all been implicated in elevated levels of homocysteine, and elevated levels of homocysteine may be successfully reduced by folate, vitamin B_{12}, and/or pyridoxine therapy

F. Sedentary lifestyle: exercise is inversely related to cardiovascular mortality; sedentary people also tend to be obese

G. Stress
1. Chronic stress promotes the long-term development of CAD
2. Acute stress increases catecholamine levels, myocardial oxygen consumption, and dysrhythmia potential
3. Personality type A with aggression may also contribute

H. Obesity: body weight more than 120% of ideal body weight; ideal body weight is desirable
1. Obesity also contributes to hypertension, hyperlipidemia, glucose intolerance, and sedentary lifestyle
2. Midline fat is of greater risk than hip and thigh fat (apple versus pear)

I. Oral contraceptives: increase risk of MI especially in smokers; increases BP; smoking cessation is desirable for all people but especially in women who use oral contraceptives

III. Protective factors
A. Exercise (HR 50%-80% of predicted maximal HR for 20-60 minutes, 3-5 times/week)
1. Elevates HDL
2. Decreases BP and resting HR
3. Decreases body fat
4. Increases endogenous tissue plasminogen activator (tPA) levels

B. Stress management: daily stretching, breathing exercises, meditation, prayer, yoga

C. Estrogen: increases HDL and may decrease platelet aggregation

D. High-fiber, low fat diet: reduces total cholesterol

E. Alcohol (1-2 beverages per day): increases HDL and may decrease platelet aggregation; overall health benefit diminishes after 1 to 2 alcoholic beverages per day

F. ASA (81-325 mg daily): prevents platelet aggregation; decreases inflammation (one postulated cause of CAD)

G. Folic acid (0.65-1 mg daily): prevents hyperhomocystinemia

H. Antioxidants (vitamins C [1 g] and vitamin E [400-800 IU] daily): prevent oxygen-free radical damage

I. Loving relationships: decrease the overall incidence of CAD, although mechanisms are unclear (loneliness has been identified for years as contributing factor to CAD); pets also have a beneficial effect by decreasing stress and depression

Pathologic Consequences of Atherosclerosis, Arteriosclerosis

I. Angina pectoris
II. Myocardial infarction
III. Heart failure (e.g., ischemic cardiomyopathy)
IV. Dysrhythmias caused by ischemia
V. Sudden death

Angina Pectoris

Definition: Transient chest pain associated with myocardial ischemia

Etiology

I. Factors that decrease supply
A. Arteriosclerosis/atherosclerosis
B. Coronary artery spasm
C. Aortitis
D. Dysrhythmias
E. Anemia
F. Shock

II. Factors that increase demand
A. Hypertension
B. Aortic valve disease
C. Tachydysrhythmias
D. Heart failure (HF)
E. Hyperthyroidism

Pathophysiology

I. A temporary imbalance exists between myocardial oxygen supply and myocardial oxygen demand, which causes ischemia
A. Common precipitating factors: 5Es + smoking
1. Exercise: volume work (e.g., walking, running, swimming)

2. Exertion: pressure work (e.g., lifting, pushing, Valsalva maneuver)
3. Emotion: catecholamine release
4. Eating: shunting of blood to gut
5. Exposure to cold: vasoconstriction
6. Smoking
   a) Nicotine increases heart rate and blood pressure
   b) Carbon monoxide decreases oxygen-carrying capacity of hemoglobin
II. Ischemia leads to anaerobic metabolism and accumulation of lactic acid, causing chest pain
III. Angina is associated with a coronary artery occlusion of 75% or more

Clinical Presentation

I. Subjective
   A. Substernal chest discomfort that usually lasts 1 to 4 minutes (but may last up to 15 minutes) and subsides with rest and/or nitroglycerin (NTG)
      1. Discomfort may be described as burning, squeezing, tightness, pressure, heaviness, indigestion, aching
      2. Pain may radiate to shoulders, back, arms, jaw, neck, epigastrium
      3. Precipitating factors: 5Es + smoking
   B. Dyspnea
   C. Nausea/vomiting
   D. Anxiety
   E. Weakness
II. Objective
   A. Tachycardia
   B. Hypotension or hypertension
   C. Tachypnea
   D. Levine's sign: clenched fist held over sternum
   E. Pallor
   F. Diaphoresis
   G. S_4
III. Diagnostic
   A. Serum
      1. Isoenzymes: negative for cardiac damage
      2. Lipid profile (fasting): to identify hyperlipidemia as a risk factor
      3. Fasting glucose: to identify diabetes mellitus or glucose intolerance as a risk factor
   B. Electrocardiogram
      1. ST segment depression in unstable angina
      2. ST segment elevation in Prinzmetal's angina
      3. Ventricular dysrhythmias may be present
   C. Graded exercise stress test: may or may not be positive; sensitivity lower with women
   D. Cardiac catheterization: coronary artery occlusion 75% or greater; may be negative in Prinzmetal's angina but develop occlusion from spasm
   E. Echocardiography: may show segmental wall motion defects
   F. Myocardial perfusion scan with thallium 201: cold areas indicating ischemia
IV. Types (Table 3-9)

Nursing Diagnoses

I. Chest Pain related to myocardial ischemia
II. Alteration in Cardiopulmonary Tissue Perfusion related to coronary artery occlusion
III. Activity Intolerance related to chest pain or fear of chest pain, adverse effects of medication (e.g., beta-blockers)
IV. Knowledge Deficit related to unfamiliarity with disease process, therapy, and required lifestyle changes

Collaborative Management

I. Relieve chest pain
   A. Nitroglycerin (NTG)
      1. Usually sublingual tablets or metered-dose spray
      2. Intravenous nitroglycerin may be used in unstable angina
      3. NTG is most valuable in increasing oxygen supply if good collateral circulation exists (diseased coronary arteries do not dilate well because they are relatively immobilized by calcium deposits in the media)
   B. Calcium channel blockers (Table 3-10) (e.g., nifedipine [Procardia]); especially for Prinzmetal's angina
   C. Morphine sulfate may be required for unstable angina
II. Increase oxygen supply
   A. Oxygen via nasal cannula: 5 L/min during ischemic pain unless contraindicated by chronic lung disease; in patients with chronic lung disease use pulse oximetry to guide oxygen administration (aim for an SpO_2 of 90%)
   B. NTG in doses greater than 1 μg/kg/min causes arterial as well as venous dilation; since diseased coronary arteries are calcified and immobilized, NTG works best to increase supply in patients who have good collateral circulation
   C. Calcium channel blockers or NTG if angina caused by coronary artery spasm
   D. Blood transfusion if angina caused by anemia
   E. Dysrhythmias management
      1. Tachydysrhythmias decrease the time for coronary artery filling and may decrease cardiac output
      2. Bradydysrhythmias increase the time for coronary artery filling but may decrease cardiac output
   F. Platelet aggregation inhibitors (e.g., ASA, ticlopidine [Ticlid], clopidogrel [Plavix]) to prevent platelet aggregation; heparin may be prescribed to prevent clotting or extension of a clot
   G. Intraaortic balloon pump may be used in unstable angina; IABP increases coronary artery perfusion pressure
III. Decrease oxygen demand
   A. Removal of provoking factors
      1. Activity cessation immediately when chest pain occurs

Table 3-9 Types of Angina

Stable	• Unchanging frequency, duration, and severity • Predictable to the patient • ST segment depression may occur during pain
Types of Unstable Angina	**Description**
• De novo angina	• Angina of new onset
• Crescendo angina: angina that has increased in frequency, intensity, or duration • Preinfarction: angina of prolonged duration that occurs even at rest	• Associated with progression of CAD • Less exertion to cause pain or pain at rest • Greater severity • Longer duration • More difficult to relieve and may not be relieved with nitroglycerin • May have ST segment depression during pain
• Wellen's syndrome: critical proximal LAD stenosis	• Associated with critical proximal LAD stenosis • Characteristic ECG changes that appear even in a pain-free state 　• ST segment isoelectric or elevated no more than 1 mm in V_1-V_3 　• Symmetrical T-wave inversion in V_2-V_3 　• No loss of normal R-wave progression in V_1-V_3 　• No pathologic Q-waves • Normal or slightly elevated enzymes • Emergency cardiac catheterization is indicated
• Prinzmetal's (also called *variant* or *vasospastic*)	• Associated with coronary artery spasm 　• Pain occurs at rest 　• May be caused by tobacco, alcohol, or cocaine • Pain lasts longer than usual anginal pain: 10 minutes or more • ST segment elevation during pain

Table 3-10 Effects of Calcium Channel Blockers

Type of Calcium Channel Blocker	Coronary Arterial Dilation	Peripheral Arterial Dilation	AV Nodal Depression	SA Nodal Depression	Effect on LV Contractility
Dihydropyridine type (e.g., nifedipine [Procardia] or nicardipine [Cardene])	+	+++	0	0	0
Diphenylalkylamine type (diltiazem [Cardizem])	+	++	↓	↓	↓
Benzothiazepine type (verapamil [Calan])	+	+	↓	↓	↓↓

Adapted from: Grauer K, Cavalaro D: *ACLS: certification preparation and a comprehensive review,* ed 3, St Louis, 1993, Mosby Lifeline.

　2. Bed rest during pain; semi-Fowler's position usually most comfortable for the patient
B. NTG as prescribed
　1. NTG in doses less than 1 µg/kg/min is a predominantly venous dilator; it decreases myocardial workload and myocardial oxygen consumption by decreasing preload
　2. NTG in doses greater than 1 µg/kg/min is an arterial as well as venous dilator; it decreases myocardial workload and myocardial oxygen consumption by decreasing afterload and preload
C. Beta-blockers (Table 3-11) as prescribed
　1. Beta-blockers decrease myocardial workload and myocardial oxygen demand by decreasing HR and contractility
　2. Beta-blockers are contraindicated in Prinzmetal's angina; blocking beta receptors leaves alpha receptors unopposed and perpetuates vascular spasm
D. Calcium channel blockers (Table 3-10) as prescribed
　1. Calcium channel blockers dilate arteries and veins, decreasing myocardial workload and myocardial oxygen consumption by decreasing preload and afterload
　2. Calcium channel blockers are the drugs of choice for Prinzmetal's angina since they are excellent antispasmotics

3-11	Beta-Blockers	
Noncardioselective	**Cardioselective**
Propranolol (Inderal)	Acebutolol (Sectral)
Nadolol (Corgard)	Atenolol (Tenormin)
Timolol (Blocadren)	Metoprolol (Lopressor)
Pindolol (Visken)	Esmolol (Brevibloc)
Carteolol (Cartrol)	Betaxolol (Betoptic)
Penbutolol (Levatol)	Bisoprolol (Zebeta)
Labetalol (Normodyne) (α and β)	
Carvedilol (Coreg) (α and β)	

E. Control dysrhythmias: tachydysrhythmias increase myocardial workload and myocardial oxygen consumption
F. Decrease catecholamine release
   1. Establish and maintain a calm, quiet environment
   2. Keep the patient and family informed
   3. Restrict stimulants
IV. Monitor for complications
   A. Progression to myocardial infarction (MI)
   B. Dysrhythmias
   C. Mitral regurgitation caused by ischemia and dysfunction of papillary muscles
   D. Heart failure
V. Additional treatments
   A. Identify risk factors and encourage modification to decelerate arteriosclerotic/atherosclerotic process
   B. Percutaneous coronary interventions (Table 3-12) are utilized to open the lumen of diseased coronary artery (or arteries) and restore blood flow
   C. Coronary artery bypass graft (Table 3-13) is utilized to provide arterial or venous conduits to redirect coronary blood flow around occluded coronary arteries
   D. Transmyocardial revascularization
      1. Used in patient with inoperable, class IV angina; patient must have an ejection fraction of at least 20%
      2. High-powered carbon dioxide laser used to create 15 to 30 transmural channels that direct nonarterial oxygenation to the ischemic myocardium
      3. Performed through left anterolateral thoracotomy without slowing of the functioning heart or transvenously

Myocardial Infarction
Etiology
I. Arteriosclerosis/atherosclerosis
II. Coronary artery thrombosis
III. Coronary artery spasm
IV. Cocaine-induced: excessive sympathetic stimulation causes tachycardia, hypertension, arterial vasoconstriction and spasm; coronary artery spasm may cause MI especially non–Q-wave infarction
V. Combination of these factors: most MIs are caused by atherosclerosis and thrombosis
VI. Other less commonly seen causes
   A. Severe, prolonged hypotension
   B. Chest trauma (e.g., myocardial contusion)
   C. Trauma to coronary artery or arteries
   D. Aortic stenosis or insufficiency
   E. Thyrotoxicosis
   F. Blood dyscrasias
   G. Aortic dissection
   H. Arteritis
   I. Carbon monoxide poisoning

Pathophysiology
I. Prolonged imbalance between myocardial oxygen supply and demand
II. Inadequate oxygenation causes anaerobic metabolism
III. Anaerobic metabolism causes lactic acidosis
IV. Prolonged ischemia causes electrical and mechanical death of myocardium
   A. Electrical death causes Q-waves on ECG
   B. Mechanical death causes loss of contractility and poor wall motion on echocardiogram
V. Contractility and compliance is decreased, causing left ventricular dysfunction
   A. Decrease in contractility may cause S_3
   B. Decrease in compliance causes S_4
VI. Ischemia, injury, and acidosis cause electrical irritability; this condition potentially leads to PVCs, ventricular tachycardia, ventricular fibrillation
VII. Healing takes approximately 2 to 3 months; a firm, white scar is formed but it does not contract or conduct electrical impulses

Classifications
I. Q-wave versus non–Q-wave: presence of Q wave correlates to mass loss of myocardium
   A. Non–Q-wave infarctions: partial occlusions or early reperfusion
      1. Spontaneous reperfusion: cessation of spasm or endogenous tPA (remember that exercise increases endogenous tPA levels)
      2. Therapeutic reperfusion: thrombolytics or percutaneous coronary intervention (PCI)
   B. Acute coronary syndrome: term used to refer to unstable angina or non–Q-wave MI
II. Left versus right ventricular: Table 3-14 describes wall of MI along with coronary artery affected, indicative ECG leads, and anticipated complications
   A. Left ventricular myocardial infarction (LVMI): most MIs are LV
      1. Anterior LV: 42%
      2. Septal LV: 10%
      3. Lateral LV: 10%
      4. Inferior LV: 33%
      5. Posterior LV: 5%
   B. Right ventricular myocardial infarction (RVMI)
      1. Concurrent with inferior LVMI; one third of all inferior MIs have concurrent RV infarction

Text continued on p. 131

Table 3-12

Table 3-12 Percutaneous Coronary Interventions

Procedures	• Percutaneous transluminal coronary angioplasty (PTCA): inflation of a balloon-tipped catheter in an area of coronary artery stenosis from plaque; plaque is pushed back against the wall of the vessel and fractured (controlled trauma)
	• Coronary artery stent: use of a stainless steel wire coil that acts as a scaffolding device to support a coronary artery and maintain patency after PTCA; previously used only in case of acute closure, more than 60% of PTCA patients now get stents
	• Coronary atherectomy: removal of plaque from coronary artery by a high-speed diamond-tipped (rotational) or shaving (directional) device
	  • Directional coronary atherectomy (DCA): a directional device shaves pieces of the atheroma into the catheter tip
	  • Coronary rotational ablation (Rotablator): a diamond-coated burr drills through the atheroma and pulverizes the plaque
	  • Transluminal extraction catheter (TEC): a motorized cutting head shaves the atheroma from the arterial wall and suctions out the pieces
	• Excimer laser coronary atherectomy (ELCA): use of a laser to vaporize the atheroma

Indications	• Unstable or chronic angina • Acute or postacute MI • Postcoronary artery bypass graft with postoperative angina • Patient must be surgical candidate (in case of coronary artery dissection)
Contraindications	• Left main CAD (unless there is a patent bypass around it, referred to as *protected*) • Stenosis of coronary artery at orifice • Variant angina • Critical valvular disease
Action	• The goal of percutaneous coronary interventions is to reduce the degree of coronary artery stenosis; the intervention is considered successful if the degree of stenosis is reduced to 20%-30% without serious complications
Assessment	• Vital signs: BP, HR, respiratory rate, T • ECG: monitor closely for ST segment elevation • Sheath insertion site • Neurovascular status of affected limb • Any complaints of chest pain • Any complaints of back pain
Nursing Diagnoses	• Altered Cardiopulmonary Tissue Perfusion related to thrombosis, acute closure, or spasm • Potential for Chest Pain related to myocardial ischemia • Altered Peripheral Tissue Perfusion related to arterial trauma, mechanical occlusion by sheath, vasospasm, hematoma, swelling • Back Pain related to immobilization • Activity Intolerance related to immobilization and deconditioning • Altered Protection related to arterial sheath, anticoagulation • Anxiety related to acute health alteration and recommended lifestyle changes • Knowledge Deficit related to procedure, therapy, recommended lifestyle changes

Brief summary of specific nursing management	• Assess puncture site frequently to detect bleeding and/or hematoma formation
	  • Control systolic BP to less than 150 mm Hg and diastolic BP less than 90 mm Hg with antihypertensives as prescribed
	  • Monitor platelet count and aPTT (patient will have received platelet aggregation inhibitors and heparin to prevent reocclusion)
	  • Immobilize groin by restraining with sheet stretched over knee on affected side and tucked on each side of bed rather than restraining ankle
	  • Perform neurovascular checks to detect peripheral ischemia related to femoral artery thrombosis
	• Monitor for clinical indications of retroperitoneal hemorrhage: postural tachycardia and/or hypotension; back and/or flank pain; Grey Turner's sign; decrease in Hgb, Hct (unfortunately there are no early indications)
	• Keep affected limb straight and immobile; head of bed should be elevated no more than 30 degrees as long as the sheath is in place and for 4-8 hours after removal
	• Assist with removal or remove sheath (depending on hospital protocol)
	  • Usually next morning after heparin has been discontinued for 2-4 hours and ACT is less than 150 seconds; heparin is usually restarted several hours after sheath removal
	  • Pain control and sedation (e.g., local infiltration with lidocaine and/or IV morphine, midazolam [Versed], or lorazepam [Ativan])
	  • Apply pressure to where the sheath entered the artery, which is about 1 inch above the skin entry site
	  • Manual pressure or mechanical pressure devices (e.g., C-clamp, FemoStop) may be used
	  • Pressure is held for at least 30 minutes or until hemostasis is achieved
	  • Control of bleeding must be maintained while peripheral pulses are still palpated

Continued

Table 3-12 Percutaneous Coronary Interventions—cont'd

Complications	• Coronary artery dissection: due to catheter trauma; necessitates emergent coronary artery bypass graft
	• Cardiac tamponade: due to cardiac perforation
	• Dysrhythmias: due to ischemia or reperfusion
	• Pseudoaneurysm: due to catheter dissection of artery
	• Hemorrhage or hematoma: due to anticoagulated state
	• Retroperitoneal hemorrhage or hematoma
	• Femoral artery puncture site hemorrhage or hematoma
	• Embolic complications (e.g., myocardial infarction, cerebral infarction, peripheral emboli)
	• Acute reocclusion or closure: due to:
	  • Trauma to intima initiating clotting cascade
	  • ASA, GP IIb/IIIa platelet receptor blockers (e.g., abciximab [ReoPro], eptifibatide [Integrilin], tirofiban HCl [Aggrastat]), and heparin are used to prevent thrombosis; ASA and ticlopidine (Ticlid) or clopidogrel (Plavix) are maintained after the procedure
	    • Monitor aPTT; usually maintained at 45-70 seconds
	  • Coronary artery spasm
	    • Nitroglycerin infusion and/or calcium channel blockers are frequently used
	    • **Note:** new onset chest pain or ST segment changes should be reported immediately
	• Chronic restenosis: due to intimal hyperplasia
	• Hypotension, bradycardia (vagal reaction): due to increased parasympathetic nervous system during sheath removal; atropine is effective

Table 3-13 Coronary Artery Bypass Grafting (CABG)

Procedures	• Types of bypasses
	  • Arterial bypass (preferred because of better long-term patency rates)
	    • Internal thoracic (also called *internal mammary*) arteries
	    • Gastroepiploic arteries
	    • Inferior epigastric arteries
	    • Radial arteries
	  • Vein grafts
	    • Saphenous veins
	    • Brachial veins
	• Surgical approaches
	  • Median sternotomy
	  • Lateral thoracotomy (minimally invasive direct [MIDCABG])
	    • May be used for proximal LAD and select lesions of RCA or circumflex (single vessel disease)
	    • Cardiopulmonary bypass not required
	    • Thoracoscopy may be used
	  • Port access
	    • Small anterior thoracotomy and a few 1-cm port incisions are made on the lateral aspect of the chest
	    • Cardiopulmonary bypass achieved through the femoral artery and vein cannulation
	    • Cross-clamping of the aorta achieved by endoaortic balloon clamp
	    • May be used with multiple vessel disease

Indications	• Left main artery disease or three-vessel disease • Double-vessel disease if one of vessels is proximal LAD • Single- or double-vessel disease with angina unresponsive to medical therapy • CAD with ejection fraction less than 35% • Emergent conditions such as unstable angina, acute MI with persistent pain or shock, or coronary artery dissection during PCI
Action	• The goal of coronary artery bypass graft is to provide arterial or venous conduits to redirect coronary blood flow around occluded coronary arteries
Assessment	• Vital signs: HR, BP, respiratory rate, temperature • Hemodynamic parameters: RAP, PAP, PAOP, CO, CI, SVR, PVR, LVSWI, RVSWI • Oxygenation parameters: Sao_2, Svo_2; arterial blood gases • Serum electrolytes • Mediastinal and pleural tube drainage • Complaints of incisional pain, chest pain, dyspnea • Incision for bleeding, separation, or redness and induration

Table 3-13	Coronary Artery Bypass Grafting (CABG)—cont'd
Nursing Diagnoses	• Risk for Decreased Cardiac Output related to myocardial stunning, dysrhythmias, conduction block, silent ischemia, cardiac tamponade • Risk for Fluid Volume Deficit related to hemorrhage, third-spacing • Risk for Alteration in Myocardial Tissue Perfusion related to graft occlusion, myocardial ischemia • Chest Pain related to surgical incision • Risk for Alteration in Cardiopulmonary, Cerebral, Renal, Peripheral Tissue Perfusion related to emboli, pump failure • Risk for Impairment in Gas Exchange related to anesthesia, pain, immobility, atelectasis, ARDS • Impairment in Skin Integrity related to chest incision, invasive procedures, leg incisions • Risk for Injury related to epicardial pacing, intracardiac catheters • Sleep Pattern Disturbance related to noise, frequent interruptions, medications • Anxiety related to acute health alteration and recommended lifestyle changes • Knowledge Deficit related to unfamiliarity with disease process, therapy, and recommended lifestyle changes

Brief summary of specific nursing management	• Relieve pain
	  • Administer narcotics and sedatives for relief of incisional pain
	  • Provide instruction regarding splinting during coughing and turning
	  • Report ischemic pain; titrate NTG for relief of ischemic pain
	• Monitor closely for hemodynamic changes: titrate drug therapy to optimize cardiac output and minimize myocardial oxygen consumption
	  • Pharmacologic support of this patient often includes dobutamine, dopamine, nitroglycerin, nitroprusside
	  • Vasopressors may be used to increase coronary artery perfusion pressure and maintain patency of grafts; monitor for excessive afterload and myocardial oxygen consumption as well as excessive vasoconstriction and peripheral hypoperfusion
	• Monitor closely for hemorrhage: mediastinal tube, pleural tubes, incision
	  • Utilize autotransfusion if appropriate
	  • Administer intravenous fluids, blood, and/or blood products as prescribed
	  • Maintain patency of mediastinal and pleural tubes
	• Monitor closely for changes in perfusion
	  • Note any complaints of chest pain, ST segment elevation, dysrhythmias
	  • Note any changes in appearance or volume of urine
	  • Note any changes in level of consciousness or neurologic function
	  • Note any changes in Sao_2, PAP, PVR
	  • Note any changes in bowel sounds, abdominal distention, abdominal pain
	• Monitor the ECG for dysrhythmias or blocks
	  • Administer antidysrhythmics as prescribed
	  • Utilize epicardial pacing wires for symptomatic bradycardias or blocks
	• Monitor electrolytes and replace as prescribed
	• Monitor for complications

Complications	• Potential complications during surgery
	  • Cerebral or myocardial infarction
	  • Hemorrhage: greater risk with internal thoracic artery implant
	  • Inability to wean from cardiopulmonary bypass: intraaortic balloon pump and/or VAD used
	• Potential complications during immediate postoperative period
	  • Low cardiac output/hypotension
	  • Hemorrhage
	  • Cardiac tamponade
	  • Dysrhythmias
	  • MI
	  • Hypertension
	  • Acute respiratory failure (e.g., atelectasis, ARDS)
	  • Renal failure
	  • Electrolyte imbalance (e.g., hypokalemia, hypocalcemia, hypomagnesemia)
	  • Graft closure

Table 3-14

Myocardial Infarction Summary

Coronary Artery	Location of Infarction	Indicative ECG Leads	Anticipated Complications

Left main coronary artery	Extensive anterior	V_1-V_6	• Sudden cardiac death
			• Dysrhythmias, especially:
			  • Sinus tachycardia
			  • Atrial dysrhythmias
			  • Ventricular dysrhythmias
			  • Blocks
			    • First-degree AV block
			    • Second-degree AV block Mobitz type II
			    • Third-degree AV block with ventricular escape
			    • Bundle branch block
			• Ventricular rupture
			• Ventricular septal defect
			• Ventricular aneurysm
			• Heart failure
			• Cardiogenic shock

Left anterior descending artery	Septal	V_1, V_2	• Dysrhythmias, especially:
			  • Sinus tachycardia
			  • Atrial fibrillation
			  • Ventricular dysrhythmias
			  • Blocks
			    • First-degree AV block
			    • Second-degree AV block Mobitz type II
			    • Third-degree AV block with ventricular escape
			    • Bundle branch block
			• Ventricular septal rupture

	Anterior	V_3, V_4	• Dysrhythmias, especially:
			  • Sinus tachycardia
			  • Atrial fibrillation
			  • Ventricular dysrhythmias
			  • Blocks
			    • First-degree AV block
			    • Second-degree AV block Mobitz type II
			    • Third-degree AV block with ventricular escape
			    • Bundle branch block
			• Ventricular aneurysm
			• Heart failure
			• Cardiogenic shock

Left circumflex artery	Lateral	High: I, aVL Low: V_5, V_6	• Dysrhythmias • Heart failure

Right coronary artery	Inferior	II, III, aVF	• Dysrhythmias, especially:
			  • Sinus bradycardia
			  • Sinus arrest
			  • Junctional rhythms
			  • Ventricular dysrhythmias
			  • Blocks
			    • SA blocks
			    • First-degree AV block
			    • Second-degree AV block Mobitz type I
			    • Third-degree AV block usually with AV junctional escape
			    • Bundle branch block
			• Papillary muscle rupture with acute mitral regurgitation
			• Heart failure

	Posterior	Reciprocal changes in V_1, V_2 indicative changes in V_7-V_9	• Dysrhythmias, especially:
			  • Sinus bradycardia
			  • Sinus arrest
			  • Junctional rhythms
			  • Ventricular dysrhythmias
			  • Blocks
			    • First-degree AV block
			    • Second-degree AV block Mobitz type I
			    • Third-degree AV block usually with AV junctional escape
			• Papillary muscle rupture with acute mitral regurgitation

Table 3-14	Myocardial Infarction Summary—cont'd		
Coronary Artery	**Location of Infarction**	**Indicative ECG Leads**	**Anticipated Complications**
	Right ventricular	V_{4R}-V_{6R}	• Dysrhythmias, especially: • Sinus bradycardia • Sinus arrest • Junctional rhythms • Ventricular dysrhythmias • Blocks • First-degree AV block • Second-degree AV block Mobitz type I • Third-degree AV block usually with AV junctional escape • Bundle branch block • Papillary muscle rupture with acute tricuspid regurgitation • Right ventricular failure

2. Rarely isolated: isolated RVMI more common in patients with right ventricular hypertrophy (e.g., COPD)
3. Smaller infarct due to decreased oxygen requirements of right ventricle
4. Almost always transmural

III. Factors affecting mortality
  A. Age
  B. Left ventricular ejection fraction
  C. Number of occluded vessels
  D. Previous history of MI
  E. Presence of cardiogenic shock: associated with loss of 40% of LV muscle mass; may be from one MI or several cumulative MIs
  F. **Note:** females have twice the mortality of males; probably related to the fact that they tend to be older and have more significant risk factors (e.g., diabetes mellitus, hypertension) when they develop their MIs

Clinical Presentation

I. Subjective
  A. Pain: 75% to 85% of all patients with MI have pain
    1. Provocation: emotional or physical stress; may occur at rest
    2. Palliation: not relieved by oxygen, rest, and/or nitrates; relieved by narcotics and/or reperfusion (thrombolytics or PCI)
    3. Quality
      a) Frequently described as pressure on the chest
      b) May also be described as knifelike, stabbing, burning, or indigestion
      c) May feel like their usual anginal pain but more severe
      d) Atypical pain common in women
      e) If described as tearing or ripping, consider dissecting aortic aneurysm
    4. Region/radiation
      a) Primary location is usually chest but may be epigastric (especially with inferior MI)
      b) Radiation is usually to the left arm, left elbow, left shoulder, both arms, or jaw
      c) If radiating to back, consider dissecting thoracic aortic aneurysm
    5. Severity: from vague, slight discomfort to severe pain; more intense than the patient's typical anginal pain
    6. Timing
      a) Most MIs occur within 3 hours of awakening
      b) The pain is continuous from onset with a duration of 30 minutes or more
      c) Pain that comes and goes for as long as several days before the actual MI is referred to as a *stuttering MI* pattern; intermittent pain before continuous pain is preinfarction angina
  B. Silent MI: as many as 25% of all patients with MI have no pain
    1. More likely in the elderly or diabetic patient
    2. Clues suggesting possible silent MI: new onset heart failure or acute change in mental status, unexplained abdominal pain, unexplained dyspnea or fatigue
  C. Associated symptoms
    1. Nausea and vomiting: seen more often in inferior or posterior MI
    2. Dyspnea or orthopnea: seen more often in anterior MI
    3. Diaphoresis
    4. Palpitations
    5. Apprehension

II. Objective
  A. Heart rate and rhythm
    1. Tachycardia: seen more often in anterior MI
    2. Bradycardia: seen more often in inferior MI
  B. Normotension, hypotension, hypertension
    1. Hypertension: seen more often in anterior MI
    2. Hypotension: seen more often in inferior MI
    3. Equality in arms: inequality in arms indicates possible dissecting thoracic aortic aneurysm

C. Tachypnea

D. Elevated temperature: may occur 48 to 72 hours after MI

E. Levine's sign: clenched fist held over sternum

F. May have JVD: indicative of RVF; commonly seen in RV infarction

G. May have abnormal PMI: downward and lateral displacement

H. Heart sound changes
1. May have diminished heart sounds: related to decreased contractility
2. May have S_4: indicative of left ventricular noncompliance; common for first 24 hours
3. May have S_3: early sign of LVF
4. May have pericardial friction rub: indicative of pericarditis
5. May have systolic murmur of mitral regurgitation (high-pitched, blowing, holosystolic murmur loudest at apex, which radiates to the axilla); may indicate LVF or papillary muscle dysfunction or rupture
6. May have murmur of ventricular septal rupture (high-pitched, harsh, holosystolic murmur loudest at lower left sternal border)

I. May have carotid, aortic, or femoral bruits

J. May have clinical indications of hypoperfusion (Table 2-6)

K. May have clinical indications of heart failure
1. LVF (e.g., S_3, crackles, dyspnea) in left ventricular infarction
2. RVF (e.g., JVD, hepatomegaly, peripheral edema) in right ventricular infarction

III. Laboratory
A. Leukocyte count: increased (usually 12,000 to 15,000 mm^3) at 48 to 72 hours
B. Erythrocyte sedimentation rate (ESR): increased at 48 to 72 hours
C. Diagnostic studies for cell injury (Table 3-15)
1. Increased serum enzymes
a) CK: elevation (usually twice normal in MI) occurs 4 to 6 hours after MI, peaks 24 hours later, and returns to normal after about 3 days; early CK peak is an indication of successful reperfusion

b) LDH: elevation occurs within 24 hours after MI, peaks at 72 hours, and returns to normal within 2 weeks; may be particularly valuable for evaluation of patients who delay seeking medical attention for 2 or more days
2. Positive serum isoenzymes
a) CK: positive CK-MB (>4%) is indicative of MI; highly specific test for MI
(1) Electrophoresis technique: traditional CK-MB; not usually diagnostic for 8 to 24 hours after onset of pain
(2) Immunoassay technique: more sensitive earlier (within 4 hours) than electrophoresis technique; sometimes referred to as a *stat MB*
b) LDH: normally LDH_2 greater than LDH_1; LDH_1 greater than LDH_2 (referred to as *flipped LDH*) indicative of MI; does not occur until 48 to 72 hours after the onset of pain
3. Increased serum muscle proteins
a) Myoglobin: muscle protein; high sensitivity but low specificity; excellent early negative predictive value
b) Troponin: contractile protein
(1) Cardiac troponin I (cTnI): found only in cardiac muscle; more specific but later rise and peak
(2) Cardiac troponin T (cTnT): found in cardiac muscle as well as skeletal muscle; less specific than I, especially in patients with renal failure, but earlier rise and peak

IV. ECG
A. As a diagnostic tool for acute MI: most helpful when clearly abnormal
1. If initial ECG nondiagnostic, repeat ECGs should be done every 30 minutes until pain cessation or the ECG is clearly diagnostic and definitive therapy can be initiated
2. ECG diagnosis of MI has multiple problems
a) Lag time of hours (or even days) may exist before diagnostic ECG changes

Table 3-15 Laboratory Diagnostic Tests for Acute MI

Test	Normal Values	Time to Rise (After Injury)	Peak (After Injury)	Return to Normal (After Injury)
CK	Men: 55-170 U/L Women: 30-135 U/L	4-6 hours	24 hours	3-4 days
CK-MB	0% of total CK	6-10 hours	18 hours	2-3 days
LDH	90-200 IU/L	24-48 hours	72 hours	8-14 days
LDH$_1$	17%-25% of total LDH	8-24 hours	72 hours	8-14 days
Myoglobin	<85 ng/ml	1-4 hours	6-10 hours	24 hours
Cardiac troponin I (cTnI)	<1.5 ng/ml	4-6 hours	18 hours	7 days
Cardiac troponin T (cTnT)	<0.1 ng/ml	3-4 hours	24 hours	2-3 weeks

become evident; first ECG diagnostic only 50% of the time
   b) Changes may be subtle
   c) Previous ECG may not be available for comparison
   d) Changes may be obscured by a competitive condition
      (1) LBBB or ventricular pacemaker obscures anterior MI
      (2) WPW obscures anterior MI
      (3) Left anterior hemiblock obscures interior MI
      (4) Left posterior hemiblock obscures lateral MI
      (5) Ventricular hypertrophy may obscure anterior or lateral MI
   e) 15 or 18 leads are used to prevent missing an infarction in a traditionally "electrically silent" area of the heart; sensitivity and inclusion for reperfusion therapy is increased through the use of right ventricular and posterior leads
      (1) 18-lead ECG: 12 standard, 3 right ventricular leads, 3 posterior leads
      (2) 15-lead ECG: 12 standard + V_{4R} + V_8 + V_9
   B. ECG indicators (see Electrocardiography section and Figure 2-37)
   C. Locations, indicative leads, coronary artery affected (see Electrocardiography section and Table 2-12)
   D. Determination of the age of the MI (see Electrocardiography section and Table 2-13)
V. Echocardiography
   A. Normal wall motion: strong predictor of nonischemic pain
   B. Reduced wall motion: strong predictor of acute occlusion
   C. May show mechanical complications (e.g., ventricular septal defect, papillary muscle rupture)
VI. Chest X-ray: may show cardiomegaly or indications of heart failure
VII. Cardiac catheterization: will likely show coronary artery occlusion; percutaneous coronary intervention (PCI) may be performed after diagnosis
VIII. Radionuclide studies
   A. Technetium-99 pyrophosphate scan: infarcted areas show up as "hot spots"
   B. Thallium-201 scan: ischemic or infarcted areas show up as "cold spots"

Nursing Diagnoses
I. Chest Pain related to coronary artery occlusion and resultant myocardial ischemia, infarction
II. Alteration in Cardiopulmonary Tissue Perfusion related to coronary artery occlusion
III. Risk for Decreased Cardiac Output related to alterations in contractility, dysrhythmias, rupture of cardiac structure (e.g., papillary muscle rupture and ventricular septal rupture)
IV. Risk for Activity Intolerance related to decreased cardiac output, decrease in tissue oxygen delivery
V. Sleep Pattern Disturbance related to pain, dyspnea, noise, interruptions related to care
VI. Risk for Ineffective Individual Coping related to acute health alteration, recommended lifestyle changes
VII. Anxiety related to acute health alteration and recommended lifestyle changes
VIII. Knowledge Deficit related to unfamiliarity with disease process, therapy, and recommended lifestyle changes

Collaborative Management
I. Manage cardiopulmonary arrest if needed
   A. Ventricular fibrillation frequently occurs within 1 hour: early identification of clinical indications of MI and hospitalization is very important
   B. Manage airway, oxygenation, and circulation using BCLS, ACLS
II. Monitor ECG, vital signs, physical examination, and hemodynamic parameters for changes
   A. Safely and accurately monitor the patient's hemodynamic parameters as indicated; indications for hemodynamic monitoring in acute MI include the following:
      1. Persistent chest pain
      2. Persistent tachycardia
      3. Significant hypertension or hypotension
      4. Significant left ventricular or right ventricular failure
      5. Intravenous inotropes or vasoactive agents
      6. New systolic murmur
   B. Utilize hemodynamic parameters in evaluating clinical status for changes and responses to prescribed therapies
III. Reduce size of myocardial infarction: myocardial salvaging techniques
   A. Treat pain promptly and adequately: decreases catecholamine release and myocardial oxygen demand
      1. Morphine sulfate: 2 to 4 mg every 5 minutes until pain relief
         a) Actions: decreases preload by venous dilation; decreases catecholamine release by pain relief (which decreases heart rate and afterload); decreases anxiety and restlessness
         b) Cautions: inferior MI; right ventricular MI
      2. Nitroglycerin IV: may be given prophylactically at 25 to 100 μg/min for 24 to 48 hours; dosage may be reduced at night to decrease chance of nitrate tolerance
         a) Actions
            (1) Decreases preload to decrease myocardial oxygen demand
            (2) Dilates epicardial coronary vessels to increase myocardial oxygen supply
            (3) Augments the analgesic effect of morphine

b) Caution: may cause reflex tachycardia; beta-blockers may be needed

3. Reperfusion therapies (e.g., thrombolytics, PCI): relieve pain by reestablishing blood flow and aerobic metabolism

4. IABP: may be used for intractable pain because it increases coronary artery perfusion pressure (Figs. 3-18 and 3-19 and Table 3-16)

B. Increase myocardial oxygen supply

1. Administer oxygen at 2 to 6 L/min per nasal cannula for 24 to 48 hours
   a) Probably has little effect on the arterial oxygen content of otherwise normal individuals; it may significantly improve oxygenation of an ischemic myocardium in patients with hypoxemia from pulmonary edema
   b) Even in the absence of pulmonary edema or other complications, some patients develop modest hypoxemia early during the course of acute MI

2. Treat anemia if present: maintain Hgb greater than 12 g/dl if possible

3. Maintain coronary artery perfusion pressure
   a) Use caution in administering NTG and other vasoactive agents because they may decrease CAPP by decreasing the aortic root pressure
   b) NTP is contraindicated during ischemic pain because it may cause coronary artery steal and decrease coronary artery perfusion pressure

4. Control dysrhythmias
   a) Tachydysrhythmias decrease the time for coronary artery filling and may decrease cardiac output
   b) Bradydysrhythmias increase the time for coronary artery filling but may decrease cardiac output

5. Administer calcium channel blockers or NTG for coronary artery spasm

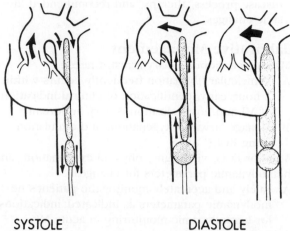

SYSTOLE   **DIASTOLE**

Figure 3-18   Mechanics of the intraaortic balloon pump. The balloon is deflated immediately prior to systole and remains deflated during systole; the balloon is inflated at the beginning of diastole and remains inflated until immediately before the next systole. (From Kinney MR, Packa DR, Dunbar SB: *AACN's clinical reference for critical-care nursing,* ed 3, St Louis, 1994, Mosby.)

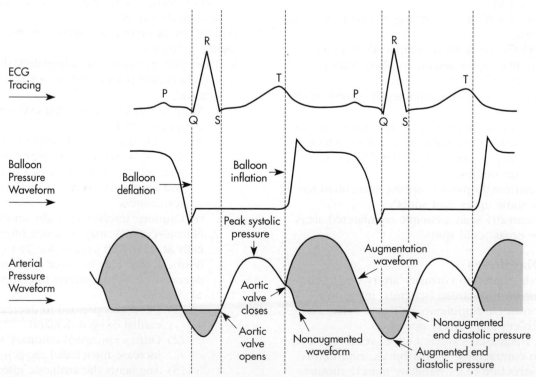

Figure 3-19   Inflation and deflation of the intraaortic balloon *(center)* timed with either ECG waveform *(top)* or arterial pressure waveform *(bottom).* (From Holloway NM: *Nursing care of the critically ill adult,* ed 3, 1988, Addison-Wesley.)

Table 3-16	**Intraaortic Balloon Pump**
Indications	• Unstable angina refractory to medical therapy • Cardiogenic shock or severe left ventricular failure • Refractory ventricular dysrhythmias • Acute mitral regurgitation (e.g., papillary muscle rupture post-MI) • Acute ventricular septal rupture (e.g., post-MI) • Preoperative, perioperative, and/or postoperative support with coronary artery bypass graft or other major surgery • Weaning from cardiopulmonary bypass • During percutaneous coronary arteriography and PCI • As a bridge to cardiac transplantation
Contraindications	• Aortic valve regurgitation • Aortic aneurysm • Aortic dissection • Severe bilateral peripheral vascular disease (e.g., absent femoral pulse) • Coagulopathy • Not recommended for patients with chronic end-stage heart disease who are not awaiting a cardiac transplant • Not recommended for patients with irreversible brain damage or terminal condition

Actions (Fig. 3-18)	• Balloon is inflated during diastole
	  • Increases myocardial oxygen supply
	  • Increases coronary artery blood flow by displacing blood retrograde toward the aortic arch and increasing diastolic blood pressure
	  • Increases blood flow to the renal arteries and lower extremities by displacing blood antegrade toward the renal and lower extremities arteries
	• Balloon is deflated immediately prior to systole
	  • Decreases myocardial oxygen demand
	  • Decreases left ventricular afterload by decreasing systolic BP

Insertion and mechanics	• Catheter with 40 ml balloon is inserted via femoral artery (Note: the catheter may be inserted via iliac, subclavian, or axillary artery if the femoral artery is not an option) • Balloon is positioned in descending thoracic aorta between left subclavian and renal arteries; the tip of the catheter should be at the second to third ICS just distal to the left subclavian artery by chest X-ray • Helium to inflate the balloon is shuttled into and out of the balloon by a pump, which is housed in a console at the bedside • The balloon occludes 80% of the aortic diameter when inflated

Timing (Fig. 3-19)	• By ECG
	  • Inflated after the T-wave
	  • Deflated prior to QRS
	• By arterial waveform
	  • Inflated at the dicrotic notch
	  • Deflated at the end-diastolic dip immediately prior to systole
	• Inflation and deflation are usually triggered by ECG, but fine timing is done by the nurse using the arterial waveform

Assessment	• HR: a normalization of heart rate is desirable • BP: a decrease in systolic BP, an increase in diastolic BP, and an increase in MAP are the usual desirable effects • CO/CI: an increase in cardiac output/index is desirable • PAP/PAOP: a decrease in PAP and PAOP is desirable • A decrease in the amplitude of v-wave on the PAOP waveform is desirable in patients with mitral regurgitation or ventricular septal rupture • Sao_2: an increase in Sao_2 is desirable • Svo_2: an increase in Svo_2 is desirable • Urine output: an increase in urine output is desirable • Complaints of chest pain: a decrease in chest pain is desirable • ECG: a decrease in the presence or frequency of dysrhythmias is desirable • Neurovascular status of affected limb: the presence of palpable pulses and a warm limb with normal capillary refill is desirable
Nursing Diagnoses	• Decreased Cardiac Output related to balloon or pump malfunction, timing errors, catheter kink, leak, rupture • Risk for Altered Peripheral Tissue Perfusion related to presence of femoral artery catheter, catheter malposition, thrombosis or embolus, arterial spasm • Altered Protection related to anticoagulation • Impaired Physical Mobility related to bedrest, extremity restriction • Risk for Infection related to invasive catheters, devices • Anxiety related to insertion of IABP, critical illness, critical care environment

Continued

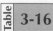

Brief summary of nursing management	• Assess the parameters described previously • Ensure optimal timing of balloon inflation and deflation • Titrate pharmacologic therapies to augment the mechanical therapy of the IABP • Ensure positioning of the patient with head of bed elevation <30 degrees and avoidance of hip flexion • Observe for complications and provide appropriate management for the prevention of complications

Complications: prevention and treatment	• Thrombosis causing lower extremity ischemia
	  • Insertion precautions
	    • Use the smallest sheath that will allow the catheter to be advanced through it
	    • Select the limb with the best pulse
	  • Dextran 40 as prescribed as an antiplatelet aggregation agent
	  • Restraint of affected leg to prevent displacement of the balloon and trauma to intima of artery
	  • Neurovascular assessment of the affected limb every hour
	  • If limb ischemia is noted: treatment may include any of the following:
	    • Removal of catheter with placement of the sheath and catheter in the other femoral artery if the IABP is still needed
	    • Fogarty thrombectomy
	    • Femorofemoral graft
	    • Lidocaine or papaverine: to decrease arterial spasm
	• Catheter displacement causing renal or left upper extremity ischemia
	  • Elevation of head of bed no more than 30 degrees to prevent displacement of the balloon
	  • Restraint of affected limb to prevent displacement of the balloon
	  • Close monitoring of urine output
	  • Neurovascular assessment of left arm every hour
	  • Notification of physician of significant changes in urine output or left arm perfusion
	• Emboli
	  • Dextran 40 as prescribed as an antiplatelet aggregation agent
	  • Heparin may be prescribed
	  • Avoidance of allowing the balloon to remain static (noninflating) for more than 30 minutes; clots may form in the folds of the balloon and be embolized when the balloon is then reinflated
	• Infection
	  • Sterile dressing changes daily or every other day
	  • Close monitoring of the site for erythema, edema, induration, warmth
	• Aortic dissection
	  • Attention to complaints of back pain, vital sign changes
	  • Removal of catheter and repair of aorta if dissection occurs
	• Anemia
	  • Attention to presence of petechiae or ecchymosis, platelet counts
	  • Discontinuance of heparin
	  • Blood and/or blood products may be prescribed
	• Balloon complications
	  • Leak
	    • Attention to increase in volume or frequency of refilling
	    • Replacement of catheter if leak occurs to prevent gas embolism
	  • Rupture
	    • Attention to blood in catheter
	    • Replacement of catheter if rupture occurs to prevent entrapment
	• Timing complications
	  • Inflation is too early: aortic valve closes too early and stroke volume is decreased
	  • Inflation is too late: diastolic augmentation is decreased
	  • Deflation is too early: less increase in coronary artery perfusion pressure and less of a decrease in afterload
	  • Deflation is too late: increase in afterload
	• Inadequate pumping: usually due to dysrhythmias
	  • Timing method changed from ECG to arterial line

Weaning	• Indications
	  • CI >2.0 L/min/m^2
	  • PAP, PAOP normal
	  • MAP >70 mm Hg
	  • SVR <1400 dynes/sec/cm^{-5}
	  • Absence of anginal pain
	  • Absence of clinical indications of hypoperfusion (Table 2-6)
	• Methods
	  • May be done by decreasing the frequency (e.g., from every cardiac cycle to every other cardiac cycle to every third cardiac cycle)
	  • May be done by decreasing the volume in the balloon with each inflation (e.g., decreased by 25% with each weaning step)

6. Utilize intraaortic balloon pump as prescribed (see Table 3-16)
7. Administer thrombolytics, anticoagulants to
   reestablish patency of the infarction-related
   artery (IRA) (Table 3-17 and Table 3-18)
   a) These procedures are preceded and followed by ASA and heparin; GP IIb/IIIa
   platelet receptor blockers (e.g., abciximab
   [ReoPro], eptifibatide [Integrilin],
   tirofiban HCl [Aggrastat]) are also frequently used especially after stent
   placement
   (1) ASA (160-325 mg initially and daily) or
   another antiplatelet drug (e.g., ticlopidine [Ticlid], clopidogrel [Plavix]) to
   decrease platelet aggregation and
   clot extension
   (2) Heparin for 24 to 48 hours to maintain aPTT 45 to 70 seconds; initial
   dosing should be weight-based, then
   infusion is adjusted by aPTT results
   (a) Bolus: 60 to 80 U/kg
   (b) Infusion: 12 to 18 U/kg/hr
   (3) Warfarin for at least 3 months in patients with any of the following:
   (a) Anterior Q-wave MI
   (b) Heart failure

(c) Severe left ventricular dysfunction
(d) Atrial fibrillation
(e) Previous embolic event
8. Assist in prompt preparation of high-risk patients for emergent (also called *rescue*) PTCA
   or other interventional procedure if thrombolytics are contraindicated or unsuccessful
9. Concurrent use of PCI and thrombolytics
   a) The rationale for a combination therapy
   approach is based on the pathophysiology
   of CAD
   b) Usual approaches
   (1) Thrombolytic therapy, along with
   heparin and ASA
   (a) Actions
   (i) Thrombolytic therapy targets
   the fibrin component of
   the clot
   (ii) ASA targets the platelet
   (b) Limitations
   (i) Failure to achieve reperfusion
   in a large proportion of
   patients
   (ii) Risk of reocclusion
   (2) PCI
   (a) Action: targets the atherosclerotic
   plaque

Table 3-17   Thrombolytic Agents Used in Acute MI

	Streptokinase	Recombinant tPA (rt-PA) (alteplase) Recombinant PA (r-PA) (reteplase)
Dose	1.5 million U over 30-60 minutes	• 15 mg bolus, then 0.75 mg/kg over 30 minutes (50 mg maximum), then 0.5 mg/kg over 60 minutes (35 mg maximum) with alteplase (Activase) • 10 U over 2 minutes, repeated after 30 minutes with reteplase (Retavase)
Half-life	20 minutes but effects last 48-72 hours because of fibrinogen depletion	5 minutes for alteplase 15 minutes for reteplase
90-Minute Expected Reperfusion Rate	50%-60%	70%-85%
Fibrin Specificity	No	Yes
Anticoagulant Effect	Yes; depletes fibrinogen for up to 72 hours; ASA given but heparin no longer recommended	No; ASA and heparin required to prevent reocclusion
Allergic Reactions	Yes	No
Hypotensive Effects	++	+
Contraindications (see Table 3-18 for general contraindications for thrombolytics)	Prior streptokinase or streptococcal infection within 6-9 months (some references say up to 5 years)	None specific to rt-PA or r-PA
Cost	+ (~$500)	+++++ (~$2500 for alteplase or reteplase)

Note: The difference in reperfusion rates between streptokinase and recombinant thrombolytics (rt-PA and r-PA) is less pronounced in patients more than 75 years old, inferior MI, and patients presenting more than 4 hours after the onset of pain

Table 3-18	Thrombolytic Therapy

Actions	• Activate plasminogen to plasmin, the active agent that breaks down clots (speeds up the normal fibrinolytic process to allow early reperfusion)
	• Limit cellular necrosis and decrease infarction size
	• Decrease mortality, morbidity
	  • Short-term: reestablishing arterial patency
	  • Long-term: maintaining ejection fraction

Thrombolytic agents (see Table 3-17 for comparison between SK and recombinant thrombolytics [rt-PA and r-PA])	• Streptokinase (SK)
	• Recombinant tissue plasminogen activator (rt-PA)
	  • Alteplase (Activase)
	• Recombinant plasminogen activator (r-PA)
	  • Reteplase (Retavase)
	• Urokinase (rarely used in acute MI but frequently used in peripheral arterial occlusion)

Indications	• History strongly suggestive of MI • ST segment elevation of at least 1 mm in at least 2 contiguous leads (no data supports the use of thrombolytics without ST segment elevation) or new LBBB • Pain of less than 6 hours or still having pain (Note: as long as the patient is having pain, salvageable myocardial is assumed since dead myocardium does not metabolize aerobically or anaerobically and neither lactic acid nor pain would be produced)
Absolute Contraindications	• Active internal bleeding • History of hemorrhagic stroke, intracranial neoplasm, AV malformation, or cerebral aneurysm • Intracranial or intraspinal surgery or trauma within 2 months • Known bleeding disorder (e.g., thrombocytopenia, hemophilia) • Suspected aortic aneurysm or acute pericarditis • Systolic BP ≥200 mm Hg and/or diastolic BP ≥120 mm Hg • Prolonged (more than 10 minutes) or traumatic CPR • Pregnancy • Streptokinase is contraindicated if the patient has received streptokinase or had a streptococcal infection within the last 6-9 months, but recombinant thrombolytics (rt-PA and r-PA) can still be used
Relative Contraindications	• Major surgery or trauma within 10 days • Recent gastrointestinal or genitourinary bleeding • Cerebrovascular disease • Oral anticoagulant therapy • Systolic BP ≥180 mm Hg and/or diastolic BP ≥110 mm Hg • Significant liver dysfunction • Septic thrombophlebitis • Subacute bacterial endocarditis • High likelihood of left heart thrombus (e.g., mitral stenosis with atrial fibrillation, ventricular aneurysm, left atrial myxoma) • Diabetic hemorrhagic retinopathy • Advanced age (more than 70-75 years old) with consideration of physiologic age, severity of concomitant diseases, mental status • Any condition when bleeding would be a significant hazard or would be difficult to manage (e.g., recent femoral artery puncture or sheath)

Clinical indications of reperfusion	• Pain cessation
	• ST segment return to baseline
	• Reperfusion dysrhythmias
	  • Sinus bradycardia
	  • Idioventricular rhythm, accelerated idioventricular rhythm
	  • AV blocks
	  • Ventricular irritability: PVCs, ventricular tachycardia, ventricular fibrillation
	• CK washout: early or markedly elevated CK peak

Assessment	• Heart rate • Blood pressure • ECG rhythm; note reperfusion dysrhythmias • Clinical indications of reperfusion • Bleeding (e.g., puncture points, gums, saliva, sputum, gastric secretions, stool, urine) • Complaints of chest pain, back pain, or headache

Table 3-18	**Thrombolytic Therapy—cont'd**
Nursing Diagnosis	• Altered Protection related to dissolution of stable protective clots by thrombolytics, delay in coagulation caused by heparin therapy • Risk for Decreased Cardiac Output related to reperfusion dysrhythmias • Risk for Alteration in Cardiac Tissue Perfusion related to reocclusion • Knowledge Deficit related to unfamiliarity with disease process, therapy, and recommended lifestyle changes

Brief summary of nursing management	• Administer adjuvant therapy: recombinant thrombolytics (rt-PA and r-PA) are followed by ASA and heparin (SK causes significant fibrinogen depletion, and heparin is not indicated due to increased bleeding risk)
	• Monitor for clinical indications of reperfusion; notify physician if these indications are not seen so that emergent PCI can be scheduled
	• Avoid punctures: arterial, IV, IM, SC
	  • Apply pressure until hemostasis is achieved if punctures are required after thrombolytics initiated
	  • Insert multiple (usually 2-3) IV catheters prior to initiation of thrombolytic therapy; one of these catheters may be used for venous sampling
	• Monitor stool, urine, emesis, sputum, and saliva for blood
	• Monitor for complications

Complications	• Hemorrhage
	  • At site of vascular puncture: 80% incidence
	  • GI or GU bleeding: 15%-20% incidence
	  • Intracranial bleed: 1% incidence
	    • Monitor for clinical indications (e.g., headache, change in LOC, focal neurologic signs)
	    • Discontinue thrombolytic and anticoagulant; protamine, cryoprecipitate, and/or platelets may be given
	    • Obtain CT of head as requested
	    • If fluid level seen, surgery may be performed
	• Reocclusion: monitor for new pain and/or ST segment changes
	• Allergic reactions to streptokinase
	  • Monitor for urticaria, fever, bronchospasm, dyspnea, stridor, or dysrhythmias
	  • Administer diphenhydramine (Benadryl) and/or hydrocortisone (Solu-Cortef) as prescribed in attempt to prevent allergic reaction
	• Reperfusion dysrhythmias: usually transient
	  • Administer antidysrhythmics or perform cardioversion or defibrillation as indicated for sustained ventricular tachycardia or ventricular fibrillation (prophylactic lidocaine is no longer recommended with thrombolytic therapy)
	  • Administer atropine or apply transcutaneous pacemaker for symptomatic bradycardia or block

    (b) Limitations
      (i) Availability of interventional cardiology facility, especially in rural areas
      (ii) Availability of services on very short notice at all times of the night and day
  c) New possibilities
    (1) Glycoprotein (GP) IIb/IIIa inhibitors (potent form of antiplatelet agent) and reduced-dose thrombolytic therapy
    (2) GP IIb/IIIa inhibitors plus rescue angioplasty after failed thrombolytics
    (3) PCI plus GP IIb/IIIa inhibitors
    (4) PCI plus thrombolytic therapy
C. Decrease myocardial oxygen consumption
  1. Administer beta-blockers as prescribed to decrease heart rate and contractility to decrease myocardial oxygen consumption
    a) Actions
      (1) Decrease incidence of dysrhythmias and increase ventricular fibrillation threshold
      (2) Block the effects of catecholamines (cardioprotection)
      (3) Reduce infarct size and severity of HF
    b) Agents: metoprolol (Lopressor) 5 mg IV every 2 minutes × 3 is usually given, but atenolol (Tenormin) or esmolol (Brevibloc) may be used
    c) Contraindications
      (1) Heart rate less than 50/min
      (2) Second- or third-degree AV block
      (3) Systolic BP less than 100 mm Hg
      (4) Heart failure
      (5) Bronchospasm
        (a) No beta-blockers should be given to a patient with active bronchospasm
        (b) Cardioselective beta-blockers (e.g., metoprolol or esmolol) may be given to a patient with a history of bronchospastic lung

disease (e.g., asthma) but noncardioselective beta-blockers (e.g., propranolol) should not be given

(6) Cocaine-induced MI

2. Administer ACE inhibitors (e.g., captopril [Capoten], enalapril [Vasotec]) or angiotensin II blockers (e.g., losartan [Cozaar], valsartan [Diovan], telmisartan [Micardis]) as prescribed to attenuate ventricular remodeling

   a) Action: block the vasoconstriction and sodium and water retention associated with activation of the renin-angiotensin-aldosterone system

   b) Indications in acute MI: anterior or large inferior MI or evidence of HF

   c) ACE inhibitors block the conversion of angiotensin I to angiotensin II; angiotensin-blockers block angiotensin II and do not block the breakdown of bradykinin so are less likely to cause cough

   d) Caution: hypotension

3. Administer vasodilators (Table 3-19) as prescribed

   a) Venous vasodilators (usually nitroglycerin) to decrease preload

   b) Arterial vasodilators (usually nitroprusside) to decrease afterload

   c) Caution: hypotension; careful titration necessary to decrease myocardial oxygen consumption but to prevent hypoperfusion

4. Provide physical and emotional rest

   a) Maintain bed rest for 24 hours then gradually increase activity as long as patient is hemodynamically stable; allow rest after meals, personal hygiene, toileting, and physical therapy

   b) Prevent Valsalva maneuver

     (1) Teach patient to exhale when turning in bed

     (2) Administer stool softeners as prescribed

     (3) Provide bedside commode for elimination

   c) Explain procedures thoroughly: monitor alarms, equipment, visiting hours, reasons for procedures

   d) Keep family informed regarding patient's progress and status

   e) Provide for patient's comfort

     (1) Provide prompt pain control: analgesics

     (2) Provide nausea control: antiemetics; provide mouth care after emesis

     (3) Provide for physical comfort: temperature, lighting, noise control

   f) Instruct patient regarding relaxation techniques; encourage utilization of these techniques; utilize calming music, white noise, or nature sounds to aid in relaxation

Table 3-19	Vasodilators		
Drug		**Arteries**	**Veins**
Hydralazine (Apresoline)		yes	no
Nitroglycerin (Tridil)		only if >1 μg/kg/min	yes
Morphine sulfate		minimal	yes
Nitroprusside (Nipride)		yes	yes
Prazosin (Minipress)		yes	yes
Nifedipine (Procardia)		yes	yes
Nicardipine (Cardene)		yes	yes

   g) Provide appropriate nutrition: clear liquid to soft diet, usually low (2-3 g/day) sodium

     (1) Caffeine: may have up to 4 to 5 caffeinated beverages per 24 hours as long as dysrhythmias do not occur

     (2) Iced water: no restriction

   h) Administer anxiolytics as prescribed: usually diazepam (Valium), lorazepam (Ativan), or alprazolam (Xanax)

   i) Note common emotional responses seen in acute MI and treat appropriately (Table 3-20)

D. Monitor for, prevent, and treat complications (Table 3-21)

E. Collaborative management specific to RV infarctions

1. Assess for clinical indications of RVMI, especially in the patient with acute inferior MI

   a) ECG changes in V_{4R}, V_{5R}, V_{6R}

   b) Increased RAP, decreased PAOP

   c) Decreased CO, CI, MAP, increased SVR

   d) Right-sided S_4

   e) Clinical indications of RVF: jugular venous distention (JVD), hepatojugular reflux, right-sided S_3, murmur of tricuspid insufficiency

   f) Minimal to absent pulmonary congestion

2. Administer therapy specific to right ventricular infarction

   a) Maintain adequate filling volumes

     (1) Measure right atrial and pulmonary artery occlusive pressures; patients with significant right ventricular infarction usually require hemodynamic monitoring

     (2) Administer volume: usually in the form of colloids (e.g., dextran, plasma protein fraction, albumin); fluids administered until PAOP is increased by more than 5 mm Hg but PAOP and RAP should not exceed 20 mm Hg

     (3) Avoid use of diuretics and/or venous vasodilators; if dilators are needed, selective arterial dilators should be

Table 3-20	Emotional Responses Seen in Acute Myocardial Infarction	
Response	**Indications**	**Collaborative Management**
Anxiety	• Increased verbalization • Inability to concentrate • Restlessness, apprehension • Sleep disturbances • Tremors • Tachycardia, mild hypertension	• Be consistent with patient assignment • Provide orientation to unit, procedures, equipment, etc. • Assess usual coping mechanisms • Invite patient to ask questions • Keep family informed about patient's condition • Encourage participation in rehabilitation program
Denial	• Avoidance of discussion of heart attack • Discussions kept on a social, humorous level • Minimization of severity (e.g., "little heart attack") • Noncompliance with activity and diet restrictions; smoking • Overly cheerful demeanor • Repetition of same questions to different staff members	• Listen but do not reinforce denial • Assess consequences of denial: denial decreases in-hospital mortality but increases incidence of sudden cardiac death after discharge • Assess the threat causing the need for denial • Provide counseling if patient still in denial at time of discharge • Encourage participation in rehabilitation program
Depression	• Listlessness, disinterest • Expressions of hopelessness, pessimism • Abbreviated verbal responses (e.g., monosyllable answers) • Slowness in movement and speech • Withdrawn behavior • Anorexia • Sad look, crying	• Voice your observations (e.g., "you look sad") • Let patient know that it is normal to feel this way • Encourage verbalization of feelings • Allow and encourage crying • Encourage participation in rehabilitation program
Anger	• Open opposition to treatment regimen • Expressions of disappointment or frustration • Passive-aggressive behavior • Sarcasm • Voicing of anger, screaming, cursing	• Acknowledge angry or hostile feelings • Explore cause of anger • Let patient know that these feelings are normal • Let spouse and family know that anger is normal • Be matter-of-fact about expressions of anger • Encourage participation in rehabilitation program
Aggressive sexual behavior	• Frequent seductive comments • Frequent initiation of sexually related conversation • Frequent boasts about past sexual interests and prowess • Flirtatious compliments • Attempts to hold, fondle, or kiss parts of nurse's body • Deliberate exposure of genitals	• Be honest and simply tell patient that this behavior makes you uncomfortable if it does • Accept compliments with simple "thank you" • Arrange sexual counseling for patient and spouse • Encourage participation in rehabilitation program

used (e.g., hydralazine [Apresoline]) so that preload is not decreased
(4) Maintain contractility: inotropes (e.g., dobutamine) are usually needed

Heart Failure

Definitions

I. Heart failure: condition in which one or both ventricles cannot pump sufficient blood to meet the metabolic needs of the body; characterized by one or both of the following:
   A. Clinical indications of intravascular and interstitial volume overload (e.g., dyspnea, crackles, edema)
   B. Clinical indications of tissue hypoperfusion (e.g., fatigue, exercise intolerance)

II. Pulmonary edema: fluid in the alveolus, which impairs gas exchange by impairing the diffusion between alveolus and capillary; may be cardiac versus noncardiac
   A. Cardiac pulmonary edema is caused by acute left ventricular failure
   B. Noncardiac pulmonary edema is most commonly caused by acute respiratory distress syndrome (ARDS)
   C. Cardiac versus noncardiac pulmonary edema is frequently clinically differentiated using hemodynamic parameters
      1. Elevated PAP, elevated PAOP = cardiac

Table 3-21 **Complications of Myocardial Infarction**

Complication	Clinical Indications	Prevention/Treatment
Dysrhythmias and conduction system defects	• Change in rhythm or conduction on rhythm strip or multiple-lead ECG • Indications of hypoperfusion may be evident (see Table 2-6)	• Close monitoring for changes in rhythm or conduction • Beta-blocker as a cardioprotective agent as prescribed • Magnesium, potassium, or calcium to correct electrolyte imbalance as prescribed • Antidysrhythmic agents as indicated and prescribed (lidocaine is used most often) • Application of external pacemaker or insertion of transvenous pacemaker as indicated (see Table 3-5) • Cardioversion or defibrillation as indicated

Heart failure	• Tachycardia, tachypnea
	• Clinical indications of LVF
	  • Dyspnea, orthopnea, cough
	  • S_3
	  • Crackles in lung bases
	• Clinical indications of RVF
	  • Jugular venous distention
	  • Hepatomegaly, splenomegaly
	  • Peripheral edema
	• Chest X-ray shows pulmonary venous congestion, cardiomegaly
	• Increased RAP, PAP, PAOP (PAOP usually >20 mm Hg)
		• Oxygen
		• Sodium and fluid restriction
		• ACE inhibitors (e.g., captopril, enalapril)
		• Diuretics (e.g., furosemide, bumetanide)
		• Vasodilators (e.g., nitroglycerine, nitroprusside)
		• Inotropic agents (e.g., digoxin, dobutamine, amrinone or milrinone)
		• Intraaortic balloon pump
		• Ventricular assist device

Cardiogenic shock	• Tachycardia, tachypnea, hypotension • Clinical indications of LVF • Clinical indications of RVF • Clinical indications of hypoperfusion (see Table 2-6) • Urine output <0.5 ml/kg/hr • Cool to cold skin • Diminished to absent bowel sounds • Lethargy to confusion to coma • Chest X-ray shows pulmonary venous congestion, cardiomegaly • Decreased CO/CI (usually <2 L/min/m²) • Increased PAOP (usually >18 mm Hg) • Increased SVR (usually >2000 dynes/sec/cm⁻⁵)	• Oxygen • Sodium and fluid restrictions • ACE inhibitors (e.g., captopril, enalapril) • Inotropic agents (e.g., digoxin, dobutamine, amrinone or milrinone) • Diuretics (e.g., furosemide, bumetanide) • Vasodilators (e.g., nitroglycerin, nitroprusside) • IABP • Emergent revascularization: thrombolytics; PCI; CABG • Ventricular assist device
Papillary muscle dysfunction/rupture	• New holosystolic murmur loudest at apex • Clinical indications of LVF • Clinical indications of hypoperfusion (see Table 2-6) • Increased PAP, PAOP • Large *v*-waves on PAOP waveform • Echocardiography shows mitral regurgitation	• Vasodilators (e.g., nitroglycerine, nitroprusside) • IABP • Surgical replacement of mitral valve with concurrent CABG
Ventricular septal rupture	• New holosystolic murmur loudest at lower left sternal border (LLSB) • Chest pain, dyspnea • Syncope • Increased PAP, PAOP • Increased Svo_2 • Increased CO/CI by thermodilution method of measurement (inaccurate) • Clinical evidence of hypoperfusion (see Table 2-6)	• Vasodilators (e.g., nitroglycerine, nitroprusside) • IABP • Surgical correction of ventricular septal defect with concurrent CABG

Table 3-21 **Complications of Myocardial Infarction—cont'd**

Complication	Clinical Indications	Prevention/Treatment

Cardiac rupture	• Clinical indications of hypoperfusion (see Table 2-6)
	• Clinical indications of cardiac tamponade
	  • Jugular venous distention
	  • Muffled heart sounds
	  • Hypotension
	  • Increased RAP, PAP, PAOP with equalization within 5 mm Hg
	• Sinus tachycardia or pulseless electrical activity
	• Eventual cardiopulmonary arrest
		• Pericardiocentesis
		• CPR; internal cardiac massage may be necessary
		• Surgical repair may be attempted (survival is rare)

Ventricular aneurysm	• Diffuse PMI, left ventricular heave • Atrial fibrillation or ventricular dysrhythmias • Persistent ST segment elevation • Chest X-ray shows left ventricular dilation • Echocardiography shows dyskinesia, left ventricular dilation • Clinical indications of LVF may be present • Clinical indications of systemic emboli may be present: cerebral emboli; peripheral emboli with acute arterial occlusion	• Antidysrhythmics (e.g., lidocaine, amiodarone) • Anticoagulants (e.g., heparin followed by warfarin) • Treatment of HF: ACE inhibitors; diuretics; vasodilators; inotropes • Surgical resection may be performed • Ablative procedures may be necessary for recurrent ventricular dysrhythmias
Pericarditis	• Fever • Chest pain that worsens with deep breath and lessens with sitting up and leaning forward • Pericardial friction rub • Elevated WBC, sedimentation rate • Diffuse ST segment elevation across the precordial leads • Chest X-ray may show pericardial effusion	• Nonsteroidal antiinflammatory drugs (e.g., ibuprofen, indomethacin) • Discontinuance of anticoagulants • Close monitoring for clinical indications of cardiac tamponade
Dressler's syndrome (also referred to as *postmyocardial infarction syndrome*): late pericarditis that is thought to be autoimmune	• Fever • Chest pain that worsens with deep breath and lessens with sitting up and leaning forward • Pericardial friction rub • Elevated WBC, sedimentation rate • Diffuse ST segment elevation across the precordial leads • Chest X-ray may show pericardial effusion	• Corticosteroids (e.g., prednisone)

Sudden cardiac death	• Cardiopulmonary arrest	• Preventive measures include:
		  • Risk factor modification
		  • Antiplatelet aggregation therapy (e.g., ASA)
		  • Beta-blockers for Q-wave MIs
		  • Diltiazem for non–Q-wave MIs
		  • HMG CoA reductase inhibitors (statins)
		  • Encouragement of family members to learn CPR
		• Treatment: CPR; ACLS modalities

pulmonary edema where fluid is pushed from the pulmonary capillary into the interstitium and finally into the alveolus due to increased pulmonary capillary hydrostatic pressure

2. Elevated PAP, normal PAOP = noncardiac pulmonary edema where fluid leaks from the pulmonary capillary into the interstitium and alveolus due to damage to the alveolar-capillary membrane

Etiology (see Table 3-22)
Pathophysiology

I. Systolic versus diastolic dysfunction
  A. Systolic dysfunction (pump problem): inability of the ventricle to shorten against a load; the left ventricle loses its ability to contract normally against progressive increases in afterload
    1. Possible causes: myocardial infarction, myocardial contusion, myocarditis, dilated

Table 3-22	Etiologic Factors of Heart Failure	
LVF	**RVF**	
• Hypertension	• LVF	
• CAD/LV infarction	• CAD/RV infarction	
• Dysrhythmias	• Dysrhythmias	
• Volume overload	• Volume overload	
• Valvular disease: mitral or aortic	• Valvular disease: mitral or pulmonic	
• Ventricular septal defect	• Ventricular septal defect	
• Cardiomyopathy	• Cardiomyopathy	
• Coarctation of aorta	• Myocardial contusion	
• Myocarditis	• Pulmonary hypertension	
• Cardiac tamponade	• Passive: mitral valve disease	
	• Active: hypoxemia, pulmonary embolus	
Biventricular Failure		
• Increased demand	• Electrolyte imbalance	
• Thyrotoxicosis	• Hyponatremia	
• Anemia	• Hypokalemia	
• Pregnancy	• Hypocalcemia	
• Systemic infection	• Hypomagnesemia	
• Beriberi	• Hypophosphatemia	
• Paget's disease		

    cardiomyopathy, aortic regurgitation, electrolyte imbalance, dysrhythmias

    2. Hemodynamics: decreased contractility; EF less than 40%; increased cardiac volumes and pressures

    3. Clinical indications: displaced PMI, JVD, S_3, crackles, dyspnea

    4. Pharmacology: arterial vasodilators, ACE inhibitors, diuretics, inotropes

  B. Diastolic dysfunction (filling problem): an impairment in left ventricular filling at near normal or mildly elevated left atrial and ventricular pressures; due to decrease in ventricular compliance; small changes in volume are associated with a disproportionate increase in pressure

    1. Possible causes: myocardial ischemia, hypertrophic cardiomyopathy, hypertension, ventricular hypertrophy, hypervolemia, constrictive pericarditis or cardiac tamponade, valvular heart disease, aging

    2. Hemodynamics: increased contractility, normal EF, increased cardiac pressures, normal or slightly increased cardiac volumes

    3. Clinical indications: S_4, crackles, dyspnea

    4. Pharmacology: beta-blockers, calcium channel blockers, venous vasodilators

II. Compensatory mechanisms: in the short term these mechanisms compensate for the failing heart, but in the long term all of these factors trigger a process of pathologic growth and remodeling

A. Sympathetic nervous system stimulation

    1. Increase in heart rate, contractility, and conductivity initially increases cardiac output

      a) Coronary artery blood flow is eventually reduced by diastolic shortening caused by tachycardia

      b) Dysrhythmias may occur

    2. Vasoconstriction increases preload and afterload and therefore blood pressure

      a) Myocardial oxygen consumption increases

      b) Ventricular dilation and hypertrophy may occur

B. Activation of renin-angiotensin-aldosterone system

    1. Sodium and water retention and peripheral vasoconstriction increase blood volume and preload

      a) Myocardial oxygen consumption increases

      b) Pulmonary and peripheral edema may eventually occur

      c) Ventricular dilation and hypertrophy may occur

C. Hypertrophy

    1. More myofibrils increase cross-bridge cycling, and more mitochondria increase supply of ATP

      a) Disproportionate number of ATP-consuming myofibrils to ATP-producing mitochondria eventually results

      b) Decreased endocardial perfusion and increased wall stress may eventually occur

D. Interstitial remodeling

    1. Collagen formation may initially reduce ventricular dilation

    2. Compliance is eventually decreased and diastolic dysfunction results

    3. Force transmission through ventricular wall is eventually decreased

Clinical Presentation (see Table 3-23)

I. Additional diagnostics

  A. BUN and creatinine: may be elevated

  B. Echocardiography: chamber dilation, atrial and/or ventricular hypertrophy, valve dysfunction, septal or ventricular free wall motion abnormality, decreased ejection fraction (usually <40%)

  C. Multiple-gated acquisition (MUGA) scan: wall motion abnormalities, decreased ejection fraction

  D. CT and MRI: may show chamber, valve, or cardiac wall abnormalities

  E. Cardiac catheterization: increase in cardiac pressures; may show valvular abnormalities with pressure gradient

II. New York Heart Association functional classification

  A. Class I: patients with cardiac disease but without resulting limitation of physical activity; ordinary physical activity does not cause undue fatigue, palpitation, dyspnea, or angina

Table 3-23	**Clinical Manifestation of Heart Failure**
LVF	**RVF**
• Tachypnea, dyspnea, orthopnea, PND	• Jugular venous distention
• Tachycardia	• Hepatojugular reflux
• Left-sided S_3	• Dependent pitting edema
• Displaced PMI, heave at apex	• Heave at sternum
• Crackles, wheezes	• Hepatomegaly/ splenomegaly
• Cough, frothy sputum, hemoptysis	• Anorexia, nausea, vomiting, abdominal pain
• Pulsus alternans	• Ascites
• Oliguria	• Nocturia
• Weakness, fatigue	• Weakness, fatigue
• Mental confusion	• Weight gain
• Murmur of MR	• Murmur of TR
ABGs: decreased Pao_2, Sao_2	• Right-sided S_3
Hemodynamics: elevated PA, PAOP; decreased CO/CI	Hemodynamics: elevated CVP, RAP
Abnormal chest X-ray	Abnormal liver function studies
• Cardiomegaly	• ALT
• Engorged pulmonary vasculature	• AST
• Kerley B lines	• LDH
• Pleural effusion	ECG
ECG	• Right atrial enlargement
• Left atrial enlargement	• Right ventricular hypertrophy
• Left ventricular hypertrophy	• Atrial dysrhythmias
• Atrial dysrhythmias	

B. Class II: patients with cardiac disease resulting in slight limitation of physical activity; they are comfortable at rest; ordinary physical activity results in fatigue, palpitation, dyspnea, or angina

C. Class III: patients with cardiac disease resulting in marked limitation of physical activity; they are comfortable at rest; less than ordinary activity causes fatigue, palpitation, dyspnea, or angina

D. Class IV: patients with cardiac disease resulting in inability to carry on any physical activity without discomfort; symptoms of cardiac insufficiency or angina may be present even at rest; if any physical activity is attempted, discomfort is increased

Nursing Diagnoses
I. Decreased Cardiac Output related to alterations in preload, afterload, contractility, or heart rate
II. Impaired Gas Exchange related to intraalveolar fluid
III. Fluid Volume Excess related to maladaptive compensatory mechanism secondary to decreased cardiac output
IV. Altered Protection caused by Electrolyte Balance related to increased body fluid, decrease

in renal perfusion, diuretic therapy, sodium restriction
V. Activity Intolerance related to decreased cardiac output, decrease in tissue oxygen delivery, deconditioning
VI. Sleep Pattern Disturbance related to dyspnea, anxiety, nocturia
VII. Anxiety related to acute health alteration and recommended lifestyle changes
VIII. Knowledge Deficit related to unfamiliarity with disease process, therapy, and recommended lifestyle changes

Collaborative Management
I. Treat the cause if possible
II. Improve oxygenation
   A. Oxygen by nasal cannula at 2 to 6 L/min to maintain Spo_2 of 95% unless contraindicated
   B. Intubation, mechanical ventilation with positive end-expiratory pressure (PEEP) may be required
   C. Elimination of accumulated fluid: diuretics
III. Decrease myocardial oxygen consumption
   A. Physical and emotional rest
      1. Maintain bed rest for 24 hours then gradually increase activity after 24 hours; allow rest after meals, personal hygiene, toileting, physical therapy, etc.
      2. Prevent Valsalva maneuver
         a) Teach patient to exhale when turning in bed
         b) Administer stool softeners as prescribed
         c) Provide bedside commode for elimination
      3. Explain procedures thoroughly: monitor alarms, equipment, visiting hours, reasons for procedures
      4. Keep family informed regarding patient's progress and status
      5. Provide for physical comfort: temperature, lighting, noise control
      6. Instruct patient regarding relaxation techniques; encourage utilization
      7. Provide appropriate nutrition: soft, low-sodium (2-3 g/day) diet
      8. Administer anxiolytics as prescribed: usually diazepam (Valium), lorazepam (Ativan), or alprazolam (Xanax)
   B. Beta-blockers as prescribed; usually used for Class II, III HF
      1. Beta-blockers act as cardioprotective agents to protect the heart from excessive catecholamines; they have also been shown to decrease left ventricular mass and volume, change the shape of the ventricle from spherical to elliptical, increase exercise capacity
      2. Carvedilol (Coreg) is a noncardioselective alpha- and beta-blocker; it is the first FDA-approved beta-blocker for heart failure

3. Monitor closely for decompensation as beta-blocker therapy is initiated

IV. Manage dysrhythmias

A. Atrial

1. Treat the HF since conversion to NSR is most likely as atrial stretch is decreased
2. Administer digoxin to decrease ventricular rate by increasing refractoriness of AV node

B. Ventricular

1. Administer antidysrhythmics as prescribed (e.g., lidocaine); lidocaine does not decrease contractility as procainamide and bretylium can
2. Treat the HF to improve tissue perfusion

C. Dual-chamber pacemaker with rate modulation: beneficial for patients with severe heart failure with poor activity tolerance; increases heart rate in response to physical activity

V. Decrease preload

A. Positioning: high Fowler's, legs dependent

B. Sodium and fluid restrictions

1. Fluid restriction to less than 1500 ml/24 hr
2. Sodium restriction to less than 2.5 g/24 hr

C. Diuretics (usually loop diuretics [e.g., furosemide]) to decrease pulmonary congestion and preload; overuse will decrease blood volume, decrease CO, and lead to organ hypoperfusion and prerenal azotemia

D. Venous vasodilators: NTG, morphine

E. Phlebotomy: only if patient is polycythemic

F. Dialysis: if the patient is in renal failure

VI. Decrease afterload

A. Nitroprusside: particularly helpful for hypertensive patients

B. Calcium channel blockers

C. ACE inhibitors or angiotensin II blockers: especially if HF and normal sinus rhythm

D. Pulmonary vasodilators: aminophylline; furosemide

E. Intraaortic balloon pump: may be used in severe cases (see Table 3-16)

1. Intraaortic balloon pump is especially helpful for patients who have very high afterload that is refractory to arterial vasodilators or who are too hypotensive to utilize arterial dilators to reduce afterload

VII. Increase contractility

A. Cardiac glycosides (e.g., digoxin); especially if HF and supraventricular tachycardia

1. Action: increases ejection fraction and exercise tolerance
2. Narrow therapeutic/toxic ratio (Table 3-24)

B. Sympathetic stimulants (e.g., dobutamine); especially helpful if HF in presence of acute MI; parenteral only

C. PDE inhibitors (e.g., amrinone, milrinone); used only if no response to digitalis, diuretics, vasodilators; parenteral only

D. Ventricular assist device (VAD): used in severe

Table 3-24	**Digitalis Toxicity: Summary**	
Normal Digoxin Level	**0.8-2.4 ng/ml**	
Clinical manifestations of digitalis toxicity	GI • Anorexia • Nausea • Vomiting Neurologic • Headache • Restlessness • Visual changes Cardiovascular • Sinus bradycardia, block, or arrest • PAT with AV block • Junctional tachycardia • AV blocks: 1st, 2nd type I, 3rd • PVCs: bigeminy, trigeminy, quadrigeminy • Ventricular tachycardia: especially bidirectional • Ventricular fibrillation	

Treatment of digitalis toxicity	Discontinue digitalis: digoxin, digitoxin
	Treat the cause, if possible
	• Correct electrolyte imbalance (frequently hypokalemia)
	• Corect acid-base imbalance
	• Correct hypoxemia
	• Correct ischemia
	Treat dysrhythmias
	• For symptomatic bradydysrhythmias and blocks
	  • Atropine
	  • External pacemaker
	• For symptomatic tachydysrhythmias
	  • Lidocaine
	  • Propranolol if no conduction problems
	  • Defibrillation for ventricular fibrillation
	  • **Note:** elective cardioversion is not used for patients with digitalis toxicity
	• For life-threatening rhythm that does not respond to therapy
	  • Digoxin immune FAB (Digibind)	

cases, especially if patient is a candidate for cardiac transplantation (see Table 3-25)

E. Surgical approaches: most suited for dilated cardiomyopathy

1. Dynamic cardiomyoplasty

a) Latissimus dorsi muscle (LDM) wrapped around the heart and stimulated by electrical impulses to contract with each heartbeat

b) Indicated if LVEF less than 40% and LVEDP less than 35 mm Hg and patient is not a candidate for cardiac transplantation

Table 3-25 **Ventricular Assist Device**

Indications	• Pending recovery: persistent heart failure despite aggressive therapy but with potential for recovery if the heart is given time to rest
	  • Inability to wean from cardiopulmonary bypass
	  • Cardiogenic shock refractory to pharmacologic or IABP therapy
	• Bridge to transplant: end-stage heart disease awaiting suitable donor for cardiac transplant
	• Physiologic indications despite pharmacologic support or IABP therapy
	  • MAP <60 mm Hg
	  • Systolic BP <90 mm Hg
	  • PAOP or RAP >20-25 mm Hg
	  • Urine output <20 ml/hr
	  • CI <2 L/min/m^2
	• May be used with IABP

Contraindications	• Irreversible, extensive heart disease; no possibility of being weaned from VAD and patient not a candidate for cardiac transplant • Prolonged cardiac arrest with resultant neurologic damage • Multiple organ failure • Significant complications or disease (e.g., chronic renal failure, cancer with metastasis, severe hepatic disease, significant blood dyscrasias, severe COPD)
Actions	• Maintains circulation with flow assistance • Decreases myocardial workload to promote ventricular recovery

Insertion and mechanics	• LVAD
	  • Outflow circuit anastomosed to patient aorta or femoral artery
	  • Inflow circuit anastomosed to left atrium or ventricle
	  • Left atrium is usually used in the pending recovery patient
	  • Left ventricle is usually used in the bridge to transplant patient
	• RVAD
	  • Outflow circuit anastomosed to patient's pulmonary artery
	  • Inflow circuit anastomosed to right atrium
	• Bi-VAD
	  • Both ventricles are supported; the main advantage here is that with either LVAD or RVAD the unassisted ventricle may fail
	• Implanted device
	  • The pump unit may be implanted into the abdominal wall
	  • Controller unit and power source are attached to the pump unit by a percutaneous lead

Assessment	• HR: a normalization of heart rate is desirable • BP: an increase in MAP is desirable • CO/CI: an increase in cardiac output/index is desirable • Thermodilution CO will not be accurate in patients with RVAD; use Fick formula (calculation of CO using mixed venous oxygen saturation and arterial oxygen saturation) • PAP/PAOP: a decrease in PAP and PAOP is desirable • Sao$_2$: an increase in Sao$_2$ is desirable • Svo$_2$: an increase in Svo$_2$ is desirable • Urine output: an increase in urine output is desirable • Complaints of chest pain: a decrease in chest pain is desirable • ECG: a decrease in the presence or frequency of dysrhythmias is desirable • Neurovascular status of affected limb: the presence of palpable pulses and a warm limb with normal capillary refill is desirable
Nursing Diagnoses	• Decreased Cardiac Output related to pump failure, dysrhythmias, mechanical problems with the VAD • Risk for Impaired Gas Exchange related to pulmonary vascular congestion or pulmonary infection • Risk for Fluid Volume Deficit related to third-spacing, coagulopathies • Risk for Infection related to invasive catheters, devices, open thorax • Anxiety related to insertion of VAD, noise from device, critical illness, critical care environment
Brief summary of nursing management	• Assess the parameters described above • Titrate pharmacologic therapies to augment the mechanical therapy of the VAD • Adjust fluid balance by administering colloids, crystalloids, or diuretics as prescribed • Prevent hazards of immobility: turn side to side when hemodynamics are stabilized; passive range of motion; utilize special mattresses and beds as indicated • Observe for complications and provide appropriate management for the prevention of complications • Provide emotional support to the patient and family; utilize social services, pastoral care, and support groups as indicated

Continued

Table 3-25	Ventricular Assist Device—cont'd

Complications	• Thromboembolism: heparin may be prescribed
	• Hemolysis
	• Bleeding
	  • Monitor ACT while on heparin
	  • Monitor for bleeding
	  • Administer blood and blood products as indicated
	  • Prevent tubing disconnection; all connections should be clearly visible and securely connected
	• Infection
	  • Monitor CBC, body temperature, and heart rate
	  • Monitor for pain, tenderness, heat, redness at exit site, and abdominal pump pocket
	  • Assess breath sounds and chest X-ray; pneumonia is common because of immobilization; ventilatory assistance is required with some VADs
	• Cerebral emboli
	• Respiratory failure
	• Renal failure
	• Air embolus
	• Mechanical failure

Weaning	• The following parameters with VAD off are required prior to weaning the patient from the VAD:
	  • MAP >60 mm Hg
	  • RAP (RVAD) or PAOP (LVAD) <25 mm Hg
	  • CI >2.0 L/min/m^2
	• The VAD flow is decreased
	• Anticoagulation is recommended during weaning
	• VAD removal is done in the OR

c) Requires thoracotomy but does not require cardiopulmonary bypass
   (1) Cardiac drugs restarted after extubation
   (2) Electrical stimulation of muscle wrap begins about 2 weeks after surgery
   (3) Clinical improvement may not be evident for 6 months or more
2. Partial left ventriculectomy (also referred to as the *Batista heart failure procedure*)
   a) Resection of a wedge of left ventricular wall to restore the volume-mass-diameter relationship of the left ventricle; mitral and/or tricuspid valve may be replaced concurrently
   b) Indicated if LV end-diastolic diameter more than 7 cm, NYHD Functional class III or IV; may be awaiting cardiac transplantation
3. Cardiac transplantation: especially for cardiomyopathy (see Chapter 11)

VIII. Provide collaborative management specific to RVF (cor pulmonale)
   A. Oxygen at 2 L/min: usually required continuous 24 hr/day
   B. Aminophylline or other pulmonary vasodilators as prescribed
   C. Anticoagulants if cause of RVF is pulmonary embolism
   D. Thrombolytics if cause of RVF is pulmonary embolism and patient has significant RVF or refractory hypoxemia

IX. Monitor for complications
   A. Deep-vein thrombosis/pulmonary embolism
   B. Progressive deterioration
   C. Dysrhythmias: common cause of sudden death
   D. Complications of therapy
      1. Fluid and electrolyte imbalance: hypokalemia, hypocalcemia, hypomagnesemia due to diuretic therapy
      2. Digitalis toxicity

Cardiomyopathy

Definition: Disorder involving the structure and function of the myocardium (Fig. 3-20)

Dilated (Previously Called *Congestive*)

I. Etiology
   A. Idiopathic
   B. Infection, especially viral (e.g., coxsackievirus B, arbovirus)
   C. Toxins (e.g., doxorubicin [Adriamycin], daunorubicin [Cerubidine]), alcohol, lead, arsenic, cobalt)
   D. Electrolyte, vitamin, or nutrient deficiency
      1. Hypokalemia
      2. Hypocalcemia
      3. Hypophosphatemia
      4. Thiamine deficiency
   E. Pregnancy
   F. Neuromuscular disorders (e.g., myasthenia gravis, multiple dystrophy)

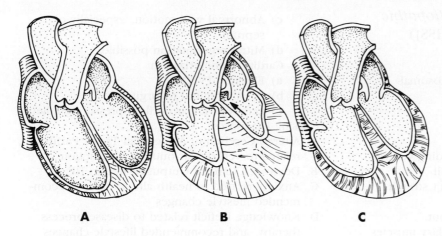

Figure 3-20 Cardiomyopathies. **A,** Dilated. **B,** Hypertrophic. **C,** Restrictive. (From Kinney MR, Packa DR, Dunbar SB: *AACN's clinical reference for critical-care nursing,* ed 3, St Louis, 1993, Mosby.)

G. Connective tissue disorders (e.g., lupus, scleroderma)
H. Infiltrative disorders (e.g., sarcoidosis, amyloidosis)
I. Hyperthyroidism
II. Pathophysiology
  A. Damage to myofibrils
  B. Decreased contractility
  C. Preload and afterload increased by stimulation of the renin-angiotensin-aldosterone system
  D. Gross dilation of heart, often affecting all four chambers
  E. Refractory HF
III. Clinical presentation
  A. Subjective
    1. Fatigue
    2. Chest pain
    3. Palpitations
    4. Syncope
    5. Symptoms of HF: dyspnea, edema
  B. Objective
    1. Orthostatic BP changes
    2. May have murmurs of tricuspid and/or mitral regurgitation
    3. Signs of biventricular failure
      a) LVF: S_3, crackles, PMI displaced laterally
      b) RVF: JVD, peripheral edema, hepatomegaly
  C. Diagnostic
    1. Chest X-ray
      a) Cardiomegaly
      b) Pulmonary congestion
      c) Possibly pleural effusion
    2. Electrocardiography
      a) Biventricular hypertrophy, biatrial enlargement
      b) Dysrhythmias: atrial fibrillation common
    3. Echocardiography
      a) Decreased ventricular wall motion
      b) Decreased ejection fraction
      c) Enlarged chamber size
      d) Abnormal wall motion
    4. Cardiac catheterization
      a) Elevated LVEDP, PAOP, PAP

      b) Decreased cardiac output
      c) Decreased ejection fraction
      d) Mitral valve abnormality
      e) RVEDP, RAP may be elevated if RVF present
IV. Nursing diagnoses
  A. Decreased Cardiac Output related to decreased contractility
  B. Impaired Gas Exchange related to intraalveolar fluid
  C. Activity Intolerance related to decreased tissue oxygenation
  D. Anxiety related to health alteration and recommended lifestyle changes
  E. Knowledge Deficit related to disease process, therapy, and recommended lifestyle changes
V. Collaborative management
  A. Provide care as for HF
    1. Oxygen by nasal cannula at 2 to 6 L/min to maintain SpO_2 of 95% unless contraindicated
    2. ACE inhibitors (e.g., captopril)
    3. Vasodilators (e.g., nitrates)
    4. Diuretics (e.g., furosemide)
    5. Inotropes (e.g., digoxin)
  B. Decrease myocardial oxygen consumption
    1. Activity restrictions
    2. Sodium restrictions
    3. Physical comfort: temperature, lighting, noise control
    4. Anxiolytics as prescribed and indicated: usually diazepam (Valium), lorazepam (Ativan), or alprazolam (Xanax)
  C. Monitor for complications
    1. Dysrhythmias
      a) Atrial fibrillation: digoxin
      b) Ventricular dysrhythmias: antidysrhythmic agents (e.g., lidocaine)
    2. Systemic emboli: anticoagulation frequently prescribed especially for patients with ejection fractions less than 30%
  D. Assist in preparation of the patient for cardiac transplantation if he or she is a candidate

Hypertrophic (Previously called *Idiopathic Hypertrophic Subaortic Stenosis* [IHSS])

I. Etiology
  A. Idiopathic
  B. Heredity: genetically transmitted autosomal-dominant trait
  C. Neuromuscular disorders
  D. Hypoparathyroidism
II. Pathophysiology
  A. Hypertrophy of heart muscle, including ventricular septum and ventricular free wall
  B. Rigid, noncompliant ventricles won't stretch to fill
  C. Decreased preload and cardiac output
  D. Mitral regurgitation caused by papillary muscles and mitral valve pulled out of alignment
  E. With severe hypertrophy, left ventricular outflow tract obstruction, especially when contractility is increased by increase in circulating catecholamines
  F. Decrease in blood flow to coronary arteries (angina) and brain (syncope)
  G. Sudden cardiac death may result
III. Clinical presentation
  A. Subjective
    1. Dyspnea, orthopnea, PND
    2. Chest pain
    3. Palpitations
    4. Syncope
  B. Objective
    1. PMI displaced laterally
    2. Crackles
    3. S_3
    4. S_4
    5. Murmurs
      a) Subaortic stenosis: systolic ejection murmur loudest along left sternal border; increases with Valsalva maneuver, decreases with squatting position
      b) Mitral regurgitation: holosystolic blowing murmur loudest at apex radiates to axilla
  C. Diagnostic
    1. Chest X-ray
      a) Left atrial dilation
      b) Cardiomegaly
      c) Pulmonary congestion
    2. Electrocardiography
      a) Left atrial enlargement and left ventricular hypertrophy, ST and T-wave abnormalities
      b) Dysrhythmias
        (1) Atrial fibrillation frequently seen
        (2) Ventricular dysrhythmias may be seen
      c) Blocks: left anterior hemiblock frequently seen
    3. Echocardiography
      a) Left atrial enlargement
      b) Increased thickness of the interventricular septum and narrowing of left ventricular outflow tract

      c) Abnormal wall motion, especially of septum
      d) Mitral regurgitation possible
    4. Cardiac catheterization
      a) Elevated LVEDP
      b) Possibly mitral regurgitation
      c) Left ventricular outflow pressure gradient
IV. Nursing Diagnoses
  A. Altered Cerebral or Myocardial Tissue Perfusion related to ventricular outflow obstruction
  B. Decreased Cardiac Output related to HF
  C. Anxiety related to health alteration and recommended lifestyle changes
  D. Knowledge Deficit related to disease process, therapy, and recommended lifestyle changes
V. Collaborative management
  A. Prevent obstruction of the left ventricular outflow tract
    1. Administer beta-blockers and/or calcium channel blockers as prescribed
    2. Do not give inotropes
  B. Maintain adequate filling volumes
    1. Administer intravenous fluids as prescribed
    2. Do not give nitrates
    3. Be cautious with diuretics
  C. Monitor for complications
    1. Dysrhythmias
      a) Atrial: digoxin is not used because it may increase outflow tract obstruction; diltiazem or verapamil may be used
      b) Ventricular: antidysrhythmics (e.g., lidocaine)
    2. Systemic emboli: anticoagulants frequently prescribed, especially for patients with ejection fractions less than 30%
  D. Assist in preparation of the patient for surgical procedures
    1. Percutaneous laser myoplasty
    2. Ventriculomyotomy with mitral valve replacement
    3. Cardiac transplantation

Restrictive

I. Etiology
  A. Idiopathic
  B. Infiltrative disorders (e.g., sarcoidosis, amyloidosis)
  C. Endomyocardial fibrosis
  D. Glycogen deposition
  E. Radiation
  F. Lymphoma
  G. Connective tissue disorders (e.g., scleroderma)
II. Pathophysiology
  A. Fibrous tissue infiltrates myocardium, endocardium, and subendocardium
  B. Heart becomes noncompliant and can't stretch, fill, or contract well
  C. Decreased preload and contractility
  D. Decreased CO
  E. HF

III. Clinical presentation
  A. Subjective
    1. Chest pain
    2. Fatigue, weakness
    3. Dyspnea, orthopnea, PND
  B. Objective
    1. JVD
    2. Hepatomegaly
    3. Peripheral edema
    4. S₃
    5. Crackles
  C. Diagnostic
    1. Chest X-ray
      a) Cardiomegaly
      b) Pulmonary congestion
      c) Possibly pleural effusion
    2. Electrocardiography
      a) Low QRS voltage
      b) AV blocks are common
    3. Echocardiography
      a) Atrial enlargement
      b) Enlarged ventricular outside dimension but small ventricular chamber
    4. Cardiac catheterization: elevated LVEDP, RVEDP, PAOP, RAP
IV. Nursing diagnoses
  A. Decreased Cardiac Output related to inability of the heart to stretch and fill
  B. Activity Intolerance related to pump failure
  C. Anxiety related to health alteration and recommended lifestyle changes
  D. Knowledge Deficit related to disease process, therapy, and recommended lifestyle changes
V. Collaborative management
  A. Treat the cause: may include steroids
  B. Provide care as for HF
    1. Oxygen by nasal cannula at 2 to 6 L/min to maintain SpO₂ of 95% unless contraindicated
    2. ACE inhibitors (e.g., captopril)
    3. Vasodilators (e.g., nitrates)
    4. Diuretics (e.g., furosemide)
    5. Inotropes (e.g., digoxin)
  C. Monitor for complications
    1. Dysrhythmias
      a) Atrial fibrillation: digoxin
      b) Ventricular dysrhythmias: antidysrhythmic agents (e.g., lidocaine)
    2. AV blocks: pacemaker may be needed
    3. Systemic emboli: anticoagulants frequently prescribed, especially for patients with ejection fractions less than 30%
  D. Assist in preparation of the patient for cardiac transplantation if he or she is a candidate

Indications for Cardiac Transplantation
(for More Information About Organ Transplantation, see Chapter 11)
  I. Heart disease
    A. Severe functional limitations
    B. Poor prognosis

  C. Not surgically correctable
  D. Unresponsive to medical therapy
  E. Pulmonary vascular resistance (PVR) normal or reversible with therapy (if pulmonary hypertension is severe and irreversible, the patient may be a candidate for a heart-lung transplant)
 II. Age of 65 years or less
III. Lack of intrinsic disease in other organ systems that would limit long-term survival or be worsened by immunosuppressive therapy
 IV. Favorable psychosocial profile
  V. Blood negative for HIV and HBV

Acute Inflammatory Heart Disease
Pericarditis
  I. Definition: inflammatory process involving the visceral or parietal pericardium
 II. Etiology
  A. Idiopathic
  B. Myocardial infarction
    1. Acute: usually occurs within 7 days; related to inflammation and the healing process
    2. Dressler's syndrome: occurs later (usually 2 weeks or more); thought to be an autoimmune response
  C. Trauma
  D. Postcardiotomy or postthoracotomy
  E. Connective tissue diseases (e.g., lupus, scleroderma, rheumatoid arthritis)
  F. Infection (e.g., tuberculosis)
  G. Neoplasms
  H. Dissecting thoracic aortic aneurysms
  I. Radiation therapy
  J. Uremia
  K. Hypothyroidism
  L. Drugs (e.g., procainamide, hydralazine, minoxidil, phenytoin, daunorubicin, isoniazid, penicillin, phenylbutazone)
III. Pathophysiology
  A. Inflammation of pericardium is usually a manifestation of a generalized disease process
  B. Fibrin, leukocytes, platelets may be deposited on the serous pericardium, causing constrictive pericarditis
  C. Increased capillary permeability due to inflammation may cause fluid leak into pericardial space; cardiac tamponade is possible
    1. As little as 50 to 100 ml may cause cardiac tamponade if the fluid accumulation is acute and rapid (e.g., trauma, postcardiotomy)
    2. As much as 2 L may not cause cardiac tamponade if the fluid accumulation is chronic and slow (e.g., uremia with pleural effusion)
  D. Either constrictive pericarditis or cardiac tamponade decreases diastolic filling of the heart, causing systemic and/or pulmonary venous congestion, decreased cardiac output, and cardiac index, leading to shock

IV. Clinical presentation
  A. Subjective
    1. Precordial or left pleuritic chest pain
      a) Persistent sharp or stabbing pain
      b) Radiates to the left shoulder, neck, or abdomen
      c) Aggravated by inspiration, cough, and supine position
      d) Relieved by sitting up and/or leaning forward (referred to as *Mohammed's sign*)
    2. Dyspnea
    3. Cough
    4. Hemoptysis
  B. Objective
    1. Tachypnea
    2. Tachycardia
    3. Fever
    4. Heart sound changes
      a) Pericardial friction rub
      b) Muffled heart sounds if pericardial effusion or cardiac tamponade occur
      c) Pericardial knock (loud, early-diastolic sound heard best at lower LSB) may be heard if constrictive pericarditis occurs
  C. Diagnostic
    1. Serum
      a) WBC: increased
      b) Sedimentation rate: increased
      c) CK-MB: negative
      d) ANA: positive if due to connective tissue disease
      e) Blood cultures: positive if due to infection
    2. Chest X-ray
      a) Cardiomegaly
      b) Pericardial effusion
      c) Pulmonary infiltrates
    3. Electrocardiography
      a) Diffuse concave ST elevation in all leads except aVL, aVR, and V_1; upright T-waves; no Q-waves
      b) Low voltage
      c) Dysrhythmias: atrial fibrillation, atrial flutter, premature atrial contractions, paroxysmal atrial tachycardia
    4. Echocardiography: pericardial effusion may be seen
V. Nursing Diagnoses
  A. Ineffective Breathing Patterns related to guarding due to chest pain
  B. Pain related to pericardial inflammation
  C. Risk for Decreased Cardiac Output related to decreased preload and contractility with cardiac tamponade
VI. Collaborative management
  A. Relieve pain and discomfort
    1. Semi-Fowler's or high Fowler's positions
    2. Nonsteroidal antiinflammatory drugs (NSAIDs)
      a) Indomethacin (Indocin)
      b) Ibuprofen (Motrin)
      c) Aspirin
    3. Steroids if no response to NSAIDs or if effusion present
    4. Narcotic analgesics if necessary
  B. Administer drugs and therapies for treatment of cause
    1. Antibiotics if bacterial
    2. Steroids if connective tissue disorder
    3. Dialysis for uremia
    4. Withdrawal of suspect drugs
  C. Discontinue anticoagulants as prescribed
    1. If anticoagulants must be continued, use heparin because it is much easier to reverse (with protamine) than dicumarol
    2. If anticoagulants are not discontinued, monitor the patient closely for clinical indications of cardiac tamponade
  D. Monitor for complications
    1. Dysrhythmias
      a) Atrial: digoxin, cardioversion
      b) Ventricular: lidocaine
    2. Constrictive pericarditis
    3. Cardiac tamponade: see Cardiac Tamponade section
    4. Heart failure
  E. Assist in preparation of patient for surgical procedures
    1. Pericardiocentesis and biopsy if cause unclear or if purulent pericarditis suspected
    2. Pericardial stripping

Myocarditis

I. Definition: inflammation of the myocardium
II. Etiology
  A. Viral infections (e.g., coxsackievirus A and B, poliomyelitis, influenza, rubella, rubeola, adenoviruses, echoviruses)
  B. Bacterial infections (e.g., diphtheria, tuberculosis, typhoid fever, tetanus, and staphylococcal, pneumococcal, and gonococcal infections)
  C. Parasitic infections (e.g., trypanosomiasis, toxoplasmosis)
  D. Helminthic infections (e.g., trichinosis)
  E. Fungal infections (e.g., *Candida*); usually seen in patients with immunosuppression
  F. Hypersensitivity reactions (e.g., rheumatic fever, postcardiotomy syndrome)
  G. Radiation therapy to the chest
  H. Chronic alcoholism
III. Pathophysiology
  A. Two stages
    1. Acute stage: usually lasts 5 to 7 days; myocyte destruction caused by causative agent or toxin
    2. Chronic stage: usually lasts 1 week to 2 months; autoimmune-mediated myocyte destruction
    3. Recovery or progression to dilated cardiomyopathy may occur

B. Damage to myocardium may be diffuse to focal
 1. Diffuse injury frequently causes heart failure
 2. Focal injury may cause necrosis of portions of the conduction system and blocks

IV. Clinical presentation
 A. Subjective
  1. Chest soreness or burning: increased by inspiration and supine position
  2. Easy fatigability
  3. Syncope
  4. Sudden, unexplained dyspnea, orthopnea, PND
 B. Objective
  1. Fever
  2. Crackles
  3. Heart sound changes
   a) Distant heart sounds
   b) S₃, S₄
   c) Murmur of mitral regurgitation may be heard
   d) Pericardial friction rub may be heard
 C. Diagnostic
  1. Serum
   a) WBC: increased
   b) CK-MB: may be elevated
   c) Sedimentation rate: elevated
  2. Chest X-ray
   a) Cardiomegaly
   b) Pleural or pericardial effusion
   c) Pulmonary congestion
  3. Electrocardiography
   a) Diffuse ST segment and T-wave abnormalities
   b) Low voltage
   c) Left axis deviation
   d) Dysrhythmias: supraventricular or ventricular
   e) Blocks: AV or bundle branch blocks
  4. Endomyocardial biopsy: done for definitive diagnosis
   a) Lymphocyte infiltration
   b) Myocyte necrosis

V. Nursing Diagnoses
 A. Decreased Cardiac Output related to HF
 B. Activity Intolerance related to HF
 C. Anxiety related to health alteration and recommended lifestyle changes
 D. Knowledge Deficit related to disease process, therapy, and recommended lifestyle changes

VI. Collaborative management
 A. Decrease myocardial oxygen consumption
  1. Bed rest and activity restrictions until fever and cardiac symptoms subside
  2. Oxygen by nasal cannula at 2-6 L/min to maintain Sao₂ of 95% unless contraindicated
  3. Sodium restrictions
  4. Physical comfort: temperature, lighting, noise control

  5. Anxiolytics as prescribed: usually diazepam (Valium), lorazepam (Ativan), or alprazolam (Xanax)
 B. Provide care as for HF
  1. Oxygen at 2 to 6 L/min via nasal cannula as indicated by pulse oximetry and/or arterial blood gases
  2. ACE inhibitors (e.g., captopril)
  3. Vasodilators (e.g., nitrates)
  4. Diuretics (e.g., furosemide)
  5. Inotropes
   a) Dobutamine usually used initially
   b) Digitalis may be used, especially if supraventricular tachydysrhythmias are present
   c) Amrinone (Inocor) or milrinone (Primacor) may be used
 C. Administer drugs and therapies for treatment of cause
  1. Antibiotics for bacterial infections
  2. Amphotericin B for fungal infections
  3. Steroids for connective tissue diseases (steroids are contraindicated in early infectious viral myocarditis because they may enhance myocardial damage by increasing tissue necrosis and viral replication)
  4. Withdrawal of offending agent
 D. Monitor for complications
  1. Dysrhythmias
   a) Atrial: may be treated with digoxin or cardioversion (these patients are very sensitive to digitalis and prone to digitalis toxicity)
   b) Ventricular: usually treated with lidocaine, cardioversion, or defibrillation
  2. Blocks: temporary or permanent pacemaker frequently required
  3. Pericarditis: monitor closely for clinical indications of cardiac tamponade
  4. Systemic emboli: anticoagulants may be prescribed; if so, monitor closely for clinical indications of cardiac tamponade
  5. Dilated cardiomyopathy

Infective Endocarditis

I. Definition: inflammation of the endocardium, usually occurring in the membranous lining of the heart valves; may also involve cardiac prosthesis
II. Etiology
 A. Predisposing factors include the following:
  1. Congenital or acquired valvular heart disease
   a) Rheumatic heart disease
   b) Congenital heart disease, including septal defects
   c) Mitral valve prolapse
  2. Cardiac surgery: especially valve repairs or replacements
  3. Invasive tests or monitoring
   a) Intracardiac catheters (e.g., cardiac catheterization, pulmonary artery catheter, transvenous pacing catheters)

b) Intravenous catheters (e.g., central vein catheter, dialysis shunt)

c) Gastrointestinal or genitourinary procedures (e.g., bladder catheterization)

d) Gynecologic or obstetric surgeries

4. Skin, bone, or pulmonary infections

5. Poor oral hygiene

6. Dental procedures

7. IV drug use

8. Immunosuppressed state (e.g., AIDS, cancer, diabetes mellitus, burns, hepatitis, immunosuppressive drugs, or steroids)

B. Causative agents

1. Group A nonhemolytic *Streptococcus*

2. *Streptococcus pneumoniae* (pneumococcus)

3. *Staphylococcus aureus*

4. *Staphylococcus epidermidis*

5. *Streptococcus viridans*

6. *Streptococcus faecalis* (enterococci)

7. *Pseudomonas aeruginosa*

8. *Aspergillus fumigatus*

9. *Serratia marcescens*

10. *Candida albicans*

III. Pathophysiology

A. May be either acute or subacute

1. Acute infective endocarditis: normal valves; severe systemic infection; progresses rapidly and causes severe valvular destruction; usually caused by *Staphylococcus aureus*

2. Subacute endocarditis: damaged valves; progresses more slowly; outcome usually good with adequate treatment; usually caused by *Streptococcus viridans*

B. Bacteria and/or blood products adhere to structural irregularities in the cardiac valves

C. Lesions form as a result of bacterial colonization

1. These lesions, called *vegetations,* contain bacteria, red blood cells, platelets, fibrin, collagen, and necrotic tissue

D. Valvular tissue damaged by the vegetations

E. Valve becomes incompetent and may later scar to become stenotic

F. Other problems include allergic vasculitis and embolization of vegetations and bacteria

IV. Clinical presentation

A. Subjective

1. Infectious symptoms (e.g., fever, chills, diaphoresis, malaise, anorexia, myalgias, arthralgias)

2. May have symptoms of HF: dyspnea, orthopnea, PND

B. Objective

1. Embolic or allergic vasculitis signs

a) Splinter hemorrhages

b) Petechiae: conjunctiva, chest, abdomen, oral mucosa

c) Janeway lesions: flat, painless erythematous lesion on palms, soles of feet, or extremities

d) Roth's spots: round white lesions on retina

e) Osler's nodes: painful nodules on fingers, toes

2. New or changed murmur

3. May have signs of HF: S_3, crackles, JVD, hepatomegaly, peripheral edema

C. Diagnostic

1. Serum

a) WBC: increased

b) Sedimentation rate: elevated

c) Blood cultures: positive

D. Chest X-ray

1. Cardiomegaly

2. Pulmonary congestion

E. Electrocardiography

1. Dysrhythmias

a) Atrial: supraventricular tachydysrhythmias, including PAT, atrial fibrillation, atrial flutter

b) Ventricular: PVCs

2. Blocks: AV blocks or bundle branch blocks

F. Echocardiography: vegetations and valve dysfunction

V. Nursing diagnosis

A. Risk for infection related to valve disease, causative organism

B. Risk for Decreased Cardiac Output related to valvular damage and resultant valve regurgitation

C. Risk for Altered Tissue Perfusion related to emboli

D. Knowledge Deficit related to unfamiliarity with disease process, therapy, and recommended lifestyle changes

VI. Collaborative management

A. Prevent endocarditis

1. People with valvular heart disease should receive prophylactic antibiotics prior to intrusive procedures (e.g., dental procedures, cardiac catheterization)

2. Good hygiene, especially oral, may also help to prevent endocarditis, especially in susceptible persons

3. Intrusive procedures should be avoided if possible

4. Injection of contaminated substances (e.g., "street" drugs) should be avoided

B. Decrease myocardial oxygen consumption

1. Bed rest and activity restrictions until fever and cardiac symptoms subside

2. Oxygen by nasal cannula at 2 to 6 L/min to maintain Spo_2 of 95% unless contraindicated

3. Sodium restrictions

C. Control and treat infection

1. Blood cultures

2. Antibiotics as prescribed

a) Antibiotic therapy for endocarditis is usually for 6 to 8 weeks duration

b) Long-term antibiotic therapy generally requires central venous catheter placement

D. Control hyperthermia
  1. Antipyretics (e.g., ASA, acetaminophen)
  2. Cooling measures
E. Maintain hydration: oral or intravenous fluid as indicated
F. Monitor for complications
  1. Systemic emboli: anticoagulants may be prescribed
    a) Monitor for clinical manifestations
      (1) Neurologic: visual field defects, hemiplegia, aphasia, change in level of consciousness, seizures
      (2) Cardiac: chest pain, ECG indicators of ischemia, injury, or infarction
      (3) Pulmonary: tachypnea, dyspnea, hemoptysis, pleuritic chest pain
      (4) Renal: hematuria, flank pain, oliguria
      (5) Splenic: pain in upper left quadrant, abdominal rigidity
      (6) Peripheral vascular: pain, pallor, pulselessness, paresthesia, paralysis, polar (coldness)
  2. Bacterial or mycotic aneurysm: localized abnormal expansion of a vessel due to destruction of part or all of the vessel wall by growth of bacteria or fungus
  3. Pericarditis or myocarditis
  4. Dysrhythmias or blocks: antidysrhythmics or pacemaker used
  5. HF: inotropes may be needed
G. Assist in preparation of patient for surgery for valve repair or replacement if indicated

Valvular Heart Disease

Definition: An acquired or congenital disorder of a cardiac valve; characterized by stenosis (obstruction) or regurgitation (backward flow) of blood

Mitral Regurgitation (Insufficiency, Incompetence)

I. Etiology
  A. Trauma
  B. Rheumatic heart disease (RHD) or other form of endocarditis
  C. Papillary muscle dysfunction or rupture, or rupture of chordae tendineae
  D. Congenital malformation of mitral valve
  E. Mitral valve prolapse (MVP) (also referred to as *Barlow's syndrome* or *floppy mitral valve syndrome*)
  F. LV dilation from LVF
  G. Hypertrophic cardiomyopathy
  H. Marfan's syndrome
  I. Calcification of mitral valve leaflets
II. Pathophysiology
  A. Portion of LV volume is ejected back into the LA during ventricular systole because of incompetent mitral valve
    1. Increased left atrial pressure

  2. Increased pulmonary artery pressure
  3. Pulmonary hypertension
  4. Right ventricular failure (and eventually hypertrophy)
  B. Since the mitral valve does not close, blood enters the left ventricle during the entire phase of diastole (including isovolumetric relaxation); this leakage leads to left ventricular failure (and eventually hypertrophy)
III. Clinical presentation
  A. Subjective
    1. Dyspnea, orthopnea, PND; may have cough
    2. Chest pain may occur but is not common
    3. Palpitations may occur
    4. Weakness, fatigue
    5. Anxiety
  B. Objective
    1. Tachycardia
    2. Diaphoresis
    3. Confusion
    4. PMI displaced laterally; may be more diffuse
    5. Crackles may be present
    6. Heart sound changes
      a) S$_2$ may be widely split
      b) S$_3$, S$_4$ may be heard
      c) Holosystolic murmur: high-pitched, blowing, loudest at apex, and radiates to axilla
    7. Signs of RVF: JVD, hepatomegaly, peripheral edema
  C. Hemodynamic parameters: PAOP waveform shows large *v*-waves
  D. Diagnostic
    1. Chest X-ray
      a) Cardiomegaly
      b) Left atrial enlargement
      c) Left ventricular hypertrophy
      d) Pulmonary congestion may be present
    2. Electrocardiography
      a) Left atrial enlargement
      b) Left and/or right ventricular hypertrophy
      c) Dysrhythmias: most frequently atrial fibrillation
    3. Echocardiography
      a) Thickening, prolapse, and calcification of mitral valve
      b) Right ventricular, left atrial, and left ventricular enlargement
    4. Cardiac catheterization
      a) Increased left atrial and ventricular pressures
      b) Regurgitation of blood from the left ventricle to the left atrium

Mitral Stenosis

I. Etiology
  A. RHD
  B. Endocarditis
  C. Congenital
  D. Tumors of left atrium (e.g., atrial myxoma)
  E. Calcification of mitral annulus

II. Pathophysiology
    A. Mitral valve will not open well because of progressive fibrosis, scarring, calcification, or fusion of commissures
    B. LA pressure increases
    C. Dilation of LA (may cause atrial fibrillation)
    D. Pulmonary hypertension
    E. Pulmonary edema may occur
    F. Right ventricular hypertrophy
    G. RVF

III. Clinical presentation
    A. Subjective
        1. Dyspnea, orthopnea, PND, crackles
        2. Cough, hemoptysis
        3. Fatigue, weakness
        4. Palpitations
        5. Dysphagia
        6. Hoarseness
        7. Syncope may occur
        8. Chest pain may occur but is rare
    B. Objective
        1. Ruddy face (mitral facies)
        2. RV heave palpable at sternum
        3. Heart sound changes
            a) Loud S_1: referred to as *closing snap*
            b) Loud P_2
            c) Opening snap
            d) Middiastolic murmur: harsh, rumbling, loudest at apex; may have associated thrill
        4. Signs of RVF: JVD, hepatomegaly, peripheral edema
    C. Hemodynamic parameters: PAOP waveform shows large *a*-waves
    D. Diagnostic
        1. Chest X-ray
            a) Left atrial enlargement
            b) Pulmonary congestion
            c) Right ventricular hypertrophy
            d) Mitral valve calcification
        2. Electrocardiography
            a) Left atrial enlargement (frequently referred to as *P-mitrale*)
            b) Right ventricular hypertrophy
            c) Dysrhythmias: most frequently atrial fibrillation
        3. Echocardiography
            a) Abnormal movement and thickening of valve leaflets and narrowing of mitral valve orifice
            b) Left atrial enlargement
            c) Right ventricular hypertrophy
        4. Cardiac catheterization
            a) Elevated pressure gradient across mitral valve
            b) Elevated LAP, PAP, PAOP

Aortic Regurgitation (Insufficiency, Incompetence)

I. Etiology
    A. RHD
    B. Calcification
    C. Congenital malformation (e.g., bicuspid aortic valve)
    D. Endocarditis
    E. Syphilis
    F. Marfan's syndrome
    G. Hypertension
    H. Connective tissue disease (e.g., lupus erythematosus)
    I. Aortic dissection
    J. Trauma

II. Pathophysiology
    A. Incompetent aortic valve allows blood from the aorta to reenter left ventricle during diastole
    B. LVEDV and LVEDP increase
    C. Left ventricle dilates and fails
    D. Left atrium dilates
    E. Pulmonary hypertension; pulmonary edema may occur
    F. Low aortic root pressure decreases coronary artery filling pressure, causing myocardial ischemia

III. Clinical presentation
    A. Subjective
        1. Fatigue
        2. Cough
        3. Symptoms of HF: dyspnea, orthopnea, PND
        4. Exertional chest pain
        5. Syncope
        6. Palpitations
    B. Objective
        1. Musset's sign: nodding of the head with each systole
        2. Widened pulse pressure
        3. Water-hammer (also called *Corrigan's*) pulse: rapid rise that collapses suddenly
        4. PMI displaced laterally and downward
        5. Hill's sign: popliteal is greater than brachial BP by 40 mm Hg or more
        6. Quincke's sign: visible capillary pulsation of nailbeds when fingertip is pressed
        7. Signs of HF: S_3, crackles, JVD, hepatomegaly, peripheral edema
        8. Heart sound changes
            a) Diastolic murmur: high-pitched, blowing, decrescendo, loudest at base, may radiate to the apex; may have associated thrill
            b) May have aortic ejection click
            c) Systolic murmur: may have systolic ejection murmur
    C. Diagnostic
        1. Chest X-ray
            a) Left atrial enlargement
            b) Left ventricular hypertrophy
            c) Pulmonary congestion
        2. Electrocardiography
            a) Sinus tachycardia
            b) Left ventricular hypertrophy
            c) Left atrial enlargement
        3. Echocardiography
            a) Poor aortic valve motion
            b) Thickening of aortic valve

c) Left ventricular hypertrophy
d) Left atrial enlargement
4. Cardiac catheterization
   a) Elevated LAP, LVEDP
   b) Regurgitation from aorta to left ventricle

Aortic Stenosis

I. Etiology
  A. RHD
  B. Calcification
  C. Congenital bicuspid valve
  D. Aortic coarctation
II. Pathophysiology
  A. Incomplete aortic valve opening
  B. Increased afterload
  C. Increased left ventricular workload
  D. Left ventricle hypertrophy
  E. LVF
  F. Left atrial enlargement
  G. Pulmonary hypertension; pulmonary edema may occur
  H. RVF
  I. Low aortic root pressure decreases coronary artery filling pressure, causing myocardial ischemia
III. Clinical presentation
  A. Subjective
    1. Chest pain, especially on exertion
    2. Syncope, especially on exertion
    3. Symptoms of LVF: dyspnea, orthopnea, PND
    4. Fatigue, weakness
    5. Palpitations
  B. Objective
    1. Narrow pulse pressure
    2. PMI displaced laterally and/or downward
    3. Signs of LVF: S_3, crackles
    4. Heart sound changes
      a) May have split S_1
      b) Paradoxical split of S_2
      c) Systolic ejection murmur: harsh, crescendo/decrescendo, loudest at aortic area radiating to the neck
      d) May have aortic ejection click
  C. Diagnostic
    1. Chest X-ray
      a) Calcification of aortic valve may be seen
      b) Cardiomegaly
      c) Left atrial enlargement
      d) Left ventricular hypertrophy
      e) Pulmonary congestion
      f) Right ventricular hypertrophy
    2. Electrocardiography
      a) Left atrial enlargement (P-mitrale)
      b) Left ventricular hypertrophy
      c) Dysrhythmias: most frequently atrial fibrillation
      d) Blocks: AV blocks, left bundle branch block
    3. Echocardiography
      a) Aortic valve leaflet thickening and decreased movement of the leaflets

b) Calcification of aortic valve
c) High-pressure gradient between left ventricle and aorta
d) Left ventricular hypertrophy
e) Possibly right ventricular hypertrophy
4. Cardiac catheterization
   a) Significant pressure gradient
   b) Elevated LAP, LVEDP

Nursing Diagnoses

I. Decreased Cardiac Output related to HF
II. Altered Protection related to anticoagulant therapy
III. Activity Intolerance related to HF
IV. Anxiety related to health alteration and recommended lifestyle changes
V. Knowledge Deficit related to disease process, therapy, and recommended lifestyle changes

Collaborative Management

I. Decrease myocardial oxygen consumption
  A. Oxygen by nasal cannula at 2 to 6 L/min to maintain SpO_2 of 95% unless contraindicated
  B. Sodium restrictions
  C. Physical comfort: temperature, lighting, noise control
  D. Anxiolytics as prescribed: usually diazepam (Valium), lorazepam (Ativan), or alprazolam (Xanax)
II. Provide care for HF
  A. Oxygen at 2 to 6 L/min via nasal cannula as indicated by pulse oximetry and/or arterial blood gases
  B. ACE inhibitors (e.g., captopril)
  C. Vasodilators (e.g., nitrates)
  D. Diuretics (e.g., furosemide)
  E. Inotropes
    1. Digitalis may be used, especially if supraventricular tachydysrhythmias are present
    2. Dobutamine, amrinone, or milrinone may be used
III. Monitor for complications
  A. Dysrhythmias: usually atrial fibrillation
  B. Blocks: permanent pacemaker may be necessary
  C. Emboli (mural thrombi): potential for pulmonary, cerebral, renal, splenic, mesenteric embolus; antiembolic measures, including anticoagulation
  D. Endocarditis: prophylactic antibiotics prior to any invasive or dental procedures for prevention

Surgical Repair or Replacement of the Affected Valve

I. Valvuloplasty: repair of a valve utilizing a balloon-tipped intracardiac catheter; procedure similar to PTCA
II. Commissurotomy: surgical separation of the thickened adherent leaves of a stenoses valve (usually mitral)
III. Valve repair: repair of a valve; fibrous pericardium is frequently used

IV. Valve replacement
   A. Types of valve replacement
      1. Homografts: human cadaver valves that have been specially treated for surgical use; last approximately 5 to 8 years
      2. Heterograft: valve from an animal, usually a pig or cow, that has been prepared for surgical use; last approximately 5 to 8 years
      3. Artificial grafts: stainless steel, carbon, or other durable material; last approximately 10 to 15 years
   B. Postoperative management as for CABG with close monitoring for AV nodal blocks
   C. Homografts or heterografts do not require long-term anticoagulation; artificial grafts require long-term anticoagulation

Hypertensive Crises
Definitions
   I. Hypertension: elevation in blood pressure above 140/90 mm Hg on at least three separate occasions
   II. Hypertensive urgencies: develop over days to weeks and are characterized by a marked elevation in diastolic BP but usually are not associated with any clinical manifestations of end-organ damage
   III. Hypertensive crisis: hypertensive emergencies severe enough to cause the threat of immediate vascular necrosis and end-organ damage; usually greater than 180/120 mm Hg or MAP more than 150 mm Hg
   IV. Hypertensive emergencies: develop over hours to days; BP must be lowered within minutes to an hour to reduce potential complications of new or progressive end-organ damage

Etiology
   I. Primary or secondary
      A. Primary
         1. Untreated or inadequately treated essential (idiopathic) hypertension
            a) Risk factors: family history, African-American race, stress, obesity, high-fat and/or sodium diet, sedentary lifestyle, aging, tobacco use, oral contraceptives
            b) Poor compliance frequently a factor in hypertensive crisis; factors closely related to poor compliance include the following:
               (1) Lack of symptoms
               (2) Side effects
               (3) Cost
      B. Secondary
         1. Renal disease
            a) Increased renin-angiotensin levels
               (1) Renin-secreting tumor
               (2) Renovascular disease
            b) Acute glomerulonephritis
            c) Chronic pyelonephritis
         2. Eclampsia of pregnancy
         3. CNS injuries
            a) Head injury
            b) Spinal cord injury: autonomic dysreflexia

causes hypertension with bradycardia in patients with spinal cord injury T6 or above in response to noxious stimuli
         4. Burns
         5. Drug side effects: oral contraceptives, steroids, cocaine, amphetamines, decongestants
         6. Drug interactions: MAO inhibitors and tyramine; disulfiram (Antabuse) and alcohol
         7. Drug withdrawal: clonidine, beta-blockers, alcohol
         8. Pheochromocytoma
         9. Polycythemia
        10. Coarctation of the aorta
        11. Pituitary or adrenocortical hyperfunction (e.g., Cushing's syndrome, primary hyperaldosteronism)
        12. Vasculitis
        13. Scleroderma or other connective tissue disease
   II. Types of hypertensive crises
      A. Hypertensive urgencies
         1. Hypertension associated with coronary artery disease
         2. Severe hypertension following kidney transplant
         3. Postoperative hypertension
         4. Uncontrolled hypertension in the patient who requires emergency surgery
         5. Accelerated hypertension: DBP more than 120 mm Hg
         6. Malignant hypertension: DBP more than 140 mm Hg
      B. Hypertensive emergencies: develop over hours to days; BP must be lowered within minutes to an hour to reduce potential complications of new or progressive end-organ damage
         1. Acute aortic dissection
         2. Acute left ventricular failure with pulmonary edema
         3. Pheochromocytoma crisis
         4. MAO inhibitor and tyramine interaction
         5. Intracranial hemorrhage
         6. Eclampsia
         7. Hypertensive encephalopathy: BP more than 250/150 mm Hg

Pathophysiology
   I. Hypertension produces changes in the arterioles and decreases blood flow to vital organs; severe hypertension causes necrosis of the intima and media of the arteries
   II. Organ ischemia occurs from platelet aggregation, intravascular coagulation, arteriolar spasm, and edema
   III. Target organs most likely to be damaged by hypertensive crises
      A. Heart: increased afterload, hypertensive cardiovascular disease (HCVD), left ventricular hypertrophy and failure, angina, myocardial infarction
      B. Kidney: decreased renal perfusion, proteinuria, renal failure

C. Retina: hemorrhages, blindness
D. Brain: hypertensive encephalopathy
   1. Excessive cerebral hydrostatic pressure
   2. When cerebral perfusion pressure exceeds 150 mm Hg, cerebral autoregulation fails
   3. Increased capillary pressure and permeability
   4. Vasospasm, ischemia, cerebral edema and hemorrhage

Clinical Presentation

I. Accelerated or malignant hypertension
   A. Irritability, cognitive alterations
   B. Headache, especially in the morning
   C. Epistaxis
   D. Blurred vision, diplopia
   E. Retinopathy with exudates
   F. Severe impairment of renal function
      1. Serum BUN and creatinine may be elevated
      2. Nocturia
      3. Pressure-related diuresis
      4. Hematuria may be present
   G. Chest pain may be present
   H. Signs of left ventricular hypertrophy: PMI displaced to left, S_4, ECG indicators of LVH
   I. Signs of LVF may be present: dyspnea, left ventricular heave, S_3, crackles
II. Hypertensive encephalopathy
   A. Severe occipital or anterior headache
   B. Nausea, vomiting
   C. Visual disturbances (e.g., blurred vision, reduced visual acuity, photophobia, temporary loss of vision)
   D. Retinopathy, papilledema
   E. Signs of left ventricular failure/pulmonary edema: dyspnea, orthopnea, PND, S_3, crackles
   F. Altered mental status: confusion and agitation progressing to lethargy and coma
   G. Transitory focal neurologic signs (e.g., cranial nerve palsy, sensory or motor deficits, aphasia), positive Babinski reflex
III. Diagnostic
   A. Serum
      1. Potassium: hypokalemia occurs in primary hyperaldosteronism
      2. BUN, creatinine may be elevated
      3. Lipid profile to evaluate additional cardiac risk
   B. Urine: hematuria or proteinuria may be present
   C. Chest X-ray
      1. Cardiomegaly may be present
      2. Widening of mediastinum suggests dissecting thoracic aortic aneurysm
   D. Electrocardiography: may show left atrial enlargement, left ventricular hypertrophy
   E. CT of brain: may show cerebral edema and/or hemorrhage

Nursing Diagnoses

I. Altered Cardiopulmonary, Cerebral, and Renal Tissue Perfusion related to uncontrolled hypertension, adverse effects of antihypertensive therapy (e.g., hypotension)

II. Anxiety related to threat to or change in health status
III. Risk for Ineffective Management of Therapeutic Regimen related to complexity of regimen, cost of medication, side effects of therapy
IV. Knowledge Deficit related to unfamiliarity with disease process, therapy, and recommended lifestyle changes

Collaborative Patient Management

I. Maintain airway, ventilation, oxygenation
   A. Oxygen at 2 to 6 L/min via nasal cannula
   B. Airway maintenance: oropharyngeal airway if level of consciousness is altered
   C. Intubation, mechanical ventilation may be required
II. Decrease myocardial oxygen consumption
   A. Activity restriction initially
   B. Sodium restriction to less than 2-3 g/24 hr
   C. Smoking cessation
   D. Physical comfort: temperature, lighting, noise control
   E. Anxiolytics as prescribed: usually diazepam (Valium), lorazepam (Ativan), or alprazolam (Xanax)
III. Decrease blood pressure gradually
   A. Blood pressure decreased too aggressively may cause neurologic damage by significantly decreasing cerebral perfusion pressure; MAP should by decreased by 20% to 30% during the first 24 hours
   B. Antihypertensive agents
      1. Vasodilators
         a) Nitroprusside (Nipride): mixed arterial and venous vasodilator
            (1) Monitor for methemoglobinemia
               (a) Conversion of normal hemoglobin to methemoglobin, which cannot carry oxygen
               (b) Monitor for decrease in Spo_2 and clinical indications of hypoxia
               (c) Evaluate methemoglobin levels if methemoglobinemia is suspected
               (d) Discontinue NTP and administer 1% methylene blue as prescribed
            (2) Monitor of nitroprusside-induced intrapulmonary shunt
               (a) Caused by increased blood flow to the lung and resultant ventilation-perfusion mismatch
               (b) Monitor for decrease in Spo_2 and clinical indications of hypoxia
            (3) Monitor for thiocyanate/cyanide toxicity
               (a) Clinical indications include: metabolic acidosis, dyspnea, confusion, hyperreflexia, seizures, loss of consciousness
               (b) Treatment may include amyl nitrate, sodium nitrate, or sodium thiosulfate

(c) Fenoldopam mesylate (Corlopam): arterial vasodilator with dopaminergic stimulation

(d) Nitroglycerin (NTG): venous vasodilator at doses of less than 1 µg/kg/min; mixed arterial and venous vasodilator when dose more than 1 µg/kg/min; particularly helpful in patients with chest pain

(e) Hydralazine (Apresoline): arterial vasodilator; monitor closely for significant reflex tachycardia

(f) Nicardipine (Cardene): mixed arterial and venous vasodilator; only predominantly vascular calcium channel blocker available for IV use

(g) Nifedipine (Procardia): mixed arterial and venous vasodilator; oral agent only; sublingual use no longer recommended due to precipitous drop in BP and hypoperfusion consequences

2. Sympathetic blockers
   a) Alpha-blockers block vasoconstriction
      (1) Especially helpful if hypertension due to autonomic dysreflexia
      (2) Example: phentolamine (Regitine)
   b) Beta-blockers block the reflex tachycardia associated with vasodilators
      (1) Especially helpful if hypertension due to pheochromocytoma
      (2) Contraindicated if bradycardia or pulmonary edema present
      (3) Examples: esmolol (Brevibloc): rapid-acting, cardioselective beta-blocker
   c) Alpha- and beta-blockers: block both vasoconstriction and tachycardia
      (1) Especially helpful if hypertension is due to pheochromocytoma
      (2) Example: labetalol (Normodyne): alpha- and noncardioselective beta-blocker

3. ACE inhibitors
   a) Captopril (Capoten): oral agent
   b) Enalapril (Vasotec): only ACE inhibitor currently available for IV use

C. Administer diuretics: usually loop diuretics (e.g., furosemide)
   1. Use of diuretics is controversial since these patients may have had significant diuresis related to excessive glomerular filtration rate

IV. Assist in preparation of patient for surgical procedures to treat cause of hypertension if appropriate
A. Angioplasty may be done for renovascular disease
B. Adrenalectomy is done for pheochromocytoma after tachycardia and hypertension have been adequately controlled

V. Monitor for complications
A. Cerebral infarction

B. Myocardial infarction
C. Heart failure/pulmonary edema
D. Dissection of aorta
E. Renal failure

Peripheral Vascular Insufficiency and Vascular Surgery

Definition: Partial or total occlusion of an artery by atherosclerosis/arteriosclerosis obliterans

Etiology

I. Arteriosclerosis/atherosclerosis (same risk factors as referred to in discussion of Coronary Artery Disease)
II. Hypertension
III. Arteritis

Pathophysiology

I. Arteriosclerosis/atherosclerosis
II. Most significant occlusion usually occurs at bifurcations (Fig. 3-21)
III. Damage to intima with progressive deterioration and thrombus formation

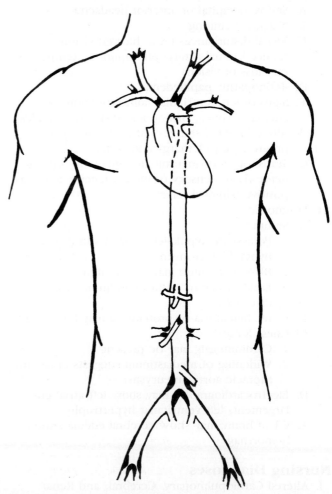

Figure 3-21 Common sites for atherosclerotic plaque deposition. (Drawing by Ann M. Walthall.)

IV. Partial or complete occlusion

V. Ischemic symptoms occur with 75% occlusion

VI. Necrosis occurs as occlusion approaches 100%

Clinical Presentation

I. Occlusive disease of terminal aorta and iliac

  A. Subjective

    1. Intermittent claudication in thigh, hip: pain increases with exercise and decreases with rest

    2. Impotence

  B. Objective

    1. Cool lower extremities

    2. Hair loss over lower extremities

    3. Decreased or absent iliac or femoral pulses

    4. Bruit or thrill over iliac area

II. Occlusive disease of femoral and popliteal arteries

  A. Subjective

    1. Intermittent claudication in lower leg progressing to pain at rest

    2. Decreased sensation or paresthesia of lower extremities

  B. Objective

    1. Coolness of lower extremities

    2. Hair loss over lower extremities

    3. Pallor, mottling of lower extremities

    4. Nonhealing ulcers on toes or points of trauma

    5. Decreased motor strength in lower extremities

    6. Decreased or absent femoral and popliteal pulses

    7. Bruit or thrill over femoral or popliteal area

  C. Diagnostic: angiography, Doppler flow studies show partial to complete obstruction

Nursing Diagnoses

I. Risk for Altered Peripheral Perfusion related to graft occlusion, hematoma, or bleeding

II. Risk for Infection related to surgery, invasive procedures

III. Pain related to surgery, ischemia

IV. Activity Intolerance related to intermittent claudication

V. Anxiety related to health alteration and recommended lifestyle changes

VI. Knowledge Deficit related to disease process, therapy, and recommended lifestyle changes

Collaborative Management

I. Decrease peripheral oxygen requirements

  A. Activity cessation when pain occurs

  B. Bed rest during acute occlusion

  C. Maintenance of normothermia

  D. Prevention of trauma

  E. Instruction regarding need for regular exercise (e.g., walking), smoking cessation, low-fat/low-sodium diet, BP and serum glucose control

II. Administer appropriate pharmacologic agents to improve peripheral blood flow

  A. Platelet aggregation inhibitors (e.g., ASA, ticlopidine [Ticlid]; clopidogrel [Plavix])

  B. Agents that increase the flexibility of the red blood cells: pentoxifylline (Trental)

  C. Anticoagulants: heparin, dicoumarol

  D. Thrombolytics: urokinase, streptokinase, rt-PA

III. Assist in preparation of the patient for procedures aimed at decreasing occlusion

  A. Balloon angioplasty

  B. Laser techniques

IV. Assist in preparation of the patient for surgery aimed at improving flow (Fig. 3-22)

  A. Thromboendarterectomy: excision of thickened layer of artery; aortoiliac, aortofemoral, or femoral-popliteal thromboendarterectomy

  B. Bypass: graft is anastomosed proximal and distal to the occlusion; graft may be Dacron, Teflon, autogenous veins usually saphenous, or bovine heterografs; aortoiliac, aortofemoral, or femoral-popliteal bypass

  C. Sympathectomy: interruption of sympathetic tract; decreases local vascular resistance to improve local blood flow

  D. Amputation: removal of limb performed only when attempts to revascularize the limb have failed

V. Postoperative Management

  A. Maintain adequate flow and pressure at graft site

    1. Maintain and control systolic BP under 120 mm Hg or as prescribed

      a) Nitroprusside (NTP)

      b) Nicardipine (Cardene)

      c) Analgesics as indicated

    2. Prevent emboli by using antiembolic techniques

      a) Dextran 40 often used as platelet aggregation inhibitor

      b) Heparin may also be used

    3. Avoid any pressure on incision sites

      a) Elevate HOB no greater than 45 degrees for first 72 hours

      b) Encourage foot and leg exercises

      c) Mobilize from lying to standing; avoid sitting position, flexing or crossing of legs after femoral artery revascularization

  B. Assess for clinical indications of hypoperfusion

    1. Perform neurovascular assessment of extremities hourly; monitor for: pain, pallor, pulselessness, paresthesia, paralysis, polar (cold)

    2. Measure Doppler pressures and calculate ankle-brachial index (ABI)

      a) Report any decrease in ABI of 0.15 or more

      b) Do not measure Doppler pressure if the bypass is performed to the most distal arteries of the leg (painful for the patient and may cause graft compression)

  C. Treat pain

    1. Administer analgesics as indicated

    2. Position for comfort

  D. Prevent skin breakdown related to ischemia, immobility

    1. Inspect skin, bony prominences, and affected extremities frequently

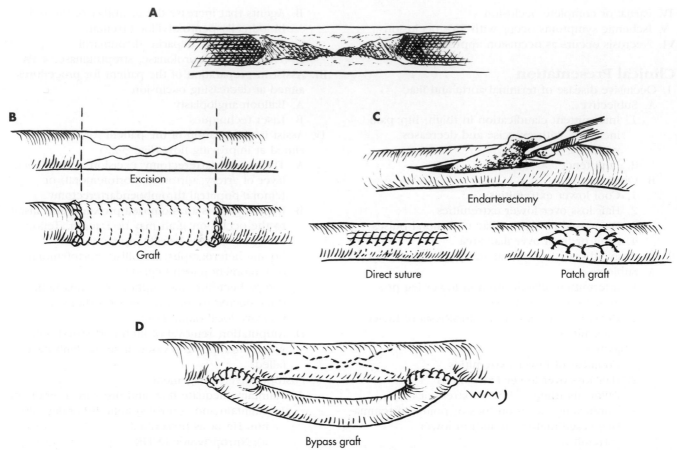

Figure 3-22 Surgical procedures for peripheral vascular disease. **A,** Occluded vessel. **B,** Excision and circumferential graft. **C,** Endarterectomy with direct suture or patch graft. **D,** Bypass graft. (Drawing by Wendy M. Johnson.)

2. Reposition often
3. Use eggcrate, alternating air mattress, or special bed depending on other risk factors
4. Keep heels elevated off bed
E. Monitor for postoperative complications
   1. Hemorrhage
   2. Infection
      a) Assess incision, wounds for indications of infection
      b) Monitor WBC and body temperature
      c) Provide aseptic wound care
      d) Administer antibiotics as prescribed
   3. Arterial thrombosis
   4. Cerebral embolus (blood or plaque)

Aortic Aneurysm
Definition: A localized dilation of the wall of a blood vessel
I. Types (Fig. 3-23)
   A. False: does not involve all layers of the artery; pulsating hematoma
   B. True: involves all layers of the arterial wall; usually saccular arising from a distinct portion of the wall
   C. Saccular: outpouching from an artery that results from localized thinning and stretching of the media

D. Fusiform: involves the total circumference of the artery with diffuse dilation
E. Dissecting: a cavity is formed by dissection by blood between the layers of the arterial wall
F. Rupture: arterial wall ruptures and leaks arterial blood into the mediastinum if thoracic or into abdominal cavity if abdominal

Etiology
I. Arteriosclerosis/atherosclerosis
II. Congenital weakness of the aorta
III. Hypertension
IV. Pregnancy: especially third trimester
V. Coarctation of the aorta
VI. Syphilis
VII. Severe systemic infection (e.g., bacterial aneurysm, mycotic aneurysm)
VIII. Marfan's syndrome
IX. Trauma: especially blunt trauma with acceleration-deceleration injury
X. Arterial cannulation; intraaortic balloon pump

Pathophysiology
I. Arteriosclerosis/atherosclerosis initially affects the intima
II. Hemorrhage into the plaque subsequently affects medial layer and causes weakness and dilation of

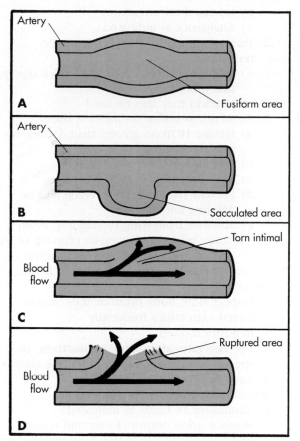

Figure 3-23 Types of aneurysms. **A,** Fusiform. **B,** Saccular. **C,** Dissecting. **D,** Ruptured. (From Thelan LA, et al: *Critical care nursing: diagnosis and management,* ed 2, St Louis, 1994, Mosby.)

the vessel; expanding hematoma compresses or occludes the arteries that branch off the aorta

III. Hematoma formation in the medial layer causes longitudinal separation of the layers of the aorta (dissection)
  A. As the heart contracts, more blood enters the false lumen and the dissection expands
  B. Blood leaking into the pericardial sac may cause cardiac tamponade

IV. The resultant thin-walled channel can easily rupture and hemorrhage into mediastinal, pleural, or abdominal cavities

Clinical Presentation

I. Subjective: may be asymptomatic
II. Objective
  A. Normal to high BP; hypotension suggests cardiac tamponade or aortic rupture
  B. Pulsatile mass
  C. Increased aortic diameter on palpation
  D. Bruit over aorta
III. Specific to ascending thoracic aorta
  A. May be asymptomatic
  B. Dyspnea
  C. Chest pain
  D. Clinical indications of aortic regurgitation: diastolic murmur, LVF, widened pulse pressure

IV. Specific to aortic arch
  A. Dyspnea
  B. Stridor
  C. Cough
  D. JVD
  E. Hoarseness
  F. Weak voice
V. Specific to descending thoracic arch
  A. Dull chest pain and upper back pain
  B. Hoarseness
VI. Specific to dissecting TAA
  A. Sudden, sharp, tearing or ripping pain in chest radiating to shoulders, neck, or back
  B. Hypotension
  C. Dyspnea
  D. Syncope
  E. Leg weakness, transient paralysis
  F. May have BP and pulse difference between arms or between arms and legs
  G. Clinical indications of cardiac tamponade (see Cardiac Tamponade section)
VII. Specific to abdominal aorta
  A. Dull abdominal and back pain
  B. Nausea and vomiting
  C. Abdominal bloating
  D. Pulsation in abdomen
VIII. Specific to ruptured AAA
  A. Severe, sudden, dull, continuous abdominal pain radiating to low back, hips, scrotum; unaffected by movement
  B. Feeling of abdominal fullness
  C. Nausea and vomiting
  D. Syncope and shock
  E. Pulsation in abdomen: periumbilical area
IX. Diagnostic
  A. Serum: hemoglobin and hematocrit may be decreased
  B. Chest X-ray
    1. Mediastinal widening in thoracic aneurysm
    2. Aortic calcification
  C. Electrocardiography
    1. May show left ventricular hypertrophy
    2. May show nonspecific ST-T-wave changes
    3. Absence of ECG indicators of MI
  D. Aortogram: lumen of aorta; size and location of aneurysm
  E. CT scan, MRI: presence and location of aneurysm
  F. Transesophageal echocardiography: presence, size, shape of aneurysms of ascending thoracic aorta
  G. Ultrasound: presence, size, shape, and location of aneurysm
  H. Flat plate of abdomen (KUB): outline of abdominal aortic aneurysm

Nursing Diagnoses

I. **Risk for Altered Tissue Perfusion** related to aneurysm dissection and decreased peripheral blood flow
II. **Risk for Decreased Cardiac Output** related to aneurysm dissection or rupture

III. Fluid Volume Deficit related to vascular disruption
IV. Risk for Impaired Skin Integrity related to decreased peripheral blood flow
V. Anxiety related to health alteration and recommended lifestyle changes
VI. Knowledge Deficit related to disease process, therapy, and recommended lifestyle changes

Collaborative Management

I. Control pain
   A. Administer narcotics as required in rupture or dissection
   B. Use extreme caution if patient is hypotensive
II. Maintain and control mean arterial pressure at approximately 80 to 90 mm Hg if dissection occurs
   A. If patient is hypertensive
      1. Nitroprusside (NTP)
      2. Labetalol (Normodyne)
   B. If patient is hypotensive
      1. IV access: 2 large-bore, short IV catheters; type and crossmatch for blood
      2. Normal saline or lactated Ringer's by rapid infusion until blood is available; colloids (e.g., albumin, hetastarch, or dextran) may also be used
      3. Blood and blood products as prescribed
III. Decrease tissue oxygenation requirements
   A. Activity restriction
   B. Oxygen by nasal cannula at 2 to 6 L/min to maintain Spo_2 of 95% unless contraindicated
   C. Intubation and mechanical ventilation may be necessary
   D. Physical comfort: temperature, lighting, noise control
   E. Anxiolytics as prescribed: usually diazepam (Valium), lorazepam (Ativan), or alprazolam (Xanax)
IV. Assist in preparation of patient for surgical repair
   A. Surgical procedure: resection of aneurysm and circumferential (fusiform aneurysm) or patch graft (saccular aneurysm)
      1. Generally repaired when 5 to 6 cm in diameter
      2. Concurrent aortic valve repair or replacement may be needed for ascending thoracic aneurysms; repair of thoracic aortic aneurysm may require cardiopulmonary bypass
      3. Indications for immediate surgical repair
         a) Involvement of ascending aorta; aortic insufficiency
         b) Failure of drug therapy to control progression of dissection as evidenced by continued pain and progressive symptoms
         c) Cardiac tamponade
         d) Compromise of a major branch of aorta
         e) Indications of cerebral or cardiac ischemia
V. Postoperative management
   A. Maintain adequate flow and pressure at graft site
      1. Maintain and control systolic BP under 120 mm Hg
         a) Nitroprusside (NTP)

b) Labetalol (Normodyne)
c) Analgesics as indicated
   2. Prevent emboli by using antiembolic techniques
      a) Dextran 40 often used as platelet aggregation inhibitor
      b) Heparin may also be used
   3. Avoid any pressure on incision sites
      a) Elevate HOB no greater than 45 degrees for first 72 hours
      b) Elevate legs 20 to 30 degrees
      c) Encourage foot and leg exercises
      d) Prevent patient from crossing legs or bending knees
      e) Mobilize from lying to standing; avoid sitting position, flexing or crossing of legs after femoral artery revascularization
   B. Prevent skin breakdown related to ischemia, immobility
      1. Inspect skin, bony prominences, and affected extremities frequently
      2. Reposition often
      3. Use eggcrate, alternating air mattress, or special bed depending on other risk factors
      4. Keep heels elevated off bed
   C. Maintain adequate hydration
      1. Administer IV fluids as indicated
      2. Monitor urine output closely and report urine output of less than 0.5 ml/kg/hr
   D. Monitor for postoperative complications
      1. Hemorrhage, hypovolemia, hematoma; monitor for all of the following:
         a) Hypotension
         b) Tachycardia
         c) Clinical manifestations of hypoperfusion
         d) Decreased RAP, PAP, PAOP
      2. Myocardial ischemia, infarction; monitor for all of the following:
         a) Chest pain
         b) Dyspnea
         c) Decreased cardiac output
         d) Dysrhythmias
         e) ECG: ST segment changes
      3. Cerebral ischemia, infarction; monitor for all of the following:
         a) Change in LOC
         b) Pupillary change
         c) Aphasia
         d) Motor or sensory changes
      4. Pulmonary ischemia, infarction; monitor for all of the following:
         a) Dyspnea
         b) Chest pain
         c) Pleural friction rub
         d) Hypoxemia
      5. Renal ischemia, infarction; monitor for all of the following:
         a) Flank pain
         b) Decreased urine output
         c) Changes in BUN or creatinine
         d) Hematuria

6. Mesenteric ischemia, infarction; monitor for all of the following:
   a) Watery, bloody diarrhea (often described as *currant jelly diarrhea*)
   b) Abdominal pain
   c) Change in bowel sounds
7. Splenic ischemia, infarction; monitor for all of the following:
   a) LUQ pain radiating to left shoulder
   b) Abdominal rigidity
8. Spinal cord ischemia, infarction; monitor for all of the following:
   a) Paralysis of lower extremities
   b) Bowel/bladder paralysis
9. Arterial thrombosis
   a) Perform neurovascular assessment of extremities hourly; monitor for: pain, pallor, pulselessness, paresthesia, paralysis, polar (cold)
   b) Measure Doppler pressures and calculate ankle-brachial index (ABI); report any decrease in ABI of 0.15 or more

Cardiovascular Trauma
Blunt Cardiac Trauma

I. Definition: blunt trauma to the heart; myocardial contusion occurs when petechiae and ecchymosis are present in the myocardium
II. Etiology
   A. Usually acceleration/deceleration injury sustained in motor vehicle collision; sternum may hit steering wheel or dashboard; injury may also be caused by shoulder strap of seatbelt
   B. Other accidents: motorcycle collisions, auto-pedestrian collisions
   C. Kicking of chest by large animal (e.g., horse, cow, human)
   D. Assault with blunt instrument
   E. Industrial crush injury
   F. Explosion
   G. Vigorous CPR
III. Pathophysiology
   A. Blunt trauma may cause bruising, bleeding into myocardium
   B. RBCs extravasate around myocardial fibers
   C. Subpericardial and subendocardial myocardial fibers become edematous and may fragment; necrosis may even occur in severe cases
   D. Right ventricle primary site of injury because it is directly under the sternum
   E. Decreased right ventricular contractility causes increase in right ventricular end-diastolic volume and decrease in right ventricular ejection fraction
   F. Decrease in RV ejection fraction decreases preload to the left ventricle
   G. Dilation of RV shifts interventricular septum to the left, compromising left ventricular compliance
   H. Increase in PVR frequently seen, increasing RV afterload and further decreasing RV ejection fraction
   I. Damage to cardiac valves may occur, especially mitral and aortic, because LV pressures are higher
IV. Clinical presentation
   A. Subjective
      1. Precordial angina-like chest pain
         a) Frequently increases with inspiration, cough, and movement
         b) Unresponsive to nitroglycerin but frequently responsive to oxygen, antiinflammatory agents, or narcotics
      2. Dyspnea
      3. Palpitations
   B. Objective
      1. Tachycardia
      2. Ecchymosis may be present on anterior chest
      3. Clinical indications of RVF: JVD, peripheral edema, hepatomegaly
   C. Diagnostic
      1. Serum: CK-MB and cardiac troponin may be positive depending on the severity of the injury
      2. Electrocardiography with right ventricular leads
         a) ST segment changes, T-wave inversion; Q-waves may be seen if injury is severe or if a coronary artery is lacerated or thromboses
         b) QT interval may be prolonged
         c) Dysrhythmias
            (1) Atrial dysrhythmias: PACs, atrial fibrillation, atrial flutter
            (2) Ventricular dysrhythmias: PVCs, ventricular tachycardia, ventricular fibrillation
            (3) Blocks: AV blocks, bundle branch blocks
      3. Echocardiography
         a) Decreased regional wall motion (especially right ventricular)
         b) Increased end-diastolic wall thickness
         c) Decreased RV ejection fraction
         d) May show complications (e.g., apical thrombi, pericardial effusion, cardiac tamponade)
      4. Radionuclide studies may be done: decreased RV ejection fraction
V. Nursing diagnoses
   A. Decreased Cardiac Output related to HF, tamponade, hemorrhage
   B. Risk for Altered Peripheral Tissue Perfusion related to emboli
   C. Impaired Gas Exchange related to pulmonary edema
   D. Activity Intolerance related to HF
   E. Anxiety related to health alteration and recommended lifestyle changes
   F. Knowledge Deficit related to disease process, therapy, and recommended lifestyle changes

VI. Collaborative management
  A. Decrease myocardial oxygen demand
    1. Bed rest
    2. Oxygen by nasal cannula at 2 to 6 L/min to maintain SpO$_2$ of 95% unless contraindicated
    3. Anxiolytics as prescribed and indicated
  B. Treat pain
    1. Morphine sulfate usually used
    2. Antiinflammatory agents may also be helpful
  C. Treat dysrhythmias
    1. Atrial: digitalis, cardioversion
    2. Ventricular: usually lidocaine
    3. Blocks: atropine and/or external pacemaker
  D. Assist in assessment for other thoracic injuries (e.g., fractured ribs, sternum, clavicle)
  E. Monitor for complications
    1. Ventricular rupture
    2. Cardiac tamponade
    3. Coronary artery thrombosis
    4. Valve rupture
    5. Conduction defects
    6. Heart failure
    7. Ventricular aneurysm
    8. Cardiogenic shock: monitor for clinical manifestations of hypoperfusion
    9. Systemic emboli
      a) Sequential compression devices may be used on the legs
      b) Anticoagulation avoided unless intramural thrombi are present

Penetrating Cardiac Trauma

I. Definition: puncture of the heart with a sharp object or rib
II. Etiology
  A. Violence (e.g., knife wound, gunshot wound, ice pick)
  B. Industrial accident (e.g., scaffolding)
  C. Motorcycle collision (e.g., handlebar impalement)
  D. Sports injury
  E. Explosion
  F. Crush injury
III. Pathophysiology
  A. Puncture of the heart (usually RV) with sharp object or rib
  B. Loss of blood into the pericardial space or into the mediastinum
  C. Cardiac tamponade or shock may occur
IV. Clinical presentation
  A. Subjective: chest pain
  B. Objective
    1. Visible wound; object causing penetration may be seen
    2. Bleeding from chest
    3. Hypotension
    4. Clinical indications of hypoperfusion (see Table 2-6)
    5. Clinical indications of cardiac tamponade (see Cardiac Tamponade section)

  C. Hemodynamic parameters
    1. Decrease in RAP, PAP, PAOP if hemorrhage; increase in RAP, PAP, PAOP if cardiac tamponade
    2. Decrease in CO, CI
    3. Decrease in SvO$_2$
  D. Diagnostic: hemoglobin and hematocrit decreased
V. Nursing diagnoses
  A. Decreased Cardiac Output related to HF
  B. Impaired Gas Exchange related to pulmonary edema
  C. Activity Intolerance related to HF
  D. Anxiety related to health alteration and recommended lifestyle changes
  E. Knowledge Deficit related to unfamiliarity with disease process, therapy, and recommended lifestyle changes
VI. Collaborative management
  A. Manage cardiopulmonary arrest if indicated: manage airway, oxygenation, circulation using BCLS, ACLS if needed
  B. Control hemorrhage
    1. Do not remove an impaled object; objects may be stabilized with IV bags, dressings
    2. Apply pressure to site if the object has been removed and the wound is bleeding
    3. Apply pressure around site if the object has not already been removed and the wound is bleeding
    4. Assist with insertion of chest tube for hemothorax or pneumothorax
    5. Assist with pericardiocentesis for cardiac tamponade
  C. Improve oxygen delivery
    1. Oxygen by nasal cannula at 2 to 6 L/min to maintain SpO$_2$ of 95% unless contraindicated
    2. Intubation and mechanical ventilation may be necessary
    3. IV access: 2 large-bore, short IV catheters; blood for type and crossmatch
    4. Normal saline or lactated Ringer's by rapid infusion until blood is available; colloids (e.g., albumin, hetastarch, or dextran) may also be used
    5. Blood and blood products as prescribed
  D. Assist in preparation of the patient for exploratory thoracotomy
  E. Monitor for complications
    1. Hemorrhagic shock
    2. Cardiac tamponade
    3. Hemothorax
    4. Pneumothorax

Great Vessel Injury

I. Definition: injury or tear to great vessel or vessels, usually the aorta but possibly the pulmonary artery

II. Etiology
   A. Acceleration-deceleration injury (e.g., motor vehicle collision)
   B. Compression injury
   C. Penetrating trauma
III. Pathophysiology: disruption of major vessel integrity causes loss of effective circulating blood volume leading to shock
IV. Clinical presentation
   A. Subjective
      1. Chest or back pain
      2. Dyspnea
      3. Dysphagia or hoarseness
      4. Sensory or motor changes in lower extremities
   B. Objective
      1. Tachycardia
      2. Blood pressure changes
         a) Hypertension or hypotension
         b) Difference between left and right arms
         c) Difference (greater than normal) between upper and lower extremities
      3. Tracheal shift
      4. Clinical indications of hypoperfusion
      5. Harsh systolic murmur may be audible along the precordium
   C. Hemodynamic parameters
      1. Decrease in RAP, PAP, PAOP
      2. Decrease in CO, CI
      3. Decrease in Svo_2
   D. Diagnostic
      1. Serum: hemoglobin and hematocrit decreased
      2. ECG: may show dysrhythmias or ST-T-wave changes indicative of ischemia
      3. Chest X-ray
         a) Mediastinal widening
         b) Loss of aortic knob shadow
      4. Aortogram: will show extravasation of dye
V. Nursing diagnoses
   A. Fluid Volume Deficit related to hemorrhage
   B. Risk for Decreased Cardiac Output related to cardiac tamponade
   C. Anxiety related to health alteration and recommended lifestyle changes
   D. Knowledge Deficit related to disease process, therapy, and recommended lifestyle changes
VI. Collaborative management
   A. Manage cardiopulmonary arrest if needed: manage airway, oxygenation, circulation using BCLS, ACLS if needed
   B. Improve oxygen delivery
      1. Oxygen by nasal cannula at 2 to 6 L/min to maintain Spo_2 of 95% unless contraindicated
      2. Intubation and mechanical ventilation may be necessary
      3. IV access: 2 large-bore, short IV catheters; blood for type and crossmatch
      4. Normal saline or lactated Ringer's by rapid infusion until blood is available; colloids

(e.g., albumin, hetastarch, or dextran) may also be used
      5. Blood and blood products as prescribed
   C. Control bleeding: antihypertensive may be needed to keep MAP less than 90 mm Hg
   D. Assist in preparation of the patient for exploratory thoracotomy as soon as possible; it is not possible to truly stabilize this patient except in the operating room with injury repair
   E. Monitor for complications
      1. Hemorrhagic shock
      2. Cardiac tamponade
      3. Hemothorax
      4. False aneurysm

Cardiac Tamponade
Definition
I. When fluid (blood, effusion fluid, pus) in the pericardial space compromises cardiac filling and cardiac output
II. Hemodynamic consequences of pericardial fluid

Etiology
I. Blunt or penetrating injury to heart
II. Postcardiotomy
   A. If mediastinal tube is occluded or after removal of mediastinal tube
   B. After removal of epicardial pacing wires
III. Postmyocardial infarction
   A. Pericarditis especially in the anticoagulated patient
   B. Cardiac rupture
IV. Iatrogenic causes: perforation of the myocardium by transvenous pacemaker wires, invasive catheters, intracardiac injection, cardiac needle biopsy
V. Post-CPR, electrical cardioversion
VI. Anticoagulant therapy
VII. Rupture of great vessels
VIII. Dissecting aortic aneurysms
IX. Malignancy and/or radiation therapy
X. Connective tissue disease: rheumatoid arthritis, lupus erythematosus, scleroderma
XI. Metabolic disease: renal failure, hepatic failure, myxedema
XII. Infection: viral, bacterial, fungal
XIII. Drugs: procainamide (Pronestyl), hydralazine (Apresoline), minoxidil (Loniten), daunorubicin (Cerubidine), methyldopa (Aldomet), sulfasalazine (Azulfidine), isoniazid (INH), methysergide (Sansert), sargramostim (Leukine), tetracycline derivatives

Pathophysiology
I. Accumulation of fluid or blood in pericardial space (as little as 100 ml or as much as 2 L)
II. When intrapericardial pressure is very high and approaches atrial pressures and ventricular diastolic pressure, the transmural cardiac pressure falls, leading to inability of the heart to fill

III. End-diastolic volume (preload) decreases
IV. Contractility decreases
V. Stroke volume decreases
VI. Cardiac output decreases
VII. LVF, RVF, shock

Clinical Presentation

I. Subjective
   A. Precordial fullness or pain
   B. Dyspnea
   C. Anxiety or feeling of impending doom
II. Objective
   A. Usually tachycardia but may be pulseless and present as pulseless electrical activity (PEA)
   B. Hypotension, narrowed pulse pressure
   C. Increased JVD: may not be seen if patient is hypotensive
   D. Absent PMI
   E. Heart sound changes
      1. Pericardial friction rub may be heard
      2. Distant, muffled, or absent heart sounds
   F. Beck's triad: hypotension, distended neck veins, muffled heart sounds
III. Hemodynamic parameters
   A. Increased RAP (CVP), PAd, PAOP
   B. Pulsus paradoxus on arterial waveform or by auscultation
   C. Equalization of left and right-heart filling pressures with hemodynamic monitoring: RAP, PAd, PAOP within 5 mm Hg of each other
   D. Change in PAOP waveform: large a-wave, large v-wave (M sign)
   E. Decrease in CO/CI
   F. Decrease in Svo_2
IV. Diagnostic
   A. Chest X-ray
      1. Widened mediastinum
      2. Dilated superior vena cava
   B. Electrocardiography
      1. May have ST segment elevation if pericarditis is cause
      2. Electrical alternans: alternating large and small QRSs
      3. Bradycardia may indicate impending PEA
      4. Ventricular dysrhythmias
   C. Echocardiogram: 2D or transesophageal
      1. Echo-free space will be evident between the pericardium and myocardium
      2. Shift of interventricular septum from right to left
      3. Transesophageal echocardiogram: helpful in differentiating severe right ventricular contusion from acute tamponade
   D. CT of chest
   E. Fluoroscopy of chest: may be used during pericardiocentesis

Nursing Diagnoses

I. Decreased Cardiac Output related to decreased preload and decreased contractility

II. Fluid Volume Deficit related to hemorrhage into pericardial space
III. Anxiety related to health alteration and recommended lifestyle changes
IV. Knowledge Deficit related to disease process, therapy, and recommended lifestyle changes

Collaborative Management

I. Maintain airway, ventilation, oxygenation, and perfusion
   A. Airway, oxygenation, circulation support using BCLS, ACLS if needed
   B. 100% oxygen by face mask; intubate and mechanically ventilate as indicated
   C. Circulating volume replacement
      1. Initiate 2 large-bore IVs: replace vascular volume as necessary
         a) Normal saline: 200 to 500 ml over 10 to 15 minutes
         b) Fresh frozen plasma, dextran, or albumin may also be used
         c) Blood replacement may also be necessary
   D. Inotropes (e.g., dobutamine) as prescribed
II. Administer drugs or therapies related to cause
   A. Protamine or vitamin K if patient is on anticoagulants
   B. Dialysis for patients with renal failure
   C. Antibiotics if purulent effusion
III. Prepare to assist with pericardiocentesis (Fig. 3-24)
   A. Place patient in semi-Fowler's position
   B. Apply ECG machine and electrode necessary
      1. Apply limb leads
      2. Attach chest lead wire to the exploring needle with an alligator clamp; when needle touches epicardium, ST segment elevation is seen
   C. Have emergency equipment available, including transcutaneous pacemaker
   D. Assist with administration of local anesthetic
   E. Assist with placement of pericardial catheter if indicated
   F. Monitor for complications
      1. Laceration of coronary artery or conduction system
      2. Myocardial puncture
      3. Pneumothorax
      4. Dysrhythmias
      5. Hypotension
IV. Assist in preparation of patient for surgical intervention
   A. Pericardiocentesis may not resolve the tamponade if effusion is posterior; surgical drainage is indicated if purulent or hemorrhagic effusion
   B. Surgical opening of pericardial space may be necessary
   C. Emergency thoracotomy may be necessary for chest trauma
   D. Pericardial window procedure may be done for recurrent tamponade

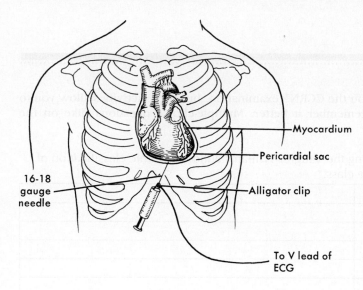

Myocardium

Pericardial sac

16-18 gauge needle

Alligator clip

To V lead of ECG

Figure 3-24   Pericardiocentesis. (From Sheehy SB, Lombardi JE: *Manual of emergency care,* ed 4, St Louis, 1994, Mosby.)

LEARNING ACTIVITIES

Note: Remember that you won't see questions like these on the CCRN® examination, but these activities allow you to approach the content from a different perspective to remember it better. Multiple-choice questions (like on the CCRN® examination) are on the CD-ROM.

1. **DIRECTIONS:** Complete the following table by identifying the Vaughn-Williams antidysrhythmic classification of the following drugs. Some drugs are of more than one class.

Propranolol (Inderal)	
Verapamil (Calan)	
Lidocaine (Xylocaine)	
Quinidine	
Flecainide (Tambocor)	
Ibutilide (Corvert)	
Procainamide (Pronestyl)	
Esmolol (Brevibloc)	
Sotalol (Betapace)	
Bretylium (Bretylium)	
Adenosine (Adenocard)	
Diltiazem (Cardizem)	

2. **DIRECTIONS:** Complete the following table to identify the NAPSE code for the pacemaker that would have the capabilities of the others together.

AOO		VVI		a.
VVI		VAT		b.
AAI	VAT		VVI	c.

3. **DIRECTIONS:** Analyze the following ECG rhythm strips. Identify the type of pacemaker and if a pacemaker malfunction has occurred.

a.

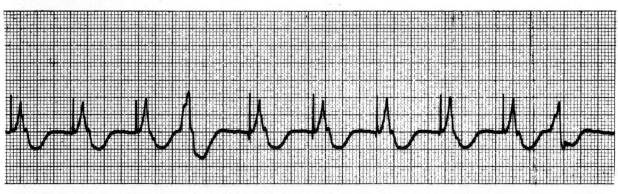

Interpretation:_____

b.

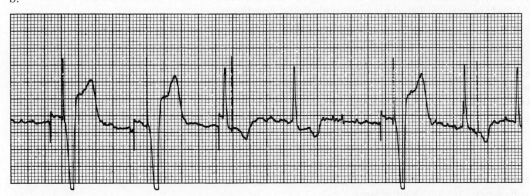

Interpretation:_____

c.

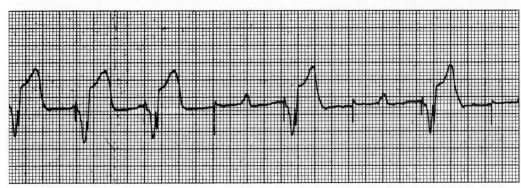

Interpretation:_____

4. **Directions:** Complete the following table differentiating cardiac risk factors as nonmodifiable or modifiable by the individual at risk.

Nonmodifiable	Modifiable

5. **Directions:** Match the following treatments for acute MI with rationales for use. More than one rationale may apply.

____1. Thrombolytics
____2. Percutaneous coronary interventions such as angioplasty, atherectomy
____3. ACE inhibitors
____4. Nitroglycerin
____5. Calcium channel blockers
____6. Beta-blockers
____7. ASA
____8. Heparin

a. Increases myocardial oxygen supply by reestablishing patency of the infarct-related artery.
b. Decreases myocardial oxygen demand by blocking the effects of catecholamines.
c. Increases myocardial oxygen supply by reducing spasm.
d. Decreases myocardial oxygen demand by reducing preload.
e. Prevents extension of a clot by decreasing platelet aggregation.
f. Prevents extension of a clot by preventing the conversion of prothrombin to thrombin.
g. Prevents ventricular dilation and adverse remodeling of the myocardium.
h. Used for secondary prevention after Q-wave MI.
i. Used for secondary prevention after non–Q-wave MI.

6. **DIRECTIONS:** Identify the physical findings from the following list that are seen in these pathologic conditions. More than one physical finding may be listed for each pathologic condition.

_____ 1. Right ventricular failure
_____ 2. Left ventricular failure
_____ 3. Myocardial infarction
_____ 4. Pulmonary embolism
_____ 5. Tension pneumothorax
_____ 6. Cardiac tamponade
_____ 7. Valvular dysfunction
_____ 8. Pericarditis
_____ 9. Endocarditis
_____10. Hyperlipidemia
_____11. Chronic arterial insufficiency
_____12. Chronic venous insufficiency

a. Jugular venous distention
b. Displaced PMI
c. S_3 at apex
d. S_3 at sternum
e. S_4 at apex
f. S_4 at sternum
g. Murmur
h. Pericardial friction rub
i. Muffled heart sounds
j. Splinter hemorrhages
k. Intermittent claudication
l. Xanthelasma
m. Peripheral edema
n. Peripheral pallor
o. Peripheral rubor
p. Fever
q. Crackles in lung bases
r. Corneal arcus
s. Hepatomegaly
t. Pulsus paradoxus

7. **DIRECTIONS:** Identify whether the following causes or clinical findings are associated with left or right ventricular failure. Some may be associated with biventricular failure.

Causes	Left	Right
Aortic stenosis		
Cardiac tamponade		
Cardiomyopathy		
Mitral stenosis		
Left ventricular MI		
Right ventricular MI		
Pulmonary embolism		
Pulmonary hypertension		
Systemic hypertension		

Sign/Symptom	Left	Right
Abnormal liver function studies		
Ascites		
Atrial dysrhythmias		
Crackles audible over lungs		
Dyspnea		
Elevated PAOP		
Elevated RAP		
Hepatomegaly		
Jugular venous distention		
Mental confusion		
Murmur of mitral regurgitation		
Murmur of tricuspid regurgitation		
Orthopnea		
Peripheral edema		
S_3, S_4 at apex		
S_3, S_4 at sternum		
Weight gain		

8.

a.

Two primary effects of IABP:

(1) _____

(2) _____

b.

Two major contraindications of IABP:

(1) _____

(2) _____

c.

The balloon is inflated during which phase of the cardiac cycle?

_____

d.

The balloon is deflated immediately before which phase of the cardiac cycle?

_____

e.

List two complications of displacement of the balloon in the aorta

(1) _____

(2) _____

9.   **DIRECTIONS:** Identify the labeled portions of the IABP waveform.

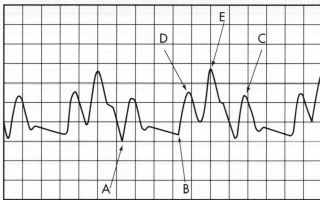

A. _____

B. _____

C. _____

D. _____

E. _____

10. **DIRECTIONS:** Identify the following signs, symptoms, causes, or treatments as associated with dilated, hypertrophic, or restrictive cardiomyopathy. You may identify more than one type of cardiomyopathy for each feature.

Feature	Dilated	Hypertrophic	Restrictive
Associated with alcoholism or infection			
Do not give inotropes			
Clinical presentation: syncope, chest pain, sudden death			
Clinical presentation similar to HF			
May be candidate for cardiac transplantation			
Atrial fibrillation common			
Treatment includes beta-blockers and calcium channel blockers			
Do not give diuretics or nitrates			
Associated with infiltrative and connective tissue disorders			
Treated with digoxin, diuretics, ACE inhibitors			
Associated with genetically transmitted autosomal-dominant trait			
AV blocks are common			
Hemiblock is common			
Treatment may include steroids			

11. **DIRECTIONS:** Identify the following signs, symptoms, causes, or treatments as associated with pericarditis, myocarditis, or endocarditis. You may identify more than one type of cardiomyopathy for each feature.

Feature	Pericarditis	Myocarditis	Endocarditis
Associated with MI			
May cause cardiomyopathy			
Causes splinter hemorrhages, petechiae			
Treated with antiinflammatory drugs			
Sudden onset of HF			
Causes pericardial friction rub			
Valve replacement may be necessary			
Usually associated with viral infection			
Associated with cardiac surgery			
Definitive diagnosis requires biopsy			
May cause systemic emboli			
Monitor closely for cardiac tamponade			
Causes murmur			
Associated with uremia			
Associated with ST segment elevation			
Treated with antibiotics			
Increased incidence in patients with rheumatic heart disease			

12. **DIRECTIONS:** Complete the following table regarding antihypertensive agents.

Description	Drug
IV calcium channel blocker used for hypertension	
IV beta-blocker that also blocks alpha receptors	
IV vasodilator that may cause coronary artery steal and intra-pulmonary shunt	
IV vasodilator that is particularly helpful in patients with chest pain	
IV ACE inhibitor	
Oral ACE inhibitor that was first ACE inhibitor	
Two oral calcium channel blockers used for hypertension	
IV vasodilator that causes significant reflex tachycardia	

13. **DIRECTIONS:** Identify the following vasoactive agents as arterial dilators, venous dilators, or vasopressors.

Drug	Arterial Dilator	Venous Dilator	Vasopressor
Amrinone (Inocor)			
Dobutamine (Dobutrex)			
Dopamine (Intropin)			
Hydralazine (Apresoline)			
Minoxidil (Loniten)			
Morphine sulfate			
Nifedipine (Procardia)			
Nitroglycerin (<1 µg/kg/min)			
Nitroglycerin (>1 µg/kg/min)			
Nitroprusside (Nipride)			
Norepinephrine (Levophed)			
Phentolamine (Regitine)			
Phenylephrine (Neo-Synephrine)			
Prazosin (Minipress)			
Vasopressin (Pitressin)			

14. **DIRECTIONS:** Complete the following crossword puzzle dealing with critical care pharmacology. Use generic names.

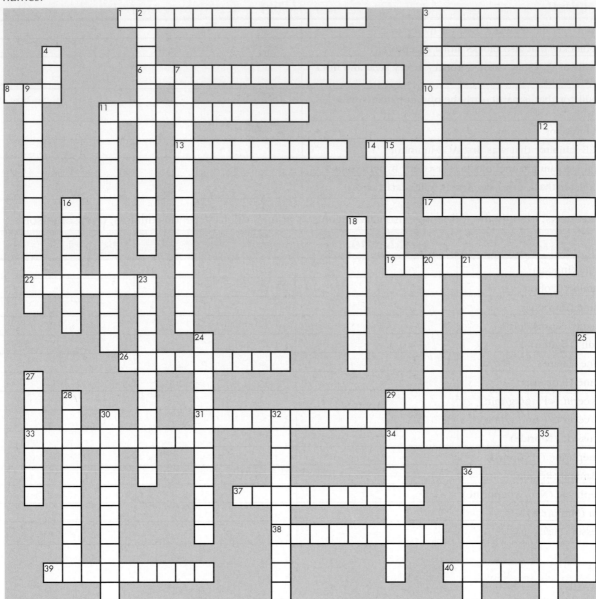

Across

1. Predominantly arterial nitrate-type vasodilator
3. Alpha- and beta-blocker used for hypertension
5. Class IV antidysrhythmic; may be used for secondary prophylaxis in non–Q-wave MIs
6. Drug used in peripheral vascular disease to increase the flexibility of the RBC
8. Thrombolytic; does not cause fibrinogen depletion (abbrev.)
10. ACE inhibitor; may cause rash or cough
11. Noncardioselective beta-blocker
13. Electrolyte; frequently included in postoperative fluid replacement
14. Alpha-blocker; frequently used for sympathomimetic infiltration to prevent tissue necrosis
17. Class III antidysrhythmic; used for acute onset atrial fibrillation
19. Calcium channel blocker; frequently used in variant angina
22. Low-molecular-weight form used as an antiplatelet aggregation agent; high-molecular-weight form used as a colloid-type volume expander
26. Class III antidysrhythmic; causes nausea, vomiting, hypotension
29. Sympathomimetic; #1 drug in cardiac arrest
31. Class III antidysrhythmic; major side effect is pulmonary fibrosis
33. Alpha- and beta-blocker used in heart failure
34. Nucleoside used for PSVT; breaks reentrant mechanism
37. Cardioselective beta-blocker; used for primary and secondary prevention after MI
38. Electrolyte; indicated in torsades de pointes
39. Class IV antidysrhythmic; frequently used for PSVT
40. Analgesic of choice in MI; venous vasodilator

Down

2. Pure beta stimulant
3. Class II antidysrhythmic; #1 antidysrhythmic in ventricular tachycardia or fibrillation
4. Antiplatelet agent used for primary and secondary prevention of MI (abbrev.)
7. Alpha-dominant sympathomimetic
9. Class IA antidysrhythmic; may cause prolongation of the QT interval
11. Alpha-selective sympathomimetic

12. Phosphodiesterase inhibitor; more potent and fewer adverse effects than amrinone
15. Parenteral anticoagulant
16. Cardiac glycoside; used for heart failure and to decrease the ventricular rate in atrial fibrillation or flutter
18. Benzodiazepine anxiolytic
20. Class IC antidysrhythmic; used for refractory ventricular dysrhythmias

21. Sympathomimetic; effects dependent on dose
23. Calcium channel blocker used for hypertension, which is available IV
24. Arterial dilator administered by IV injection; used in hypertension
25. Thrombolytic; may cause anaphylaxis in patients who have previously received it
27. Electrolyte; used in hyperkalemia, hypermagnesemia
28. Loop diuretic

30. New arterial dilator used in hypertension; also causes dopaminergic stimulation
32. Sympathomimetic inotrope most frequently used for cardiogenic shock
34. Parasympatholytic; used in symptomatic bradycardia or blocks
35. ACE inhibitor now available in IV form
36. Cardioselective beta-blocker with very short half-life

LEARNING ACTIVITIES ANSWERS

1.

Propranolol (Inderal)	II
Verapamil (Calan)	IV
Lidocaine (Xylocaine)	IB
Quinidine	IA
Flecainide (Tambocor)	IC
Ibutilide (Corvert)	III
Procainamide (Pronestyl)	IA
Esmolol (Brevibloc)	II
Sotalol (Betapace)	II, III
Bretylium (Bretylium)	III
Adenosine (Adenocard)	nonclassified
Diltiazem (Cardizem)	IV

2.

AOO		VVI	a. DVI
VVI		VAT	b. VDD
AAI	VAT	VVI	c. DDD

3. a. Interpretation: VVI with normal function; complex #4 is a PVC and it is sensed appropriately.
   b. Interpretation: DVI function with failure to sense; complex #3 shows atrial pacing with an intrinsic ventricular complex that is not sensed.
   c. Interpretation: VVI with intermittent failure to capture; after the third paced complex, there is a nonconducted pacing spike; after the fourth paced complex, there is a nonconducted pacing spike.

4.

Nonmodifiable	Modifiable
Heredity Advancing age Male sex	Hypertension Diabetes mellitus or glucose intolerance Hyperlipidemia Hyperhomocystinemia Sedentary lifestyle Stress Obesity Cigarette smoking Oral contraceptives (especially in smokers)

5.
a	1.	Thrombolytics
a	2.	Percutaneous coronary interventions such as angioplasty, atherectomy
d, g	3.	ACE inhibitors
c, d	4.	Nitroglycerin
c, d, i	5.	Calcium channel blockers
b, h	6.	Beta-blockers
e, h, i	7.	ASA
e, f	8.	Heparin

6.
a, b, d, g, m, s	1.	Right ventricular failure
b, c, g, q	2.	Left ventricular failure
e	3.	Myocardial infarction
f	4.	Pulmonary embolism
a, b	5.	Tension pneumothorax
a, i, t	6.	Cardiac tamponade
g	7.	Valvular dysfunction
h, p	8.	Pericarditis
g, j, p	9.	Endocarditis
l, r	10.	Hyperlipidemia
k, n	11.	Chronic arterial insufficiency
m, o	12.	Chronic venous insufficiency

7.

Causes	Left	Right
Aortic stenosis	✓	
Cardiac tamponade	✓	✓
Cardiomyopathy	✓	
Mitral stenosis	✓	✓
LVMI	✓	
RVMI		✓
Pulmonary embolism		✓
Pulmonary hypertension		✓
Systemic hypertension	✓	

7. cont'd

Sign/Symptom	Left	Right
Abnormal liver function studies		✓
Ascites		✓
Atrial dysrhythmias	✓	✓
Crackles audible over lungs	✓	
Dyspnea	✓	
Elevated PAOP	✓	
Elevated RAP		✓
Hepatomegaly		✓
Jugular venous distention		✓
Mental confusion	✓	
Murmur of mitral regurgitation	✓	
Murmur of tricuspid regurgitation		✓
Orthopnea	✓	
Peripheral edema		✓
S₃, S₄ at apex	✓	
S₃, S₄ at sternum		✓
Weight gain		✓

8. a. Two primary effects of IABP:
   (1)   increases coronary artery perfusion pressure
   (2)   decreases afterload
   b. Two major contraindications of IABP:
   (1)   aortic insufficiency
   (2)   aortic aneurysm
   c. The balloon is inflated during which phase of the cardiac cycle?
   diastole
   d. The balloon is deflated immediately before which phase of the cardiac cycle?
   systole
   e. List two complications of displacement of the balloon in the aorta:
   (1)   ischemia of left arm
   (2)   renal ischemia

9. A. Assisted aortic end-diastolic pressure
   B. Unassisted aortic end-diastolic pressure
   C. Assisted systole
   D. Unassisted systole
   E. Diastolic augmentation

10.

Feature	Dilated	Hypertrophic	Restrictive
Associated with alcoholism or infection	✓		
Do not give inotropes		✓	
Clinical presentation: syncope, chest pain, sudden death		✓	
Clinical presentation similar to HF	✓		✓
May be candidate for cardiac transplantation	✓	✓	✓
Atrial fibrillation common	✓	✓	
Treatment includes beta-blockers and calcium channel blockers		✓	
Do not give diuretics or nitrates		✓	
Associated with infiltrative and connective tissue disorders	✓		✓
Treated with digoxin, diuretics, ACE inhibitors	✓		✓
Associated with genetically transmitted autosomal-dominant trait		✓	
AV blocks are common			✓
Hemiblock is common		✓	
Treatment may include steroids			✓

11.

Feature	Pericarditis	Myocarditis	Endocarditis
Associated with MI	✓		
May cause cardiomyopathy		✓	
Causes splinter hemorrhages, petechiae			✓
Treated with antiinflammatory drugs	✓		
Sudden onset of HF		✓	
Causes pericardial friction rub	✓		
Valve replacement may be necessary			✓
Usually associated with viral infection		✓	
Associated with cardiac surgery	✓		✓
Definitive diagnosis requires biopsy		✓	
May cause systemic emboli		✓	✓
Monitor closely for cardiac tamponade	✓		
Causes murmur			✓
Associated with uremia	✓		
Associated with ST segment elevation	✓		
Treated with antibiotics		✓	✓
Increased incidence in patients with rheumatic heart disease		✓	✓

12.

Description	Drug
IV calcium channel blocker used for hypertension	Nicardipine (Cardene)
IV beta-blocker that also blocks alpha-receptors	Labetalol (Normodyne)
IV vasodilator that may cause coronary artery steal and intrapulmonary shunt	Nitroprusside (Nipride)
IV vasodilator that is particularly helpful in patients with chest pain	Nitroglycerin (Tridil)
IV ACE inhibitor	Enalapril (Vasotec IV)
Oral ACE inhibitor that was first ACE inhibitor	Captopril (Capoten)
Two oral calcium channel blockers used for hypertension	Nifedipine (Procardia); diltiazem (Cardizem)
IV vasodilator that causes significant reflex tachycardia	Hydralazine (Apresoline)

13.

Drug	Arterial Dilator	Venous Dilator	Vasopressor
Amrinone (Inocor)	✓	✓	
Dobutamine (Dobutrex)	✓	✓	
Dopamine (Intropin)			✓
Hydralazine (Apresoline)	✓		
Minoxidil (Loniten)	✓		
Morphine sulfate		✓	
Nifedipine (Procardia)	✓	✓	
Nitroglycerin (<1 μg/kg/min)		✓	
Nitroglycerin (>1 μg/kg/min)	✓	✓	
Nitroprusside (Nipride)	✓	✓	
Norepinephrine (Levophed)			✓
Phentolamine (Regitine)	✓	✓	
Phenylephrine (Neo-Synephrine)			✓
Prazosin (Minipress)	✓	✓	
Vasopressin (Pitressin)			✓

14.

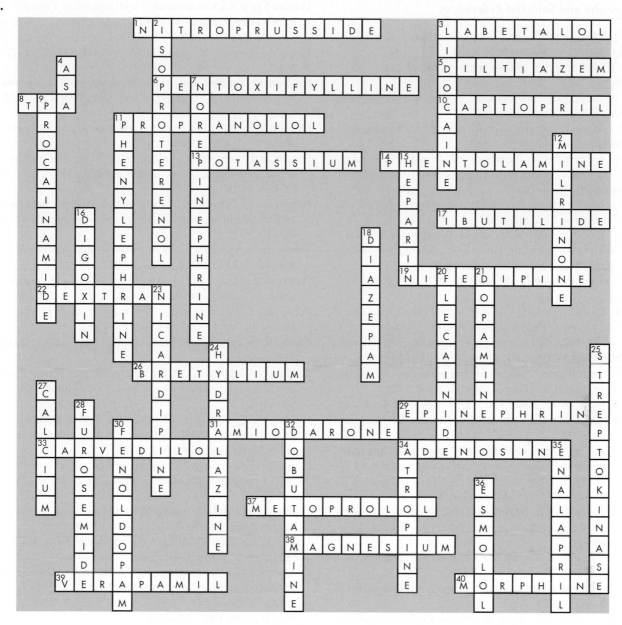

Bibliography and Selected References

Adams J, Miracle V: Cardiac biomarkers: past, present, and future, *Am J Crit Care* 7(6):418, 1998.

Aehlert B: ACLS: quick review study guide, St Louis, 1994, Mosby.

Ahrens S: Managing heart failure: a blueprint for success, *Nursing95* 95 (12):27, 1995.

Alspach J, editor: *Core curriculum for critical care nursing,* ed 5, Philadelphia, 1998, WB Saunders.

Anderson J, Gonzales R: Transmyocardial laser revascularization: old theory, new technology, *Critical Care Nursing Quarterly* 20 (4):53, 1998.

Baig M et al: The pathophysiology of advanced heart failure, *Heart and Lung* 28 (2):87, 1999.

Ballard J, Wood L, Lansing A: Transmyocardial revascularization: criteria for selecting patients, treatment, and nursing care, *Critical Care Nurse* 17 (1):42, 1997.

Beare P, Myers J: *Adult health nursing,* ed 2, St Louis, 1994, Mosby.

Boggs R, Wooldridge-King M: *AACN procedure manual for critical care,* ed 3, Philadelphia, 1993, WB Saunders.

Bove L et al: Nursing care of patients undergoing dynamic cardiomyoplasty, *Critical Care Nurse* 15 (6):96, 1995.

Callahan L, Frohlich G: Understanding nonsurgical coronary revascularization procedures, *AJN* 95(3):52H, 1995.

Carroll K et al: Risks associated with removal of ventricular epicardial pacing wires after cardiac surgery, *Am J Crit Care* 7 (6):444, 1998.

Casey K, Bedker D, Roussel-McElmeel P: Myocardial infarction: review of clinical trials and treatment strategies, *Critical Care Nurse* 18 (2):39, 1998.

Chernow B, editor: *The pharmacologic approach to the critically ill patient,* ed 3, Baltimore, 1994, Williams & Wilkins.

Clochesy J et al: *Critical care nursing,* ed 2, Philadelphia, 1996, WB Saunders.

Cramer C: Hypertensive crisis from drug-food interaction, *AJN* 97 (5):32, 1997.

Cuddy R: Hypertension: keeping dangerous blood pressure down, *Nursing95* 25 (8):35, 1995.

Cummins R, Graves J: *ACLS Scenarios: Core Concepts for Case-Based Learning,* St Louis, 1996, Mosby Lifeline.

Dabbs A, Chambers C, Macauley K: Complications after placement of an intracoronary stent: nursing implications, *Am J Crit Care* 7 (2):117, 1998.

Daniel J, Dattolo J: Minimally invasive cardiac surgery: surgical techniques and nursing considerations, *Critical Care Nursing Quarterly* 20 (4):29, 1998.

Dracup D, Dunbar S, Baker D: Rethinking heart failure, *AJN* 95 (7):23, 1995.

Dracup K, Bryan-Brown C: Reducing patient delay in seeking treatment, *Am J Crit Care* 6 (6):415, 1997.

Dracup K, Cannon C: Combination treatment strategies for management of acute myocardial infarction: new directions with current therapies, *Critical Care Nurse* (Supplement) April 1999:3, 1999.

Dugan K: Caring for patients with pericarditis, *Nursing98* 28 (3):50, 1998.

Dukovcic A, Daleiden-Burns A, Shawl F: Percutaneous cardiopulmonary support for high-risk angioplasty, *Critical Care Nursing Quarterly* 20 (4):16, 1998.

Dunbar S et al: Factors associated with outcomes 3 months after implantable cardioverter defibrillator insertion, *Heart and Lung* 28 (5):303, 1999.

Edgar W, Ebersole N, Mayfield M: MIDCAB, *AJN* 99 (7):46, 1999.

Eichhorn E: Our new understanding of heart failure: the role of beta-blockers in treatment, *Cleve Clin J Med* 65 (8):428, 1998.

Flynn M, Bonini S: Blunt chest trauma: case report, *Critical Care Nurse* 19 (5):68, 1999.

Futterman L, Lemberg L: Inflammation in plaque rupture: an active participant or an invited guest?, *Am J Crit Care* 7 (2):153, 1998.

Futterman L, Lemberg L: Low-molecular-weight heparin: an antithrombotic agent whose time has come, *Am J Crit Care* 8 (1):520, 1999.

Futterman L, Lemberg L: Homocysteine and coronary artery disease, *Am J Crit Care* 6 (1):72, 1997.

Futterman L, Lemberg L: Hypertension, stroke, and noncompliance: an avoidable triad, *Am J Crit Care* 5 (3):227, 1996.

Futterman L, Lemberg L: Sudden cardiac death-preventable-reversible, *Am J Crit Care* 6 (6):472, 1997.

Gahart B, Nazareno A: *1999 Intravenous Medications,* St Louis, 1999, Mosby.

Gawlinski A, Hamwi D: *Acute care nurse practitioner clinical curriculum and certification review,* Philadelphia, 1999, WB Saunders.

Goldsmith ST, Dick C: Differentiating systolic from diastolic heart failure: pathophysiologic and therapeutic considerations, *Am J Med* 95 (6):645, 1993.

Gonzalez-Aler de Solis M, Hendrix L: Acute methemoglobinemia: a nursing perspective, *Critical Care Nurse* June 95:33, 1995.

Goodwin M et al: Early extubation and early activity after open heart surgery, *Critical Care Nurse* 19 (5):18, 1999.

Grauer K, Cavalaro D: *ACLS-A Comprehensive Review,* Ed. 3, St Louis, 1993, Mosby Lifeline.

Gregory S, Stockman L: Reducing the risks from postprocedure anticoagulant therapy, *Nursing97* 27 (8):32cc1, 1997.

Guzzetta C, Dossey B: *Cardiovascular nursing: holistic practice,* St Louis, 1992, Mosby.

Gysi J, Smull E: Speeding thrombolytic therapy, *Nursing97* 27 (5):32cc, 1997.

Hahn S, Jang I, O'Donnell C: Antithrombotic therapy for acute coronary syndrome, Part 1: STE-MI, *Journal of Critical Illness* 13 (12):772, 1998.

Halpern N: Today's strategies for treating postoperative hypertension, *The Journal of Critical Illness* 10 (7):478, 1995.

Hambach C: Opening a window on pericardial effusion, *Nursing98* 28 (8):32cc1, 1998.

Hayes D: Understanding coronary atherectomy, *AJN* 96 (12):38, 1996.

Hayes E, L'Ecuyer K: A standard of care for radial artery grafting, *Am J Crit Care* 7 (6):429, 1998.

Hochman J et al: A new regimen for heparin use in acute coronary syndromes, *Am Heart J* 138 (2):313, 1999.

Holcomb S: When a myocardial infarction gets complicated, *Nursing97* 27 (8):32cc8, 1997.

Homes L, Hollabaugh S: Using the continuous quality improvement process to improve the care of patients after angioplasty, *Critical Care Nurse* 17 (6):56, 1997.

Howes P: Treating intermittent claudication, *AJN* 98 (12):16A, 1998.

Katz AM: Cardiomyopathy of overload. A major determinant of prognosis in congestive heart failure, *N Engl J Med* 322 (2):100, 1990.

Keen J, Searingen P: *Mosby's critical care nursing consultant,* St Louis, 1997, Mosby.

Kinney M et al: *AACN clinical reference for critical care nursing,* ed 4, St Louis, 1998, Mosby.

Kline-Rogers E, Martin J, Smith D: New era of reperfusion in acute myocardial infarction, *Critical Care Nurse,* 19 (1):21, 1999.

Knight L et al: Caring for patients with third-generation implantable cardioverter defibrillators: from decision to implant to patient's return home, *Critical Care Nurse* 17 (5):46, 1997.

Kuncl N, Nelson K: Antihypertensive drugs: balancing risks and benefits, *Nursing97* 27 (8):46, 1997.

Lai S, Cohen M: Promoting lifestyle changes, *AJN* 99 (4):63, 1999.

Lazzara D, Pfersdorf P, Sedlacek M: Femoral compression, *Nursing97* 27 (12):54, 1997.

Levin T et al: Right ventricular MI: when to suspect, what to do, *Journal of Critical Illness* 10 (1):14, 1995.

Lewandowski D: Congestive heart failure, *AJN* 95 (5):36, 1995.

Lewandowski D: Myocarditis, *AJN* 99 (8):44, 1999.

Lewis A: Cardiovascular emergency! *Nursing99* 29 (6):49, 1999.

Lilley L, Guanci R: A cautious look at heparin, *AJN* 95 (9):14, 1995.

Lindsay G, Gaw A, editors: *Coronary heart disease prevention: a handbook for the health care team,* New York, 1997, Churchill Livingstone.

Littrell K et al: Myocardial infarction and the nondiagnostic ECG: strategies to meet the challenges, *Journal of Emergency Nursing* 21:287, 1995.

Livorsi-Moore J, Gulanick M, Rosko P: Port access: another advance in cardiovascular surgery, *AJN* 99 (7):52, 1999.

Logan P: What you need to know about interventional cardiology, *Nursing95* 25 (9):32II, 1995.

Macari J, Bryant M: Coronary artery stenting 1998, *AJN* 98 (Supplement):S43, 1998.

Mancini M, Kaye W: AEDs: changing the way you respond to cardiac arrest, *AJN* 99 (5):26, 1999.

Marino P: *The ICU book,* ed 2, Baltimore, 1998, Williams and Wilkins.

Mayer D, Docktor W: Abciximab, a novel platelet-blocking drug: pharmacology and nursing implications, *Critical Care Nurse* 18 (2):29, 1998.

McAlpine L: The left anterior small thoracotomy technique: a new approach for coronary artery bypass grafting, *Critical Care Nurse* 17 (5):40, 1997.

McClarren-Curry C, Shaughnessy K: Acute thoracic aortic dissection: how to diffuse a time bomb, *Nursing99* 29 (1):32cc1, 1999.

McKinney B: Solving the puzzle of heart failure, *Nursing99* 29 (5):33, 1999.

Mehan C, Hayden A: Transmyocardial revascularization: a case study, *Critical Care Nursing Quarterly* 20 (4):60, 1998.

Mims B et al: *Critical care skills: a clinical handbook,* Philadelphia, 1996, WB Saunders.

Mizell J, Maglish B, Matheny R: Minimally invasive direct coronary artery bypass graft surgery, *Critical Care Nurse* 17 (3):46, 1997.

Moccia J: Unmasking pericarditis, *Nursing97* 27 (12):32cc1, 1997.

Morse D, Campbell R, Riddle M: Transmyocardial revascularization: a case study, *Am J Crit Care* 7 (6):426, 1998.

Moseley M, Oenning V, Melnik G: Methemoglobinemia, *AJN* 99 (5):47, 1999.

Moser D: Maximizing therapy in the advanced heart failure patient, *J Cardiovasc Nurs* 10(2):29, 1996.

Moser D: Correcting misconceptions about women and heart disease, *AJN 97* (4):26, 1997.

Murphy M: Use of measurements of myoglobin and cardiac troponins in the diagnosis of acute myocardial infarction, *Critical Care Nurse,* 19 (1):58, 1999.

Nass N, Solomon S: What role for ACE inhibitors in acute MI? *Journal of Critical Illness* 12 (12):789, 1997.

Nelson L, Hoffman R: How to manage acute MI when cocaine is the cause, *Journal of Critical Illness* 10 (1):39, 1995.

Newman P: Blunt cardiac injury, *New Horizons* 7 (1):26, 1999.

Newton J: Angina pectoris: a cry from the heart, *Nursing98* 28 (8):58, 1998.

Noureddine S: Research review: use of activated clotting time to monitor heparin therapy in coronary patients, *Am J Crit Care* 4 (4):272, 1995.

O'Connor C et al: Current and novel pharmacologic approaches in advanced heart failure, *Heart and Lung* 28 (4):227, 1999.

Opie L: *Drugs for the heart,* ed 4, Philadelphia, 1995, WB Saunders.

Owen A: Tracking the rise and fall of cardiac enzymes, *Nursing95* 25 (5):35, 1995.

Parikh A, Shah P: Diagnosing unstable angina: what to look for, how to assess MI risk, *Journal of Critical Illness* 11 (1):9, 1996.

Patel V, Moliterno D: Invasive versus conservative management of non-Q-wave myocardial infarction, *Cleve Clin J Med* 66 (2): 100, 1999.

Patterson S, Citro K, Gillum N: Percutaneous myocardial revascularization: new treatment option for patients with angina, *Critical Care Nurse* 19 (5):27, 1999.

Penney C: Learning how to remove femoral sheaths, *Nursing95* 25 (5):32QQ, 1995.

Pettinicchi T: Hypertensive crisis, *Nursing96* 26(8):25, 1996.

Phillips J: Abdominal aortic aneurysm, *Nursing98* 28 (5):35, 1998.

Piano M, Bondmass M, Schwertz D: The molecular and cellular pathophysiology of heart failure, *Heart and Lung* 27 (1):3, 1998.

Platek Y, Atzori M: PTMR, *AJN* 99 (7):64, 1999.

Possanza C: Coronary artery bypass grafts: tapping into the radial artery, *Nursing97* 27 (10): 32cc6, 1997.

Raimer F, Thomas M: Clot stoppers: using anticoagulants safely and effectively, *Nursing95* 25 (3):35, 1995.

Reger T, Vargus G: The return of the radial artery in CABG, *AJN* 99 (9):26, 1999.

Rice K, Walsh E: Navigating a bottleneck surgically, *Nursing98* 28 (2):39, 1998.

Rice K, Walsh E: Navigating a bottleneck, *Nursing98* 28 (2):33, 1998.

Rickenbacker P, Haywood G, Fowler M: Selecting candidates for cardiac transplantation, *Journal of Critical Illness* 10 (3):199, 1995.

Riegel B, Tomason T, Carlson B: Nursing care of patients with acute myocardial infarction: results of a national survey, *Critical Care Nurse* 17 (5):23, 1997.

Robinson A: Getting to the heart of denial, *AJN* 99 (5):38, 1999.

Ross G, DeJong M: Pericardial tamponade, *AJN* 99 (2):35, 1999.

Sabo J, Mehan C: Partial ventriculectomy: new hope for patients, *AJN 98* (Supplement):S49: 1998.

Sansevero A, Ruddy Y: Managing aortic dissections: a critical care challenge, *Critical Care Nurse* 16 (5):44, 1996.

Scherck K: Recognizing a heart attack: the process of determining illness, *Am J Crit Care* 6 (4):267, 1997.

Shaffer R: Keeping pace with permanent pacemakers, part II, *Nursing99* 29 (7):32cc8, 1999.

Sims J, Miracle V: Using the ECG to detect myocardial infarction, *Nursing99* 29 (8):41, 1999.

Spodick D: The technique of pericardiocentesis, *Journal of Critical Illness* 10 (11): 807, 1995.

Strimike C, Wojcik J: Putting in a plug for faster hemostasis, *Nursing97* 27 (7):32cc, 1997.

Strimike C: Caring for a patient with an intracoronary stent, *AJN* 95 (1):40, 1995.

Stromberg A et al: Factors influencing patient compliance with therapeutic regimens in chronic heart failure: a critical incident technique analysis, *Heart and Lung* 28 (5):334, 1999.

Thelan L et al: *Critical care nursing: diagnosis and management,* ed 3, St Louis, 1998, Mosby.

Tietjen C et al: Treatment modalities for hypertensive patients with intracranial pathology: options and risks, *Critical Care Medicine* 24 (2):311, 1996.

Turjanica M: Anatomy of a code, *Nursing98* 28 (1):35, 1998.

Turner D, Turner L: Right ventricular infarction: detection, treatment, and nursing implications, *Critical Care Nurse* February 95:22, 1995.

Vaca K, Daake C, Lambrechts D: Nursing care of patients undergoing thoracoscopic minimally invasive bypass grafting, *Am J Crit Care* 6 (4):281, 1997.

Valle B, Lemberg L: Regression of coronary artery disease: the role of plaque biology, *Am J Crit Care* 4(6): 481, 1995.

Valle B, Valle G, Lemberg L: Volume control: a reliable option in the management of "refractory" congestive heart failure, *Am J Crit Care* 4 (2):169, 1995.

Wallace C: Nitroglycerin tolerance, *AJN* 98 (11):16CC, 1998.

Wallace C: Dual-chamber pacemakers in the management of severe heart failure, *Critical Care Nurse* 18 (2):57, 1998.

Wolff C, Scott C, Banks T: The radial artery: an exciting alternative conduit in coronary artery bypass surgery, *Critical Care Nurse* 17 (5):34, 1997.

Woods A: Managing hypertension, *Nursing99* 29 (3):41, 1999.

Woods S et al: *Cardiac nursing,* ed 3, Philadelphia, 1995, JB Lippincott Company.

Zevola D, Maier B: Improving the care of cardiothoracic surgery patients through advanced nursing skills, *Critical Care Nurse,* 19 (1):34, 1999.

Zevola D et al: Clinical pathways and coronary artery bypass surgery, *Critical Care Nurse* 17 (6):20, 1997.

Pulmonary System: Physiology, Assessment, and Ventilatory Support

Selected Concepts in Anatomy and Physiology

General Information

I. The pulmonary system consists of lungs, conducting air passages, muscles of ventilation, central nervous system control, thoracic cage, and alveoli (Fig. 4-1)

II. Functions of the pulmonary system include the following:
   A. Allows interchange of gases between the atmosphere and the bloodstream
   B. Assists in maintenance of acid-base balance
   C. Contributes to phonation
   D. Acts as a reservoir for blood for the left atrium and ventricle
   E. Assists in metabolism

Functional Anatomy

I. Conducting airways: nose to terminal bronchioles
   A. Where gas flows but no gas exchange occurs between the alveoli and the blood
      1. Consists of branching tubes with diminishing diameter
      2. Accounts for approximately 2 ml/kg of inspired tidal volume (this volume is termed *anatomic deadspace*)
   B. Upper airway (Fig. 4-2): nose or mouth to external opening of vocal cords; serves as a passageway for food and inspired gas
      1. Mouth: not as effective as the nose in conditioning the inspired air
         a) Smaller surface area
         b) No ciliated epithelium to trap dust or bacteria from inspired air
      2. Nose
         a) Structure
            (1) Mucous membrane lining contains cilia and mucus-producing cells
            (2) Rich supply of blood vessels lies under the mucous membranes to provide warmth
            (3) Skeletal rigidity maintains patency during inspiration
            (4) Turbinates increase surface area
            (5) Four sinuses surround and drain into the nasal cavity: frontal, maxillary, ethmoid, sphenoid
            (6) Septum divides the nose into two fossac
            (7) Small inlet with larger outlet allows air to have maximal contact with the nasal mucosa
         b) Functions
            (1) Warms inspired gas to body temperature
            (2) Humidifies inspired gas to relative humidity of approximately 80% to 100% at body temperature; accounts for insensible water loss of 400 ml/24 hr
            (3) Protects the lower airway from foreign material; filters inspired air of particles 5 μ or larger
            (4) Prevents inspiration of potentially dangerous environmental gases
            (5) Assists in production of sound in phonation
            (6) Provides sense of olfaction: olfactory area located in the superior turbinate (sniffing directs air toward this area)
         c) More resistance (2-3 times) than the mouth
            (1) Dyspneic patients are more likely to breath through their mouth
      3. Pharynx: posterior nasal cavity to esophagus
         a) Structure
            (1) Nasopharynx: between posterior nasal cavity to soft palate; contains the pharyngeal tonsils and eustachian tube
               (a) Pharyngeal tonsils (also called *adenoids*): dense concentration of lymphatic tissue; guards entryway into respiratory and GI tracts

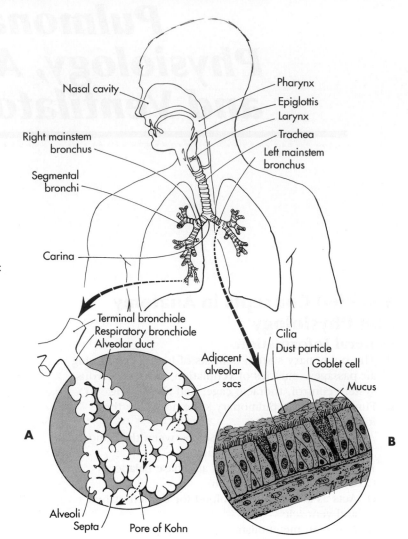

Figure 4-1 The respiratory system. **A,** Acinus. **B,** Mucociliary escalator. (From Price SA, Wilson LM: *Pathophysiology: clinical concepts of disease processes,* ed 5, St Louis, 1997, Mosby.)

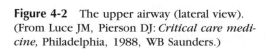

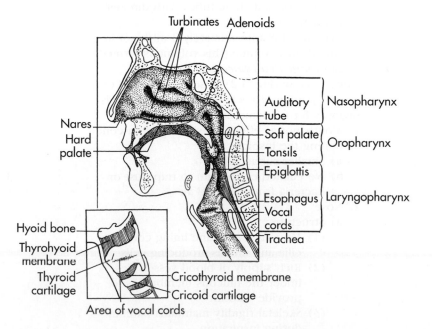

Figure 4-2 The upper airway (lateral view). (From Luce JM, Pierson DJ: *Critical care medicine,* Philadelphia, 1988, WB Saunders.)

(b) Eustachian tube: connection to the middle ear; opens during swallowing to equalize pressure in the middle ear
  (i) Middle ear pain or infection may develop during upper respiratory infection if eustachian tube closes
  (ii) Nasal intubation may block eustachian tubes and cause otitis media
(2) Oropharynx: between the soft palate and base of tongue
  (a) Contains the palatine and lingual tonsils
  (b) Center of the gag reflex, which defends the lower airway against aspiration; gag reflex controlled by cranial nerves IX (glossopharyngeal) and X (vagus)
  (3) Laryngopharynx (also called the *hypopharynx*): from base of tongue to the epiglottis
b) Functions
  (1) Swallowing: uvula and soft palate move posteriorly and superiorly to keep food and liquid from entering the nasopharynx
  (2) Protection: area is rich in lymphatic tissue
4. Larynx: upper portion of the trachea; connects the laryngopharynx with the trachea
  a) Structure: consists of thyroid cartilage, vocal cords, and cricoid cartilage
    (1) Epiglottis: flexible cartilage attached to the thyroid cartilage, which overhangs the larynx like a lid; prevents food from entering the larynx and trachea during swallowing
    (2) Thyroid cartilage: largest laryngeal cartilage
      (a) Contains the vocal cords
      (b) Also referred to as the *Adam's apple*
    (3) Vocal folds: two pairs of membranes that protrude into the lumen of the larynx; controlled by recurrent laryngeal nerve, a branch of the vagus nerve
      (a) False vocal cords: upper pair; play no part in vocalization
      (b) True vocal cords: lower pair
        (i) Form a triangular opening between them that leads to the trachea
        (ii) Change shape and vibrate in response to contraction of muscles in the larynx to result in phonation

(c) Glottis: passage through the vocal cords
(4) Cricothyroid membrane: avascular structure that connects the thyroid and cricoid cartilage; cricothyrotomy, an emergency opening of the airway, is performed at this membrane
(5) Cricoid cartilage: complete ring located below the thyroid cartilage
b) Functions
  (1) Allows speech
  (2) Prevents aspiration through the valve action of the epiglottis
  (3) Allows for cough reflex and Valsalva maneuver
C. Lower airway (Fig. 4-3): below larynx; conducts air to the gas exchange surface
  1. Structure
    a) Trachea: first portion of tracheobronchial tree
      (1) Consists of 16 to 20 C-shaped rings; 10 to 12 cm long
      (2) The esophagus and trachea share a common wall; erosion through this wall (tracheoesophageal fistula) may be caused by an overinflated endotracheal tube (ET) or tracheostomy tube cuff
    b) Carina: bifurcation of trachea into left and right mainstem bronchi
      (1) The carina is rich in parasympathetic nervous system fibers and cough receptors
      (2) Suctioning may cause bradycardia and hypotension due to stimulation of carina with the suction catheter
    c) Bronchi
      (1) Right mainstem bronchus is almost straight (25 degrees) off trachea and larger in diameter than the left (40 to 60 degrees); aspiration of liquid or food, foreign bodies, suction catheter, and ET tube go to right preferentially
      (2) Conducting airways branch from mainstem bronchi → lobar bronchi; from lobar bronchi → segmental bronchi; from segmental bronchi → subsegmental bronchi, and so on
        (a) These branches are called *generations* or *levels* (Fig. 4-4): mainstem (first level), lobar (second), segmental (third), subsegmental (fourth through ninth), bronchioles (tenth through fifteenth)
      (3) Bronchi are supported by cartilage and smooth muscle
      (4) Mast cells lie just beneath the

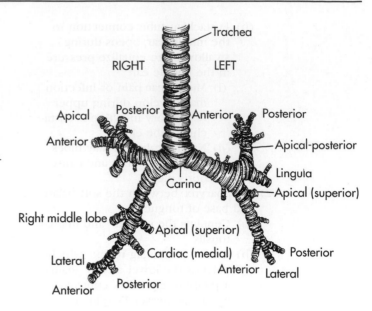

Figure 4-3   The lower airway. (Modified from Frownfelter DL, editor: *Chest physical therapy and pulmonary rehabilitation,* Chicago, 1978, Mosby.)

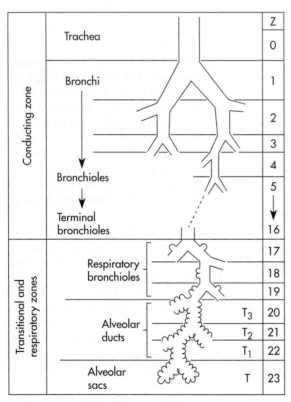

Figure 4-4   Airway generations.

bronchial epithelium near the smooth muscle and blood vessels

d) Function
  (1) The lower airway conducts, warms, cleanses, and humidifies air
  (2) The bronchi are responsible for most of total airway resistance in a healthy person
  (3) Mast cells secrete histamine and other mediators of the inflammatory process when stimulated by antigen-antibody response

2. Terminal bronchioles
  a) Structure
    (1) Sixteenth branch
    (2) One mm in diameter; fibrous, elastic smooth muscle with no cartilage; no mucous glands or cilia
  b) Function
    (1) Terminal bronchioles are particularly sensitive to CO_2 and dilate in response to increased CO_2 levels
    (2) Bronchospasm may narrow lumen and increase airway resistance

II. Lung
  A. Lobes separated by fissures
    1. Right: three lobes
    2. Left: two lobes
      a) The upper left lobe is divided by a fissure
      b) The lower portion of the left upper lobe is referred to as the *lingula;* it is approximately the same size as the right middle lobe
  B. Segments
    1. Right: ten segments
    2. Left: eight segments
  C. Subsegments
  D. Lobules
    1. Primary functional units of lung
    2. Consists of terminal bronchiole, alveolar ducts, alveolar sacs, alveoli, and pulmonary circulation
  E. Gas exchange units (Fig. 4-5): respiratory bronchioles to alveoli
    1. Acinus: a term used to refer to the terminal respiratory unit distal to the terminal bronchioles; has an alveolar-capillary membrane for gas exchange
    2. Respiratory bronchioles
      a) Structure
        (1) Composed of the seventeenth though twentieth branches

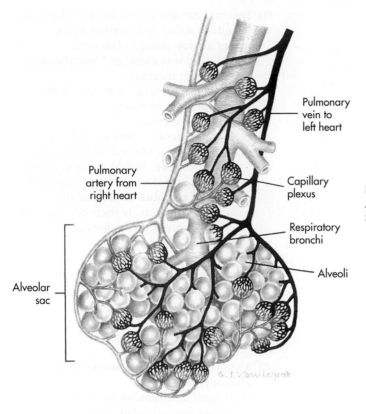

Figure 4-5   The acinus. (From Wilson SF, Thompson VM: *Mosby's clinical nursing series: respiratory disorders,* St Louis, 1990, Mosby.)

(2) Less than 1 mm in diameter; bronchioles less than 1 mm are subject to collapse when compressed

b) Function

(1) Increasing number of alveoli are attached

(2) Gas exchange takes place here

3. Alveolar ducts, alveolar sacs, and alveoli

a) Structure

(1) Alveolar ducts: twentieth through twenty-second levels

(2) Alveolar sacs: level 23

(3) Alveoli: three hundred million alveoli

(a) 1 to 2 millimicrons in size

(b) One half of alveoli in ducts and one half in alveolar sacs in grapelike clusters of 15 to 20 alveoli

(c) Contain pores of Kohn: openings between alveoli in intraalveolar septa

(i) Thought to allow collateral ventilation

(ii) May also contribute to movement of microorganisms between alveoli and rapid transmission of infection

(4) Lined with alveolar epithelium: site of diffusion of oxygen and carbon dioxide between inspired air and blood

(5) Type I pneumocytes

(a) Cover 90% of total alveolar surface

(b) Flat, large, squamous cells and very susceptible to injury

(c) Responsible for integumentary air-blood barrier; cytoplasmic junctions very tight and impermeable to water under normal circumstances

(6) Type II pneumocytes

(a) These small, cuboidal, granular cells cover only 5% total alveolar surface

(b) They produce, store, and secrete surfactant, a lipoprotein that lines the inner aspect of the alveolus

(i) Surfactant decreases surface tension of the fluid lining the alveoli and prevents alveolar collapse at the end of expiration, especially at low volumes

(ii) It is especially important in inferior portions of lung where alveoli are small and distending pressures are low

(iii) A deficiency of surfactant causes alveolar collapse, poorly compliant lungs, and alveolar edema

(iv) The half-life of surfactant is only 14 hours; injury to these cells quickly results in massive atelectasis

(c) If type I pneumocytes are injured, type II pneumocytes increase mitosis to replicate and form a cuboidal cell line and may differentiate to type I

F. Alveolar-capillary membrane
  1. Structure
     a) Lines respiratory bronchioles to alveoli
     b) Surface area of 1 m²/kg body weight and 0.5 μ in thickness
     c) Diffusion pathway (Fig. 4-6): gases travel through the pathway from alveolus to blood (oxygen) or blood to alveolus (carbon dioxide)
        (1) Alveolar epithelium
        (2) Epithelial basement membrane
        (3) Interstitial space
        (4) Capillary basement membrane
        (5) Capillary endothelium
  2. Function
     a) Immense surface area and thinness of membrane allow for rapid gas exchange by diffusion
     b) Pulmonary capillary endothelial cells produce and degrade prostaglandins, metabolize vasoactive amines, convert angiotensin I to angiotensin II, and at least partly produce coagulation factor VIII

G. Defense mechanisms
  1. Upper airway
     a) Nasal cilia
     b) Sneeze: reaction to irritation in the nose
     c) Cough: reaction to irritation in the upper airway distal to the nose
        (1) Vocal cords close and intrathoracic pressure increases
        (2) Sudden opening of glottis allows propulsion of mucus
     d) Mucociliary escalator
        (1) Combination of mucus and cilia
        (2) Particles not filtered by nasal cilia (smaller than 5 mm) are trapped in mucus and then propelled upward by the pulsatile motion of the cilia; this mucus is then coughed and expectorated or swallowed
     e) Lymphatics
  2. Lower airway
     a) Cough: especially at level of carina
     b) Mucociliary escalator
     c) Lymphatics
  3. Alveoli
     a) Immune system
     b) Lymphatics
     c) Alveolar macrophages: mononuclear phagocytes
        (1) Engulf and remove bacteria and other foreign substances
        (2) Move from alveolus to alveolus through the pores of Kohn
  4. Loss of normal defense mechanisms
     a) Disease
     b) Injury
     c) Anesthesia
     d) Corticosteroids
     e) Smoking
     f) Malnutrition
     g) Ethanol

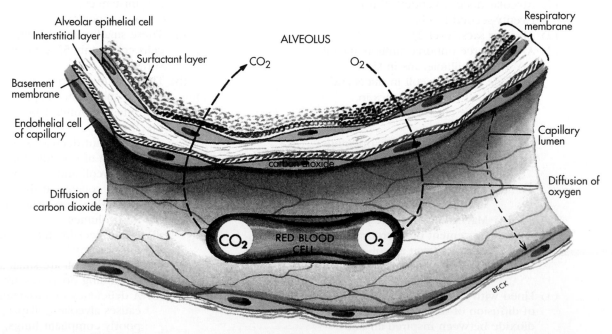

Figure 4-6 The diffusion pathway. (From Lewis SM, Collier IC: *Medical-surgical nursing,* ed 3, St Louis, 1992, Mosby.)

h) Uremia

i) Hypoxia or hyperoxia

j) Artificial airways

III. Lymphatics

A. Structure: surround lobule

B. Functions

1. Remove interstitial fluid to keep lung free of excess fluid

a) Normal lymph drainage is approximately 20 ml/hr; may be 200 ml/hr in pulmonary edema

b) When interstitial lymphatic vessels become enlarged through increased fluid filtration such as pulmonary edema, horizontal linear opacities referred to as *Kerley-B lines* are seen on chest X-ray

2. Remove inhaled particles from distal areas of lung

IV. Circulation (Fig. 4-7)

A. Pulmonary circulation: low pressure, low resistance system

1. Lungs receive the full cardiac output (approximately 5 L/min)

2. RV → main pulmonary artery → left and right pulmonary arteries → arterioles → capillaries, which spread over the surface of the alveoli → red blood cells (RBCs) move through in single file to allow the diffusion of gases and the attachment of oxygen to hemoglobin

a) A corresponding arteriole and venule exists for every bronchiole

b) The network of capillaries is very dense and frequently described as a sheet of blood

c) The pulmonary capillaries are very small and barely accommodate erythrocyte passage

3. Veins move out of lung toward the pleura

a) Numerous veins gradually form four pulmonary veins that empty into the left atrium

b) The venous system serves as an immense reservoir of blood for the left atrium and left ventricle

4. Mean pressure in pulmonary artery: 10 to 20 mm Hg

a) Pulmonary hypertension (PA_m >20 mm Hg)

(1) Passive pulmonary hypertension

(a) Mitral stenosis

(b) Left ventricular failure

(2) Constriction of the pulmonary circulation is caused by:

(a) Decreased alveolar oxygen concentration (called *hypoxemic pulmonary hypertension*)

(b) Acidosis

(c) Chemicals: epinephrine, norepinephrine, angiotensin II

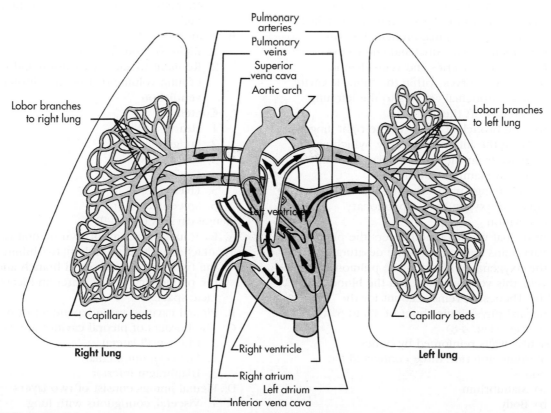

Figure 4-7   The pulmonary circulation. (From Wilson SF, Thompson VM: *Mosby's clinical nursing series: respiratory disorders,* St Louis, 1990, Mosby.)

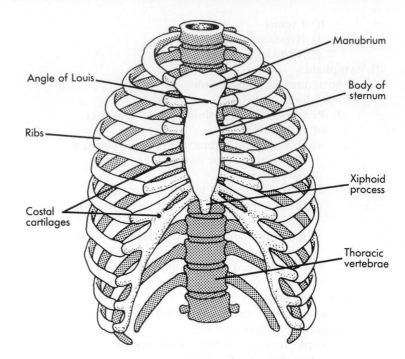

Figure 4-8 The thoracic cage. (From Scanlan CL et al: *Egan's fundamentals of respiratory care*, ed 6, St Louis, 1990, Mosby.)

(3) Obstruction in pulmonary circuit: pulmonary embolus
  b) Dilation of the pulmonary circulation caused by:
    (1) Oxygen
    (2) Isoproterenol
    (3) Aminophyllin
B. Bronchial circulation
  1. This system consists of the nutrient and oxygen circulation for the tracheobronchial tree down to terminal bronchioles, visceral pleura, interstitial and connective tissue, some arteries and veins, lymph nodes, and nerves within the thoracic cavity
    a) Two bronchial arteries to the left lung: directly off the aorta
    b) One bronchial artery to the right lung: from the intercostal artery, which originates from the right subclavian or internal mammary artery
  2. Gas exchange units are supplied with nutrients and oxygen by the pulmonary circulation
  3. Bronchial venous blood enters the pulmonary veins and causes some desaturation of the oxygenated blood in the pulmonary vein; this venous blood and the blood from the Thebesian veins account for the normal physiologic shunt of 3% to 5%
V. Thoracic cage (Fig. 4-8)
  A. Muscular walls reinforced by bones
    1. Sternum anterior: three connected flat bones
      a) Manubrium
      b) Body
      c) Xiphoid

2. Spine posterior: 12 pairs of ribs are attached to the vertebrae
3. Ribs anterior, lateral, and posterior
  a) Seven pairs of ribs, called *true ribs,* are attached to sternum
  b) Five pairs of ribs are attached to the rib above it
4. Clavicles superior
5. Diaphragm: inferior border of the thoracic cage
  B. Properties
    1. Rigid to protect the lungs
    2. Resilient to allow expansion and reduction of lung volume that occurs during ventilation
  C. Contents
    1. Heart
    2. Lungs
    3. Esophagus
    4. Great vessels
    5. Liver
    6. Spleen
VI. Pleural cavities (Fig. 4-9)
  A. Each lung hangs in its own pleural cavity attached only at the hilum; the hilum is where the two mainstem bronchi branch and where the pulmonary vessels enter and leave the thoracic space
  B. Pleural cavities are independent of one another
  C. The borders of pleural cavities are as follows:
    1. Chest wall lateral
    2. Mediastinum medial
    3. Diaphragm inferior
  D. Pleural linings consist of two layers
    1. Visceral: contiguous with lung
    2. Parietal: contiguous with chest wall

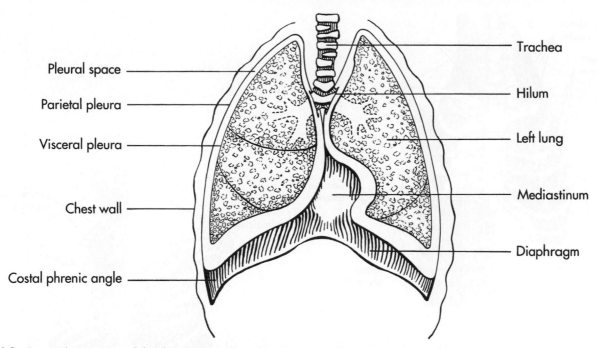

Figure 4-9   Internal structures of the thorax, including pleural cavities. (From Dettenmeier PA: *Pulmonary nursing care*, St Louis, 1992, Mosby.)

3. Pleural space
   a) Contains a few ml of serous fluid, which acts as a lubricant and adhesive between the visceral and parietal pleura as they slide along each other with each ventilatory cycle
   b) Maintains a negative intrapleural pressure of approximately −5 mm Hg below atmospheric pressure; this pressure becomes more negative (−10 mm Hg) during inspiration; loss of this negative intrapleural pressure (e.g., pneumothorax) causes the lung to collapse

VII. Mediastinum: center of thoracic cavity; contains the following:
   A. Heart and great vessels
   B. Trachea and mainstem bronchi
   C. Esophagus
   D. Phrenic, vagus, and other nerves
   E. Lymph nodes and ducts
   F. Thymus gland

VIII. Muscles of ventilation (Fig. 4-10)
   A. Inspiratory
      1. Diaphragm
         a) Innervation occurs via phrenic nerves (C3-C5)
         b) The diaphragm consists of two hemidiaphragms connected by a central membranous tendon; this tendon is contiguous with the fibrous pericardium
         c) Contraction flattens the diaphragm
            (1) Increases size of thorax superior-inferior
            (2) Normally accounts for 70% of tidal volume during quiet breathing
         d) Relaxation makes the diaphragm dome shaped and decreases the volume of the thoracic cavity
      2. External intercostals
         a) Innervation occurs from T1-T11
         b) Contraction raises the ribs, increasing the size of the thorax anteroposteriorly
      3. Accessory muscles of inspiration
         a) Scalene
            (1) Located in the neck; stretch from the first cervical vertebra to the first and second ribs
            (2) Enlarge the upper rib cage
         b) Sternocleidomastoid
            (1) Located in the neck; stretch from the manubrium and clavicle to the mastoid process and occipital bone
            (2) Elevate the sternum to increase the anteroposterior and transverse diameter of the chest
         c) Not used in normal resting ventilation but used during exercise and in respiratory distress; also used in the inspiratory phase of sneeze or cough
   B. Expiratory
      1. Expiration is normally passive
         a) It occurs when diaphragm and external intercostals relax and return to resting position
         b) The natural tendency of the lungs is to collapse, because they are made of elastic tissue; elastance is the quality of the lungs to recoil after inspiration
      2. Accessory muscles of expiration: internal oblique, external oblique, rectus

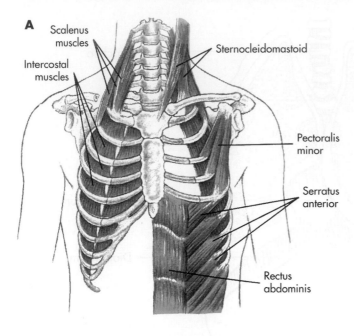

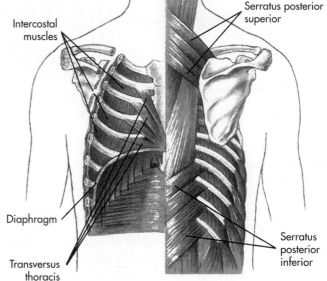

Figure 4-10 Muscles of ventilation. **A,** Anterior. **B,** Posterior. (From Thelan LA et al: *Critical care nursing: diagnosis and management,* ed 3, St Louis, 1998, Mosby.)

abdominis, internal intercostal, and transverse abdominis
  a) These muscles are used when increased levels of ventilation are needed
  b) They are also important in forceful expiration, coughing, and sneezing
  c) They increase pressure in the abdominal cavity and compress the abdominal viscera against the diaphragm
  d) They also depress the lower ribs and pull down the anterior portion of the lower chest

IX. Neuroanatomy
  A. Medulla: central chemoreceptors sensitive to cerebrospinal fluid (CSF) pH ($\uparrow$ $Paco_2 \rightarrow$ acidosis)
    1. Primary control of ventilation is by these central chemoreceptors and $Paco_2$ and pH levels
    2. They respond to minimal changes in $Paco_2$ very quickly
    3. Adjustment of alveolar ventilation occurs
      a) Increase in $Paco_2$ causes an increase in the rate and depth of ventilation
      b) Decrease in $Paco_2$ causes a decrease in the rate and depth of ventilation
  B. Arterial chemoreceptors in aortic arch and carotid bodies: sensitive to pH, Pao_2
    1. These peripheral chemoreceptors and Pao_2

levels provide secondary control of ventilation
    2. They will not respond to $Paco_2$ levels until a 10 mm Hg change is seen
    3. They respond when Pao_2 falls below 60 mm Hg; particularly important in patients with chronically elevated levels of $Paco_2$
  C. Pons: controls rhythmic ventilation
    1. Apneustic center stimulates inspiratory center
    2. Pneumotaxic center inhibits inspiratory activity
  D. Stretch receptors in alveoli (Hering-Breuer reflex): inhibits further inspiration to prevent overdistension of alveoli; may cause bronchodilation, tachycardia, vasodilation
  E. Proprioceptors in muscles and tendons: increase ventilation in response to body movements
  F. Baroreceptors in aortic arch and carotid bodies: increase in BP inhibits ventilation
  G. Juxtacapillary receptors (also called *pulmonary J-receptors*): stimulated by increase in interstitial fluid volume; may cause laryngeal constriction, hypotension, bradycardia, mucous production, dyspnea
  H. Chest wall pain receptors
    1. Lung parenchyma has no pain receptors
    2. Parietal pleura does have pain receptor;

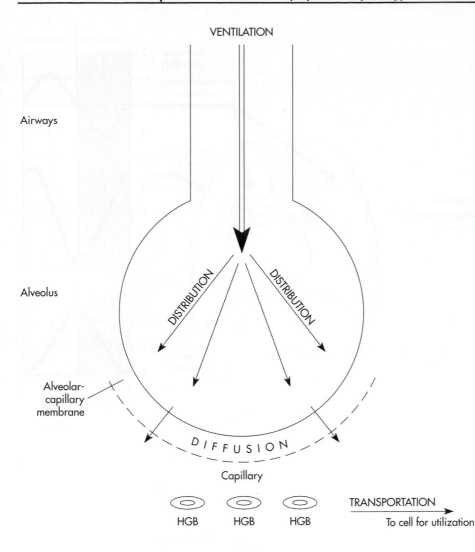

VENTILATION

Airways

Alveolus

DISTRIBUTION   DISTRIBUTION

Alveolar-
capillary
membrane

D I F F U S I O N

Capillary

HGB   HGB   HGB

TRANSPORTATION

To cell for utilization

Figure 4-11 Respiratory process: ventilation, distribution, diffusion, transportation, cellular utilization. (Drawing by Ann M. Walthall.)

transmits impulses via intercostal nerves and thoracic ganglia
I. Irritant receptors: stimulated by pulmonary edema, chemical or mechanical irritation; may cause bronchospasm, cough, mucus production
J. Modifying influences: drugs; brain trauma, edema, or increased ICP; chronic hypercapnia

Physiology (Fig. 4-11)

I. Ventilation: movement of air between atmosphere and alveoli and distribution of air within the lungs to maintain appropriate concentrations of oxygen and carbon dioxide in the alveoli
   A. Process (Fig. 4-12)
      1. Inspiration (inhalation): the movement of atmospheric air into the alveoli
         a) Message from medulla travels down phrenic nerve to diaphragm
         b) Diaphragm and external intercostals contract
         c) Size of thorax increases
         d) Lungs are stretched and intrapulmonary pressure is decreased to less than atmospheric pressure (-1 cm H_2O)
         e) Air movement into lungs to equalize the difference between atmospheric and alveolar pressure
      2. Expiration (exhalation): movement of air from alveoli to the atmosphere
         a) Relaxation of diaphragm and external intercostals
         b) Recoil of lungs to their resting size and a concomitant increase in alveolar pressure above atmospheric pressure ($+1$ cm H_2O)
         c) Air movement out of lungs to equalize the pressure difference
   B. Efficiency of ventilation: evaluated by Pa_{CO_2}
      1. Pa_{CO_2} greater than 45 mm Hg indicates hypoventilation
      2. Pa_{CO_2} less than 35 mm Hg indicates hyperventilation
   C. Lung volumes (Fig. 4-13 and Table 4-1)
      1. Alveolar ventilation is the part of total ventilation participating in gas exchange; it is the most important portion of minute ventilation; minute ventilation minus dead-space ventilation

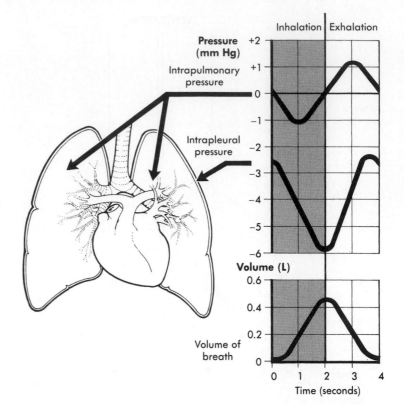

Figure 4-12 Pressure changes during ventilation. (From Thelan LA et al: *Critical care nursing: diagnosis and management,* ed 3, St Louis, 1998, Mosby.)

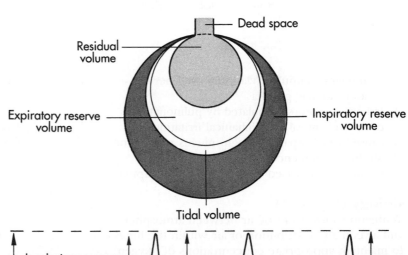

Figure 4-13 Lung volumes and capacities: upward deflection reflects inspiration and downward deflection reflects expiration. (From Dettenmeier PA: *Pulmonary nursing care,* St Louis, 1992, Mosby.)

Table 4-1	Lung Volumes, Capacities, and Mechanics	
Volume	**Definition**	**Normal**
Tidal Volume (V_T)	The volume of air moved in and out of the lungs with each normal breath	7 ml/kg or approximately 500 ml
Inspiratory reserve volume (IRV)	The volume of air that can be maximally inspired above the normal inspiratory level	3000 ml
Expiratory reserve volume (ERV)	The volume of air that can be maximally exhaled beyond the normal expiratory level	1000 ml
Residual volume (RV)	The volume of air remaining in the lungs at the end of a maximal expiration	1000 ml
Inspiratory capacity (IC)	V_T + IRC; the volume of air that can be maximally inspired from a normal expiratory level	3500 ml
Functional residual capacity (FRC)	RV + ERV; volume of air remaining in the lungs at the end of normal expiration	2000 ml
Vital capacity (VC)	V_T + IRC + ERV; the volume of air that can be maximally expired after a maximal inspiration	4500 ml
Total lung capacity (TLC)	V_T + IRC + ERV + RV; the volume of air that the lungs can hold with maximal inspiration	5500-6000 ml
Respiratory rate or frequency (f)	The number of breaths per minute	12-20
Minute ventilation ($\mathring{V}_E$)	$V_T \times$ f; the volume of air expired per minute	5-10 L
Dead space (V_D)	$V_D/V_T = Paco_2 - Peco_2/Paco_2$ $Paco_2$ (arterial); $Peco_2$ (exhaled) the volume or percentage of the V_T that does not participate in gas exchange; includes the volume of air in the conducting pathways (anatomic dead space) plus the volume of alveolar air that is not involved in gas exchange due to pathology (alveolar dead space)	V_D/V_T ratio is normally less than 0.4; V_D/V_T >0.6 is usually an indication for mechanical ventilation
Alveolar ventilation (V_A)	$V_T - V_D$; the volume of tidal air that is involved in alveolar gas exchange	350 ml
Forced vital capacity (FVC)	The volume of air in a forceful maximal expiration	Normally same as VC: 4500 ml
Forced expiratory volume (FEV)	The volume of air exhaled in a given time period; FEV_1: the volume of air exhaled in 1 second; FEV_3: the volume of air exhaled in 3 seconds	FEV_1: >75% of VC FEV_3: >95% of VC

2. Deadspace ventilation (Fig. 4-14) is the volume of air that does not participate in gas exchange
   a) Anatomic deadspace is the volume of air in conducting airways and it does not participate in gas exchange; approximately 2 ml/kg of tidal volume
   b) Alveolar (pathologic) deadspace is the volume of air in contact with nonperfused alveoli
   c) Physiologic deadspace is anatomical plus alveolar deadspace
      (1) Calculated by: $\dfrac{V_D}{V_T} = \dfrac{Paco_2 - Peco_2}{Paco_2}$
      (2) Normal: 0.2 to 0.4

D. Work of breathing = work of deforming the elastic system + work of producing airflow through the airways (Fig. 4-15)
   1. The work of breathing is usually negligible: 2% to 3% of total energy expenditure by the body
   2. Compliance
      a) Measure of expandability of lungs and/or thorax
      b) $C = \dfrac{\text{Change in volume}}{\text{Change in pressure}}$
         (1) Static compliance: affected by changes in compliance of chest wall or lung
         (2) Dynamic compliance: affected by

changes in compliance of chest wall or lung or airway resistance
  (3) Points to be used in calculation of static and dynamic compliance (Fig. 4-16, Table 4-2)
c) Factors affecting static compliance
  (1) Chest wall changes
    (a) Kyphoscoliosis
    (b) Flail chest
    (c) Thoracic pain with splinting
    (d) Obesity
  (2) Lung changes
    (a) Atelectasis
    (b) Pneumonia
    (c) Pulmonary edema
    (d) Pulmonary fibrosis
    (e) Pleural effusion
    (f) Pneumothorax
d) Additional factors affecting dynamic compliance
  (1) As above and airway resistance changes
3. Airway resistance
  a) Pressure differential required to produce a unit flow change; affected by airway caliber and length

b) Factors affecting airway resistance (and dynamic compliance)
  (1) Bronchospasm
  (2) Mucus
  (3) Artificial airways
  (4) Water condensation in ventilator tubing
  (5) Mucosal edema
  (6) Bronchial tumor
II. Perfusion: movement of blood through the pulmonary capillaries
  A. Pulmonary vasculature: resistance varied to accommodate the blood flow that it receives
  B. Distribution of perfusion
    1. Related to gravity and intraalveolar pressures
      a) Gravity causes the pressure in the capillaries in the bases to be higher than the pressure in the capillaries in the apices; preferential blood flow to the gravity-dependent areas of the lungs
      b) The intraalveolar pressures are generally equal throughout the lungs
      c) This equality creates the potential for intraalveolar pressure to exceed capillary hydrostatic pressure in some areas of the lung, causing absence of blood flow to these areas
    2. Zones (Fig. 4-17)
      a) Zone 1: nondependent portion of the lung; potential for no perfusion
      b) Zone 2: middle portion of the lung; varying blood flow
      c) Zone 3: gravity-dependent area of the lung; receives constant blood flow; pulmonary artery catheters ideally are placed in zone 3 for accurate reflection of left atrial pressure by the PAOP
    3. Hypoxemic pulmonary vasoconstriction
      a) Localized
        (1) Protective mechanism that decreases blood flow to an area of poor ventilation so that blood can be shunted to areas of better ventilation

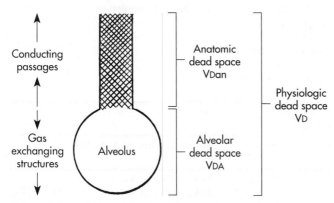

Figure 4-14   Physiologic deadspace: anatomic deadspace and alveolar deadspace. (Drawing by Wendy W. Johnson.)

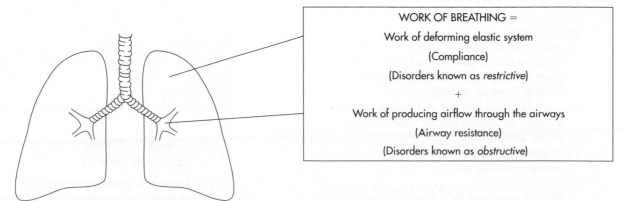

Figure 4-15   The work of breathing.

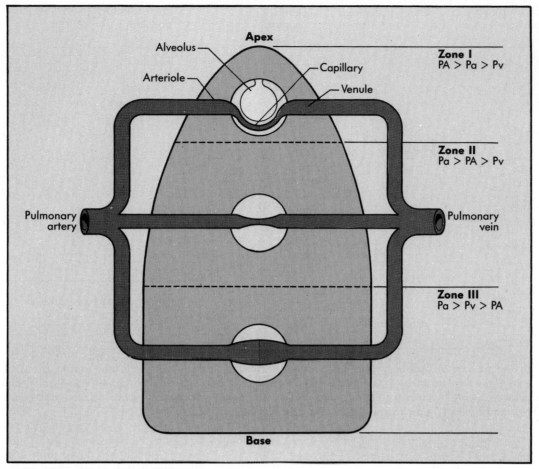

Figure 4-16 Zones of distribution of perfusion: relationship of alveolar pressure and gravitational forces to pulmonary vascular pressures and blood flow. The upright lung can be divided into three zones. In zone I, the upper third of the lung, alveolar pressure exceeds pulmonary venous and pulmonary artery pressures. In zone II, the middle third of the lung, the pulmonary artery pressure is greater than alveolar pressure, which is greater than pulmonary venous pressure. In zone III, the lower third of the lung, pulmonary artery pressure is greater than pulmonary venous pressure, which is greater than alveolar pressure. **Note:** pulmonary artery catheters are positioned in zone III for accurate measurement of PAWP as a reflection of left atrial pressure. (From McCance KL, Huether SE: *Pathophysiology: the biologic basis for disease in adults and children,* St Louis, 1990, Mosby.)

Table 4-2   Types Of Compliance

Type	Formula	Normal	Significance
Static compliance	$\dfrac{\text{Tidal volume}}{\text{Plateau pressure} - \text{PEEP}}$	50-100 ml/cm H_2O	Affected by changes in compliance of chest wall or lung
Dynamic compliance	$\dfrac{\text{Tidal volume}}{\text{Peak pressure} - \text{PEEP}}$	35-55 ml/cm H_2O	Affected by changes in compliance of chest wall or lung or airway resistance

    (2) Stimulated by decreased alveolar oxygen levels

  b) Generalized

    (1) If all alveoli have low oxygen levels as occurs with alveolar hypoventilation, hypoxemic pulmonary vasoconstriction may be distributed over the lungs

    (2) Increases pulmonary vascular resistance (PVR) and PAP

    (3) Right ventricular hypertrophy and failure (cor pulmonale) may result

C. Ventilation (V)/perfusion (Q) ratio

  1. Normal (Fig. 4-18): alveolar minute ventilation = 4 L; normal cardiac output (100% goes to lungs) = 5 L; normal V/Q ratio = 0.8

  2. Pathologic mismatch (Fig. 4-19)

    a) Deadspace: V greater than Q; V/Q ratio greater than 0.8

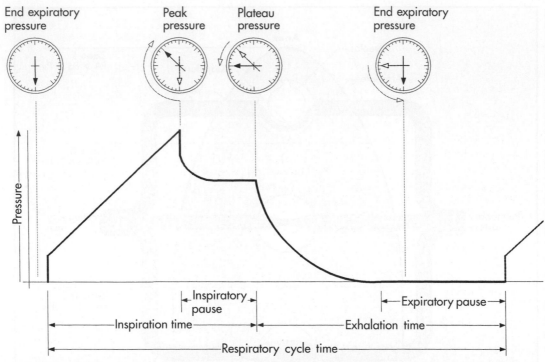

Figure 4-17 Airway pressure in a patient on positive pressure ventilation. Plateau pressure is used to calculate static compliance. Peak pressure is used to calculate dynamic compliance. The difference between static and dynamic compliance represents airway resistance. Remember that PEEP levels are subtracted from the plateau or peak pressures before calculation of compliance. (From Dupuis, YG: *Ventilators: theory and clinical application,* ed 2, St Louis, 1992, Mosby.)

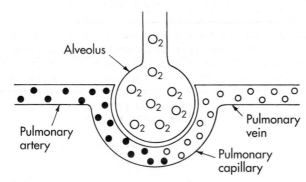

Figure 4-18 Normal ventilation/perfusion ratio. Normal alveolar ventilation per minute is approximately 4 L, and normal perfusion (cardiac output) is approximately 5 L/min; normal ventilation/perfusion ratio is 0.8. (From Kinney MR, Packa DR, Dunbar SB: *AACN's clinical reference for critical-care nursing,* ed 4, St Louis, 1998, Mosby.)

b) Shunt: Q greater than V; V/Q ratio less than 0.8
  (1) Pao_2 less than 60 mm Hg with an FIo_2 of 0.5 or greater suggests clinically significant shunt
  (2) There are several methods of estimating shunt (Table 4-3)
c) Silent: no V or Q
3. Positional mismatch (Fig. 4-20)
  a) Greatest ventilation in superior areas
  b) Greatest perfusion in inferior areas

  c) Rationale for "good lung down"; improve ventilation to the "bad lung" (e.g., atelectasis, pneumonia, pneumothorax, lobectomy) and optimize perfusion to the "good lung"
III. Distribution: movement of inspired air into lobes, segments, and lobules
  A. Transpulmonary pressure or distending pressure equals alveolar pressure minus pleural pressure
    1. Alveolar pressure is the pressure that reaches the alveoli after resistance has been overcome
    2. Pleural pressure is determined by gravity
  B. Closing volume is lung volume present when a significant number of small alveoli close
IV. Diffusion: movement of gases between the alveoli, plasma, and RBCs
  A. Gases diffuse from areas of higher concentration to areas of lower concentration regardless of medium until concentration is the same throughout the chamber
  B. Dalton's law of partial pressure (Fig. 4-21): In a mixture of gases, the pressure exerted by each gas is independent of the other gases and directly corresponds to the percentage of the total mixture that it represents
    1. Barometric pressure at sea level is 760 mm Hg
      a) Components and pressures in the atmosphere

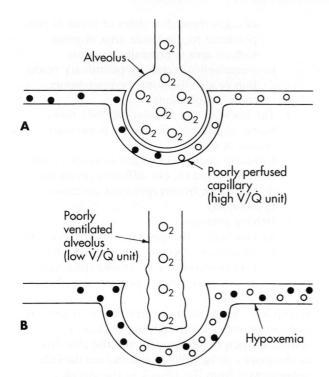

Figure 4-19 Abnormal ventilation/perfusion ratio. **A,** High V/Q ratio with ventilation exceeding perfusion; also called a *deadspace unit.* **B,** Low V/Q ratio with perfusion exceeding ventilation; also called a *shunt unit.* (From Kinney MR, Packa DR, Dunbar SB: *AACN's clinical reference for critical-care nursing,* ed 4, St Louis, 1998, Mosby.)

Table 4-3	Methods Of Estimating Intrapulmonary Shunt		
Parameter	**Formula**		**Normal**
a/A ratio	(Pao_2/PAo_2)		Normal >0.8 Moderate 0.5 to 0.8 Significant 0.25 to 0.5 Critical <0.25
A:a gradient	$PAo_2 - Pao_2$		<10 mm Hg A:a gradient × 0.05 = approximate % shunt
Pao_2/FIo_2 ratio	$\dfrac{Pao_2}{FIo_2}$		>300 300 = ~15% shunt 200 = ~20% shunt
Respiratory index	$\dfrac{PAo_2 - Pao_2}{Pao_2}$		<1.0
Clinical shunt	$\dfrac{CcO_2 - Cao_2}{CcO_2 - Cvo_2}$		3%-5%
Alternate clinical shunt equation	$\dfrac{(Hgb \times 1.34)(1 - Sao_2) + (0.003) Pao_2 - Pao_2}{(Hgb \times 1.34)(1 - Svo_2) + (0.003) Pao_2 - Pvo_2}$		3%-5%

Note: PAo_2 is calculated as: $FIo_2 (760 - 47) - (Paco_2/0.8)$
Key: *Pao₂,* arterial oxygen tension; *PAo₂,* alveolar oxygen tension; *C꜀o₂,* pulmonary capillary oxygen content; *Cₐo₂,* arterial oxygen content; *Cᵥo₂,* venous oxygen content; *FIo₂,* fraction of inspired oxygen (written as a decimal); *Pb,* barometric pressure (760 mm Hg at sea level, adjust for higher altitudes); *Paco₂,* arterial carbon dioxide tension
47 is the pressure of water vapor at sea level and is subtracted from barometric pressure
0.8 is the usual respiratory quotient

(1) Oxygen represents 21% of 760 mm Hg and exerts 158 mm Hg
(2) Nitrogen represents 78% of 760 mm Hg and exerts 596 mm Hg
(3) Carbon dioxide represents 0.5% of 760 mm Hg exerts 0.2 mm Hg

b) During inspiration the upper airway warms and humidifies atmospheric air, increasing the pressure of water vapor to 47 mm Hg; the partial pressures of the other gases must decrease because the total cannot exceed barometric

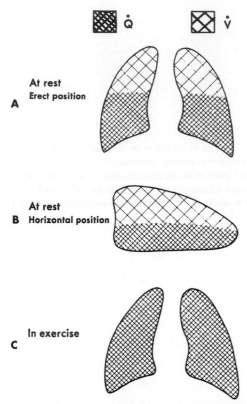

Figure 4-20 Positional changes in ventilation and perfusion. **A,** While sitting or standing, the upper lobes are ventilated best and the lower lobes are perfused best. **B,** While lying on one side, the superior lung is ventilated best and the inferior lung is perfused best. **C,** In exercise, ventilation and perfusion are increased and optimally matched throughout. (From Wade JF: *Comprehensive respiratory care,* St Louis, 1982, Mosby.)

pressure of 760 mm Hg; example: (760 [barometric pressure] −47 [pressure of water vapor at body temperature]) × 0.21 (FIo_2 of room air) = 150 mm Hg

    c) As the inspired gas mixes with gas that was not expired, the concentrations of CO_2 and O_2 change again

    d) Alveolar air is high in oxygen pressure and low in carbon dioxide pressure, and the pulmonary capillary blood is high in carbon dioxide pressure and low in oxygen pressure

    e) This differential in partial pressure of oxygen and carbon dioxide causes the gases to move across the alveolar-capillary membrane toward the lower side of the respective pressure gradients (e.g., oxygen moves from the alveolus to the capillary and carbon dioxide moves from the capillary to the alveolus)

C. Determinants of diffusion
  1. Surface area available for gas transfer
    a) Fick law of diffusion: the rate of transfer

of a gas through a sheet of tissue is proportional to the tissue area; alveolar surface area is normally immense
    b) Negatively affected by pulmonary resection (e.g., lobectomy or pneumonectomy, emphysema)
  2. Thickness of the alveolar-capillary membrane; negatively affected by pulmonary edema or fibrosis
  3. Diffusion coefficient of gas: CO_2 20 × more diffusible than O_2 (so diffusion problems do not cause hypercapnia but do cause hypoxemia)
  4. Driving pressure
    a) Fraction of the gas × barometric pressure
    b) Negatively affected by low inspired fraction of oxygen (e.g., smoke inhalation) or low barometric pressure (e.g., high altitudes)

V. Transport of gases in blood: movement of oxygen and carbon dioxide through the circulatory system; oxygen being moved from the alveolus to the tissues to be utilized and carbon dioxide being moved from the tissues to the alveolus for exhalation
A. Oxygen
  1. Mode of transport
    a) Hgb: 97% of oxygen is combined with hemoglobin; represented by the Sao_2
      (1) One molecule of hemoglobin can carry four molecules of oxygen
      (2) The amount of oxygen that the hemoglobin actually carries depends on the affinity of the hemoglobin for oxygen
      (3) There is normally more affinity at the lung level and less affinity at the tissue level
      (4) Ability of hemoglobin to deliver oxygen to the tissues is negatively affected by:
        (a) Anemia
        (b) Abnormal hemoglobin (e.g., methemoglobinemia, carboxyhemoglobin, or hemoglobin S [sickle cell])
    b) Plasma: 3% of oxygen is dissolved in the plasma; represented by the Pao_2
  2. Oxyhemoglobin dissociation curve: shows the relationship between Pao_2 and hemoglobin saturation (Fig. 4-22)
    a) Critical point: Pao_2 60 mm Hg
      (1) Pao_2 above 60: horizontal limb of curve; increase in Pao_2 above 60 mm Hg results in minimal increases in oxygen saturation
      (2) Pao_2 below 60: vertical limb of curve; decrease in Pao_2 below 60 mm Hg results in dramatic decreases in oxygen saturation

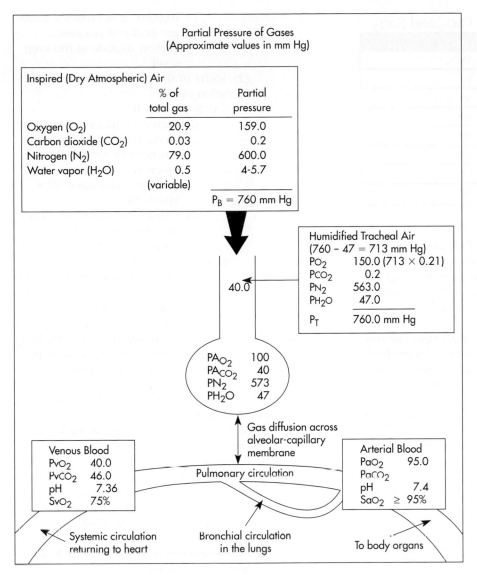

Figure 4-21   Dalton's law of partial pressure.

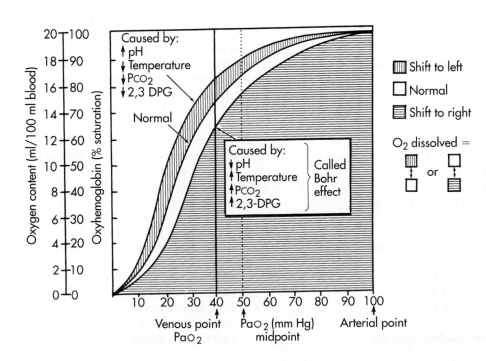

Figure 4-22   Oxyhemoglobin dissociation curve. Normal curve optimizes pickup of oxygen at the lung and dropoff of oxygen at the tissue level; left shift increases the affinity between oxygen and hemoglobin, which optimizes pickup of oxygen at the lung level but impairs dropoff of oxygen at the tissue level; right shift decreases affinity between oxygen and hemoglobin, which impairs pickup of oxygen at the lung level but optimizes dropoff of oxygen at the tissue level. (From Dettenmeier PA: *Pulmonary nursing care,* St Louis, 1992, Mosby.)

Table 4-4	Correlation Between Pao_2 and Sao_2	
Pao_2 (in mm Hg)	**Sao_2 (in %)**	
100	98	
90	97	
80	95	
70	93	
60	90	
50	85	
40	75	
30	57	

b) Correlation between Pao_2 and Sao_2 with a normal curve (see Table 4-4)
  (1) P_{50}: the partial pressure of oxygen at which hemoglobin is 50% saturated with a pH of 7.40; usually Pao_2 of 27 mm Hg
    (a) When the P_{50} decreases, affinity of hemoglobin and oxygen is increased; this relationship means that it is easier to pickup oxygen at the lung level but more difficult to dropoff oxygen at the tissue level
    (b) When the P_{50} increases, affinity of hemoglobin and oxygen is decreased; this relationship means that it is more difficult to pickup oxygen at the lung level but easier to dropoff oxygen at the tissue level
c) Affinity between hemoglobin and oxygen
  (1) Bohr effect: controls the reaction between hemoglobin and oxygen and carbon dioxide
    (a) Oxygenated hemoglobin is a stronger acid than deoxygenated hemoglobin
      (i) This change in pH facilitates the release of oxygen from the hemoglobin at the tissue level
      (ii) As the hemoglobin gives up the oxygen, it becomes a weaker acid and picks up carbon dioxide for transport back to the lung
    (b) Deoxygenated hemoglobin is a weaker acid than oxygenated hemoglobin
      (i) This change in pH facilitates the attraction of oxygen to the hemoglobin at the lung level
      (ii) As the hemoglobin picks up

oxygen, it becomes a stronger acid and releases carbon dioxide at the lung level
  (2) Shifts of the oxyhemoglobin dissociation curve
    (a) Shifts to left
      (i) Increases affinity of Hgb for oxygen; therefore, hemoglobin is more saturated for a given Pao_2 and less oxygen is unloaded for a given Pao_2
      (ii) Caused by alkalemia, hypothermia, hypocapnia, decreased 2,3-DPG
    (b) Shifts to right
      (i) Decreases affinity of Hgb for oxygen; therefore, hemoglobin is less saturated for a given Pao_2 and more oxygen is unloaded for a given Pao_2
      (ii) Caused by acidemia, hyperthermia, hypercapnia, increased 2,3-DPG
    (c) Discussion of 2,3-DPG (Box 4-1)
3. Oxygen capacity
  a) Maximal amount of oxygen the blood can carry
  b) Formula: $Hgb \times 1.34$
    (1) Hemoglobin in g/dl
    (2) 1.34 represents the amount of oxygen one gram of hemoglobin can carry; it is a constant
4. Oxygen content in arterial blood (Cao_2)
  a) Actual amount of oxygen that arterial blood is carrying
  b) O_2 capacity $\times$ O_2 saturation; amount of oxygen dissolved in the plasma ($.0031 \times Pao_2$) may be added but is such a minute factor in most situations that it is inconsequential unless the patient is hyperoxemic (e.g., hyperbarbic oxygen therapy)
  c) Formula: $Hgb \times 1.34 \times Sao_2$
    (1) Hemoglobin in g/dl
    (2) 1.34 represents the amount of oxygen one gram of hemoglobin can carry; it is a constant
    (3) Saturation as a decimal (e.g., 95% is 0.95)
  d) Normal: 18 to 20 ml/dl (~20 ml/dl)
5. Oxygen content in venous blood (Cvo_2)
  a) Actual amount of oxygen in venous blood
  b) Formula: $1.34 \times Hgb \times Svo_2$
    (1) Hemoglobin in g/dl
    (2) 1.34 represents the amount of oxygen 1 g of hemoglobin can carry; it is a constant

---

**4-1   Important Information About
2,3-Diphosphoglycerate (2,3-DPG)**

What is it?
- A substance in the erythrocyte that affects the affinity of hemoglobin for oxygen
- A chief end product of glucose metabolism and a link in the biochemical feedback control system that regulates the release of oxygen to the tissues

What does it do to the oxyhemoglobin dissociation curve?
- Increased amounts of 2,3-DPG shift the curve to the right
- Decreased amounts of 2,3-DPG shift the curve to the left

What causes amounts of 2,3-DPG to increase or decrease?
- Increased
  - Chronic hypoxemia (e.g., high altitude, congenital heart disease)
  - Anemia
  - Hyperthyroidism
  - Pyruvate kinase deficiency
- Decreased
  - Massive (~10 U) transfusion of banked blood
  - Hypophosphatemia
  - Hypothyroidism
  - Hexokinase deficiency

            (3) Saturation as a decimal (e.g., 95% is 0.95)
        c) Normal: 12 to 16 ml/dl (~15 ml/dl)
  B. CO_2: most transported as bicarbonate
      1. Carbonic acid and water in the presence of carbonic anhydrase form bicarbonate in the erythrocyte
      2. Five percent is dissolved in plasma ($Paco_2$)
      3. Five percent is combined with hemoglobin as carbaminohemoglobin; CO_2 attaches to hemoglobin at a different bonding site than oxygen
  C. Diffusion between systemic capillary bed and body tissues: pressure gradients allow diffusion
      1. Haldane effect: in the tissue, as O_2 leaves hemoglobin, increased CO_2 is able to be picked up by hemoglobin; in the lungs, the binding of oxygen with hemoglobin tends to displace CO_2
      2. Oxygen diffusion to peripheral tissues is affected by the following:
        a) Quantity and rate of blood flow
        b) Difference in capillary and tissue oxygen pressures
        c) Capillary surface area
        d) Capillary permeability
        e) Intracapillary distance
VI. Oxygen delivery to the tissue
  A. Oxygen delivery (DO_2): volume of oxygen delivered to the tissues each minute
      1. Product of cardiac output and arterial oxygen content
        a) Cardiac output is a product of HR and

stroke volume; stroke volume is affected by preload, afterload, and contractility
        b) Arterial oxygen content is a product of hemoglobin and arterial saturation
      2. Formula: $CO \times Hgb \times Sao_2 \times 13.4$
        a) Cardiac output in L/min
        b) Hemoglobin in g/dl
        c) Saturation as a decimal (e.g., 95% is 0.95)
      3. Normal DO_2: 900 to 1100 ml/min (~1000 ml/min)
      4. DO_2I: DO_2 divided by body surface area; considers body size
        a) Formula for DO_2I: $CI \times Hgb \times Sao_2 \times 13.4$
            (1) Cardiac index in L/min/m^2
            (2) Hemoglobin in g/dl
            (3) Saturation as a decimal (e.g., 95% is 0.95)
        b) Normal: 550 to 650 ml/min/m^2 (~600 ml/min/m^2)
  B. Oxygen consumption (VO_2): volume of oxygen consumed by the tissues each minute
      1. Determined by comparing the oxygen content in the arterial blood to the oxygen content in the mixed venous blood (e.g., drawn from the distal tip of the pulmonary artery catheter)
      2. Formula: $CO \times Hgb \times 13.4 \times (Sao_2 - Svo_2)$
      3. Normal VO_2: 200 to 300 ml/min (~250 ml/min)
      4. VO_2I: VO_2 divided by body surface area; considers body size
        a) Formula for VO_2I: $CI \times Hgb \times 13.4 \times (Sao_2 - Svo_2)$
        b) Normal: 110 to 160 ml/min/m^2 (~150 ml/min/m^2)
  C. Oxygen extraction ratio (O_2ER)
      1. Evaluation of the amount of oxygen that is extracted from the arterial blood as it passes through the capillaries; ratio of the difference between the content of oxygen in the arterial blood and the content of oxygen in venous blood to the content of oxygen in the arterial blood
      2. Formula: $Cao_2 - Cvo_2 \div Cao_2$
      3. Normal: 22% to 30% (~25%)
  D. Oxygen extraction index (O_2EI)
      1. Estimation of O_2ER calculated using only saturations
      2. Formula: $Sao_2 - Svo_2 \div Sao_2$
      3. Normal: 20% to 27% (~25%)
  E. Oxygen reserve in venous blood
      1. Determined by mixed venous oxygen saturation
      2. Normal: 60% to 80% (~75%)
      3. Note that normal Sao_2 is 99% and Svo_2 is 75% (the tissues used 25%); note that normal Cao_2 is 20 ml/dl and Cvo_2 is 15 ml/dl (the tissues used 25%); note that normal DO_2 is 1000 ml/min and VO_2 is

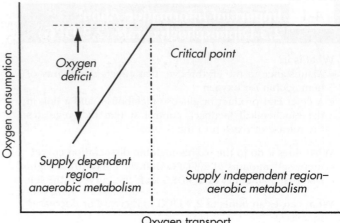

Figure 4-23   Critical oxygen delivery point. A critical level of oxygen delivery exists whereby oxygen delivery and consumption are interdependent of each other. Once this critical oxygen delivery point is exceeded, oxygen consumption becomes dependent on oxygen delivery. (From Dantzker and Scharf: *Cardiopulmonary critical care,* Philadelphia, 1998, Saunders.)

250 ml/min (the tissues used 25%); there is normally a 75% oxygen reserve

F. Critical oxygen delivery (DO_2) point (Fig. 4-23)
   1. A critical level of oxygen delivery exists where oxygen delivery and consumption are independent
   2. When the critical oxygen delivery point is exceeded, oxygen consumption depends on oxygen delivery
      a) If Svo_2 improves with increase in DO_2, oxygen delivery and consumption are independent
      b) If Svo_2 does not improve with increase in DO_2, oxygen consumption depends on oxygen delivery

VII. Cellular respiration: utilization of oxygen by the cell
   A. Estimated by the amount of carbon dioxide produced and the oxygen consumed
      1. Respiratory quotient (RQ): ratio of these two values
         a) Normally 0.8 but changes occur according to the nutritional substrate being utilized; primary carbohydrate metabolism changes the ratio to 1.0 because carbohydrate metabolism produces more carbon dioxide than does the metabolism of protein or fat
         b) Simplified Krebs cycle: food is converted by the body to H_2O and CO_2 and cellular energy (ATP)
      2. Variables affecting oxygen consumption
         a) Increased oxygen consumption
            (1) Increased work of breathing
            (2) Hyperthermia
            (3) Trauma
            (4) Sepsis
            (5) Anxiety
            (6) Hyperthyroidism
            (7) Muscle tremors or seizures
         b) Decreased oxygen consumption
            (1) Hypothermia
            (2) Sedation

            (3) Neuromuscular blockade
            (4) Anesthesia
            (5) Hypothyroidism
            (6) Inactivity
   B. Oxygen is utilized by the mitochondria in the production of cellular energy; oxygen deficit may result in lethal cell injury if prolonged

VIII. Metabolic functions of the lung
   A. Synthesis of interferon and tumor-inhibiting factor
   B. Production, conversion, or removal of many vasoactive substances in the pulmonary circulation; bradykinin, serotonin, heparin, histamine, prostaglandins E, F, and certain polypeptides

Pulmonary Assessment
Interview

I. Chief complaint: why the patient is seeking help and duration of the problem; possible symptoms related to pulmonary disorders, which may be identified as chief complaint, may include any of the following:
   A. Dyspnea or shortness of breath
      1. Onset
      2. Duration
      3. Frequency
      4. Timing: time of day, weather or season, activity, eating, talking, deep breathing
      5. Position (e.g., orthopnea)
      6. Severity
         a) Subjective scale
            (1) Grade 1: shortness of breath with mild exertion, such as running a short distance or climbing a flight of stairs
            (2) Grade 2: shortness of breath while walking a short distance at a normal pace on level grade
            (3) Grade 3: shortness of breath with mild daily activity such as shaving or bathing

(4) Grade 4: shortness of breath while sitting at rest

(5) Grade 5: shortness of breath while lying down

b) Effect on ability to do activities of daily living (ADL)

c) Frequently accentuated by anxiety

7. Palliation: what is effective in relieving dyspnea

8. Accompanying symptoms
   a) Cough
   b) Chest pain
   c) Wheezing

B. Cough
   1. Onset
   2. Duration
   3. Frequency
   4. Timing: time of day, weather or season, activity, eating, talking, deep breathing
   5. Position
   6. Pattern: regular or occasional
   7. Dry or productive
   8. Accompanying symptoms
      a) Sputum production
      b) Hemoptysis
      c) Chest pain
      d) Wheezing
      e) Dyspnea

C. Sputum production
   1. Duration
   2. Frequency
   3. Amount: use household measurements (e.g., teaspoons, tablespoons, shot glass, Dixie cup, iced tea glass)
   4. Color
   5. Consistency
   6. Odor
   7. Hemoptysis
   8. Usual treatment (e.g., expectorants, cough drops, a cigarette)

D. Hemoptysis
   1. May be related to tuberculosis, lung cancer, bronchiectasis, pneumonia, pulmonary embolism
   2. Character
      a) Grossly bloody
      b) Blood-tinged
      c) Blood-streaked
      d) Hematest positive
   3. Hemoptysis: frothy, alkaline, accompanied by sputum (hematemesis is nonfrothy, acidic, dark red or brown, accompanied by food particles)

E. Chest pain: (information regarding Differentiation of Chest Pain is located in Table 2-4)
   1. P
      a) Provocation: pulmonary pain is frequently provoked by trauma, coughing, deep breathing, or movement
      b) Palliation: pulmonary pain may be relieved by sitting upright or by narcotics

2. Q
   a) Quality: pulmonary pain is most frequently sharp and increased by coughing, inspiration, movement
3. R
   a) Region: pulmonary pain is usually located at lateral chest
   b) Radiation: pulmonary pain may radiate to shoulder, neck
4. S
   a) Severity: pulmonary pain is usually moderate but may be severe
5. T
   a) Timing
      (1) Onset: pulmonary pain onset is usually gradual
      (2) Duration: pulmonary pain duration is usually days to weeks

F. Wheezing
   1. Onset
   2. Duration
   3. Timing: time of day, weather or season, activity, eating, talking, deep breathing, position
   4. Identified triggers (e.g., dust, pollen, propellants)
   5. Usual treatment

G. Nasal or sinus problems
   1. Epistaxis
   2. Nasal stuffiness
   3. Postnasal drip
   4. Sinus pain

H. Hoarseness: may be related to cancer of larynx

I. Ascites: may be related to cor pulmonale

J. Abdominal pain: may be related to cor pulmonale

K. Edema or weight gain: may be related to cor pulmonale

L. Fatigue or weakness: may be related to cor pulmonale

M. Fever: may be related to pulmonary infections

N. Night sweats: may be related to tuberculosis

O. Anorexia: may be related to cor pulmonale, dyspnea, or drug side effects (e.g., xanthine bronchodilators)

P. Weight loss: may be related to dyspnea, fatigue (preventing food preparation), or hypermetabolism

Q. Sleep disturbances: may be related to dyspnea or coughing

II. History of present illness
   A. PQRST
   B. Associated symptoms

III. Past medical history
   A. Childhood diseases
      1. Frequent respiratory infections
      2. Allergies
      3. Asthma
      4. Scarlet fever
   B. Past illnesses
      1. Recurrent respiratory infections

2. Pneumonia
3. Cystic fibrosis
4. Asthma
5. Chronic obstructive pulmonary disease
   a) Chronic bronchitis
   b) Emphysema
6. Tuberculosis
7. Lung cancer
8. Pulmonary fibrosis: frequently related to occupational lung disease
   a) Pneumoconiosis (coal worker's lung disease)
   b) Asbestosis
   c) Silicosis
9. Fungal disease (e.g., histoplasmosis)
10. Pulmonary embolism
11. Pneumothorax
12. Granulomatous diseases (e.g., sarcoidosis)
13. Connective tissue disorders (e.g., lupus, scleroderma)
14. Immunosuppression
15. Cor pulmonale: right ventricular hypertrophy and/or failure as a result of pulmonary disease

C. Past injury: chest trauma
D. Past surgical procedures: thoracotomy
E. Allergies and type of reaction
F. Past diagnostic studies
   1. Allergy testing
   2. Tuberculin and/or fungal skin tests
   3. Chest X-ray
   4. Pulmonary function studies
   5. Bronchoscopy
   6. Laryngoscopy

IV. Family history
A. Asthma
B. Emphysema: particularly alpha$_1$-antitrypsin deficiency-related emphysema
C. Tuberculosis
D. Cystic fibrosis
E. Cancer

V. Social history
A. Work environment
   1. Occupation
   2. Environmental hazards: chemicals, vapors, dust, pulmonary irritants, allergens
   3. Use of protective devices
B. Home environment
   1. Allergens: pets, plants, trees, molds, dust mites
   2. Type of heating
   3. Use of air conditioner and/or humidifier
C. Recreational habits: exposure to inhalants and allergens
D. Exercise habits
E. Tobacco use: present and past
   1. Type of tobacco
   2. Duration and amount
      a) Cigarettes: record as pack-years (number of packs per day times the number of years the patient has been smoking)
      b) Chewing or rubbing tobacco: type and amount per day
      c) Marijuana: joints per day
   3. Efforts to quit: previous and current desire to quit
   4. Second-hand smoke exposure
F. Fluid consumption
   1. Volume of water/day
   2. Caffeine-containing beverages
   3. Alcohol-containing beverages: alcoholic beverages/day or week
G. Eating habits
   1. Quality and quantity of meals
   2. Number of meals/day
   3. Pulmonary symptoms during meals: dyspnea, cough, wheezing

VI. Medication history
A. Prescribed drug, dosage, frequency, time of last dose
B. Nonprescribed drugs
   1. Over-the-counter drugs, including herbs
   2. Substance abuse
C. Patient understanding of drug actions, side effects; knowledge of how to use and clean inhaler if prescribed

Landmarks (see Fig. 2-25)

I. Anatomic
A. Clavicle
B. Sternum
C. Ribs
D. Intercostal spaces
E. Angle of Louis: sternal angle between manubrium and body of sternum
F. Xiphoid process
G. Costal margin
H. Costal angle

II. Imaginary
A. Midsternal line
B. Midclavicular line (MCL)
C. Anterior axillary line (AAL)
D. Midaxillary line (MAL)
E. Posterior axillary line (PAL)
F. Scapular line
G. Midspinal line

III. Location of lungs (Fig. 4-24)
A. The apex of the lungs extends 2 to 4 cm above the inner third of the clavicle
B. The inferior border anteriorly is at the sixth rib at the MCL and at the eighth rib at the MAL, posteriorly at T10 on expiration and at T12 with deep inspiration
C. Fissure dividing upper and lower lobes is at T3 posteriorly
D. Upper lobes primarily anterior; lower lobes primarily posterior
E. Trachea bifurcates at the Angle of Louis anteriorly or T4 posteriorly

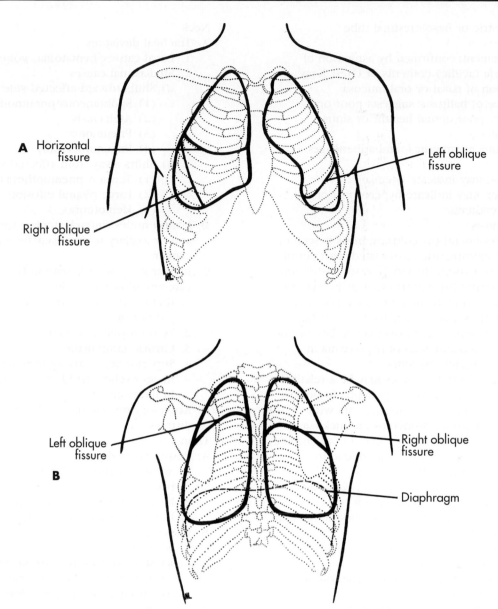

Figure 4-24   Location of the lungs. **A,** Anterior. **B,** Posterior. (From Wilkins RL, Sheldon RL, Krider SJ: *Clinical assessment in respiratory care,* St Louis, 1994, Mosby.)

Inspection and Palpation

I. Vital signs
  A. BP
  B. HR
  C. Respiratory (ventilatory) rate
  D. Temperature
  E. Height
  F. Weight
II. General survey
  A. Apparent health status: compare apparent age relative to chronologic age
  B. Level of consciousness: note restlessness and/or confusion (frequently the first sign of hypoxia)
  C. Increased work of breathing: note use of accessory muscles
  D. Speech pattern: note pausing midsentence to take a breath

  E. Presence of injury, abrasion, deformity
  F. Nutritional status
  G. Stature/posture
III. Mouth or nose
  A. Pursed-lip breathing: may be instinctive, or the patient may have been taught to use this technique during times of dyspnea
  B. Artificial airway
    1. Type
    2. Size
    3. Placement (e.g., cm mark at teeth for oral endotracheal tube)
    4. Cuff pressure (measured with a cuff pressure gauge or sphygmomanometer with three-way stopcock)
  C. Oxygen therapy: administration device and flow rate or FIo_2

D. Nasogastric or nasointestinal tube
  1. Size
  2. Placement: confirmed by aspiration of gastric (acidic) contents or chest X-ray
E. Condition of nasal or oral mucosa
F. Presence of halitosis: suggests poor oral hygiene, poor dental health, or sinus infection

IV. Skin, mucous membranes, and appendages
  A. Color
    1. Pallor: may indicate anemia
    2. Rubor: may indicate hypercapnia or polycythemia
    3. Cyanosis
       a) Peripheral (or cold) cyanosis is seen on fingertips, toes; associated with peripheral hypoperfusion or vasoconstriction
       b) Central (or warm) cyanosis is seen on lips, mucous membranes; associated with 5 g deoxygenated hemoglobin
          (1) Central cyanosis may be late or impossible sign of hypoxemia in anemic patients
          (2) Central cyanosis may be a relatively early sign of hypoxemia in polycythemic patients; patients with chronic bronchitis are nicknamed "blue bloaters"; blue due to chronic cyanosis and bloaters due to chronic RVF
       c) In dark-skinned patients, cyanosis appears as an ashen color
    4. Cherry-red: may indicate carbon monoxide intoxication
    5. Tobacco stains on fingertips
  B. Scars: especially thoracic
  C. Petechiae: may indicate any of the following:
    1. Fat embolism
    2. Blood dyscrasias affecting platelets
       a) Disseminated intravascular coagulation (DIC)
       b) Platelet aggregation inhibitors (e.g., ASA)
    3. Cirrhosis
  D. Edema: may be associated with cor pulmonale
  E. Nailbeds
    1. Color: note cyanosis
    2. Clubbing
       a) Indicates chronic decrease in oxygen supply to body tissues
          (1) Especially indicative of restrictive lung diseases (e.g., pulmonary fibrosis, lung cancer)
          (2) Also indicative of right-to-left cardiac shunting (e.g., cyanotic heart disease)
          (3) May be seen in late obstructive lung disease
       b) Normal angle between nailbed and nail less than 180 degrees
       c) Early clubbing: angle = 180 degrees
       d) Late clubbing: angle >180 degrees

V. Neck
  A. Tracheal deviation
    1. Local causes: hematoma, goiter
    2. Mediastinal causes
       a) Shifts toward affected side
          (1) Spontaneous pneumothorax
          (2) Atelectasis
          (3) Pneumonia
          (4) Pneumonectomy
       b) Shifts away from affected side
          (1) Tension pneumothorax
          (2) Large pleural effusion
          (3) Hemothorax
  B. Lymph nodes (infraclavicular, supraclavicular, and/or axillary nodes): may be enlarged in lung cancer
  C. Jugular neck vein distention (JVD): may indicate any of the following:
    1. Right ventricular failure (e.g., cor pulmonale)
    2. Tension pneumothorax
    3. Cardiac tamponade
    4. Superior vena cava syndrome: edema of neck, eyelids, hands also seen; may occur in lung cancer
  D. Accessory muscle use: indicates respiratory distress

VI. Thorax
  A. Posture: tripod position
    1. Sitting up and leaning forward (e.g., over bedside table)
    2. Position for optimal ventilation
    3. Indicates respiratory distress
  B. Contour
    1. Normal
       a) Slope of ribs: ribs are normally at 45 degree angle to vertebrae
       b) Costal angle: normally less than 90 degrees
       c) Anterior-posterior diameter: normally one half of lateral diameter; ratio of anterior-posterior to lateral diameter 1:2
       d) Symmetrical
    2. Abnormalities
       a) Pectus excavatum (funnel chest)
          (1) Sternum pushed inward
          (2) May cause hypoventilation, restrictive lung disease
       b) Pectus carinatum (pigeon chest)
          (1) Sternum pushed outward
          (2) May cause hypoventilation, restrictive lung disease
       c) Scoliosis
          (1) S curvature to spine
          (2) May cause hypoventilation, restrictive lung disease
       d) Kyphosis (hunchback)
          (1) Frequently occurs with aging due to osteoporosis
          (2) May cause hypoventilation, restrictive lung disease

e) Increased A-P diameter: indicates obstructive pulmonary disease

C. Intercostal spaces
1. Retraction of interspaces during inspiration
   a) Tracheal obstruction
   b) Asthma
2. Bulging of interspaces during expiration
   a) Asthma
   b) Tension pneumothorax
   c) Pleural effusion

D. Chest movement
1. Impaired movement
   a) Thoracic pain with splinting
   b) Restrictive lung disease
2. Unequal expansion
   a) Massive unilateral atelectasis
   b) Massive pleural effusion
   c) Pneumonia
   d) Pneumothorax
   e) Pulmonary resection: lobectomy, pneumonectomy
   f) Right mainstem intubation (no movement on left)
   g) Flail chest
3. Respiratory excursion: normally 3 to 6 cm during normal breathing

E. Respiratory rate, rhythm, quality
1. Rate and rhythm (Table 4-5)
2. Type
   a) Abdominal: males or supine females
   b) Thoracic or costal: upright females
3. Inspiration to expiration (I:E) ratio
   a) Normally 1:2 with expiration lasting twice as long as inspiration
   b) Obstructive lung diseases cause prolonged expiratory time with ratios 1:3 or greater

F. Chest wall
1. Point of maximal impulse
   a) Normally palpated at fifth LICS at MCL
   b) Frequently shifted medially in patients with chronic lung disease and pulmonary hypertension due to right ventricular hypertrophy
   c) May be shifted in either direction with mediastinal shift depending on side and type of condition
2. Heave: right ventricular heave may be felt at the sternum or in epigastric area due to right ventricular hypertrophy and/or failure
3. Tenderness: may be caused by any of the following:
   a) Fracture
   b) Tumor
   c) Costochondritis
4. Fremitus
   a) Vocal fremitus
      (1) Evaluated by asking the patient to say "99" while the patient's thorax is palpated with the ball of the examiner's hand

(2) Decreased vocal fremitus
   (a) Thick chest wall
   (b) Bronchial obstruction
   (c) Pleural effusion
   (d) Pleural thickening
   (e) Pneumothorax
   (f) Emphysema
(3) Increased vocal fremitus
   (a) Over large airways
   (b) Pneumonia
   (c) Tumor
   (d) Pulmonary fibrosis
   (e) Pulmonary infarction
   b) Pleural friction fremitus: grating sensation that occurs with pleural inflammation
   c) Rhonchal fremitus: vibration felt with movement of secretions through the tracheobronchial tree
5. Subcutaneous emphysema (air in subcutaneous tissue)
   a) Assess for subcutaneous emphysema around tracheostomy, chest tube, or stab wound
   b) Assess for subcutaneous emphysema after bronchoscopy
6. Chest tubes (Table 5-1 in Chest Surgery and Chest Tubes section)
7. Central venous catheters
   a) Location
   b) Patency
   c) Rate and type of solutions
8. Wounds

VII. Abdomen
A. Liver
1. May be palpable in patients with normal liver but hyperinflated lungs as liver is pushed downward
2. May be enlarged and tender due to cor pulmonale
B. Abdominal muscles (accessory muscles of expiration): frequently used by patients with obstructive lung disease to help push the air out of the lungs

VIII. Mechanical ventilator parameters
A. Mode (e.g., control, assist-control, intermittent mandatory ventilation, etc.)
B. Tidal volume
C. Rate
D. FIO_2
E. PEEP
F. Peak inspiratory pressure and calculated dynamic compliance
G. Plateau pressure and calculated static compliance

IX. Clinical indications of respiratory distress (Box 4-2)

X. Clinical indications of hypoxemia/hypoxia
A. Hypoxemia (decreased oxygen in the blood): noted by PaO_2 less than 80 mm Hg and SaO_2 less than 95% on ABGs or SpO_2 less than 95%

Table 4-5	Respiratory Rhythms	
Rhythm	**Description**	**Possible Causes**
Eupnea	Rate 12-20/min and normal depth of ventilation; regular with occasional sigh	• Normal
Bradypnea	Slow (<10/min), regular ventilation	• Depression of respiratory center with opium, alcohol, or tumor • Sleep • Increased intracranial pressure • CO_2 narcosis • Metabolic alkalosis
Tachypnea	Rapid (>30/min) ventilation; depth may be normal or decreased	• Restrictive lung disease • Pneumonia • Pleurisy • Chest pain • Fear • Anxiety • Respiratory insufficiency
Hypopnea	Shallow ventilation, normal rate	• Deep sleep • Heart failure • Shock • Meningitis • Central nervous system depression • Coma
Hyperpnea	Deep ventilation; rate may be normal or increased	• Exercise • Hypoxia • Fever • Hepatic coma • Midbrain or pons lesions • Acid-base imbalance • Salicylate overdosage
Cheyne-Stokes	Increasing and decreasing rate and depth of ventilation followed by apnea lasting 20-60 seconds	• Intracranial hypertension • Heart failure • Renal failure • Meningitis • Cerebral hemisphere damage • Drug overdosage
Kussmaul	Deep, gasping, rapid (usually >35/min) ventilation	• Metabolic acidosis (e.g., diabetic ketoacidosis, renal failure) • Peritonitis
Apneustic	Prolonged gasping inspiration followed by short inefficient expiration	• Lesion of pons
Cluster	Periods of apnea alternating with a series of breaths of equal depth; breathing may be slow and deep or rapid and shallow	• Meningitis • Encephalitis • Lesion of lower pons, upper medulla • Intracranial hypertension
Ataxic	Lack of any pattern to ventilation	• Brainstem lesion
Obstructive	I:E ratio of 1:4 or greater	• Asthma • Emphysema • Chronic bronchitis
Apnea	Cessation of ventilation for longer than 15 seconds	• Central nervous system damage • Sleep

B. Hypoxia (decreased oxygen in the tissues): noted by clinical indications of hypoxia (Box 4-3) and increased serum lactate level

XI. Clinical indications of hypercapnia (increased CO_2 in the blood): noted by increased $Paco_2$ on ABGs and clinical indications of hypercapnia (Box 4-4)

Percussion

I. Description of percussion tones (Table 4-6)

II. Thorax

   A. Percussion tones normally heard

      1. Lung: resonant

      2. Diaphragm: flat

      3. Heart: dull

<table>
<tr><td>

> **BOX**
>
> ## 4-2   Clinical Indications of Respiratory Distress
>
> Pursed lip breathing
> Tripod positioning
> Intercostal retractions
> Use of accessory muscles
> Speaking only one or two words between breaths
> Cough

</td></tr>
</table>

> **BOX**
>
> ## 4-3   Clinical Indications of Hypoxia
>
> Restlessness → Confusion → Lethargy → Coma
> Tachycardia → Dysrhythmias
> Tachypnea
> Use of accessory muscles
> Mild hypertension (early) → hypotension (late)
> Cyanosis may be present (depending on hemoglobin level)

> **BOX**
>
> ## 4-4   Clinical Indications of Hypercapnia
>
> Tachycardia → dysrhythmias
> Hypotension
> Bradypnea
> Headache
> Facial rubor (plethora)
> Irritability
> Confusion
> Inability to concentration → somnolence → coma

B. Abnormal percussion tones over thorax
  1. Hyperresonant: asthma, emphysema, pneumothorax
  2. Dull: atelectasis, pneumonia, tumor
  3. Flat: pleural effusion
C. Diaphragmatic excursion
  1. Evaluated by percussing the position of the diaphragm at expiration and then during full inspiration
  2. Normal diaphragmatic excursion is 3 to 5 cm
  3. May be decreased by:
    a) Increased intrathoracic volume: emphysema
    b) Increased intraabdominal volume and pressure as might occur with any of the following:
      (1) Ascites
      (2) Hepatomegaly
      (3) Pregnancy
      (4) Gaseous abdominal distention
    c) Decreased chest excursion and tidal volume: thoracic or abdominal pain
    d) Phrenic nerve injury
III. Abdomen
  A. Liver
    1. Normal liver span in the right MCL is 6 to 12 cm
  2. Hepatomegaly (liver span greater than 12 cm in right MCL) may be seen in cor pulmonale
    a) Assessment by percussion is necessary before specifying hepatomegaly since patients with hyperinflated lungs may have a palpable normal liver

Auscultation
I. Method of lung auscultation
  A. Use diaphragm
  B. Ask patient to take deep breaths through his or her mouth
  C. Listen to at least one full breath at each location
  D. Compare symmetrical areas
II. Breath sounds
  A. Intensity
    1. Increased
      a) Hyperventilation
      b) Anything that decreases the distance between the lung and your stethoscope (e.g., thin chest wall)
    2. Decreased
      a) Hypoventilation
        (1) Emphysema
        (2) Thoracic pain
        (3) Atelectasis
        (4) Pulmonary fibrosis
      b) Anything that increases the distance between the lung and your stethoscope
        (1) Muscular or obese chest
        (2) Pneumothorax (may be diminished or absent)
        (3) Hemothorax (may be diminished or absent)
        (4) Pleural effusion
    3. Absent
      a) Severe bronchospasm
      b) Massive atelectasis
      c) Pneumonectomy
      d) Pneumothorax
      e) Hemothorax
      f) Malpositioned endotracheal tube (absent breath sounds over left lung)
  B. Quality
    1. Descriptions and normal locations (Fig. 4-25 and Table 4-7)
    2. Implications
      a) Bronchial in areas other than normal location: consolidation (e.g., atelectasis, pneumonia, tumor)
      b) Bronchovesicular in areas other than normal location: partial consolidation, partial aeration
  C. Adventitious sounds (Table 4-8): pathologic extra sounds that may be heard at points in the ventilatory cycle or throughout the ventilatory cycle
  D. Voice sounds: abnormal and indicative of consolidation
    1. Bronchophony: increase in clarity of voice sounds
      a) Ask patient to say "99"

Table 4-6 **Percussion Tones**

Tone	Intensity	Pitch	Duration	Quality	Normal Location
Tympany	Loud	High	Medium	Drumlike	Stomach, bowel
Hyperresonance	Loud	Low	Long	Booming	Hyperinflated lungs
Resonance	Medium	Low	Long	Hollow	Normal lung
Dullness	Soft	High	Medium	Thudlike	Liver, spleen, heart
Flatness	Soft	High	Short	Extreme dullness	Muscle, bone

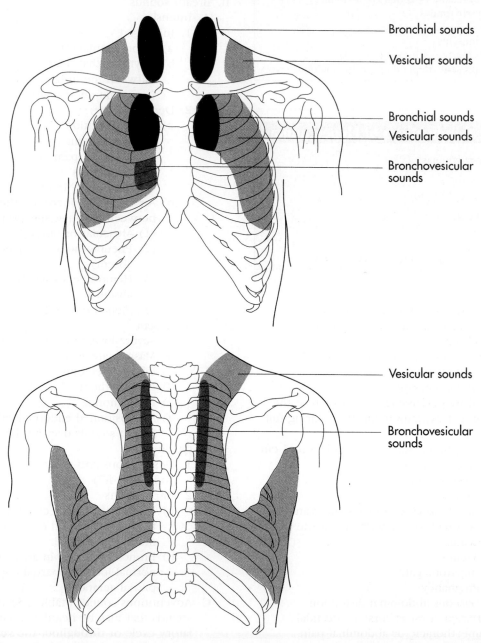

Figure 4-25 Quality of breath sounds: normal locations. (From Barkauskas VH et al: *Health and physical assessment,* St Louis, 1994, Mosby.)

Table 4-7	Breath Sounds: Quality				
Quality	I:E Ratio	Intensity	Pitch	Quality	Normal Location
Bronchial	I < E	Loud	High	Hollow	Trachea
Bronchovesicular	I = E	Medium	Medium	Breezy	Mainstem bronchi
Vesicular	I > E	Soft	Low	Swishy	Peripheral lung

Table 4-8	Breath Sounds: Adventitious Sounds			
Sound	Alternative Terms	Phase	Description	Cause

Stridor	Croupy	Inspiratory	High-pitched whistle audible without a stethoscope	• Upper airway obstruction
				  • Epiglottis
				  • Foreign body
				  • Laryngospasm
				  • Laryngeal edema

Crackles	Rales	Inspiratory	Discontinuous crackling sound; similar to rubbing hair between fingers	• Pulmonary edema • Atelectasis • Pulmonary fibrosis
Rhonchi	Gurgles; sonorous rhonchi	Expiratory	Continuous gurgling sound	• Fluid or mucus in airways

Wheezes	Whistles; sibilant rhonchi	Inspiratory or expiratory	High-pitched whistling sound	• Decrease in airway lumen
				  • Bronchospasm
				  • Mucus plug
				  • Tumor

Pleural Friction Rub		Inspiratory and expiratory	Grating or scratching sound	• Pulmonary infarction • Pleurisy • Tuberculosis • Lung cancer

   b) Voice sounds are normally muffled
   c) If voice sounds are clear over a particular area, bronchophony is present
2. Egophony: "e" to "a" conversion of voice sounds
   a) Ask patient to say "e"
   b) Muffled "e" should be heard over normal lung
   c) If "a" is heard over a particular area, egophony is present
3. Whispered pectoriloquy: increase in clarity of whispered sounds
   a) Ask the patient to whisper "99"
   b) Whispered sounds are normally muffled
   c) If whispered sounds are clear over a particular area, whispered pectoriloquy is present

Bedside Assessment of Pulmonary Function

I. Bedside parameters (also referred to as *ventilatory mechanics*)
   A. Spirometry: measured with Wright respirometer
      1. Tidal volume
         a) Amount of air moved in and out each breath
         b) Normal: 5 to 7 ml/kg

         c) Tidal volume less than 5 ml/kg indicates need for artificial airway and/or mechanical ventilation; tidal volume greater than 5 ml/kg indicates that the patient can be weaned and/or extubated
      2. Vital capacity
         a) Maximal amount of air that can be exhaled after a maximal inspiration
         b) Normal: 10 to 15 ml/kg
         c) Vital capacity less than 10 ml/kg indicates need for artificial airway and/or mechanical ventilation; vital capacity greater than 10 ml/kg indicates that the patient can be weaned and/or extubated
      3. Minute ventilation
         a) Tidal volume × ventilatory frequency
         b) Normal: 5 to 10 L/min
      4. Maximal voluntary ventilation (MVV)
         a) Volume of air moved into and out of the lungs with maximal effort over a short period (usually 10-15 seconds)
         b) Normal is 170 L/min (**Note:** one quarter this total is actually measured in the 15-second period; patients are not asked to ventilate at this intensity for an entire minute)
         c) Reflects the status of the ventilatory

muscles, compliance of the lung and thorax, and airway resistance; may provide a quick assessment of the patient's ventilatory reserve prior to surgery

B. Maximal inspiratory pressure (MIP): measured with negative inspiratory pressure meter
1. Also referred to as *negative inspiratory force* (NIF)
2. Normal is greater than (more negative than) −60 to 80 cm H_2O
3. MIP of less than −25 cm H_2O indicates need for artificial airway and/or mechanical ventilation; MIP of greater than −25 cm H_2O indicates that the patient can be weaned and/or extubated

II. Capnography
A. Continuous noninvasive method for evaluating the adequacy of CO_2 exchange in the lungs
1. Measurement of expired carbon dioxide tension
2. Display of the carbon dioxide waveform from breath to breath
B. Indications
1. Verification of tracheal intubation
a) Esophageal intubation is reflected by decreased $P_{et}CO_2$ or an abnormal waveform
b) Inexpensive, disposable, colorimetric CO_2 indicators are frequently used for this purpose; they do not display waveform
2. Verification of adequacy of chest compression during CPR
a) In the absence of pulmonary blood flow, $P_{et}CO_2$ decreases rapidly because no CO_2 is being returned to the lungs
b) $P_{et}CO_2$ is decreased when chest compressions are inadequate and $P_{et}CO_2$ increases when effectiveness of compression is increased
3. Evaluation of ventilation and $PaCO_2$
a) This use is limited in critically ill patients since the relationship between $PaCO_2$ and $P_{et}CO_2$ is affected by changes in pulmonary dead space and perfusion
b) $PaCO_2 − P_{et}CO_2$ gradient may be used as an indication of changes in pulmonary deadspace
C. Description
1. The CO_2 in the expired air is measured; the end tidal ($P_{et}CO_2$) is assumed to represent alveolar gas and may be used to estimate the $PaCO_2$; since this relationship is dependent on the ventilation-perfusion ratios throughout the lung, this assumption may be particularly erroneous in critically ill patients
D. Normal value: the $P_{et}CO_2$ is usually 1 to 4 mm Hg below the $PaCO_2$
1. Increased $P_{et}CO_2$ assumes hypoventilation
2. Decreased $P_{et}CO_2$ assumes hyperventilation
E. Implication: changes in $P_{et}CO_2$ indicates that the patient requires prompt assessment and arterial blood gases for analysis

III. Pulse oximetry (SpO_2)
A. Continuous noninvasive method of monitoring arterial oxygen saturation
B. Indications
1. Recovery from anesthesia
2. Assessment of adequacy of oxygenation (does not adequately evaluate ventilation since $PaCO_2$ increases with hypoventilation but PaO_2 and SaO_2 do not decrease until much later)
C. Description
1. Sensor with light source is placed on the fingertip, toe, bridge of nose, forehead, or earlobe
2. The amount of arterial hemoglobin that is saturated with oxygen is determined by beams of light passed through the tissue
D. Normal value: greater than 95%; moderate to severe hypoxemia should be suspected if less than 90%; causes of decreased SpO_2 include the following:
1. Decrease in SaO_2 and PaO_2
2. Decrease in cardiac output
E. Limitations
1. Inadequate pulsations may result from the following:
a) Significant hypotension
b) Vasopressor use
c) Severe hypothermia
d) Arterial compression
2. Tends to overestimate SaO_2 by 2% to 5%; accuracy of SpO_2 below 70% is questionable; the lower the SaO_2, the larger the difference between it and the SpO_2
3. Does not accurately reflect oxygen tissue delivery in patients with anemia
4. Abnormal hemoglobins
a) Carboxyhemoglobin
(1) Results in false high oxygen saturation reading (hemoglobin is saturated but with carbon monoxide)
(2) Smokers may have elevated carboxyhemoglobin levels
b) Methemoglobin
(1) Results in true low oxygen saturation reading
(2) Methemoglobin is a form of hemoglobin that cannot carry oxygen
(3) May be related to the administration of nitrates, nitrites, sulfonamides, local anesthetics
5. Intravenous dyes: result in inaccurate oxygen saturation readings
6. Increased bilirubin (greater than 20 mg%): results in inaccurately low readings
7. Ambient light: may affect accuracy
8. Edema: may result in inaccurately low readings
9. Nail polish: blue, green, gold, black, or brown nail polish needs to be removed
F. Implication: changes in SpO_2 indicate that the

patient requires prompt assessment and arterial blood gases for analysis

IV. Transcutaneous Pao_2 ($P_{tc}O_2$) monitoring
   A. Continuous noninvasive method of monitoring Pao_2
   B. Indications: as for pulse oximetry
   C. Description
      1. Sensor is placed on the skin; electrode has a heating element to warm skin and cause capillaries to dilate and increase blood flow
   D. Normal value: greater than 80 mm Hg; moderate to severe hypoxemia should be suspected if less than 60 mm Hg
   E. Limitations
      1. Affected by skin blood flow, thickness, temperature, skin oxygen consumption, subcutaneous emphysema, edema
      2. Tends to underestimate Pao_2
      3. Less reliable in adults than in infants
   F. Implications
      1. Pao_2 will always be equal to or greater than $P_{tc}O_2$
      2. Changes in $P_{tc}O_2$ indicate that the patient requires prompt assessment and arterial blood gases for analysis

V. Mixed venous oxygen saturation (Svo_2)
   A. Oxygen saturation of the blood as it returns to the lung for reoxygenation; reflects how well the body's demand for oxygen is met by the amount of oxygen supplied
   B. Normal Svo_2: 60% to 80%
   C. Complete discussion of Svo_2 monitoring in Hemodynamic Monitoring section of Chapter 2

Diagnostic Studies

I. Serum chemistries
   A. Sodium: normal 136 to 145 mEq/L
   B. Potassium: normal 3.5 to 5.0 mEq/L
   C. Chloride: normal 96 to 106 mEq/L
   D. Calcium: normal 8.5 to 10.5 mg/dl
   E. Phosphorus: normal 3.0 to 4.5 mg/dl
   F. Magnesium: normal 1.5 to 2.5 mEq/L or 1.8 to 2.4 mg/dl
   G. Glucose: normal 70 to 110 mg/dl
   H. BUN: normal 5 to 20 mg/dl
   I. Creatinine: normal 0.7 to 1.5 mg/dl
   J. Lactate: 1 to 2 mmol/L

II. Arterial blood gases
   A. pH: normal 7.35 to 7.45
   B. $Paco_2$: normal 35 to 45 mm Hg
   C. HCO_3^-: normal 22 to 26 mEq/L
   D. Pao_2: normal 80 to 100 mm Hg
   E. Sao_2: greater than 95%

III. Hematology
   A. Hematocrit: normal 40% to 52% for males; 35% to 47% for females
   B. Hemoglobin: normal 13 to 18 g/dl for males; 12 to 16 g/dl for females
   C. White blood cells (WBC): normal 3,500 to 11,000 mm^3

D. D-dimer: normal negative

IV. Sputum analysis: may be obtained by morning specimen by cough, induced tracheobronchial aspiration, transtracheal aspiration, or bronchoscopy
   A. Characteristics: color, odor, viscosity, presence of blood
   B. Culture and sensitivity tests: identifies infecting organism and effective antibiotic agent
   C. Gram stain: differentiates between gram-negative or gram-positive bacteria
   D. Acid-fast stain: determines presence of acid-fast bacilli (tuberculosis)
   E. Cytology studies: determines presence of malignant cells

V. Pleural fluid analysis
   A. Total protein: differentiates between exudative pleural effusion and transudative pleural effusion
   B. Gram stain: differentiates between gram-negative or gram-positive bacteria
   C. Acid-fast stain: determines presence of acid-fast bacilli (tuberculosis)
   D. Cytology studies: determines presence of malignant cells

VI. Skin tests
   A. Type I hypersensitivity tests ("allergy tests")
   B. Type II hypersensitivity tests: purified protein derivative (PPD) for tuberculosis
   C. Fungal diseases

VII. Other diagnostic studies (Table 4-9)

Acid-Base Balance and Arterial Blood Gas Interpretation
Physiology Review

I. Acid: a substance that can give up an H^+ ion; acids are produced by the body as a result of cellular metabolism
   A. Volatile (e.g., carbonic acid)
      1. Exhalable
      2. Results from aerobic metabolism of glucose
      3. Eliminated by the lungs
   B. Nonvolatile (also called *fixed*) (e.g., sulfuric, phosphoric, uric)
      1. Nonexhalable and cannot be converted into a gas
      2. Results from aerobic metabolism of protein and fat and anaerobic metabolism of glucose
      3. Eliminated by the kidney
   C. Elimination or neutralization necessary

II. Acidemia: the condition of the blood with a pH of below 7.35

III. Acidosis: the process that causes the acidemia

IV. Base: a substance that can accept an H^+ (the primary base in the body is bicarbonate)

V. Alkalemia: the condition of the blood with a pH of above 7.45

VI. Alkalosis: the process that causes the alkalemia

Table 4-9 DIAGNOSTIC STUDIES

Study	Evaluates	Comments
Bronchography	• Detects obstruction or malformation of the tracheobronchial tree	• Patient inspires radiopaque substance and then X-rays are taken • Inquire about possibility of pregnancy
Chest X-ray	• Detects lung pathology (e.g., pneumonia, pulmonary edema, atelectasis, tuberculosis, etc.) • Determines size and location of lung lesions and tumors • Verifies placement of endotracheal tube, central venous catheters, chest tubes	• Noninvasive test with minimal radiation exposure • Inquire about possibility of pregnancy • Posteroanterior (PA) and lateral films are done most commonly, but in critical care areas anteroposterior (AP) portable films are frequently necessary due to inability to transport patient • Lateral decubitus films aid in identification of pleural effusion
Exercise testing	• Identify early disability • Differentiate between cardiac and pulmonary disease	• Monitor for changes in Spo_2 during exercise • Monitor closely for exercise-induced hypotension or ventricular dysrhythmias
Laryngoscopy, bronchoscopy, mediastinoscopy	• Obtain cytology specimen or biopsy • Identify tumors, obstructions, secretions, foreign bodies in tracheobronchial tree • Locate a bleeding site • May be used therapeutically to remove secretions, foreign bodies, other contaminants	• Patient is sedated prior to the procedure, usually with a benzodiazepine (e.g., diazepam, midazolam) • Monitor the patient for subcutaneous emphysema after study; indicates tracheal or bronchial tear • Monitor for hemoptysis; some blood in sputum is normal after biopsy, but frank hemoptysis requires immediate attention
Lung biopsy • Transthoracic needle lung biopsy • Open lung biopsy	• Obtain specimen for cytology evaluation	• Transthoracic needle biopsy performed under fluoroscopy; inquire about possibility of pregnancy • Open lung biopsy requires thoracotomy
Magnetic resonance imaging (MRI)	• Distinguishes tumors from other structures (e.g., tumor, pleural thickening, fibrosis)	• Noninvasive test • Contraindicated for patients with pacemakers or implanted metallic devices
Pulmonary angiography	• Detects changes in lung tissue (e.g., masses) • Diagnoses abnormalities in pulmonary vasculature, including thrombi and emboli • Identifies congenital abnormalities of the circulation	• Invasive test • Inquire about possibility of pregnancy • Contrast media injected into pulmonary artery: ensure adequate hydration after study • Monitor arterial puncture point for hematoma or hemorrhage
Pulmonary function studies (see Table 4-1 for lung volumes and parameters with normals) • Spirometry: volumes and capacities • RV, FRC, TLC requires nitrogen washout technique • Ventilatory mechanics • Flow-volume loop studies • Diffusing capacity	• Measures lung volumes, capacities, and flow rates • Identifies features of restrictive or obstructive lung disease • Evaluates responsiveness to bronchodilator therapy • Aids in evaluation of surgical risk • Documents a disability or cause of dyspnea	• Noninvasive study • Frequently repeated after bronchodilator therapy
Sleep studies	• Diagnose and differentiate between obstructive sleep apnea, central sleep apnea, and cardiac sleep apnea	• Restrict caffeine prior to testing • Usually done during normal sleep hours

Table 4-9	DIAGNOSTIC STUDIES—cont'd	
Study	**Evaluates**	**Comments**
Thoracentesis (may include pleural biopsy)	• Obtain pleural fluid and/or tissue specimen • May be used therapeutically to remove pleural fluid	• Monitor patient for indications of pneumothorax • Monitor for leakage from puncture point
Thoracic computed tomography (CT)	• Defines lesions, masses, cavities, or shadows seen on a normal chest X-ray • Evaluates tracheal or bronchial narrowing • Aids in planning radiation therapy	• X-rays taken at different angles
Ultrasonography	• Evaluates pleural disease • Visualizes diaphragm and detects disease around diaphragm (e.g., subphrenic hematoma or abscess)	• Noninvasive test
Ventilation scan Lung perfusion scan Ventilation/perfusion (V/Q) scan	• Diagnoses ventilation and/or perfusion abnormalities, including emphysema, pulmonary emboli	• Invasive test: radioisotope inspired and injected intravascularly • Inquire about possibility of pregnancy • Nuclear scan study: assure patient that amount of radioactive material is minimal

VII. pH
   A. Indirect measurement of hydrogen ion concentration
   B. Reflection of the balance between carbonic acid (acid regulated by the lungs) and bicarbonate (base regulated by the kidneys)
   C. Inversely proportional to hydrogen ion concentration
      1. Increase in H^+ concentration: lower pH, more acid
      2. Decrease in H^+ concentration: higher pH, more base
   D. Must be maintained within a narrow range to allow functioning of enzymatic systems in the body
      1. pH below 6.8 or above 7.8 is incompatible with life
      2. Note that this is a 0.6 change toward acidosis but only a 0.4 change toward alkalosis (from midline normal of 7.4); this is because the shift of the oxyhemoglobin dissociation curve caused by alkalosis affects tissue oxygenation more adversely than does the shift caused by acidosis
VIII. Henderson-Hasselbalch equation
   A. pH is determined by the logarithm of the ratio of bicarbonate concentration to arterial Pa_{CO_2}
      1. $pH = \dfrac{pK \text{ (constant of 6.1)} + \log HCO_3}{Pa_{CO_2}}$
   B. Ratio of 20 bicarbonate: 1 carbonic acid maintains normal pH (Fig. 4-26)

Acid-Base Regulation
I. Chemical buffers
   A. Weak acid and strong base
   B. Immediate response when a change in acid-base status occurs by combining with excess acid or base
   C. Buffer systems
      1. Bicarbonate-carbonic acid buffer system
         a) The most important buffer system
         b) Bicarbonate is generated by the kidney and aids in the elimination of H^+
         c) $\underset{\text{Lungs}}{\underline{CO_2 + H_2O \Leftrightarrow H_2CO_3 \Leftrightarrow \underset{\text{Kidneys}}{\underline{H^+ + HCO_3}}}}$
      2. Phosphate system: aids in excretion of H^+ by the kidney
      3. Ammonium: H^+ is added to ammonia (NH_3) in the renal tubule to form ammonium (NH_4); allows greater excretion of H^+ by the kidney
      4. Hemoglobin and other proteins: aids in buffering extracellular fluid
II. Respiratory system
   A. Regulates the excretion or retention of carbonic acid
      1. If pH decreases, the rate and depth of ventilation increases
      2. If pH increases, the rate and depth of ventilation decreases
   B. Responds within minutes: fast but weak
III. Renal system
   A. Regulates the excretion or retention of bicarbonate and the excretion of hydrogen and nonvolatile acids
      1. If pH decreases, the kidney retains bicarbonate
      2. If pH increases, the kidney excretes bicarbonate
   B. Responds within 48 hours: slow but powerful

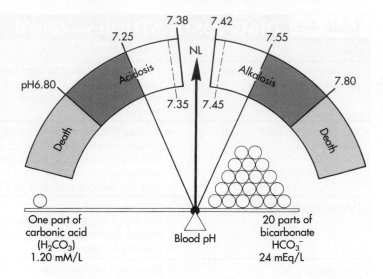

Figure 4-26 Acid-base balance. 20 parts of bicarbonate are required to buffer 1 part carbonic acid; pH is normally maintained within the narrow range of 7.35 to 7.45; pH below 6.8 or above 7.8 is incompatible with life. (From Price SA, Wilson LM: *Pathophysiology: clinical concepts of disease processes*, ed 4, St Louis, 1994, Mosby.)

Acid-Base Imbalances (Table 4-10)

I. Acidemia: pH below 7.35
   A. Acidosis: the process causing acidemia
      1. Caused by acid gain
         a) If acid is volatile (reflected by increase in Pa_{CO_2}): respiratory acidosis
         b) If acid is nonvolatile (reflected by decrease in HCO_3^-): metabolic acidosis
      2. Caused by base loss (reflected by decrease in HCO_3^-): metabolic acidosis
      3. Anion gap is used to differentiate between metabolic acid gain or base loss as cause of metabolic acidosis
         a) Calculated: $(Na^+ + K^+) - (Cl^- + HCO_3^-)$
         b) Normal: 5 to 15
         c) If anion gap is normal (5-15): metabolic acidosis is due to a base loss
         d) If anion gap is increased (>15): metabolic acidosis is due to acid gain
         e) More information on anion gap found in Chapter 9

II. Alkalemia: pH above 7.45
   A. Alkalosis: the process causing alkalosis
      1. Caused by acid loss
         a) If acid is volatile (reflected by decrease in Pa_{CO_2}): respiratory alkalosis
         b) If acid is nonvolatile (reflected by increase in HCO_3^-): metabolic alkalosis
      2. Caused by base gain (reflected by increase in HCO_3^-): metabolic alkalosis

III. Compensation
   A. Respiratory acidosis
      1. The kidneys reabsorb more bicarbonate or excrete more H^+
      2. The bicarbonate and base excess levels increase
      3. This change is slow and may take as long as 2 to 3 days
   B. Respiratory alkalosis
      1. The kidneys excrete more bicarbonate
      2. The bicarbonate and base excess levels decrease

Table 4-10	Acid-Base Imbalances		
Imbalance	**pH**	**Primary Change**	**Compensatory Change**
Respiratory Acidosis	<7.35	↑ Pa_{CO_2}	↑ HCO_3^-
Metabolic Acidosis	<7.35	↓ HCO_3^-	↓ Pa_{CO_2}
Respiratory Alkalosis	>7.45	↓ Pa_{CO_2}	↓ HCO_3^-
Metabolic Alkalosis	>7.45	↑ HCO_3^-	↑ Pa_{CO_2}

↑, = increased; ↓, = decreased

      3. This change is slow and may take as long as 2 to 3 days
   C. Metabolic acidosis
      1. The lungs increase the rate and depth of ventilation
      2. The Pa_{CO_2} level decreases
      3. This change is rapid, usually within minutes to hours
   D. Metabolic alkalosis
      1. The lungs decrease the rate and depth of ventilation
      2. The Pa_{CO_2} level increases
      3. This change is rapid, usually within minutes to hours
   E. Correction versus compensation
      1. Correction may be a physiologic process or the result of appropriate therapeutic measures (Table 4-13 for Discussion of Acid-Base Imbalances); correction is achieved when the pH is normal and both indicators (Pa_{CO_2}, HCO_3^-) are normal
      2. Compensation is a physiologic process; the pH is normal and both indicators are abnormal
         a) Partial compensation: pH is still abnormal but the secondary parameter is outside normal range in the direction to move the pH toward normal

Table 4-11	Mixed Acid-Base Disorders	
Mixed Disorder	**Clinical Example**	
Mixed Acidosis	Cardiac and respiratory arrest	
Mixed Alkalosis	Compensated respiratory acidosis (e.g., COPD) being excessively mechanically ventilated	
Respiratory Acidosis and Metabolic Alkalosis	Patient with COPD receiving diuretics	
Respiratory Alkalosis and Metabolic Acidosis	Hepatic and renal failure	

Table 4-12	Arterial Blood Gas Normal Values	
pH	**7.35-7.45**	
$Paco_2$	35-45 mm Hg	
HCO_3^-	22-26 mEq/L	
Pao_2	80-100 mm Hg	

b) Full compensation: pH is normal and the secondary parameter is outside normal range in the direction to move the pH toward normal

IV. Mixed disorders (Table 4-11)
   A. More than one disorder may coexist
   B. The degree of respiratory component versus metabolic component can be calculated utilizing these formulas
      1. As the $Paco_2$ changes by 10 torr (from normal of 40), it is associated with a change in pH of 0.08 in the opposite direction
      2. As the pH changes by 0.15 (from normal of 7.40), it is associated with a change in base of 10 mEq/L
   C. Compensation cannot exist in mixed disorders since each system is independently abnormal and cannot help the other

Analysis of Arterial Blood Gases

I. Purposes of arterial blood gases
   A. Evaluate ventilation: $Paco_2$
   B. Evaluate acid-base status: pH; to determine the cause of the acid-base imbalance, determine which parameter is abnormal
      1. Respiratory: $Paco_2$
      2. Metabolic: HCO_3^-
   C. Evaluate oxygenation: Pao_2, Sao_2
II. Parameters and normals (Table 4-12)
   A. pH: negative logarithm of hydrogen ion concentration in arterial blood
      1. Normal pH is 7.35 to 7.45
      2. Levels below 7.35 indicate acidosis
      3. Levels above 7.45 indicate alkalosis
   B. $Paco_2$: partial pressure of carbon dioxide in arterial blood
      1. Normal $Paco_2$ is 35 to 45 mm Hg
      2. Levels below 35 indicate respiratory alkalosis or respiratory compensation for a metabolic acidosis
      3. Levels above 45 indicate respiratory acidosis or respiratory compensation for a metabolic alkalosis
   C. HCO_3^-: bicarbonate ion level in arterial blood
      1. Normal HCO_3^- is 22 to 26 mEq/L

   2. Levels below 22 indicate metabolic acidosis or metabolic compensation for respiratory alkalosis
   3. Levels above 26 indicate metabolic alkalosis or metabolic compensation for respiratory acidosis
   D. Base excess (BE): difference between acid and base levels in arterial blood
      1. Normal BE is +2 to −2
      2. Levels below −2 (actually a base deficit) indicate metabolic acidosis or metabolic compensation for respiratory alkalosis
      3. Levels above +2 indicate metabolic alkalosis or metabolic compensation for respiratory acidosis
   E. Pao_2: partial pressure of oxygen in arterial blood
      1. Normal Pao_2 is 80 to 100 mm Hg
      2. Levels above 100 indicate hyperoxemia
      3. Levels below 80 indicate mild hypoxemia
      4. Levels below 60 indicate moderate hypoxemia
      5. Levels below 40 indicate severe hypoxemia
   F. Sao_2: saturation of hemoglobin by oxygen
      1. Normal Sao_2 is 95% or greater
      2. Levels below 95% indicate mild desaturation of hemoglobin
      3. Levels below 90% indicate moderate desaturation of hemoglobin
      4. Levels below 75% indicate severe desaturation of hemoglobin
III. Steps in analysis
   A. Is pH acidotic, alkalotic, or normal?
   B. Which parameter is abnormal?
      1. $Paco_2$: respiratory
      2. HCO_3^-: metabolic
   C. If pH is normal, is it leaning? If so, consider compensation; rules of compensation:
      1. Compensation causes a leaning pH: the pH leans toward the **initial** disorder
      2. One parameter change must help the other
      3. The body never overcompensates; a normal nonleaning pH with two abnormal indicators suggests a mixed disorder (e.g., one alkalotic process + one acidotic process)
   D. Assess oxygenation
      1. Pao_2 less than 80 mm Hg is hypoxemia
      2. Pao_2 less than 60 mm Hg on room air is usually an indication for oxygen administration
      3. Acceptable Pao_2 should be adjusted for age; one method is to subtract 1 mm Hg for each year greater than 60 years from 80 mm Hg;

this gives acceptable Pao_2 on room air for a patient of that age

IV. Technical problems that may affect accuracy of arterial blood gas values
   A. Too much heparin: decrease in $Paco_2$, decrease in HCO_3^-, increase in base excess
   B. Air bubble: increase in pH, decrease in $Paco_2$, increase in Pao_2
   C. Not chilled immediately: decrease in pH, decrease in Pao_2, increase in $Paco_2$
   D. Inadequate discard volume when drawing from catheter with flush solution: decreased $Paco_2$

Discussion of Acid-Base Imbalances
(Table 4-13)

Airway Management
Etiology of Airway Obstruction
I. Upper airway
   A. Relaxation of tongue against hypopharynx: primary cause of obstruction in unconscious patient
   B. Foreign body aspiration
      1. Aspiration of food: primary cause of obstruction in conscious patient
      2. Vomitus
      3. Dentures
   C. Tumor
   D. Hematoma
   E. Laryngeal spasm, edema
   F. Vocal cord paralysis
   G. Infection (e.g., epiglottis)
   H. Trauma (e.g., fractured trachea)
II. Lower airway
   A. Foreign bodies
   B. Secretions
   C. Hemorrhage
   D. Pneumonia
   E. Space-occupying lesions, tumors
   F. Bronchospasm

Assessment
I. Partial obstruction
   A. Presence of air movement
   B. Restlessness, agitation, anxiety
   C. Respiratory distress: tracheal tug, intercostal retractions, use of accessory muscles
   D. Cyanosis
   E. Coughing
   F. Altered speech
   G. Inspiratory sounds: snoring, stridor
   H. Breath sound changes: wheezes, rhonchi
II. Complete obstruction
   A. Lack of air movement
   B. Extreme anxiety in conscious patient
   C. Respiratory distress: tracheal tug, intercostal retractions, use of accessory muscles
   D. Cyanosis
   E. Inability to speak, cough, or produce any sound

F. Universal sign of choking: patient clutches throat with hand
G. Unconsciousness within seconds

Collaborative Management of Airway Obstruction and/or Respiratory Distress
I. Positioning: maintain optimal airway and thoracic position
   A. Head-tilt, chin-lift: optimal airway position
      1. Also called *sniffing position*
      2. True hyperextension to be avoided
      3. Contraindicated if cervical spine fracture possible (instead use jaw thrust)
   B. Position for optimal chest excursion: semi-Fowler's to high Fowler's position
II. Removal of obstruction
   A. Removal of visible obstruction
      1. Use of fingers to remove only visible foreign body
      2. Use of Magill forceps but care must be taken to prevent pushing the obstruction deeper into the airway
   B. Heimlich maneuver
      1. Subxiphoid thrusts to relieve upper airway obstruction
      2. Avoidance of abdominal thrusts (use chest thrusts) in any of the following situations:
         a) Patient is too obese for you to get your arms around him or her
         b) Patient has had recent abdominal surgery
         c) Patient is pregnant
   C. Recovery position: side-lying on left side
III. Deep breathing: sustained inspiratory effort
   A. Purpose
      1. Increases air in the alveoli, preventing atelectasis
      2. Makes coughing more effective
   B. Incentive spirometry: provides graded incentives for sustained inspiration
IV. Removal of secretions
   A. Cough: forceful expiration to dislodge and remove secretions from the tracheobronchial tree
      1. Indications
         a) Breath sound changes: especially rhonchi; wheezes caused by mucus plugs may also clear with coughing
         b) Between postural drainage position changes but never in a head down position
         c) While coughing should be encouraged in the above identified situations, routine coughing may increase the incidence of atelectasis; preventive measures (e.g., postoperative patients) should focus on deep breathing with sustained inspiration rather than forced expiration
      2. Technique for effective coughing
         a) Assist patient to comfortable position
         b) Instruct patient to do the following:
            (1) Inhale deeply

Table 4-13	Discussion of Acid-Base Imbalances		
Imbalance	**Etiology**	**Clinical Presentation**	**Collaborative Management**
Respiratory acidosis: pH low; Paco$_2$ high	Hypoventilation • Airway obstruction • CNS depression from drugs, injury, or disease • Chest wall injury (e.g., flail chest) • Obstructive lung disease (e.g., chronic bronchitis, emphysema, late asthma) • Restrictive lung disease (e.g., kyphoscoliosis, obesity hypoventilation syndrome) • Oxygen-induced hypoventilation in patients with chronic hypercapnia • Neuromuscular abnormality (e.g., Guillain-Barré syndrome, myasthenia gravis, multiple sclerosis) • Atelectasis, pneumonia • Pulmonary edema • Respiratory arrest	Initially • Sympathetic nervous system stimulation symptoms (e.g., tachycardia, tachypnea, diaphoresis) Later • Bradypnea • Hypotension • Dysrhythmias • Confusion • Headache • Blurred vision • Flushed face (plethora) • Somnolence leading to coma (these late symptoms are also referred to as *CO$_2$ narcosis*)	Increase ventilation and treat cause • Maintain patent airway • Position for optimal ventilation • Implement bronchial hygiene measures • Administer drug therapy (e.g., bronchodilators, mucolytics, antibiotics) • Mechanical ventilation may be necessary • If patient is on mechanical ventilation, increase rate or tidal volume
Respiratory alkalosis: pH high; Paco$_2$ low	Hyperventilation • Anxiety or hysteria • Thoracic pain • Early asthma • Pneumothorax • Pulmonary embolism • Early salicylate intoxication • Hyperthyroidism • Hepatic failure • Fever • Gram-negative septicemia • CNS infection or injury • Excessive mechanical ventilation	• Tachycardia • Palpitations • Dry mouth • Anxiety • Profuse perspiration • Paresthesia around mouth and extremities • Dizziness, vertigo, syncope • Increased muscle irritability, twitching • Tetany • Inability to concentrate • Seizures • Coma	Decrease ventilation and treat cause • Provide reassurance and maintain a calm attitude • Administer sedatives (frequently given intravenously) • Ask patient to breathe into and out of a paper bag or use a rebreathing mask • If patient is on mechanical ventilation, decrease rate or tidal volume
Metabolic acidosis: pH low; HCO$_3^-$ low	Acid gain (increased anion gap) • Tissue hypoxia (e.g., shock [lactic acidosis]) • Ketoacidosis (diabetic ketoacidosis or starvation) • Renal failure • Drugs and toxins (e.g., salicylates; methanol, ethylene glycol) Bicarbonate loss (normal anion gap) • Bile drainage • Pancreatic fistula • Diarrhea • Acetazolamide (Diamox) therapy	• Nausea, vomiting, abdominal discomfort • Weakness • Tremors • Malaise • Headache • Tachypnea progressing to Kussmaul's • Hypotension • Dysrhythmias • Confusion • Lethargy → coma	• Treat cause as appropriate • Improve oxygenation and/or perfusion (lactic acidosis) • Give insulin (DKA) • Dialysis (renal failure) • Antidiarrheals (diarrhea) • Administer buffer • Bicarbonate IV or orally for pH 7.0 or less
Metabolic alkalosis: pH high; HCO$_3^-$ high	Acid loss • Nasogastric suction or severe vomiting • Potassium-wasting diuretic therapy • Steroid therapy • Cushing's disease • Hyperaldosteronism • Hepatic disease • Hypokalemia, hypochloremia Bicarbonate gain • Dosing with bicarbonate • Excess infusion of lactated Ringer's	• Bradypnea • Nausea, vomiting, diarrhea • Paresthesia around mouth and extremities • Confusion • Dizziness • Increased muscle irritability • Tetany • Seizures • Coma	• Treat cause • Replace potassium and/or chloride • Administer carbonic anhydrase inhibitor • Acetazolamide (Diamox) • Administer buffer • Arginine monohydrochloride • Ammonium chloride • Weak HCl acid solution

(2) Cough two to three times with mouth open

(3) Expectorate any sputum

(4) Inhale slowly and deeply

3. Special techniques

a) Huff coughing is forced expiration with glottis open; may be helpful for patients with COPD to keep airways open

b) Augmented coughing requires an assistant to deliver a subxiphoid thrust during expiration; may be necessary for patients with abdominal muscle weakness or paralysis

B. Suctioning of oropharynx: removal of secretions from the oropharynx through the use of a suction catheter and negative pressure

1. Performed before deflation of endotracheal tube cuff to prevent oropharyngeal secretions from draining into tracheobronchial tree

2. Performed routinely after suctioning of tracheobronchial tree to prevent accumulation of oropharyngeal secretions that can be silently aspirated around endotracheal tube cuff

3. Yankauer suction device usually used; if suction catheter that was used to suction the tracheobronchial tree is used, suction oropharynx only **after** suctioning the tracheobronchial tree and rinsing the catheter

C. Suctioning of tracheobronchial tree: removal of secretions from the tracheobronchial tree through the use of a suction catheter and negative pressure

1. Clinical indications for the need to suction

a) Sympathetic nervous system stimulation (tachycardia, tachypnea)

b) Decrease in BP

c) Dyspnea

d) Noisy or shallow ventilation

e) Rhonchi

f) Obvious visible secretions

g) Excessive coughing during inspiratory cycle of ventilator

h) High pressure alarm on ventilator

i) Clinical indications of hypoxia (Box 4-3), hypercapnia (Box 4-4)

2. Technique for suctioning the tracheobronchial tree utilizing principles to prevent complications

a) Suction only if indicated and limit number of passes to minimum required

b) The outer diameter of the catheter should be no more than one half the inner diameter of the ET tube or tracheostomy

c) Special adaptor or closed suction system are especially helpful for patients on therapeutic PEEP because these patients frequently have significant oxygen desaturation during suctioning

d) Special curved-tip catheter (Coudé catheter) is required to enter the left mainstem bronchus; it is usually adequate to use a regular suction catheter to suction the right mainstem bronchus and the trachea because the coughing stimulated effectively clears the left mainstem bronchus into the trachea

e) Sterile technique is used if suctioning through an endotracheal tube or tracheostomy; aseptic technique is used if suctioning nasotracheally

(1) Two gloves should be used

(2) Goggles should be worn to protect the nurse's eyes

f) Explain procedure to the patient; protect the patient's eyes

g) Hyperoxygenation (100% oxygen) and hyperinflation (1.5 times usual tidal volume) for 5 to 6 breaths before and after suctioning

(1) Ideally should be done with the ventilator

(a) Hyperoxygenation can be provided by temporarily increasing the FIo_2 to 1.0 (100%); many mechanical ventilators provide 2 or 3 minutes of 100% oxygen by pushing a button

(b) Hyperinflation can be provided by setting the sigh volume at 1½ times the inspired tidal volume and then using the manual sigh button

(2) Can be done with manual resuscitation bag with two people (e.g., one person suctioning and one person manually ventilating); one-hand ventilation with a manual resuscitation bag does not provide hyperinflation

(3) Hyperinflation should be omitted if the patient has high peak airway pressure (indicating poor compliance) or if a clinically significant increase in mean arterial pressure accompanies hyperinflation

(4) Hyperinflation may not be necessary when a closed suction system is used, but more research is needed; hyperoxygenation is necessary

h) If doing nasotracheal suctioning, place patient in "sniffing" position while sitting up or place towel roll between shoulders if patient is supine

i) Lubricate catheter with saline if endotracheal tube or tracheostomy; use water-soluble lubricant if nasotracheal

j) Monitor Spo_2 during suctioning for oxygen desaturation

k) Monitor ECG during and after suctioning

for vagal stimulation (bradycardia) as well as dysrhythmias related to hypoxemia (PVCs)

l) Advance catheter to point of obstruction, then pull back slightly before applying suction; apply suction intermittently during withdrawal of catheter

m) Limit suctioning to 10 seconds; hyperoxygenate and hyperinflate between passes

n) Avoid excessive negative pressure; keep pressure 100 mm Hg or less unless closed suction system; 120 mm Hg is recommended if closed suction system

o) Liquefy secretions through humidification and hydration

   (1) Instillation of saline (also referred to as *saline lavage*) has been proven ineffective and potentially harmful; contributes to hypoxemia and nosocomial pneumonia

   (2) If increased oral or parenteral fluids cannot be given (e.g., renal failure), either of the following treatments may be prescribed:

     (a) Saline by inhalation (small particle size allows deeper penetration into tracheobronchial tube and liquefies mucus)

     (b) Acetylcysteine (Mucomyst) given by inhalation (breaks down disulfide bonds to liquefy mucus); a bronchodilator is frequently required with acetylcysteine

p) Rinse catheter and appropriately discard disposable catheter; if closed suction system, rinse the catheter after pulling it out of the airway by injecting saline into irrigation port while applying suction (this is irrigation not lavage) then close irrigation port and suction valve

q) Stop suctioning if: change in heart rate, ECG rhythm, or skin color; significant change in SpO_2 or SvO_2

r) Hyperoxygenate and hyperinflate after suctioning for 5 to 6 breaths

s) Assess breath sounds after suctioning to evaluate effectiveness

3. Advantages of closed suction system

a) Continued oxygenation and reduction in loss of PEEP, so decreased incidence of hypoxemia

b) Decreased cost and nursing time

c) Decreased chance of aerosolization of secretions, which protects patient's and nurse's eyes

d) Decreased risk of introducing bacteria into airway

D. Chest physiotherapy (chest PT)

1. Indication: prevention and treatment of respiratory complications

2. Postural drainage (PD): sequential positioning of the patient

a) Purpose: utilize gravity to drain secretions from peripheral areas into the major bronchi or trachea so that they can be coughed and expectorated or suctioned

b) Technique

   (1) Administer bronchodilator prior to PD if prescribed

   (2) Turn off enteral feedings for 30 minutes prior to postural drainage; ensure that cuff of endotracheal or tracheostomy tube is inflated

   (3) Place patient in position to drain selected segment of lung or alternate through the following positions:

     (a) Left side with hips higher than head

     (b) Right side with hips higher than head

     (c) Supine with hips higher than head

     (d) Prone with hips higher than head

   (4) Maintain each position for 10 to 30 minutes

   (5) Cough between position changes but never in a head-down position

   (6) Avoid PD for at least 1½ hours after meals

c) Contraindications

   (1) Obesity

   (2) Rib fracture, flail chest

   (3) Spinal fracture

   (4) Pulmonary hemorrhage

   (5) Pulmonary embolism

   (6) Pneumothorax

   (7) Tuberculosis

   (8) Lung abscess or malignancy

   (9) Asthma, acute bronchospasm

   (10) Bleeding disorder

   (11) Osteoporosis

   (12) Seizures

   (13) Intracranial hypertension

   (14) Acute myocardial infarction

3. Percussion: clapping the chest with cupped hands

a) Purpose: mechanically dislodge secretions from the bronchial walls into the major bronchi or trachea so that they can be coughed and expectorated or suctioned

b) Technique

   (1) Cup hands as if holding water

   (2) Tap chest with cupped hands, listening for a cupping not slapping sound

   (3) Avoid: spine, liver, kidneys, spleen, female patient's breasts

c) Contraindications

   (1) Known bleeding disorder

   (2) Lung cancer

   (3) Pneumothorax

(4) Extreme caution after thoracotomy or in elderly patients with osteoporosis
4. Vibration: vibration of areas of the chest with either an open hand or a vibrating device
   a) Purpose: loosen secretions from the bronchial walls into the major bronchi or trachea so that they can be coughed and expectorated or suctioned
   b) Technique
      (1) Hold hand flat against chest and vibrate hand during expiration
      (2) Hand vibrator may also be used
   c) Contraindications: as for percussion
V. Artificial airways
   A. General principles
      1. Provide humidification because natural humidification mechanisms are bypassed
      2. Use aseptic technique with upper airway artificial airways; use sterile technique with lower airway artificial airways
      3. Suction as indicated; postural drainage, percussion, vibration may also be needed
      4. Provide method of communication; this is the most significant stressor experienced by intubated patients
         a) Picture communication board, alphabet board, or magic slate, or felt-tip pen or marker and paper may be used; avoid pencils and ballpoint pens, which require more pressure
         b) Fenestrated or Passy-Muir tracheostomy tubes may be used in some patients; these allow air to leak over the vocal cords
         c) Lip reading is usually not an acceptable method, especially if oral tube is in place
   B. Selection of appropriate artificial airway (Table 4-14)
   C. Summary of artificial airways (Table 4-15)
      1. Upper airway artificial airways (Fig. 4-27)
         a) Oropharyngeal airway
         b) Nasopharyngeal airway
         c) Cricothyrotomy
      2. Lower airway artificial airways (Figure 4-28)
         a) Endotracheal tube
            (1) Nasotracheal tube
            (2) Orotracheal tube
         b) Tracheostomy
   D. Endotracheal intubation
      1. Indications
         a) Tidal volume less than 5 ml/kg
         b) Vital capacity less than 10 ml/kg
         c) Maximal inspiratory pressure less negative than −20 cm H_2O
         d) Inability to adequately cough and clear airway
         e) Loss of protective reflexes
         f) Need for sealed airway (e.g., mechanical ventilation, risk for aspiration)
      2. Insertion of endotracheal tube
         a) Prepare the oxygen delivery system to be used after intubation: usually T-piece with

Table 4-14	Selection of Appropriate Artificial Airway	
Problem	**Preferred Artificial Airway**
Tongue against hypopharynx	Oropharyngeal or nasopharyngeal
Need for frequent nasotracheal suctioning	Nasopharyngeal
Inability to open mouth (e.g., seizure)	Nasopharyngeal
Complete upper airway obstruction when endotracheal intubation is impossible (e.g., laryngeal edema or spasm, tracheal fracture)	Cricothyrotomy or tracheostomy
Need for sealed airway (e.g., mechanical ventilation or potential for aspiration)	Endotracheal tube or tracheostomy
Need for long-term lower airway access and sealed airway	Tracheostomy

nebulizer or mechanical ventilator; manual resuscitation bag with reservoir bag with 100% oxygen may be used during cardiac arrest or until mechanical ventilator is ready
   b) Collect supplies and select tube size
      (1) Tube: females usually 7.5 to 8.0; males usually 8.0 to 8.5
      (2) Equipment to insert and secure tube: laryngoscope with straight (Miller) and curved (MacIntosh) blades with working lights, stylet, Magill forceps, lubricant, syringe, and tape or device for stabilization of tube
      (3) Suction equipment, including suction catheter and Yankauer suction device
   c) Monitor ECG, Spo_2 during intubation
   d) Hyperoxygenate with 100% oxygen for at least 2 minutes
   e) Place patient in head tilt–chin lift position
   f) Intubation should be performed by the most qualified person available who has been trained in endotracheal intubation and who often performs the procedure (usually physician or nurse anesthetist)
   g) Intubation should be completed within 30 seconds; if not, attempts should be ceased and the patient should again be hyperoxygenated
   h) Confirm placement of endotracheal tube
      (1) Feel air movement through tube
      (2) Assess bilateral chest excursion
      (3) Auscultate bilateral breath sounds; if breath sounds are audible on the right but not on the left, right mainstem

Table 4-15	Summary Of Artificial Airways		
Type of Airway	**Advantages**	**Disadvantages**	**Miscellaneous**
Oropharyngeal airway	• Easy to insert • Inexpensive • Effectively holds tongue away from pharynx	• Improper insertion technique can push tongue back and occlude airway • Easily dislodged • Poorly tolerated by conscious patients as it may stimulate gag reflex • Causes increased oral secretions • Contraindicated in patients with trauma to lower face, recent oral surgery, loose or avulsed teeth	• Determine appropriate size: with flange at teeth, end of airway should not extend beyond the angle of the jaw • Large adult: usually 100 mm (size 5) • Medium adult: usually 90 mm (size 4) • Small adult: usually 80 mm (size 3) • Insert by holding tongue down with tongue blade and sliding into place; alternative method: insert upside down and turn over when into pharynx; take care not to traumatize palate • Do not use as a bite block; likely to cause vomiting and potential aspiration in conscious patients • Remove, wash, and give mouth care every 4-8 hours; check mucous membranes for ulcerations
Nasopharyngeal airway (also called a *trumpet airway*)	• Easy to insert • Inexpensive • Effectively holds tongue away from pharynx • May be used in conscious or unconscious patients • Prevents trauma to nasal mucosa during nasotracheal suctioning • May be inserted when mouth cannot be opened (e.g., during seizures, jaw fractures)	• May cause nosebleeds, pressure necrosis, or sinus infection • Kinks and clogs easily • Contraindicated in patients predisposed to nosebleeds, nasal obstruction, bleeding disorder, or sepsis, and in patients with basal skull fracture	• Determine appropriate size: 1 inch longer than nose to earlobe; lumen smaller than naris • Large adult: usually 8-9 internal diameter • Medium adult: usually 7-8 internal diameter • Small adult: usually 6-7 internal diameter • Insert with bevel against septum • Use viscous Xylocaine as a lubricant for insertion to decrease discomfort • Do not use in patients receiving anticoagulants • Provide humidification of inspired air • Confirm placement by visualizing the tip of the airway next to the uvula • Rotate naris to naris every 8 hours
Cricothyrotomy	• Provides immediate airway access, especially helpful if complete upper airway obstruction	• May cause bleeding • Only temporary; very small opening if established with large needle; larger if airway opened with scalpel and small tracheostomy tube used	• Provide humidification of inspired air • Use large-bore over-the-needle catheter; adaptor required to attach to manual resuscitation bag • Physician may use scalpel and insert small tracheostomy tube • Monitor for bleeding, subcutaneous emphysema

Continued

Table 4-15	Summary Of Artificial Airways—cont'd		
Type of Airway	**Advantages**	**Disadvantages**	**Miscellaneous**
Endotracheal tube (general)	• Provides relatively sealed airway for mechanical ventilation, prevention of aspiration • Permits easy suctioning • Prevents gastric distention with air during CPR	• Requires skilled personnel for insertion • Splints epiglottis open and prevents effective cough • Causes loss of physiologic PEEP since epiglottis is splinted open; patient should receive 3-5 cm PEEP to reestablish physiologic PEEP • May kink and clog • Causes aphonia • May cause laryngeal or tracheal damage • Contraindicated in patients with laryngeal obstruction caused by tumor, infection, or vocal cord paralysis	• Determine appropriate size • Females: usually 7.5-8.0 internal diameter • Males: usually 8.0-8.5 internal diameter • Tube may need to be 0.5-1.0 smaller if to be inserted nasally • Provide humidification of inspired air • Mark tube at corner of mouth or at naris to assess any movement • Use minimal occlusive volume or minimal leak volume for cuff inflation; ensure that cuff pressure does not exceed 18 mm Hg (if pressure >18 mm Hg required to achieve seal, tube is too small and needs to be replaced with larger tube) • Confirm placement by chest X-ray: tip of tube should be 3-5 cm above carina • Provide mouth care every 4 hours; observe oral or nasal mucosa for signs of ulcerations or necrosis • Position to prevent kinking; utilize mechanical ventilator's support arms to support ventilator tubing
Oral (specific) endotracheal tube	• Easier insertion than nasal intubation • Permits larger tube than nasal intubation	• Less stable and comfortable than nasal tube • May stimulate gag reflex • May be bitten or chewed • May cause necrosis at corner of mouth • Increases oral secretions; makes mouth care more difficult • Contraindicated in patients with acute unstable cervical spine injury due to need for neck extension (blind nasotracheal intubation may be attempted in these patients)	• Reposition tube from one side of the mouth to the other and retape when indicated; avoid unnecessary manipulation of tube
Nasal (specific) endotracheal tube	• More comfortable for patient than oral endotracheal tube • Permits good oral hygiene • Can't be bitten or chewed	• More difficult insertion than oral intubation • May cause pressure necrosis or sinus infection • Requires smaller size • Contraindicated in patients with nasal obstruction, fractured nose, sinusitis, bleeding disorder, basal skull fracture	• Monitor for clinical indications of sinus infection: fever, increased pharyngeal drainage, halitosis, leukocytosis, sinus pain or headache

Table 4-15	Summary Of Artificial Airways—cont'd		
Type of Airway	**Advantages**	**Disadvantages**	**Miscellaneous**
Tracheostomy	• Provides long-term airway access • Minimizes risk of vocal cord damage from an endotracheal tube during long-term airway maintenance • Decreases dead space and decreases work of breathing • Provides a relative seal to prevent aspiration • Allows the patient to eat, swallow • Allows easier suctioning • Permits Valsalva maneuver and effective cough • Is more comfortable for patient • Is less likely to be dislodged than endotracheal tube • Bypasses upper airway obstruction	• Requires surgery, but may be done percutaneously if ET tube is in place • Causes aphonia • May cause false passage anterior to trachea in patients with thick necks • May cause erosion of innominate artery with tip of tube or low stoma • Causes scar • May cause tracheocutaneous or tracheoesophageal fistula	• Usually considered if artificial airway is required longer than 3 weeks • Determine appropriate size: usually 5-6 • Requires humidification of inspired air • Preferred if airway obstruction (e.g., tumor or laryngeal edema or spasm) • Provide tracheostomy care that includes cleaning stoma and tube every 8 hours with saline; keep stoma dry (if 4×4 used, change often if secretions present) • Keep obturator, extra tracheostomy tube, and tracheal spreader at bedside

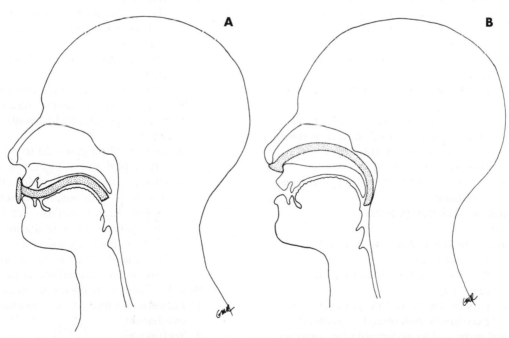

Figure 4-27   Upper airway artificial airways. **A,** Oropharyngeal airway. **B,** Nasopharyngeal airway. (From Sheehy SB: *Emergency nursing: principles and practice,* ed 3, St Louis, 1992, Mosby.)

intubation has occurred; pull the tube back slightly and then recheck breath sounds

   (4) Use a capnometer to confirm consistent exhalation of CO_2

   (5) Auscultate over epigastrium: air movement should not be audible

   (6) Confirm tube positioning by chest

X-ray; distal tip of tube should be 3 to 5 cm above the carina

i) Inflate the cuff using either minimal occlusive volume or minimal leak volume (see section on Cuffs)

j) Tape tube in place

   (1) Secure tape to minimize pressure areas on the face; tape with tension to

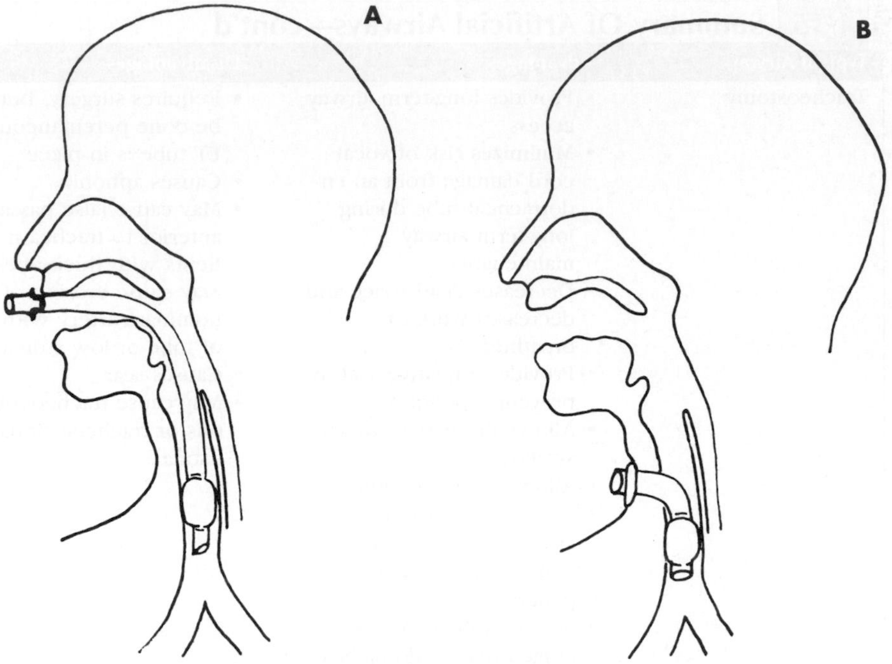

Figure 4-28 Lower airway artificial airways. **A,** Endotracheal tube. **B,** Tracheostomy tube. (From Phipps WJ et al: *Medical-surgical nursing: concepts and clinical practice,* ed 5, St Louis, 1995, Mosby.)

both sides to avoid excessive pressure on one corner of mouth if oral tube
   - (2) If a commercial stabilization device is used, monitor oral mucosa carefully for evidence of excessive pressure
   - k) Note the depth marking on the side of the tube
       - (1) Usually at 19 to 23 cm for an average adult
       - (2) Cut tube so that only 5 to 7 cm of tube extends beyond mouth or nose to decrease airway resistance and potential for kinking
   - l) Attach oxygen delivery system or mechanical ventilator
- E. Extubation of intubated patients
   1. Criteria
       - a) Patient awake and oriented or able to keep airway open
           - (1) Protective reflexes must be intact (e.g., gag)
           - (2) Patient should not be paralyzed or excessively narcotized or sedated
       - b) Vital signs stable; acceptable hemoglobin and hemodynamics
       - c) ABGs within acceptable limits after a trial of 30 minutes on nebulizer (T-piece) at 40% oxygen: Pao_2 60 mm Hg or greater, Sao_2 90% or greater, $Paco_2$ 35 to 45 mm Hg or consistent with patient's normal values
       - d) Acceptable bedside ventilatory parameters:
           - (1) Tidal volume 5 ml/kg or greater
           - (2) Vital capacity 10 ml/kg or greater
           - (3) Maximal inspiratory pressure (MIP) of -20 cm H_2O or greater
   2. Technique
       - a) Have postextubation oxygen delivery system ready; intubation kit should also be available
       - b) Suction trachea, then pharynx
       - c) Deflate cuff
       - d) Remove tube during expiration
       - e) Apply oxygen delivery system
       - f) Encourage patient to cough, suction if needed
       - g) Repeat blood gases 20 to 30 minutes after extubation and as indicated thereafter
       - h) Observe for laryngospasm: stridor, dyspnea, tachypnea; treatment may include high humidity, steroids, racemic epinephrine, or reintubation
       - i) Monitor patient's tolerance to extubation by clinical observation, ventilatory measurements, arterial blood gas studies
- F. Weaning patients from tracheostomy tube
   1. Indications same as for endotracheal extubation
   2. Techniques
       - a) Progression to a smaller size uncuffed (or cuff not inflated) tracheostomy tube: allows the patient to use his or her upper airway and the opening of the tracheostomy tube
       - b) Change to fenestrated tube: opening at the top of the tube allows air to leak upward so that the patient can use the upper airway (and can speak)
       - c) Deflate cuff: allows the patient to use his

or her upper airway and the opening of the tracheostomy tube
  d) Tracheostomy button: closes the opening in the trachea and allows the patient to use his or her upper airway with minimal obstruction
G. Cuffs
  1. Cuffs in current use are high-volume, low-pressure cuffs; these cuffs distribute the low pressure over a larger area of the trachea and decrease the incidence of tracheal ischemia and stenosis; laryngectomy patients may have uncuffed (and longer) laryngectomy tubes
  2. Cuffed tubes provide a **relative** seal for patients receiving mechanical ventilation and aid in prevention of aspiration; note that cuffs do not establish an absolute seal, and silent aspiration of oropharyngeal or gastric secretions is common in critically ill patients
  3. Inflate cuff using minimal occlusive volume or minimal leak volume
    a) Minimal occlusive volume
      (1) Listen over trachea with stethoscope
      (2) Inflate cuff until no air leak is audible during the inspiratory cycle of the ventilator or lung inflation with a manual resuscitation bag
    b) Minimal leak volume
      (1) Listen over trachea with stethoscope
      (2) Inflate cuff until no air leak is audible during the inspiratory cycle of the ventilator or lung inflation with a manual resuscitation bag
      (3) Remove 0.1 cm of air or until a minimal leak is audible during the inspiratory cycle of the ventilator
  4. Intracuff pressure should not exceed capillary filling pressure (18 mm Hg or 25 cm H_2O); measure and record cuff pressure every 4 to 8 hours; measurement of cuff pressure is done with a cuff pressure gauge or a mercury manometer and three–way stopcock
  5. Routine deflation is not necessary with high-volume, low-pressure cuffs and may contribute to nosocomial pneumonia by allowing oropharyngeal secretions to drain into the tracheobronchial tree
H. Complications of airway intubation
  1. Physiologic alterations created by airway diversion
    a) Inadequate humidification of inspired air
    b) Increased risk of nosocomial pneumonia caused by accumulation of secretions
      (1) Increased mucus is caused by tube since it is a foreign body
      (2) Ciliary movement is impaired
    c) Aphonia
    d) Ineffective cough: endotracheal tubes

splint the epiglottis open, preventing effective intrathoracic pressure to achieve an effective cough (patients can cough fairly effectively with a tracheostomy because the epiglottis is not splinted open)
    e) Loss of physiologic PEEP: endotracheal tubes splint the epiglottis open and remove physiologic PEEP (tracheostomy tubes do not do this); physiologic PEEP is reestablished with 3 to 5 cm H_2O of PEEP for intubated patients
  2. During placement
    a) Endotracheal intubation
      (1) Trauma: damage to teeth, mucous membranes, perforation or laceration of pharynx, larynx, trachea
      (2) Aspiration
      (3) Laryngospasm, bronchospasm
      (4) Tube malposition: esophageal or endobronchial intubation
      (5) Hypoxia, anoxia if attempts are prolonged
    b) Tracheostomy
      (1) Barotrauma: pneumothorax, pneumomediastinum
      (2) Hemorrhage
      (3) Tracheoesophageal fistula
      (4) Laryngeal nerve injury
      (5) Cardiopulmonary arrest
  3. While tube is in place
    a) Tube obstruction or displacement
    b) Cuff rupture
    c) Disconnection between tracheal tube and ventilator, including self-extubation
    d) Pressure necrosis
      (1) At corners of mouth if oral endotracheal tube
      (2) At superior nasal concha if nasal endotracheal tube
    e) Local infection; otitis media; sinus infection with nasotracheal tubes
    f) Bronchospasm
    g) Leaks due to broken cuff balloon
    h) Trauma: laryngeal injury, tracheal ischemia, necrosis, dilation
  4. Postextubation
    a) Endotracheal tube
      (1) Acute laryngeal edema
      (2) Hoarseness (common)
      (3) Aspiration if swallowing is impaired
      (4) Stenosis of larynx or trachea (late complication)
    b) Tracheostomy
      (1) Difficulties with decannulation of a tracheostomy
      (2) Tracheoesophageal fistula
      (3) Tracheoinnominate artery fistula
      (4) Tracheocutaneous fistula
      (5) Tracheal stenosis

Oxygen Therapy

Definitions

I. Hypoxemia
  A. Decrease in arterial blood oxygen tension
  B. Diagnosis by arterial blood gases
  C. Decrease in Pao_2 and Sao_2
    1. Mild hypoxemia: Pao_2 less than 80 mm Hg (Sao_2 95%)
    2. Moderate hypoxemia: Pao_2 less than 60 mm Hg (Sao_2 90%)
    3. Severe hypoxemia: Pao_2 less than 40 mm Hg (Sao_2 75%)
II. Hypoxia
  A. Decrease in tissue oxygenation
  B. Diagnosis by clinical indications of hypoxia (see Box 4-3)
  C. Affected by Pao_2 and Sao_2, hemoglobin, cardiac output, patent vessels, cellular demand

Etiology

I. Hypoxemia
  A. Low inspired oxygen concentration (e.g., high altitudes)
  B. Hypoventilation (e.g., asthma)
  C. V/Q mismatching (e.g., pulmonary embolism)
  D. Shunt (e.g., acute respiratory distress syndrome)
  E. Diffusion abnormalities (e.g., pulmonary fibrosis)
II. Hypoxia
  A. Hypoxemic hypoxia: secondary to a gas exchange problem (e.g., ventilation-perfusion mismatch, shunt, diffusion abnormalities)
  B. Anemic hypoxia: secondary to reduced oxygen-carrying capacity of the blood (e.g., anemia, carbon monoxide poisoning, methemoglobinemia)
  C. Circulatory hypoxia: secondary to a reduced blood flow in the body or a reduction in cardiac output (e.g., shock)
  D. Histotoxic hypoxia: secondary to the inability of the cells to utilize oxygen (e.g., cyanide poisoning)

Pathophysiology

I. Decrease in Pao_2 initially stimulates the sympathetic nervous system (SNS)
II. Increase in oxygen extraction reduces oxygen reserve and Svo_2
III. As Pao_2 becomes critically low, tissue oxygenation becomes inadequate and hypoxia occurs
IV. Nutrient metabolism changes from aerobic to anaerobic, which results in 20 times less ATP than aerobic metabolism and lactic acid as a waste product
V. Acidosis and decreased cellular energy results

Assessment

I. Evidence of altered perfusion
  A. Tachycardia
  B. Hypotension
  C. Changes in skin color and temperature
II. Evidence of anaerobic metabolism: lactic acidosis (serum arterial lactate level >2 mmol/L)

III. Evidence of organ dysfunction
  A. Cerebral: altered sensorium
  B. Myocardial: decreased cardiac output; dysrhythmias
  C. Renal: decreased urine output
IV. Parameters of oxygen delivery
  A. Pao_2, Sao_2, Spo_2
  B. Hemoglobin, hematocrit
  C. Cardiac output, cardiac index
V. Hemodynamic monitoring parameters
  A. Cardiac output
  B. Venous oxygen saturation (Svo_2)
    1. Measured: by Svo_2 port of a fiberoptic oximetric PA catheter or by mixed venous blood gas analysis
    2. Normal: 60% to 80%

Indications for Oxygen Therapy

I. Hypoxemia: Pao_2 less than 60 mm Hg; Sao_2 less than 90%
II. Increased myocardial workload (e.g., HF, hypertensive crisis, MI)
III. Decreased cardiac output (e.g., shock)
IV. Increased oxygen demand (e.g., sepsis)
V. Decreased oxygen-carrying capacity (e.g., carbon monoxide poisoning, sickle cell disease, anemia)
VI. Prior to procedures that may cause hypoxemia (e.g., suctioning)

Principles of Oxygen Therapy

I. Airway is always the first priority; oxygen is useless without an adequate airway
II. Oxygen is a potent drug that should be administered as prescribed; may be prescribed as flow rate, oxygen concentration (expressed as a percentage), or fraction of inspired oxygen (FIo_2) (expressed as a decimal)
III. The objective is to improve tissue oxygenation
  A. Maintain Pao_2 at least 60 mm Hg and Sao_2 at 90%; serial serum lactate levels are also helpful in monitoring progression or improvement of hypoxia and degree of anaerobic metabolism
  B. Determine the effectiveness of oxygen therapy; oxygen therapy is ineffective for shunt; alveoli must be opened (also referred to as *alveolar recruitment*) to get the oxygen to the alveolar-capillary membrane; PEEP is frequently required in these cases
IV. If high concentrations are necessary, limit duration to prevent oxygen toxicity
  A. Frequent ABGs are mandatory if FIo_2 is above 0.40
  B. Exact concentration of inspired O_2 should be measured with O_2 analyzer
V. FIo_2 can be estimated by counting the number of reservoirs
  A. Nose and pharynx (1) provides less than 40%; example: nasal cannula
  B. Nose and pharynx + mask (2) provides 40% to 60%; example: simple face mask
  C. Nose and pharynx + mask + reservoir bag (3)

provides 60% to 80%; example: partial rebreathing mask

    D. Nose and pharynx + mask + reservoir bag + one-way valves (3 + decrease in dilution) delivers 80% to 100%; example: nonrebreathing mask

VI. Safety guidelines

    A. Keep oxygen source at least 10 ft from open flame; keep oxygen source away from heat or direct sunlight

    B. Do not allow smoking in a room with supplemental oxygen

    C. Do not use electrical appliances within 5 ft of oxygen source

    D. Do not use petroleum-based products around oxygen source; use only water-soluble lubricants, creams

    E. Turn the oxygen off when not in use

    F. Secure the oxygen tanks to prevent accidental dropping

High-flow Versus Low-flow O_2 Delivery Systems

I. Low-flow oxygen delivery systems

    A. Do not provide total inspired gas; remainder of patient's inspiratory volume is met by patient breathing varying amounts of room air

    B. FIO_2 dependent on rate and depth of ventilation and fit of device

        1. If minute ventilation increases, oxygen concentration decreases since the amount of room air (diluent) increases in relation to the amount of oxygen via the oxygen delivery system

        2. If minute ventilation decreases, oxygen concentration increases

    C. Does not necessarily mean low FIO_2

    D. Devices

        1. Nasal cannula

        2. Simple face mask

        3. Partial rebreathing mask

        4. Nonrebreathing mask

II. High-flow oxygen delivery systems

    A. Provide the entire inspired gas by high flow of gas or entrainment of room air

    B. Provide a predictable FIO_2

    C. Does not necessarily mean high FIO_2

    D. Devices

        1. Venturi mask

        2. T-piece: may be high or low flow depending on flow rate

        3. Tracheostomy collar: may be high or low flow depending on flow rate

        4. Mechanical ventilator

Oxygen Delivery Systems (Table 4-16)
Hazards of Oxygen Therapy

I. Oxygen-induced hypoventilation

    A. Greatest risk if $PaCO_2$ greater than 50 mm Hg since low PaO_2 becomes primary stimulus to breath

        1. Airway obstruction

        2. COPD

        3. Respiratory center depression

    B. Prevention: use O_2 with caution but remember low PaO_2 not FIO_2 is stimulus to breath; use only enough oxygen to bring PaO_2 up to approximately 60 mm Hg or SaO_2 up to approximately 90%

II. Absorptive atelectasis

    A. Causes: high concentrations of oxygen (an absorbable gas) washes out the nitrogen (a nonabsorbable gas) that normally holds the alveoli open at the end of expiration and the effects of oxygen on pulmonary surfactant

    B. Prevention: do not administer oxygen that is not indicated

III. Oxygen toxicity

    A. Cause: too high a concentration over too long a period (hours to days)

    B. Pathophysiology

        1. Overproduction of oxygen-free radicals

        2. Large numbers of oxygen-free radicals overwhelms the supply of neutralizing enzymes

        3. Injury to capillary endothelium and increase in interstitial edema

        4. Injury to type I pneumocytes and intraalveolar edema

        5. Proliferation of type II pneumocytes

        6. Thickening of alveolar-capillary membrane

        7. Scarring and pulmonary fibrosis

    C. Clinical indications

        1. Early

            a) Substernal chest pain that increases with deep breathing

            b) Dry cough and tracheal irritation

            c) Dyspnea

            d) Upper airway changes (e.g., nasal stuffiness, sore throat, eye and ear discomfort)

            e) Anorexia, nausea, vomiting

            f) Fatigue, lethargy, malaise

            g) Restlessness

        2. Late

            a) Chest X-ray changes: atelectasis, patches of pneumonia

            b) Progressive ventilatory difficulty: decreased vital capacity, decreased compliance, hypercapnia

            c) Increased intrapulmonary shunt: increasing A:a gradient and decreased PaO_2/FIO_2 ratio; hypoxemia

    D. Prevention:

        1. Use the lowest FIO_2 possible to maintain a PaO_2 of at least 60 mm Hg (SaO_2 90%)

            a) Limit duration of 1.0 FIO_2 to 24 hours if at all possible

            b) Limit the use of FIO_2 above 0.60 to 2 to 3 days if at all possible

        2. Assess arterial blood gases frequently if FIO_2 is above 0.40 to ensure that high concentration is still required

Table 4-16 | **Summary of Oxygen Delivery Systems**

System	Advantages	Disadvantages	Miscellaneous
Nasal cannula 1-6 L/min delivers 24%-44% oxygen (4% increase with each liter)	• Safe and simple • Comfortable • Effective for low oxygen concentration • Allows eating and talking • Inexpensive	• Contraindicated in nasal obstruction • Causes drying and irritation of nasal mucosa • May cause necrosis at ears • Cannot be used when patient has nasal obstruction • Variable concentrations of oxygen depending on tidal volume, respiratory rate, flow rate, and nasal patency	• Ensure that flow rates do not exceed 6 L/min • Provide humidification if flow rates exceed 4 L/min • Use gauze pads under cannula at tops of ears to prevent pressure ulceration • Give oral and nasal care every 8 hours; moisten lips, nose with water-soluble lubricant
Simple face mask 6-10 L/min delivers 40%-60% oxygen	• Delivers high oxygen concentration • Doesn't dry mucous membranes of nose and mouth • Can be used in patients with nasal obstruction	• Hot, confining, uncomfortable • Tight seal necessary • Frequently poorly tolerated in dyspneic patient • Interferes with eating and talking • May cause CO_2 retention if flow rate is < 6 L/min • Variable concentrations of oxygen depending on tidal volume, respiratory rate, and flow rate • Can't deliver less than 40% • Potential for oxygen toxicity • Impractical for long-term therapy	• Place pads between mask and bony facial parts • Wash and dry face every 4 hours • Clean mask every 8 hours • Ensure flow rate of at least 6 L/min • Check ABGs frequently • Monitor for clinical indications of oxygen toxicity
Partial rebreathing mask 6-10 L/min delivers 35%-60%	• Delivers high oxygen concentrations • Doesn't dry mucous membranes	• As for face mask • May cause CO_2 retention if reservoir bag is allowed to collapse	• Ensure that bag does not totally deflate during inhalation (increase flow rate) • Keep mask snug • Check ABGs frequently • Monitor for clinical indications of oxygen toxicity
Nonrebreathing mask 6-10 L/min delivers 60%-100%	• As for other masks • One-way valves prevent rebreathing of CO_2 and increases oxygen concentrations	• As for other masks except does not cause CO_2 retention	• As for partial rebreathing mask • Check ABGs frequently • Monitor for clinical indications of oxygen toxicity
Venturi mask 4 L/min delivers 24%-28% 8 L/min delivers 35%-40%	• Delivers accurate oxygen concentration depending on flow rate and diluter jet inserted despite changes in patient's respiratory pattern • Oxygen concentration can be changed • Doesn't dry mucous membranes	• FIo_2 can be lowered if mask doesn't fit snugly, if tubing is kinked, if oxygen intake ports are blocked, or if less than recommended liter flow is used • Hot, confining, uncomfortable • Tight seal necessary • Frequently poorly tolerated in dyspneic patient • Interferes with eating and talking	• Check ABGs frequently • Monitor for clinical indications of oxygen toxicity • As for other masks

Table 4-16	Summary of Oxygen Delivery Systems—cont'd		
System	**Advantages**	**Disadvantages**	**Miscellaneous**
Tracheostomy collar 21%-70% 10 L or to provide visible mist	• Does not pull on tracheostomy • Elastic ties allow movement of mask away from tracheostomy without removing it	• Oxygen diluted by room air • Increased likelihood of infection and skin irritation around stoma because of high humidity • Condensation can collect in the tubing and drain into patient's airway, especially during turning	• Ensure that oxygen is warmed and humidified • Empty condensation from tubing frequently; empty into water trap or container for appropriate discard; do not empty water back into humidifier
T-piece or tube flow rate set at 2.5 times patient's minute ventilation to deliver 21%-100%	• Delivers variable concentrations • Less moisture around tracheostomy than with tracheostomy collar	• May cause CO_2 retention at low-flow rates • Weight of T-piece can pull on tracheostomy tube • Condensation can collect in the tubing and drain into patient's airway, especially during turning	• Requires heated nebulizer • Use extension on open side to act as a reservoir and increase oxygen concentration as prescribed • Empty condensation from tubing frequently • Check ABGs frequently • Monitor for clinical indications of oxygen toxicity
Mechanical ventilation 21%-100%	• Delivers predictable, constant concentrations of oxygen • Supports ventilation as well as oxygenation • Addition of positive end-expiratory pressure (PEEP) augments the driving pressure of oxygen; this aids in the achievement of acceptable Pao_2 levels at lower oxygen concentrations	• Requires skilled personnel • Requires electricity and backup power generator (plug into red outlet) • Condensation can collect in the tubing and drain into patient's airway, especially during turning	• Requires heated humidifier • Empty condensation from tubing frequently • Check ABGs frequently • Monitor for clinical indications of oxygen toxicity

3. Utilize PEEP to increase the driving pressure of oxygen; use of PEEP achieves:
   a) The same Pao_2 at a lower FIo_2
   b) A better Pao_2 at the same FIo_2
4. Remember that hypoxia is far more common than O_2 toxicity and must be corrected; **actual** hypoxemia should never be allowed to persist because of concern regarding **potential** oxygen toxicity

Hyperbaric Oxygenation

I. Definition: administration of high concentration (usually 100%) oxygen under greatly increased pressure (usually 2-3 atmospheres)
II. Indications: carbon monoxide poisoning, air embolism, radiation therapy, gas gangrene, burns, decubiti
III. Actions: can cause a 22-fold increase in Pao_2, which increases the amount of oxygen dissolved in the blood to enhance tissue oxygenation
IV. Complications: oxygen toxicity, absorptive atelectasis, acute respiratory distress syndrome

Mechanical Ventilation
Indications for Mechanical Ventilation

I. Acute ventilatory failure with respiratory acidosis not relieved by ordinary methods
II. Hypoxemia despite maximum oxygen therapy
III. Relief of hypoxemia causes increased CO_2 retention
IV. Apnea
V. Physiologic indications
   A. Vital capacity less than 10 ml/kg or twice predicted tidal volume
   B. Unable to achieve maximal inspiratory force of −20 cm H_2O
   C. Pao_2 less than 60 mm Hg with FIo_2 greater than 0.6
   D. Arterial $Paco_2$ below 30 or above 50 mm Hg (hypercapnia must be accompanied by acidosis to be an indication for mechanical ventilation)
   E. Deadspace/tidal volume ratio (V_D/V_T) greater than 0.60
   F. Respiratory rate greater than 30 to 35/min

Types of Ventilators

I. Negative pressure ventilators
  A. Types: iron lung, chest cuirass, poncho style, body wrap
  B. Ventilatory process
    1. Negative pressure generated outside of body, excluding the upper airway
    2. Negativity transmitted to intrapleural and intraalveolar spaces
    3. Pressure gradient occurs and air moves into lungs
    4. Expiration passively occurs by removing negative pressure around the chest wall
  C. Uses
    1. Restricted to nonpulmonary (e.g., neuromuscular) problems
    2. Long-term ventilator support without an artificial airway
    3. Used primarily in home or rehabilitation settings
  D. Advantages
    1. Artificial airway not required
    2. Normal breathing mechanics maintained; avoids harmful changes in intrathoracic pressure caused by positive pressure ventilators
  E. Disadvantages
    1. Not helpful for patients with lung disease
    2. Not possible to precisely regulate tidal volume and alveolar ventilation
    3. Large size required (e.g., iron lung)
    4. Restriction of patient movement
    5. Patient care difficult since body is enclosed in ventilator
    6. Difficulty obtaining a seal around chest
    7. May cause venous pooling in the abdomen, leading to decreased cardiac output particularly in hypovolemic patients
II. Positive pressure ventilators
  A. Ventilatory process
    1. Inspiration is created by positive pressure being pushed into the airway
    2. Expiration occurs passively when the positive pressure stops
  B. Cycling classifications
    1. Pressure-cycled: deliver inspiratory flow until preset pressure is met
     a) Advantages
      (1) Relatively inexpensive
      (2) Mobile
      (3) Run on compressed air or oxygen
     b) Disadvantages
      (1) Tidal volume varies dependent on compliance of the lung and the integrity of the ventilatory circuit
      (2) Sealed airway (e.g., cuffed endotracheal tube or tracheostomy tube) is required
      (3) Positive intrathoracic pressure decreases venous return to the right side of the heart and may decrease

cardiac output, especially in hypovolemic patients
      (4) Barotrauma (e.g., pneumothorax, pneumomediastinum, subcutaneous emphysema) may occur
    2. Volume-cycled: deliver inspiratory flow until preset volume is met
     a) Advantages: delivers the set tidal volume regardless of changes in lung compliance
     b) Disadvantages
      (1) Sealed airway is required
      (2) Positive intrathoracic pressure decreases venous return to the right side of the heart and may decrease cardiac output, especially in hypovolemic patients
      (3) Barotrauma may occur
  C. Modes: refers to how the machine senses or signals the initiation of inspiration (Fig. 4-29 and Table 4-17)
  D. Expiratory maneuvers
    1. Positive end-expiratory pressure (PEEP)
     a) Definition: maintenance of pressure above atmospheric at airway opening at end-expiration
      (1) Physiologic: 3 to 5 cm
      (2) Therapeutic: more than 5 cm (there is no true upper limit but the higher the level, the greater the chance of barotrauma)
      (3) Best (or optimal) PEEP: PEEP that provides SaO_2 of at least 90% without compromising cardiac output (remember that tissue oxygen delivery is affected by SaO_2, Hgb, and CO; if SaO_2 is increased but CO is decreased, no true gains in tissue oxygen delivery are achieved, and tissue oxygen delivery may even be decreased)
      (4) Auto-PEEP (also called *occult PEEP* or *intrinsic PEEP*) (Fig. 4-30)
       (a) The development of PEEP as a result of obstructed or impeded exhalation
       (b) Generally seen as undesirable
       (c) Adds to therapeutic PEEP
       (d) Can be measured by occluding the ventilator circuit expiratory outlet at end-expiratation
     b) Actions of PEEP
      (1) Increases the driving pressure of oxygen
       (a) Improves the PaO_2 without increasing the FIO_2
       (b) Allows the use of lower FIO_2 to achieve the same PaO_2, thereby decreasing risk of oxygen toxicity
      (2) Decreases surface tension to prevent alveolar collapse at end-expiration
      (3) Decreases intrapulmonary shunt by

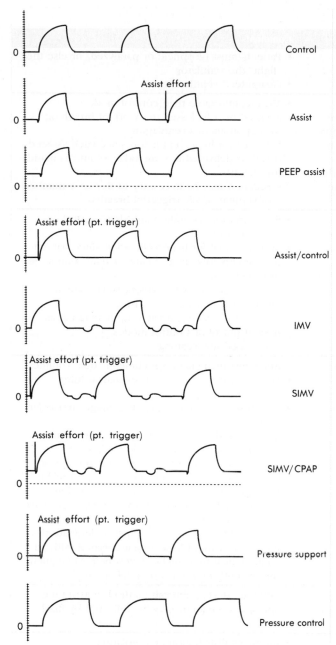

Figure 4-29 Common modes of mechanical ventilation. (From McPherson SP, Spearman CB: *Respiratory therapy equipment,* St Louis, 1990, Mosby.)

opening alveoli that are collapsed (referred to as *alveolar recruitment*); increases functional residual capacity

c) Uses of PEEP
  (1) Acute respiratory distress syndrome (ARDS) (also referred to as *noncardiac pulmonary edema*)
  (2) Cardiac pulmonary edema
  (3) Acute respiratory failure with persistent hypoxemia
  (4) Physiologic PEEP is used in intubated patients to mimic the positive end-expiratory pressure exerted by the closed glottis

d) Adverse effects of PEEP
  (1) Hemodynamic consequences of positive pressure ventilation is accentuated
    (a) Decreased venous return
    (b) Increased right ventricular afterload
    (c) Decreased left ventricular distensibility
    (d) Decreased cardiac output
  (2) Barotrauma
  (3) Increased intracranial pressure (ICP)
e) Contraindications of therapeutic PEEP
  (1) Untreated hypovolemia
  (2) Hypovolemic, neurogenic, anaphylactic, or septic shock
  (3) Extreme caution in patients with COPD
f) Nursing management to maintain PEEP
  (1) Monitor vital signs and hemodynamic parameters closely
  (2) Maintain prescribed levels of PEEP; patients with an inspiratory effort pull a negative pressure and negate the level of PEEP; these patients require sedation and/or muscle paralysis to maintain the therapeutic effects of PEEP
    (a) Sedation: diazepam (Valium) or lorazepam (Ativan) may be used
    (b) Analgesics: morphine intermittently or infusion may be needed, especially in patients who have chest trauma or surgery
    (c) Muscle paralysis (e.g., pancuronium [Pavulon], vecuronium [Norcuron], atracurium [Tracrium])
      (i) Sedatives and/or analgesics must always be given with these agents
      (ii) Inform the patient that the effect is temporary
      (iii) Patient does not have blink reflex; protect the cornea by instilling saline or artificial tears into each eye at least every 4 hours
      (iv) May cause residual muscle weakness; use peripheral nerve stimulation unit to evaluate level of paralysis (Fig. 4-31)
      (v) Discontinue muscle paralytics at least 24 hours prior to weaning
2. Continuous positive airway pressure (CPAP): nonventilator technique for maintaining positive pressure during spontaneous ventilation

Table 4-17 | Modes of Mechanical Ventilation

Mode	Description	Comments
Control	Preset volume delivered at a preset rate; circuit is closed between these mandatory breaths	• Patients must be apneic or paralyzed, or else they "fight" the ventilator • Guaranteed ventilation
Assist/control (also called *assisted mandatory ventilation*)	Preset volume is delivered for each patient inspiratory effort of set amount; if the patient fails to initiate a minimum number of breaths per minute by generating a specified amount of negative pressure, the ventilator will initiate the breaths at the preset volume and rate	• More comfortable than control mode • Assisted breaths lessen the work of breathing over spontaneous ventilation • Potential for hyperventilation since each assisted breath is delivered at same tidal volume as mandatory breaths • Sedation may be necessary to decrease number of spontaneously triggered breaths
Synchronized intermittent mandatory ventilation (SIMV)	Preset volume delivered at preset rate; patient may take additional breaths of any tidal volume from the open circuit between these mandatory breaths; mandatory breaths are synchronized so that they do not interrupt the patient's own ventilatory efforts	• Better muscle reconditioning than control or assist/control • Less potential for hyperventilation since patient-initiated breaths are at whatever tidal volume he or she chooses • May be more work for patient since patient-initiated breaths are not assisted • Does not decrease cardiac output as much as Assist/Control or Control modes • Often used for weaning
Pressure support ventilation (PSV)	Preset positive pressure is initiated by the patient's inspiratory effort; tidal volume and rate is patient-controlled minimal level; augments or assists spontaneous breaths	• Augments inadequate spontaneous tidal volumes • Lower mean airway pressures than volume ventilation • Use of respiratory muscles discourages muscular atrophy • May be used with IMV or alone; if used alone, patient must be spontaneously breathing • There is no preset respiratory rate, and apnea occurs if the patient does not initiate a breath; newer models provide a volume ventilation backup (called *volume-assured pressure support ventilation* [VAPSV]) • Low level (5-10 cm H_2O) helps to eliminate the increased work of breathing associated with an endotracheal tube; higher levels help to augment the patient's own intrinsic tidal volume
Bi-PAP	Preset positive pressure delivered during inspiration and expiration; each level may be set independently	• Often used as an interim method to avoid mechanical ventilation; may be delivered by mask
Inverse ratio ventilation (IRV)	Inspiratory time is greater than expiratory time; I:E ratio of 2:1 or greater; may be volume controlled or pressure controlled	• Improves distribution of ventilation • Prevents collapse of alveoli • Increased mean airway pressure • May decrease cardiac output • Makes the patient uncomfortable; patients usually require sedation to decrease discomfort and anxiety; muscle paralysis may be required along with sedation • May cause auto-PEEP, which when added to therapeutic PEEP increases risk of barotrauma • Increases Pao_2 and Sao_2 • Do not use in patients with COPD
Pressure-controlled/ inverse ratio ventilation (PC/IRV)	Combination of pressure support ventilation and inverse ratio ventilation; tidal volume is delivered by pressure	• Improves oxygenation and allows reduction of FIo_2 • May be used in ARDS with refractory hypoxemia • As for PSV and IRV

Table 4-17   Modes of Mechanical Ventilation—cont'd

Mode	Description	Comments
High-frequency ventilation (HFV)	Preset (very low) volumes delivered at preset (very high) rates; ventilation and oxygenation are achieved by gas diffusion and convection • High-frequency positive pressure ventilation (HFPPV): 60-120 bpm • High-frequency jet ventilation (HFJV): 120-600 bpm • High-frequency oscillation ventilation (HFO): 500-1200 oscillations per minute	• May be used in some cases of chest trauma or bronchopleural fistula; has not been proven to be effective in ARDS • Causes lower airway and intrathoracic pressures than traditional mechanical ventilation; may decrease the incidence of barotrauma and decreased cardiac output • Muscle paralysis and/or sedation usually required • May cause increased oral secretions • Auscultation of heart and lung sounds is difficult • Requires special ventilator
Independent lung ventilation (ILV) (also called *differential lung ventilation*)	• Ventilation technique that ventilates each lung separately • Separate modes and tidal volumes may be used for each lung	• Used for unilateral pathology or thoracic trauma • Requires double lumen tube, separate ventilators to each lumen, and a synchronizer • Patient requires sedation and/or paralysis

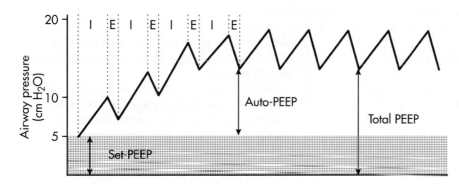

Figure 4-30   Auto-PEEP as is frequently seen in inverse ratio ventilation. Insufficient expiratory time permits the trapping of gases in the lung. This trapped gas creates pressure, which is known as auto-PEEP. This PEEP is added to therapeutic PEEP for total PEEP. (From Pierce L: *Guide to mechanical ventilation and intensive respiratory care,* Philadelphia, 1995, Saunders.)

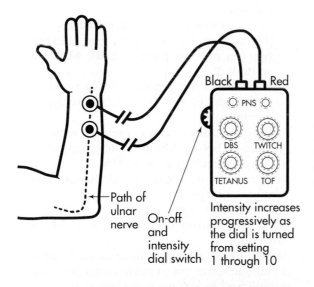

Figure 4-31   Peripheral nerve stimulator. Note placement of electrodes along ulnar nerve. If train of four is used, one or two twitches of the thumb is a desirable result. Absence of any thumb twitch indicates overparalysis (reduce dosage of paralytic agent). Three or four twitches of the thumb indicates underparalysis (increase dosage of paralytic agent). (From Thelan LA et al: *Critical care nursing: diagnosis and management,* ed 3, St Louis, 1998, Mosby.)

a) May be used by mask as an interim treatment to prevent the need for intubation or for sleep apnea
   (1) Monitor for skin breakdown on face because CPAP mask must fit tightly
   (2) Monitor closely for gastric distention
   (3) Do not use in patients without airway protective reflexes
b) May be used to wean a patient from PEEP

Mechanical Ventilator Parameters

I. Minute ventilation: 6 to 10 L/min
   A. Tidal volume: 5 to 15 ml/kg body weight though the current trend is to stay between 5 to 10 ml/kg to avoid volutrauma and barotrauma
   B. Respiratory rate: varies according to ventilator flow rate, I:E ratio, and whether ventilator is on control or assist mode; usually 8 to 16/min

II. FIO$_2$
   A. Initially 1.0 for 20 minutes, especially if cardiac arrest
   B. Adjusted so that Pao$_2$ is 60 mm Hg
   C. Use lowest FIO$_2$ that achieves desired Pao$_2$
   D. PEEP may be added to maintain acceptable Pao$_2$ with lower FIO$_2$ to reduce the risk of oxygen toxicity

III. Sensitivity: if assist mode is used
   A. Amount of inspiratory effort required to initiate an assisted breath
   B. Usually set at −1 to −2 cm H$_2$O

IV. Sigh
   A. Volume: 1.5 to 2 times the inspired tidal volume
   B. Frequency: 10 to 15 times/hr
   C. Infrequently used if patient is receiving large tidal volumes or PEEP

V. Humidification
   A. Continuous humidification is required with inspired air warmed to body temperature; temperature usually maintained at 32° to 37° C and humidity at 100%
   B. Nebulizers are emptied and refilled at least every 8 hours
   C. Water condensation is emptied frequently into a water trap or container for discard

VI. Flow rate
   A. Usually 40 to 80 L/min but adjusted so that inspiratory volume can be completed in time allowed, based on desired respiratory rate and I:E ratio
      1. Slower the flow rate, better distribution in normal lung
      2. Faster the flow rate, better for patients with COPD
   B. Patient comfort is also a consideration: does the patient feel like he or she is getting enough air?

VII. I:E ratio
   A. Usually 1:1.5 or 1:2
   B. Inverse ratio ventilation: more time for inspiration than expiration

VIII. Alarm settings: all alarms should be ON
   A. High-pressure alarm: set alarm 10 to 20 cm H$_2$O above the patient's peak inspiratory pressure
      1. Causes for high-pressure alarm
         a) Increased airway resistance: secretions, bronchospasm, kink in tubing, displacement of artificial airway, patient coughing during inspiration, patient biting on ET tube, water condensation in tubing
         b) Decreased compliance: pneumothorax (sudden increase), development of pulmonary edema, atelectasis, pneumonia, ARDS (gradual increase)
   B. Low-exhaled-volume alarm: set alarm at 50 to 100 ml below inspired tidal volume; causes for low-exhaled-volume alarm:

      1. Disconnection
      2. Cuff leak
      3. Leak in circuitry
      4. Overbreathing: occurs when the patient deeply inspires as the ventilator delivers inspiration; the ventilator senses low pressure; this patient may require sedation to prevent recurrent ventilator alarms
   C. Apnea: ON
      1. Patient fatigue
      2. Overmedication
      3. Decrease in level of consciousness
   D. Low FIO$_2$: ON
      1. Oxygen disconnect
      2. Break in inspiratory circuit

IX. Power: the mechanical ventilator must be pulled into a grounded electrical outlet that is backed up by the emergency generator; this outlet is usually red

Assessment

I. Pulmonary
   A. Airway: type, size, position, cuff pressure
   B. Chest excursion, use of accessory muscles
   C. Breath sounds
   D. Secretions: amount, color, consistency, odor
   E. Ventilatory mechanics: patient's own tidal volume, vital capacity, minute ventilation, maximal inspiratory pressure, respiratory rate
   F. Ventilator parameters
      1. Mode: as set
      2. Tidal volume as set and exhaled
      3. Respiratory rate: ventilator and patient initiated
      4. FIO$_2$: confirmed with oxygen analyzer
      5. PEEP: airway pressure at the end of expiration (on pressure gauge not just what it is set to be)
      6. Peak inspiratory pressure: airway pressure at the peak of inspiration; calculate dynamic compliance
      7. Plateau pressure: airway pressure with an inflation hold; calculate static compliance
      8. Alarms: check that all are ON
   G. Ventilator circuitry: leaks, condensation, temperature of inspired air
   H. Pulse oximetry: Spo$_2$
   I. Chest X-ray: usually done daily unless chronic situation
   J. Arterial blood gases: usually done daily, 20 to 30 minutes after any ventilator changes, and as indicated by change in patient status
      1. Table 4-18 describes mechanical ventilator parameter changes to make in response to ABGs

II. Cardiovascular
   A. Heart rate
   B. ECG rhythm
   C. Heart sounds
   D. Blood pressure: direct (arterial catheter) or indirect (auscultated)

Table 4-18	Mechanical Ventilator Parameter Changes to make According to Arterial Blood Gases	
If $Paco_2$ is >45 mm Hg (or above the patient's normal if patient has COPD)	• Increase ventilation • Increase rate • Increase tidal volume (if it does not currently exceed 15 ml/kg)
If $Paco_2$ is <35 mm Hg (unless therapeutic hypocapnia is being maintained [e.g., increased ICP])	• Decrease ventilation • Decrease rate • Decrease tidal volume • If patient on Assist/Control mode: change mode from AC to IMV • Consider sedation • Some physicians may add mechanical deadspace (tubing that acts as a rebreathing device)
If Pao_2 is <60 mm Hg	• Increase Fio_2 • Add or increase PEEP (especially if Fio_2 is already >0.5)
If Pao_2 is >100 mm Hg	• Decrease Fio_2 • Decrease PEEP

  E. Hemodynamic parameters: RAP, PAP, PAOP, CO/CI, SVR/SVRI, PVR/PVRI, Svo_2
III. Neurologic
   A. Level of consciousness
   B. Airway reflexes: gag, swallowing, corneal
IV. Renal/Metabolic
   A. Urine output
   B. Urine specific gravity
   C. Serum electrolytes
 V. Gastrointestinal
   A. Abdominal distention
   B. Bowel sounds
   C. Guaiac testing: NG aspirate, vomitus, stools
VI. Nutritional status
   A. Daily weight
   B. Total protein, albumin, and serum transferrin levels
   C. Calorie counts and nutrient balance
VII. Immunologic
   A. Temperature
   B. Sputum cultures
   C. WBC count
VIII. Psychologic
   A. Complaints of pain or anxiety
   B. Clinical indicators of pain or anxiety

Potential Complications of Positive Pressure Ventilation (Table 4-19)
Weaning
   I. Definition: the gradual withdrawal of ventilatory support for patients who have been mechanically ventilated for more than 24 hours

 II. Indications
   A. Resolution or improvement of disease process that necessitated mechanical ventilation
   B. Patient's strength, nutritional status, and consciousness are adequate
   C. Stable and acceptable hemodynamics and hemoglobin
   D. Patient does not require more than 5 cm of PEEP or Fio_2 greater than 0.50 to maintain acceptable Pao_2 (Pao_2 60 mm Hg)
   E. $Paco_2$ less than 45 mm Hg or equal to the patient's baseline $Paco_2$
   F. Tidal volume greater than 5 ml/kg
   G. Vital capacity greater than 10 ml/kg or twice predicted tidal volume
   H. Minute ventilation less than 10 L/min
   I. Maximal inspiratory pressure more negative than −20 cm H_2O
   J. Respiratory rate less than 25 breaths per minute
   K. Patient is psychologically prepared and cooperative; the mechanical ventilator may provide security, so it may be helpful to leave it in room with patient for 24 hours after weaning
III. Methods
   A. General guidelines
      1. Position for optimal ventilation: usually semi-Fowler's to high Fowler's
      2. Avoid depressing the patient's ventilatory drive and muscle strength by avoiding sedatives and muscle paralytics; treat pain but do not overnarcotize
      3. Reduce carbohydrates if indicated; equivalent calories can be provided in the form of fats
         a) Utilize Pulmocare if being fed enterally: high fat and protein but low carbohydrates
         b) Decrease glucose and increase fat (Intralipids) if being fed parenterally
      4. Do not attempt to wean the patient at night
      5. Complementary therapies such as biofeedback and music may be helpful
      6. Monitor closely for clinical indicators of fatigue and ventilatory failure; these symptoms indicate the need to abort weaning efforts at this time
         a) Decreased level of consciousness
         b) Systolic BP increased or decreased by 20 mm Hg
         c) Heart rate increased by 30 bpm or greater
         d) PVCs more than 6/min, couplets, or runs of ventricular tachycardia
         e) ST segment changes
         f) Respiratory rate more than 30/min or less than 10/min
         g) Use of accessory muscle of ventilation
         h) Paradoxical chest wall motion
         i) Complaints of dyspnea, fatigue, or pain
         j) Spo_2 less than 90%
         k) Increase in $Paco_2$ of 5 to 8 mm Hg and/or pH of less than 7.30

| Table 4-19 | Complications of Mechanical Ventilation | | | |

Complication	Causes	Prevention	Clinical Presentation	Treatment

Decreased cardiac output	• Increased intrathoracic pressures that
	  • decrease venous return to the right side of the heart
	  • increase RV afterload
	  • decrease LV distensibility
		• Ensure adequate preload prior to mechanical ventilation
		• Avoid excessive tidal volumes
		• Adjust PEEP carefully
			• Tachycardia, hypotension
			• Cool, clammy skin
			• Decrease in urine output
			• Change in level of consciousness
				• Administer fluids to increase preload
				• Administer inotropes as prescribed

Fluid retention	• Decrease in insensible loss via respiratory system • Overhydration by humidification • Decreased urine output due to ADH and aldosterone secretion	• Avoid decrease in cardiac output, which stimulates renin-angiotensin-aldosterone system	• Weight gain • Intake greater than output • Crackles • Decreased compliance	• Utilize previous therapies to prevent decrease in cardiac output
Barotrauma: pneumothorax; pneumomediastinum; subcutaneous emphysema; bronchopleural fistula	• Caused by excessive intraalveolar pressure; overdistended alveolus ruptures, forcing air into interstitial tissue • Increased chance if patient on PEEP, high tidal volume, elderly, or has COPD	• Avoid excessive tidal volumes • Adjust PEEP carefully	• Chest pain, dyspnea • Sudden increase in peak inspiratory pressure • Decreased breath sounds and chest movement on affected side • Tracheal shift • Hypotension, JVD if tension pneumothorax • Clinical indications of hypoxia • Decreased SpO_2 • Chest X-ray changes	• Decrease tidal volume or PEEP if possible to decrease mean airway pressure • Utilize high-frequency ventilation especially if bronchopleural fistula • If pneumothorax suspected: take patient off ventilator and manually ventilate with a manual resuscitation bag • Assist with insertion of chest tube for pneumothorax
Atelectasis	• Airway obstruction • Small tidal volumes or lack of sighing • Infrequent turning of patient	• Use larger tidal volumes or periodic sighing • Turn frequently • Provide adequate humidification • Perform tracheal suctioning as indicated • Provide chest physical therapy (PT) as indicated • Reposition frequently	• Diminished breath sounds • Crackles • Abnormal chest X-ray • Increased A:a gradient • Decreased compliance	• Increase tidal volume or provide periodic sighing • Provide chest PT
Hypercapnia; hypocapnia	• Inadequate or excessive ventilation • Hypermetabolism may contribute to hypercapnia	• Initiate ventilation with tidal volume at 5-15 ml/kg and rate of 8-12 • Make ventilator changes after initial ABGs	• Increased (>45 mm Hg) or decreased (<35 mm Hg) $PaCO_2$	• Hypercapnia: increase tidal volume or rate • Hypocapnia: decrease rate or tidal volume; change to IMV or PSV
Oxygen toxicity	• Too high a concentration of O_2 over too long a time	• Maintain FIO_2 below 0.50 if possible • **REMEMBER:** hypoxemia is far more common than O_2 toxicity and must be corrected	• Substernal distress • Paresthesias in extremities • Anorexia, nausea, vomiting • Fatigue, lethargy, malaise	• Decrease O_2 concentration as soon as possible • Provide supportive management

Table 4-19

Table 4-19 Complications of Mechanical Ventilation—cont'd

Complication	Causes	Prevention	Clinical Presentation	Treatment
Oxygen toxicity—cont'd			• Restlessness • Dyspnea, progressive respiratory difficulty • Decreased compliance • Increased A:a gradient	
Aspiration	• Stomach contents • Tube feedings • Oral secretions • Gastric distention • Impaired gastric emptying • Gastroesophageal reflux	• Maintain cuff inflation using minimal occlusive volume • Keep head of bed elevated during and after tube feedings • Check for gastric retention at least every 4 hours • Check NG tube placement at least every 4 hours	• Increased tracheal secretions • Fever • Rhonchi, wheezes • Clinical indications of hypoxemia/hypoxia • Infiltrate on chest X-ray	• Provide supportive management • Administer antibiotics as prescribed • Administer steroids as prescribed
GI effects: stress ulcer, ileus, gastric dilation	• Hyperacidity • Endogenous or exogenous steroids • Gastric or mesenteric ischemia • Inadequate nutrition	• Utilize enteral feedings • Administer antacids; H_2-receptor antagonists (e.g., cimetidine [Tagamet]); barrier agents (e.g., sucralfate [Carafate]) as prescribed	• NG aspirate, vomitus, or stools positive for blood • Decreased bowel sounds • Gastric distention • Increased gastric retention	• Note effect of hemoglobin loss of tissue oxygenation; blood administration may be necessary • Administer antacids, H_2-receptor antagonists, sucralfate as prescribed
Infection	• Immunosuppression • Artificial airways bypass normal upper airway defense mechanisms • Ventilatory equipment: warm, moist environment is good for bacterial growth • Suctioning procedure • Silent aspiration of GI bacteria when H_2 antagonists or antacids used for ulcer prophylaxis • Cross-contamination may be cause	• Use good handwashing techniques • Use sterile technique for suctioning • Provide aseptic airway management, tubing changes, etc. • Avoid change in usual acidic gastric pH • Keep head of bed elevated during tube feedings • Keep ET tube or trach cuff inflated to 18 mm Hg • Drain humidifier condensation into water trap or container and not back into humidifier	• Tachycardia, tachypnea • Fever • Crackles, rhonchi, or wheezes • Hypoxemia • Change in color or character of sputum • Positive cultures • Infiltrate on chest X-ray	• Administer antibiotic specific to culture
Patient-ventilator asynchrony (patient "fighting" ventilator)	• Incorrect ventilator setup for the patient's needs • Acute change in patient's status • Obstructed airway • Ventilator malfunction • Anxiety	• Ensure proper setup of ventilator equipment; monitor settings every hour • Monitor peak inspiratory pressure • Suction as indicated • Talk to patient, keep him or her informed • Administer anxiolytics as indicated	• Anxiety, agitation • Increase in peak inspiratory pressure • Ventilator alarm sounding • Change in pulse oximetry or ABGs	• Perform rapid check of patient and ventilator • Disconnect patient from ventilator and provide manual ventilation via manual resuscitation bag • Check vital signs, breath sounds, pulse oximetry • Assess ABGs • Suction airway • Check patency of endotracheal or tracheostomy tube

Continued

Table 4-19	Complications of Mechanical Ventilation—cont'd			
Complication	**Causes**	**Prevention**	**Clinical Presentation**	**Treatment**
Anxiety	• Loss of autonomy over vital body function (breathing) • Inability to communicate • Sensory overload (e.g., alarms, repeated interruptions for vital signs, noise of ventilator) • Sensory deprivation (e.g., separation from family, work, meaningful activities) • Discomfort (e.g., arterial punctures, endotracheal tube, nasogastric tube, Foley catheter, etc.)	• Explain to patient why he or she can't speak; provide method of communication • Explain all procedures thoroughly; keep patient informed regarding progress and plans • Add familiar objects to patient's environment (e.g., family photos, cards) • Have calendar, clock in room; have window shades or curtains open to orient patient to light and dark • Allow uninterrupted time for rest and sleep • Put eyeglasses and hearing aide on patient if appropriate • Encourage expression of fears • Be available; answer call bell promptly • Promote as much independence as possible • Provide emotional support to the family • Avoid uncomfortable or painful procedures if possible (e.g., arterial catheter instead of arterial punctures)	• High pressure alarm because the patient is breathing out of synch with ventilator • Tachycardia • Tachypnea, excessive triggering of ventilator is on assist/control, potentially causing hypocapnia and respiratory alkalosis • Complaints of being "nervous"	• Stay with patient during times of extreme anxiety • Use therapeutic touch (e.g., hold hand) • Utilize soft restraints only as necessary to prevent self-extubation • Encourage family visitation and participation if appropriate
Inability to wean	• COPD: occurs when $Paco_2$ is corrected instead of pH • Malnutrition: catabolism and muscle breakdown • Neuromuscular blocking agents: disuse syndrome	• Correct pH instead of $Paco_2$ in patients with COPD • Provide adequate calories to prevent catabolism; adequate protein and high calories are given; adequate calories must be given to prevent the protein from being utilized for energy; calories given are predominantly fat because CHO metabolism produces more CO_2 • Avoid neuromuscular blocking agents if possible; limit duration of use	• Increased $Paco_2$, increased ventilatory rate, tachycardia with weaning efforts	• COPD: allow $Paco_2$ to increase so that the kidney will hold on to bicarbonate to compensate; keep Pao_2 close to patient's normal (e.g., 60-65 mm Hg) • Provide adequate protein and calories; avoid high-carbohydrate feedings during weaning • Discontinue neuromuscular blocking agents several days prior to weaning

B. T-piece method
1. Place patient on T-piece with O_2 10 percent higher than when on ventilator or as prescribed; gradually increase the amount of time that patient is off the ventilator; CPAP frequently used with T-piece
2. Advantage: may be able to wean patient more quickly than IMV method
3. Disadvantage: recurrent ventilatory failures discourage and frighten the patient
C. IMV method
1. Gradually reduce IMV rate
2. Advantages
   a) Provides exercise for ventilatory musculature
   b) More physiologic Pa_{CO_2} may be achieved
   c) Large ventilator-provided breaths help to prevent atelectasis
   d) Safer than trial-and-error method
   e) Good acceptance by patients
3. Disadvantages: may take longer than T-piece method
D. Pressure support method
1. Gradually decrease the amount of pressure support assisting the patient
2. Advantages
   a) Patient comfort frequently greater with PSV
   b) Work of breathing less than with IMV or T-piece method
E. CPAP
1. May be used for patients whose Pa_{O_2} is PEEP-dependent; the patient is weaned from the ventilator by one of the previous methods but left on CPAP to provide the improved driving pressure needed to maintain an adequate Pa_{O_2}

LEARNING ACTIVITIES

1. **DIRECTIONS:** Complete the following crossword puzzle to review pulmonary anatomy and physiology.

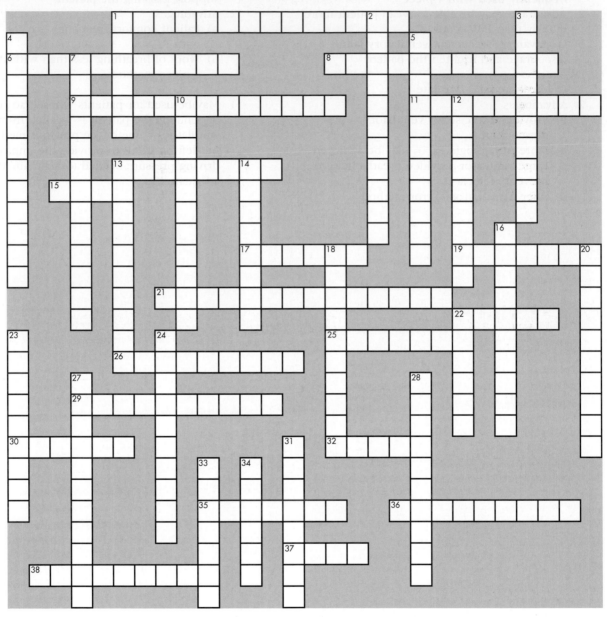

Across

1. Lowest portion of the pharynx
6. Active phase of ventilation
8. First bronchial branch that is part of the gas exchange unit is the _____ bronchiole
9. Relationship between Pao$_2$ and hemoglobin saturation is illustrated on the _____ dissociation curve
11. Main accessory muscles of expiration include the internal intercostal and _____ muscles
13. Pleural layer contiguous with chest wall
15. Pores of _____ are openings between the alveoli
17. Primary responsibility of the cardiac and pulmonary systems is to ensure the delivery of _____ to the tissues
19. Passage or opening through the vocal cords
21. Receptors that are stimulated by an increase in interstitial fluid volume
22. Hairlike projections that move mucus with entrapped particles upward to be coughed out
25. Area of upper lobe of the left lung, which corresponds to the middle lobe of the right lung
26. Ability of the lung to recoil
29. Passive phase of ventilation
30. Type of compliance that reflects compliance of the lung and chest wall
32. When deoxygenated blood comes in contact with nonventilated alveoli; V < Q
35. Type of compliance that reflects compliance and airway resistance

36. Pleural layer contiguous with lung
37. Structure that is primarily responsible for warming, humidifying, and filtering inspired air
38. Nutrient circulation of the lung is supplied by this artery

Down
1. First portion of the trachea
2. Eustachian tubes open into the _____
3. Structures that increase the surface area in the nose

4. Cellular organelles that use oxygen to make ATP
5. Most carbon dioxide is transported in the blood as _____
7. Receptors that increase ventilation rate in response to body movement
10. Center of thoracic cavity
12. Primary muscle of inspiration
13. Surfactant is produced by the type II _____
14. Type of deadspace that describes air in the alveoli that is not perfused

16. Change in pressure for a given change in volume
18. Flexible cartilage attached to the thyroid cartilage; closes to protect the larynx
20. Lipoprotein that decreases intraalveolar surface tension
22. Bifurcation of the trachea
23. Process by which oxygen and carbon dioxide move across the alveolar-capillary membrane
24. Phagocyte located in the alveolus
27. Movement of air into and out of the lungs

28. Type of deadspace that describes the air in conducting pathways
31. Last branch of the conducting airways is the _____ bronchiole
33. Central chemoreceptors are located in this area of the brain
34. Dense concentration of lymphatic tissue that protects entryways to respiratory and GI tracts

2.   DIRECTIONS: Fill in the primary and accessory muscles of inspiration and expiration.

	Primary	Accessory
Inspiration		
Expiration		

3.   DIRECTIONS: Identify whether the following factors cause a shift of the oxyhemoglobin curve to the left or right.

	Left	Right
Increased 2,3-DPG		
Hypothermia		
Hypercapnia		
Hyperthermia		
Acidosis		
Decreased 2,3-DPG		
Hypocapnia		
Alkalosis		
Hypophosphatemia		
Massive blood transfusion		

4. **DIRECTIONS:** Identify the following conditions as restrictive or obstructive. Remember: If compliance of the lung or chest wall is affected, the condition is restrictive; if airway resistance is affected, the condition is obstructive.

	Restrictive	Obstructive
Obesity hypoventilation syndrome		
Asthma		
Pneumothorax		
Atelectasis		
Pneumonia		
Kyphoscoliosis		
Pulmonary edema		
Mucus plugs		
Lung cancer (bronchial)		
Lung cancer (parenchymal)		
Tuberculosis		
Chronic bronchitis		
Artificial airway		
Bronchospasm		

5. **DIRECTIONS:** Identify the primary breath sound change that occurs in the following conditions.

Condition	Breath Sound Change or Changes
Emphysema	
Atelectasis	
Pneumonia	
Chronic bronchitis	
Pneumothorax	
Pulmonary fibrosis	
Asthma	
Pulmonary edema	
Pleurisy	
Hemothorax	
Pleural effusion	
Pulmonary embolism	

6. **DIRECTIONS:** Identify normal values for the following parameters.

Tidal volume	
Vital capacity	
Maximal inspiratory pressure	
Pao_2	
Sao_2	
Svo_2	
DO_2	
VO_2	
O_2ER	

7. **DIRECTIONS:** Identify the acid-base imbalance likely to occur in each of these situations.

a.	A patient is admitted to your unit with epidural analgesia being delivered. Her ventilatory rate is 8/min.	
b.	A patient has had large volumes of NG drainage for the last several shifts.	
c.	A postoperative patient has a history of COPD. He is now having problems with retained secretions.	
d.	A postoperative patient has a history of HF. She has been on diuretics before and after surgery.	
e.	A postoperative thoracotomy patient is complaining of chest pain and has a respiratory rate of 32/min. She is complaining of tingling around her mouth and fingertips.	
f.	A postoperative patient has large volumes of ileal drainage from the new ileostomy.	

8. **DIRECTIONS:** Analyze the following arterial blood gases. Identify any acid-base imbalance, any partial or total compensation, and the presence of hypoxemia. Assume all patients to be under 60 years of age.

	pH	$Paco_2$	HCO_3	Pao_2	Answer
1.	7.30	54	26	64	
2.	7.48	30	24	96	
3.	7.30	40	18	85	
4.	7.50	40	33	92	
5.	7.35	54	30	55	
6.	7.21	60	20	48	
7.	7.54	25	30	95	
8.	7.40	58	33	72	
9.	7.40	30	18	89	

9. **DIRECTIONS:** Match the oxygen delivery system with the oxygen concentration range that it can deliver.

____a. Nasal cannula   1. 21%-100%
____b. Simple face mask   2. 24%-40%
____c. Partial rebreathing mask 3. 24%-44%
____d. Nonrebreathing mask   4. 35%-60%
____e. Venturi mask   5. 40%-60%
____f. T-piece   6. 60%-80%
____g. Mechanical ventilator   7. 60%-100%

10. **DIRECTIONS:** Identify if the following factors will cause a high-pressure or low-exhaled-volume alarm.

	High-Pressure	**Low–Exhaled-Volume**
Cuff leak		
Bronchospasm		
Need for suctioning		
Disconnect		
Water condensation in tubing		
Pneumothorax		
ARDS		

11. **DIRECTIONS:** Identify the values for the following parameters, which indicate that the patient may be successfully weaned from mechanical ventilation.

a.	Spontaneous tidal volume_____
b.	Spontaneous vital capacity_____
c.	Maximal inspiratory pressure_____
d.	Pao$_2$ of at least _____ on an FIo$_2$ of no greater than _____ with no more than _____ cm H$_2$O PEEP.

12. **DIRECTIONS:** Identify three physiologic effects of PEEP.

a. _____

b. _____

c. _____

LEARNING ACTIVITIES ANSWERS

1.

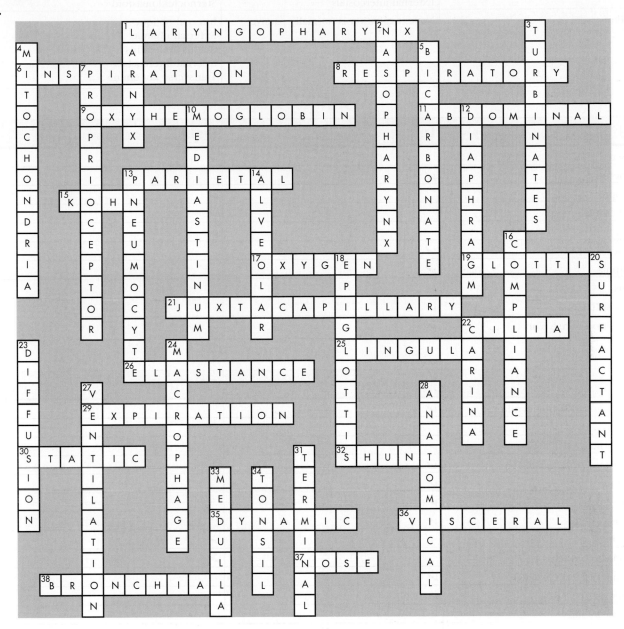

2.

	Primary	Accessory
Inspiration	Diaphragm External intercostals	Scalene Sternocleidomastoid
Expiration	None; expiration is normally passive	Internal oblique External oblique Rectus abdominis Internal intercostals Transverse abdominis

3.

	Left	Right
Increased 2,3-DPG		✔
Hypothermia	✔	
Hypercapnia		✔
Hyperthermia		✔
Acidosis		✔
Decreased 2,3-DPG	✔	
Hypocapnia	✔	
Alkalosis	✔	
Hypophosphatemia	✔	
Massive blood transfusion	✔	

4.

	Restrictive	Obstructive
Obesity hypoventilation syndrome	✔	
Asthma		✔
Pneumothorax	✔	
Atelectasis	✔	
Pneumonia	✔	
Kyphoscoliosis	✔	
Pulmonary edema	✔	
Mucus plugs		✔
Lung cancer (bronchial)		✔
Lung cancer (parenchymal)	✔	
Tuberculosis	✔	
Chronic bronchitis		✔
Artificial airway		✔
Bronchospasm		✔

5.

Condition	Breath Sound Change or Changes
Emphysema	• Diminished breath sounds
Atelectasis	• Diminished breath sounds • Bronchial or bronchovesicular breath sounds • Crackles
Pneumonia	• Diminished breath sounds • Bronchial or bronchovesicular breath sounds
Chronic bronchitis	• Rhonchi • Wheezes may also be present
Pneumothorax	• Diminished or absent breath sounds
Pulmonary fibrosis	• Diminished breath sounds • Crackles
Asthma	• Wheezes • Rhonchi
Pulmonary edema	• Crackles • Wheezes (referred to as *cardiac asthma*) may be present
Pleurisy	• Pleural friction rub
Hemothorax	• Diminished or absent breath sounds
Pleural effusion	• Diminished breath sounds
Pulmonary embolism	• Crackles • Pleural friction rub if pulmonary infarction develops

6.

Tidal volume	7 ml/kg
Vital capacity	>15 ml/kg
Maximal inspiratory pressure	> (more negative than) –60 cm H_2O
Pao_2	80-100 mm Hg
Sao_2	>95%
Svo_2	60%-80%
DO_2	~1000 ml/min
VO_2	~250 ml/min
O_2ER	~25%

7.

a.	Respiratory acidosis
b.	Metabolic alkalosis
c.	Respiratory acidosis (but with elevated bicarbonate; chronic compensated respiratory acidosis with decompensation)
d.	Metabolic alkalosis
e.	Respiratory alkalosis
f.	Metabolic acidosis

8.

	pH	PaCO$_2$	HcO$_3$$^-$	PaO$_2$	Answer
1.	7.30	54	26	64	Respiratory acidosis with mild hypoxemia
2.	7.48	30	24	96	Respiratory alkalosis
3.	7.30	40	18	85	Metabolic acidosis
4.	7.50	40	33	92	Metabolic alkalosis
5.	7.35	54	30	55	Compensated respiratory acidosis with moderate hypoxemia
6.	7.21	60	20	48	Mixed disorder: respiratory and metabolic acidosis with moderate hypoxemia
7.	7.54	25	30	95	Mixed disorder: respiratory alkalosis and metabolic alkalosis
8.	7.40	58	33	72	Mixed disorder: respiratory acidosis and metabolic alkalosis; Note: compensation causes the pH to lean toward either end of the normal pH range; the nonleaning pH indicates that this is a mixed disorder rather than compensation
9.	7.40	30	18	89	Mixed disorder: respiratory alkalosis and metabolic acidosis; Note: compensation causes the pH to lean toward either end of the normal pH range; the nonleaning pH indicates that this is a mixed disorder rather than compensation

9.

__3__ a. nasal cannula
__5__ b. simple face mask
__4__ c. partial rebreathing mask
__7__ d. nonrebreathing mask
__2__ e. Venturi mask
__1__ f. T-piece
__1__ g. mechanical ventilator

10.

	High Pressure	Low Exhaled Volume
Cuff leak		✔
Bronchospasm	✔	
Need for suctioning	✔	
Disconnect		✔
Water condensation in tubing	✔	
Pneumothorax	✔	
ARDS	✔	

11.   a. Spontaneous tidal volume: at least 5 ml/kg
   b. Spontaneous vital capacity: at least 10 ml/kg
   c. Maximal inspiratory pressure > (more negative than) −20 cm H$_2$O
   d. PaO$_2$ of at least 60 mm Hg on an FIO$_2$ of no greater than 0.50 with no more than 5 cm H$_2$O PEEP

12.   a. Increases the driving pressure of oxygen
   b. Decreases surface tension
   c. Decreases intrapulmonary shunt (alveolar recruitment)

Bibliography and Selected References

Ackerman M, Mick D: Instillation of normal saline before suctioning in patients with pulmonary infections: a prospective randomized controlled trial, *Am J Crit Care* 7 (4):261, 1998.

Alspach J, editor: *Core curriculum for critical care nursing,* ed 5, Philadelphia, 1998, WB Saunders.

Ambrose M: Chronic dyspnea: controlling a perplexing symptom, *Nursing98* 28 (5):41, 1998.

Anderson J: Management of four arterial blood gas problems in adult mechanical ventilation: decision-making algorithms and rationale for their use, *Critical Care Nurse* 16 (3):62, 1996.

Baden H et al: High-frequency oscillatory ventilation with partial liquid ventilation in a model of acute respiratory failure, *Crit Care Med* 25 (2):299, 1997.

Barkauskas V et al: *Health and physical assessment,* St Louis, 1994, Mosby.

Beare P, Myers J: *Adult health nursing,* ed 3, St Louis, 1998, Mosby.

Bell S: Use of Passy-Muir tracheostomy speaking valve in mechanically ventilated neurological patients, *Critical Care Nurse* 16 (1):63, 1996.

Belli M: Bronchoscopy, *AJN* 99 (7):24AA, 1999.

Boggs R, Wooldridge-King M: *AACN procedure manual for critical care,* ed 3, Philadelphia, 1993, WB Saunders.

Bolton P, Kline K: Understanding modes of mechanical ventilation, *AJN* 94(6):36, 1994.

Carlson-Catalano J et al: Clinical validation of ineffective breathing pattern, ineffective airway clearance, and impaired gas exchange. *Image* 30 (3):243, 1998.

Clochesy J et al: *Critical care nursing,* ed 2, Philadelphia, 1996, WB Saunders.

Dettenmeier P: *Pulmonary nursing care,* St. Louis, 1992, Mosby.

Fort P et al: High-frequency oscillatory ventilation for adult respiratory distress syndrome: a pilot syndrome, *Crit Care Med* 25 (6):937, 1997.

Froese A et al: High-frequency oscillatory ventilation for adult respiratory distress syndrome: let's get it right this time! *Crit Care Med* 25 (6):906, 1997.

Gallagher J: Taking the pressure off mechanically ventilated patients, *Nursing97* 27 (5):32ccl, 1997.

Gawlinski A, Hamwi D: *Acute care nurse practitioner clinical curriculum and certification review,* Philadelphia, 1999, WB Saunders.

Grap M: Pulse oximetry, *Critical Care Nurse* 18 (1):94, 1998.

Grap MJ et al: Endotracheal suctioning: ventilator vs manual delivery of hyperoxygenation breaths, *Am J Crit Care* 5 (3):192, 1996.

Guyton D, Barlow M, Besselievre T: Influence of airway pressure on minimum occlusive endotracheal tube cuff pressure, *Crit Care Med* 25 (1):91, 1997.

Hagler D, Traver G: Endotracheal saline and suction catheters: sources of lower airway contamination, *Am J Crit Care* 3 (6):444, 1994.

Hanneman S: Weaning from short-term mechanical ventilation, *Critical Care Nurse* 19 (5):86, 1999.

Horne C, Derrico D: Mastering ABGs, *AJN* 99 (8):26, 1999.

Jensen L, Onyskiw J: Meta-analysis of arterial oxygen saturation monitoring by pulse oximetry in adults, *Heart Lung* 27 (6):387, 1998.

Johannigman J et al: Ventilatory support of the critically injured patient, *New Horizons* 7 (1):116, 1999.

Kalweit S: Inhaled nitric oxide in the ICU, *Critical Care Nurse* 17 (4):26, 1997.

Keen J, Swearingen P: *Mosby's critical care nursing consultant,* St Louis, 1997, Mosby.

Kersten L: *Comprehensive respiratory nursing,* Philadelphia, 1989, WB Saunders.

Kinney M et al: *AACN clinical reference for critical care nursing,* ed 4, St Louis, 1998, Mosby.

Knebel A et al: Weaning from mechanical ventilatory support: refinement of a model, *Am J Crit Care* 7 (2):149, 1998.

Lewis P et al: The effect of turning and backrub on mixed venous oxygen saturation in critically ill patients, *Am J Crit Care* 6 (2):132, 1997.

Marino P: *The ICU book,* ed 2, Baltimore, 1998, Williams & Wilkins.

Mathews P: Ventilator-associated infection, part I, *Nursing97* 27 (2):59, 1997.

Mathews P: Ventilator-associated infection, part II, *Nursing97* 27 (3):50, 1997.

McGowan C: Noninvasive ventilatory support: use of bi-level positive airway pressure in respiratory failure, *Critical Care Nurse* 18 (6):47, 1998.

Menzel L: Factors related to the emotional responses of intubated patients to being unable to speak, *Heart Lung* 27 (4):245, 1998.

Mims B et al: *Critical care skills: a clinical handbook,* Philadelphia, 1996, WB Saunders.

O'Hanlon-Nichols T: The adult pulmonary system, *AJN* 98 (2):39, 1998.

Owen A: Respiratory assessment revisited, *Nursing98* 28 (4):48, 1998.

Pranikoff T et al: Mortality is directly related to the duration of mechanical ventilation before the initiation of extracorporeal life support for severe respiratory failure, *Crit Care Med* 25 (1):28, 1997.

Price S, Wilson L: *Pathophysiology: clinical concepts of disease processes,* ed 5, St Louis, 1997, Mosby.

Raffin et al: Indices of hypoxemia in patients with acute respiratory distress syndrome: reliability, validity, and clinical usefulness, *Crit Care Med* 25 (1):6, 1997.

Raymond S: Normal saline instillation before suctioning: helpful or harmful? A review of the literature, *Am J Crit Care* 4 (4):267, 1995.

Rodriguez R, Light R: Capnography in the ICU, *Journal of Critical Illness* 13 (6):372, 1998.

Rodriguez R, Light R: Pulse oximetry in the ICU: uses, benefits, limitations, *Journal of Critical Illness* 13 (4):247, 1998.

Roizen M, Fleisher L: *Essence of anesthesia practice,* Philadelphia, 1997, WB Saunders.

Rowlee S: Monitoring neuromuscular blockade in the intensive care unit: the peripheral nerve stimulator, *Heart Lung* 28 (5):352, 1999.

Simmons C: How frequently should endotracheal suctioning be undertaken? *Am J Crit Care* 6 (1):4, 1997.

Smatlak P, Knebel A: Clinical evaluation of noninvasive monitoring of oxygen saturation in critically ill patients, *Am J Crit Care* 7 (5):370, 1998.

St. John R: Airway management, *Critical Care Nurse* 19 (4):70, 1999.

Stone D et al: *Perioperative care: anesthesia, medicine, and surgery,* St Louis, 1998, Mosby.

Tamurri L: Assisting your patient's breathing with noninvasive ventilation, *Nursing98* 28 (10):32hnl, 1998.

Tasota F, Wesmiller S: Balancing act: keeping blood pH in equilibrium, *Nursing98* 8 (12):35, 1998.

Thelan L et al: *Critical care nursing: diagnosis and management,* ed 3, St Louis, 1998, Mosby.

Varon J, Fromm R: *The ICU handbook of facts, formulas, and laboratory values,* St Louis, 1997, Mosby.

Pulmonary System: Pathologic Conditions

CHAPTER 5

Chest Surgery and Chest Tubes
Surgical Procedures

I. Thoracotomy: opening into the thorax or pleural cavity

II. Exploratory thoracotomy: opening the thorax to perform a biopsy or locate bleeding

III. Lobectomy: removal of one or more lobes of the lung

IV. Segmental resection: removal of segment(s) of a lobe

V. Wedge resection: removal of a small peripheral section of the lung without regard to segments

VI. Pneumonectomy: removal of an entire lung; indicated when tumor is centrally located at hilus or bronchus

VII. Thoracoplasty: surgical collapse of a portion of chest wall by multiple rib resections to decrease volume in hemithorax; may be used after pulmonary resection if lung cannot reexpand to fill thoracic space or after pneumonectomy: reduces the size of the thoracic cavity on the operative side and decreases the chance of mediastinal shift toward that side

VIII. Decortication of lung: removal of fibrinous membrane covering visceral and parietal pleura

IX. Bullectomy: removal of cysts or bullae in lung

X. Pneumoplasty (lung volume reduction surgery): resection of hyperinflated areas of lung to allow more normal function of diaphragm and expansion of more normal areas of the lung

XI. Closed thoracostomy: insertion of chest tube through intercostal space into pleural space; tube is connected to underwater-seal drainage system

XII. Open thoracostomy: insertion of chest tube during rib resection; usually used in empyema when pleural space is fixed

XIII. Thymectomy: removal of the thymus; usually performed for myasthenia gravis

XIV. Chest trauma surgery: repair of penetrating or nonpenetrating trauma; drainage of pleural cavity and control of hemorrhage

XV. Removal of mediastinal masses: removal of cysts, tumors, abscesses from mediastinum

XVI. Tracheal resection: resection of a portion of the trachea with end-to-end anastomosis; removal of stenotic area of trachea or tumor

XVII. Esophagogastrectomy: resection of a part of the esophagus and upper portion of the stomach with end-to-end anastomosis; colon interposition using a portion of the large intestine may be performed as an alternative to end-to-end anastomosis; for cancer of esophagus or corrosive esophagitis

Chest Tubes (also called *Thoracostomy Tube* or *Thoracic Catheter*)

I. Indications for chest tube drainage
   A. Pneumothorax
      1. Greater than 20%
      2. On mechanical ventilator
   B. Hemothorax
      1. Greater than 500 ml
      2. On mechanical ventilator
   C. Pneumohemothorax
      1. Surgically induced during thoracotomy
      2. Traumatic
   D. Pleural effusion

II. Purposes of chest tubes
   A. Pleural tubes
      1. To remove free air: tube placed anterior and superior (usually at second ICS at MCL); pneumothorax: air in the pleural space
      2. To drain intrapleural space: tube placed lateral and inferior (usually at fifth or sixth ICS at midaxillary line)
         a) Hemothorax: blood in the pleural space
         b) Pleural effusion: fluid in the pleural space; may be transudate or exudate

(1) Transudate: occurs if there is a rise in pulmonary venous pressure (e.g., HF) or hypoproteinemia (e.g., malnutrition, cirrhosis); tends to accumulate at the base of the lungs

(2) Exudate: occurs as a result of increased capillary permeability or impaired lymphatic absorption (e.g., involvement of the pleura by inflammation or malignancy); the fluid has a higher specific gravity and protein content than a transudate

c) Empyema (also called *pyothorax*): pus in the pleural space

d) Chylothorax: chyle (lymph fluid and triglyceride fat) in the pleural space

e) Hydrothorax: water (e.g., IV fluid) in the pleural space

3. To reestablish negative pressure in the pleural space

B. Mediastinal tubes: to drain air and blood from the mediastinum after cardiac or other mediastinal surgery

III. Chest drainage system
A. Components
1. Drainage collection bottle or chamber collects liquid drainage
2. Water-seal bottle or chamber provides a one-way valve to allow air to escape but does not allow atmospheric air to go into the pleural space
3. Suction control bottle or chamber controls the amount of suction
B. Systems (Fig. 5-1)
1. Three-bottle system
a) The drainage collection bottle is the bottle closest to the patient; this bottle is connected to the water-seal bottle
b) The water-seal bottle is filled so that the tube from the chest tube is submerged 2 cm under the water
c) The water-seal bottle must have a vent open at the top of the bottle to allow air to escape if not attached to suction
d) The third bottle is the suction control bottle
(1) It has one tube to connect it to the water-seal bottle

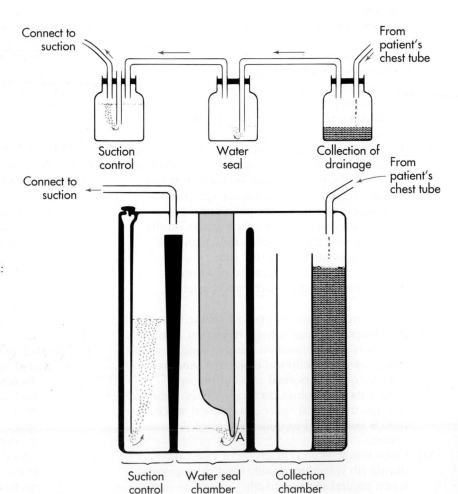

Figure 5-1 Comparison of a commercially available chest tube drainage system with a three bottle system. (From Thelan LA et al: *Critical care nursing: diagnosis and management,* ed 3, St. Louis, 1998, Mosby.)

(2) Another tube connects it to the suction device (usually wall suction but it may be a free-standing Emerson-type suction device)

(3) The third tube is submerged under water to the prescribed suction amount in cm of water (usually 20 cm H_2O); this bottle also has an air vent

(4) Suction is adjusted so that a gentle bubbling occurs in this bottle

(a) Remember that vigorous bubbling makes it evaporate more quickly so you must keep refilling it

(b) The actual amount of suction is determined by the depth that the tube is submersed minus the depth of the water-seal tube

2. All-in-one system (e.g., Atrium, Pleur-evac, Sentinel Seal, Thora-Klex, Thora-Seal III)

a) More convenient

b) Only the water-seal and drainage collection chambers may be used, or all three will be used if suction is desired

c) In a wet system: adjust the amount of suction by filling the water level in the suction control chamber; adjust wall suction so that gentle bubbling occurs in the suction control chamber

(1) Again, remember the actual amount of suction is the height of suction control chamber minus the height of the water-seal chamber

d) In a dry system: adjust the amount of suction until the indicator appears

IV. Autotransfusion

A. Definition: the reinfusion of the patient's own blood; consists of collecting, filtering, and reinfusing the patient's own blood

B. Indications for autotransfusion of blood from a chest drainage system

1. Chest trauma

2. Chest surgery

3. Consider autotransfusion if volume in chamber is 400 ml within 4 hours and hematocrit is less than 30%

C. Advantage: eliminates risk of potentially fatal transfusion reactions and transmission of blood-borne diseases

D. Contraindications

1. Malignancy

2. Sepsis

3. Coagulopathies

4. Contamination of blood with urine or feces

5. Traumatic wounds more than 4 hours after injury

E. Method

1. Large-bore chest tube is connected to a closed drainage system

2. The blood passes through a filter into a collection bag

3. Collection bag may contain a preservative (usually citrate phosphate dextrose [CPD])

4. When filled, this bag is removed, inverted, and infused into the patient intravenously

F. Complications

1. Disturbances in coagulation: thrombocytopenia, DIC

2. Acute renal failure caused by hemolysis and hemoglobinuria

3. Emboli

4. Sepsis

5. Spread of malignancy

6. Citrate toxicity: hypocalcemia

Assessment (Table 5-1)
Nursing Diagnoses

I. Ineffective Breathing Pattern related to incisional pain, inadequate lung expansion

II. Impaired Gas Exchange related to alveolar hypoventilation

III. Pain related to thoracic incision

IV. Anxiety related to acute change in health status

V. Anticipatory Grieving related to diagnosis of malignancy (if thoracotomy performed for lung cancer)

Collaborative Management

I. Control pain

A. Analgesics to relieve pain and encourage deep breathing

1. Intravenous analgesia: by regularly scheduled IV injection or by patient-controlled analgesia

2. Interpleural analgesia: local anesthetic (e.g., bupivacaine [Marcaine]) injected into pleural space

3. Epidural analgesia: opiate and/or local anesthetic injected into epidural space

4. Nonsteroidal antiinflammatory agent (e.g., ibuprofen [Motrin]) to augment the pain relief of narcotics

B. Instruction related to how to splint chest when coughing

II. Maintain airway patency and adequate oxygenation and ventilation

A. Position the patient for optimal ventilation/perfusion matching: head of bed elevated to 30 to 45 degrees; good lung down optimizes ventilation to encourage reexpansion and optimizes perfusion to the nonaffected "good" lung; exception: pneumonectomy patients are positioned on their operative lung or back

B. Encourage deep breathing and incentive spirometry; encourage coughing if indicated; note that air is removed from the pleural space by the positive pressure of expiration and the negative pressure of the suction device; deep breathing is very important in lung reexpansion

Table 5-1	Assessment Parameters for the Patient with a Chest Tube	
Parameter	**Note**
Patient	• Ventilatory effort • Chest discomfort or pain • Anxiety • Level of understanding • Cough • Sputum production
Breathing	• Rate • Regularity • Depth • Breath sounds (disconnection of suction source from suction control chamber is required for accurate assessment of breath sounds)
Insertion site	• Intactness of dressing • Drainage on dressing or around insertion site • Subcutaneous emphysema around insertion site
Tubing	• Tight, taped connections • Absence of kinks, compressions, or dependent loops
Drainage collection chamber	• Volume (normal 50-100 ml/hr for first few hours, then 10-20 ml/hr) • Type: color, consistency, odor • Bottle below chest level
Water seal chamber	• Filled to 2 cm or prescribed amount • Fluctuations with respirations • Any bubbling • If not on suction: air vent open
Suction control chamber	• Filled to prescribed amount (usually –20 cm H_2O) • Gentle, continuous bubbling
Suction source	• If no control bottle: suction set at ordered level • If control bottle: suction set so gentle, continuous bubbling occurs

C. Perform nasotracheal suctioning only if the patient is unable to clear secretions; do not vigorously suction patients after pneumonectomy because this procedure may cause bronchial stump leak

D. Treat bronchospasm with bronchodilators as prescribed

E. Assess daily chest X-ray to monitor reexpansion

F. Monitor for gastric distention; NG tube may be utilized

G. Administer oxygen as indicated by arterial blood gases and Spo_2

H. If still receiving mechanical ventilation after surgery: wean and extubate as soon as possible

because positive pressure ventilation increases risk of air leak

III. Maintain water-seal drainage system and patency of chest tubes

A. Check functioning of system at least hourly

B. Tape all connections

C. Position tubing to prevent kinks and dependent loops

D. Maintain suction at prescribed level

E. Note loss of fluctuation in water-seal bottle or chamber; the primary risk of an occluded tube is tension pneumothorax and mediastinal shift

F. Milk or strip chest tube only as indicated

1. Milking is hand-over-hand squeezing of the chest tube; stripping is clamping with the thumb and forefinger of the nondominant hand while pulling the tube between the thumb and forefinger of the dominant hand followed by release of the thumb and forefinger of the nondominant hand

2. Indications to milk or strip the chest tube
   a) No fluctuation in water-seal chamber
   b) Absence of kink or compressions
   c) Lung not yet expanded according to morning chest X-ray

3. Milking or stripping chest tubes creates negative pressure within the pleural space; while it may help to move a clot along, it may create trauma to the pleura
   a) Milking should be attempted first because it is more gentle
   b) If stripping is necessary, strip short sections

G. Never drain chest tubes back into the patient's chest

H. Clamping the tube

1. Clamp tube only if:
   a) The chest drainage system must be lifted above the level of the chest (e.g., putting patient in helicopter for transport) so that chest drainage does not drain back into the pleural space; clamp as briefly as possible
   b) There has been a minimal leak and the chest drainage system breaks; clamp as briefly as possible while the next system is set up
   c) The drainage collection bottle needs to be emptied or the system changed and the next bottle or system is ready; clamp as briefly as possible

2. If a significant air leak has persisted and the chest drainage system breaks: Submerse the tube about 2 cm into a bottle of sterile water or saline; if a bottle of sterile water or saline is not available, put tap water into a clean Styrofoam cup and submerse the tube about 2 cm into the cup; if no water or saline is available, the patient is better off with an open pneumothorax than a tension pneumothorax

IV. Monitor for common complications
  A. Hemorrhage/shock
    1. Replace blood and fluid volume as prescribed; thoracic surgery patients generally receive less fluid than nonthoracic surgery patients in early postoperative period to prevent ARDS and pulmonary edema
    2. Monitor for clinical indications of hypoperfusion (see Box 2-6)
  B. Infection
    1. Utilize sterile technique while dressing the insertion site, setting up the chest drainage system, and draining or replacing the system
    2. Monitor for fever
    3. Assess incision and chest tube insertion site for redness, induration, drainage; culture drainage if purulent
    4. Monitor sputum and chest drainage for indications of infection; culture as necessary
    5. Administer antibiotics as prescribed
  C. Tension pneumothorax
    1. Maintain patency of chest tube and functioning of water-seal drainage system
    2. Avoid clamping chest tube except for reasons previously identified
    3. Monitor for clinical indications of tension pneumothorax: dyspnea, chest pain, tracheal shift away from affected side, hyperresonance to percussion, decreased breath sounds on affected side
  D. Dysrhythmias: especially atrial dysrhythmias
  E. Pulmonary edema: related to capillary leak and pulmonary hypertension; use caution with fluid resuscitation
  F. ARDS: aspiration pneumonitis, ARDS devastating after pneumonectomy
  G. Pulmonary embolism
    1. Encourage deep breathing and incentive spirometry
    2. Patient should sit on edge of bed the evening of surgery, be out of bed into chair within 24 to 36 hours, and ambulate as soon as possible
  H. Bronchopleural fistula: usually related to empyema
  I. Empyema
  J. Frozen shoulder: impairment in shoulder mobility
    1. Perform passive range of motion to shoulder on operative side initially
    2. Administer analgesia to allow motion
    3. Encourage active range of motion and use of arm for self-care activities
V. Assist with removal of chest tube
  A. Usually removed when there has been no air leak from anterior tube or less than 100 ml/24 hr for posterior tube
  B. Frequently clamped for up to 24 hours before removal
  C. Instruct the patient to hold his or her breath at the end of expiration when requested

  D. Apply occlusive dressing after the physician removes the tube at the end of expiration
  E. Monitor the patient for dyspnea, chest pain, asymmetrical chest excursion, or diminished breath sounds that indicate tension pneumothorax

Acute Respiratory Failure
Definition
I. Failure of the respiratory system to provide for the exchange of oxygen and carbon dioxide between the environment and tissues in quantities sufficient to sustain life
II. Hypoxemic normocapnic respiratory failure (type I): low Pao_2 with normal $Paco_2$
III. Hypoxemic hypercapnic respiratory failure (type II): low Pao_2 with high $Paco_2$

Etiology
I. Type I respiratory failure
  A. Pneumonia
  B. Pulmonary edema
  C. Pulmonary fibrosis
  D. Pleural effusion
  E. Pneumothorax
  F. Asthma
  G. Atelectasis
  H. Aspiration pneumonitis
  I. ARDS (early)
  J. Smoke inhalation
  K. Pulmonary embolism
  L. Kyphoscoliosis
  M. Fat embolism
II. Type II respiratory failure (may also be called *acute ventilatory failure*)
  A. COPD with acute exacerbation
  B. Status asthmaticus
  C. CNS depressant drugs
  D. Anesthesia
  E. Neuromuscular blocking drugs
    1. Muscle paralytics
    2. Aminoglycosides
    3. Organophosphate poisoning
  F. Head trauma
  G. Poliomyelitis
  H. Amyotrophic lateral sclerosis
  I. Spinal cord injury
  J. Guillain-Barré syndrome
  K. Myasthenia gravis
  L. Multiple sclerosis
  M. Muscular dystrophy
  N. Morbid obesity
  O. Chest trauma
  P. Surgery: especially thoracic, abdominal, flank incision
  Q. Sleep apnea
  R. Tracheal obstruction
  S. Epiglottis

T. Cystic fibrosis

U. Near-drowning

Pathophysiology (Table 5-2)

I. Hypoventilation

II. Ventilation-perfusion mismatching

III. Shunting

IV. Diffusion defects

Clinical Presentation

I. Subjective

A. History of precipitating factor

B. Clinical indications of respiratory distress (see Box 3-2)

C. Clinical indications of hypoxia (see Box 3-3)

D. Clinical indications of hypercapnia (see Box 3-4)

II. Objective

A. Clinical indications of respiratory distress (see Box 3-2)

B. Hypoxemia: decrease in SpO_2, SaO_2, PaO_2

C. Clinical indications of hypoxia (Box 3-3)

D. Clinical indications of hypercapnia (Box 3-4)

III. Diagnostic

A. Arterial blood gas changes

1. PaO_2 less than 50 to 60 mm Hg

2. $PaCO_2$ more than 50 mm Hg with a pH of less than 7.30

B. Chest X-ray: may identify cause

Nursing Diagnosis

I. Impaired Gas Exchange related to V/Q mismatching, intrapulmonary shunt

II. Ineffective Breathing Patterns related to increased work of breathing and fatigue

III. Ineffective Airway Clearance related to retained secretion

IV. Risk for Infection related to invasive procedures, poor airway clearance

V. Altered Nutrition: Less than Body Requirements related to lack of exogenous nutrients, increased nutrient requirements

VI. Activity Intolerance related to imbalance between oxygen supply and oxygen demand

VII. Anxiety related to change in health status

Collaborative Management

I. Treat the cause

II. Maintain airway and ventilation

A. Positioning

1. Head of bed elevated to 30 to 45 degrees

2. Overbed table for patient to lean on

3. "Good lung down" if unilateral lung condition exists

4. Prone position especially in ARDS

B. Hydration: 2 to 3 L/24 hr unless contraindicated by cardiac or renal disease

1. Oral fluids: noncaffeinated

2. Intravenous fluids: usually D_5NS

C. Bronchial hygiene and chest physiotherapy

1. Inspiratory maneuvers: deep breathing, incentive spirometry

2. Analgesics in doses adequate to allow patient to breath deeply and cough as indicated

3. Encouragement of the patient to cough if rhonchi are audible; suctioning if the patient is unable to clear airways

4. Postural drainage, percussion, vibration may be used

5. Bronchoscopy may be necessary if airway clearance techniques are inadequate

6. Intubation and mechanical ventilation may be necessary if $PaCO_2$ continues to rise and acidosis develops

a) The goal of mechanical ventilation is to normalize the pH, not necessarily the $PaCO_2$

b) It is not appropriate to normalize the $PaCO_2$ in patients with COPD and chronic hypercapnia (this treatment causes metabolic alkalosis, eventual excretion of sodium bicarbonate, and weaning difficulties)

D. Drug therapy

1. Bronchodilators may be indicated

a) Beta$_2$-adrenergic agonists (these agents are preferred over nonrespiratory-selective beta stimulants such as epinephrine and isoproterenol because they cause fewer cardiovascular side effects)

(1) Terbutaline (Brethine)

(2) Albuterol (Proventil)

(3) Isoetharine HCl (Bronkosol)

(4) Metaproterenol (Alupent)

b) Xanthines (e.g., aminophylline, theophylline)

2. Expectorants (e.g., guaifenesin [Robitussin], potassium iodide [SSKI]) may be used but hydration is most important

3. Mucolytics (e.g., acetylcysteine [Mucomyst]) may be used to decrease the tenacity of the mucus; frequently causes bronchospasm so should be given with a bronchodilator

4. Sedatives: generally avoided unless patient is very agitated

5. Antitussives: generally avoided

III. Optimize oxygen delivery and decrease oxygen consumption

A. Oxygen as indicated for hypoxemia

1. Nasal cannula or mask; masks are contraindicated in hypercapnic patients because the high concentration of oxygen provided by these delivery systems would likely eliminate the hypoxic drive

2. Flow rate or oxygen concentration to keep SpO_2 approximately 95% unless contraindicated; in patients with chronic hypercapnia, adjust flow rate or oxygen concentration to keep SpO_2 approximately 90%

B. Positive end-expiratory pressure (PEEP): may be necessary to maintain adequate SaO_2, PaO_2

C. Rest periods especially after meals or activities

D. Quiet, restful environment

Table 5-2	Mechanisms of Hypoxemia			
Mechanism	**Pathophysiology**	**Etiology**	**Diagnosis**	**Treatment**

Hypoventilation	Hypoventilation causes CO_2 retention and hypoxemia	• Damage to/depression of the neurologic control of ventilation
		  • head injury
		  • cerebral thrombosis or hemorrhage
		  • CNS depressant drugs
		  • oxygen-induced hypoventilation
		• Neuromuscular defects in the ventilatory mechanism
		  • myasthenia gravis
		  • multiple sclerosis
		  • muscular dystrophy
		  • Guillain-Barré syndrome
		  • poliomyelitis
		  • spinal cord injuries
		  • botulism
		  • tetanus
		  • neuromuscular blocking drugs
		• Obstructive lung conditions
		  • asthma
		  • chronic bronchitis
		  • emphysema
		  • airway obstruction
		  • cystic fibrosis
		• Restrictive lung conditions
		  • kyphoscoliosis
		  • obesity hypoventilation syndrome
		  • recent thoracic, abdominal, or flank incision
		  • lung cancer
		  • flail chest
		  • pleural effusion
		  • pneumothorax
			• Physical examination
			  • neurologic status may be altered
			  • abnormal chest wall motion
			  • abnormal breath sounds
			  • clinical indications of hypoxemia, hypercapnia
			• ABG: hypoxemia with increased $Paco_2$ and normal A:a gradient
			• May have abnormal chest X-ray, PFTs
				• Improve oxygenation by increasing alveolar ventilation (e.g., positioning, bronchial hygiene, drug therapy)
				• Specific therapy is dependent on the specific etiology

V/Q mismatching	Low V/Q units, with perfusion in excess of ventilation, result in hypoxemia because the blood traversing these alveolar units is not fully oxygenated
	High V/Q units, with ventilation in excess of perfusion, result in oxygenated alveolar units that are not perfused
		• Regional ventilation abnormalities
		  • asthma
		  • chronic bronchitis
		  • emphysema
		  • atelectasis
		  • pneumonia
		  • bronchospasm
		  • mucus plugs
		  • foreign bodies
		  • tumor
		• Regional perfusion abnormalities
		  • pulmonary embolism
		  • decreasd cardiac output/index
		  • excessive PEEP
			• Physical examination
			  • abnormal chest wall motion
			  • abnormal breath sounds
			  • clinical indications of hypoxemia
			• ABG: hypoxemia with a widened A:a gradient; $Paco_2$ dependent on ventilation status
			• Abnormal chest X-ray, PFTs, and/or V/Q scan
				• Oxygen
				• Specific therapy dependent on the specific etiology

Continued

Table 5-2	Mechanisms of Hypoxemia—cont'd			
Mechanism	**Pathophysiology**	**Etiology**	**Diagnosis**	**Treatment**

Shunt	Blood transverses from the right heart to the left heart without being oxygenated: anatomic shunt is when the blood bypasses the alveolar-capillary unit and physiologic shunt is when the blood goes through the alveolar-capillary unit but it is nonfunctional	Anatomic shunts
		• Normal anatomic shunts: bronchial, pleural, Thebesian veins
		• Intrapulmonary shunts: pulmonary A-V fistula
		• Intracardiac shunts: tetralogy of Fallot
		• Other pathologic shunts (e.g., shunts associated with neoplasms)
		Physiologic shunts
		• Alveolar collapse
		  • atelectasis
		  • pneumothorax
		  • hemothorax
		  • pleural effusion
		• Alveoli filled with a fluid or foreign material
		  • cardiac pulmonary edema
		  • noncardiac pulmonary edema (e.g., near-drowning, ARDS)
		  • pneumonias
			• Physical examination
			  • abnormal breath sounds
			  • clinical indications of hypoxemia
			• ABG: hypoxemia with a normal or decreased $Paco_2$
			  • widened A:a gradient
			  • shunt >6%
			• May have abnormal chest X-ray, PFTs
				• Oxygen administration has little or no effect
				• Specific therapy dependent on the specific etiology
				• PEEP is frequently used for physiologic shunt

Diffusion abnormalities	Increased diffusion pathway: diffusion between alveolar oxygen and pulmonary capillary blood is impaired; blood exiting the gas exchange unit is hypoxemic
	Decreased diffusion area: decrease in alveolar-capillary membrane surface area available for diffusion and/or loss of pulmonary capillary bed
		Increased diffusion pathway
		• Accumulation of fluid
		  • pulmonary edema: cardiac or noncardiac
		• Accumulation of collagen in the pulmonary interstitium
		  • pulmonary fibrosis
		  • sarcoidosis
		  • collagen-vascular disease
		Decreased diffusion area
		• Pulmonary resection (e.g., lobectomy, pneumonectomy)
		• Destructive lung diseases
		  • emphysema
		  • tumor
		  • obliterative pulmonary vascular diseases
			• History and physical examination findings are compatible with the diagnosis
			• ABG: hypoxemia with normal or low Pco_2
			  • widened A:a gradient
			  • further decrease in Pao_2 with exercise
			• PFTs: decreased diffusing capacity for CO
			• Chest X-ray may show cause
				• Oxygen
				• Home oxygen therapy is frequently indicated

E. Treatment of fever: antipyretics, cooling blankets

F. Blood administration: may be necessary to provide adequate tissue delivery of oxygen if hemoglobin is low

G. Fluid administration, inotropes, intraaortic balloon pump, etc.: may be necessary to provide adequate tissue delivery of oxygen if cardiac output/index is low

IV. Treat infection if present
  A. Antibiotics
  B. Bronchial hygiene techniques

V. Monitor for complications
  A. Dysrhythmias

B. Pulmonary infections: pneumonia

C. Pulmonary edema

D. Pulmonary embolism

E. Barotrauma (e.g., pneumothorax)

F. Pulmonary fibrosis

G. Oxygen toxicity

H. Renal failure

I. Acid-base imbalance
  1. Respiratory acidosis
  2. Metabolic alkalosis: when $Paco_2$ is normalized rather than the pH

J. Electrolyte imbalance

K. GI complications: abdominal distention, ileus, ulcer, hemorrhage

L. Thromboembolism

M. Disseminated intravascular coagulation (DIC)

N. Sepsis, septic shock

O. Psychologic responses: psychosis, depression

Acute Respiratory Distress Syndrome

Definition: A syndrome of acute respiratory failure characterized by noncardiac pulmonary edema and manifested by refractory hypoxemia caused by intrapulmonary shunt

Etiology: Risk increases if more than one risk factor occurs simultaneously

I. Direct injury

  A. Chest trauma: pulmonary contusion

  B. Near-drowning

  C. Hypervolemia, pulmonary edema

  D. Inhalation of toxic gases and vapors

    1. Smoke

    2. Chemicals

    3. Oxygen toxicity

  E. Pneumonia: viral, bacterial, or fungal

  F. Aspiration pneumonitis

  G. Radiation pneumonitis

  H. Pulmonary embolism: thrombotic, air, fat, amniotic fluid

  I. Radiation

  J. Drugs: bleomycin

II. Indirect injury

  A. Sepsis: most likely cause

  B. Shock or prolonged hypotension

    1. Septic shock

    2. Hypovolemic shock

    3. Anaphylactic shock

    4. Cardiogenic shock

    5. Neurogenic shock

  C. Multisystem trauma, especially multiple fractures

  D. Burns

  E. Cardiopulmonary bypass

  F. Disseminated intravascular coagulation (DIC)

  G. Toxemia of pregnancy

  H. Acute pancreatitis

  I. Diabetic coma

  J. Head injury

  K. Drug overdosage: heroin, methadone, barbiturates, aspirin, thiazide diuretics

  L. Multiple blood transfusions

  M. Abdominal trauma

Pathophysiology

I. Time from acute injury to alveolar-capillary membrane to the onset of symptoms is usually 12 to 48 hours

II. Acute phase

  A. Acute lung injury reduces normal perfusion to the lungs, causing platelet aggregation and stimulation of the inflammatory-immune system

  B. Release of mediators of the inflammatory process

  C. These mediators activate or stimulate neutrophils, macrophages, and other cells to release toxic substances that cause microvascular injury

  D. Acute and diffuse injury to endothelium and epithelium surface of lung

  E. Damage to pulmonary capillary membrane and increase in capillary permeability occurs

  F. Capillary leak allows proteins and fluids to spill into the interstitium and alveolar spaces; pulmonary lymphatic drainage capacity is overwhelmed and alveolar flooding occurs

  G. Pulmonary edema results and causes interference with oxygen diffusion and inactivation of surfactant; damage to type II pneumocytes results in decreased production of surfactant

  H. Alveolar collapse and massive atelectasis occur and decrease functional residual capacity and lung compliance

  I. Profound hypoxemia related to extensive shunting

  J. Vasoconstrictive mediators cause increased pulmonary vasoconstriction and pulmonary hypertension

III. Chronic phase (fibroproliferative phase)

  A. Type I pneumocytes are destroyed and replaced by type II pneumocytes, which proliferate

  B. Interstitial space expands by edema fluid, fibers, and proliferating cells

  C. Hyaline membranes are formed (probably from transudated plasma proteins), which increase the thickness of the alveolar-capillary membrane and therefore the diffusion pathway

  D. Pulmonary fibrosis may occur

Clinical Presentation

I. Phases of ARDS (Table 5-3)

II. Criteria used in ARDS diagnosis

  A. Presence of a predisposing condition

  B. Severe oxygenation defect: hypoxemia is the hallmark of ARDS

    1. Pao_2 less than 60 mm Hg on Fio_2 more than 0.50

    2. Pao_2/Fio_2 ratio less than or equal to 200

  C. Chest X-ray: diffuse bilateral parenchymal infiltrates

  D. Static compliance: significantly less than the normal of 50 to 100 ml/cm H_2O (usually 15 to 25 ml/cm H_2O)

  E. PAOP: less than 18 mm Hg

  F. No other explanation for the previous findings

III. Recommended criteria for acute lung injury and ARDS: American-European Consensus Conference on ARDS (1992) (Table 5-4)

IV. Hemodynamic parameters

  A. PAOP differentiates cardiac from noncardiac pulmonary edema

    1. ARDS (noncardiac pulmonary edema) causes elevated PAP with normal PAOP

Table 5-3   **Phases of ARDS**

Parameter	Phase I	Phase II	Phase III	Phase IV
Heart rate	Tachycardia	Tachycardia	Tachycardia	Bradycardia
Cardiac index	Normal	Increased	Increased	Decreased
Tidal volume/ minute ventilation	Increased	Increased	Normal or decreased	Decreased
$Paco_2$	Decreased	Decreased	Normal or increased	Increased
Acid-base	Respiratory Alkalosis	Respiratory Alkalosis	Metabolic (and possibly Respiratory) Acidosis	Respiratory and Metabolic Acidosis
Pao_2 on room air	Normal	Normal or slightly decreased (~60 mm Hg)	Significantly decreased (~40 mm Hg)	Severely decreased (~25 mm Hg)
Shunt	<6%	10%	20%	>30%
Compliance	Normal	Slightly decreased	Moderately decreased	Severely decreased
Pulmonary clinical manifestations	Dyspnea	Dyspnea, fatigue, retractions	Dyspnea, fatigue, retractions, cyanosis	Dyspnea, fatigue (may have had respiratory arrest), cyanosis, rusty sputum
Breath sounds	Clear	Fine crackles	Coarse crackles and/or wheezes	Crackles, rhonchi, and/or wheezes
Chest X-ray	Normal	Patchy infiltrates usually in dependent areas	Diffuse infiltrates	Consolidation
Other signs/ symptoms			Dysrhythmias, decreasing sensorium	Dysrhythmias, hypotension, decreasing sensorium

Table 5-4   **Recommended or Criteria for Acute Lung Injury and ARDS (American-European Consensus Conference on ARDS, 1992)**

	Oxygenation: Pao_2/Fio_2 ratio	Frontal Chest X-ray	PAOP
Acute lung injury	<300 mm Hg (regardless of PEEP)	Bilateral infiltrates	<18 mm Hg or no clinical evidence of left atrial enlargement
Acute respiratory distress syndrome (ARDS)	≤200 mm Hg (regardless of PEEP)	Bilateral infiltrates	<18 mm Hg or no clinical evidence of left atrial enlargement

    2. Cardiac pulmonary edema causes elevated PAP and PAOP
  B. Pulmonary vascular resistance (PVR) is increased because of hypoxemic pulmonary vasoconstriction
V. Diagnostic
  A. May give clues to cause
  B. Arterial blood gases (see Table 5-3): refractory hypoxemia (hypoxemia despite high concentration of oxygen); Pao_2 of less than 60 mm Hg despite Fio_2 0.5 or greater for 24 hours
  C. Sputum analysis: tracheal protein/plasma protein ratio more than 0.7 (cardiac pulmonary edema <0.5)
  D. Pulmonary function studies
    1. Lung volumes decreased: tidal volume, vital capacity
    2. Functional residual capacity decreased
    3. Static and dynamic compliance decreased

  E. Chest X-ray
    1. Bilateral diffuse interstitial and alveolar infiltrates
    2. Ground glass appearance
    3. "White-out" due to massive atelectasis
    4. Heart size is normal (one factor that differentiates ARDS from cardiac pulmonary edema)

Nursing Diagnoses

  I. Impaired Gas Exchange related to V/Q mismatching, intrapulmonary shunt
  II. Ineffective Breathing Patterns related to increased work of breathing and fatigue
  III. Alteration in Cardiac Output related to decreased preload caused by PEEP
  IV. Risk for Infection related to invasive procedures, poor airway clearance
  V. Altered Nutrition: Less than Body Requirements related to lack of exogenous nutrients, increased nutrient requirements

VI. Activity Intolerance related to imbalance between oxygen supply and oxygen demand

VII. Anxiety related to change in health status

Collaborative Management

I. Prevention
   A. Identify the high-risk patient
      1. Monitor pulse oximetry for drop in SpO_2
      2. Monitor serial arterial blood gas values for drop in PaO_2, SaO_2
      3. Monitor peak inspiratory pressure, static and dynamic compliance in patients on mechanical ventilator
   B. Utilize standard infection control measures
   C. Treat precipitating factors (e.g., antibiotics if infection is present)
   D. Provide nutritional support
      1. Enteral feeding prevents villous atrophy and increases the blood flow; helps to retard transmigration of bacteria or lipopolysaccharides, which play a significant role in sepsis and MODS
      2. Selective gut decontamination may be used in patients who cannot be fed enterally to prevent bacterial translocation from the GI tract

II. Maintain airway and ventilation
   A. Positioning for optimal ventilation
      1. Elevate head of bed 30 to 45 degrees
      2. Turn frequently; oscillation therapy may be used
      3. Prone or semiprone position has been shown to improve oxygenation
   B. Bronchial hygiene and chest physiotherapy
      1. Cough and/or suction as indicated
      2. Chest physiotherapy may be indicated
   C. Airway maintenance: intubation is indicated to deliver mechanical ventilation and PEEP when FIO_2 more than 0.50 is required to maintain acceptable oxygenation or as patient fatigues
   D. Mechanical ventilation
      1. Modes: pressure control/inverse ratio ventilation or high-frequency jet ventilation may be used
      2. Tidal volume: limitation of peak inspiratory pressure and reduction of regional lung overdistention by the use of low tidal volumes with permissive hypercapnia may reduce ventilator-induced lung injury and improve outcome in severe ARDS
         a) Avoid large tidal volumes (an ARDS lung is like a "baby lung"); tidal volume should be 4 to 8 ml/kg since excessive volume forced into a small aerated lung can cause volutrauma
         b) The $PaCO_2$ is allowed to gradually increase as minute ventilation is reduced (this condition is referred to as *permissive hypercapnia*)
            (1) Bicarbonate may be used is pH if less than 7.15
            (2) Permissive hypercapnia is contraindicated if the patient has a concurrent head injury and, potentially, intracranial hypertension
   E. CPAP or PEEP
      1. Decreases surface tension: keeps alveoli open
      2. Aids in reopening collapsed alveoli (referred to as *alveolar recruitment*); this effect reduces intrapulmonary shunt and increases functional residual volume
      3. Increases the driving pressure of oxygen: allows achievement of same PaO_2 on a lower FIO_2 or a higher PaO_2 on the same FIO_2; therefore, decreases risk of oxygen toxicity
      4. Usual level is 5 to 15 cm H_2O but higher levels may be needed to maintain SaO_2 and PaO_2
   F. Aerosolized surfactant (colfosceril [Exosurf] or beractant [Survanta]): decreases surface tension and helps to prevent alveolar collapse; benefit has not been proven in adults

III. Improve oxygen delivery and decrease oxygen consumption
   A. Oxygen therapy
      1. May require high concentrations (up to 100%) with nonrebreathing mask prior to intubation and mechanical ventilation
      2. FIO_2 should be maintained as low as possible to prevent oxygen toxicity; positive pressure (CPAP or PEEP) increases driving pressure, allowing the use of a lower FIO_2 to maintain an acceptable oxygenation (e.g., PaO_2 60 mm Hg; SaO_2 of 90%)
         a) CPAP may be administered via mask prior to intubation
         b) Mechanical ventilation with PEEP; sedation and/or muscle paralysis may be necessary to maintain PEEP
         c) Utilize closed suction system or PEEP valve on a manual resuscitation bag prior to and after suctioning (these patients are usually very PEEP-dependent and will quickly desaturate when PEEP is temporarily discontinued)
   B. Decrease intraalveolar fluid
      1. CPAP or PEEP: increases intraalveolar pressure to aid in prevention of further fluid sequestration into the alveoli
      2. Diuretics
         a) May be given to prevent further fluid sequestration into the alveoli
         b) Guided by PAOP: maintain PAOP at ~12 mm Hg
      3. Avoidance of overhydration, which may occur in trauma patients
   C. Maintain cardiac output and tissue oxygenation
      1. Volume as indicated by PAOP readings: maintain PAOP ~12 mm Hg
      2. Crystalloids versus colloids
         a) Colloids leak across the alveolar-capillary

membrane as readily as crystalloids in this patient due to damage to the alveolar-capillary membrane

b) There is no advantage of one over the other in these patients; balanced amounts may be used, or crystalloids may be used because they have a cost benefit

3. Inotropes as indicated by LVSWI and CI
a) Dobutamine is usually the first choice
b) CI more than 4.5 L/min/m$_2$ may be used as the goal (supranormal oxygen delivery goal of >600 ml/min/m$_2$)

4. Hemodynamic monitoring, including Svo$_2$, to guide therapy
a) Volume or diuretics
b) Inotropic therapy
c) Best PEEP (PEEP that increases Pao$_2$ and Sao$_2$ but does not decrease CI)

5. Blood administration: indicated if hemoglobin is less than 10 to 12 g/dl

6. Liquid ventilation with perfluorocarbons: experimental
a) Increases pulmonary end-expiratory volume and compliance in atelectasis
b) Reduces lung inflammation

7. Extracorpeal membrane oxygenation (ECMO): a form of cardiopulmonary bypass in which the blood is removed from the patient, passed through large membrane lungs, and then placed back into circulation
a) Risks are decreasing
b) May be used as a salvage therapy in patients with life-threatening respiratory failure without multiple organ dysfunction

D. Decrease oxygen consumption
1. Eliminate unnecessary activity
2. Provide rest periods after meals, other activities that increase oxygen consumption
3. Decrease anxiety: anxiolytics, sedatives
4. Treat fever: antipyretics, cooling blankets

IV. Decrease pulmonary hypertension
A. Vasodilators
1. NTP dilates all vessels, interferes with hypoxic vasoconstriction, and may lead to increased intrapulmonary shunting since perfusion is increased in relation to ventilation
2. Nitric oxide is synthesized by vascular endothelium and acts as a natural **local** vasodilator; when administered by inhalation, it dilates vessels only to ventilated areas and acts as a potent bronchodilator
a) Note: NTG and NTP work by a nitric oxide-activated pathway
b) May have best results when used at an earlier, less severe stage of acute lung injury
c) Dosage of nitric oxide: 0.01 to 100 ppm;

low dosages seem to have best effects; average 20 to 40 ppm
d) Adverse effect: methemoglobinemia; monitor methemoglobin levels
3. Prostaglandin E$_1$ may also be used

V. Modify mediator release and effect (experimental)
A. Corticosteroids: may be helpful during the fibroproliferative phase
B. Antiinflammatory agents: anticytokines, antioxidants, antiinflammatory agents

VI. Provide nutritional support to prevent respiratory muscle atrophy
A. Enteral nutrition: helps to prevent translocation of bacteria from the GI tract to the lymphatics and blood vessels
B. High-protein and high-calorie diet rich in omega 3 and omega 6
C. Multivitamin and mineral replacement: vitamins A, C, E, zinc, selenium
D. Glutamine-rich and alanine-rich diet may be particularly helpful in reducing endotoxemia

VII. Monitor for complications
A. Secondary infections: nosocomial pneumonia
B. Sepsis
C. Shock
D. Multiple organ dysfunction syndrome (MODS)
E. Heart failure
F. Airway trauma
G. Dysrhythmias
H. Pulmonary embolism
I. Pulmonary fibrosis
J. Barotrauma
K. GI hemorrhage
L. Disseminated intravascular coagulation
M. Renal failure

Pneumonia
Definition: Acute infection of the lung parenchyma, including alveolar spaces and interstitial tissue
Etiology
I. Causative agents
A. Bacteria
1. Community-acquired pneumonia (CAP)
a) *Streptococcus pneumoniae*
b) *Staphylococcus aureus*
c) *Haemophilus influenzae*
d) *Klebsiella pneumoniae*
e) *Legionella pneumophila*
f) *Bacteroides fragilis*
g) *Mycobacterium tuberculosis*
2. Hospital-acquired (nosocomial) pneumonia
a) *Staphylococcus aureus*
b) *Streptococcus faecalis*
c) *Escherichia coli*
d) *Pseudomonas aeruginosa*
e) *Proteus mirabilis*
f) *Klebsiella pneumoniae*
g) *Enterobacter* species

B. Viruses
   1. *Influenza A*
   2. *Adenovirus*
C. Fungi
   1. *Histoplasma capsulatum*
   2. *Coccidioides immitis*
D. Parasites
E. Mycoplasma: *Mycoplasma pneumoniae*

II. Predisposing factors
   A. Advanced age
   B. History of smoking
   C. Surgery, especially if the following:
      1. Thoracic, abdominal, or flank incisions
      2. Long anesthesia time
      3. Prolonged hospitalization
      4. Mechanical ventilation
   D. Decreased level of consciousness
   E. Artificial airways
   F. Chronic illness
      1. COPD
      2. Diabetes mellitus
      3. Cardiovascular disease
      4. Malignancy
   G. Malnutrition: alcoholism, malignancy, eating disorder, poverty
   H. Immunocompromise
      1. Patients with neutropenia resulting from acute leukemia or cytotoxic agents usually have gram-negative bacilli as a source
      2. Severely immunocompromised patient may also develop pneumonia caused by:
         a) Gram-negative aerobic bacteria
            (1) *Haemophilus influenzae*
            (2) *Klebsiella pneumoniae*
            (3) *Legionella pneumophila*
            (4) *Escherichia coli*
            (5) *Pseudomonas aeruginosa*
            (6) *Proteus mirabilis*
            (7) *Klebsiella pneumoniae*
            (8) *Enterobacter* species
         b) Viruses
            (1) *Cytomegalovirus*
            (2) *Varicella-zoster*
            (3) *Herpes simplex*
         c) Fungi
            (1) *Candida albicans*
            (2) *Aspergillus fumigatus*
            (3) *Cryptococcus neoformans*
         d) Protozoa: *Pneumocystis carinii*
   I. Chronic immobility
   J. Nosocomial pneumonia
      1. Concurrent antibiotic therapy: predisposes the patient to colonization with resistant gram-negative bacilli of the oropharynx
      2. Aspiration of oropharyngeal or gastric secretions; H_2-receptor antagonists and antacids contribute to nosocomial pneumonia by altering the normal extremely acidic pH of the stomach, allowing proliferation of bacteria in the stomach, which then migrate upward to be silently aspirated into the lungs

   3. Bypassing of normal respiratory defense mechanisms (e.g., artificial airway); saline lavage during suctioning of endotracheal tube or tracheostomy has been implicated in increased incidence of nosocomial pneumonia
   4. Hematogenous spread from another site

Pathophysiology

I. Causative agent is inhaled or enters the pharynx through direct contact
II. Alveoli become inflamed and edematous
III. Alveolar spaces fill with exudate and consolidate
IV. Alveoli are not ventilated, but they are perfused: ventilation-perfusion mismatch, shunt
V. Diffusion of O_2 obstructed, causing hypoxemia; hypercapnia may occur
VI. Stimulation of goblet cells increases mucus, which causes increased airway resistance and increased work of breathing
VII. Acute respiratory failure
VIII. Abscesses may form and rupture into the pleural space to form pneumothorax and/or empyema

Clinical Presentation

I. Subjective
   A. Frequently begins with cold or flulike symptoms; infectious symptoms: chills, fever, malaise, tachycardia, headache, myalgia
   B. Chest pain (frequently pleuritic-type pain)
   C. Confusion: especially in elderly patients
II. Objective
   A. Tachycardia
   B. Tachypnea
   C. Fever
   D. Productive cough; sputum mucoid, rusty, blood, or purulent; may have foul odor
   E. Diaphoresis
   F. Cyanosis may be seen (dependent on hemoglobin and Sao_2 levels)
   G. Splinting of chest; decreased chest excursion
   H. Use of accessory muscles
   I. Increased tactile fremitus
   J. Clinical indications of dehydration
   K. Dullness to percussion over areas of consolidation
   L. Breath sound changes: diminished, bronchial breath sounds, crackles and/or rhonchi, rub may be audible
   M. Voice sounds: egophony, bronchophony, whispered pectoriloquy
III. Diagnostic
   A. Serum
      1. WBC
         a) Elevated with shift to left if bacterial but may be normal in elderly patient, immunocompromised patient, or in overwhelming infection
         b) Normal or decreased if viral
      2. Arterial blood gases: decreased Pao_2 with clinical indications of hypoxemia; $Paco_2$ may be increased, decreased, or normal depending on ventilation

B. Blood culture: positive for specific organism in bacteremia
C. Sputum culture: positive for specific organism if bacterial; acid-fast: to rule out tuberculosis
D. Chest X-ray
   1. Localized segmental or lobar consolidation
   2. Multiple infiltrates
   3. Viral pneumonias cause diffuse changes
   4. Pleural effusion may indicate empyema

Nursing Diagnosis
   I. Impaired Gas Exchange related to V/Q mismatching, intrapulmonary shunt
   II. Ineffective Breathing Patterns related to increased work of breathing and fatigue
   III. Ineffective Airway Clearance related to retained secretions, increased viscosity of secretions
   IV. Risk for Fluid Volume Deficit related to increased sensible loss from hyperventilation, fever, oxygen therapy, decrease fluid intake
   V. Risk for Infection related to inadequate primary defenses, invasive procedures, chronic disease, poor airway clearance
   VI. Altered Nutrition: Less than Body Requirements related to lack of exogenous nutrients, increased nutrient requirements
   VII. Activity Intolerance related to imbalance between oxygen supply and oxygen demand, dyspnea
   VIII. Anxiety related to change in health status
   IX. Ineffective Individual and Family Coping related to hospitalization, critical illness

Collaborative Management
   I. Prevent nosocomial pneumonia or spread of infection
      A. Use good handwashing techniques
      B. Provide meticulous oral, nasal, and airway care
      C. Suction oropharynx to prevent drainage of secretions around endotracheal or tracheostomy cuff
      D. Use sterile suctioning techniques if endotracheal; aseptic if nasotracheal
      E. Empty water condensation in ventilator or nebulizer tubing into water trap or container; never empty back into humidifier reservoir
      F. Change ventilator tubing according to hospital policy (usually every 48-72 hours)
      G. Change closed suction system every 24 hours
   II. Maintain airway and improve ventilation
      A. Positioning
         1. Elevate head of bed to 30 to 45 degrees
         2. Turn from "good lung down" to back
      B. Organism-specific antibiotics; broad-spectrum antibiotics may be used until culture and sensitivity is back from laboratory
      C. Hydration: 2 to 3 L/24 hr unless contraindicated by cardiac or renal disease
         1. Oral fluids: noncaffeinated
         2. Intravenous fluids: usually D_5NS
      D. Bronchial hygiene and chest physiotherapy
         1. Inspiratory maneuvers: deep breathing, incentive spirometry

2. Humidified air and/or oxygen
3. Encouragement to cough or suctioning if the patient is unable to clear airways
4. Postural drainage, percussion, vibration if necessary
5. Bronchodilators as prescribed
6. Expectorants (e.g., guaifenesin [Robitussin], potassium iodide [SSKI]) may be used but hydration is most important; water is the best expectorant
7. Mucolytics (e.g., acetylcysteine [Mucomyst]) may be used to decrease the tenacity of the mucus
8. Sedatives: generally avoided unless patient is very agitated
9. Antitussives: generally avoid
   E. Bronchoscopy may be necessary if airway clearance techniques are inadequate
   F. Intubation and mechanical ventilation may be necessary, if $PaCO_2$ continues to rise and acidosis develops; the goal of mechanical ventilation is to normalize the pH, not necessarily the $PaCO_2$
   III. Optimize oxygen delivery and decrease oxygen consumption
      A. Oxygen
         1. Nasal cannula or mask; masks are contraindicated in hypercapnic patients because the high concentration of oxygen provided by these delivery systems would likely eliminate the hypoxic drive
         2. Flow rate or oxygen concentration to keep SpO_2 approximately 95% unless contraindicated; in patients with chronic hypercapnia, adjust flow rate or oxygen concentration to keep SpO_2 approximately 90%
      B. Rest periods, especially after meals or activities
      C. Treatment of fever: antipyretics, cooling blankets
   IV. Treat chest pain
      A. Analgesics in adequate doses but still allow patient to breath deeply and cough as indicated
      B. Positioning on unaffected side or back
   V. Monitor for complications
      A. Acute respiratory failure
      B. Pleural effusion
      C. Empyema
      D. Lung abscess
      E. Septic shock

Aspiration Lung Disorder
Definition: Lung injury related to the inhalation of stomach contents, saliva, food, or other foreign material into the tracheobronchial tree
Etiology (Risk Factors)
   I. Altered consciousness and/or gag reflex
      A. Anesthesia
      B. CNS disorders: cerebral infarction or hemorrhage, seizures, neuromuscular diseases

II. Altered anatomy
   A. Endotracheal tube keeps the epiglottis splinted open
   B. Tracheostomy tube impairs swallowing mechanism
   C. GI tamponade (e.g., Sengstaken-Blakemore tube)
   D. Facial, neck, or oral trauma
III. GI conditions
   A. Esophageal abnormalities
   B. Hiatal hernia with gastroesophageal reflux
   C. Decreased GI motility or obstruction
   D. Vomiting
IV. Enteral nutritional support
   A. Nasogastric tube causes incompetence of the gastroesophageal sphincter
   B. Increased residual content in patients receiving enteral feedings
   C. Improper positioning of patients, especially if on enteral feedings

Pathophysiology

I. Oropharyngeal secretions are most commonly aspirated
II. Aspiration of large particles can obstruct major airways, cause asphyxia, and potentially result in death
III. Aspiration of smaller particles causes segmental atelectasis and subacute inflammatory pulmonary reaction with extensive hemorrhage
   A. Clear acidic liquid causes chemical burn and destruction of the type II pneumocytes; frequently referred to as *aspiration pneumonitis*
      1. Fluid and blood accumulate in the interstitium and the alveoli
      2. Decreased lung compliance and decreased alveolar ventilation
      3. Hypoxemia, bronchospasm, and hemorrhage with pulmonary edema and necrosis
   B. Clear nonacidic liquid causes reflex airway closure, pulmonary edema, surfactant changes; contaminated material may cause massive infection
   C. Aspiration into the right lung is more common than aspiration into the left lung due to the straighter angle of the right mainstem bronchus off the trachea

Clinical Presentation

I. Subjective
   A. Dyspnea
   B. Cough
   C. Chest pain: pleuritic in nature
   D. Anxiety
II. Objective
   A. Tachycardia
   B. Tachypnea
   C. Fever
   D. Increased work of breathing: use of accessory muscles, intercostal retractions
   E. Productive cough or suctioned material
      1. Foul-smelling sputum
      2. Food, stomach contents may be seen in

secretions suctioned from lungs; enteral feedings test positive for glucose
      3. Pink, frothy sputum may occur with acidic aspiration
   F. Breath sounds
      1. Stridor if obstruction of the upper airway occurs
      2. Diminished breath sounds
      3. Adventitious sounds: crackles, rhonchi, wheezing
   G. Hypoxemia (decreased SpO_2, SaO_2, PaO_2) and clinical indications of hypoxia (see Box 4-3)
   H. Compliance: decreased static and dynamic compliance; increased peak inspiratory pressures
III. Diagnostic
   A. Serum
      1. WBC increased
      2. Arterial blood gases
         a) PaO_2 and SaO_2 decreased
         b) $PaCO_2$ may be normal, decreased, or increased depending on ventilation pattern (e.g., may be low due to hyperventilation or high due to hypoventilation)
   B. Sputum: culture and sensitivity
   C. Chest X-ray
      1. Bilateral patchy infiltrates or atelectasis
      2. Pulmonary edema may be present

Nursing Diagnosis

I. Risk for Aspiration related to impaired swallowing ability, altered consciousness, impaired protective reflexes, delayed gastric emptying, artificial airway
II. Impaired Gas Exchange related to V/Q mismatching, intrapulmonary shunt, intraalveolar fluid
III. Ineffective Breathing Patterns related to airway obstruction, increased work of breathing and fatigue
IV. Ineffective Airway Clearance related to retained secretion
V. Risk for Infection related to aspiration of foreign material, inadequate primary defenses, invasive procedures, chronic disease, and poor airway clearance
VI. Altered Nutrition: Less than Body Requirements related to lack of exogenous nutrients, increased nutrient requirements
VII. Anxiety related to change in health status

Collaborative Management

I. Prevention
   A. Maintain appropriate positioning
      1. Place unconscious patient in side-lying position
      2. Avoid flat position, especially in patients receiving enteral feedings; keep head of bed elevated to 30 to 45 degrees continuously for patients on continuous feedings and during and for at least 30 minutes after intermittent feedings
         a) Stop continuous enteral feedings at least 30 minutes prior to any procedure that requires that the head of bed must be lowered

b) If the head of bed cannot be elevated, position the patient on his or her right side as much as possible to facilitate movement of gastric contents through the pylorus and to allow drainage of emesis out of the mouth rather than be aspirated

3. Do not restrain in such a way that the patient cannot protect the airway if vomiting occurs

B. Maintain proper functioning of nasogastric tube utilized for gastric suctioning
   1. Check placement by the following
      a) Aspirating gastric contents: ensure with litmus paper that pH is acidic
      b) Inject air into stomach with a bulb syringe while listening for bubbling at the epigastrium
   2. Check placement if gastric secretions decrease in volume

C. Prevent aspiration in patients with artificial airways
   1. Ensure inflation of tracheostomy cuff during meals and suction mouth and oropharynx before deflating the cuff
   2. Suction secretions that accumulate above an endotracheal tube or tracheostomy tube cuff whenever suctioning tube and prior to any cuff deflation (remember that the cuff is not absolutely occlusive and silent aspiration occurs)

D. Select appropriate tube and site for enteral feeding
   1. Patients with altered pharyngeal reflexes should be fed into the intestine via duodenal or jejunal tubes
   2. Small-lumen feeding tubes cause less gastroesophageal incompetence than do larger lumen nasogastric tubes
      a) Tubes that do not go through the gastroesophageal sphincter (e.g., percutaneous endoscopic gastrostomy [PEG] or needle jejunostomy tubes) are best for long-term enteral feeding
   3. The only consistently reliable method to confirm placement of small-lumen feeding tubes is by X-ray

E. Monitor for gastric retention in patients on gastric enteral feedings
   1. Check for retention before each feeding if intermittent enteral feedings are being administered and every 4 hours if continuous enteral feedings are being administered
   2. If more than 100 ml are aspirated, hold feeding for 1 hour and then recheck for retention; metoclopramide (Reglan) may be prescribed to increase gastric motility
   3. Aspiration of small-lumen feeding tubes is difficult because they tend to collapse with suction; increase in abdominal girth, absent bowel sounds, and nausea are signs of gastric retention that indicate that the feeding should be stopped in patients with these tubes

F. Closely monitor secretions suctioned or expectorated
   1. Glucose testing may be performed to confirm presence of enteral feeding in sputum
   2. Antacids and histamine$_2$-receptor antagonists alter the pH of gastric secretions, decreasing the risk of acid aspiration; NOTE: This change means that bacteria that are normally killed by the acid environment of the stomach are not killed but proliferate; these bacteria may be silently aspirated, causing nosocomial pneumonia

G. Keep appropriate equipment at bedside
   1. Airway suctioning equipment
   2. Wirecutters for patients with wired jaws
   3. Scissors for patient with GI tamponade

II. Maintain airway, ventilation, and oxygenation if aspiration does occur
   A. Place bed in a slight Trendelenburg position and the patient in a right lateral decubitus position
   B. Suction airway immediately
   C. Stop the enteral feeding if appropriate
   D. Assist with bronchoscopy for removal of large particles if indicated
   E. Administer oxygen therapy if hypoxemia occurs
   F. Monitor arterial blood gases and pulse oximetry closely: a decrease in Sao$_2$ and Pao$_2$ may indicate the development of acute respiratory distress syndrome
   G. Assist with intubation and mechanical ventilation with PEEP as indicated
   H. Administer antibiotics as prescribed (prophylactic antibiotics are not recommended, but antibiotics specific to positive sputum or blood cultures are indicated)
   I. Prepare patient for pulmonary resection if abscess develops
   J. Administer bronchodilators as indicated

III. Decrease inflammatory response if aspiration does occur
   A. Suction airway immediately
   B. Place patient in a side-lying position
   C. Administer corticosteroids after acid aspiration if prescribed (controversial)

IV. Monitor for complications
   A. Acute respiratory failure
   B. Acute respiratory distress syndrome
   C. Pneumonia
   D. Lung abscess
   E. Empyema

Status Asthmaticus
Definitions

I. Asthma: a recurrent, reversible airway disease characterized by increased airway responsiveness to a variety of stimuli that produce airway narrowing

II. Status asthmaticus: exacerbation of acute asthma characterized by severe airflow obstruction that is not relieved after 24 hours of maximal doses of traditional therapy

Etiology

I. Extrinsic: when a specific allergy can be related to the attack
   A. Dust mites
   B. Pet dander
   C. Pollen
   D. Mold
   E. Smoke
   F. Propellants
   G. Air pollution
   H. Preservatives (e.g., bisulfites)
   I. Food
   J. Cold or hot air
   K. Aspirin or nonsteroidal noninflammatory drugs (NSAIDs)
   L. Beta-blockers
II. Intrinsic: when the attack is seemingly unrelated to a specific allergen
   A. Respiratory infection
   B. Stress
   C. Exercise
   D. Gastroesophageal reflux
   E. Aspiration

Pathophysiology

I. Extrinsic trigger (e.g., inhalation of a substance to which the patient is allergic) or intrinsic trigger (e.g., stress)
II. Extrinsic triggers cause IgE to be released; IgE stimulates the mast cells in the pulmonary submucosa to release histamine and slow-reacting substance of anaphylaxis (SRS-A); intrinsic triggers impact on the balance between sympathetic and parasympathetic branches of the autonomic nervous system
III. Histamine causes swelling and inflammation of the smooth muscle of the larger bronchi and mucous membrane swelling
IV. SRS-A causes swelling of the smooth muscle of the smaller bronchi and release of prostaglandins, which enhance the effects of histamine
V. Histamine causes excessive secretion of mucus, which further narrows the airway lumen; tachypnea increases insensible water loss via the respiratory tract, leading to thick tenacious mucus
VI. Airway narrowing is greatest during expiration; the work of breathing is increased and fatigue occurs, impairing ventilation; air trapping causes hyperinflation of alveoli
VII. Excessive mucus in smaller airways causes ventilation/perfusion mismatching and shunt
VIII. Acute respiratory failure with hypoxemia and respiratory acidosis eventually occurs if the attack is not promptly reversed
IX. Intrathoracic pressures are elevated and venous return to the right ventricle is decreased, cardiac output falls, and cardiopulmonary arrest may occur

Clinical Presentation

I. Subjective
   A. Anxiety
   B. Dyspnea
   C. Chest tightness
   D. Fatigue
   E. Insomnia
   F. Anorexia
II. Objective
   A. Tachycardia
   B. Tachypnea
   C. Cough with thick tenacious sputum production
   D. Use of accessory muscles
   E. Intercostal retractions
   F. Prolonged expiration
   G. Diaphoresis
   H. Peak expiratory flow rate below 80% of patient's personal best (frequently below 50% of patient's personal best)
   I. Clinical indications of dehydration: poor skin turgor, dry mucous membranes, increased specific gravity of urine
   J. Breath sound changes: rhonchi, wheezing
   K. Pulsus paradoxus may be seen in critical stages
   L. Absence of rhonchi and wheezes may occur in critical stages; indication of absence of airflow
III. Diagnostics
   A. Serum
      1. WBC count may be increased if infection is the cause
      2. Eosinophil count may be increased if patient is not receiving steroids
      3. Hematocrit may be increased due to dehydration
      4. Serum electrolytes: potassium and/or magnesium may be low during an acute attack
      5. Serum theophylline: if therapeutic 10 to 20 μg/dl; if patient has not been taking the drug, serum theophylline level will be less than therapeutic
      6. Arterial blood gases (Table 5-5)
   B. Sputum
      1. Increased viscosity, may have positive culture
      2. Eosinophil stain: increase in number of eosinophils indicates allergic reaction
   C. Pulmonary function studies (may be impossible to do during attack because the patient is so dyspneic)
      1. Decreased tidal volume and vital capacity
      2. Increased residual volume
      3. FEV_1 and FEV_3 are diminished with improvement after bronchodilators
   D. ECG: sinus tachycardia
   E. Chest X-ray
      1. Normal or hyperinflated lungs with flattened diaphragms
      2. Helpful to rule out foreign body, aspiration, pulmonary edema, pulmonary embolus, pneumonia

Nursing Diagnosis

I. Ineffective Breathing Patterns related to increased airway resistance, increased work of breathing and fatigue

Table 5-5	Asthma: ABG Analysis			
Stage	Pao$_2$	Paco$_2$	pH	Acid-Base Imbalance
I	Normal	Decreased	Increased	Respiratory alkalosis
II	Decreased	Decreased	Increased	Respiratory alkalosis and mild to moderate hypoxemia
III	Very low	Normal	Normal	Significant hypoxemia
IV	Extremely low	Elevated	Decreased	Respiratory acidosis and critical hypoxemia

II. Impaired Gas Exchange related to alveolar hypoventilation
III. Ineffective Airway Clearance related to excessive mucus production, increased viscosity of mucus, decreased ability to expectorate
IV. Risk for Infection related to retained secretions
V. Risk for Fluid Volume Deficit related to increased insensible loss due to hyperventilation
VI. Risk for Infection related to inadequate primary defenses, invasive procedures, chronic disease, poor airway clearance
VII. Altered Nutrition: Less than Body Requirements related to lack of exogenous nutrients, increased nutrient requirements
VIII. Activity Intolerance related to imbalance between oxygen supply and oxygen demand
IX. Anxiety related to change in health status
X. Knowledge Deficit related to disease process, self-care, prescribed therapies

Collaborative Management

I. Assess predisposing factors; eliminate and/or treat cause
   A. Antibiotics to promptly treat infection
   B. Avoidance of exposure to pulmonary irritants and pollutants
   C. Avoidance of drugs or foods that may trigger an attack
   D. Cromolyn sodium (inhaled nonsteroidal antiinflammatory agent) for prevention (not helpful during an acute attack)
II. Maintain airway and improve ventilation
   A. Head of bed elevation to 30 to 45 degrees; overbed table for patient to lean on
   B. Bronchodilators to relax bronchial smooth muscle
      1. Patient has usually administered long-acting (e.g., Salmeterol [Serevent]) and/or short-acting (e.g., metaproterenol [Alupent], albuterol [Proventil], isoetharine [Bronkosol]) beta$_2$-adrenergic agonists via metered-dose inhaler prior to hospitalization
      2. Short-acting beta$_2$-agonists are usually given by nebulizer or metered-dose inhaler acutely; an intermittent positive pressure breathing (IPPB) system should be avoided except in patients with very poor inspiratory effort who cannot distribute medication adequately because IPPB systems can cause pneumothorax, especially in this high-risk group
      3. Xanthines (e.g., theophylline, aminophylline) may be given intravenously for refractory attack
         a) Xanthines were previously classified as class I agents but are now classified as class III
         b) Obtain a theophylline level for patients who have been receiving xanthines at home
         c) Monitor closely for indications of theophylline toxicity
            (1) GI: anorexia, nausea, vomiting
            (2) Cardiac: dysrhythmias
            (3) Neurologic: restlessness, seizures
      4. Anticholinergic (e.g., ipratropium bromide [Atrovent]) may be used in severe attacks to augment the effects of beta$_2$-agonists; may be especially helpful for asthma stimulated by an intrinsic trigger
      5. Magnesium may be prescribed as a smooth muscle relaxant, although its efficacy has not been fully established; given as IV infusion; monitor blood pressure and deep tendon reflexes
   C. Steroids to decrease mucosal swelling and release of histamine by the mast cells; potentiate the bronchodilators
      1. Patient has usually administered steroids (e.g., beclomethasone [Vanceril], Flunisolide [Aerobid], triamcinolone [Azmacort]) via metered-dose inhaler prior to hospitalization
         a) Steroids by inhalation avoid the systemic effects of steroid administration
      2. Prednisone and prednisolone may be administered orally
         a) Initial large doses are titrated downward over days to weeks
         b) Alternate day dosing decreases the potential for adrenal suppression
      3. In status asthmaticus, steroids may be initially administered intravenously (e.g., methylprednisolone [Solu-Medrol]) or orally
   D. Expectorants (e.g., guaifenesin [Robitussin], potassium iodide [SSKI]) may be used but hydration is most important; water is the best expectorant
   E. Mucolytics (e.g., acetylcysteine [Mucomyst]) are generally contraindicated because of the adverse effect of bronchospasm

F. Bronchial hygiene and chest physiotherapy
   1. Deep breathing
   2. Effective coughing
   3. Suctioning only if coughing is ineffective
   4. Postural drainage, percussion, vibration may be necessary
G. Sedatives: generally avoided unless patient is very agitated
H. Antitussives: generally avoided
I. Noninvasive ventilatory methods (CPAP, Bi-PAP) may be administered using a mask
J. Intubation and mechanical ventilation may be necessary if $Paco_2$ continues to rise and acidosis develops
   1. The goal of mechanical ventilation is to normalize the pH, not necessarily the $Paco_2$
   2. Avoid high inspiratory pressure and PEEP if possible since this patient is at high risk for barotrauma
III. Optimize oxygen delivery and decrease oxygen consumption
   A. Oxygen as indicated; usually given by nasal cannula; adjust flow rate to keep Spo_2 ~90%
   B. Relaxation techniques
   C. Rest periods especially after meals or activities
IV. Provide adequate rehydration
   A. Oral fluids: noncaffeinated
   B. Intravenous fluids: usually D_5NS
V. Monitor for complications
   A. Acute respiratory failure
   B. Pneumonia
   C. Pneumothorax
   D. Dysrhythmias
   E. Hypovolemia

Pulmonary Embolism/Infarction

Definition: Obstruction of blood flow to one or more arteries of the lung by a thrombus lodged in a pulmonary vessel; other types of emboli include fat, air, amniotic fluid, tumor, and foreign body (e.g., catheter fragment)
   I. Massive: more than 50% occlusion of pulmonary blood flow; caused by occlusion of a lobar artery or larger artery
   II. Submassive: less than 50% occlusion of pulmonary blood flow; in patients with preexisting heart or lung disease, hemodynamic deterioration occurs with less than 50% pulmonary vascular obstruction

Etiology

I. Risk factors for thrombus formation (Virchow's triad)
   A. Hypercoagulability
      1. Malignancy: especially breast, lung, pancreas, or GI or GU tracts
      2. Oral contraceptives high in estrogen: especially in smokers

   3. Dehydration and hemoconcentration
   4. Fever
   5. Sickle cell anemia
   6. Pregnancy and postpartum period
   7. Polycythemia vera
   8. Abrupt discontinuance of anticoagulants
   9. Sepsis
B. Alterations in the vessel wall
   1. Trauma
   2. IV drug use
   3. Aging
   4. Vasculitis
   5. Varicose veins
   6. Diabetes mellitus
   7. Atherosclerosis
   8. Inflammatory process
C. Venous stasis
   1. Prolonged bedrest or immobilization
   2. Obesity
   3. Advanced age
   4. Burns
   5. Pregnancy
   6. Postpartum period
   7. Heart failure
   8. Myocardial infarction
   9. Bacterial endocarditis
   10. Recent surgery, especially legs, pelvis, or abdomen
   11. Thrombus formation in heart (AF)
   12. Cardioversion
II. Risk factors for fat embolism
   A. Osteomyelitis
   B. Sickle cell anemia
   C. Multiple long-bone fractures, especially pelvis, femur
   D. Trauma to adipose tissue or liver
   E. Burns
III. Risk factors for air embolism
   A. Recent surgical procedure
   B. Insertion of deep vein catheter
   C. Cardiopulmonary bypass
   D. Hemodialysis
   E. Endoscopy

Pathophysiology

I. More than 90% of thrombi develop in the deep veins of the lower extremities; superficial thrombophlebitis poses little risk unless the associated clot extends into the major deep veins; this condition would be suggested by swelling of the leg
II. Thrombus formation enhances platelet adhesiveness and causes release of serotonin (vasoconstrictor)
III. Factors contributing to dislodgment of thrombi
   A. Intravascular pressure changes
      1. Sudden standing (e.g., initial ambulation)
      2. Valsalva maneuver (e.g., coughing, sneezing, vomiting)
      3. Fluid challenges
      4. Massaging legs
   B. Natural mechanism of clot dissolution: 7 to 10 days after clot develops

IV. Consequences
   A. Clot moves to pulmonary vessels, where it stops in the first vessel because it is too large to occlude
   B. Ventilation continues but perfusion is decreased: ventilation-perfusion mismatch; increased alveolar deadspace
   C. No gas exchange takes place, so alveolar CO_2 decreases which causes bronchoconstriction and alveolar shrinking so that less inspired air goes into nonperfused alveoli and more inspired air goes into perfused alveoli
   D. Cessation of blood flow damages type II pneumocytes and leads to a decrease in surfactant
   E. Loss of surfactant causes atelectasis, interstitial fluid movement into the alveolus, and decreased lung compliance
   F. Increased airway resistance and decreased lung compliance increase work of breathing
   G. Pulmonary arterial obstruction and pulmonary vasoconstriction caused by hypoxemia increase pulmonary vascular resistance
   H. Increased PVR causes pulmonary hypertension, increased right ventricular afterload
   I. Right ventricular failure (acute cor pulmonale) may result
   J. Pulmonary infarction may occur, causing hemorrhage, consolidation, and necrosis
      1. Pleural effusion or lung abscess may occur
      2. Some degree of pulmonary fibrosis may occur as the lung heals
      3. Occurs only in approximately 10% of cases of pulmonary embolism due to dual blood supply to the lung (pulmonary and bronchial)
V. Fat emboli: cause interactions with platelets and free fatty acids; release of vasoactive substances
VI. Air emboli: as little as 10 to 100 ml of air may be lethal; clotting of small blood vessels may occur as a result of activation of the clotting cascade

Clinical Presentation
I. Small embolus: patient is asymptomatic
II. Small to medium embolus
   A. Anxiety
   B. Dyspnea
   C. Tachypnea
   D. Tachycardia
   E. Chest pain
   F. Cough
   G. Accentuated P_2 (pulmonic component of S_2; the second component of S_2)
   H. Right-sided S_3 or S_4 (audible at sternum)
   I. Breath sound changes: crackles
III. Large to massive: massive PE is when 50% of pulmonary artery bed is occluded
   A. Feeling of impending doom
   B. Dyspnea
   C. Tachypnea
   D. Tachycardia

   E. Chest pain
   F. Mental clouding and/or syncope
   G. Cyanosis
   H. Clinical indications of RVF: JVD, hepatomegaly, murmur of tricuspid regurgitation, right ventricular heave
   I. Hypotension or sudden shock
   J. May present as pulseless electrical activity (PEA)
IV. If pulmonary infarction develops (hours to days after embolism), the patient will also have:
   A. Fever
   B. Pleuritic chest pain
   C. Hemoptysis
   D. Pleural friction rub
V. If fat embolus: may have no symptoms for 12 to 48 hours
   A. Subjective
      1. Restlessness, confusion
      2. Dyspnea
      3. Confusion, delirium
   B. Objective
      1. Tachypnea
      2. Tachycardia
      3. Fever
      4. Petechiae on conjunctivae, anterior chest, neck, axilla
      5. Breath sound changes: stridor, wheezes
      6. Lethargy, coma
      7. Seizures
      8. Hypoxemia: decreased SpO_2, SaO_2, PaO_2
      9. Clinical indications of hypoxia (see Box 4-3)
VI. If air embolus:
   A. Subjective
      1. Lightheadedness
      2. Weakness
      3. Dyspnea
      4. Palpitations
   B. Objective
      1. Pallor
      2. Tachycardia
      3. Churning noise ("Mill wheel murmur") may be audible
      4. Hypoxemia: decreased SpO_2, SaO_2, PaO_2
      5. Clinical indications of hypoxia (see Box 4-3)
VII. Hemodynamic monitoring
   A. Elevated CVP and RAP
   B. Elevated PA pressures with normal PAOP (increased PAd-PAOP gradient)
   C. Elevated PVR
   D. Decreased CO/CI in massive PE
VIII. Diagnostics
   A. Serum
      1. If thrombotic: Hgb, Hct may be elevated if cause is polycythemia
      2. If fat embolism, laboratory data may include:
         a) Thrombocytopenia
         b) Elevated fibrin split products
         c) Elevated sedimentation rate
         d) Elevated lipase
         e) Elevated triglycerides

f) Increased free fatty acids
g) Decreased hemoglobin
3. ABGs
   a) If thrombotic:
      (1) Decreased Pao_2, Sao_2, Svo_2; Pao_2 less than 50 mm Hg in a patient with previously normal ABGs indicates more than 50% obstruction of pulmonary blood flow and that pulmonary hypertension is present
      (2) Decreased $Paco_2$
      (3) Respiratory alkalosis initially; may have metabolic acidosis if severe hypoxemia; respiratory acidosis may develop with significant atelectasis or fatigue
   b) If fat or air embolism:
      (1) Decreased Pao_2, Sao_2
      (2) Increased $Paco_2$
      (3) Respiratory acidosis; may have metabolic acidosis if severe hypoxemia
B. ECG
   1. Dysrhythmias
      a) Sinus tachycardia
      b) Atrial dysrhythmias, especially atrial fibrillation are common
      c) Ventricular dysrhythmias may occur in hypoxemia
   2. Blocks: new RBBB may be seen
   3. Tall, peaked P-waves in lead II (P-pulmonale)
   4. Right axis deviation may be seen (QRS complex negative in I, positive in aVF)
   5. Right ventricular strain: ST segment elevation in V_1, V_2
   6. Helpful to rule out MI as cause of signs/symptoms
C. Chest X-ray
   1. If thrombotic:
      a) Initially normal
      b) After 24 hours: small infiltrates may be seen secondary to atelectasis; elevated hemidiaphragm on affected side; decreased pulmonary vascularity
      c) If pulmonary infarction: infiltrates and pleural effusion may be seen
   2. If fat embolism:
      a) Diffuse extensive interstitial and alveolar infiltrates
D. Echocardiography
   1. Shows right ventricular dilation and hypokinesis
   2. May show tricuspid regurgitation
   3. May show bulging of interventricular septum into LV, which reduces LV size with D-shaped LV
E. V/Q scan
   1. Most important noninvasive diagnostic study for PE
   2. Shows perfusion defect with normal ventilation

3. Positive predictive value of high-probability V/Q scan is 96% when supported by high clinical suspicion of PE
4. Intermediate or low-probability V/Q scan with positive D-dimer is indication for pulmonary angiography; positive D-dimer is an indication that the fibrinolytic system has been activated (e.g., clot)
F. Pulmonary angiography
   1. The definitive diagnostic study for PE
   2. Shows cutoff of a vessel or a filling defect within 24 to 72 hours

Nursing Diagnosis

I. Impaired Gas Exchange related to V/Q mismatching, alveolar deadspace
II. Ineffective Breathing Patterns related to increased work of breathing and fatigue
III. Decreased Cardiac Output related to acute pulmonary hypertension and right ventricular failure
IV. Risk for Infection related to inadequate primary defenses, invasive procedures, chronic disease, poor airway clearance
V. Altered Nutrition: Less than Body Requirements related to lack of exogenous nutrients, increased nutrient requirements
VI. Activity Intolerance related to imbalance between oxygen supply and oxygen demand
VII. Altered protection related to thrombolytics and/or anticoagulants
VIII. Anxiety related to change in health status
IX. Knowledge Deficit related to disease process, self-care, prescribed therapies

Collaborative Management

I. Prevent emboli formation
   A. Ambulation when possible
   B. Range-of-motion exercises for nonambulatory patients
   C. Elastic stockings or sequential compression devices for high-risk patients; care must be taken to prevent constriction and tourniquet effect of stockings
   D. Repositioning frequently; avoid extreme knee or hip flexion
   E. Deep breathing exercises
   F. Mini-heparin (usually 5000 U subcutaneously every 12 hours) or dextran 40 (usually 500 ml/24 hr) may be ordered; low-molecular-weight heparin may be used
   G. Adequate fluid intake
   H. Careful venipuncture and IV care
      1. Avoidance of venipunctures in legs
      2. Atraumatic venipuncture; avoid multiple sticks
II. Prevent dislodgment of clot
   A. Avoidance of Valsalva maneuver
   B. Steady IV flow rates
   C. Avoidance of leg massage
III. Maintain adequate airway, ventilation, and oxygenation
   A. Oxygen to maintain Spo_2 95% or greater

unless contraindicated; if patient has history of COPD, administer oxygen to maintain SpO_2 ~90%; high concentrations of oxygen via nonrebreathing mask may be needed to maintain the desired oxygen saturation

  B. Analgesics to prevent splinting and encourage deep breathing

  C. Quiet, restful environment

  D. Intubation and mechanical ventilation may be needed if patient becomes fatigued

IV. Arrest thrombosis and reestablish perfusion

  A. Baseline clotting profile

  B. Thrombolytic therapy: indicated for massive PE with refractory hypoxemia or right ventricular failure

    1. Actions

      a) Dissolves recent clots promptly

      b) Speeds pulmonary tissue reperfusion

      c) Reverses right ventricular failure

      d) Improves pulmonary capillary blood volume

    2. Agents

      a) Tissue plasminogen activator (rt-PA): 100 mg over 2 hours

      b) Streptokinase: 250,000 U over 30 minutes followed by 100,000 U/hr for next 24 hours

      c) Urokinase: 4,400 U/kg over 10 to 20 minutes followed by 4,400 U/kg/hr for 12 to 24 hours

    3. Contraindications and nursing management: see the MI section of Chapter 3

    4. Follow thrombolytic with anticoagulant

  C. Heparin

    1. Action: prevents further clot deposition

    2. Dose: 60 to 80 U/kg initially, followed by 12 to 18 U/kg/hr to maintain aPTT 1.5 to 2 × laboratory control; higher doses may be necessary initially due to low antithrombin III levels after PE

    3. Heparin therapy is usually maintained for approximately 7 to 10 days

  D. Oral anticoagulants: started 3 to 4 days before parenteral anticoagulants are discontinued; continued for up to 6 months; maintain PT at 1.5 × laboratory control (INR 1.5)

  E. Pulmonary embolectomy: indicated for patient with massive PE who is decompensating and cannot be stabilized or cannot receive thrombolytic or anticoagulant therapy

    1. Complication rates for pulmonary embolectomy are very high (30% mortality); requires cardiopulmonary bypass

    2. Experimental method: suction catheter embolectomy with percutaneously inserted catheter

  F. Surgical interruption of inferior vena cava: indicated for recurrent PE or if anticoagulants are contraindicated (remember that this treatment is effective in protecting the lung from

successive emboli but does not do anything about the current PE)

    1. Vena caval umbrella

    2. Greenfield filter

    3. Bird's nest filter (does not require precise axial orientation)

  G. Pulmonary vasodilators (e.g., isoproterenol, nitroglycerin, prostaglandins) may be administered to reverse pulmonary vasoconstriction

  H. Volume expansion may be required to maintain systolic BP of 90 mm Hg

  I. Inotropes (e.g., dobutamine) may be used to increase right ventricular contractility and cardiac output

V. Monitor for complications

  A. Pulmonary infarction

  B. Cerebral infarction

  C. Myocardial infarction

  D. Right ventricular failure

  E. Dysrhythmias or blocks

    1. Atrial dysrhythmias are common if RVF occurs

    2. Ventricular dysrhythmias may occur in hypoxemia

    3. RBBB may occur but is usually transient

  F. Hepatic congestion and necrosis

  G. Pneumonia

  H. Pulmonary abscess

  I. Acute respiratory distress syndrome

  J. Disseminated intravascular coagulation

  K. Shock

  L. Complications of therapy

    1. Bleeding related to thrombolytic or anticoagulant therapy

    2. Oxygen toxicity related to high concentrations of oxygen

VI. Specific to fat embolism

  A. Prevention: early immobilization of long bone fractures

  B. Oxygen via nasal cannula at 5 L/min unless contraindicated; 100% nonrebreathing mask may be necessary

  C. Chest physiotherapy

  D. Intubation and mechanical ventilation may be necessary

  E. Steroids (e.g., cortisone) to decrease inflammatory response

  F. Fluids may be necessary

  G. Osmotic diuretics: if pulmonary edema is present

VII. Specific to air embolism

  A. Prevention: Trendelenburg position for the insertion of central venous catheters or treatment of chest trauma; use of Luer-Lok connections

  B. Left lateral decubitus position with head down (referred to as *Durant's maneuver*) if air embolus suspected

  C. Attempts may be made to aspirate the air embolus

  D. External cardiac compressions push air out of the right ventricle into the pulmonary circulation, fragmenting the air bolus into smaller air bubbles

E. Oxygen via 100% nonrebreathing mask; hyperbaric oxygen is indicated if and when available for large air emboli

F. Pressure dressing to IV site at the time of venous catheter removal

Chest Trauma
Pulmonary Contusion

I. Definition: damage to the lung parenchyma that results in localized edema and hemorrhage

II. Etiology

  A. Blunt trauma: high-speed motor vehicle collision is most common

  B. Crush injuries

  C. Chest compressions during cardiopulmonary resuscitation

  D. Frequently associated with flail chest

III. Pathophysiology

  A. Blunt trauma causes deceleration injury to chest wall and compression of thoracic cavity

  B. Diminished thoracic size compresses lung tissue, and decompression causes capillary rupture and subsequent hemorrhage

  C. Initial hemorrhage due to bruising, pulmonary tears, lacerations

  D. Then interstitial and alveolar edema at site of contusion

  E. Finally massive interstitial edema with general inflammation

  F. Damaged or closed alveolar-capillary units cause ventilation/perfusion mismatch and shunt

  G. Increased pulmonary vascular resistance (PVR), decreased lung compliance, decreased pulmonary blood flow occurs

  H. Atelectasis may occur due to retained secretions and infection

  I. Severe pulmonary lacerations may cause concurrent hemothorax

  J. Pulmonary contusion may accompany flail chest and may be masked by the obvious ventilation difficulties seen in flail chest

IV. Clinical presentation (may be delayed 24 to 48 hours)

  A. Subjective

    1. Anxiety, restlessness

    2. Dyspnea

    3. Chest tenderness

  B. Objective

    1. Tachycardia

    2. Tachypnea

    3. Increased work of breathing: use of accessory muscles, tripod position

    4. Ecchymosis at site of impact

    5. Ineffective cough, guarding

    6. Hemoptysis

    7. Dullness to percussion on affected side

    8. Breath sound changes: crackles, wheezes

C. Diagnostic

  1. Arterial blood gases

    a) Pao_2 decreased

    b) $Paco_2$ may be normal or decreased depending on ventilation pattern (e.g., may be low due to hyperventilation)

  2. Chest X-ray

    a) Changes may take 2 to 24 hours to develop on chest X-ray: patchy, poorly defined areas of increased parenchymal density reflecting intraalveolar hemorrhage; linear and irregular infiltrates in the bronchioles

    b) If severe, extensive areas of increased parenchymal density within one or both lungs

    c) Diaphragm may be lower on affected side because injured lung is bigger

    d) To differentiate ARDS from pulmonary contusion:

      (1) Pulmonary contusion is usually localized and occurs near the site of external trauma

      (2) ARDS causes diffuse bilateral changes

  3. CT scan: assesses damage to pulmonary parenchyma and pleural cavity

V. Nursing diagnosis

  A. Impaired Gas Exchange related to V/Q mismatching, intrapulmonary shunt

  B. Ineffective Breathing Patterns related to chest pain

  C. Ineffective Airway Clearance related to retained secretions

  D. Risk for Fluid Volume Excess related to altered permeability of alveolar-capillary membrane

  E. Pain related to pleural injury, chest wall injury, rib fracture, and inflammation

  F. Risk for Infection related to inadequate primary defenses, invasive procedures, chronic disease, and poor airway clearance

  G. Altered Nutrition: Less than Body Requirements related to lack of exogenous nutrients, increased nutrient requirements

  H. Activity Intolerance related to imbalance between oxygen supply and oxygen demand

  I. Anxiety related to change in health status

VI. Collaborative management

  A. Establish and maintain airway, ventilation, and oxygenation

    1. Oxygen per nasal cannula at 5 L/min unless contraindicated; if patient has history of COPD, administer oxygen to achieve an oxygen saturation of ~90% by pulse oximetry

    2. Analgesics in doses adequate to allow patient to breath deeply and cough as indicated

    3. Chest physiotherapy

      a) Suctioning if patient cannot cough adequately to clear airways

b) Bronchoscopy may be necessary if airway clearance techniques are inadequate

4. Endotracheal intubation and mechanical ventilation with PEEP may be necessary
   a) Synchronous independent lung ventilation may be necessary to prevent the detrimental effects of PEEP on the normal alveoli (e.g., increased alveolar pressure and decreased blood flow); requires double-lumen endotracheal tube and two mechanical ventilators

5. Positioning with good lung down

6. Careful fluid administration to prevent pulmonary edema
   a) Goal is usually to maintain RAP ~4 mm Hg and PAOP ~10 mm Hg
   b) Diuretics may also be given

7. Steroids currently are not recommended

B. Control pain
   1. Narcotics given on a regular schedule
   2. Intercostal nerve block
   3. Epidural analgesic

C. Monitor for complications
   1. Pneumonia: very common complication
      a) Prophylactic antibiotics are not recommended; antibiotics are indicated only if infection is present
      b) Culture sputum as indicated
   2. Lung abscess
   3. Empyema
   4. Pulmonary edema
   5. Pulmonary embolism
   6. Acute respiratory distress syndrome

Closed (Noncommunicating) Pneumothorax (Also Called *Simple Pneumothorax*) (Fig. 5-2)

I. Definition: air enters the intrapleural space through the lung, causing partial or total collapse of the lung

II. Etiology
   A. Primary: related to congenital bleb (common in endomorphic males, age 20 to 40 years)
   B. Secondary
      1. Emphysematous bullous

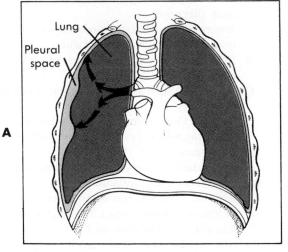

Spontaneous pneumothorax

A

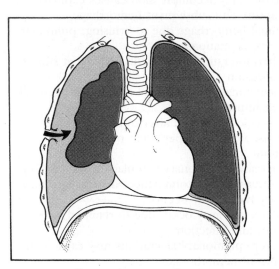

Traumatic pneumothorax

B

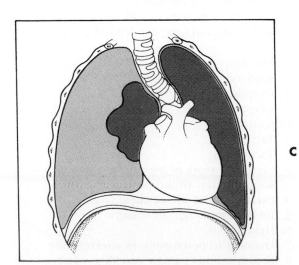

Tension pneumothorax

C

Figure 5-2 Pneumothorax: **A,** Closed. **B,** Open. **C,** Tension. (From Wilson, Thompson: *Respiratory disorders—Mosby's clinical nursing series,* St. Louis, 1990, Mosby.)

2. Tuberculosis
3. Lung cancer
C. Traumatic
   1. Blunt trauma with rib fracture
      a) Motor vehicle collision
      b) Falls
      c) Blows to chest
      d) Blast injuries
   2. Cardiopulmonary resuscitation
   3. Positive pressure mechanical ventilator
D. Iatrogenic causes: central venous catheterization via subclavian or low jugular vein puncture; intracardiac injection; thoracentesis; positive pressure ventilation

III. Pathophysiology
A. Lung laceration by rib fracture or needle; compression of the lung at the height of inspiration when alveolar pressure is high; rupture of weak alveolus, bleb, or bullous
B. Disruption of normal negative intrapleural pressure
C. Lung collapse
D. Decreased surface area for exchange of gases
E. Acute respiratory failure

IV. Clinical presentation
A. Subjective
   1. Dyspnea
   2. Chest pain: sudden, sharp, may be referred to corresponding shoulder, across chest, or abdomen
B. Objective
   1. Tachycardia
   2. Tachypnea
   3. Cough: dry, nonproductive
   4. Asymmetrical chest excursion with limited motion of affected hemithorax
   5. Subcutaneous emphysema possible
   6. Decreased fremitus on affected side
   7. Hyperresonance to percussion on affected side
   8. Diminished to absent breath sounds on affected side
   9. Clinical indications of hypoxemia may be present
   10. If patient on mechanical ventilator: dramatic increase in peak inspiratory pressures and decrease in compliance; high-pressure alarm
C. Diagnostic
   1. Arterial blood gases
      a) Pao_2 decreased
      b) $Paco_2$ increased
   2. Chest X-ray
      a) Air in pleural space and lung collapse
      b) May show mediastinal shift

V. Nursing diagnosis
A. Impaired Gas Exchange related to alveolar hypoventilation
B. Ineffective Breathing Patterns related to chest pain and decreased lung expansion
C. Pain related to pleural injury, inflammation, and presence of chest tube
D. Risk for Infection related to inadequate primary defenses, invasive procedures, chronic disease, and poor airway clearance
E. Altered Nutrition: Less than Body Requirements related to lack of exogenous nutrients, increased nutrient requirements
F. Activity Intolerance related to imbalance between oxygen supply and oxygen demand
G. Anxiety related to change in health status

VI. Collaborative management
A. Establish and maintain airway, ventilation, and oxygenation
   1. Oxygen per nasal cannula at 5 L/min unless contraindicated; if patient has history of COPD, administer oxygen to achieve an oxygen saturation of ~90% by pulse oximetry
   2. Analgesics in doses adequate to allow patient to breath deeply and cough as indicated
   3. Positioning for optimal ventilation: semi-Fowler's or Fowler's position
   4. If supine: position with good lung down
   5. Chest tube and water-seal drainage (not necessary if <10% and asymptomatic)
B. Control pain: narcotics given on a regular schedule
C. Monitor for complications
   1. Recurrent pneumothorax
      a) Avoidance of IPPB in patients with COPD
      b) If positive pressure mechanical ventilation: careful adjustment of tidal volume and PEEP; close monitoring of peak inspiratory pressures
      c) Careful placement of subclavian or jugular venous catheters
      d) Decortication may be performed for patients with recurrent spontaneous pneumothorax; involves the stripping of the parietal pleura from the apex of the lung to allow the visceral pleura to adhere to the chest wall
   2. Atelectasis
   3. Pneumonia, abscess

Tension Pneumothorax (see Fig. 5-2)

I. Definition: accumulation of air in the pleural space without means of escape, causing complete lung collapse and potential mediastinal shift
II. Etiology
A. Blunt or penetrating trauma
B. Positive pressure mechanical ventilation: especially if patient:
   1. Has emphysematous bullae or congenital blebs
   2. Is receiving large tidal volumes and/or PEEP
C. Nonfunctional (e.g., clotted or clamped) water-seal drainage system
D. Airtight dressing on an open pneumothorax
III. Pathophysiology
A. Air rushes into, but not out of, the pleural space

B. Disruption of negative intrapleural pressure; creation of a positive pressure in the pleural space
C. Ipsilateral lung collapses
D. If tear does not seal, a one-way valve effect may be produced, allowing air to enter during inspiration but not to escape during exhalation
E. Increasing positive intrapleural pressure may cause mediastinal shift, leading to compression of the contralateral lung and heart with stretching, and potential tearing of thoracic aorta and vena cava
F. Decreased right ventricular filling, decreased cardiac output
G. Acute respiratory failure and shock may occur

IV. Clinical presentation
A. Subjective
1. Dyspnea
2. Chest pain
B. Objective
1. Tachycardia
2. Tachypnea
3. Asymmetrical chest excursion with limited motion of affected hemithorax
4. Subcutaneous emphysema possible
5. Decreased fremitus on affected side
6. Hyperresonance to percussion on affected side; may even be tympanic
7. Diminished to absent breath sounds on affected side
8. Clinical indications of hypoxemia may be present
9. If mediastinal shift:
   a) Tracheal shift away from affected side
   b) Point of maximal impulse (PMI) shift away from affected side
   c) Jugular venous distention
   d) Hypotension
C. Diagnostic
1. Arterial blood gases
   a) Pao_2 decreased
   b) $Paco_2$ increased
2. Chest X-ray
   a) Air in pleural space and lung collapse on affected side
   b) May show mediastinal shift toward unaffected side

V. Nursing diagnosis
A. Potential Decrease in Cardiac Output related to mediastinal shift, cardiac compression, and tearing of great vessels
B. Impaired Gas Exchange related to alveolar hypoventilation, lung compression
C. Ineffective Breathing Patterns related to chest pain and decreased lung expansion
D. Pain related to pleural injury, inflammation, and presence of chest tube
E. Risk for Infection related to inadequate primary defenses, invasive procedures, chronic disease, and poor airway clearance
F. Altered Nutrition: Less than Body Requirements related to lack of exogenous nutrients, increased nutrient requirements

G. Activity Intolerance related to imbalance between oxygen supply and oxygen demand
H. Anxiety related to change in health status

VI. Collaborative management
A. Establish and maintain airway, ventilation, and oxygenation
1. Oxygen at 100% via nonrebreathing mask unless contraindicated; if patient has history of COPD, administer oxygen to achieve an oxygen saturation of ~90% by pulse oximetry
2. Emergency decompression with perpendicular insertion of a large-bore needle (or IV catheter [e.g., angiocath]) into second anterior interspace at the midclavicular line on the affected side until a chest tube can be inserted; a flutter valve may be placed on the needle to allow air to escape but prevent atmospheric air from entering the pleural space
3. Chest tube and water-seal drainage
4. Analgesics in doses adequate to allow patient to breath deeply and cough as indicated
5. Position for optimal ventilation: semi-Fowler's or Fowler's position
6. If supine: position with good lung down
B. Control pain: narcotics given on a regular schedule
C. Monitor for complications
1. Shock
2. Cardiopulmonary arrest
3. Atelectasis
4. Pneumonia, abscess

Open (Communicating) Pneumothorax (Also Called *Sucking Chest Wound*)
(see Fig. 5-2)

I. Definition: air enters the pleural space through the chest wall
II. Etiology: penetrating trauma
III. Pathophysiology
A. Communication between the intrathoracic space and the atmosphere results in equilibrium between intrathoracic and atmospheric pressures
B. Air movement in and out of opening in chest wall
C. If opening in chest wall is smaller than diameter of trachea, patient may tolerate condition well
D. If opening is larger, more air enters pleural space than enters lungs through trachea
E. During inspiration, the affected lung collapses resulting in ineffective gas exchange
F. May cause tension pneumothorax
IV. Clinical presentation
A. Subjective
1. Dyspnea
2. Chest pain
B. Objective
1. Tachycardia
2. Tachypnea

3. Obvious wound with noise of air moving in and out of pleural space
4. Subcutaneous emphysema is usually present
C. Other subjective, objective, and diagnostic findings as for closed pneumothorax
V. Nursing diagnosis
A. Impaired Gas Exchange related to alveolar hypoventilation
B. Ineffective Breathing Patterns related to chest pain and decreased lung expansion
C. Pain related to pleural injury, inflammation, and presence of chest tube
D. Risk for Infection related to inadequate primary defenses, invasive procedures, chronic disease, and poor airway clearance
E. Altered Nutrition: Less than Body Requirements related to lack of exogenous nutrients, increased nutrient requirements
F. Activity Intolerance related to imbalance between oxygen supply and oxygen demand
G. Anxiety related to change in health status
VI. Collaborative management
A. Establish and maintain airway, ventilation, and oxygenation
1. Oxygen per nasal cannula at 5 L/min unless contraindicated; if patient has history of COPD, administer oxygen to achieve an oxygen saturation of ~90% by pulse oximetry
2. Positioning for optimal ventilation: semi-Fowler's or Fowler's position
3. Closure of open sucking chest wound with petroleum jelly gauze at end-expiration; if symptoms of a tension pneumothorax occur, lift one edge of dressing to allow air to escape
4. Chest tube and water-seal drainage
5. Analgesics in doses adequate to allow patient to breath deeply and cough as indicated
6. Positioning for optimal ventilation: semi-Fowler's or Fowler's position; good lung down or back
7. Surgical intervention may be needed to explore and debride the wound
B. Control pain: narcotics given on a regular schedule
C. Monitor for complications
1. Tension pneumothorax
2. Atelectasis
3. Pneumonia, abscess

Hemothorax

I. Definition: accumulation of blood in pleural space, causing compression and lung collapse
II. Etiology
A. Blunt or penetrating trauma to chest wall, lung tissue, or mediastinum
B. Pleural or pulmonary neoplasm
C. Anticoagulant therapy
D. Iatrogenic causes: subclavian vein puncture (e.g., insertion of deep vein catheter), lung biopsy

III. Pathophysiology
A. Hemorrhage into pleural space compresses and collapses lung
B. Ventilation and oxygenation are impaired
C. Hemorrhage may lead to shock
IV. Clinical presentation
A. Subjective
1. Chest pain may be present
2. Dyspnea
B. Objective
1. Asymmetrical chest excursion with limited motion of affected hemithorax
2. Dullness to percussion on affected side
3. Diminished or absent breath sounds on affected side
4. May have clinical indications of shock if greater than 400 ml
C. Diagnostic
1. Serum
a) Hemoglobin and hematocrit: may be decreased, but remember that changes may occur for up to 6 hours after blood loss
b) Arterial blood gases
(1) PaO_2 decreased
(2) $PaCO_2$ increased
2. Chest X-ray
a) Fluid in pleural space and lung compression
b) Blunting of costophrenic angle if more than 250 ml
c) Hazy appearance over the lower chest
V. Nursing diagnosis
A. Decrease in Cardiac Output related to hemorrhage, loss of circulating volume
B. Altered Tissue Perfusion related to loss of hemoglobin and oxygen-carrying capacity
C. Impaired Gas Exchange related to alveolar hypoventilation, lung compression
D. Ineffective Breathing Patterns related to chest pain and decreased lung expansion
E. Pain related to pleural injury, inflammation, and presence of chest tube
F. Risk for Infection related to inadequate primary defenses, invasive procedures, chronic disease, and poor airway clearance
G. Altered Nutrition: Less than Body Requirements related to lack of exogenous nutrients, increased nutrient requirements
H. Activity Intolerance related to imbalance between oxygen supply and oxygen demand
I. Anxiety related to change in health status
VI. Collaborative management
A. Establish and maintain airway, ventilation, and oxygenation
1. Oxygen per nasal cannula at 5 L/min unless contraindicated; if patient has history of COPD, administer oxygen to achieve an oxygen saturation of ~90% by pulse oximetry
2. Chest tube with water-seal drainage may be adequate treatment if bleeding is self-limiting
3. Surgery for isolation and repair of source of hemorrhage is indicated if blood loss is

greater than 500 ml/hr for 2 hours, hemo-dynamic compromise occurs despite fluid resuscitation, or if hemoglobin and hemato-crit levels fall to severely low levels impairing tissue oxygenation

    4. Positioning for optimal ventilation: semi-Fowler's or Fowler's position

  B. Maintain perfusion and adequate circulating volume

    1. Fluids and/or blood transfusion may be necessary

    2. Autotransfusion may be indicated if blood loss is greater than 400 ml

  C. Monitor for complications

    1. Atelectasis

    2. Shock

Flail Chest (Fig. 5-3)

  I. Definition: instability of chest wall as a result of multiple rib or sternal fractures, causing paradoxi-cal movement of the chest wall during ventilation

  II. Etiology: blunt trauma

    A. Two or more ribs broken in two or more places

    B. Fractured sternum

    C. Sternotomy that hasn't healed (patients with DM have this complication most often especially if internal mammary artery has been used for CABG)

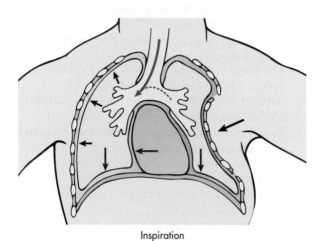

Inspiration

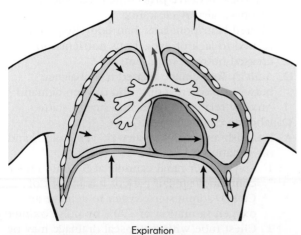

Expiration

Figure 5-3   Flail chest produces paradoxical chest excursion. On inspiration, the flail section sinks in. On expiration, the flail section bulges outward.

  III. Pathophysiology

    A. Fractured segment is free of the bony thorax and moves independently in response to intra-thoracic pressure

    1. During inspiration, atmospheric pressure exceeds intrathoracic pressure on affected side, causing chest wall to move inward

    2. On expiration, intrathoracic pressure exceeds atmospheric pressure, causing chest wall to move outward until the thorax contracts

    B. The bellows effect of the thorax is lost, intra-pleural pressure is less negative than normal

    C. Ventilation is diminished; tidal volume is de-creased causing hypercapnia and hypoxemia; at-electasis may occur

    D. Increased work of breathing causes fatigue

    E. Note related injuries: pulmonary contusion fre-quently accompanies flail chest; pneumothorax, pleural effusion may also be present

  IV. Clinical presentation

    A. Subjective

    1. Dyspnea

    2. Chest pain: related to inspiration and movement

    3. Chest tenderness

    B. Objective

    1. Tachycardia

    2. Tachypnea

    3. Diminished air movement at mouth and nose

    4. Ineffective cough

    5. Ecchymosis over thorax

    6. Paradoxical movement of flail segment

    7. Palpable detached segment, bony crepitation at fracture sites

    8. Subcutaneous emphysema possible

    9. Breath sound changes: diminished breath sounds on affected side

    C. Diagnostic

    1. Arterial blood gases

      a) Pao_2 decreased

      b) $Paco_2$ increased

    2. Spirometry: decreased tidal volume and vital capacity

    3. Chest X-ray: shows rib and/or sternal fractures

  V. Nursing diagnosis

    A. Impaired Gas Exchange related to alveolar hypoventilation

    B. Ineffective Breathing Patterns related to chest wall splinting, loss of thoracic bellows effect

    C. Ineffective Airway Clearance related to retained secretions

    D. Pain related to pleural injury, chest wall injury, rib fracture, and inflammation

    E. Risk for Infection related to inadequate primary defenses, invasive procedures, chronic disease, and poor airway clearance

    F. Altered Nutrition: Less than Body Requirements related to lack of exogenous nutrients, in-creased nutrient requirements

    G. Activity Intolerance related to imbalance between oxygen supply and oxygen demand

    H. Anxiety related to change in health status

VI. Collaborative management
  A. Establish and maintain airway, ventilation, and oxygenation
    1. Oxygen per nasal cannula at 5 L/min unless contraindicated; if patient has history of COPD, administer oxygen to achieve an oxygen saturation of ~90% by pulse oximetry
    2. Reestablishment of the thoracic bellows effect
      a) Stabilization of flail segment with hand, tape, or binder (temporary)
      b) Intubation and internal stabilization with mechanical ventilation may be necessary if patient cannot maintain adequate ventilation despite adequate analgesia
        (1) Indications: respiratory rate more than 35/min, Pao_2 less than 60 mm Hg with supplemental oxygen; $Paco_2$ more than 50 mm Hg
        (2) Mechanical ventilation may need to be maintained for 3 weeks or longer
      c) Surgical internal stabilization of rib and sternal fragments may be done, especially if thoracotomy is needed for another reason
    3. Chest physiotherapy
      a) Deep breathing and incentive spirometry
      b) Positioning for optimal ventilation: semi-Fowler's or Fowler's position
      c) Postural drainage, percussion, vibration; do not percuss over fractured areas
      d) Coughing, suctioning if coughing is ineffective and rhonchi are present
      e) Bronchoscopy may be necessary if airway clearance is inadequate
  B. Provide adequate analgesia to encourage deep breathing (and coughing if indicated)
    1. Intravenous narcotics
    2. Intercostal nerve blocks
    3. Intrapleural analgesia
  C. Assist in insertion of chest tube and establish water-seal drainage if pneumothorax also present
  D. Monitor for complications
    1. Atelectasis
    2. Pneumonia, abscess

LEARNING ACTIVITIES

1. DIRECTIONS: List 10 possible causes of acute respiratory failure.

1. _____
2. _____
3. _____
4. _____
5. _____
6. _____
7. _____
8. _____
9. _____
10. _____

2. DIRECTIONS: List five pulmonary and five nonpulmonary causes for acute respiratory distress syndrome (ARDS).

Pulmonary	Nonpulmonary
1.	1.
2.	2.
3.	3.
4.	4.
5.	5.

3. DIRECTIONS: Complete the following table describing arterial blood gas changes in asthma.

Stage	Pao$_2$	Paco$_2$	pH	Acid-Base Imbalance
I				
II				
III				
IV				

4. DIRECTIONS: Match the treatment to the pathophysiology of ARDS.

____1. pulmonary hypertension   a. PEEP
____2. intrapulmonary shunt   b. nitric oxide
____3. mediator release   c. fluid restriction and diuretics
____4. diffusion defect   d. ECMO
____5. pulmonary edema   e. exosurf
____6. alveolar collapse   f. NSAIDs

5. DIRECTIONS: List three causes of pulmonary embolism in each of the following categories.

Hypercoagulability	Alteration in Blood Vessel	Venous Stasis
1.	1.	1.
2.	2.	2.
3.	3.	3.

6. DIRECTIONS: Match the treatment to the pathology in pulmonary embolism. More than one may be used.

____1. isoproterenol   a. forward failure of left ventricle
____2. dobutamine   b. pulmonary hypertension
____3. heparin   c. occlusion of pulmonary blood supply
____4. tissue plasminogen activator (rt-PA)   d. backward failure of right ventricle
____5. fluids   e. low levels of antithrombin III

7. **DIRECTIONS:** Complete the following crossword puzzle to review pulmonary drugs and therapies.

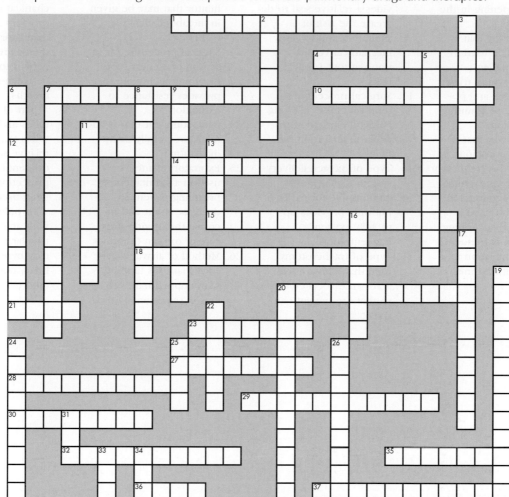

Across

1. Xanthine bronchodilator; also dilates pulmonary vasculature (generic)
4. Type of activity that decreases stress and oxygen requirements; may incorporate music, imagery, stretching, yoga
7. Type of oxygen mask that delivers the highest oxygen concentration
10. Machine that pushes air into the lungs to inflate them
12. Potent sedative frequently used in mechanically ventilated patients (generic)
14. Diagnostic study to obtain fluid from the pleural space for analysis
15. Function normally performed by the upper airway that must be provided in the care of a patient with an artificial airway
18. Drug that breaks down the disulfide bonds in mucus to liquefy the mucus (generic)
20. Beta$_2$-stimulant that may be given orally, subcutaneously, or by inhalation (generic)
21. One method of ensuring that cuff pressure is not excessive is the minimal _____ technique
23. Method of airway clearance used if the patient cannot effectively cough; used only when indicated
27. _____ drainage is a method of airway clearance that uses gravity to drain secretions into the upper airway so that they can be coughed out
28. Complication of mechanical ventilation; risk is increased when large tidal volumes or PEEP are used
29. Opening of the thorax
30. Risk of prolonged use of high concentrations of oxygen
32. Muscle paralytic that may be administered by infusion in patients on mechanical ventilation (generic)
35. Type of oxygen mask that ensures the desired oxygen concentration
36. Expiratory maneuver used in a mechanically ventilated patient to decrease shunt and increase the driving pressure of oxygen (abbrev.)
37. Intubated patients identify their major stressor as the inability to _____

Down

2. Drug used to prevent extension or recurrence of a clot in patients with pulmonary embolus (generic)
3. Drug used to prevent asthma attacks; strictly prophylactic and not used in acute attacks (generic)

5. Surgical procedure to make an opening in the trachea

6. Type of airway that should not be used in conscious patients because it would trigger the gag reflex and potentially cause vomiting and aspiration

7. Type of airway that may be used in conscious patients and is frequently used to prevent trauma to the nasal mucosa in patients who need nasotracheal suctioning

8. Steroid that is frequently given by inhalation in patients with asthma (generic)

9. Type of airway that provides a relative seal to decrease the risk of aspiration and to allow mechanical ventilation without surgical risks

11. Surgical procedure to remove a lobe of a lung

13. Forceful expiration to expel mucus from the lungs

16. Type of oxygen delivery system that is most comfortable for patients but only provides up to 44% oxygen concentration

17. Type of tracheostomy tube that allows a leak across the vocal cords so that the patient can speak

19. Carbonic anhydrase inhibitor that may be given in metabolic alkalosis (generic)

20. Surgical procedure for insertion of a chest tube

22. Breathing technique that provides resistance to expiration

24. Beta$_2$-stimulant that is administered orally or by inhalation

25. Expiratory maneuver used in a spontaneously breathing patient to decrease shunt and increase the driving pressure of oxygen (abbrev.)

26. Method of airway clearance that uses tapping with cupped hands to loosen secretions

31. Inspiratory mode of mechanical ventilation but provides a number of mandatory breaths and then allows the patient to breath between the mandatory breaths

33. A part of endotracheal tubes and tracheostomy tubes that provides a relative seal for mechanical ventilation and airway protection

34. Drug used in patients with pulmonary embolus with acute right ventricular failure or refractory hypoxemia to break down the clot (abbrev.)

LEARNING ACTIVITIES ANSWERS

1. Pneumonia
   Pulmonary edema
   Pulmonary fibrosis
   Pleural effusion
   Pneumothorax
   Asthma
   Atelectasis
   Aspiration pneumonitis
   Adult respiratory distress syndrome (early)
   Smoke inhalation
   Pulmonary embolism
   Kyphoscoliosis
   Fat embolus
   COPD with acute exacerbation
   Status asthmaticus
   CNS depressant drugs
   Anesthesia
   Neuromuscular blocking drugs
   Muscle paralytics
   Aminoglycosides
   Organophosphate poisoning
   Head trauma
   Poliomyelitis
   Amyotrophic lateral sclerosis
   Spinal cord injury
   Guillain-Barré syndrome
   Myasthenia gravis
   Multiple sclerosis
   Muscular dystrophy
   Morbid obesity
   Chest trauma
   Surgery: especially thoracic, abdominal, flank incision
   Sleep apnea
   Tracheal obstruction
   Epiglottitis
   Cystic fibrosis
   Near-drowning

2.

Pulmonary	Nonpulmonary
Chest trauma: pulmonary contusion	Sepsis (#1 cause)
Near-drowning	Shock or prolonged hypotension
Hypervolemia, pulmonary edema	Septic shock
Inhalation of toxic gases and vapors	Hypovolemic shock
Smoke	Anaphylactic shock
Chemicals	Cardiogenic shock
Oxygen toxicity	Neurogenic shock
Pneumonia: viral, bacterial, or fungal	Multisystem trauma
Aspiration pneumonitis	Burns
Radiation pneumonitis	Cardiopulmonary bypass
Pulmonary embolism: thrombotic; air; fat; amniotic fluid	Disseminated intravascular coagulation (DIC)
Radiation	Toxemia of pregnancy
Drugs: bleomycin	Acute pancreatitis
	Diabetic coma
	Head injury
	Drug overdosage: heroin; methadone; barbiturates; aspirin; thiazide diuretics
	Multiple blood transfusions

3.

b 1. pulmonary hypertension   a. PEEP
a 2. intrapulmonary shunt   b. nitric oxide
f 3. mediator release   c. fluid restriction and diuretics
d 4. diffusion defect   d. ECMO
c, a 5. pulmonary edema   e. exosurf
e, a 6. alveolar collapse   f. NSAIDs

4.

Stage	PaO$_2$	PaCO$_2$	pH	Acid-Base Imbalance
I	Normal	Decreased	Increased	Respiratory alkalosis
II	Decreased	Decreased	Increased	Respiratory alkalosis and mild to moderate hypoxemia
III	Very low	Normal	Normal	Moderate hypoxemia
IV	Extremely low	Elevated	Decreased	Respiratory acidosis and critical hypoxemia

5.

Hypercoagulability	Alteration in Blood Vessel	Venous Stasis
Malignancy: especially breast, lung, pancreas, or GI or GU tracts	Trauma	Prolonged bedrest or immobilization
Oral contraceptives high in estrogen: especially in smokers	IV drug use	Obesity
Dehydration and hemoconcentration	Aging	Advanced age
Fever	Vasculitis	Burns
Sickle cell anemia	Varicose veins	Pregnancy
Pregnancy	Diabetes mellitus	Postpartum period
Polycythemia vera	Atherosclerosis	Heart failure
Thrombocytopenia	Inflammatory process	Myocardial infarction
Abrupt discontinuance of anticoagulants		Bacterial endocarditis
Sepsis		Recent surgery especially legs, pelvis, or abdomen
		Thrombus formation in heart (AF)
		Cardioversion

6.

b 1. isoproterenol   a. forward failure of left ventricle
d, a 2. dobutamine   b. pulmonary hypertension
e 3. heparin   c. occlusion of pulmonary blood supply
c 4. tissue plasminogen activator (t-PA) d. backward failure of right ventricle
a 5. fluids   e. low levels of antithrombin III

7.

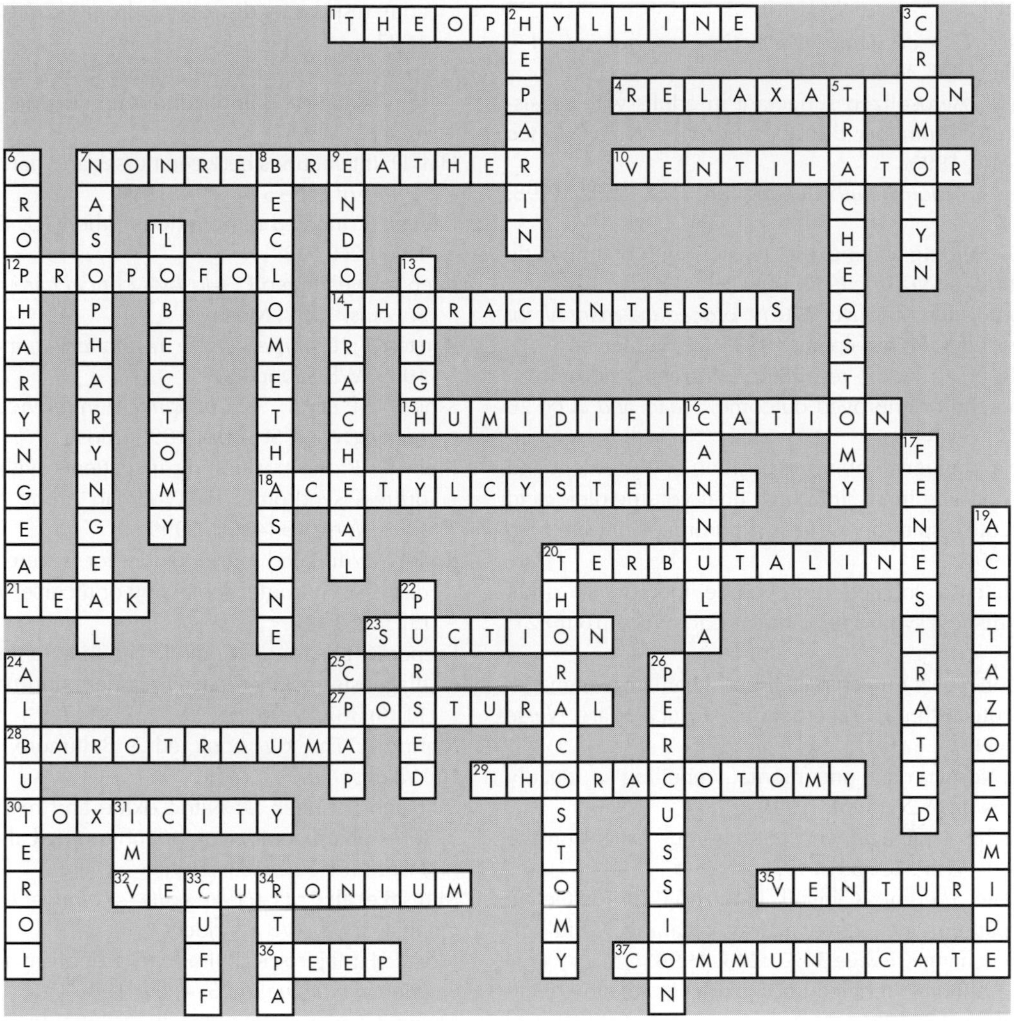

Crossword puzzle (completed):

Across
1. THEOPHYLLINE
4. RELAXATION
7. NONREBREATHER
10. VENTILATOR
12. PROPOFOL
14. THORACENTESIS
15. HUMIDIFICATION
18. ACETYLCYSTEINE
20. TERBUTALINE
21. LEAK
23. SUCTION
27. POSTURAL
28. BAROTRAUMA
29. THORACOTOMY
30. TOXICITY
32. VECURONIUM
35. VENTURI
36. PEEP
37. COMMUNICATE

Down
2. HEPARIN
3. CROMOLYN
5. TRACHEOSTOMY
6. OROPHARYNGEAL
8. BRONCHODILATOR
9. ENDOTRACHEAL
11. LOBECTOMY
13. CRUG...
16. ANATOMY
17. FENESTRATED
19. ACETAZOLAMIDE
22. PHREDSTOMY
24. ALBUTEROL
25. CRED
26. PERCUSSION
31. IMM
33. CUFF
34. T

Bibliography and Selected References

Alspach J, editor: *Core curriculum for critical care nursing,* ed 5, Philadelphia, 1998, WB Saunders.

Anzueto A et al: Aerosolized surfactant in adults with sepsis-induced acute respiratory distress syndrome, *N Engl J Med* 334 (22):1417, 1996.

Beare P, Myers J: *Adult health nursing,* ed 3, St Louis, 1998, Mosby.

Blank-Reid C, Reid P: Taking the tension out of traumatic pneumothoraxes, *Nursing99* 29 (4):41, 1999.

Boggs R, Wooldridge-King M: *AACN procedure manual for critical care,* ed 3, Philadelphia, 1993, WB Saunders.

Brandsletter R et al: Adult respiratory distress syndrome: a disorder in need of improved outcome, *Heart and Lung* 26 (1):3, 1997.

Broccard A et al: Influence of prone position on the extent and distribution of lung injury in a high tidal volume oleic acid model of acute respiratory distress syndrome, *Crit Care Med* 25 (1):16, 1997.

Burke-Martindale C: Inhaled nitric oxide therapy for adult respiratory distress syndrome, *Critical Care Nurse* 18 (6):21, 1998.

Burns S, Lawson C: Pharmacological and ventilatory management of acute asthma exacerbations, *Critical Care Nurse* 19 (4):39, 1999.

Calianno C: Nosocomial pneumonia: repelling a deadly invader, *Nursing96* 26 (5):32, 1996.

Canales M: Asthma management: putting your patient on the team, *Nursing97* 27 (12):33, 1997.

Carlson-Catalano J et al: Clinical validation of ineffective breathing pattern, ineffective airway clearance, and impaired gas exchange, *Image* 30 (3):243, 1998.

Charlton F, Spainhour V: Inhaled nitric oxide: its role in critical care, *AJN* 96 (5):15, 1996.

Chernow B, editor: *The pharmacologic approach to the critically ill patient,* ed 3, Baltimore, 1994, Williams & Wilkins.

Clochesy J et al: *Critical care nursing,* ed 2, Philadelphia, 1996, WB Saunders.

Dellinger R: How to provide safe anticoagulation and reduce venous stasis, *Journal of Critical Illness* 12 (8):486, 1997.

Dettenmeier P: *Pulmonary nursing care,* St Louis, 1992, Mosby.

Evans-Murray A: Adult respiratory distress syndrome after near drowning, *Critical Care Nurse* 17 (2):41, 1997.

Fort P et al: High-frequency oscillatory ventilation for adult respiratory distress syndrome—a pilot syndrome, *Crit Care Med* 25 (6):937, 1997.

Froese A et al: High-frequency oscillatory ventilation for adult respiratory distress syndrome: let's get it right this time! *Crit Care Med* 25 (6):906, 1997.

Gahart B, Nazareno A: *1999 intravenous medications,* St Louis, 1999, Mosby.

Gawlinski A, Hamwi D: *Acute care nurse practitioner clinical curriculum and certification review,* Philadelphia, 1999, WB Saunders.

Gordon P et al: Positioning of chest tubes: effects on pressure and drainage, *Am J Crit Care,* 6 (1):33, 1997.

Gowda M, Klocke R: Variability of indices of hypoxemia in adult respiratory distress syndrome, *Crit Care Med* 25 (1):41, 1997.

Grap M, Munro C: Ventilator-associated pneumonia: clinical significance and implications for nursing, *Heart and Lung* 26 (6):419, 1997.

Hall D: Interactions between nurses and patients on ventilators, *Am J Crit Care* 5 (4):293, 1996.

Kalweit S: Inhaled nitric oxide in the ICU, *Critical Care Nurse* 17 (4):26, 1997.

Keen J, Swearingen P: *Mosby's critical care nursing consultant,* St Louis, 1997, Mosby.

Kersten L: *Comprehensive respiratory nursing,* Philadelphia, 1989, WB Saunders.

Kinney M et al: *AACN clinical reference for critical care nursing,* ed 4, St Louis, 1998, Mosby.

Klein D: Prone positioning in patients with acute respiratory distress syndrome: the Vollman prone positioner, *Critical Care Nurse* 19 (4):66, 1999.

Kollet M: Inhaled nitric oxide for severe acute respiratory distress syndrome: A blessing or a curse? *Heart and Lung* 26 (5):358, 1997.

Leeper K, Shearin S, Cook T: Life-threatening PE: noninvasive diagnosis and aggressive treatment, *Journal of Critical Illness* 11 (6):367, 1996.

Marino P: *The ICU book,* ed 2, Baltimore, 1998, Williams & Wilkins.

McHugh J, Cheek D: Nitric oxide and regulation of vascular tone: pharmacological and physiological consideration, *Am J Crit Care* 7 (2):131, 1998.

Mims B et al: *Critical care skills—a clinical handbook,* Philadelphia, 1996, WB Saunders.

Moccia J, Majoros K: Pulmonary embolism: targeting an elusive enemy, *Nursing96* 26 (4):27, 1996.

Owen C: New directions in asthma management, *AJN* 99 (3):26, 1999.

Price S, Wilson L: *Pathophysiology: clinical concepts of disease processes,* ed 5, St Louis, 1997, Mosby.

Raffin et al: Indices of hypoxemia in patients with acute respiratory distress syndrome: reliability, validity, and clinical usefulness, *Crit Care Med* 25 (1):6, 1997.

Roizen M, Fleisher L: *Essence of anesthesia practice,* Philadelphia, 1997, WB Saunders.

Shah N et al: Efficacy of inhaled nitric oxide in oleic acid-induced acute lung injury, *Crit Care Med* 25 (1):153, 1997.

Shelton B: Mounting an offense against lobar pneumonia, *Nursing98* 28 (12):43, 1998.

Stone D et al: *Perioperative care: anesthesia, medicine, and surgery,* St Louis, 1998, Mosby.

Thelan L et al: *Critical care nursing: diagnosis and management,* ed 3, St Louis, 1998, Mosby.

Thies R, Hotter A: Preventing complications of ARDS therapy, *AJN* 99 (5):34, 1999.

Wiedemann H, Tai D: Adult respiratory distress syndrome: current management, future directions, *Cleve Clini J Med* 64 (7):365, 1997.

Zaccardelli D, Pattishall E: Clinical diagnostic criteria of the adult respiratory distress syndrome in the intensive care unit, *Crit Care Med* 24 (2):247, 1996.

Neurologic System: Physiology, Assessment, and Intracranial Hypertension

Selected Concepts in Anatomy and Physiology

General Information

I. Functions of the neurologic system
   A. Receiving stimuli from the internal and external environment over sensory pathways
   B. Communicating information between the body periphery and the central nervous system
   C. Processing information received at reflex or conscious levels to determine appropriate responses
   D. Transmitting information over motor pathways to organs responsible for responding to the stimuli

II. Components of the neurologic system
   A. Central nervous system (CNS)
      1. Brain
      2. Spinal cord
   B. Peripheral nervous system
      1. Cranial nerves
      2. Spinal nerves
      3. Peripheral nerves
   C. Autonomic nervous system
      1. Sympathetic nervous system (SNS)
      2. Parasympathetic nervous system (PNS)

Microscopic Anatomy and Physiology

I. Nerve cells
   A. Neuroglia (also called *glial cells*)
      1. Neuroglia are more numerous than neurons (85% of the cells in the CNS are neuroglial)
      2. These cells provide support, nourishment, and protection to the neurons
      3. Most tumors of the CNS are neuroglial because they are mitotic and can replicate themselves
      4. Types
         a) Microglia
            (1) Part of the reticuloendothelial system
            (2) Relatively rare in normal CNS tissue
            (3) Become mobile and travel to the area of damage when the neurons become damaged; microglia then enlarge and phagocytize tissue debris

         b) Oligodendroglia: responsible for myelin formation in the CNS
         c) Astrocytes
            (1) May provide nutrients and regulate chemical environment for neurons
            (2) Form the blood–brain barrier with the endothelium of the blood vessels
            (3) Provide structure and support for nerve cells
            (4) May have an indirect role in synaptic transmission
         d) Ependyma
            (1) Line the ventricles of the brain and the central canal of the spinal cord
            (2) Aid in secretion of CSF
   B. Neurons (Fig. 6-1)
      1. Transmit nerve impulses
      2. Ten billion in CNS, most are in the cerebral cortex
      3. Cannot regenerate in the CNS; can regenerate in peripheral nervous system by growing within the myelin if the cell body is intact
      4. Components
         a) Cell body (soma)
            (1) Nucleus: controls metabolic processes of cell
            (2) Cytoplasm: contains organelles to carry out metabolic functions
         b) Axons
            (1) Conduct impulses away from cell body to other neurons or to end organs
            (2) One axon per neuron
            (3) May be myelinated or unmyelinated
         c) Dendrites
            (1) Conduct impulses toward cell body, which receives nerve impulses from the axons of other neurons
            (2) May be more than one dendrite
         d) Neurofibrils: thin, threadlike fibers forming a network in the cytoplasm

293

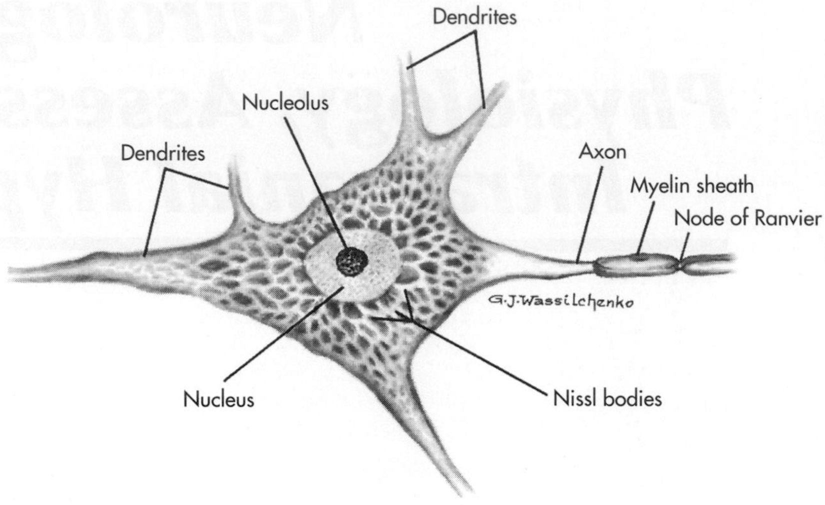

Figure 6-1 The neuron. (From Long BC, Phipps WJ, Cassmeyer VL: *Medical-surgical nursing: a nursing process approach,* ed 3, St Louis, 1993, Mosby.)

e) Nissl bodies
 (1) Specialize in protein synthesis with RNA
 (2) Maintain and regenerate neuronal processes
f) Myelin sheath
 (1) In some neurons, the axons are covered with myelin, a white lipid substance, between the nodes of Ranvier
 (2) Acts as insulation to speed conduction of impulses down the axon sheath
 (3) Accounts for white color found in parts of brain and spinal cord
 (4) Made by oligodendroglia in CNS and by Schwann cells in PNS
g) Nodes of Ranvier
 (1) Constrictions occurring periodically along the axon where it is not covered by myelin
 (2) Allows rapid conduction of impulses by saltatory conduction (node to node)
h) Neurilemma
 (1) Outer coating of the neurons in the peripheral nervous system
 (2) Provides for peripheral nerve regeneration
i) Synaptic knobs: contain vesicles that store neurotransmitter substances
5. Categorization
a) Direction of impulse formation
 (1) Afferent sensory neurons transmit impulses to the spinal cord or brain
 (2) Efferent motor neurons transmit impulses away from the brain or spinal cord
 (3) Remember SA ME (sensory afferent, motor efferent)
 (4) Interneurons transmit impulses from sensory neurons to motor neurons

b) Number of processes
 (1) Unipolar neurons have one process coming from the cell body; it bifurcates into an axon and a dendrite
 (2) Bipolar neurons have two processes (one axon and one dendrite) coming from the cell body
 (3) Multipolar neurons have one axon and more than one dendrite
c) Location
 (1) Upper motor neurons originate in the cerebral cortex and remain in the CNS
 (2) Lower motor neurons originate below the brainstem and innervate muscle
II. Neurophysiology
A. Impulse transmission (Fig. 6-2)
 1. Initiated by a stimulus: chemical, electrical, mechanical, thermal
 2. Change in permeability of the cell membrane to sodium
 3. Depolarization of the cell caused by sodium influx; initiation of an action potential
 4. Repolarization and return to normal, resting, polarized (ready) state occurs
 5. Synaptic transmission (Fig. 6-3)
 a) Unidirectional conduction of an impulse from one neuron to the next
 b) As the impulse nears the end of the axon, a release of neurotransmitter from the synaptic vesicles occurs
 c) Diffusion of neurotransmitter across the synaptic gap, changing the permeability of the cell membrane of the adjoining cell
 d) Continuation of the impulse to its end-organ or cell
 e) Types of synapses
 (1) Axosomatic: the axon of one neuron synapses with the cell body of another neuron
 (2) Axodendritic: the axon of one neuron synapses with the dendrite of another neuron

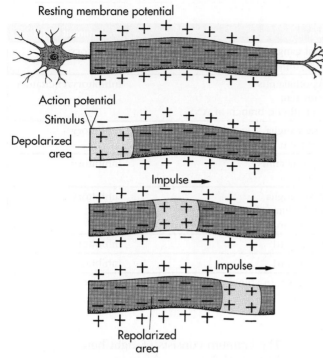

Figure 6-2 Transmission of a nerve impulse. (From Chipps EM, Clanin NJ, Campbell VG: *Neurologic disorders: Mosby's clinical nursing series,* St Louis, 1992, Mosby.)

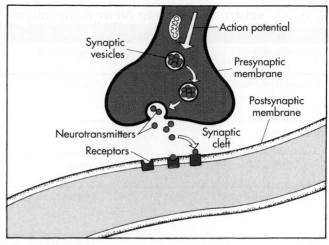

Figure 6-3 Synaptic transmission. (From Chipps EM, Clanin NJ, Campbell VG: *Neurologic disorders: Mosby's clinical nursing series,* St Louis, 1992, Mosby.)

(3) Axoaxonic: the axon of one neuron synapses with the axon of another neuron
　B. Refractory periods
　　1. Absolute: period when the nerve cannot be stimulated again
　　2. Relative: period when the nerve can only be stimulated by a strong impulse
III. Cerebral neurotransmitters (Table 6-1)
　A. Function
　　1. Neurotransmitters are released from the presynaptic vesicles and act as a chemical bridge for the transmission of impulses from one neuron to another
　　2. After synaptic transmission, the neurotransmitter is inactivated by an enzyme (e.g., cholinesterase deactivates acetylcholine)
　B. Types
　　1. Excitatory neurotransmitters promote conduction of the impulse from one cell to the next
　　2. Inhibitory neurotransmitters increase resistance to depolarization
IV. Cerebral metabolism
　A. Oxygen requirements
　　1. The brain constitutes 2% of body weight but receives 20% of the cardiac output
　　2. The brain, especially the cerebral cortex, is very susceptible to change in oxygen delivery; the brainstem is the most resistant to hypoxic damage
　　3. Anoxia causes cerebral edema and neuron death

　B. Nutrient requirements
　　1. The brain has high metabolic energy needs
　　2. Glucose is the main source of cellular energy (ATP)
　　　a) Triggered by the SNS, gluconeogenesis is a very important process because it causes the conversion of protein and fat to glucose; the brain does not require insulin to use glucose
　　　b) Hypoglycemia is associated with neurologic symptoms
　　　　(1) Confusion usually occurs if blood glucose is less than 50 mg/dl
　　　　(2) Coma occurs if blood glucose is less than 20 mg/dl
　　　c) Although hyperglycemia does not cause direct neurologic effects, the osmotic effect may cause hyperosmolality and cerebral dehydration (e.g., HHNK)
　　3. Vitamins
　　　a) Thiamine (B_1) is important in the Krebs cycle; deficiency of B_1 causes Wernicke's encephalopathy
　　　b) Vitamin B_{12} is important in the spinal cord and peripheral nervous system; a deficiency of B_{12} causes pernicious anemia and gradual deterioration of the CNS and peripheral nerves
　　　c) Pyridoxine (B_6) is a coenzyme that participates in many enzymatic reactions in the CNS; deficiency of B_6 causes neuropathy and seizures
　　　d) Niacin (nicotinic acid) is needed for the synthesis of coenzymes; deficiency of niacin causes pellagra
V. Blood–brain barrier
　A. Not a true structure but is a special permeability characteristic of brain capillaries and choroid plexus

Table 6-1 Neurologic System Neurotransmitters

Name	Type	Region	Predominant Effect
Acetylcholine	Cholinergic	• Basal ganglia pyramidal cells • Parasympathetic branch of ANS	Excitatory
Norepinephrine	Amine	• Hypothalamus • Brainstem • Sympathetic branch of ANS	Inhibitory/excitatory
Dopamine	Amine	• Basal ganglia • Brainstem	Inhibitory
Serotonin	Amine	• Hypothalamus • Brainstem	Inhibitory
Gamma-aminobutyric acid (GABA)	Amino acid	• Basal ganglia • Cerebellum • Spinal cord	Inhibitory
Glycine	Amino acid	• Spinal cord	Inhibitory
Beta endorphins	Peptide	• Spinal cord	Inhibitory
Substance P	Peptide	• Pain fibers in spinal cord	Excitatory

B. Functions
1. Acts to limit transfer of certain substances into extracellular fluid (ECF) or cerebral spinal fluid (CSF) of the brain
2. Prevents toxic substances from readily entering the extracellular space of the nervous system; may hinder the effective use of certain drug therapies in the treatment of neurologic system problems
3. May be altered by trauma, infection, intracranial tumor, brain irradiation

Macroscopic Anatomy and Physiology

I. Scalp: skin covering the cranium
  A. Made of five layers:
    1. **Skin**: thicker than anywhere else in the body
    2. **Cutaneous** tissue
    3. **Adipose** tissue
    4. **Ligament** layer referred to as *galea aponeurotica*; moves freely over the skull
    5. **Pericranium**
  B. Blood vessels located in the subcutaneous tissue
    1. The scalp is very vascular
    2. Blood vessels here do not contract well when injured
    3. Scalp laceration can result in significant blood loss
II. Skull (Fig. 6-4): bony structure of the head, consisting of the cranium and the skeleton of the face
  A. The skull is composed of an inner table and outer table separated by cancellous (spongy) bone; this structure allows for maximum strength and minimal weight
  B. The cranium is a body vault that holds and protects the brain from external forces; volume capacity is approximately 1500 ml

C. The cranium consists of eight bones
    1. Frontal: 1
    2. Parietal: 2
    3. Temporal: 2
    4. Occipital: 1
    5. Ethmoid: 1
    6. Sphenoid: 1
  D. The sphenoid bone divides the interior of the skull into three fossae (Fig. 6-5)
    1. Anterior fossa: contains the frontal lobes
    2. Middle fossa: contains the temporal, parietal, and occipital lobes
    3. Posterior fossa: contains the cerebellum
  E. The foramen magnum is a large oval-shaped opening at the base of the skull; this is the location of the connection of the brain and the spinal cord
III. Meninges (Fig. 6-6): protective coverings of the brain and the spinal cord
  A. Pia mater
    1. This delicate layer adheres to the surface of the brain and the spinal cord
    2. It follows sulci and gyri of the brain and carries branches of cerebral arteries with it
      a) Sulci: shallow grooves or invaginations on the surface of the brain (deep sulci are referred to as *fissures*)
      b) Gyri: convolutions on the surface of the brain
    3. Blood vessels of pia form the choroid plexus
  B. Arachnoid mater
    1. This is the middle layer of the meninges
    2. The subarachnoid space is between the arachnoid mater and the pia mater
      a) Contains larger blood vessels of brain
      b) Contains CSF
      c) Contains arachnoid villi (projections of arachnoid mater that serve as channels

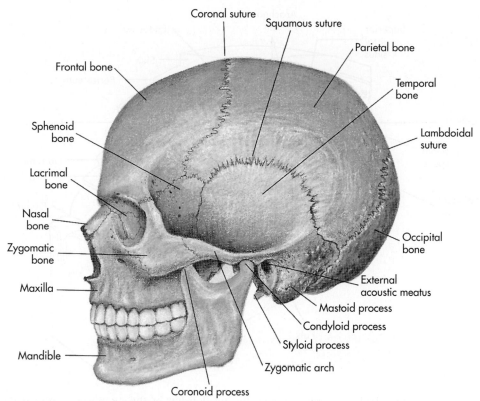

Figure 6-4   Lateral view of skull. (From Chipps EM, Clanin NJ, Campbell VG: *Neurologic disorders: Mosby's clinical nursing series,* St Louis, 1992, Mosby.)

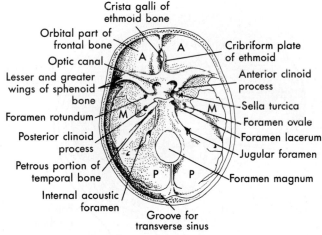

A = Anterior cranial fossa
M = Middle cranial fossa
P = Posterior cranial fossa

Figure 6-5   Bones that form the floor of the cranial cavity and the three fossae formed by these bones. (From Kinney MR, Packa DR, Dunbar SB: *AACN's clinical reference for critical-care nursing,* ed 4, St Louis, 1998, Mosby.)

for absorption of CSF into the venous system)

C. Dura mater
1. This is the outermost layer of meninges
2. Meningeal arteries and venous sinuses lie within clefts formed by separation of the inner and outer layers of dura

3. The epidural space is between the skull and the dura mater
   a) Only a potential space
   b) Site of epidural hemorrhage or hematoma
4. The subdural space is between the dura mater and the arachnoid mater
   a) Only a potential space
   b) Site of subdural hemorrhage or hematoma
5. There are several folds of the dura mater (Fig. 6-7)
   a) The falx cerebri separates the two cerebral hemispheres
   b) The falx cerebelli separates the two cerebellar hemispheres
   c) The tentorium cerebelli separates the cerebral hemispheres from the cerebellum
   d) The diaphragm sella canopies the sella turcica (where the pituitary gland is located) and encloses the pituitary gland
IV. Brain (Fig. 6-8)
  A. General information
    1. Weighs approximately 1.5 kg
    2. Divided into cerebrum, brainstem, and cerebellum
  B. Telencephalon: two cerebral hemispheres connected by the corpus callosum
    1. Cerebrum (Fig. 6-9)
      a) Structure
        (1) Outer layer of cerebral cortex is

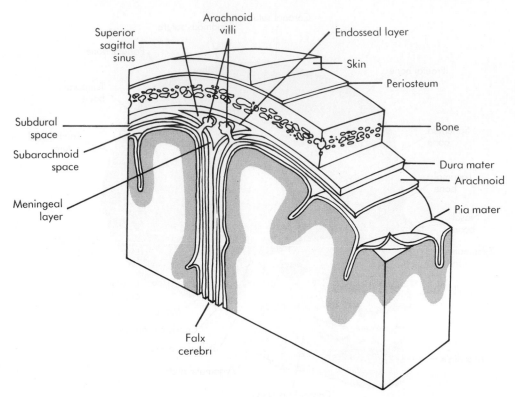

Figure 6-6 Coronal section of the skull and brain showing the relationship of the meninges. (From Barker E: *Neuroscience nursing,* St Louis, 1994, Mosby.)

Figure 6-7 Folds of the dura. (From Kinney MR, Packa DR, Dunbar SB: *AACN's clinical reference for critical-care nursing,* ed 4, St Louis, 1998, Mosby.)

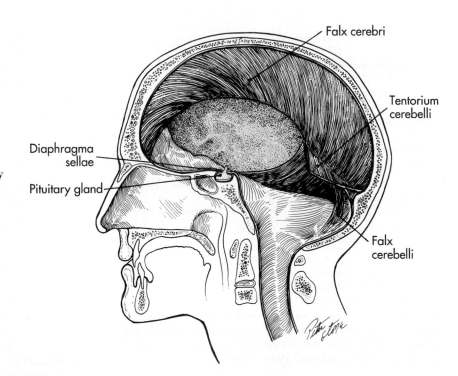

gray matter consisting of neuron cell bodies (six cell layers thick)
(2) Deeper layers of each hemisphere are white matter consisting of myelinated axons with four paired masses of gray matter known as *basal ganglia*

(3) Fissures
(a) Longitudinal fissure (also referred to as *falx cerebri*): divides the left and right cerebral hemispheres
(b) Fissure of Rolando (also referred to as *central sulcus*): divides

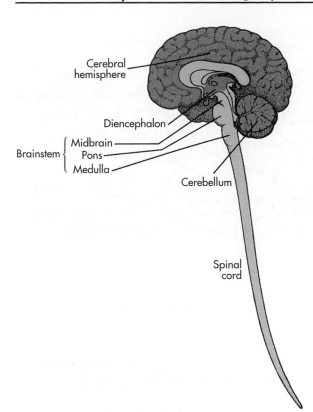

Figure 6-8   Major divisions of the CNS. (From Lewis SM, Collier IC: *Medical-surgical nursing,* ed 3, St Louis, 1992, Mosby.)

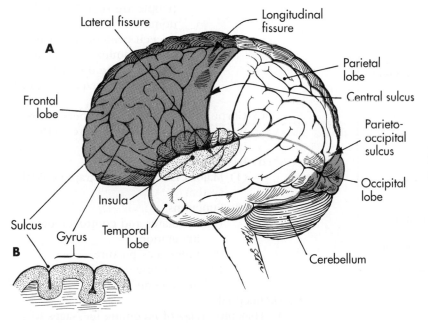

Figure 6-9   A, Lateral view of the cerebrum. **B,** Portion of the cortex in cross section showing gyrus and sulcus.

frontal lobe from parietal lobes; separates the motor and sensory strips

   (c) Fissure of Sylvius (also referred to as *lateral sulcus*): divides frontal lobe from temporal lobes

  b) Cerebral cortical areas and functions (Table 6-2 and Fig. 6-10)

    (1) Lobes

     (a) Frontal: contains the precentral gyrus (also referred to as the *motor strip*) (Fig. 6-11)

     (b) Parietal: contains the postcentral gyrus (also referred to as the *sensory strip*) (Fig. 6-11)

     (c) Temporal

     (d) Occipital

    (2) Cerebral hemispheres

     (a) Each hemisphere of the brain receives sensory information from

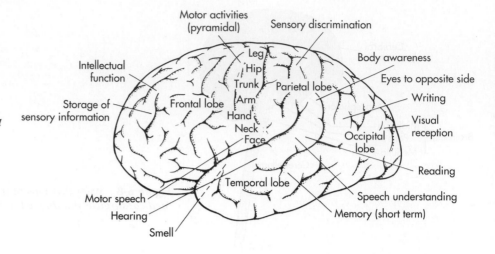

Figure 6-10 Functional areas of the cerebral cortex. (From Kinney MR, Packa DR, Dunbar SB: *AACN's clinical reference for critical-care nursing,* ed 4, St Louis, 1998, Mosby.)

Table 6-2	Cerebral Cortical Areas and Functions
Cerebral Cortical Area	**Functions**

Frontal lobe	• Personality
	• Behavior: ethical, moral, social
	• Intellectual functions
	  • Conscious thought
	  • Abstract thinking
	  • Judgment and foresight
	• Short-term memory
	• Voluntary motor function
	• Motor speech (Broca's area in dominant hemisphere)

Parietal lobe	• Localization of sensory information to the body surface • Sensory integration and discrimination • Object recognition • Position sense • Body awareness • Body image
Temporal lobe	• Emotion • Long-term memory • Processing of olfactory, gustatory, auditory input • Sensory speech (Wernicke's area in dominant hemisphere)
Occipital lobe	• Processing of visual input

the opposite side of the body and controls skeletal muscles of the opposite side
- (b) Each hemisphere has specialization
  - (i) The left cerebral hemisphere is specialized for analysis, problem solving, language, mathematics, abstract reasoning, and interpretation of symbols
  - (ii) The right cerebral hemisphere is specialized for visuospatial patterns, nonverbal communication, music, and artistic ability
- (c) Hemispheric dominance
  - (i) Ninety percent of right-handed people are left hemisphere dominant
  - (ii) Sixty percent of left-handed people are right hemisphere dominant
  - (iii) Speech centers are located in the dominant hemisphere; lesions in the dominant hemisphere frequently cause aphasia
- c) Corpus callosum: path for fibers to cross from one cerebral hemisphere to the other
- d) Basal ganglia
  - (1) Major center of the extrapyramidal system
  - (2) Functions
    - (a) Regulates and controls motor integration
    - (b) Influences posture
    - (c) Allows fine voluntary movements
- C. Diencephalon
  1. Thalamus: relay of incoming messages to appropriate areas of the brain
  2. Hypothalamus
     - a) Temperature regulation
     - b) Regulation of food and water intake
     - c) Sleep patterns
     - d) Autonomic responses
     - e) Control of hormonal secretion of pituitary gland
  3. Limbic system
     - a) Self-preservation behaviors, including aggression
     - b) Basic drives (e.g., food, sex)

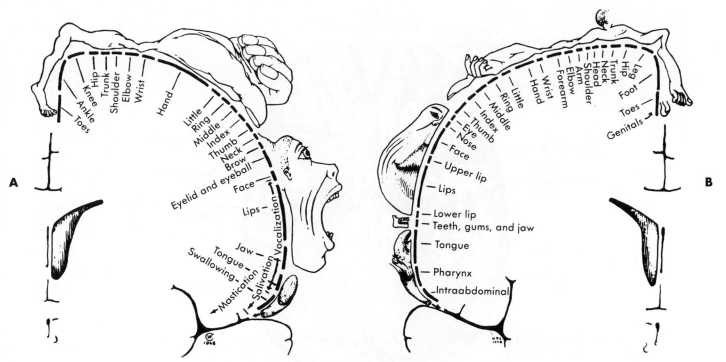

Figure 6-11 A, Motor homunculus showing areas of the motor strip devoted to specified areas of the body. **B,** Sensory homunculus showing areas of the sensory strip devoted to specified areas of the body. (From Thelan LA et al: *Critical care nursing: diagnosis and management,* ed 3, St Louis, 1998, Mosby.)

c) Affective aspect of emotional behavior
d) Some aspects of memory

D. Brainstem
1. Functions
a) Relays messages between the brain and lower levels of the nervous system
b) Is the origin of all cranial nerves except first and second
2. Divisions
a) Mesencephalon (Midbrain)
(1) Is the origin of third and fourth cranial nerves
(2) Contains motor and sensory pathways
(3) Location of reticular activating system (RAS); responsible for arousal from sleep, wakefulness, focusing of attention
b) Pons
(1) Is the origin of fifth, sixth, seventh cranial nerves
(2) Connects cerebral cortex and cerebellum
(3) Contains motor and sensory pathways
(4) Contains respiratory centers
c) Medulla oblongata
(1) Is the origin of eighth, ninth, tenth, eleventh, and twelfth cranial nerves
(2) Connects motor and sensory tracts of spinal cord to medulla

(3) Contains cardiac and respiratory centers

E. Cerebellum
1. Coordinates muscle movement with sensory input
2. Controls balance
3. Influences muscle tone in relation to equilibrium
4. Affects locomotion and posture
5. Controls nonstereotyped movements
6. Synchronizes muscle action

V. Cerebral circulation
A. The brain receives 20% of cardiac output
B. Arterial system (Fig. 6-12 and Fig. 6-13)
1. External carotid system: arises from common carotid arteries
a) Occipital arteries: supply the posterior fossa
b) Temporal arteries: supply the temporal area
c) Maxillary arteries: form the middle meningeal arteries
d) Meningeal arteries: branches of external carotid arteries that supply dura mater (internal carotid and vertebral arteries supply pia and arachnoid mater)
(1) Anterior meningeal artery: supplies anterior portion of dura
(2) Middle meningeal artery: supplies most of dura
(3) Posterior meningeal artery: supplies occipital area of dura

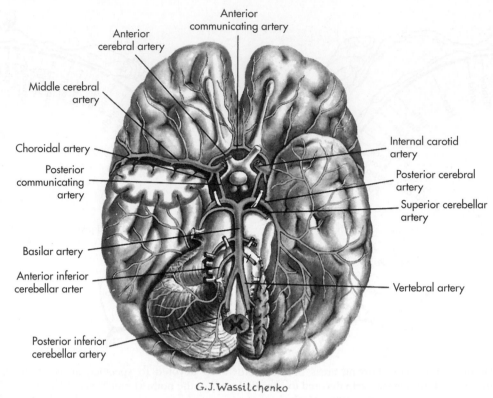

Figure 6-12 Arterial system of the brain. (From Thelan LA et al: *Critical care nursing: diagnosis and management,* ed 3, St Louis, 1998, Mosby.)

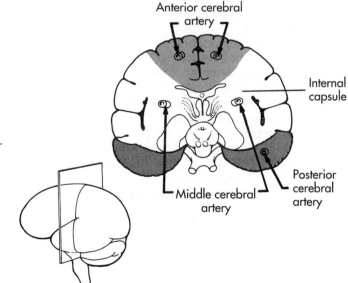

Figure 6-13 Distribution of the arterial blood supply. (From Thelan LA et al: *Critical care nursing: diagnosis and management,* ed 3, St Louis, 1998, Mosby.)

2. Internal carotid system: arises from common carotid arteries; accounts for 80% of cerebral perfusion
   a) Anterior cerebral arteries (Table 6-3)
   b) Anterior communicating artery
      (1) Connects right and left anterior cerebral arteries
      (2) Forms anterior section of circle of Willis
   c) Middle cerebral arteries (Table 6-3)

   d) Posterior communicating arteries
      (1) Connect posterior cerebral arteries with internal carotid arteries
      (2) Form posterior portion of circle of Willis
3. Vertebral system: arise from subclavian arteries and join at lower border of pons to form basilar artery
   a) Posterior cerebral arteries (Table 6-3)
   b) Basilar arteries (Table 6-3)

Table 6-3	**Cerebral Artery Distribution**
Artery	**Areas**
INTERNAL CAROTID SYSTEM (ANTERIOR CIRCULATION)	
• Anterior cerebral arteries	• Superior surface of the frontal and parietal lobes • Medial surface of cerebral hemispheres • Basal ganglia • Corpus callosum • Hypothalamus
• Middle cerebral arteries	• Lateral surfaces of parietal, frontal, and temporal lobes • Superior surface of temporal lobe • Precentral (motor) gyri • Postcentral (sensory) gyri
VERTEBRAL SYSTEM (POSTERIOR CIRCULATION)	
• Basilar arteries	• Most of brainstem • Cerebellum
• Posterior cerebral arteries	• Thalamus • Medial portion of occipital • Inferior portion of temporal • Vestibular organs • Cochlear apparatus

c) Anterior spinal artery: supplies anterior half of three quarters of spinal cord and medial aspect of brainstem

d) Posterior spinal arteries: traverses the cord along the dorsal roots

4. Circle of Willis
   a) Formed by internal carotids and vertebral arteries
   b) Permits collateral circulation if one of the carotid or vertebral arteries becomes occluded

C. Cerebral blood flow
   1. Brings oxygen and nutrients to the brain tissue for cellular energy production; waste products are removed from the blood
   2. Cerebral blood flow (CBF) varies with changes in cerebral perfusion pressure (CPP) and diameter of the cerebrovascular bed
      a) Normal cerebral blood flow is approximately 50 ml/100 g/min
      b) Normal cerebral oxygen extraction ratio is between 25% and 35%; an oxygen extraction ratio greater than 40% indicates an imbalance between oxygen supply and demand and impending cerebral ischemia
         (1) Calculated by $Sao_2 - Sjo_2 / Sao_2$, where Sao_2 is oxygen saturation of arterial blood by arterial blood gases or pulse oximetry, and Sjo_2 is the saturation of the venous blood from

the jugular vein by a fiberoptic catheter placed in the jugular bulb

3. CPP = mean arterial pressure (MAP) − mean intracranial pressure (ICP)
   a) Changes in MAP or ICP affect CPP
   b) Normal MAP is 70 to 105 mm Hg; normal ICP is 5 to 15; normal CPP is 60 to 100 mm Hg
   c) CPP less than 50 mm Hg is associated with impaired neuronal functioning

4. Autoregulation is the ability of the brain to alter the diameter of the arterioles to maintain cerebral blood flow at a constant level despite changes in CPP
   a) When ICP approaches MAP, CPP decreases to the point where autoregulation is impaired and CBF decreases
   b) Limits of autoregulation are CPP between 50 to 150 mm Hg
      (1) CPP less than 50 mm Hg (e.g., cardiopulmonary arrest, shock) causes hypoperfusion and anoxic encephalopathy
      (2) CPP more than 150 mm Hg (e.g., hypertensive crisis) causes hyperperfusion, cerebral edema, and hypertensive encephalopathy

5. Factors affecting CBF
   a) Increase in CBF
      (1) Hypercapnia
      (2) Hypoxemia
      (3) Decreased blood viscosity
      (4) Hyperthermia
      (5) Drugs: vasodilators
   b) Decrease in CBF
      (1) Hypocapnia
      (2) Hyperoxemia
      (3) Increased blood viscosity
      (4) Hypothermia
      (5) Intracranial hypertension
      (6) Drugs: anesthetics, barbiturates

D. Venous system (Fig. 6-14)
   1. The cerebrum has external veins that lie in the subarachnoid space on surfaces of hemispheres and internal veins that drain the central core of the cerebrum and lie beneath the corpus callosum
   2. Both external and internal venous systems empty into venous sinuses that lie between dural layers
      a) Superior sagittal sinus drains venous blood from the anterior portions of the brain
      b) Cavernous sinus drains venous blood from the inferior portions of the brain
      c) Transvenous sinus drains venous blood from the posterior portion of the brain
   3. The internal jugular veins collect blood from the dural venous sinuses

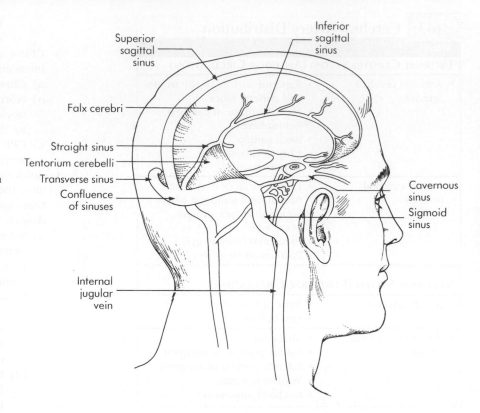

Figure 6-14 Venous system of the brain showing major dural venous sinuses and their connection to the internal jugular veins. (From Barker E: *Neuroscience nursing,* St Louis, 1994, Mosby.)

VI. Cerebrospinal fluid (CSF)
  A. Characteristics
    1. Functions
      a) Cushions brain and spinal cord
      b) Allows for compensation for changes in ICP; displacement of CSF out of the cranial cavity compensates for increases in intracranial volume to prevent an increase in intracranial pressure
    2. Volume: 120 to 150 ml
      a) Distribution: 90 ml in lumbar subarachnoid space, 25 ml in ventricles, 35 ml in rest of subarachnoid space
      b) Daily synthesis: 500 ml
    3. Pressure: 80 to 180 mm H_2O, measured at lumbar level, with patient in side-lying position
  B. CSF production and reabsorption
    1. CSF is a transudate of plasma formed by the choroid plexus in ventricles
      a) Choroid plexus: sheets of epithelial cells that project into the lumen of the ventricular spaces
      b) Majority (95%) of CSF produced in lateral ventricles
    2. CSF is absorbed via arachnoid villi, which return it to systemic circulation by the internal jugular veins; the hydrostatic pressure gradient between CSF and the venous sinus is one factor that determines CSF absorption
  C. Communication system within brain (Fig. 6-15)
    1. Ventricles: hollow spaces that are lined with ependyma; contain specialized epithe-

lium called *choroid plexus,* which produce CSF
      a) The lateral ventricles are the largest of the ventricles; one lies in each cerebral hemisphere
      b) The third ventricle lies midline between the two lateral ventricles
      c) The fourth ventricle lies in posterior fossa
    2. Pathway of CSF circulation (Fig. 6-16): lateral ventricles → foramen of Monro → third ventricle → aqueduct of Sylvius → fourth ventricle → cisterns and subarachnoid space where arachnoid villi reabsorb CSF into the systemic circulation
VII. Spine and spinal cord
  A. Structure
    1. Vertebral column: composed of 7 cervical, 12 thoracic, 5 lumbar, 5 sacral, and 4 coccygeal vertebrae
    2. Spinal cord: 42 to 45 cm extending from superior border of atlas to upper border of second lumbar vertebrae (L2); continuous with the brainstem
      a) Meninges: pia mater, arachnoid mater, dura mater
      b) Central canal: opening in the center of the spinal cord that contains CSF; communicates with the fourth ventricle
      c) Central gray horns that form an H; contain mostly cell bodies (Fig. 6-17)
        (1) The anterior (or ventral) horn of gray matter contains cell bodies of efferent or motor fibers

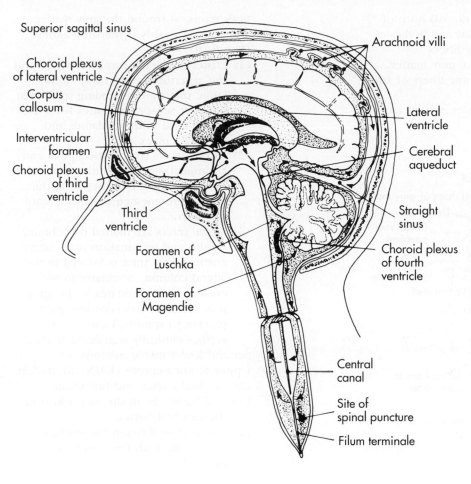

Figure 6-15 Lateral view of the ventricular system. Arrows show direction of CSF circulation. (From Kinney MR, Packa DR, Dunbar SB: *AACN's clinical reference for critical-care nursing,* ed 4, St Louis, 1998, Mosby.)

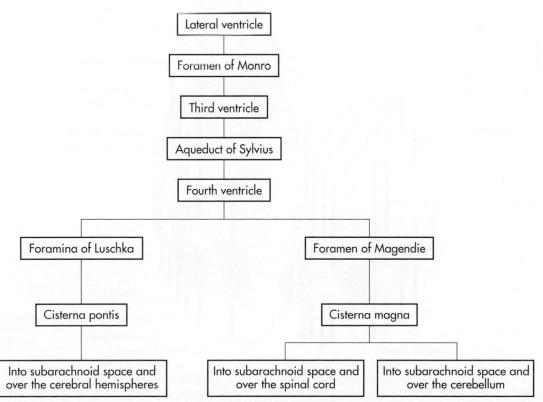

Figure 6-16 Circulation of CSF.

(2) The posterior (or dorsal) horn of gray matter contains cell bodies of afferent or sensory fibers

(3) The lateral horns of gray matter contain preganglionic fibers of autonomic system

d) Columns of white matter, which are

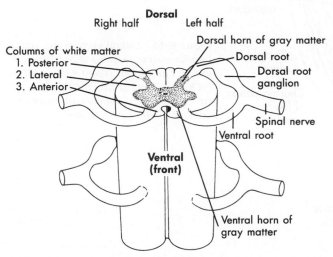

Figure 6-17 Segment of the thoracic spinal cord in cross section. (From Kinney MR, Packa DR, Dunbar SB: *AACN's clinical reference for critical-care nursing*, ed 4, St Louis, 1998, Mosby.)

fiber tracts, surround the gray matter and contain mostly myelinated axons (Fig. 6-18)

(1) Posterior tracts (dorsal columns) and the anterior and lateral spinothalamic tracts are ascending tracts that conduct sensory impulses from the spinal cord to the thalamus and cerebral cortex

(2) Lateral tracts (the corticospinal and pyramidal) are descending tracts that conduct motor impulses from the brain to motor neurons in the anterior horn

(3) Spinal tracts are named by column, origin, and termination (e.g., lateral corticospinal tract is located in the lateral column, originates in the cortex, and terminates in the spine; it is therefore a descending tract [cortex to spine]); Table 6-4 describes clinically significant tracts

3. Upper and lower motor neurons

a) Upper motor neurons (UMN): located in the cerebral cortex and brainstem

(1) Cell bodies lie in the motor area of the cerebral cortex

(2) Axons pass through the spinal cord to synapse with the lower motor neurons

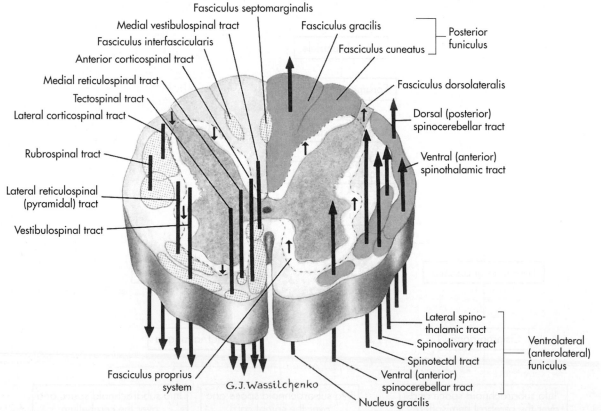

Figure 6-18 Spinal cord tracts of the white matter. (From Thelan LA et al: *Critical care nursing: diagnosis and management*, ed 3, St Louis, 1998, Mosby.)

(3) Damage to UMN causes spastic paralysis and hyperactive reflexes
  b) Lower motor neurons (LMN): located in the spinal cord
    (1) Cell bodies lie in the anterior horn of gray matter in the spinal cord
    (2) Axons directly innervate striated muscle fibers
    (3) Damage to LMN causes flaccid paralysis and areflexia

B. Function
  1. Mediates the reflex arc (Fig. 6-19)
    a) An involuntary response to a stimulus (e.g., touching hot stove causes reflex withdrawal of hand)
    b) Does not go beyond the spinal cord to the brain; does not require cerebral interpretation
    c) Components
      (1) Receptor organ

Table 6-4   Spinal Cord Tracts and Functions

Tract	Column	Direction	Functions	Sidedness
SPINOTHALAMIC				
• Lateral spinothalamic	Lateral	Ascending	• Pain • Temperature	Contralateral
• Anterior spinothalamic	Anterior	Ascending	• Light touch • Pressure • Pain • Temperature	Contralateral
• Spinotectal	Lateral	Ascending	• Tactile stimulation arousing consciousness	Contralateral
SPINOCEREBELLAR				
• Dorsal spinocerebellar	Lateral	Ascending	• Reflex proprioception • Muscle tone and synergy	Ipsilateral
• Ventral spinocerebellar	Lateral	Ascending	• Reflex proprioception • Muscle tone and synergy	Contralateral
MEDIAL LEMNISCAL SYSTEM				
• Fasciculus gracilis	Posterior	Ascending	• Position sense • Vibratory sense • Pressure • Tactile localization • Two-point discrimination	Ipsilateral
• Fasciculus cuneatus	Posterior	Ascending	• Position sense • Vibratory sense • Pressure • Tactile localization • Two-point discrimination	Ipsilateral
PYRAMIDAL				
• Lateral corticospinal	Lateral	Descending	• Voluntary movement	Contralateral
• Ventral corticospinal	Lateral	Descending	• Voluntary movement	Ipsilateral
• Corticobulbar		Descending	• Facial expression • Swallowing • Speech	Contralateral
EXTRAPYRAMIDAL				
• Rubrospinal	Lateral	Descending	• Synergy and muscle tone	Contralateral
• Lateral vestibulospinal	Anterior	Descending	• Posture and equilibrium	Ipsilateral
• Medial vestibulospinal	Anterior	Descending	• Posture and equilibrium	Contralateral
• Lateral reticulospinal	Lateral	Descending	• Muscle tone	Ipsilateral
• Medial reticulospinal	Anterior	Descending	• Muscle tone	Ipsilateral
• Tectospinal	Anterior	Descending	• Vision and hearing	Contralateral

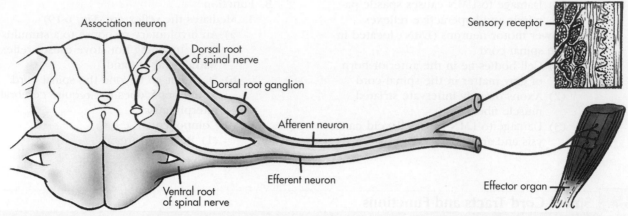

Figure 6-19 Basic diagram of a reflex arc, including the sensory receptor, afferent neuron, association neuron, efferent neuron, and effector organ. (From Lewis SM, Collier IC: *Medical-surgical nursing*, ed 3, St Louis, 1992, Mosby.)

    (2) Afferent neuron
    (3) Effector neuron
    (4) Effector organ
  2. Serves as the communicating pathway between the brain and the peripheral nervous system
VIII. Peripheral nervous system
  A. Spinal nerves consist of 31 pairs: 8 cervical (C1-C8), 12 thoracic (T1-T12), 5 lumbar (L1-L5), 5 sacral (S1-S5), and 1 coccygeal
    1. Fibers of spinal nerve
      a) Motor fibers
        (1) Originate in anterior gray column of spinal cord
        (2) Form ventral root of spinal nerve and pass to skeletal muscles
      b) Sensory fibers
        (1) Originate in spinal ganglia of dorsal roots
        (2) Peripheral branches distribute to visceral and somatic structures as mediators of sensory impulses to CNS
    2. Dermatomes: each spinal nerve innervates a specific portion of the skin identified as the dermatome for that spinal nerve (Fig. 6-20 and Table 6-5)
    3. Spinal nerves form various nerve plexi that innervate the skin and muscles throughout the body (Fig. 6-20)
      a) Cervical plexus: C1-C4
      b) Brachial plexus: C5-C8, T1
      c) Lumbar plexus: L1-L4
      d) Sacral plexus: L4-L5, S1-S4
  B. Cranial nerves (Fig. 6-21 and Table 6-6) consist of 12 pairs of nerves that carry impulses to and from the brain
IX. Autonomic nervous system (ANS)
  A. Structure
    1. ANS consists of two neuron chains that carry information from the central nervous system to peripheral effector organs

    2. Preganglionic neuron has cell body in the CNS
      a) Sympathetic branch: cell bodies are located in the spinal cord from T1 to L2
      b) Parasympathetic branch: cell bodies are located in the nuclei of cranial nerves III, VII, IX, X, or in the spinal cord from S2-S4
    3. The preganglionic neuron axon terminates on the postganglionic neuron cell bodies that are located throughout the body in autonomic ganglia
    4. The postganglionic neuron axon terminates and innervates the specific effector organs of the autonomic nervous system
    5. Neurotransmitters form a chemical bridge in transmission of a nerve impulse
      a) Sympathetic branch: epinephrine, norepinephrine
      b) Parasympathetic branch: acetylcholine
  B. Function
    1. Controls activities of the viscera at an unconscious level
    2. Consists of two parallel systems that regulate visceral organs by acting in opposing manners (Table 6-7)
      a) Sympathetic branch (also called *adrenergic*)
        (1) Dominates in crisis situations and is frequently referred to as "fight or flight" system
        (2) Innervated by physiologic or psychologic stressors
        (3) Promotes activities that prepare the body for crisis situations
      b) Parasympathetic branch (also called *cholinergic*)
        (1) Dominant in moments of calm or "steady state"
        (2) Promotes activities that restore the body's energy sources

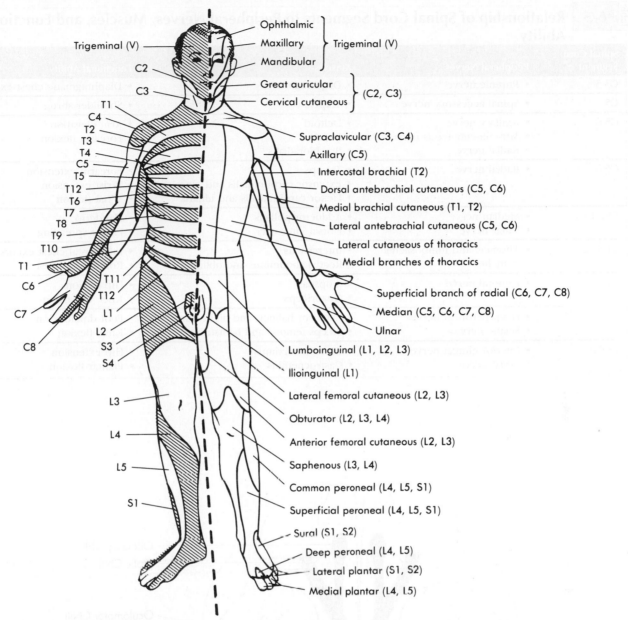

Figure 6-20 Left: dermatome distribution. Right: Peripheral distribution of cutaneous nerves. (From Long BC, Phipps WJ, Cassmeyer VL: *Medical-surgical nursing: a nursing process approach,* ed 3, St Louis, 1993, Mosby.)

Neurologic Assessment

Interview

I. Chief complaint: why the patient is seeking help and duration of the problem

  A. Symptoms related to neurologic problems

    1. Head or spinal cord trauma

      a) Sequence of events

      b) Mechanism of injury

      c) Elapsed time

      d) Extent of injury

      e) Previous treatment

      f) Current status

    2. Change in consciousness (e.g., difficulty staying awake)

    3. Headache

      a) Focal or generalized

      b) Unilateral or bilateral

      c) With or without fever

        (1) Headache with fever: infectious process (e.g., meningitis, encephalitis)

        (2) Headache without fever: intracerebral hemorrhage or tumor

      d) Time of day: early morning headache suggestive of tumor

    4. Seizures

      a) New onset

      b) Increased frequency if patient has history of epilepsy

    5. Visual changes

      a) Loss of a portion of the visual field

      b) Diplopia

Table 6-5	Relationship of Spinal Cord Segments to Peripheral Nerves, Muscles, and Functional Ability		
Spinal Cord Segment	**Peripheral Nerves**	**Muscles**	**Functional Ability**
C3-5	• Phrenic nerve	• Diaphragm	• Diaphragmatic chest excursion
C5	• Spinal accessory nerve	• Trapezius	• Shoulder shrug
C5-6	• Axillary nerve • Musculocutaneous nerve • Radial nerve	• Deltoid • Biceps • Brachioradialis	• Arm elevation • Forearm flexion
C6-8	• Radial nerve	• Triceps • Extensor carpi radialis and ulnaris • Flexor carpi radialis and ulnaris	• Forearm extension • Wrist extension • Wrist flexion
C8, T1	• Median nerve • Ulnar nerve	• Adductor pollicis • Dorsal interossei	• Handgrip • Finger spreading
T1-T12	• Thoracic and lumbosacral branches	• Intercostals • Rectus abdominus and obliques	• Intercostal chest excursion • Rotation at waist
L1-L3	• Femoral nerve	• Iliopsoas • Quadriceps	• Hip flexion • Knee extension
L2-4	• Deep peroneal nerve • Sciatic nerve	• Extensor hallucis and digitorum • Biceps femoris and hamstrings	• Foot dorsiflexion • Knee flexion
L5-S2	• Inferior gluteal nerve • Tibial nerve	• Gluteus maximus • Gastrocnemius	• Hip extension • Plantar flexion

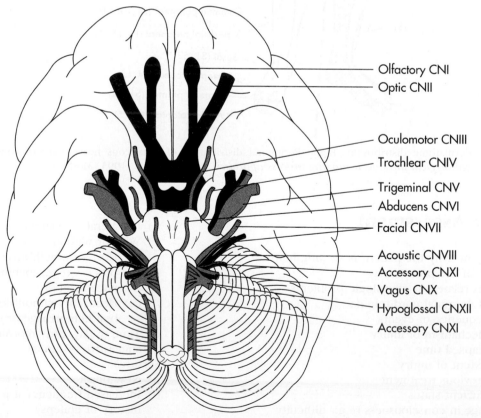

Figure 6-21 Diagram of the base of the skull showing entrance or exit of the cranial nerves. (From Barkauskas VH et al: *Health and physical assessment*, St Louis, 1994, Mosby.)

Table 6-6	**Cranial Nerve Summary**			
Number	**Name**	**Memory Jogger: Name**	**Memory Jogger: Motor/Sensory/Both**	**Functions**
I	Olfactory	On	Some	Sensory • Smell
II	Optic	Old	Say	Sensory • Vision
III	Oculomotor	Olympus'	Marry	Motor • Upward, lateral eye movement • Pupillary constriction • Eyelid elevation
IV	Trochlear	Towering	Money	Motor • Downward, medial eye movement
V	Trigeminal	Tops	But	Sensory • Sensation of scalp and face • Sensation of cornea of eye Motor • Temporal and masseter muscles
VI	Abducens	A	My	Motor • Lateral eye movement
VII	Facial	Fin	Brother	Sensory • Taste on anterior two thirds of tongue Motor • Muscles of facial expression • Eyelid closure • Lacrimal and salivary glands
VIII	Acoustic	And	Says	Sensory • Hearing • Equilibrium and balance
IX	Glossopharyngeal	German	Bad	Sensory • Taste on posterior one third of tongue • Pharynx Motor • Parotid gland
X	Vagus	Viewed	Business	Sensory • Pharynx, larynx, neck Motor • Palate, larynx, pharynx • Swallowing • Cardiac muscle • Secretory glands of pancreas and GI tract
XI	Spinal Accessory	Some	Marry	Motor • Shoulder and neck movement • Sternocleidomastoid and trapezius muscles
XII	Hypoglossal	Hops	Money	Motor • Tongue

   c) Photophobia: may be experienced with increased ICP or meningitis
6. Impaired speech (e.g., dysphasia, aphasia)
7. Change in mood (e.g., depression, euphoria, emotional lability)
8. Change in thought processes (e.g., hallucinations, delusions, illusions, paranoia)
9. Change in behavior (e.g., hygiene habits, inappropriate laughter, frequent crying)
10. Change in motor function
    a) Tremor
    b) Paresis
    c) Paralysis
11. Change in gait
12. Dizziness, syncope, vertigo
13. Change in sensory function
    a) Pain
    b) Paresthesia
    c) Anesthesia

Table 6-7	Autonomic Nervous System: Sympathetic and Parasympathetic Branch Function	
	Sympathetic (Adrenergic)	**Parasympathetic (Cholinergic)**
Eyes	• Pupils dilate	• Pupils constrict
Heart	• Heart rate increased • Contractility increased • Coronary arteries dilate	• Heart rate decreased • Contractility decreased • No effect on coronary arteries
Lungs	• Bronchodilation	• Bronchoconstriction
Liver	• Glycogenolysis and lipolysis	• Glycogenesis
GI	• Salivary flow decreased • Gastric mobility and secretion decreased • Intestinal motility decreased	• Salivary flow increased • Gastric mobility and secretion increased • Intestinal motility increased
Urinary bladder	• Bladder relaxed • Sphincter closed	• Bladder contracted • Sphincter open
Adrenal gland	• Secretes epinephrine, norepinephrine	• No effect
Skin	• Piloerection (goose pimples) • Increased perspiration	• No effect

14. Memory changes
15. Swallowing difficulties
16. Difficulties with activities of daily living (ADL)

II. History of present illness: determine PQRST
   A. P
      1. Provocation: what provokes or worsens the pain
      2. Palliation: what relieves the pain; also include what was used but did not relieve pain
   B. Q
      1. Quality: what does the pain feel like
   C. R
      1. Region: location of pain
      2. Radiation: if the pain radiates, where does the pain radiate to
   D. S
      1. Severity: how severe is the pain on a 0 to 10 scale with 0 being no pain and 10 being the most severe pain
   E. T
      1. Timing: intermittent or continuous; relationship to other events or activities

III. Past medical history
   A. Congenital disorders
      1. Spina bifida
      2. Cerebral palsy
      3. Down syndrome
   B. Childhood diseases: poliomyelitis
   C. Epilepsy
   D. Head trauma
   E. Infectious neurologic conditions
      1. Encephalitis
      2. Meningitis
   F. Neuromuscular disease
      1. Multiple sclerosis
      2. Myasthenia gravis
      3. Amyotrophic lateral sclerosis (ALS)
      4. Parkinson's disease
   G. Spinal cord injury
   H. Alzheimer's disease
   I. Cancer
   J. Cardiovascular or cerebrovascular disease
   K. Diabetes mellitus
   L. Pulmonary embolism
   M. Impairment of vision: use of eyeglasses, contact lenses, prosthesis
   N. Impairment of hearing: use of hearing aide

IV. Family history
   A. Epilepsy
   B. Diabetes mellitus
   C. Cardiovascular disease
   D. Hypertension
   E. Cerebrovascular disease
   F. Cancer
   G. Neurologic disorders
      1. ALS
      2. Huntington's disease
      3. Muscular dystrophy
      4. Neurofibromatosis
      5. Tay-Sachs disease
      6. Myasthenia gravis
      7. Multiple sclerosis
      8. Alzheimer's disease
      9. Tremor
      10. Dementia
   H. Psychiatric disorders

V. Social history
   A. Relationship with spouse or significant other; family structure
   B. Occupation: exposure to toxins (e.g., solvents, pesticides, arsenic, lead)
   C. Educational level
   D. Stress level and usual coping mechanisms
   E. Recreational habits
   F. Exercise habits
   G. Dietary habits
   H. Caffeine intake
   I. Tobacco use: record as pack-years (number of packs per day times the number of years he or she has been smoking)
   J. Alcohol use: record as alcoholic beverages consumed per month, week, or day
   K. Drug use or abuse
   L. Toxin exposure
   M. Travel
   N. Handedness: left or right

VI. Medication history
   A. Prescribed drug, dosage, frequency, time of last dose
   B. Nonprescribed drugs
      1. Over-the-counter drugs
      2. Substance abuse
   C. Patient understanding of drug actions, side effects
   D. Drugs frequently used for neurologic problems
      1. Tranquilizers
      2. Sedatives
      3. Aspirin
      4. Anticonvulsants
      5. Antihypertensives
   E. Drugs that may cause neurologic problems
      1. Tranquilizers
      2. Sedatives
      3. Aspirin
      4. Anticoagulants
      5. Alcohol

Vital Signs

I. Cushing's triad: increased systolic BP, decreased diastolic BP (widened pulse pressure), bradycardia; late sign of increased intracranial pressure
II. BP
   A. Hypotension
      1. Hemorrhage
         a) Because the cranium is an inexpansible vault, intracranial hemorrhage cannot result in hypotension because herniation would result before significant hypotension
         b) Consider other sources of bleeding (e.g., lacerated liver, ruptured spleen, thoracic trauma)
      2. General neurologic deterioration
      3. Of great concern because CPP = MAP − ICP
   B. Hypertension: systolic hypertension may be seen as a component of Cushing's triad, a late sign of intracranial hypertension
   C. Pulse pressure: difference between systolic and diastolic
      1. Normal is 30 to 40 mm Hg
      2. Increased pulse pressure is a component of Cushing's triad, a late sign of intracranial hypertension
III. Pulse
   A. Sinus bradycardia: a component of Cushing's triad, a late sign of intracranial hypertension
   B. Sinus tachycardia
      1. Hypoxia
      2. Hemorrhage
      3. General neurologic deterioration
IV. Respiratory rate and rhythm (Table 6-8)
V. Temperature
   A. Decreased (subnormal)
      1. Shock
      2. Drug overdose
      3. Metabolic coma (e.g., myxedema coma)
      4. Terminal stages of neurologic disease
   B. Increased
      1. Infection
         a) Systemic infection
         b) CNS infection
      2. Subarachnoid hemorrhage
      3. Seizures
      4. Restlessness
      5. Injury to hypothalamus: especially if inordinately elevated

General Appearance

I. Attire: appropriateness to age, environment
II. Grooming
   A. Hair
   B. Teeth
   C. Nails
   D. Hygiene
III. General behavior
   A. Demeanor
   B. Affect: facial expressions, body language
   C. Mood: euphoria, anger, depression, suicidal thoughts
IV. Posture: gestures, fidgeting, restlessness, relaxed, rigid
V. Gait: dystaxia is uncoordinated body movements
VI. Obvious physical defects
   A. Hemiparalysis
   B. Facial asymmetry
   C. Ptosis
   D. Amputations

Mental Status

I. Level of consciousness
   A. Consciousness is a state of awareness: self, environment, responses to environment
      1. Arousal
         a) Measure of being awake
         b) Function of the reticular activating system (RAS) in the midbrain
      2. Awareness
         a) Involves interpreting sensory input and giving an appropriate response
         b) Requires both an intact RAS and cerebral hemispheres
   B. Coma is the absence of awareness
      1. Causes of coma include:
         a) Structural lesion
         b) Metabolic condition
         c) Psychiatric condition
   C. LOC is the most sensitive indicator of a change in neurologic status
   D. Describe the behavior rather than using a label (e.g., lethargic, stuporous)
   E. Evaluate the degree of stimulus to get a response
      1. Verbal stimuli
         a) Call the patient by name speaking at normal voice volume
         b) Ask the patient to touch his or her nose or stick out his or her tongue
         c) Use increased volume ("yelling") if he or

Table 6-8	**Respiratory Rhythms**		
Rhythm	**Description**	**Diagram**	**Significance**
Eupnea	Regular rhythm at normal rate		• Normal
Bradypnea	Regular rhythm with rate <12/min		• CNS depression by injury, disease, or drugs
Cheyne-Stokes	Increasing rate and depth of ventilation followed by decreasing rate and depth of ventilation and then apnea		• Bilateral lesions of cerebral hemispheres • Lesion of basal ganglia • Cerebellar lesion • Lesion of upper brainstem • Metabolic condition
CNS hyperventilation	Sustained increased rate and depth of ventilation		• Lesions of lower midbrain or upper pons • May be secondary to transtentorial herniation
Apneustic	Apnea with inspiration followed by exhalation		• Lesions of mid to lower pons
Cluster (or Biot's)	3-4 breaths of identical rate and depth followed by apnea, sequence repeated		• Lesions of lower pons or upper medulla
Ataxic	No pattern to ventilation; completely irregular with mostly apnea		• Lesions of the medulla

she does not respond to normal voice volume
2. Tactile stimuli: touch or shake the patient
3. Painful stimuli: utilize only if the other methods are unsuccessful; avoid trauma and bruising caused by pinching
   a) Techniques to elicit a pain response
      (1) Central: brain responds
         (a) Pressure to trapezius muscle
            (i) Squeeze large muscle mass between thumb and index finger; do not pinch skin
         (b) Pressure to Achilles tendon
            (i) Squeeze large muscle mass between thumb and index finger; do not pinch skin
         (c) Supraorbital pressure
            (i) Push up against the supraorbital ridge with thumb; exert gentle upward pressure
            (ii) Do not push into the eye socket; injury to the eye or vagal response may occur
            (iii) Do not use this technique in patients with facial fracture or cranial fracture
         (d) Sternal rub
            (i) Rub sternum gently with knuckle
            (ii) If bruising results, discontinue using this technique
      (2) Peripheral: spine responds
         (a) Nailbed pressure
            (i) Apply pressure to the

Table 6-9	**Glasgow Coma Scale**	
Parameter	**Response**	**Score**
Eye opening	Spontaneous	4
	To speech	3
	To pain	2
	None	1
	Untestable	U
Best motor response	Obeys commands	6
	Localizes pain	5
	Withdraws from pain	4
	Abnormal flexion (decorticate posturing)	3
	Abnormal extension (decerebrate posturing)	2
	None	1
	Untestable	U
Best verbal response	Oriented	5
	Confused	4
	Inappropriate	3
	Incomprehensible	2
	None	1
	Untestable	U

nailbed using the flat surface of a pen or pencil
(ii) Useful in detecting paralysis of any of the four extremities but should not be used as the only method of evaluation of pain response
F. Glasgow coma scale (Table 6-9)
   1. Developed as a method to standardize observation of responsiveness in neurologic patients

2. Best or highest response is recorded; E (eye), M (motor), V (verbal) may be recorded separately along with a quantitative score
3. Note if certain responses cannot be evaluated because of any of the following:
   a) Endotracheal intubation or tracheostomy
   b) Aphasia
   c) Eyes swollen shut
4. Parameters
   a) Minimum: 3
   b) Maximum (normal): 15
   c) Clinically significant: change of 2 points or more

II. Orientation: patient may be alert but confused
   A. Orientation to person
      1. Ability to identify self by name (e.g., Who are you? What is your name?)
      2. Ability to identify friends, family
   B. Orientation to place
      1. Ability to identify surroundings (e.g., Where are you now?)
      2. Ability to state address (e.g., Where do you live?)
   C. Orientation to time
      1. Ability to give today's date (e.g., What is today's date?)
      2. Ability to state the year (e.g., What year is it?)
   D. Orientation to situation
      1. Ability to identify the situation (e.g., Why are you in the hospital?)

III. Speech and language
   A. Note punctuation, rhythm, stream of talk, sentence structure, appropriate use of words; speech should be fluent with expression of connected thoughts
   B. If patient cannot utilize or understand verbal communication:
      1. Can he or she understand or utilize gestures?
      2. Can he or she understand written language or write messages?
   C. Identify the presence of speech disorders
      1. Dysphonia: difficulty producing sound
      2. Dysarthria: difficulty with articulation
      3. Dysprosody: lack of inflection while talking
      4. Dysphasia: difficulty with understanding or expressing verbal language
      5. Aphasia: absence of understanding or expression of verbal language
         a) Receptive (sensory) aphasia: lesion in Wernicke's area in temporal area
         b) Expressive (motor) aphasia: lesion in Broca's area in frontal area
         c) Global: both

IV. Memory
   A. How old are you?
   B. Remote memory: Who was your first grade teacher? Where did you attend high school?
   C. Recent memory: What did you have for breakfast? What is your doctor's name?

Table 6-10	Muscle Strength Grading Scale
Grade	**Description**
0/5	No movement or muscle contraction
1/5	Trace; no movement but evidence of muscle contraction
2/5	Not greater than gravity; movement with gravity eliminated
3/5	Greater than gravity; movement against gravity
4/5	Slight weakness; movement against some resistance
5/5	Normal; movement against full resistance

V. Short-term recall: Ask the patient to repeat three or four objects after 3 to 5 minutes?
VI. General knowledge: Who is the U.S. president?
VII. Attention span: Ability of the patient to stay on a subject
VIII. Thought content: Note evidence of illusions, hallucinations, delusions, paranoia
IX. Calculation skills: Can you count backwards from 20 to 1?
X. Judgment: Why are you here? What would you do if there was a fire in the wastebasket?
XI. Abstraction: What does "a stitch in time saves nine" mean?

Motor Function
I. Muscle size
   A. Symmetry
   B. Atrophy or hypertrophy
II. Symmetrical movement and strength of extremities
   A. Movement
      1. Spontaneous movement and symmetry of movement
      2. Assumption of a position of comfort
   B. Strength (Table 6-10)
      1. Handgrips
         a) Check simultaneously
         b) Determine handedness: expect dominant side to be slightly stronger
      2. Ulnar (or palmar) drift
         a) Detection: have patient hold his or her arms out with palms up and eyes closed
         b) Normal: patient should be able to hold his or her arms even for at least 20 seconds
         c) Abnormal: the weak arm begins to drift and pronate (turn palm downward)
      3. Leg strengths: evaluated by having the patient push against your hands or hold the feet and ask the patient to pull them back toward his or her body
      4. Plegia positioning (Fig. 6-22)
III. Muscle tone
   A. Flaccidity: no resistance to passive movement; flaccid paralysis is associated with lower motor neuron lesions

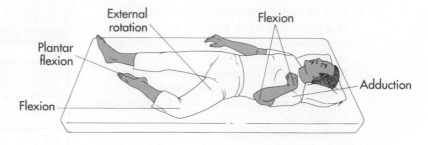

Figure 6-22 Plegia positioning. (From Beare PG, Myers JL: *Principles and practice of adult health nursing,* ed 2, St Louis, 1994, Mosby.)

Table 6-11 Locating Site Of Motor Problems

	Lower Motor Neuron	Upper Motor Neuron	
		Pyramidal Tract	**Extrapyramidal Tract**
Effect	• Flaccid paralysis • Areflexia	• Spastic paralysis with hyperactive reflexes • Positive Babinski reflex	• No paralysis • Altered muscle tone and abnormal movements
Muscle appearance	• Atrophy • Small muscular contractions (fasciculation)	• Mild atrophy from disuse	• Tremor when at rest
Muscle tone	Decreased	Increased	Increased
Muscle strength	Decreased or absent	Decreased or absent	Normal
Coordination	Absent or poor	Absent or poor	Slowed
Examples	• Poliomyelitis • ALS • Guillain-Barré syndrome	• Stroke • Spinal cord injury • Multiple sclerosis • ALS	• Parkinson's disease

B. Hypotonia: little resistance to passive movement
C. Hypertonia: increased muscle resistance to passive movement
D. Rigidity: increased muscle resistance to passive movement of a rigid limb that is uniform through both flexion and extension (paratonic rigidity may occur in coma and is a sign of diffuse cerebral dysfunction)
E. Spasticity: gradual increase in tone, causing increased resistance until tone is suddenly reduced
  1. Clonus, continued rhythmic contraction of a muscle after the stimulus has been applied, may be evident
  2. Spastic paralysis is associated with upper motor neuron lesions
F. Upper motor neuron versus lower motor neuron (Table 6-11)
IV. Coordination
  A. Point-to-point movements
    1. Finger-nose test: ask patient to touch his or her nose with a finger and with eyes closed
    2. Finger-finger test: ask patient to close his or her eyes and touch your finger with his or her finger
    3. Heel-knee test: ask patient to run the heel of one foot down the opposite leg from the knee to the foot
  B. Rapid, rhythmic alternating movements
    1. Pronation-supination test: ask patient to rapidly pronate and supinate his or her hand

    2. Patting test: ask patient to rapidly pronate and supinate his or her hand against a leg
  C. Figure eight test: ask patient to draw a figure eight in the air with his or her great toe
V. Gait
  A. Tandem gait: ask patient to walk heel-to-toe in a straight line
    1. Normal: ability to walk heel-to-toe without difficulty
    2. Abnormal: loss of balance indicates cerebellar dysfunction
  B. Abnormal gaits
    1. Spastic: leg is held stiff and moved slowly; toes and lateral aspect of foot scrape the floor as the leg is moved; this gait indicates corticospinal tract lesion
    2. Steppage: foot is lifted very high for each step with a distinctive slapping sound as it hits the floor; this gait indicates peripheral nerve injury
    3. Ataxic: feet are broad-based and steps are unsteady and staggering; this gait indicates cerebellar or dorsal column lesions
    4. Propulsive: body is bent forward, steps are short, momentum is increased, and falls are common; this gait indicates basal ganglia dysfunction (e.g., Parkinson's disease)
    5. Waddling: pelvis opposite the weight-bearing hip drops and the trunk inclines, causing a waddle; this gait indicates proximal muscle weakness (e.g., muscular dystrophy)

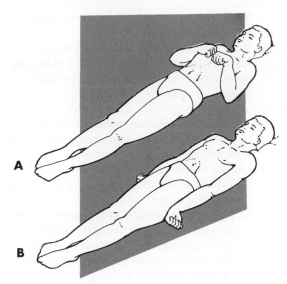

Figure 6-23   A, Abnormal flexion (decorticate) posturing. **B,** Abnormal extension (decerebrate) posturing. (From Thelan LA et al: *Critical care nursing: diagnosis and management,* ed 3, St Louis, 1998, Mosby.)

6. Scissors: thighs are held together and each foot is alternately brought forward; this gait indicates upper motor neuron lesion
VI. Station: tested by Romberg test
   A. Method: ask patient to close eyes and stand with feet together and arms extended in front
   B. Normal: patient able to stand erect and steady; slight swaying may be seen
   C. Abnormal: patient loses balance; this result indicates loss of position sense and/or cerebellar dysfunction
VII. Involuntary movements
   A. Posturing may occur spontaneously or to pain
     1. Abnormal flexion (Fig. 6-23)
       a) Also called *decorticate posturing*
       b) Arms are flexed toward the body, legs are extended
       c) Indicates cerebral lesion
     2. Abnormal extension (Fig. 6-23)
       a) Also called *decerebrate posturing*
       b) Arms are extended, wrists are externally rotated, and legs are extended
       c) Indicates midbrain or brainstem lesion
     3. Opisthotonos
       a) Also referred to as *arching*
       b) Extension of arms, legs and arching of the back and neck
       c) May indicate brainstem injury
     4. Flaccid posture: entire body is flaccid even with painful stimulation
   B. Tremor
     1. Resting: Parkinson's disease
     2. Intentional: cerebellar disease
     3. Flapping: metabolic encephalopathy (e.g., hepatic or renal failure)
     4. Physiologic: stress induced
     5. Senile: age induced

   C. Seizure: describe
     1. Preceding events: aura?
     2. Initial cry or sound
     3. Onset
       a) Initial body movements
       b) Deviation of head and eyes
       c) Chewing and salivation
       d) Posture of body
       e) Sensory changes
     4. Tonic and clonic phases
       a) Progression of body movements
       b) Skin color and airway
       c) Pupillary changes
       d) Incontinence
       e) Duration of each phase
     5. Level of consciousness during seizure
     6. Postictal phase
       a) Duration
       b) General behavior
       c) Memory of events
       d) Orientation
       e) Pupillary changes
       f) Headache
       g) Aphasia
       h) Injuries
     7. Duration of entire seizure
     8. Medications given and response

Sensory Function

I. Ability to perceive sensation
   A. Superficial sensation
     1. Light touch: wisp of cotton on skin
     2. Superficial pain: light pinprick on skin (use sterile needle and discard appropriately after testing)
     3. Skin temperature: hot and cold test tubes on skin
   B. Deep sensation
     1. Vibration: vibration of tuning fork on bony surface
     2. Position sense: position of great toe, thumb with eyes closed
     3. Deep pain: pressure on Achilles tendon, calf muscles, upper arm muscles
   C. Cortical/discriminatory sensation: requires cortical interpretation
     1. Two-point discrimination: ability to distinguish between one or two points; patient touched with two points at varying degrees of separation to see if the patient feels only one or two points
     2. Stereognosis: ability to distinguish common objects placed in the hand with eyes closed
     3. Topognosis: ability to distinguish which finger is being touched with eyes closed
     4. Graphesthesia: ability to recognize numbers or letters traced on the skin with eyes closed
     5. Tactile inattention: ability to differentiate between one or two points when being touched at one or two points on opposite sides of the body in corresponding locations

Table 6-12	Dermatomal Levels for Bedside Assessment	
Anatomic Location	**Spinal Level**	
Front of neck	C3	
Thumb	C6	
Ring and little finger	C8	
Nipple line	T4	
Umbilicus	T10	
Groin crease	L1	
Knee	L3	
Anterior ankle and foot	L5	
Lateral foot and heel	S1	
Genitalia	S3,4	

D. Ability to recognize objects through the special senses; inability referred to as *agnosia*
 1. Visual: occipital lobe
 2. Auditory: temporal lobe
 3. Tactile: parietal lobe
 4. Body parts and relationships: parietal lobe
E. Distribution of sensory loss
 1. Entire side of body: parietal or thalamic lesion
 2. Dermatomal (Table 6-12 and Fig. 6-20)
  a) Dermatome: skin area supplied by sensory fibers of a single spinal nerve
  b) Sensory loss below a dermatomal level: spinal cord lesion
  c) Sensory loss along a dermatome: spinal nerve lesion
 3. Peripheral nerve distribution (Fig. 6-20)
F. Degrees of sensory loss
 1. Anesthesia: loss of sensation
 2. Dysesthesia: impaired sensation
 3. Hyperesthesia: increased sensation
 4. Hypesthesia: decreased sensation
 5. Paresthesia: burning, tingling sensation

Cranial Nerve Function
 I. Olfactory (I)
  A. Test: patient's ability to identify familiar odors (e.g., coffee, cloves, tobacco, alcohol) tested; each nostril tested separately with eyes closed
  B. Normal: able to identify familiar odors
  C. Abnormal: unable to identify familiar odors; referred to as *anosmia*
 II. Optic (II)
  A. Visual acuity
   1. Snellen chart
    a) Ask patient to read lines of the Snellen chart from a distance of 20 feet
    b) Record the number on the lowest line that the patient can read with 50% accuracy
    c) Test with glasses or contact lenses
   2. If patient cannot see well enough to read

the Snellen chart, ask how many fingers you are holding up
   3. If the patient cannot see well enough to tell you how many fingers you are holding up, determine whether he or she can tell light from dark
  B. Visual fields
   1. Test by confrontation: comparison of patient's visual field to examiner's visual field with eye on same side covered
   2. Loss of vision or portion of visual field
    a) Unilateral blindness: lesion of eye, retina, or optic nerve
    b) Bitemporal hemianopsia: lesion of optic chiasm or lesion causing pressure on optic chiasm (e.g., pituitary tumor)
    c) Left homonymous hemianopsia: lesion of right optic tract
    d) Right homonymous hemianopsia: lesion of left optic tract
    e) Left homonymous hemianopsia with macular sparing: lesion of right geniculocalcarine tract
    f) Right homonymous hemianopsia with macular sparing: lesion of left geniculocalcarine tract
  C. Near vision
   1. Ask the patient to read newsprint at a distance of 12 inches
   2. Normal: patient should be able to read newsprint at 12 inches
  D. Funduscopic examination with ophthalmoscope to detect papilledema (Fig. 6-24)
   1. Optic disc is pushed forward
   2. Disc margins are blurry
   3. Indication of intracranial hypertension
    a) May be late in acute intracranial hypertension
    b) May be first sign in chronic intracranial hypertension (e.g., tumor)
 III. Oculomotor (III), trochlear (IV), abducens (VI)
  A. Eyelids: elevation of the eyelid is controlled by cranial nerve III; ptosis may indicate cranial nerve III injury
  B. Pupils
   1. Size
    a) Normal: 2 to 6 mm
    b) Abnormal: clinically significant change is more than 1 mm
     (1) Pinpoint (and nonreactive)
      (a) Pontine lesion
      (b) Medication effect
       (i) Opiates (e.g., morphine)
       (ii) Miotics (e.g., pilocarpine)
     (2) Midsize (2 to 6 mm) but nonreactive: midbrain lesion
     (3) Unilateral large (>6 mm) and nonreactive (may be referred to as blown or *Hutchinsonian pupil*): pressure on oculomotor nerve on same side

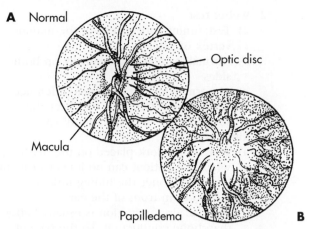

A, Normal fundus.

Figure 6-24 **A,** Normal fundus. **B,** Fundus showing papille-dema. (From Hausman et al: *Analyzing neurological status,* St Louis, 1985, Mosby.)

(4) Bilateral large (>6 mm) and nonreactive
  (a) Brainstem lesion
  (b) Medication effect
    (i) Parasympatholytics (e.g., atropine)
    (ii) Sympathomimetics (e.g., epinephrine)

2. Equality
  a) Normal: equal
  b) Abnormal: unequal (referred to as *anisocoria*)
    (1) Normal variation: 15% to 20% of the population has slightly unequal pupils (1 mm or less difference)
    (2) Abnormal: difference of more than 1 mm or change from baseline
    (3) Injury effects
      (a) Injury to parasympathetic fibers of the oculomotor nerve: ipsilateral (same side) pupil dilation
      (b) Injury to sympathetic fibers of the sympathetic fibers of the oculomotor nerves (e.g., Horner's syndrome): ipsilateral pupil constriction

3. Shape
  a) Normal: round
  b) Abnormal
    (1) Oval
      (a) May precede dilated pupil as a sign of pressure on the oculomotor nerve
      (b) Associated with intracranial pressure of 18 to 35 mm Hg
    (2) Irregular (e.g., keyhole shaped may be seen in patients after cataract removal due to concurrent iridectomy)

4. Position
  a) Normal: midposition
  b) Abnormal: eyes may deviate to the side of the injury

5. Reactivity to light
  a) Detection
    (1) Darken the room if pupils are small
    (2) Use a small, bright penlight in front of each eye
    (3) Note pupil constriction as the direct reaction
    (4) Note pupil constriction of the opposite pupil as consensual reaction
  b) Normal: brisk bilateral direct and consensual reaction to light
  c) Abnormal
    (1) Sluggish or absent reaction; indicative of any of the following:
      (a) Cranial nerve III pressure or injury
      (b) Hypothermia
      (c) Barbiturate intoxication
    (2) Hippus: pupil initially reacts briskly then followed by an exaggerated rhythmic contraction and dilation of the pupil; may be normal but may be indicative of any of the following:
      (a) Early cranial nerve III pressure or injury
      (b) Midbrain injury
      (c) Barbiturate intoxication

6. Accommodation: ability of the eyes to focus on a distant object and accommodate as the object moves closer
  a) Pupils dilate when focusing on a far object
  b) Pupils constrict when focusing on a near object

7. Ciliospinal reflex
  a) Normal: ipsilateral pupil dilation with trapezius squeeze
  b) Abnormal: no response; indicative of interruption of sympathetic fibers of oculomotor nerve

C. Range of ocular movements
  1. Patient asked to keep head straight and follow your finger with eyes; move your finger in the direction of the six cardinal positions of gaze (Fig. 6-25)
  2. Normal: both eyes move conjugately in the direction of your finger
  3. Abnormal: one or both eyes do not move to follow finger; indicative of cranial nerve injury

D. Abnormal eye movements
  1. Nystagmus: jerky eye movement that oscillates the eye back and forth quickly; may be seen in lesions of vestibular system or brainstem
  2. Dysconjugate eye movement: may indicate damage to the brainstem
  3. Conjugate eye movement: may indicate cerebral hemispheric damage

IV. Trigeminal (V)
A. Sensory branch
  1. Three branches (forehead, cheek, jaw)

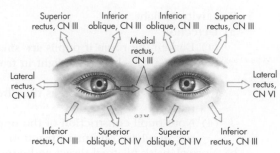

Figure 6-25 The six cardinal positions of gaze. (From Seidel HM et al: *Mosby's guide to physical examination,* ed 2, St Louis, 1991, Mosby.)

tested on both sides with a wisp of cotton (light touch), pinprick (superficial pain), hot and cold test tubes (temperature)

2. Corneal blink reflex
   a) Detection: cornea touched with a wisp of cotton
   b) Normal: bilateral blink; indicates intactness of fifth (trigeminal) and seventh (facial) cranial nerves
   c) Abnormal: decreased or absent blink; may indicate cranial nerve V injury (**Note:** contact lens wearers have diminished corneal blink reflex)

B. Motor branch
   1. Test: face inspected for muscle atrophy, tremor; the masseter muscle palpated while the patient clenches teeth; the temporal muscles palpated as the patient squeezes eyes closed
   2. Normal: symmetry of muscle strength, no atrophy or tremor
   3. Abnormal: asymmetry of muscle strength; may indicate cranial nerve V injury

V. Facial (VII)
   A. Motor branch
      1. Test: symmetry of facial expressions noted while patient raises eyebrows, frowns, smiles, closes eyelids
      2. Abnormal: asymmetry of facial expression; loss of nasolabial fold, eye remaining open; indicates cranial nerve VII injury (Bell's palsy)
   B. Sensory branch
      1. Test: ability to taste sweet, sour, salty, and bitter on anterior tongue tested
      2. Normal: ability to taste and discriminate
      3. Abnormal: inability to taste; indicates cranial nerve VII injury

VI. Acoustic (VIII)
   A. Cochlear branch: hearing acuity
      1. Whisper test
         a) Test: face turned away and examiner whispers to see if patient can hear what is whispered; Test each ear separately
         b) This test differentiates between hearing and lip reading

2. Weber test
   a) Test: tuning fork placed at the midline vertex of skull
   b) Normal: patient hears equally on both sides
   c) Abnormal: patient indicates difference between the two ears; will hear the sound better with the "good" ear
3. Rinne test
   a) Test: tuning fork placed on the mastoid; when the patient can no longer hear the sound by bone, the tuning fork is moved to in front of the ear
   b) Normal: air conduction is usually better than bone conduction, so the patient should still be able to hear the sound when the tuning fork is moved in front of the ear after the patient reports not being able to hear the sound any longer by bone
   c) Abnormal: inability to hear the sound by air after the cessation of the sound by bone; diminished air conduction is associated with middle ear infection or disease

B. Vestibular branch
   1. Not tested directly; problems may be detected by signs/symptoms such as nystagmus, vertigo, nausea, vomiting, pallor, sweating, hypotension
   2. Reflexes: vestibular branch of cranial nerve VIII and connections with cranial nerves III and VI provide information regarding integrity of the brainstem
      a) Oculocephalic reflex (also called *doll's eyes reflex*) (Fig. 6-26)
         (1) Prerequisites
            (a) Cervical spine has been radiologically cleared
            (b) Patient must be unconscious
            (c) Eyes are held open so that eye movement can be observed
         (2) Test: head rotated side to side
         (3) Normal: eyes move in the opposite direction of the head (presence of doll's eyes: like an expensive china doll); indicates supratentorial cause for the coma
         (4) Abnormal: eyes stay midline or turn to the same direction as the head (absence of doll's eyes); indicates compression in the midbrain-pontine area
      b) Oculovestibular reflex (also called *caloric testing*) (Fig. 6-26)
         (1) Prerequisites
            (a) Intact tympanic membrane
            (b) Absence of basal skull fracture
         (2) Test
            (a) Elevation of the head of the bed 30 degrees

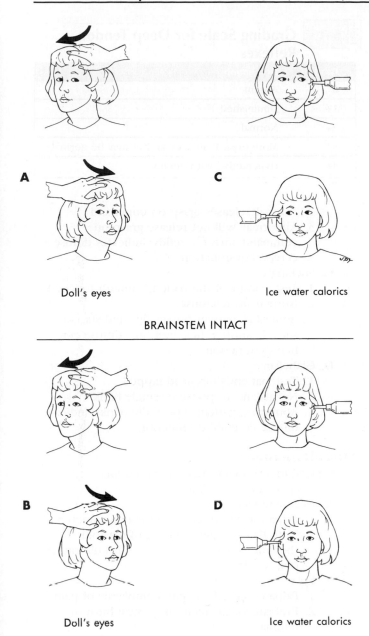

BRAINSTEM INTACT

BRAINSTEM NOT INTACT

Figure 6-26 **A,** Oculocephalic (doll's eyes) reflex with normal response: eyes move in the direction opposite the direction that the head is turned. **B,** Oculocephalic (doll's eyes) reflex with abnormal response: eyes either move in the same direction as the head is being turned or stay midline. **C,** Oculovestibular (caloric) reflex with normal response: nystagmus is present, and there may be conjugate movement toward the irrigated ear. **D,** Oculovestibular (caloric) reflex with abnormal response: no nystagmus or dysconjugate movement of the eyes. (From Beare PG, Myers JL: *Principles and practice of adult health nursing,* ed 2, St Louis, 1994, Mosby.)

(b) Injection of 20 to 50 ml of iced water into the ear canal and against the tympanic membrane
(3) Normal: nystagmus with deviation toward the irrigated ear

(4) Abnormal
   (a) No eye movement
   (b) Dysconjugate eye movement
VII. Glossopharyngeal (IX), vagus (X)
  A. Phonation
    1. Test: patient asked to say "Ah"
    2. Normal: bilateral elevation of palate
    3. Abnormal: no elevation of palate on one side
  B. Speech
    1. Test: articulation assessed; any hoarseness detected
    2. Normal: voice clear with ability to change volume and pitch
    3. Abnormal: hoarseness; indicates damage to the laryngeal branch of cranial nerve X
  C. Taste
    1. Test: ability to taste sour and bitter on posterior tongue tested
    2. Normal: ability to taste
    3. Abnormal: inability to taste sour or bitter
  D. Swallowing
    1. Test: tongue held down with a tongue blade and each side of the pharynx touched with a cotton swab
    2. Normal: involuntary swallow or gag; indicates intactness of ninth and tenth cranial nerves
    3. Abnormal: no swallow or gag (**Note:** do not give fluids; position on side; have suction equipment available)
  E. Gag
    1. Test: palate stroked with a tongue blade (**Note:** do not perform this test within 2 hours after eating)
    2. Normal: involuntary gag; indicates intactness of ninth and tenth cranial nerves
    3. Abnormal: no gag (**Note:** do not give fluids; position on side; have suction equipment available)
  F. Cough
    1. Test: hypopharynx touched with a suction catheter
    2. Normal: involuntary cough; indicates intactness of ninth and tenth cranial reflex
    3. Abnormal: no cough
  G. Carotid sinus reflex
    1. Test: not normally tested
    2. Normal: pressure over carotid sinus produces bradycardia and hypotension
VIII. Spinal accessory (XI)
  A. Sternocleidomastoid and trapezius muscles inspected for size and symmetry
  B. Patient asked to shrug his or her shoulders as you push down with your hands on his or her shoulders
  C. Patient asked to turn his or her head to each side against resistance
  D. Normal: symmetry, adequate muscle strength
  E. Abnormal: asymmetry, poor muscle strength

IX. Hypoglossal (XII)
- A. Tongue inspected for atrophy, fasciculations, alignment
- B. Tongue strength tested with your index finger when the patient pushes his or her tongue against his or her cheek
- C. Normal: no atrophy, fasciculations, midline alignment when protrudes, normal strength
- D. Abnormal: atrophy, fasciculations, or deviation from midline; decreased strength

Reflexes

I. Deep tendon (also called *muscle-stretch reflexes*)
- A. Test: tendon tapped with a reflex hammer
- B. Normal: contraction of the muscle and a jerk of affected limb
- C. Abnormal
  1. Hyporeflexia
     - a) Less than normal contraction
     - b) May be seen in hypercalcemia, hypophosphatemia, hypermagnesemia, upper motor neuron lesion
  2. Hyperreflexia
     - a) More than normal contraction; may be associated with clonus
     - b) May be seen in hypocalcemia, hyperphosphatemia, hypomagnesemia, lower motor neuron lesion
- D. Grading scale (Table 6-13)
- E. Locations and spinal levels
  1. Jaw: cranial nerve V (trigeminal)
  2. Biceps: elbow flexion, C5-6
  3. Brachioradialis: wrist extension, C5-6
  4. Triceps: elbow extension, C7-8
  5. Patellar: knee extension, L2-4
  6. Achilles: foot extension, S1-2

II. Superficial reflexes
- A. Abdominal reflexes
  1. Test: abdomen stroked toward umbilicus with blunt end of cotton-tipped applicator
  2. Normal: umbilicus moves toward the quadrant that is stroked
  3. Abnormal: no response; indicates lesion at T7-9 for upper abdomen; T11-12 for lower abdomen
- B. Cremasteric reflex
  1. Test: inner thigh stroked
  2. Normal: testis on stimulated side elevates
  3. Abnormal: no response: indicates lesion at L1-2
- C. Plantar reflex
  1. Test: sole of the foot stroked with a blunt instrument (Fig. 6-27)
  2. Normal: toes curl downward
  3. Abnormal (Babinski reflex): extension of great toe and fanning of other toes; indicates upper motor neuron lesion

III. Pathologic reflexes
- A. Babinski: described previously
- B. Grasp
  1. Test: something (frequently a finger) placed in the patient's hand

Table 6-13	Grading Scale for Deep Tendon Reflexes	
Grade	**Description**
0	Absent
1+	Diminished
2+	Normal
3+	More brisk than average but may be normal
4+	Hyperactive with clonus

  2. Normal: releases grasp on command
  3. Abnormal: will not release grasp on command; infantile reflex: indicates diffuse cerebral dysfunction
- C. Sucking
  1. Test: corner of the patient's mouth touched
  2. Normal: no response
  3. Abnormal: patient purses lips and starts to suck; infantile reflex: indicates diffuse cerebral dysfunction
- D. Glabellar
  1. Test: patient's forehead tapped
  2. Normal: no response or single blink
  3. Abnormal: patient repeatedly blinks; indicates diffuse cerebral dysfunction

Miscellaneous

I. Clinical indications of neurologic trauma
- A. Scalp: tears or swelling
- B. Head and face
  1. Palpate face, maxilla; mandible for fractures
  2. Note Battle's sign: bruising of mastoid (behind ear); indicative of basal skull fracture (Fig. 6-28)
- C. Eyes
  1. Palpate eye orbits; note complaints of pain
  2. Evaluate visual acuity if corneal burn or trauma
  3. Note raccoon eyes: bruising around eyes indicative of basal skull fracture (Fig. 6-28)
- D. Nose
  1. Palpate nose; note complaints of pain
  2. Note CSF leak: may be seen in basal skull fracture; referred to as *rhinorrhea*
     - a) Differentiation of CSF from mucus is confirmed by testing for the presence of glucose; CSF tests positive for glucose; mucus does not
     - b) CSF also leaves a "halo" on 4 × 4's or linens; this refers to blood settling in the middle with lighter-colored concentric rings around the blood (Fig. 6-28)
- E. Ears
  1. Note edema, trauma to external ear or ear canal
  2. Note blood in external ear canal or blood behind ear drum: seen in basal skull fracture
  3. Note CSF from ear: seen in basal skull fracture; referred to as *otorrhea*

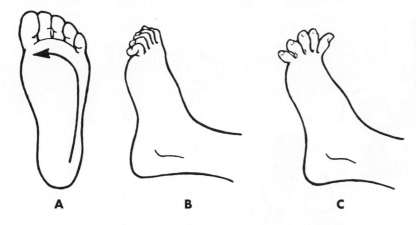

Figure 6-27 Babinski reflex. **A,** Method of stroking sole of foot. **B,** Normal response (absence of Babinski's reflex). **C,** Abnormal response (presence of Babinski's reflex).

F. Injury to teeth, tongue, gums, mucosa
G. Alteration in consciousness
H. Clinical indications of intracranial hypertension (see Intracranial Hypertension section)

II. Clinical indications of meningeal irritation
   A. Nuchal rigidity: indicative of meningeal irritation (e.g., infection or hemorrhage)
   B. Kernig's sign (Fig. 6-29)
      1. Test: patient placed on his or her back and assisted to flex thigh toward chest until hip is at 90-degree angle; then leg extended at knee
      2. Normal: ability to fully extend leg without pain
      3. Abnormal: inability to fully extend leg when thigh is flexed toward abdomen; neck pain may also occur; indicates irritation of the meninges by infection or blood
   C. Brudzinski's sign (Fig. 6-29)
      1. Prerequisite: cervical spine must be radiologically cleared
      2. Test: chin brought toward chest and head moved forward
      3. Normal: absence of neck pain and absence of involuntary adduction and flexion of knees toward body
      4. Abnormal: neck pain and involuntary adduction and flexion of legs with attempts to flex the neck; indicates irritation of the meninges by infection or blood

III. Jugular venous oxygen saturation (Sjo$_2$) monitoring
   A. Technique: fiberoptic catheter placed into the jugular vein bulb to continuously monitor the oxygen saturation of the blood returning from the brain and to intermittently sample venous blood gases; comparison between arterial oxygen saturation and jugular venous oxygen saturation allows calculation of arteriovenous oxygen difference
   B. Normal value: 55% to 70%; saturation less than 55% indicates cerebral ischemia
   C. Limitations: may not be reliable if performed unilaterally since the oxygen content of each jugular bulb may differ

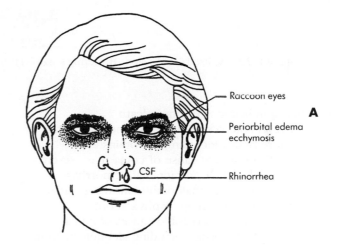

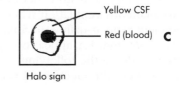

Halo sign

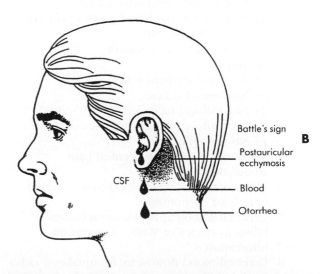

Figure 6-28 **A,** Raccoon eyes and rhinorrhea. **B,** Battle's sign with otorrhea. **C,** Halo sign. (From Barker E: *Neuroscience nursing,* St Louis, 1994, Mosby.)

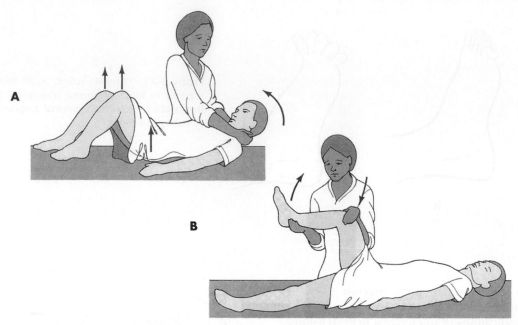

Figure 6-29 **A,** Brudzinski's sign. **B,** Kernig's sign. (From Barker E: *Neuroscience nursing,* St Louis, 1994, Mosby.)

IV. Clinical indications of brain death
   A. Irreversible cessation of all functions of the entire brain, including the brainstem
      1. Recognizable cause of coma (e.g., severe head trauma, intracranial hemorrhage, anoxic encephalopathy following cardiac arrest, drowning, asphyxiation)
      2. Potentially reversible causes of coma (sedative drugs including alcohol, neuromuscular blocking agents, hypothermia, metabolic or endocrine disturbance) excluded
      3. No spontaneous ventilation when tested for a sufficient time; usually 3 to 5 minutes of $Paco_2$ of >60 mm Hg; apnea testing is performed by doing the following
         a) Disconnect the mechanical ventilator
         b) Deliver 100% oxygen
         c) Monitor for ventilatory effort
         d) Measure arterial blood gases to confirm $Paco_2$ >60 mm Hg
         e) Reconnect the ventilator
      4. No reflexes
         a) No pupillary light reflex
         b) No corneal reflex
         c) No oculocephalic reflex (doll's eyes)
         d) No oculovestibular reflex (caloric)
         e) No gag reflex
      5. No motor response to central pain stimulation
      6. EEG: no electrical activity during a period of at least 30 minutes
      7. Cerebral angiography: no intracerebral filling in circles of Willis or at carotid bifurcation
      8. Cerebral blood flow scan: no uptake of radionuclide in brain parenchyma indicating no cerebral blood flow

Diagnostic Studies
   I. Serum
      A. Chemistries
         1. Sodium: normal 136 to 145 mEq/L
         2. Potassium: normal 3.5 to 5.5 mEq/L
         3. Chloride: normal 96 to 106 mEq/L
         4. Calcium: normal 8.5 to 10.5 mg/dl
         5. Phosphorus: normal 3.0 to 4.5 mg/dl
         6. Magnesium: normal 1.5 to 2.2 mEq/L or 1.8 to 2.4 mg/dl
         7. Glucose: normal 70 to 110 mEq/L
         8. BUN: normal 5 to 20 mg/dl
         9. Creatinine: normal 0.7 to 1.5 mg/dl
        10. Lactate: 1 to 2 mmol/L
        11. Enzymes
            a) Total CK: normal 55 to 170 U/L for males; 30 to 135 U/L for females
            b) LDH: 90 to 200 IU/L
      B. Arterial blood gases
         1. pH: normal 7.35 to 7.45
         2. $Paco_2$: normal 35 to 45 mm Hg
         3. HCO_3: normal 22 to 26 mEq/L
         4. Pao_2: normal 80 to 100 mm Hg
         5. Sao_2: greater than 95%
      C. Hematology
         1. Hematocrit: normal 40% to 52% for males; 35% to 47% for females
         2. Hemoglobin: normal 13 to 18 g/dl for males; 12 to 16 g/dl for females
         3. White blood cells (WBC): normal 3,500 to 11,000 mm^3
         4. Erythrocyte sedimentation rate: normal up to 15 mm/hr for males; up to 20 mm/hr for females
      D. Clotting profile
         1. Prothrombin time (PT): normal 12 to 15 seconds; therapeutic 1.5 to 2.5 times normal

2. Activated partial thromboplastin time (aPTT): normal 25 to 38 seconds; therapeutic 1.5 to 2.5 times normal
3. Activated clotting time (ACT): normal 70 to 120 seconds; therapeutic 150 to 190 seconds
4. Platelets: normal 150,000 to 400,000/mm^3
5. Thrombin time: normal 10 to 15 seconds
6. Bleeding time: normal 1 to 9.5 minutes
E. Toxicology
  1. Alcohol: normal 0 mg/dl
  2. Dilantin: therapeutic 10 to 20 μg/ml
II. Urine
  A. Glucose: normal negative
  B. Ketones: normal negative
  C. Specific gravity: normal 1.005 to 1.030
  D. Osmolality: normal 50 to 1200 mOsm/L
III. Cerebrospinal fluid analysis
  A. Properties
    1. Colorless, odorless; cloudy in bacterial meningitis
    2. Specific gravity: normal 1.007
    3. pH: normal 7.35
    4. Chlorides: normal 120 to 130 mEq/L
    5. Sodium: normal 140 to 142 mEq/L
    6. Glucose: normal 60% of serum glucose value; decreased in bacterial meningitis
  B. Protein: elevated in meningitis
    1. By lumbar puncture: normal 15 to 45 mg/dl
    2. By cisternal puncture: normal 10 to 25 mg/dl
    3. By ventricular puncture or catheter: normal 5 to 15 mg/dl
  C. Cells
    1. Leukocytes: normal 0 to 5/mm^3
    2. Erythrocytes: normal 0/mm^3
      a) Note: test tubes must be numbered; if first test tube bloody but others are clear, consider trauma; subarachnoid hemorrhage would cause all test tubes to be equally bloody
IV. Other diagnostic studies (Table 6-14)

Intracranial Hypertension

Etiology
I. Mass lesion
  A. Hematoma
    1. Epidural
    2. Subdural
    3. Intracerebral
  B. Neoplasm
    1. Primary brain tumor
    2. Metastatic tumor
  C. Abscess
  D. Trauma: caused by local edema, trauma (e.g., contusion may act as a mass lesion)
II. Cerebral edema: most common cause of intracranial hypertension; may be localized or generalized
  A. Cytotoxic cerebral edema
    1. Intracellular swelling of neurons and glial cells

2. Caused by any of the following:
  a) Hypoosmolality (e.g., low serum osmolality and sodium)
  b) Hypoxia (decreases ATP production, which impairs sodium-potassium pump)
  c) Cardiac arrest (cause of anoxic encephalopathy)
B. Vasogenic cerebral edema
  1. Increase in extracellular fluid caused by breakdown of blood–brain barrier; increased vascular permeability and leakage of plasma protein
  2. Begins locally, becomes generalized
  3. Caused by any of the following:
    a) Trauma (e.g., contusion)
    b) Tumors
    c) Hemorrhage
    d) Abscesses
    e) Surgical trauma (e.g., craniotomy)
III. Cerebrovascular alterations
  A. Venous outflow obstruction: caused by decreased venous return from head
    1. Neck rotation, hyperextension, hyperflexion
    2. Tracheostomy ties or cervical collar
    3. Increased intrathoracic pressure
      a) Valsalva maneuver (e.g., coughing, vomiting, straining at stool)
      b) Positive pressure mechanical ventilation
      c) Positive end-expiratory pressure
  B. Increase in cerebral perfusion pressure (caused by hypertensive crisis)
  C. Vasodilation (caused by hypercapnia, hypoxia, hyperthermia, vasoactive drugs)
IV. Increase in CSF volume (hydrocephalus)
  A. Increase in production of CSF (e.g., choroid plexus disease)
  B. Decrease in reabsorption of CSF
    1. Communicating hydrocephalus (e.g., subarachnoid hemorrhage, meningitis)
    2. Noncommunicating hydrocephalus (e.g., mass lesion, swelling as in head injury or craniotomy)

Pathophysiology
I. Intracranial volumes (Fig. 6-30)
  A. Brain tissue: approximately 80% to 88%
    1. Note: elderly patients and alcoholics or drug abusers may have cerebral atrophy; traction on bridging vessels increases the risk of intracranial bleeding; hemorrhage or hematoma may be very large before symptomatic
  B. Circulating blood: approximately 2% to 10%
  C. Cerebrospinal fluid: approximately 10%
II. Intracranial pressure: the pressure exerted by brain tissue, blood, and cerebrospinal fluid against the inside of the skull
  A. Measured as the pressure exerted by CSF within the ventricles of the brain
  B. Normal: 5 to 15 mm Hg

Table 6-14	DIAGNOSTIC STUDIES	
Study	**Purposes**	**Comments**

Angiography	• Visualizes extracranial and intracranial vasculature
	• Identifies aneurysm, AV malformation, vasospasm, vascular tumors
		• Contraindicated if patient has bleeding disorder or is receiving anticoagulants
		• May cause local hematoma, vasospasm, vessel occlusion, allergic reaction to contrast media, transient or permanent neurologic dysfunction
		• Prior to test:
		  • Keep patient NPO for 4 hours and provide sedation prior to the study
		  • Check for allergy to iodine
		• After the test:
		  • Ensure hydration post-procedure (contrast medium used)
		  • Maintain bedrest for 8-12 hours
		  • Monitor arterial puncture point for hemorrhage or hematoma
		  • Assessment neurovascular status of affected limb
		  • Monitor for indications of systemic emboli

Cisternogram	• Views CSF flow • Identifies hydrocephalus • Evaluates CSF leakage through a dural tear • Evaluates abnormality of structures at the base of the brain and upper cervical cord region	• Contraindicated in intracranial hypertension

Computed tomography (CT); Computed axial tomography (CAT)	• Views intracranial structures: size, shape, location, shifts
	• Differentiates between tumors, hemorrhage, infarction
	• Identifies hydrocephalus, cerebral edema, infectious processes, trauma, aneurysm, hematoma, AV malformation, cerebral atrophy
		• Patient must be cooperative
		• Contrast media may be used
		  • Check for allergy to iodine, seafood prior to study
		  • Patient will be NPO for 4-8 hours prior to the study
		  • Sedation may be given
		  • Monitor for signs of allergic reaction
		  • Encourage fluids

Digital subtraction angiography (DSA): brain; spine	• Visualizes the vasculature, especially carotid and larger cerebral arteries
	• Evaluates occlusive vascular disease
	• Identifies tumors, aneurysms, AV malformation, vascular abnormalities
		• May be done intravenous or intraarterial
		• If IV: less invasive with fewer complications than cerebral angiography
		• If intraarterial, care as for angiogram
		• Contrast media is used
		  • Check for allergy to iodine, seafood prior to study
		  • Patient will be NPO for 4-8 hours prior to the study
		  • Monitor for signs of allergic reaction
		  • Encourage fluids

Electroencephalography (EEG)	• Differentiates epilepsy from mass lesion • Detects focus of seizure activity • Evaluates drug intoxication • Evaluates cerebral blood flow • Localizes tumor, abscess, and other mass lesions • May be used in designation of brain death	• Stimulants, anticonvulsants, tranquilizer, antidepressants may be withheld for 24-48 hours prior to the study • Hair shampooed before and after study
Electromyography (EMG); nerve conduction velocity studies	• Detects muscle disease • Identifies peripheral neuropathies, nerve compression • Identifies nerve regeneration and muscle recovery	• Patient must be cooperative • Contraindicated in patients on anticoagulants, with bleeding disorders, or skin infection • May be uncomfortable for patient

Table 6-14	DIAGNOSTIC STUDIES—cont'd	
Study	**Purposes**	**Comments**
Electronystagmography (ENG)	• Detects nystagmus, which may aid in identification of cerebellar or vestibular problem	
Evoked potential studies	• Evaluate brain's electrical potentials (responses) to external stimuli; evaluate sensory and somatosensory neurologic pathways • Identify neuromuscular disease, cerebrovascular disease, spinal cord injury, head injury, peripheral nerve disease, tumors • Determine prognosis in severe head injury • Contribute to diagnosis of multiple sclerosis, brainstem injury	• Hair shampooed before and after study
Isotope ventriculography	• Visualizes CSF circulation system	• No CSF withdrawn • May cause meningeal irritation, aseptic meningitis
Lumbar puncture or cisternal puncture	• Obtains CSF for analysis • Measures CSF opening pressure (roughly equivalent to intracranial pressure for most patients if done recumbent and no blockage is present)	• Cisternal puncture is higher risk but may be used if there is scar tissue, which prevents lumbar puncture • Patient must be cooperative • Contraindicated in patients with intracranial hypertension because herniation may occur • Contraindicated in bleeding disorders and in patients receiving anticoagulants • Patient kept flat for 4-8 hours to prevent headache • May cause headache, low back pain, meningitis, abscess, CSF leak, puncture of spinal cord
Magnetic resonance angiography (MRA)	• As for CT except better visualization of vasculature • Identifies aneurysms, AV malformations, and vasospasm • Identifies patency of large veins, venous sinuses	• Patient must be cooperative • Cannot be performed on a patient receiving mechanical ventilation • Contraindicated in patients with any implanted metallic device, including pacemakers • Tends to overestimate degree of stenosis
Magnetic resonance imaging (MRI)	• As for CT except better visualization of vasculature • Identifies vascular lesions, tissue abnormalities, cerebral hemorrhage, cerebral infarction, epileptic foci, multiple sclerosis • Identifies brainstem abnormalities • Identifies type, location, and extent of brain injury	• More sensitive than CT scan especially for posterior fossa • Patient must be cooperative • Cannot be performed on a patient receiving mechanical ventilation • Contraindicated in patients with any implanted metallic device, including pacemakers

Myelography	• Visualizes spinal subarachnoid space
	• Detects spinal cord lesions, cord or nerve root compression
	• Detects pressure on spinal nerve roots
		• If done with oil-based iophendylate (Pantopaque)
		  • Patient must lie flat for 4-8 hours after study
		  • May cause headache, nerve root irritation, allergic reaction, adhesive arachnoiditis
		• If done with water-soluble metrizamide (Amipaque)
		  • Patient should have head of bed elevated
		  • May cause headache, nausea, vomiting, back and neck ache, chest pain, seizures, hallucinations, speech disorders, dysrhythmias, allergic reaction
		• Encourage fluids with either type of dye

Nerve conduction velocity studies	• Identifies peripheral neuropathies and nerve compression	• Needle electrodes are used

Continued

Table 6-14 DIAGNOSTIC STUDIES—cont'd

Study	Purposes	Comments
Oculoplethysmography (OPG)	• Indirectly measures ocular artery pressure • Reflects adequacy of cerebrovascular blood flow in the carotid artery	• Contraindicated in patients who have undergone eye surgery within the last 6 months, who have had lens implants or cataracts, or who have had retinal detachment • May cause conjunctival hemorrhage, corneal abrasions, transient photophobia
Pneumoencephalography	• Visualizes ventricular system and subarachnoid space • Identifies intracranial tumors • Identifies cerebral atrophy	• Care as for LP • Contraindicated in patients with intracranial hypertension • May cause headache, nausea, vomiting, autonomic dysfunction, herniation, subdural hematoma, air embolus, seizures • Patient kept flat for 12-24 hours after the study
Positron emission tomography (PET) or Single-proton emission-computed tomography (SPECT)	• Evaluates oxygen and glucose metabolism • Evaluates cerebral blood flow • Identifies cerebral ischemia, injuries, epilepsy, Alzheimer's disease	• Patient must be cooperative • Contraindicated in pregnant patients
Radioisotope brain scan	• Identifies tumors, cerebrovascular disease, cerebral infarction, trauma, infectious processes, seizures	• Generally replaced by CT scan • Reassure patient that amount of radioactive material is minimal • Patient must be cooperative • Contraindicated in pregnant patients
Regional cerebral blood flow (xenon-133 [^{133}Xe] inhalation)	• Evaluates blood flow to the cerebral cortex • Identifies cerebrovascular disease • Detects regions of increased or decreased perfusion • Determines presence of collateral blood flow • Evaluates cerebral vasospasm	• Assure patient that amount of radioactive material is minimal • Contraindicated in pregnant patients
Skull X-rays	• Detects skull fracture, facial fracture, tumor, bone erosion, cranial anomalies, air-fluid level in sinuses, abnormal intracranial calcification, and radiopaque foreign bodies	• Linear and basal fractures frequently missed by routine X-rays • Contraindicated in pregnant patients
Somnography	• Records EEG during sleep • Evaluates sleep and sleep disorders	
Spinal cord angiography	• Differentiates between spinal AV malformation, angioma, tumor, and ischemia	• As previously described for angiography • May cause thrombosis of spinal vessels, allergy to contrast agent
Spine X-rays	• Detects vertebral dislocation or fracture, degenerative disease, tumor, bone erosion, calcification • Identifies structural spinal deficits and rules out associated cervical spine injuries	• Care must be taken to prevent fracture displacement and spinal cord injury • C1-C2 view best obtained via open mouth; C6-C7 best obtained with arms pulled down • Contraindicated in pregnant patients
Suboccipital puncture	• Obtains CSF for analysis • Measures CSF pressure • Is useful when LP is contraindicated	• May cause trauma to the medulla
Transcranial Doppler	• Measures blood flow velocity through the cerebral arteries • Identifies cerebral vasospasm, emboli, vascular stenosis, brain death	
Ventriculography	• Obtains CSF for analysis • Measures CSF pressure • Is used especially when intracranial hypertension contraindicates LP	• May cause meningeal irritation, seizures, herniation, intracerebral or intraventricular hemorrhage

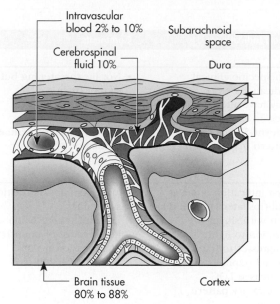

Figure 6-30   Intracranial volumes.

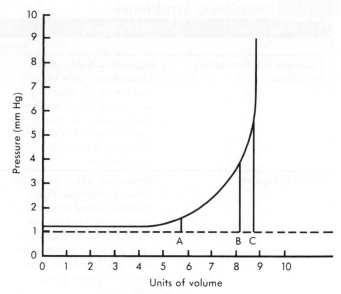

Figure 6-31   Intracranial volume-pressure curve. **A,** Pressure is normal, and increases in intracranial volume are tolerated without a resultant increase in intracranial pressure. **B,** Increases in volume can cause increases in pressure. **C,** Small increases in volume result in significant increases in pressure. (From Thelan LA et al: *Critical care nursing: diagnosis and management,* ed 3, St Louis, 1998, Mosby.)

C. Under normal circumstances, only slight fluctuation
III. Monro-Kellie hypothesis
  A. The cranium is an inexpansible vault
  B. Inside the cranium is a closed system with three fluctuating volumes
    1. Compensation is the ability of the cranium's contents to change or rearrange
    2. If the volume of one of the constituents of the intracranial cavity increases, a reciprocal decrease in volume of one or both of the others occurs
      a) Displacement of CSF from the cranium to the lumbar cistern
      b) Increased CSF reabsorption
      c) Compression of low pressure venous system; blood is shunted to venous sinuses
  C. As successive units of any of the three volumes are added to the cranium, a critical point is reached where each additional unit of volume added increases ICP dramatically and herniation occurs
    1. Volume-pressure relationship exists (Fig. 6-31)
    2. When the critical point is reached, herniation syndromes occur (Fig. 6-32 and Table 6-15)
IV. Compliance
  A. The brain's ability to tolerate increases in volume without a corresponding increase in pressure
  B. Compliance is poor if a small increase in volume causes a large increase in pressure
V. Cerebral perfusion pressure
  A. Pressure at which the brain tissue is perfused; used to estimate adequacy of cerebral blood flow (CBF)

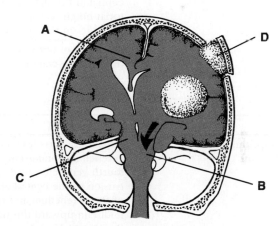

Figure 6-32   Supratentorial herniation. **A,** Cingulate. **B,** Uncal. **C,** Central. **D,** Transcalvarial. (From Thelan LA et al: *Critical care nursing: diagnosis and management,* ed 3, St Louis, 1998, Mosby.)

  B. Calculated by subtracting ICP from MAP; MAP − ICP (Fig. 6-33)
  C. Normal CPP: 60 to 100 mm Hg
  D. Abnormal CPP
    1. CPP greater than 150 mm Hg disrupts the blood–brain barrier and causes hyperperfusion and potentially cerebral edema
    2. CPP less than 50 mm Hg causes hypoperfusion and cerebral ischemia, (although CCP of 70 mm Hg is required in most head-injured patients, and some require an even higher CPP to adequately perfuse the brain)

Table 6-15	Herniation Syndromes		
Type of Herniation	**Description**	**Clinical Indications**	**Comments**
Supratentorial			
Cingulate (or subfalcine) herniation	Expanding lesion of one hemisphere shifts laterally and forces the cingulate gyrus under the falx cerebri; compression of vessels causes cerebral edema, ischemia, intracranial hypertension	• No specific clinical indications • May have altered LOC, plegia • Cheyne-Stokes respiratory pattern may be seen	• Not life-threatening but a sign of brain decompensation • If condition not controlled, uncal or central herniation will occur
Uncal herniation	Expanding lesion in middle fossa or temporal lobe causes a lateral displacement, which pushes the uncus of the temporal lobe over the edge of the tentorium; uncus may be lacerated by sharp edge of tentorium	• First indication is unilateral (ipsilateral) pupil dilation with sluggish reaction to light; progresses to fixed, dilated pupils • Decreased LOC • Respiratory pattern change • Contralateral hemiplegia progressing to posturing	• Most common herniation syndrome • Life-threatening when hemorrhage of brainstem compression occurs
Central (or transtentorial) herniation	Expanding lesions of the frontal, parietal, or occipital lobes or severe generalized edema cause downward displacement of the basal ganglia and diencephalon through the tentorial notch, causing pressure on the midbrain	• First indication is change in level of consciousness • Small, reactive pupils to fixed, dilated pupils • Respiratory pattern changes to apnea • Decorticate posturing to flaccidity	• May be preceded by cingulate or uncal herniation • Life-threatening
Transcalvarial herniation	Extrusion of cerebral tissue through the cranium	• No specific clinical indications	• May occur through an opening from a skull fracture, craniotomy site, Burr hole • Risk of infection
Infratentorial			
Upward transtentorial herniation	Expanding mass lesion of cerebellum, brainstem, or fourth ventricle causes protrusion of the central area of the cerebellum and the midbrain upward through the tentorial notch	• First symptom is unilateral (ipsilateral) pupil dilation • Obstructive hydrocephalus occurs with rapid deterioration of neurologic status	• May be life-threatening
Downward cerebellar (or tonsillar) herniation	Expanding lesion of the cerebellum exerts downward pressure, sending cerebellar tonsils through the foramen magnum; compression and displacement of the medulla oblongata occurs	• Coma • Flaccid paralysis • Respiratory and cardiac arrest occur	• May be a complication of lumbar puncture when LP is performed in presence of high ICP • Causes death

3. CPP less than 40 mm Hg is associated with cerebral blood flow that is 25% of normal
4. CPP less than 30 mm Hg causes irreversible ischemia
5. As ICP approaches MAP, cerebral blood flow decreases; when they equalize, cerebral blood flow ceases and cerebral death is inevitable

VI. Autoregulation: the intrinsic ability of the cerebral blood vessels to dilate or constrict in response to changes in the brain's environment
   A. Enables the cerebral blood vessels to maintain cerebral blood flow in response to wide fluctuation in mean arterial pressure
   B. Autoregulation fails if CPP is less than 50 or greater than 150 mm Hg

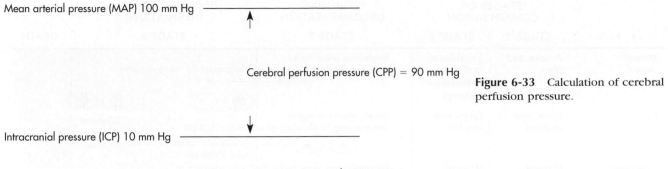

Mean arterial pressure (MAP) 100 mm Hg

Cerebral perfusion pressure (CPP) = 90 mm Hg

Figure 6-33 Calculation of cerebral perfusion pressure.

Intracranial pressure (ICP) 10 mm Hg

Normal >60 mm Hg

VII. Cerebral blood flow (CBF)
   A. Varies with changes in CPP and diameter of cerebrovascular bed
   B. Normal CBF: 50 ml/min/100 g of brain
   C. Increased ICP and decreased CPP decreases CBF; the brain receives less oxygen and nutrients, eventually causing neuronal death
VIII. Decompensation: brain loses its ability to compensate
   A. Pressure on cerebral vessels slows blood flow to the brain
   B. Diminished circulation produces ischemia and an accumulation of carbon dioxide and lactic acid
   C. Hypoxia and hypercapnia trigger cerebral vasodilation, which increases blood volume and cerebral edema
   D. Cerebral edema further increases ICP
   E. Compression of cerebral vessels occurs and causes further ischemia
   F. Cerebral circulation eventually stops and brain death occurs

Clinical Presentation

I. Change in level of consciousness
   A. Early: restlessness, confusion
   B. Late: diminishing level of consciousness, posturing
II. Cranial nerve changes
   A. Oculomotor (III)
      1. Early
         a) Ipsilateral pupil changes
            (1) Change in size, shape (oval)
            (2) Sluggish reaction to light
         b) Conjugate eye deviation
      2. Late
         a) Ipsilateral pupil changes
            (1) Dilated, nonreactive to light pupil or pupils
            (2) Ptosis
            (3) Dysconjugate eye movement with brainstem lesions
   B. Optic (II): visual changes
      1. Diplopia; blurring; decreased visual acuity; visual field deficit

2. Papilledema: more likely to occur when ICP rises slowly rather than quickly
   C. Trigeminal (V): impaired corneal reflex
   D. Glossopharyngeal (IX) and vagus (X): impaired gag and swallow reflexes
III. Motor changes: contralateral
   A. Due to compression or pressure on the corticospinal tracts
   B. Early: paresis, plegia
   C. Late: posturing
IV. Vomiting: may occur especially with lesions below the tentorium
   A. Pressure on the vomiting center in the brainstem causes projectile vomiting without nausea
V. Headache: increasing severity but inconsistent symptom
VI. Seizures may occur
VII. Reflexes: decrease in or absence of reflexes (e.g., cough, gag, corneal reflexes)
VIII. Vital sign changes
   A. Cushing's triad
      1. Due to pressure on or ischemia of vasomotor center in brainstem
      2. Components
         a) Increased systolic BP
         b) Widening pulse pressure due to diastolic BP being normal or decreased along with increased systolic BP
         c) Bradycardia
   B. Respiratory pattern changes dependent on location of injury (Table 6-8)
   C. Temperature: central hyperthermia may occur late in intracranial hypertension due to pressure on the thermoregulatory center in the hypothalamus
IX. Stages of intracranial hypertension (Fig. 6-34)
X. ICP monitoring
   A. Indications
      1. The need for ICP monitoring usually correlates with a GSC of 8 or less
      2. The following diagnoses may require ICP monitoring:
         a) Head trauma
         b) Intracerebral masses

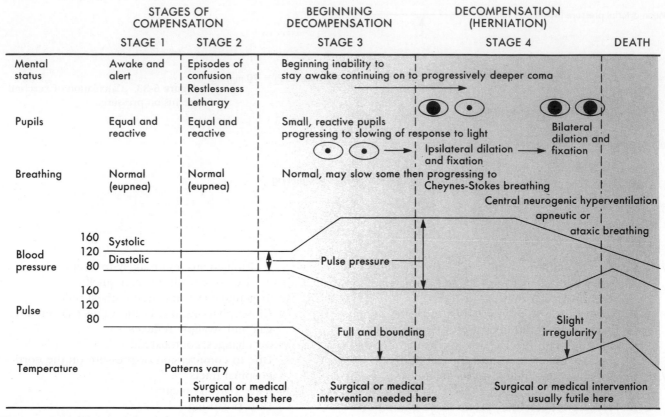

Figure 6-34 Clinical correlates of compensated and decompensated phases of intracranial hypertension. (From Beare PG, Myers JL: *Principles and practice of adult health nursing,* ed 2, St Louis, 1994, Mosby.)

c) Subarachnoid hemorrhage
d) Intracerebral hemorrhage (e.g., massive stroke)
e) Infectious processes (e.g., encephalitis, meningitis)
f) Encephalopathy
(1) Anoxic encephalopathy (e.g., post-cardiac arrest)
(2) Reye's syndrome
g) Hydrocephalus
h) Postcraniotomy
3. ICP monitoring should be used if deep sedation, paralysis, or barbiturate coma is being utilized since LOC is eliminated as an assessment parameter
B. Purposes
1. Diagnose intracranial hypertension
2. Allow drainage of CSF to decrease pressure
3. Observe effects of medical or nursing management
4. Predict outcomes: patients who sustain an ICP more than 50 mm Hg for longer than 20 minutes have a very poor prognosis
C. General information
1. CSF pressure is considered the most accurate indication of ICP
a) The most accurate devices measure the pressure of CSF and are in contact with CSF

b) This contact with CSF causes a risk of infection
c) Intraparenchymal devices: a linear relationship exists between intraventricular and intraparenchymal pressure measured with fiberoptic transducer-tipped probe (e.g., Camino catheter)
2. Several types of ICP measuring devices are used (Fig. 6-35 and Table 6-16)
a) Insertion of all of these devices is via a small burr hole made with a twist drill utilizing strict aseptic technique
3. Three types of monitoring systems are used
a) Fluid-filled system
(1) Sensor: fluid-filled catheter or bolt, which communicates the subarachnoid or intraventricular pressure to the transducer
(2) Closed fluid-filled system between the sensor and the transducer
(a) Use only preservative-free isotonic saline
(b) Do not add heparin; do not use a pressure bag or an intermittent flush device
(c) Utilize Luer-Lok connections
(d) Routine irrigation is not done; subarachnoid bolts may be irrigated if specifically ordered with

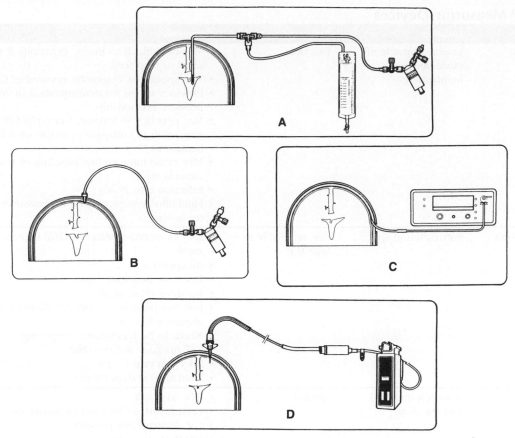

Figure 6-35   Devices for the measurement of intracranial pressure. **A,** Intraventricular catheter and system. **B,** Subarachnoid screw or bolt and system. **C,** Epidural transducer and system. **D,** Intraparenchymal transducer and system. (From Thelan LA et al: *Critical care nursing: diagnosis and management,* ed 3, St Louis, 1998, Mosby.)

approximately 0.1 ml every 2 hours; dilute antibiotic solution may be prescribed as irrigation solution

(3) Transducer: converts the pressure signal to an electrical signal that can be recorded

    (a) The transducer is positioned at level of the foramen of Monro; this correlates externally to the tragus of ear

    (b) The transducer cable is connected to the pressure module of the bedside monitor

b) Continuous drainage system (Fig. 6-36)

    (1) Drip chamber is placed at prescribed height above foramen of Monro to regulate drainage according to ICP

    (2) One-way flow valves and micropore filters on air vents are in commercial systems

c) Fiberoptic transducer

    (1) A fluid-filled system is not necessary

    (2) The catheter is plugged directly into the monitor

    (3) This system may require a special monitor

D. Measurement guidelines

1. Rezero with each head position change if fluid-filled system

2. Do not stimulate patient prior to measurements

3. Evaluate trends rather than one measurement

4. Assist with volume-pressure response (VPR) testing

    a) Inject 1 ml of preservative-free isotonic saline into the intraventricular catheter

    b) Normal: increase in ICP of 2 mm Hg or less

    c) Low compliance: increase in ICP of 3 mm Hg or more

5. If the ICP does not return normal within 4 minutes after activity, compliance is poor

E. ICP values

1. Normal: 5 to 15 mm Hg

2. Slightly elevated: 16 to 20 mm Hg

3. Moderately elevated: 21 to 40 mm Hg

4. Severely elevated: more than 40 mm Hg

F. ICP waveforms (Table 6-17)

1. Normal waveform (Fig. 6-37)

    a) P_1: upward spike with a systolic or percussion wave

Table 6-16 | **ICP Measuring Devices**

Device	Location	Accuracy	Comments
Intraventricular catheter or fiberoptic transducer	Lateral ventricle of nondominant hemisphere	Excellent	• May be difficult to insert, especially if ventricles are small or displaced • Therapeutic or diagnostic removal of CSF possible • Provides access for determination of volume-pressure relationship • May permit CSF leakage, but rapid CSF drainage may result in collapsed ventricle or subdural hematoma • May cause intracerebral bleeding or edema at cannula track • Infection rate 2%-5% • Fluid-filled system utilized if intraventricular catheter is placed
Subarachnoid bolt	Subarachnoid space	Fair; unreliable at high ICP	• Easy to insert; especially useful if ventricles are small • Inexpensive • Does not penetrate brain • Requires intact skull • Bolt can become occluded with clots or tissue; may require irrigation • Needs to be recalibrated frequently • CSF drainage not possible • Infection rate 1%-2% • Fluid-filled system utilized
Epidural sensor or transducer	Between the skull and the dura	Variable	• Easy to insert • Least invasive (does not penetrate dura or brain) • CSF drainage not possible • Infection rate <1% • Head position has no effect on pressure reading • Cannot be rezeroed once in place • Epidural pressure is slightly higher than intraventricular pressure
Intraparenchymal transducer	1 cm into brain tissue	Excellent	• Easy to insert • Unable to drain CSF or to test volume pressure response (VPR) • Catheter relatively fragile; avoid sharp kinks or pulls • Head position has no effect on pressure reading • Cannot be rezeroed once in place • Risk of intracerebral bleeding and infection

b) P_2: tidal wave; result of venous pulsations
  (1) Most clinically significant
  (2) As ICP rises, so does the P2; this change gives the waveform a rounded appearance
  (3) When the amplitude of P2 is greater than that of P1 or becomes lost in the tracing, it is indicative of a decrease in compliance
c) P_3: small, superimposed notch
2. C-waves (Fig. 6-38)
  a) Rapid, rhythmic oscillation of pressure without any relevance
  b) Small spikes as high as 20 to 25 mm Hg every 4 to 8 minutes
  c) Associated with changes in arterial BP, ventilation
3. B-waves (Fig. 6-38)
  a) Sharp, sawtooth appearance waves

b) Pressures of 20 to 50 mm Hg occurring every 30 seconds to 2 minutes
c) Related to changes in cerebral blood flow
d) Although not significant alone, may precede A-waves
4. A-waves (Fig. 6-38)
  a) Elevations on top of baseline elevation of ICP
  b) Pressures reach 50 to 100 mm Hg and last 5 to 20 minutes
  c) Pathologic waves produced by secondary changes in cerebral blood volume
  d) Require immediate treatment
G. Prevent/monitor for complications of ICP monitoring
  1. Infection (e.g., bacterial meningitis)
    a) Risk factors associated with ICP monitoring-related infection
      (1) Intracerebral hemorrhage with intraventricular blood

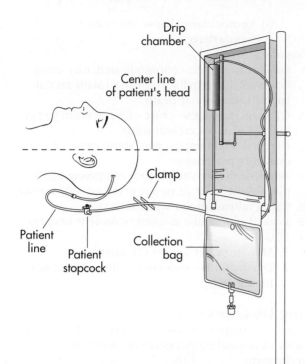

Figure 6-36 Continuous drainage system. Continuous drainage involves placing the drip chamber of the drainage system at a specified level above the foramen of Monro (usually 15 cm). The system is left open to allow continuous drainage of CSF into the chamber (which drains into a collection bag) against a pressure gradient that prevents excessive drainage and ventricular collapse. (Courtesy Codman/Johnson & Johnson Professional Inc., Raynham, Mass.)

Table 6-17 ICP Waveforms

Waveforms	Description	Significance	Comments
Normal	Low amplitude fluctuations in ICP with pressure <15 mm Hg	• Normal	
C-waves	Rapid, rhythmic oscillation of pressure Small spikes as high as 25 mm Hg every 4-8 minutes	• Not significant • Associated with changes in arterial BP, ventilation	
B-waves	Sharp, sawtooth appearance waves Pressures of 20-50 mm Hg occurring every 30 seconds to 2 minutes	• Associated with changes in cerebral blood flow • Probably not clinically significant but may precede A-waves	• Do not perform any activities that may further increase ICP • May indicate decreased compliance
A-waves or *plateau waves*	Elevations on top of baseline elevation of ICP Pressures reach 50-100 mm Hg and last 5-20 minutes	• Most significant • Pathologic waves produced by secondary changes in cerebral blood volume • Ominous sign of decreasing cerebral compliance and rapidly progressing decompensation • Usually occur only in advanced stages of intracranial hypertension	• Requires treatment • Irreversible brain damage occurs if not resolved within 15 minutes
Terminal wave	Flat wave with pressure 50-100 mm Hg	• MAP = ICP and CBF ceases • Indicative of brain death	
Damped waveform	Low-voltage wave with pressure notches	• May be caused by tubing kinks, blood in line, or stopcock positioned incorrectly	

(2) Open head trauma

(3) Postcraniotomy

(4) ICP more than 20 mm Hg

(5) Elderly patient

(6) Burr hole larger than necessary

(7) Nonsterile technique for insertion

(8) Device then penetrates dura

(9) Monitoring for more than 3 to 5 days

(10) Irrigation of ICP monitoring system

(11) Opening of system

b) Change dressing daily or according to hospital policy utilizing sterile technique

c) Maintain closed system; limit irrigation; use strict aseptic technique if system must be interrupted (e.g., VPR testing)

d) Monitoring should be maintained no longer than 3 to 5 days; if longer monitoring is required, device should be removed and replaced

e) Monitor for clinical indications of infection: fever, leukocytosis, cloudy CSF

2. Intracerebral hemorrhage, hematoma

a) Monitor for change in color of CSF, change in neurologic status

b) If continuous drainage system: do not raise or lower the head of bed; do not allow bag to be below the head

3. CSF leak

a) Use Luer-Lok connections

b) Maintain closed system

4. CSF overdrainage

a) Do not drain CSF below a pressure of 15 mm Hg unless specifically instructed

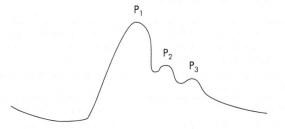

Figure 6-37   Components of a normal ICP waveform. (From Barker E: *Neuroscience nursing*, St Louis, 1994, Mosby.)

b) Ventricular collapse may cause hemorrhage

XI. Diagnostic studies

A. Lumbar puncture: contraindicated; may cause downward cerebellar herniation with medullary herniation and death

B. CT scan: may show cause of intracranial hypertension or intracerebral shifts

C. Cerebral angiography: may show cause of intracranial hypertension

D. Skull X-ray: may show cause of intracranial hypertension, shift of pineal gland or sella turcica

E. EEG: evaluates brain wave activity

F. Evoked potentials: assesses brainstem integrity

G. ECG

1. May show prolonged QT interval

2. Dysrhythmias: especially with subarachnoid hemorrhage

Nursing Diagnoses

I. Decreased Adaptive Capacity: Intracranial related to failure of normal intracranial compensatory mechanisms

II. Alteration in Cerebral Tissue Perfusion related to intracranial hypertension

III. Ineffective Breathing Patterns related to herniation

IV. Risk for Infection related to invasive procedures, traumatic wounds, surgical wounds

V. Risk for Injury related to seizure activity, inadequate protective reflexes

VI. Ineffective Individual Coping related to situational crisis, powerlessness, change in role

VII. Ineffective Family Coping related to critically ill family member

Collaborative Management

I. Monitor closely for clinical indications of intracranial hypertension; assist with insertion of ICP monitoring device if patient requires continuous monitoring

II. Recognize factors that increase ICP (Box 6-1); prevent as many of these factors as you can; space activities that increase ICP that cannot be eliminated

III. Prevent intracranial hypertension

A. Assess neurologic status frequently

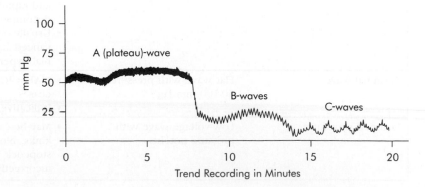

Figure 6-38   Abnormal ICP waveforms. (From Barker E: *Neuroscience nursing*, St Louis, 1994, Mosby.)

B. Maintain adequate venous drainage from head
   1. Elevate head of bed 15 to 30 degrees; this promotes venous drainage from the brain but may decrease cerebral blood flow by decreasing BP; assess patient's response to head of bed elevation and adjust accordingly
   2. Maintain head and neck in straight alignment to prevent compression of jugular veins
   3. Prevent compression of jugular veins by tracheostomy ties, cervical collar; loosen if necessary
C. Maintain patent airway and ventilation
   1. Endotracheal intubation may be necessary, especially if protective reflexes are absent
   2. Mechanical ventilation may be necessary
      a) Recognize that positive pressure mechanical ventilation increases ICP; using lower tidal volumes may minimize this effect
      b) Positive end-expiratory pressure increases ICP; using only enough PEEP to maintain adequate Pao_2 may minimize this effect

D. Teach patient to avoid Valsalva maneuver
   1. Instruct to exhale when turning in bed
   2. Instruct to cough with mouth open if coughing is necessary
   3. Avoid straining, bending, sneezing
   4. Avoid hip flexion more than 90 degrees
   5. Discourage isometric exercise
      a) Do not use footboard to prevent footdrop
      b) Use hightop tennis shoes, on for 2 hours and off for 2 hours
   6. Administer stool softeners as indicated
   7. Treat nausea with antiemetics to prevent vomiting
   8. Prevent increase in ICP associated with suctioning
      a) Suction only if necessary
      b) Limit suctioning to 10 seconds
      c) Limit negative pressure to less than 120 mm Hg
      d) Ensure that the catheter occludes no more than one half the inner diameter of the endotracheal tube
      e) Hyperoxygenate prior to, during, and after suctioning
      f) Lidocaine (0.5 to 1.5 mg/kg) may be administered IV or instilled into tracheobronchial tree via ET tube or tracheostomy tube prior to suctioning to eliminate cough reflex
      g) Do not suction via nose if head or facial trauma is evident
E. Monitor ICP during nursing care activities (e.g., turning, suctioning, enteral feedings); space activities to allow ICP to return to normal before performing another activity that may increase ICP
F. Monitor ventilation and oxygenation: hypercapnia and/or hypoxemia may cause vasodilation and increase ICP
   1. Arterial blood gases
   2. Pulse oximetry (Spo_2):
   3. Capnography ($Paco_2$):
G. Avoid overhydration but prevent dehydration
   1. Hemodynamic monitoring may be necessary
   2. Avoid hypotonic fluids (e.g., D_5W), which may contribute to cerebral edema
H. If CSF leakage is noted: do not pack nose or ears; apply mustache dressing under nose or 4×4 over ear
I. Reduce anxiety
   1. Reorient patient frequently to person, place, date, time, and situation
   2. Explain procedures thoroughly
   3. Do not conduct or allow emotionally disturbing conversations at bedside
   4. Encourage family members to touch and talk to patient; let them know that many patients report an awareness during altered levels of consciousness
J. Monitor ICP and calculate CPP; notify physician of significant changes or deteriorating trend

---

BOX 6-1   Causes of Intracranial Pressure Elevations

Ventilation and/or Oxygenation Problems
- Airway obstruction
- Hypercapnia
- Hypoxia
- Suctioning without hyperoxygenation
- Deep breathing

Position Changes
- Prone position
- Trendelenburg position
- Extreme hip flexion (>90 degrees)

Decreased Venous Return from Head
- Neck flexion, hyperextension, or rotation
- Tight tracheostomy ties or cervical collar
- Increased intrathoracic pressure
  - Positive pressure mechanical ventilation
  - Positive end-expiratory pressure
  - Valsalva maneuver
    - Straining at stool
    - Vomiting
    - Coughing
    - Suctioning
    - Isometric exercise

Increased Metabolic Rate
- Hyperthermia
- Seizure activity
- Rapid eye movement (REM) sleep

Stress
- Disturbing conversation
- Noise
- Bright lights
- Pain or noxious stimuli

Table 6-18 **Treatment for Intracranial Hypertension**

Treatment	Actions	Comments
Hyperventilation	• Reduces intracranial volume and pressure by reducing intracranial blood volume by causing vasoconstriction	• May be done initially with a manual resuscitation bag followed by mechanical ventilation with rate and tidal volume sufficient to cause a $Paco_2$ of approximately 35 mm Hg • Reducing the $Paco_2$ too low can potentially cause ischemia and/or vasodilation; this treatment is for short-term therapy only, and it is recommended that Sjo_2 monitoring be used to evaluate cerebral oxygenation • Effectiveness decreases after 24-48 hours because of renal compensation for respiratory alkalosis • Monitor arterial blood gases to evaluate $Paco_2$ and Pao_2
CSF drainage if intra-ventricular catheter in place	• Reduces intracranial volume by reducing CSF volume	• Maintain closed system and asepsis during fluid drainage; high risk for infection • Record volume of drainage • Do not overdrain; drainage is usually to ICP of 15 mm Hg • Rapid CSF drainage may cause the brain to pull away from the dura, rupturing bridging veins and possibly causing subdural hematoma
Mannitol (Osmitrol)	• Increases plasma osmolality, which pulls fluid from brain tissue and decreases cerebral edema (this increase in intravascular volume is then eliminated by the kidney) • May decrease blood viscosity and increase CBF without raising ICP	• Usually prescribed as 0.5-2 g/kg IV • Starts to work within 15 minutes; lasts 2-6 hours; may be repeated every 1-4 hours • Indwelling bladder catheter is recommended • Monitor for clinical indications of fluid overload initially, especially in patients with history of cardiovascular disease • Monitor for fluid deficit; may mask diabetes insipidus; monitor for electrolyte imbalance • Contraindicated if blood–brain barrier is not intact, may actually increase swelling • Rebound intracranial hypertension may be seen ~8-12 hours after mannitol; furosemide may be given with mannitol to reduce the incidence of rebound • Must be given with a 0.45-µ inline filter
Furosemide (Lasix)	• Reduces intracranial volume by reducing overall body fluid • Decreases CSF production (unknown mechanism)	• Usually prescribed as 0.5-1 mg/kg IV • May be administered with mannitol to reduce the incidence of rebound swelling
Barbiturate coma	• Decreases ICP by decreasing cerebral blood flow and metabolism • Decreases metabolic rate and oxygen consumption of the brain • May shunt blood from healthy brain tissue to ischemic areas	• Indicated for ICP >40 mm Hg despite aggressive therapy • Pentobarbital (Nembutal) is the preferred agent; usually prescribed as 5-10 mg/kg IV over 1-2 hours as a loading dose followed by 1-3 mg/kg/hr; maintain barbiturate level of 20-40 µg/ml • Expect 10 mm Hg decrease in ICP within 10 minutes • Monitor hepatic and renal function • Monitor cardiac status and daily weight (may decrease cardiac contractility) • Must be intubated, mechanically ventilated • Must have ICP monitor; systemic arterial and pulmonary arterial pressure monitoring is recommended • Protect the corneas by instilling artificial tears and taping eyes shut or applying moisture chamber (plastic wrap taped in place over eyes) • Discontinued when the ICP has been normal for at least 24-72 hours; patient should be on anticonvulsants prior to discontinuance as seizures may occur

Table 6-18	Treatment for Intracranial Hypertension—cont'd	
Treatment	**Actions**	**Comments**
Sedatives (e.g., morphine, propofol [Diprivan], midazolam [Versed])	• Reduces restlessness or agitation to decrease metabolic rate and oxygen consumption	• Monitor ventilatory status • May cause hypotension, which will decrease CPP; fluid administration may be necessary to maintain preload • Propofol may cause agitation; discontinue use if this occurs
Muscle paralysis (e.g., pancuronium [Pavulon], atracurium [Tracrium], vecuronium [Norcuron])	• Reduces skeletal muscle activity, metabolic rate and oxygen consumption • Controls shivering and posturing, decreasing metabolic rate and oxygen consumption	• Must be mechanically ventilated; must have ICP monitor • Protect the corneas by instilling artificial tears and taping eyes shut or applying moisture chamber • Always administer sedative with muscle paralytics • Pancuronium causes tachycardia; beta-blocker may be necessary
Dexamethasone (Decadron)	• Decreases edema and inflammation of brain tissue • May decrease CSF production • May aid in reconstruction of blood-brain barrier • Increases lactate metabolism	• Usually prescribed as 10 mg initially then 4 mg every 4-6 hours followed by diminishing doses • Of questionable effectiveness; more likely to be prescribed for brain tumor than trauma • Causes gluconeogenesis and may increase blood glucose; monitor blood glucose four times a day • May cause stress ulcer; histamine$_2$-receptor antagonists and/or antacids are usually given concurrently with steroids
Phenytoin (Dilantin)	• Does not directly decrease intracranial pressure • Prevents seizure activity, which would increase the metabolic rate and oxygen consumption of the brain	• Usually prescribed as a loading dose of up to 1 g followed by 300 mg/24 hr in divided doses • If given IV, give no faster than 50-100 mg/min
Surgical removal of skull bone flap (burr hole)	• Allows for expansion of cranial content	• Usually not done today strictly for decompression because may cause transcalvarial herniation • Strict aseptic technique is critical in prevention of infection

IV. Treat intracranial hypertension (Table 6-18)
    A. Providing therapy aimed at reducing volume of one of the three components of ICP
        1. Circulating blood volume: hyperventilation (with a manual resuscitation bag or mechanical ventilator) to maintain Paco$_2$ ~35 mm Hg
            a) This short-term therapy works by constricting the cerebral vessels; a delicate balance exists between vasoconstriction to decrease intracranial volume and pressure and vasoconstriction causing ischemia
            b) Sjo$_2$ monitoring is recommended to identify the Paco$_2$ level that does not cause cerebral ischemia
        2. Brain mass
            a) Fluid restrictions
                (1) Although it is not desirable for the patient to be hypovolemic, fluids may be restricted when ICP is elevated; focus should also be placed on improving MAP to normalize CPP
                (2) Fluids may be limited to ~70 ml/hr or to keep serum osmolality 290 to 320 mOsm/L; hypotonic solutions (e.g., D$_5$W) are avoided
                (3) Fluids are not restricted when vasospasm is an issue (e.g., subarachnoid hemorrhage); fluids (usually colloids) are increased to reduce spasm or potential for spasm
            b) Glucocorticoids
                (1) General use of glucocorticoids is no longer recommended, but they may reduce cerebral edema, especially with brain tumor; usually dexamethasone [Decadron] is prescribed as an initial dose followed by decreasing doses
                (2) Large doses of methylprednisolone are recommended early to reduce edema in acute spinal cord injury
            c) Osmotic diuretics (e.g., mannitol [Osmitrol], urea, glycerol)
                (1) Act to draw fluid out of swollen brain

(2) Contraindicated if blood–brain barrier is not intact; may actually increase swelling

(3) Loop diuretics (e.g., furosemide [Lasix]) may also be given

3. CSF: drain CSF if intraventricular catheter in place

a) Record volume of drainage

b) Do not drain to ICP less than 15 mm Hg unless specifically instructed

B. Prepare patient for surgery if indicated

1. Debride open wounds and suture scalp laceration

2. Elevate depressed skull fracture and repair dural tears

3. Evacuate epidural or subdural hemorrhage or hematoma

4. Control intracranial hemorrhage or hematoma

V. Maintain MAP and CPP

A. Assess for bleeding from chest, abdomen, pelvis, extremities

B. Control scalp bleeding by applying pressure until sutured

C. Administer IV fluids

1. Hypotonic fluids (e.g., D_5W) are avoided

2. Colloids (e.g., dextran, albumin) frequently used

3. Blood and/or blood products may be needed if significant blood loss has occurred

D. Administer inotropes and/or vasopressors as prescribed to maintain MAP and CPP; maintain CPP greater than 70 mm Hg

E. Administer antihypertensives as prescribed (labetalol [Normodyne] causes less increase in ICP than other antihypertensives)

F. Calcium channel blockers (e.g., nimodipine [Nimotop]) and/or hypervolemic hemodilution may be used for vasospasm

VI. Decrease metabolic requirements of the brain

A. Administer prophylactic anticonvulsants as prescribed

B. Maintain normothermia (<38° C [100° F])

1. Hyperthermia is aggressively treated because 1° C temperature elevation is associated with a 7% increase in metabolic rate and oxygen consumption

2. Central fever is directly attributed to brain injury and reflects hypothalamic dysfunction

a) Characterized by lack of sweating, absence of tachycardia, and may persist for days

b) Controlled best by external cooling but avoid shivering; use hypothermia blanket

(1) Turn it off when the temperature reaches 38° C as the temperature of a neurology patient tends to drift downward after a hypothermia blanket is turned off

(2) Do not allow the patient to shiver; meperidine (Demerol) may be used to decrease shivering

3. Peripheral fever is associated with infection

a) Characterized by sweating and tachycardia

b) Controlled best by antipyretics (e.g., acetaminophen [Tylenol])

C. Administer barbiturates, sedatives, or muscle paralytics as prescribed

D. Maintain calm, quiet environment; prevent loud noises, disturbing conversations

LEARNING ACTIVITIES

1.   DIRECTIONS: Complete the following crossword puzzle related to neurologic anatomy and physiology.

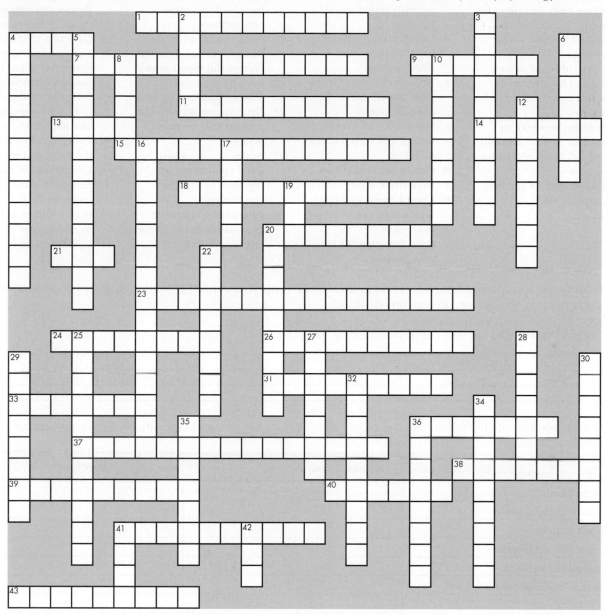

Across

1. "Fight or flight" branch of the autonomic nervous system
4. Outermost layer of the meninges is the_____ mater
7. Enzyme that breaks down acetylcholine
9. Cranial nerve that allows you to smile
11. Cranial nerve that controls the pupillary reaction
13. Convolutions on the surface of the brain
14. Coating or sheath that speeds transmission along the axon
15. Pathway for fibers between the two cerebral hemispheres (two words)
18. Division of the brain that contains the cerebral hemispheres
20. Neurons that transmit impulses to the spinal cord or brain
21. Innermost layer of the meninges is the_____ mater
23. Chemical that acts as a bridge for transmission of impulses
24. Component of the neuron that conducts impulses toward the cell body
26. Part of the brain that co-ordinates muscle movement with sensory input
31. Fold of the dura mater that separates the cerebrum hemispheres from the cerebellum
33. Posterior portion of this lobe controls voluntary motor function
36. Portion of the brainstem that controls cardiac and respiratory centers

37. "Steady state" branch of the autonomic nervous system
38. Fissure that divides the frontal lobe from the parietal lobes
39. Nerve cells that provide support, nourishment, and protection of the neurons
40. Circle of blood vessels formed by internal carotids and vertebral arteries
41. Synapse between an axon of one neuron and the cell body of another neuron
43. Middle layer of the meninges is the_____ mater

Down

2. Foramen of _____ connects the lateral ventricles with the third ventricle
3. Cranial nerve that controls sensation on the face
4. Includes the thalamus, hypothalamus, and limbic system
5. Neurotransmitter for the parasympathetic nervous system
6. Fissure that divides the frontal lobes from temporal lobes
8. Cranial nerve that controls visual acuity
10. Cranial nerve that controls lateral eye movement
12. Lobe that controls long-term memory

16. Neurons responsible for myelin formation in the CNS
17. Shallow grooves on the surface of the brain
19. Acts as a cushion for the brain and the spinal cord (abbrev.)
20. Form the blood–brain barrier with the endothelium of the blood vessels
22. Lobe that controls sensory function
25. Neurotransmitter for the sympathetic nervous system
27. Nodes of _____ allow rapid conduction of impulses by saltatory conduction
28. Four paired masses of gray matter in the deeper layers of each hemi-

sphere are called the basal _____
29. Neurons that transmit impulses away from the spinal cord or brain
30. Bat-shaped bone that divides the interior of the skull into three fossae
32. Lobe that controls vision
34. Nervous system with sympathetic and parasympathetic branches
35. Unidirectional conduction of an impulse from one neuron to the next
36. Protective coverings of the brain and spinal cord
41. Component of the neuron that conducts impulses away from cell body to other neurons or to end organs
42. Cellular energy (abbrev.)

2. **DIRECTIONS:** Your patient has had a head injury. His BP is 80/50 and his ICP is 20. Calculate his cerebral perfusion pressure. Should you be concerned? Why?

3. **DIRECTIONS:** Identify the four components of the spinal arc.
    1. _____
    2. _____
    3. _____
    4. _____

4. **DIRECTIONS:** Identify the following physiologic alterations as being associated with either sympathetic or parasympathetic.

	Sympathetic	Parasympathetic
Bronchodilation		
Coronary artery dilation		
Hypersalivation		
Increased blood glucose		
Increased perspiration		
Increased intestinal motility		
Pupil constriction		
Tachycardia		

5. **DIRECTIONS:** Identify the site of the lesion that would cause each of the following respiratory patterns.

Pattern	Site of Lesion
CNS hyperventilation	
Cheyne-Stokes	
Cluster	
Ataxic	
Apneustic	

6. **DIRECTIONS:** Name and identify how to assess the cranial nerves.

I		
II		
III		
IV		
V		
VI		
VII		
VIII		
IX		
X		
XI		
XII		

7. **DIRECTIONS:** List 10 factors that can increase intracranial pressure that can be eliminated.

1. _____
2. _____
3. _____
4. _____
5. _____
6. _____
7. _____
8. _____
9. _____
10. _____

8. **DIRECTIONS:** Identify seven interventions that can decrease intracranial pressure and identify if they decrease brain mass, CSF, or blood.

Intervention	What is decreased?
1.	
2.	
3.	
4.	
5.	
6.	
7.	

LEARNING ACTIVITIES ANSWERS

1.

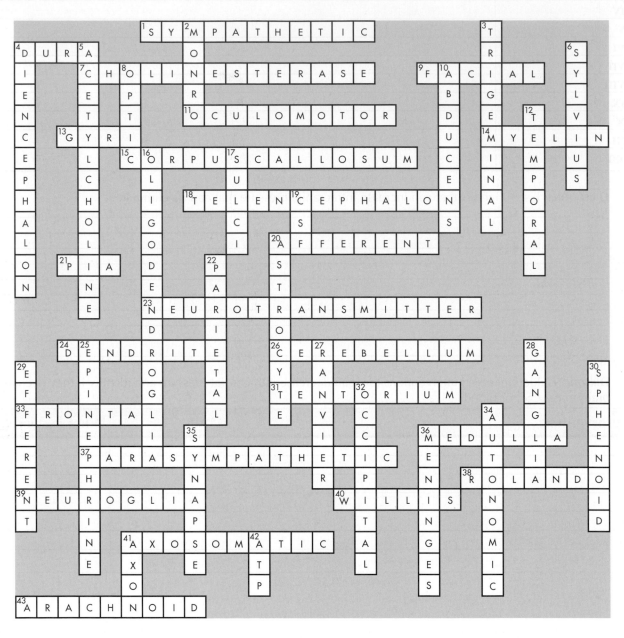

2. To calculate mean arterial pressure: [SBP + (DBP × 2)] ÷ 3: 80 + (2 × 50) = 180, then divide by 3 = 60
   To calculate cerebral perfusion pressure: MAP − ICP: 60 − 20 = 40 mm Hg
   Should you be concerned? YES! CPP <50 is associated with loss of autoregulation and hypoperfusion of the brain.

3. 1. Receptor organ
   2. Afferent neuron
   3. Effector neuron
   4. Effector organ

4.

	Sympathetic	Parasympathetic
Bronchodilation	✔	
Coronary artery dilation	✔	
Hypersalivation		✔
Increased blood glucose	✔	
Increased perspiration	✔	
Increased intestinal motility		✔
Pupil constriction		✔
Tachycardia	✔	

5.

Pattern	Site of Lesion
CNS hyperventilation	Lower midbrain or upper pons
Cheyne-Stokes	Cerebral hemispheres, basal ganglia, cerebellar lesion, or upper brainstem
Cluster	Lower pons or upper medulla
Ataxic	Medulla
Apneustic	Mid to lower pons

6.

I	Olfactory	• Evaluate the patient's ability to identify familiar odors
II	Optic	• Evaluate visual acuity using Snellen chart or newsprint • Evaluate the optic disc during funduscopic examination
III	Oculomotor	• Evaluate the ability to open eyes widely • Check size, shape, position, and reactivity of the pupils • Have patient follow your finger with his or her eyes through the six cardinal positions of gaze • Look for abnormal eye movement
IV	Trochlear	• Have patient follow your finger with his or her eyes through the six cardinal positions of gaze
V	Trigeminal	• Evaluate ability of the patient to detect light touch, superficial pain, and temperature on forehead, cheeks, and jaw • Touch the cornea with a wisp of cotton and check for bilateral blink • Palpate the strength of the masseter muscles with the patient clenching his or her teeth and the strength of the temporal muscles with the patient squeezing his or her eyes shut
VI	Abducens	• Have patient follow your finger with his or her eyes through the six cardinal positions of gaze
VII	Facial	• Ask the patient to smile and assess symmetry • Test the patient's ability to taste salt and sugar on the anterior tongue
VIII	Acoustic	• Evaluate ability of the patient to hear when speaking at normal voice tones • Note any vertigo, nystagmus, nausea, vomiting, pallor, sweating, hypotension
IX	Glossopharyngeal	• Evaluate patient's ability to speak, note any hoarseness • Look for bilateral elevation of the palate with phonation • Test the patient's ability to taste sour and bitter on the posterior tongue • Evaluate the patient's ability to swallow • Test the gag reflex by stroking the palate with a tongue blade and looking for reflex gag • Evaluate cough reflex by touching the hypopharynx with a suction catheter
X	Vagus	• As for glossopharyngeal
XI	Spinal accessory	• Ask the patient to shrug his or her shoulders as you push down on them with your hands • Palpate the sternocleidomastoid and trapezius muscles for size and symmetry
XII	Hypoglossal	• Look for midline alignment when the patient protrudes his or her tongue • Look for fasciculations of the tongue

7.   1.   Neck twisting or flexion
2.   Valsalva maneuver, including coughing, sneezing, straining at stool
3.   Airway obstruction

4. Pain or noxious stimuli
5. Disturbing conversation
6. Noise
7. Bright lights
8. Tight tracheostomy ties or cervical collar
9. Seizure activity
10. Hyperthermia

8.

Intervention	What is decreased?
1. Hyperventilation to cause respiratory alkalosis	blood
2. Fluid restrictions	brain mass
3. Dexamethasone (Decadron)	brain mass
4. Mannitol	brain mass
5. Furosemide	brain mass, CSF
6. Ventriculostomy and CSF drainage	CSF
7. Barbiturate coma	blood

Bibliography and Selected References

Alspach J, editor: *Core curriculum for critical care nursing,* ed 5, Philadelphia, 1998, WB Saunders.

Arbour R: Aggressive management of intracranial dynamics, *Critical Care Nurse* 18 (3):30, 1998.

Baker E: *Neuroscience nursing,* St Louis, 1994, Mosby.

Barkauskas V et al: *Health and physical assessment,* St Louis, 1994, Mosby.

Beare P, Myers J: *Adult health nursing,* ed 3, St Louis, 1998, Mosby.

Boggs R, Wooldridge-King M: *AACN procedure manual for critical care, ed 3,* Philadelphia, 1993, WB Saunders.

Chernow B, editor: *The pharmacologic approach to the critically ill patient,* ed 3, Baltimore, 1994, Williams & Wilkins.

Clochesy J et al: *Critical care nursing,* ed 2, Philadelphia, 1996, WB Saunders.

Crigger N: Assessing neurologic function in older patients, *AJN* 97 (3):37, 1997.

French-Sherry et al: Assessing stroke risk with carotid duplex ultrasound scanning, *Journal of Critical Illness* 13 (7):448, 1998.

Gahart B, Nazareno A: *1999 intravenous medications,* St Louis, 1999, Mosby.

Gawlinski A, Hamwi D: *Acute care nurse practitioner clinical curriculum and certification review,* Philadelphia, 1999, WB Saunders.

Ghajar J: Intracranial pressure monitoring techniques, *New Horiz* 3 (3):395, 1995.

Hudak C, Gallo B: Quick review of neurodiagnostic testing, *AJN* 97 (7):16CC, 1997.

Hudak C, Gallo B: Troubleshooting ICP lines, *AJN* 97 (6):16BB, 1997.

Keen J, Swearingen P: *Mosby's critical care nursing consultant,* St Louis, 1997, Mosby.

Kinney M et al: *AACN clinical reference for critical care nursing,* ed 4, St Louis, 1998, Mosby.

Lang E, Chesnut R: Intracranial pressure and cerebral perfusion pressure in severe head injury, *New Horiz* 3 (3):400, 1995.

Marino P: *The ICU book,* ed 2, Baltimore, 1998, Williams & Wilkins.

Marion D, Firlik A, McLaughlin M: Hyperventilation therapy for severe traumatic brain injury, *New Horiz* 3 (3):439, 1995.

Mims B et al: *Critical care skills: a clinical handbook,* Philadelphia, 1996, WB Saunders.

Minahon R, Bhardwaj A, Williams M: Critical care monitoring for cerebrovascular disease, *New Horiz* 5 (4):406, 1997.

Newell D: Transcranial Doppler measurements, *New Horiz* 3 (3):423, 1995.

O'Hanlon-Nichols T: Neurologic assessment, *AJN* 99 (6):44, 1999.

Pope W: External ventriculostomy: a practical application for the acute care nurse, *J Neurosci Nurs* 30 (3):185, 1998.

Price S, Wilson L: *Pathophysiology: clinical concepts of disease processes,* ed 5, St Louis, 1997, Mosby.

Prielipp R: Sedative and neuromuscular blocking drug use in critically ill patients with head injury, *New Horiz* 3 (3):456, 1995.

Robertson C, Cormio M: Cerebral metabolic management, *New Horiz* 3 (3):410, 1995.

Thelan L et al: *Critical care nursing: diagnosis and management,* ed 3, St Louis, 1998, Mosby.

Tonneson A: Hemodynamic management of brain-injured patients, *New Horiz* 3 (3):499, 1995.

Varon J, Fromm R: *The ICU handbook of facts, formulas, and laboratory values,* St Louis, 1997, Mosby.

Wilberger J, Cantella D: High-dose barbiturates for intracranial pressure control, *New Horiz* 3 (3):469, 1995.

Zhuang J et al: Colloid infusion after brain injury: effect on intracranial pressure, cerebral blood flow, and oxygen delivery, *Crit Care Med* 23 (1):140, 1995.

Zornow M, Prough D: Fluid management in patients with traumatic brain injury, *New Horiz* 3 (3):488, 1995.

Neurologic System: Pathologic Conditions

CHAPTER 7

Craniotomy

Surgical Procedures

I. Craniotomy: opening of the cranium to allow access to the brain (Fig.7-1)
  A. Supratentorial craniotomy is used to access the cerebral hemispheres and to accomplish any of the following:
    1. Remove intracranial tumors, hematomas, abscesses, epileptic foci
    2. Clip or ligate aneurysm or arteriovenous (AV) malformation in the anterior circulation
    3. Place ventriculovenous, ventriculopleural, or ventriculoperitoneal shunt
    4. Debride necrotic tissue; elevate and realign bone fragments
  B. Infratentorial craniotomy is used to access the brainstem and cerebellum to allow removal of cerebellar tumors and hemorrhages, acoustic neuromas, tumors of the brainstem or cranial nerves, abscesses
  C. Transsphenoidal approach (Fig. 7-2) is often used to remove the pituitary gland; referred to as a *transsphenoidal hypophysectomy*
    1. A horizontal incision is made at the junction of the inner aspect of the upper lip and gingiva and extends laterally to the canine tooth on each side
    2. The sella turcica is entered through the floor of the nose and the sphenoid sinus
    3. Transphenoidal hypophysectomy is indicated for pituitary tumor or to control pain associated with metastatic cancer
II. Craniectomy: removal of a portion of the cranium
III. Cranioplasty: repair of the cranium, usually with a synthetic material
IV. Burr holes: small holes drilled through the cranium to allow access to underlying structures; used for any of the following:
  A. Evacuation of epidural or subdural hematoma
  B. Insertion of intraventricular catheter for CSF drainage and/or ICP monitoring
  C. Insertion of another form of ICP monitoring device (e.g., subarachnoid screw)

Nursing Diagnoses

I. Anxiety related to surgical procedure
II. Fear related to surgical outcome
III. Alteration in Cerebral Tissue Perfusion related to intracranial hypertension, hydrocephalus
IV. Ineffective Airway Clearance related to increased secretions, diminished level of consciousness, inadequate protective reflexes
V. Impaired Gas Exchange related to inactivity, neurogenic pulmonary edema
VI. Risk for Fluid Volume Deficit related to decreased fluid intake, increased fluid loss, diabetes insipidus
VII. Risk for Fluid Volume Excess related to SIADH
VIII. Risk for Infection related to invasive procedures, traumatic wounds, surgical wounds
IX. Risk for Injury related to seizure activity, inadequate protective reflexes, stress ulcer
X. Ineffective Individual Coping related to situational crisis, powerlessness, change in role
XI. Ineffective Family Coping related to critically ill family member

Preoperative Collaborative Management

I. Control pain and discomfort
  A. Small doses of codeine or morphine may be prescribed
  B. Care must be taken to avoid oversedation because it eliminates LOC as an important assessment parameter
II. Prepare patient for surgery
  A. Steroids (e.g., dexamethasone [Decadron]) and/or anticonvulsants (e.g., phenytoin [Dilantin] may be initiated preoperatively
  B. Hair is washed with an antimicrobial shampoo the night before surgery; the operative area is usually shaved in the operating room (OR) or the OR holding area

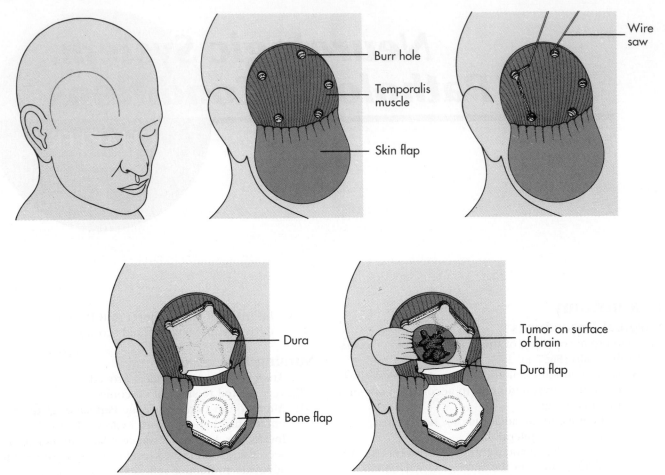

Figure 7-1 Craniotomy. (From Beare PG, Myers JL: *Principles and practice of adult health nursing,* ed 2, St Louis, 1994, Mosby.)

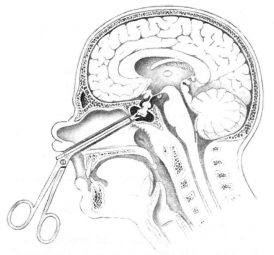

Figure 7-2 Transsphenoidal hypophysectomy. (From Thelan LA et al: *Critical care nursing: diagnosis and management,* ed 3, St Louis, 1998, Mosby.)

C. Baseline neurologic status should be carefully recorded
   1. Level of consciousness
   2. Glasgow coma score
   3. Communication deficits

   4. Cognitive deficits
   5. Motor deficits
   6. Sensory deficits
   7. Cranial nerve deficits
D. Inform the patient and family what to expect after surgery
   1. Equipment: IV catheter(s), oxygen therapy and possibly mechanical ventilation, indwelling bladder catheter, sequential compression stockings, possibly intraventricular catheter and ICP monitor
   2. Mild to moderate headache
   3. Photophobia
   4. Periorbital edema and bruising
   5. Head dressing and drain

Postoperative Collaborative Management
I. Prevent/monitor for clinical indications and treat intracranial hypertension
  A. Perform frequent neurologic assessments
    1. Compare results with preoperative status
    2. Check vision in patients having hypophysectomy
  B. Monitor for clinical indications of intracranial hypertension (may have an intraventricular catheter for monitoring ICP)

C. Teach patient to avoid causes of intracranial hypertension (see Box 6-1)

D. Prevent twisting of head or neck or flexion of neck to allow jugular vein drainage; support head, neck, shoulders when turning patient in bed

E. Control conditions that increase cerebral metabolic rate
1. Anticonvulsants for seizures
2. Antipyretics, cooling blankets for hyperthermia
3. Sedation as indicated for restlessness
4. Muscle paralytics, barbiturates to decrease the oxygen requirements of the brain (ICP monitoring is required because the most important assessment parameter [LOC] is eliminated)

F. Administer treatments for intracranial hypertension as prescribed (see Table 6-18)

G. Prevent/treat hypertension, hypotension to maintain CPP of 70 to 100 mm Hg

H. Position patient appropriately
1. If supratentorial craniotomy:
   a) Elevate head of bed 30 degrees
   b) If large mass removed, do not allow the patient to lie on operative side
2. If infratentorial craniotomy:
   a) Position flat with small pillow under nape of neck
   b) Do not allow on back for 48 hours
3. If transsphenoidal craniotomy (e.g., hypophysectomy): elevate head of bed 30 degrees
4. If insertion of interventricular shunt: position flat on nonoperative side
5. Other specific positioning may be prescribed by the surgeon

II. Maintain airway, oxygenation, ventilation
A. Encourage deep breathing; if coughing is indicated (rhonchi are audible), instruct the patient to cough with mouth open
B. Administer oxygen to maintain SpO_2 of 95% or greater unless contraindicated
C. Assess for gag and swallow reflexes; have suction equipment available

III. Maintain adequate hydration and electrolyte balance
A. Administer isotonic fluids as prescribed; avoid D_5W and other hypotonic solutions
B. Prevent overhydration, which can predispose to cerebral edema
C. Monitor closely for indications of overhydration or dehydration; evaluate urine output and urine specific gravity hourly
D. Assess head dressing hourly; notify surgeon if large amounts of drainage are noted

IV. Relieve headache
A. Inform patient to notify the nurse at the onset of headache; severe pain is not normal, notify physician
B. Administer small doses of morphine or codeine, avoiding oversedation; when the patient can take oral medications, acetaminophen with codeine is usually used

C. Decrease environmental stimuli

D. Apply cool compresses to decrease periorbital edema; dressing may be clipped if too tight (clip on side opposite surgical site)

V. Prevent injury
A. Institute seizure precautions
1. Have suction equipment available
2. Have extra pillows available that can be placed between patient and siderails
3. Assess onset, progression, and postictal period if seizure occurs
4. Administer anticonvulsants as prescribed
B. Perform passive ROM and reposition the patient every 2 hours
C. Perform frequent skin assessment
D. Instill artificial tears every 2 hours to prevent corneal abrasions in patients who do not blink; a moisture chamber may be created using plastic wrap
E. Orient to time and place often; encourage family participation in reality orientation
F. Apply restraints only if indicated for self-protection

VI. Prevent/monitor for infection
A. Administer prophylactic and/or therapeutic antibiotics as prescribed
B. Monitor head dressing and drains for purulent drainage; assess wound during aseptic dressing changes for redness, swelling, induration, drainage
C. Do not put tubes (e.g., suction catheter, nasogastric tube) into nose if patient has transsphenoidal approach; warn the patient not to blow or pick nose
D. Note drainage of CSF (CSF leak increases risk of intracranial infection)
1. Assessment
   a) Rhinorrhea
   b) Otorrhea
   c) Excessive swallowing
2. Management
   a) Moustache dressing for rhinorrhea
   b) 2×2 dressing over ear for otorrhea; sterile uribag may also be used
E. Monitor for and control hyperthermia: treat temperatures of more than 38° C (100.4° F) with hypothermia blanket and/or acetaminophen

VII. Monitor for complications
A. Intracranial hypertension: cerebral edema usually peaks about 48 to 72 hours
B. Cerebral ischemia, infarction
C. Cerebral hemorrhage
D. CSF leak (CSF leak is normal for up to 72 hours after transsphenoidal hypophysectomy)
E. CNS infection: encephalitis, meningitis
1. Clinical indications of CNS infection: headache, photophobia, nuchal rigidity, positive Kernig's and Brudzinski's signs, fever
2. Treatment: antibiotics

F. Seizures
G. Diabetes insipidus
  1. Clinical indications of diabetes insipidus: thirst, polydipsia, polyuria (4-20 L/day), specific gravity of urine 1.005 or less, increased serum sodium, hyperosmolality
  2. Treatment: fluid replacement; vasopressin (ADH)
H. Syndrome of inappropriate antidiuretic hormone (SIADH)
  1. Clinical indications of SIADH: decreased urine output, weight gain, confusion and lethargy, specific gravity of urine 1.035 or greater, decreased serum sodium (high potential for seizures)
  2. Treatment: fluid restriction, diuretics, hypertonic (3%) saline may be necessary
I. Hydrocephalus: often transient due to swelling
J. Deep-vein thrombosis (DVT): prevention methods include the following:
  1. Sequential compression devices rather than graduated elastic stockings because these patients are at high risk for DVT; best applied prior to surgery
  2. Low-dose heparin may be prescribed; low-molecular-weight heparin may be used
K. Stress ulcer (often referred to as *Cushing's ulcer*)

Closed Head Injuries

Etiology: Blunt or penetrating trauma (risk is decreased by helmets, airbags, seatbelts)
  I. Motor vehicle collision
  II. Falls
  III. Violence: assault
  IV. Sports-related accidents (e.g., boxing, football)
  V. Industrial accidents

Pathophysiology
  I. Focal injury
    A. Contusion
      1. Partial or complete dysfunction of CNS functioning that persists for less than 24 hours
      2. Trauma causes the brain to strike the internal surfaces of the skull and orbital roof, resulting in bruising and petechial hemorrhages
      3. Laceration of the brain may occur
      4. Areas of infarction and necrosis may occur as a result of vascular injury, leading to oozing of blood into the injured area
      5. Subpial and intracerebral extravasation of blood
      6. Hemorrhage and edema may act as intracranial mass and cause intracranial hypertension
      7. Injury may be at site of impact (coup) and/or opposite site (contrecoup)
  II. Diffuse injury
    A. Concussion: transient state of partial or complete paralysis of cerebral functioning with complete recovery within 12 hours; stretching of nerve fibers with subsequent failure of conduction, no structural alteration
      1. Mild: no loss of consciousness or memory loss
      2. Classic: loss of consciousness or memory loss
    B. Diffuse injury with loss of consciousness exceeding 24 hours: axonal disruption widespread throughout the cerebral hemispheres and anatomic interruption of neuronal pathways
    C. Diffuse axonal injury (DAI): severe mechanical disruption of axons and neuronal pathways in both cerebral hemispheres, diencephalon, and brainstem
  III. Secondary injury (**Note:** remember that the actual physical damage that occurs at the time of injury cannot be changed, so optimal outcome depends on avoiding or minimizing secondary injury to the brain caused by these systemic or intracranial causes)
    A. Systemic causes
      1. Hypotension
      2. Hypoxia
      3. Anemia
      4. Hyperthermia
      5. Hypercapnia or hypocapnia
      6. Electrolyte imbalance
      7. Hyperglycemia or hypoglycemia
      8. Acid-base imbalance
      9. Systemic inflammatory response syndrome (SIRS)
    B. Intracranial causes
      1. Intracranial hypertension
      2. Mass lesions
      3. Cerebral edema
      4. Vasospasm
      5. Hydrocephalus
      6. Infection
      7. Seizures

Clinical Presentation
  I. Concussion: may present with focal neurologic deficit or alteration in LOC that clears within 6 to 12 hours or less
    A. Subjective
      1. History of precipitating event
      2. Unconsciousness for 10 to 15 minutes
      3. Headache
      4. Scalp tenderness or pain at injury site
      5. Dizziness
      6. Visual changes
      7. Sluggishness
      8. Nausea/vomiting
      9. Memory loss
        a) Retrograde or antegrade amnesia may occur
        b) Posttraumatic amnesia, related to the events of the injury and events immediately preceding the injury, usually lasts less than 5 minutes

B. Objective
   1. Confusion, restlessness, irritability
   2. Disorientation
II. Contusion: signs vary depending on severity of trauma and area of brain involved; neurologic deficit persists less than 24 hours
   A. Subjective
      1. History of precipitating event
      2. Memory loss
   B. Objective
      1. Change in LOC
      2. Motor or sensory dysfunction
      3. Cranial nerve dysfunction
      4. Focal neurologic signs (e.g., hemiparesis, hemiplegia may be seen)
      5. Seizures
      6. Clinical indications of intracranial hypertension may be seen
III. Diffuse injury
   A. Subjective: history of precipitating event
   B. Objective
      1. Loss of consciousness may last days to weeks and is usually followed by long periods of retrograde and posttraumatic amnesia
      2. The patient usually has purposeful movements, withdrawal from pain, restlessness
      3. Permanent residual deficits in memory, cognitive and intellectual functioning occur; permanent residual psychologic or personality changes are common
IV. Diffuse axonal injury: coma, brainstem dysfunction
   A. Immediate and prolonged periods of unconsciousness
   B. Posturing: decorticate, decerebrate
   C. Death rates are high and many of these patients may persist in a vegetative state, which is characterized by return of wakefulness (eyes open and sleep patterns observed) but without observable signs of cognition
   D. Profound residual deficits
V. Diagnostic
   A. CT scan, MRI: may show cerebral edema, areas of petechial hemorrhages with severe contusions, hemispheric shift
   B. EEG: may show brainwave abnormalities
   C. Skull X-ray: may show fracture or hemispheric shift
   D. Cerebral angiography: may show aneurysm, vasospasm
   E. Evoked potentials: may show prolongation of transmission of impulses through the brainstem

Nursing Diagnoses

I. Decreased Adaptive Capacity: Intracranial related to failure of normal intracranial compensatory mechanisms
II. Alteration in Cerebral Tissue Perfusion related to intracranial hypertension
III. Ineffective Airway Clearance related to increased secretions, altered LOC, inadequate protective reflexes
IV. Ineffective Breathing Pattern related to inadequate airway, altered LOC
V. Pain related to injury
VI. Risk for Fluid Volume Deficit related to decreased fluid intake, increased fluid loss, diabetes insipidus, osmotic diuretics
VII. Risk for Fluid Volume Excess related to fluid resuscitation, SIADH
VIII. Risk for Infection related to invasive procedures, traumatic wounds, surgical wounds
IX. Risk for Injury related to seizure activity, inadequate protective reflexes
X. Impaired Physical Mobility related to injury, paresis or plegia, bed rest, altered LOC
XI. Sensory/Perceptual Alterations related to altered LOC
XII. Ineffective Individual Coping related to situational crisis, powerlessness, change in role
XIII. Ineffective Family Coping related to critically ill family member

Collaborative Management

I. Perform a complete assessment for primary and secondary injuries
   A. Remember that an adult head injury patient is not hypotensive due to blood loss from a closed head injury, so look for other causes of hypotension
   B. Remember that hypotension decreases CPP, increases mortality dramatically, and contributes to secondary brain injury
II. Maintain airway, ventilation, oxygenation
   A. Assume that the patient has a spinal injury until radiologic clearance of spine: do not tilt or hyperextend the head; use jaw-thrust technique to maintain open airway
   B. Use oral or nasopharyngeal airway until lateral spine X-rays rule out fracture
      1. Do not use nasopharyngeal airway or nasal suctioning if facial or skull fracture is present
      2. Do not use oral airways in conscious patients because they stimulate the gag reflex
   C. Assist with rapid-sequence intubation if intubation is required
   D. Administer oxygen as needed to maintain SpO_2 95% or greater unless contraindicated
   E. Prevent aspiration: position patient on side, have suction equipment available
III. Prevent/monitor for clinical indications and treat intracranial hypertension (see Intracranial Hypertension section in Chapter 6)
IV. Maintain CPP of at least 70 mm Hg
   A. Identify cause of hypotension if present
   B. Utilize volume replacement, inotropes, and/or vasopressors as prescribed
   C. Utilize therapies for intracranial hypertension (see Table 6-18)
V. Prepare for surgery if indicated
VI. Prevent/monitor for complications
   A. Vasogenic cerebral edema

B. Neurogenic pulmonary edema
1. Pathophysiology: thought to be due to massive sympathetic discharge
2. Clinical presentation: pulmonary edema with normal PAP and PAOP
3. Collaborative management
   a) Elevate head of bed 30 degrees, avoiding hip flexion
   b) Administer codeine as prescribed for sedation
   c) Administer osmotic diuretics (e.g., mannitol) as prescribed
   d) Utilize mechanical ventilation and PEEP as necessary to maintain ventilation and oxygenation
C. Postconcussion syndrome: persistent headache, inability to concentrate, memory problems, decreased problem-solving ability, irritability, emotional lability, depression, decreased libido, dizziness, tinnitus, diplopia, photophobia, decreased energy level, equilibrium disturbances
D. Seizures
E. Diabetes insipidus (DI)
F. Syndrome of inappropriate antidiuretic hormone (SIADH)
G. Stress ulcers (often referred to as *Cushing's ulcers*)
H. Residual neurologic deficits
I. Persistent coma

Skull Fractures
Etiology
I. Motor vehicle collision
II. Falls
III. Violence: assault, gunshot wounds, knife wounds
IV. Sports-related accidents (e.g., boxing, football)
V. Industrial accidents

Pathophysiology (Fig. 7-3)
I. Linear fractures (account for 80% of skull fractures)
A. Fracture with no displacement of bone
B. May interrupt major vascular channels

1. Linear fractures of the temporal-parietal bones may tear the middle meningeal artery, leading to epidural hematoma
2. Linear fractures of the occipital bone may tear the occipital artery, leading to epidural hematoma
II. Depressed
A. Fracture that depresses outer table of skull
B. May cause brain laceration
C. May cause intracranial hematoma
III. Basal
A. Fracture of base of skull
B. May cause injury to one or more cranial nerves or cause tearing of the dura with CSF leak

Clinical Presentation
I. Linear
A. Subjective
1. History of precipitating event or condition
2. Scalp tenderness
B. Objective
1. Swollen, ecchymotic area on scalp
2. May have scalp laceration (**Note:** because of the mobility of the scalp, the fracture may not lie directly beneath laceration)
II. Depressed
A. Subjective
1. History of precipitating event or condition
2. Headache
B. Objective
1. May have altered level of consciousness with focal neurologic deficits
2. May have scalp laceration
   a) Open fracture: scalp laceration present
   b) Closed fracture: no scalp laceration present
3. Hemiparesis, hemiplegia
4. Seizures
5. Depressed frontal fracture may cause cranial nerve I (olfactory) deficit (loss of the sense of smell is referred to as *anosmia*)
6. Depressed temporal may cause cranial nerve VII (facial) or VIII (acoustic) deficits; may see

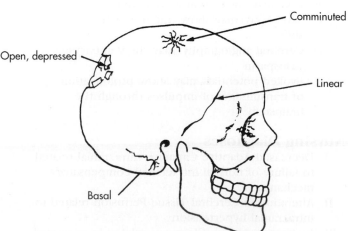

Figure 7-3 Types of skull fractures. (From Barker E: *Neuroscience nursing,* St Louis, 1994, Mosby.)

ipsilateral facial paralysis (VII) or hearing or equilibrium problems (VIII)

III. Basal
  A. Subjective
    1. History of precipitating event or condition
  B. Anterior fossa
    1. May have rhinorrhea; usually lasts 2 to 3 days
    2. May have bilateral ecchymotic eyes (referred to as *raccoon eyes*); takes 3 to 4 hours after injury to develop
    3. May have injury to CNI (olfactory), causing anosmia
    4. May have facial fractures
  C. Middle fossa
    1. May have otorrhea or rhinorrhea
    2. May have CSF or blood behind the tympanic membrane if the tympanic membrane remains intact; may cause hearing deficit
    3. May have ecchymosis over mastoid bone (referred to as *Battle's sign*); takes 4 to 6 hours after injury to develop
    4. May have cranial nerve injuries
  D. Posterior fossa
    1. May have epidural hematoma, which may result in signs of intracranial hypertension
    2. May have cerebellar, brainstem, or cranial nerve signs
      a) Visual changes
      b) Tinnitus
      c) Facial paralysis
      d) Conjugate eye deviation

IV. Diagnostic
  A. Skull X-ray
    1. Linear or depressed skull fractures may be seen on plain films
    2. Basal skull fracture is difficult to confirm on X-ray; pneumocephalus, opacity of the mastoid or sphenoid sinus, or an air-fluid level in one of the sinuses may be seen
  B. CT, MRI: may visualize depressed fractures

Nursing Diagnoses

I. Decreased Adaptive Capacity: Intracranial related to failure of normal intracranial compensatory mechanisms

II. Alteration in Cerebral Tissue Perfusion related to intracranial hypertension

III. Ineffective Airway Clearance related to increased secretions, altered LOC, inadequate protective reflexes

IV. Ineffective Breathing Pattern related to inadequate airway, altered LOC

V. Pain related to injury

VI. Risk for Fluid Volume Deficit related to scalp laceration, decreased fluid intake, increased fluid loss, diabetes insipidus

VII. Risk for Fluid Volume Excess related to fluid resuscitation, SIADH

VIII. Risk for Infection related to invasive procedures, traumatic wounds, surgical wounds, dural defect

IX. Risk for Injury related to seizure activity, inadequate protective reflexes

X. Impaired Physical Mobility related to injury, paresis or plegia, bed rest, altered LOC

XI. Sensory/Perceptual Alterations related to altered LOC

XII. Ineffective Individual Coping related to situational crisis, powerlessness, change in role

XIII. Ineffective Family Coping related to critically ill family member

XIV. Alteration in Cerebral Tissue Perfusion related to intracranial hypertension

Collaborative Management

I. Prevent/monitor for clinical indications and treat intracranial hypertension (see Intracranial Hypertension section in Chapter 6)

II. Maintain airway, ventilation, oxygenation
  A. Assume that the patient has a spinal injury until radiologic clearance of spine: do not tilt or hyperextend the head; use jaw-thrust technique to maintain open airway
  B. Use oral or nasopharyngeal airway until lateral spine X-rays rule out fracture
    1. Do not use nasopharyngeal airway or nasal suctioning if facial or skull fracture is present
    2. Do not use oral airways in conscious patients because they stimulate the gag reflex
  C. Assist with rapid-sequence intubation if intubation is required
  D. Administer oxygen as needed to maintain Spo_2 95% or greater unless contraindicated
  E. Prevent aspiration: position patient on side; have suction equipment available

III. Linear
  A. Monitor for clinical indications of intracranial hypertension or neurologic deficit
  B. No specific treatment required in the absence of neurologic symptoms

IV. Depressed
  A. Monitor for clinical indications of intracranial hypertension or neurologic deficit
  B. Protect brain under cranial defect from injury; position patient away from cranial defect
  C. Prevent/monitor for intracranial infection from open fracture
    1. Ensure meticulous cleansing and debridement of associated scalp laceration
    2. Surgical intervention is indicated if the skull depression is greater than the thickness of the skull (5-7 mm) and should be done emergently if scalp laceration or brain laceration is present
    3. Note indications of infection: fever, leukocytosis, redness, swelling, purulent drainage from wound
    4. Obtain culture if appropriate
  D. Monitor for hemorrhage; removal of bone fragment from a venous sinus may result in hemorrhage; blood must be available

V. Basal
  A. Prevent CNS infection
    1. Detect rhinorrhea/otorrhea; if present:
      a) Do not obstruct flow: use mustache dressing or 2×2
      b) Elevate head of bed 30 degrees
    2. Avert further tearing of dura by discouraging sneezing, blowing nose, Valsalva maneuver; instruct patient to cough with mouth open and to exhale when turning rather than holding the breath
    3. Do not use nasal O_2, nasogastric tube, nasopharyngeal tube, nasotracheal tube
VI. Monitor for complications
  A. Linear: epidural hematoma
  B. Depressed
    1. Laceration of brain tissue by brain fragments
    2. Intracerebral hemorrhage or contusion
    3. CNS infection (e.g., meningitis, encephalitis)
  C. Basal
    1. Intracerebral hemorrhage
    2. CNS infection (e.g., meningitis, abscess)
    3. Cranial nerve injury
    4. Carotid cavernous fistula
      a) Rare but serious complication
      b) Occurs when blood escapes from the carotid artery into the cavernous sinus
      c) Clinical indications include bruit and pulsation of orbit over affected eye, exophthalmos, headache, visual disturbances

Intracranial Hematomas

Etiology: Usually trauma
  I. Subdural hematoma (SDH)
    A. May occur spontaneously, particularly if patient has coagulation disorder or is taking anticoagulants
    B. Is prevalent in older patients with cerebral atrophy and alcoholics; may be bilateral
    C. May also be due to purulent effusion
  II. Epidural hematoma (EDH): often associated with linear skull fractures that cross major vascular channels
  III. Intracerebral hematoma (ICH)
    A. May occur as result of gunshot wound or stab wound, laceration of brain from a depressed

skull fracture, severe acceleration-deceleration injury
  B. Intracerebral bleeding caused by aneurysm, AV malformation, vascular tumor, or rupture of a vessel due to hypertension is described as a *hemorrhagic stroke* and will be discussed in the section on Hemorrhagic Stroke

Pathophysiology (Fig. 7-4)
  I. Subdural hematoma
    A. Usually venous bleeding; arterial origin is rare
    B. Accumulates below dura mater
    C. Classification
      1. Acute SDH: clinical indications occur within 48 hours after injury
      2. Subacute SDH: clinical indications occur within 2 weeks after injury
      3. Chronic SDH: clinical indications may occur weeks to months after injury
        a) Fibroblasts accumulate around and encapsulate the hematoma
        b) Hemolysis of the clot liberates plasma proteins; this reaction causes the encapsulated area to have a high osmotic pressure
        c) This hyperosmolality causes an influx of water and swelling of the mass
  II. Epidural hematoma
    A. Usually arterial bleeding; associated with tearing of arteries from skull fractures
      1. Linear fractures of the temporal-parietal bones may tear the middle meningeal artery, leading to epidural hematoma
      2. Linear fractures of the occipital bone may tear the occipital artery, leading to epidural hematoma
    B. May be due to venous bleeding; associated with fractures that cross major vascular channels such as the superior sagittal or transverse sinus (posterior fossa EDHs are usually of venous origin)
    C. Accumulates above the dura mater
  III. Intracerebral hematoma: hematoma into brain mass itself: may be due to bleeding caused by missile injury (e.g., gunshot wound or knife) or severe acceleration-deceleration force that causes bleeding into deep cerebral tissues

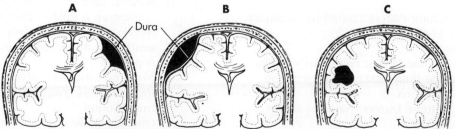

Figure 7-4 Types of hematomas. **A,** Subdural. **B,** Epidural. **C,** Intracerebral. (From Chipps EM, Clanin NJ, Campbell VG: *Neurologic disorders: Mosby's clinical nursing series,* St Louis, 1992, Mosby.)

Clinical Presentation

I. SDH
   A. Subjective
      1. History may include precipitating event or condition (in chronic SDH the patient may not be able to link the injury to any particular event either because he or she cannot remember or because no true precipitating event occurred [spontaneous])
      2. Headache
      3. Increasing irritability progressing to confusion progressing to decreased LOC
   B. Objective
      1. Decreased LOC
      2. Ipsilateral oculomotor paralysis
      3. Contralateral hemiparesis/hemiplegia

II. EDH
   A. Subjective
      1. History of precipitating event or condition
      2. History of short period of unconsciousness followed by lucid interval and then rapid deterioration
      3. Headache
   B. Objective
      1. Increasing irritability progressing to confusion progressing to decreased LOC
      2. Ipsilateral oculomotor paralysis
      3. Contralateral hemiparesis/hemiplegia

III. ICH
   A. Subjective
      1. History of precipitating event or condition
   B. Objective
      1. Varies with area of brain involved, size of hematoma, and rate of blood accumulation
      2. May or may not show clinical indications of intracranial hypertension

IV. Diagnostic
   A. Skull and cervical spine X-rays: may reveal associated skull or spine fractures
   B. LP: **contraindicated** by intracranial hypertension
   C. CT scan: will show an area of increased density; may show midline shift
   D. MRI: shows hematoma
   E. Cerebral angiogram: may reveal avascular area with displacement or stretching of vessels

Nursing Diagnoses

I. Decreased Adaptive Capacity: Intracranial related to failure of normal intracranial compensatory mechanisms
II. Alteration in Cerebral Tissue Perfusion related to intracranial hypertension, hydrocephalus
III. Ineffective Airway Clearance related to increased secretions, altered LOC, inadequate protective reflexes
IV. Ineffective Breathing Pattern related to inadequate airway, altered LOC
V. Pain related to injury
VI. Risk for Fluid Volume Deficit related to decreased fluid intake, increased fluid loss, diabetes insipidus
VII. Risk for Fluid Volume Excess related to fluid resuscitation, SIADH
VIII. Risk for Infection related to invasive procedures, traumatic wounds, surgical wounds
IX. Risk for Injury related to seizure activity, inadequate protective reflexes
X. Impaired Physical Mobility related to injury, paresis or plegia, bed rest, altered LOC
XI. Sensory/Perceptual Alterations related to altered LOC
XII. Ineffective Individual Coping related to situational crisis, powerlessness, change in role
XIII. Ineffective Family Coping related to critically ill family member

Collaborative Management

I. Detect and treat cranial, intracranial, and extracranial injuries
II. Prevent/monitor for clinical indications and treat intracranial hypertension (see Intracranial Hypertension section in Chapter 6)
III. Maintain airway, ventilation, oxygenation
   A. Assume that the patient has a spinal injury until radiologic clearance of spine
      1. Do not tilt or hyperextend the head; use jaw-thrust technique to maintain open airway
      2. Use oral or nasopharyngeal airway until lateral spine X-rays rule out fracture; do not use nasopharyngeal airway or nasal suctioning if facial or skull fracture is present
   B. Do not use oral airways in conscious patients because they stimulate the gag reflex
   C. Assist with rapid-sequence intubation if intubation is required
   D. Administer oxygen as needed to maintain SpO_2 95% or greater unless contraindicated
   E. Prevent aspiration: position patient on side; have suction equipment available
IV. Prevent further bleeding; osmotic diuretics are generally not used because the tamponade effect of the hematoma helps stop the bleeding
V. Prepare patient for surgery: generally burr hole and clot evacuation, although small hematomas may be observed through serial CT scans to verify hematoma's gradual reabsorption
   A. EDH: mortality increases dramatically if surgery is delayed
   B. SDH: mortality increases dramatically if surgery is delayed
   C. ICH: surgery is indicated if ICH is large or neurologic status deteriorates
VI. Detect and treat postoperative rebleed and/or cerebral edema; monitor closely for clinical indications of intracranial hypertension or deterioration of neurologic status
   A. Head of bed is usually elevated 20 to 30 degrees for acute and subacute subdural and epidural hematoma

B. Physician may request that head of bed be flat and patient positioned on side after surgery for removal of chronic SDH

VII. Prevent seizure activity: administer anticonvulsants prophylactically or therapeutically as prescribed

VIII. Monitor for complications
  A. Intracranial hypertension
  B. Hydrocephalus
  C. CNS infection
  D. DI
  E. SIADH
  F. Seizures

Hemorrhagic Stroke

Definition: Neurologic deficit caused by interruption of blood flow to the brain caused by vessel rupture

Etiology

I. Intracerebral hemorrhage
  A. Trauma: described in section on intracranial hematomas
  B. Hypertensive rupture of a cerebral vessel
  C. May also be caused by vascular intracerebral tumor, thrombolytics, anticoagulants, bleeding disorders

II. Subarachnoid hemorrhage: hemorrhage into the subarachnoid space
  A. Cerebral aneurysm: weakened bulging area on an intracranial blood vessel; accounts for the majority of subarachnoid hemorrhages
    1. Most cerebral aneurysms are small (2-6 mm but can be as large as 6 cm), saccular aneurysms and most occur at bifurcations in Circle of Willis
      a) Saccular (berry) aneurysms: usually congenital defects
      b) Fusiform aneurysms: from atherosclerosis
      c) Mycotic aneurysms: from necrotic vasculitis and septic emboli (rare)
      d) Traumatic aneurysms: from skull fracture disrupting vessel (very rare)
  B. AV malformation
    1. A tangle of abnormal arteries and veins: arteries feed directly into veins without a capillary bed
    2. Always congenital
    3. May occur in other circulatory systems, including the spinal cord

Pathophysiology

I. Aneurysm
  A. Congenital weakness of cerebral artery
  B. The aneurysm may act as a mass lesion if intact and large
  C. Weakness of an artery and high pressure (90% of ruptured aneurysms are associated with hypertension) lead to hemorrhage
  D. A clot initially forms in and around the rupture site and temporarily inhibits continuing hemorrhage; increase in ICP and pressure from local tissues may stop bleeding
  E. Blood leakage into the subarachnoid space and in contact with meninges causes meningeal irritation
  F. As clots hemolyze, spasmogenic substances are released
  G. Cerebral vascular spasm often occurs and contributes to ischemia or infarction
  H. Intracerebral hemorrhage causes pressure on cerebral tissues and nerves, leading to loss of function and death of neurons

II. AV malformation
  A. Congenital tangle of arteries and veins
  B. Steals blood from other areas because it is an area of low resistance
  C. Causes ischemia of surrounding tissue
  D. Hemorrhage may occur

Clinical Presentation

I. Subjective
  A. History
    1. Hypertension present in 90% of cases of ruptured aneurysm
    2. Most patients have had a "warning leak" days or weeks prior to bleed
      a) Headache
      b) Generalized, transient weakness
      c) Fatigue
      d) Ptosis, diplopia, blurred vision
  B. Sudden, severe headache
    1. Often described as "the worst headache of my life"
    2. Sudden: described as a "thunder clap" or "like being hit in the head"
    3. Localized progressing to generalized
    4. May radiate to neck and back
  C. Nausea and vomiting may be present in severe bleed

II. Objective
  A. Restlessness progressing to altered LOC
    1. Loss of consciousness is common in hemorrhage from aneurysm
    2. Loss of consciousness is uncommon in hemorrhage from AVM
  B. If hemorrhage into ventricles
    1. Nuchal rigidity
    2. Photophobia
    3. Kernig's sign, Brudzinski's sign
    4. Hyperthermia
  C. Neurologic deficit
  D. Seizures
  E. Site and size determine specific clinical presentation
  F. Hunt and Hess aneurysm grading system (Table 7-1)

III. AVM specifically
  A. May have bruit and report a constant swishing sound in the head with each heartbeat

Table 7-1	**Hunt and Hess Aneurysm Grading System**					
Grade	**0**	**I**	**II**	**III**	**IV**	**V**
Description	No bleed	Minimal bleed	Mild bleed	Moderate bleed	Moderate → severe bleed	Severe bleed
LOC	Alert	Alert	Awake	Drowsy	Stupor	Coma; moribund appearance
Headache	None	Minimal	Mild → moderate	Moderate → severe	Moderate → severe	Moderate → severe
Nuchal rigidity	None	Slight	Yes	Yes	Yes	Yes
Neuro deficit	None	No	Minimal (e.g., cranial nerve palsy)	Mild (e.g., hemiparesis)	Moderate (e.g., hemiplegia)	Severe (e.g., posturing)

Hunt WE, Hess RM: Surgical risks as related to time of intervention in the repair of intracranial aneurysms, *J Neurosurg* 28:14, 1968.

B. Motor/sensory defects
C. Aphasia
D. Dizziness, syncope
IV. Diagnostic
  A. Serum: PT, aPTT may be abnormal
  B. ECG
    1. Changes that may occur with SAH
      a) Flattened, peaked, or inverted T-wave
      b) Presence of U-wave
      c) QT prolongation
    2. Dysrhythmias are common; torsades de pointes has been associated with SAH
  C. LP: performed only if CT is nondiagnostic and no clinical indications of intracranial hypertension are present
    1. Reveals bloody CSF, elevated protein in acute SAH; it is important to number the test tubes
      a) If only test tube #1 is bloody: traumatic tap
      b) If all test tubes are bloody: bloody tap
    2. Reveals xanthochromic (dark amber) CSF if hemorrhage occurred several days (>5 days) ago
  D. Transcranial Doppler: aids in diagnosing vasospasm
  E. CT: identifies aneurysm, size, location, extent of subarachnoid or intracerebral hemorrhage; detects presence of hydrocephalus
  F. MRI
    1. May reveal small aneurysms that are not visualized with CT or angiogram
    2. May reveal ICH and intraventricular blood
    3. May show vasospasm
  G. Cerebral angiogram: will illustrate size, shape, and location of aneurysm; may show vasospasm

Nursing Diagnoses
I. Decreased Adaptive Capacity: Intracranial related to failure of normal intracranial compensatory mechanisms

II. Alteration in Cerebral Tissue Perfusion related to cerebral hemorrhage, vasospasm, rebleed, intracranial hypertension, hydrocephalus
III. Ineffective Airway Clearance related to increased secretions, altered LOC, inadequate protective reflexes
IV. Ineffective Breathing Pattern related to inadequate airway, altered LOC
V. Pain related to meningeal irritation by blood
VI. Risk for Fluid Volume Deficit related to decreased fluid intake, increased fluid loss, diabetes insipidus
VII. Risk for Fluid Volume Excess related to fluid resuscitation, SIADH
VIII. Risk for Infection related to invasive procedures, traumatic wounds, surgical wounds
IX. Risk for Injury related to seizure activity, inadequate protective reflexes
X. Impaired Physical Mobility related to injury, paresis or plegia, bed rest, altered LOC
XI. Sensory/Perceptual Alterations related to altered LOC
XII. Ineffective Individual Coping related to situational crisis, powerlessness, change in role
XIII. Ineffective Family Coping related to critically ill family member

Collaborative Management
I. Maintain airway, ventilation, oxygenation
  A. Maintain airway
    1. Oropharyngeal or nasopharyngeal airway may be needed to hold tongue away from hypopharynx in obtunded patient
    2. Endotracheal intubation may be needed in patients without airway protective reflexes
  B. Maintain oxygenation and ventilation
    1. Administer oxygen as needed to maintain SpO_2 95% or greater unless contraindicated
    2. Initiate mechanical ventilation as needed for hypoventilation

C. Prevent aspiration
   1. Position patient on side
   2. Have suction equipment available
II. Prevent/monitor for clinical indications and treat intracranial hypertension (see Intracranial Hypertension section in Chapter 6)
III. Prevent/monitor for delayed ischemia following SAH
   A. Identify vasospasm by worsening of neurologic status: vasospasm occurs anytime from the third day postbleed to 2 to 3 weeks after the initial bleed (peak incidence 7-14 days)
      1. Administer calcium channel blockers: nimodipine (Nimotop) and nicardipine (Cardene) are lipid-soluble and able to cross the blood–brain barrier
      2. Maintain triple-H therapy (hypertension, hypervolemia, hemodilution) as prescribed; monitor closely for rebleeding, pulmonary edema, coagulopathy
         a) Hypertension
            (1) The most debated of the three; some physicians use only hypervolemia and hemodilution
            (2) The goal is usually to maintain the systolic BP of 120 to 150 mm Hg prior to clipping and 160 to 200 mm Hg after clipping
            (3) Vasodilators (e.g., labetalol (Normodyne), nitroprusside [Nipride], hydralazine [Apresoline]) may be needed if patient is hypertensive
            (4) Vasopressors (e.g., dopamine [Intropin], norepinephrine [Levophed]) may be needed if patient is hypotensive
         b) Hypervolemia and hemodilution
            (1) Colloids (e.g., albumin, dextran) are usually used, but crystalloids may also be used
            (2) The goal is to maintain a PAOP of 15 to 20 mm Hg and hematocrit of 30% to 33%
      3. Prepare patient for cerebral balloon angioplasty if requested
IV. Minimize potential for rebleed and promote stabilization of patient: rebleed occurs most often within 24 hours or at 7 to 10 days after bleed
   A. Decrease environmental stimuli (these interventions may be referred to as *aneurysm precautions*)
      1. Provide a quiet, dimly lit private room
      2. Enforce bed rest with head of bed elevated 15 to 30 degrees
      3. Instruct patient to avoid Valsalva maneuver (e.g., cough with mouth open, exhale when turning in bed, not straining at stool)
      4. Instruct visitors that the patient should not be upset in any way; limit number of visitors and duration of visits

   5. Do not perform any rectal procedures (e.g., rectal temperature, enemas)
   6. Provide sedation (usually phenobarbital) if patient is restless
   B. Administer analgesics for headache, but avoid oversedation that would impair assessment
   C. Administer antihypertensives (e.g., labetalol [Normodyne], nitroprusside [Nipride], hydralazine [Apresoline]), as prescribed (**Note:** labetalol is the least likely to cause an increase in ICP)
   D. Administer aminocaproic acid (Amicar) if prescribed (**Note:** aminocaproic acid is an antifibrinolytic previously commonly used to prevent the breakdown of the clot but is rarely currently used because it increases the incidence of vasospasm and systemic clotting)
   E. Prepare patient for surgery
      1. Surgery is indicated within 48 hours for grade I, II, or III aneurysm
      2. Surgery is usually delayed for patients with grade IV or V aneurysm
V. Monitor patient's postoperative condition closely
   A. Types of procedures
      1. Aneurysm (Fig. 7-5)
         a) Surgical
            (1) Clipping: occlusion of the neck of the aneurysm with a ligature or metal clip; most common treatment, especially if a well-defined neck is visible
            (2) Wrapping or coating: reinforcement of the sac with muscle, fibrin foam, or solidifying polymer
            (3) Ligation: proximal ligation of a feeding vessel
         b) Endovascular procedures
            (1) Coiling: embolization coils are placed within the aneurysmal dome to cause thrombosis
            (2) Intravascular balloon placement: silicone microballoon is placed into the aneurysm and detached

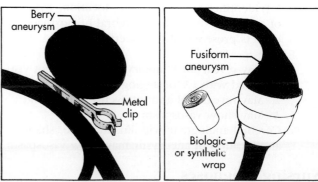

Figure 7-5 Clipping and wrapping of aneurysms. (From Chipps EM, Clanin NJ, Campbell VG: *Neurologic disorders: Mosby's clinical nursing series,* St Louis, 1992, Mosby.)

2. AVM
   a) Surgical excision
   b) Embolization of the AVM with Silastic beads
3. Intracerebral hemorrhage
   a) Surgical removal of clot depends on the size and location of the clot, the patient's ICP, and neurologic status
   b) Surgical removal of hematoma is indicated if it is large and causes shift of structures or if intracranial hypertension is unresponsive to medical treatment
   B. Provide postoperative management as described in Craniotomy section
   C. Monitor for signs of intracranial hypertension or rebleeding
VI. Monitor for complications
   A. Vasospasm
   B. Rebleeding
   C. Cerebral edema and intracranial hypertension
   D. Hydrocephalus: may require ventriculoperitoneal shunt
   E. SIADH
   F. Seizures: prophylactic anticonvulsants are often prescribed because the increase in BP during seizure activity could be detrimental

Ischemic Stroke

Definition: Sudden, severe disruption of the cerebral circulation with a subsequent loss of neurologic function caused by thrombus or embolus

I. Transient ischemic attack (TIA) (sometimes referred to as a *ministroke*): episode of neurologic impairment, attributed to focal cerebral ischemia, resolves within 24 hours (Table 7-2)
II. Reversible ischemic neurologic deficit (RIND): focal cerebral ischemic event lasting longer than 24 hours; complete resolution usually requires 1 to 3 days but always resolves within 3 to 4 weeks
III. Progressing thrombotic stroke: focal neurologic impairment attributed to thrombosis in an artery serving the brain and exhibiting a stepwise worsening of the neurologic deficit over minutes, hours, or days following presentation
IV. Completed thrombotic stroke: stable (for at least 24 hours) focal neurologic impairment attributed to thrombosis in an artery serving the brain; the deficit persists, by definition, longer than 3 weeks
V. Lacunar stroke: special subset of thrombotic stroke seen almost exclusively in hypertensive patients; well-localized infarction with resultant characteristic neurologic abnormalities

Etiology

I. Thrombosis
   A. Atherosclerosis
   B. Hypertension
   C. Hypercoagulability (e.g., polycythemia)
II. Embolism
   A. Mural thrombi
      1. Dysrhythmia (e.g., atrial fibrillation)
      2. Ventricular aneurysm
   B. Carotid artery atherosclerosis
   C. Bacterial endocarditis
   D. Prosthetic cardiac valves
III. Air or fat embolus (see Chapter 5)

Pathophysiology

I. Risk factors include the following:
   A. Family history
   B. Hypertension
   C. Smoking
   D. Hyperlipidemia
   E. Obesity
   F. Sedentary lifestyle
   G. Substance abuse: alcohol, drugs
   H. Oral contraceptives
   I. Dysrhythmias
   J. Hypercoagulability
II. Occlusive vascular disease (thrombosis or embolus) causes decreased oxygen to cerebral tissue, causing ischemia and leading to infarction
III. Cerebral edema often occurs; intracranial hypertension and persistent ischemia causes progressive damage to the penumbra, the ischemic brain tissue surrounding the infarction

Clinical Presentation

I. Subjective
   A. May have history of any of the following:
      1. Transient ischemic attack (TIA)
      2. Reversible ischemic neurologic deficit (RIND)
      3. Hypertension
      4. CV disease
      5. Arteriosclerosis
      6. DM
   B. Sudden onset of signs and symptoms
      1. Thrombotic stroke usually occurs at night
      2. Embolic stroke is more likely to occur when the patient is active

Table 7-2	Symptoms Occurring During Transient Ischemic Attacks	
Carotid Occlusion (hemispheric)	**Vertebral-Basilar Occlusion (nonhemispheric)**	
Ipsilateral monocular visual defect (amaurosis fugax) or homonymous hemianopsia	Bilateral visual defect; diplopia	
Contralateral sensory or motor defects	Bilateral sensory or motor defects	
Dysphasia; aphasia (if dominant hemisphere affected)	Dysarthria	
Ipsilateral headache Seizure activity	Occipital headache	
	Vertigo, syncope (drop attack), dizziness, ataxia	
	Dysphagia	
	Confusion, memory loss	

Table 7-3	**Clinical Indications Related to Vascular Occlusion**		
Anterior Cerebral Artery	**Middle Cerebral Artery**	**Posterior Cerebral Artery**	**Vertebral or Basilar Artery**
Impaired gait	Hemiplegia of face and arm on contralateral side	Cortical blindness	Weakness of tongue
Contralateral paralysis of leg and foot	Contralateral sensory deficit	Memory deficits	Ipsilateral facial numbness and weakness
Personality changes: flat affect, inappropriate emotional responses	Aphasia if dominant hemisphere affected	Perseveration (abnormal persistence of a response)	Dizziness
Mental impairment	Homonymous hemianopsia	Homonymous hemianopsia	Nystagmus
Urinary incontinence	Apraxia, agnosia, neglect if nondominant hemisphere affected		Dysarthria
			Dysphagia
			Ataxia
			"Locked-in" syndrome (quadriplegia and mutism with intact consciousness)

II. Objective
   A. Varies depending on area of vessel involved and extent of injury (Table 7-3)
III. Diagnostic
   A. Serum lipids: may be elevated
   B. ECG: may show dysrhythmias as a possible cause of cerebral emboli; Holter monitor may identify dysrhythmia
   C. EEG: identifies areas of decreased cellular function; identifies changes in the brain's electrical waveforms and seizure activity
   D. Echocardiography: may show intracardiac source for cerebral emboli (e.g., ventricular aneurysm, bacterial endocarditis)
   E. Skull X-ray: rules out traumatic injury
   F. LP: may be done to differentiate hemorrhagic from thrombotic stroke if no signs of intracranial hypertension are present
   G. Doppler carotid studies: may show carotid artery stenosis
   H. Transcranial Doppler: may be used to differentiate thrombotic versus hemorrhagic stroke
   I. CT
      1. Identifies the location and characteristics of stroke
      2. Identifies the presence or absence of gross hemorrhage
      3. Identifies the presence or absence of a mass lesion
      4. May show distortion or shift of ventricles
   J. MRI: identifies changes in the cranial or spinal structures
   K. Cerebral angiography: identifies occlusion, stenosis, aneurysms, hemorrhage in arterial system

Nursing Diagnoses

   I. Decreased Adaptive Capacity: Intracranial related to failure of normal intracranial compensatory mechanisms
   II. Alteration in Cerebral Tissue Perfusion related to thrombus, embolus, vasospasm, or intracranial hypertension
   III. Risk for Aspiration related to impaired swallowing, inadequate protective reflexes

   IV. Ineffective Airway Clearance related to increased secretions, altered LOC, inadequate protective reflexes
   V. Ineffective Breathing Pattern related to inadequate airway, altered LOC
   VI. Risk for Fluid Volume Deficit related to decreased fluid intake, increased fluid loss, diabetes insipidus
   VII. Risk for Fluid Volume Excess related to fluid resuscitation, SIADH
   VIII. Risk for Infection related to invasive procedures, traumatic wounds, surgical wounds
   IX. Risk for Injury related to seizure activity, inadequate protective reflexes
   X. Impaired Swallowing related to neuromuscular impairment
   XI. Altered Nutrition: less than body requirements related to decreased protein/calorie intake, hypermetabolism
   XII. Impaired Physical Mobility related to injury, paresis or plegia, bed rest, altered LOC
   XIII. Impaired Verbal Communication related to dysphasia, aphasia, intubation
   XIV. Sensory/Perceptual Alterations related to altered LOC
   XV. Body Image Disturbance related to actual change in body function and appearance
   XVI. Ineffective Individual Coping related to situational crisis, powerlessness, change in role
   XVII. Ineffective Family Coping related to critically ill family member

Collaborative Management

   I. Maintain airway, ventilation, oxygenation
      A. Maintain airway
         1. Oropharyngeal or nasopharyngeal airway may be needed to hold tongue away from hypopharynx in obtunded patient
         2. Endotracheal intubation may be needed in patients without airway protective reflexes
      B. Maintain oxygenation and ventilation
         1. Administer oxygen as needed to maintain Spo_2 95% or greater unless contraindicated
         2. Initiate mechanical ventilation as needed for hypoventilation

C. Prevent aspiration
1. Position patient on side
2. Have suction equipment available
II. Decrease metabolic requirements
A. Enforce bed rest initially
B. Administer minor tranquilizers as prescribed; be cautious to prevent oversedation
C. Administer stool softeners as prescribed
III. Maintain cerebral perfusion
A. Correct possible causes
1. Assist in electrical or pharmacologic conversion of atrial fibrillation or administer anticoagulants to prevent mural thrombi
2. Administer antihypertensives to control blood pressure; hypotension must be avoided
B. Administer platelet aggregation inhibitors (e.g., ASA, ticlopidine [Ticlid], clopidogrel [Plavix]) as prescribed (used especially in patients with carotid artery stenosis)
C. Administer anticoagulants as prescribed (especially if emboli are of cardiac origin)
D. Administer thrombolytics as prescribed
1. Indications
a) Presentation within 3 hours of acute ischemic stroke symptoms
b) Baseline CT to exclude intracranial hemorrhage and other risk factors for intracranial hemorrhage
c) Absence of contraindications; as in Table 3-18 with the addition of seizure at the onset of stroke
2. Dosing guidelines for alteplase (Activase)
a) Dose: 0.9 mg/kg with maximum dose of less than or equal to 90 mg
b) Bolus: 10% of this total dose over 1 minute
c) Infusion: remaining 90% of this total dose administer over 60 minutes
3. Management
a) Monitor vital signs and neurologic status
b) Maintain BP less than or equal to 185 mm Hg systolic and less than or equal to 110 mm Hg diastolic
c) Do not administer anticoagulants or platelet aggregation inhibitors for 24 hours after thrombolytic
E. Prepare patient for surgical procedures such as endarterectomy or bypass grafts (for patients with signs of cerebrovascular insufficiency who have not had completed stroke)
1. Provide postcarotid endarterectomy care
a) Monitor patients for embolic or thrombotic complications: changes in neurologic status
b) Monitor patients for injury to cranial nerves, especially:
(1) CN VII: ask patient to smile
(2) CN IX, X: check gag, swallowing reflexes; note any hoarseness
(3) CN XI: put your hands on the patient's shoulders and ask him or her to shrug against your hands
(4) CN XII: ask the patient to stick out his or her tongue and check for midline alignment
c) Monitor for hematoma or hemorrhage at carotid operative site; measuring neck circumference hourly for the first 8 hours may be helpful to detect expanding posterior hematoma
IV. Prevent/monitor for clinical indications and treat intracranial hypertension (see Intracranial Hypertension section in Chapter 6)
V. Assess patient's ability to communicate and establish means of communication; consult speech therapist as soon as possible in dysphasic or aphasic patients
VI. Protect patient from injury
A. Patient may have postural imbalance related to hemiparesis/hemiplegia; provide assistance during ambulation
B. Confusion and disorientation as well as memory deficits may occur concomitantly with aphasia; orient patient often, explain care
C. Seizures may occur; prophylactic anticonvulsants are often prescribed
VII. Maintain fluid and electrolyte balance
A. Maintain adequate hydration without overhydration
B. Assess gag and swallow reflexes before PO fluids; enteral feedings may be required initially
VIII. Prevent deformities, decubiti, hazards of immobility
A. Reposition every 2 hours
B. Perform passive ROM exercises every 2 hours; assist with active ROM exercises when indicated
IX. Maximize independence in ADL; allow the patient to do whatever he or she can independently
X. Provide emotional support and encourage participation in support groups
XI. Monitor for complications
A. Persistent neurologic trauma
B. Cerebral edema
C. Spastic paralysis may cause contractures
D. Seizures
E. Pneumonia

Spinal Cord Injury
Etiology
I. Trauma
A. Motor vehicle collision
B. Falls
C. Diving into shallow water or hitting a submersed object
D. Violence: assault, gunshot wounds, knife wounds
E. Sports-related accidents (e.g., boxing, football)
F. Industrial accidents
G. Thrill-seeking behavior
H. Increased risk with alcohol, drugs

II. Disease processes
   A. Tumors
   B. Ruptured spinal AV malformation
   C. Infectious process (e.g., abscess)
   D. Hematoma

Pathophysiology

I. Mechanisms of injury (Fig. 7-6)
   A. Hyperflexion
      1. Chin is forced to the chest
      2. Occurs most often in cervical region

3. Results from sudden deceleration
4. Results in ligament tears, stretching of the spinal cord, dislocated or subluxation of intervertebral disks or bone fragments compressing the spinal cord or spinal nerve roots
   B. Hyperextension: also called *whiplash*
      1. Head is thrown back
      2. Occurs most often in cervical region
      3. Results from the forces of acceleration-deceleration
      4. Results in backward and downward move-

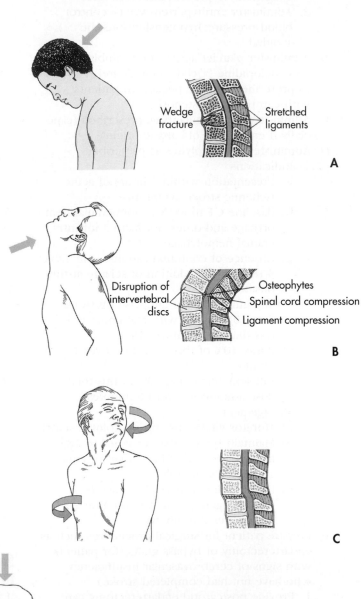

Figure 7-6 Mechanisms of spinal cord injury. **A,** Hyperflexion. **B,** Hyperextension. **C,** Flexion-rotation. **D,** Compression. (From Beare PG, Myers JL: *Principles and practice of adult health nursing,* ed 2, St Louis, 1994, Mosby.)

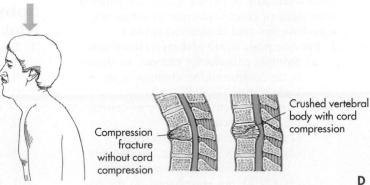

ment, which stretches the spinal cord, disrupts intervertebral disks, and tears ligaments

C. Rotation injury
1. Spinal cord is rotated
2. Can involve all parts of the vertebral column
3. Results from rotational forces tearing spinal ligaments
4. Results in displacement of intervertebral disks and compression of spinal nerve roots

D. Vertical compression
1. Vertebral column is compressed
2. Occurs primarily in area of T12-L2
3. Results from a force applied downward from the head
4. Results in burst vertebra and intervertebral disks; bony fragments may impinge on the spinal cord

E. Penetrating trauma
1. Can occur at any level
2. Results from the spinal cord being injured by a penetrating object (e.g., bullet or knife)
3. Results in complete or incomplete transection of the spinal cord

II. Injuries to the vertebrae
A. Simple fracture
1. Single break affecting the spinous or transverse process of the vertebrae
2. Spinal cord is not usually compressed, and the alignment of the vertebrae is not altered

B. Compressed fracture
1. Vertebral body is compressed anteriorly
2. Cord compression may occur

C. Comminuted fracture
1. Vertebral body shatters into many fragments
2. Fragments may injure cord

D. Dislocated vertebrae
1. May result in nonalignment of vertebral column with injury to the cord
2. Partial dislocation is referred to as *subluxation*

III. SCI results from compression, contusion, or transection of spinal cord
A. This condition causes interruption of blood supply and damage to blood vessels
B. Hemorrhage into the central gray matter within 4 hours of trauma
C. Platelet thrombi accumulate in the injured vessels, and water and protein extravasate from them
D. Norepinephrine and other vasoactive mediators may accumulate in the spinal cord and produce ischemia
E. Necrosis of the central gray matter within 4 hours of trauma
F. Vasogenic edema spreads into the surrounding white matter
G. Neuronal and axonal degeneration occurs within 8 hours
H. Neuron death occurs
I. Cerebral perfusion pressure may be decreased by spinal shock

Clinical Presentation: Depends on type and extent of lesion
I. Subjective
A. History of precipitating event or condition
II. Objective
A. Level of lesion: cervical and lumbar are more common than thoracic
1. C1-2: ventilatory cessation and immediate death
2. C3-5: quadriplegia with total loss of ventilatory function; mechanical ventilator dependent (Remember the phrase: C3, 4, 5 keeps the diaphragm alive)
3. C5-6: quadriplegia with gross arm movements; sparing of diaphragm leads to diaphragmatic breathing; no intercostal or abdominal muscles to assist in coughing
4. C6-7: quadriplegia with biceps muscles intact but no function of intrinsic hand muscles; diaphragmatic breathing; no intercostal or abdominal muscles to assist in coughing
5. C7-8: quadriplegia with triceps and biceps intact, but no function of intrinsic hand muscles; diaphragmatic breathing; no intercostal or abdominal muscles to assist in coughing
6. T1-L2: paraplegia with loss of varying amounts of intercostal and abdominal muscle; the lower the injury, the more intercostal function available
7. Below L2: cauda equina injury; mixed picture of motor-sensory loss, bowel and bladder dysfunction

B. Complete versus incomplete (Fig. 7-7)
1. Complete lesion: loss of sensory and motor function below level of lesion; irreversible
2. Incomplete syndromes (Table 7-4)

C. Spinal shock (occurs within minutes of the injury and may last from several days to months)
1. Results from the loss of inhibition of the descending tracts
2. Clinical presentation
a) Loss of all motor, sensory, and reflex responses
b) Bradycardia and hypotension
c) Loss of autonomic control
d) Transient reflex depression below the level of the injury
e) Flaccid paralysis of all skeletal muscle below the injury
f) Paralytic ileus
g) Urinary and fecal retention
h) Impairment in temperature regulation (vasodilation and inability to shiver): poikilothermia
i) Priapism may occur
3. May last from several days to months; when spinal shock is over, any or all of the following may occur:
a) Flexor spasms caused by cutaneous stimulation

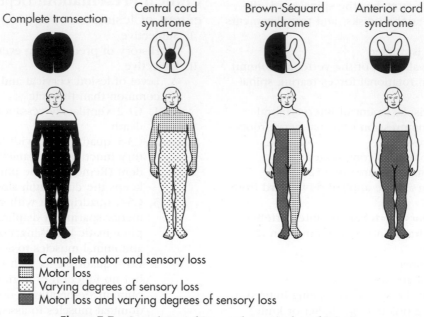

Complete transection   Central cord syndrome   Brown-Séquard syndrome   Anterior cord syndrome

■ Complete motor and sensory loss
▦ Motor loss
▒ Varying degrees of sensory loss
▨ Motor loss and varying degrees of sensory loss

Figure 7-7 Complete and incomplete spinal cord injuries.

Table 7-4 Incomplete Spinal Cord Lesions

Type of Lesion	Motor Loss	Sensory Loss	Type of Injury
Central cord syndrome	• Weakness of all extremities but greater motor loss in upper extremities	• Varies depending on the number of undamaged spinal cord tracts	• Hyperextension
Brown-Séquard syndrome	• Ipsilateral motor loss below lesion	• Ipsilateral loss of position and vibratory sense • Contralateral loss of pain and temperature	• Rotational with dislocation of fracture fragments • Penetrating (e.g., knife or gunshot wound) • Tumor
Anterior cord syndrome	• Complete motor loss below lesion	• Loss of pain and temperature below lesion (sparing of proprioception, vibratory sense, and touch)	• Hyperflexion

b) Reflex bowel and bladder emptying
c) Hyperactive deep-tendon reflexes

III. Diagnostic
A. Serum: ABGs to evaluate ventilatory and oxygenation status
B. Bedside ventilatory parameters: tidal volume, vital capacity, minute ventilation, maximal inspiratory pressure
C. Spinal X-rays: to confirm the type and location of vertebral fracture, dislocation, or degeneration; tumors or congenital abnormalities may be visualized
D. EMG: to measure evoked potentials
E. Myelogram: to detect occlusion of spinal subarachnoid space, cord or nerve root compression
F. CT: to visualize fractures; reflects compromise of the spinal canal or nerve roots by bony fragments

G. MRI: to identify extent of spinal cord damage, degree of cord contusion; demonstrates presence of blood, edema, necrosis, disk herniation, tumor

Nursing Diagnoses

I. Alteration in Spinal Cord Tissue Perfusion related to spinal cord edema and pressure
II. Alteration in Tissue Perfusion related to spinal shock and peripheral vasodilation
III. Ineffective Breathing Patterns related to ventilatory muscle paralysis
IV. Ineffective Airway Clearance related to ventilatory muscle paralysis, ineffective cough, bed rest
V. Risk for Infection related to invasive procedures, traumatic wounds, urinary stasis, immobility
VI. Altered Nutrition: less than body requirements related to decreased protein/calorie intake, hypermetabolism

VII. Impaired Physical Mobility related to paralysis
VIII. Alteration in Thermoregulation related to poikilothermism
IX. Urinary Retention related to bladder atony
X. Risk for Impairment in Skin Integrity related to paralysis, immobilization
XI. Risk for Autonomic Dysreflexia related to cervical or high thoracic spinal cord injury
XII. Self-Care Deficits related to decreased motor function due to tumor growth and pressure
XIII. Body Image Disturbance related to actual change in body function and appearance
XIV. Ineffective Individual Coping related to situational crisis, powerlessness, change in role
XV. Ineffective Family Coping related to critically ill family member

Collaborative Management

I. Prevent further damage to spinal cord
   A. Immediate immobilization by taping patient to backboard and applying a Philadelphia cervical collar; do not flex, extend, or rotate the neck
   B. Immobilization for stabilization of fracture
      1. Methods
         a) Cervical traction with Gardner-Wells, Cone, Vinke, or Crutchfield tongs inserted through skull's outer table with traction applied
         b) Halo traction with plaster or fiberglass jacket may be applied
            (1) Protect the skin under jacket
            (2) Keep wrench at bedside in case jacket would need to be removed for CPR
         c) Surgery may be performed
            (1) Decompression laminectomy
            (2) Closed or open fracture reduction
            (3) Cervical spinal fusion: especially if more than one vertebra is involved; a bone graft is usually taken from the iliac
            (4) Harrington rods: for thoracic injury
         d) Halo traction and cervical spinal fusion both allow the patient to be up in a chair earlier so that severe orthostatic BP changes are avoided
      2. Log roll patient from side to side
      3. Special beds may be utilized
   C. Prevent further spinal cord edema
      1. High-dose steroids may be used: 30 mg/kg of methylprednisolone over 15 minutes; pause for 45 minutes; maintenance dose at 5.4 mg/kg/hr for 23 hours
         a) Actions: protects the neuromembrane from further destruction and improves blood flow to injured site
         b) Contraindications
            (1) Injury more than 8 hours old
            (2) Injury below L2
            (3) Injury to cauda equina

   c) Stress ulcer prophylaxis
      (1) Administer histamine$_2$-receptor antagonists and/or antacids
      (2) Check NG aspirate, vomitus, stools for blood
   2. Administer osmotic diuretics (e.g., mannitol) as prescribed
   3. Therapeutic hypothermia may also be used to decrease oxygen consumption
II. Maintain airway, ventilation, oxygenation
   A. Assume that the patient has a spinal injury until radiologic clearance of spine: do not tilt or hyperextend the head; use jaw-thrust technique to maintain open airway
   B. If artificial airway is needed before cervical spine has been radiologically cleared, insert nasopharyngeal airway or nasotracheal tube without hyperextended neck
   C. Maintain oxygenation and ventilation
      1. Administer oxygen as needed to maintain Spo$_2$ 95% or greater unless contraindicated
      2. Initiate mechanical ventilation as needed for hypoventilation
   D. Prevent aspiration
      1. Tilt patient to side
      2. Have suction equipment available
III. Treat pain and discomfort
   A. Administer analgesics and/or muscle relaxants as prescribed
   B. Handle paralyzed limbs gently
IV. Monitor for and treat spinal shock
   A. Monitor for clinical indications of spinal shock
   B. Administer colloids (e.g., albumin) as prescribed to maintain blood pressure; avoid hypotonic (e.g., D$_5$W) solutions because they may increase cord edema
   C. Administer atropine as prescribed for bradycardia
   D. Perform intermittent urinary catheterization
V. Prevent/treat complications
   A. Cardiovascular
      1. Hypotension
         a) Be cautious with fluid replacement to avoid further cord injury; colloids are usually used
         b) Administer inotropes or vasopressors as prescribed to maintain blood pressure and perfusion
      2. Bradycardia
         a) Administer atropine if patient is symptomatic
         b) Treat hypothermia with warm blankets, radiant heaters
      3. Temperature regulation problems (poikilothermia): ensure warm environment but cool patient if hyperthermic
      4. Deep-vein thrombosis/pulmonary embolism
         a) Prophylactic anticoagulation: usually 5,000 U of heparin administered subcutaneously every 12 hours
         b) Passive range of motion every 2 hours

c) Antiembolic stockings or sequential compression stockings may also be needed

B. Autonomic dysreflexia

1. Does not occur until spinal shock is over and only occurs in patients with injuries at T6 or above

2. Etiology: caused by massive sympathetic discharge stimulated by sensory input (noxious stimuli) that cannot traverse the spinal cord to communicate with the brain; the feedback system between the sympathetic nervous system and the parasympathetic nervous system is disrupted and the brain can no longer modify the response; common examples of noxious stimuli include the following:

a) Full bladder

b) Full sigmoid colon, impaction

c) Skin pain: heat, cold, pressure

d) Labor

3. Clinical presentation

a) Subjective

(1) Throbbing headache

(2) Nausea

(3) Blurred vision

(4) Nasal congestion

(5) Flushing of the face and neck

(6) Anxiety

b) Objective

(1) Hypertension: may be as high as 300/150 mm Hg

(2) Bradycardia

(3) Diaphoresis, flushing above the lesion, especially on the forehead

(4) Pallor, coldness below the lesion

4. Collaborative management

a) Either place patient in sitting position or elevate head of bed

b) Eliminate cause

(1) Check bladder for distention and urinary catheter for kinking or occlusion; insert new catheter lubricated with Xylocaine if catheter is occluded or indwelling urinary catheter is not in place

(2) Check rectum for impaction; if impaction is present, instill dibucaine (Nupercainal) or Xylocaine ointment prior to any attempt to remove impaction

(3) Check for skin problems

c) Administer antihypertensives as prescribed

(1) Phentolamine (Regitine): alpha-blocker

(2) Nitroglycerin paste

(3) Nifedipine (Procardia) (**Note:** the use of nifedipine sublingually is no longer recommended because hypoperfusion may result from the dramatic drop in BP that often occurs when nifedipine is administered sublingually)

(4) Hydralazine (Apresoline) intravenous

(5) Nitroprusside (Nipride) IV infusion

(6) Labetalol (Normodyne): contraindicated because it will worsen bradycardia

d) Monitor for complications

(1) Intracerebral hemorrhage

(2) Myocardial infarction

(3) Seizures

(4) Retinal hemorrhage

C. Pulmonary

1. Hypoventilation

a) Assess function of diaphragm in high cervical injuries

b) Assess pulmonary ventilatory parameters: tidal volume, vital capacity

c) Monitor arterial blood gases and pulse oximetry

d) Assist with intubation and mechanical ventilation if needed

2. Pneumonia

a) Encourage inspiratory maneuvers (e.g., incentive spirometry)

b) Encourage coughing if rhonchi are audible

c) Suction if coughing is ineffective; utilize precautions to prevent hypoxemia (e.g., hyperinflation and hyperoxygenation) prior to and after suctioning

3. Aspiration

a) Utilize nasogastric tube for gastric decompression if bowel sounds are absent

b) Elevate head of bed 30 to 45 degrees during meals or during and after enteral feedings

4. Pulmonary edema: avoid overinfusion of fluids, especially crystalloids

D. Gastrointestinal

1. Gastric distention, paralytic ileus

a) Monitor bowel sounds

b) Connect nasogastric tube to intermittent suction if paralytic ileus occurs

2. Cushing's ulcer

a) Administer antacids and histamine$_2$ receptor antagonists

b) Initiate gastric lavage as needed for bleeding

c) Replace volume as prescribed; blood administration may be needed

3. Constipation

a) Encourage high-fiber foods when able to eat oral foods; fiber additives or high-fiber formula may be used for enteral feedings

b) Encourage fluids

c) Administer stool softeners, mild cathartics

d) Utilize suppositories, digital stimulation for colon evacuation

E. Urinary

1. Urinary tract infection (UTI)

a) Utilize intermittent catheterization (preferred over indwelling bladder catheterization) after the need for assessment of hourly urine output is over

b) Monitor for changes in the appearance of the urine (e.g., cloudiness, foul odor) that indicate UTI

c) Encourage fluids, especially those that acidify the urine (e.g., cranberry juice)

2. Renal or urinary tract calculi: encourage fluids, especially those that acidify the urine (e.g., cranberry juice)

F. Musculoskeletal
1. Decubiti
   a) Turn every 2 hours; keep skin clean and dry
   b) Perform passive ROM of the paralyzed limbs every 2 hours; encourage the patient to perform active ROM of functional limbs
2. Contracture
   a) Maintain proper positioning
   b) Utilize orthopedic appliances to maintain joints in functional position
3. Muscle spasm
   a) Administer muscle relaxants as prescribed for spasm
   b) Handle paralyzed limbs gently to prevent stimulating spasm

G. Metabolic
1. Acid-base imbalance
   a) Monitor arterial blood gases
   b) Correct cause of acid-base imbalance (e.g., improve perfusion, improve ventilation, replace lost electrolytes)
2. Electrolytes
   a) Monitor serum electrolytes
   b) Correct cause of electrolyte imbalance (e.g., discontinue NG suction as soon as possible; avoid hypotonic solutions)

H. Psychologic
1. Body image change; grieving
   a) Deal honestly with patient and family
   b) Maintain positive attitude
   c) Provide consistency of care
2. Powerlessness
   a) Allow patient to participate in care and decision making
   b) Define and set appropriate limits of behavior
   c) Provide consistency of care
   d) Encourage family participation in care

Brain Tumor

Etiology: Multifactorial or unknown
I. Congenital
II. Hereditary factors

Pathophysiology
I. Although one half of brain tumors are benign, death may occur by exerting pressure on vital centers
   A. Malignant tumors cause progressive deterioration of the patient's condition, leading to death; may be primary or metastatic

B. Benign CNS tumors may produce malignant effects because of their anatomic location and surgical inaccessibility
1. Benign CNS tumors may cause death because they take up space in the cranial vault and cause intracranial hypertension and herniation
2. Some benign CNS tumors may convert to malignant
II. Space-occupying lesions destroy brain tissue and nerve structures and produce intracranial hypertension
III. They may cause cerebral ischemia or edema, intracranial hypertension, seizures, focal neurologic deficits, hydrocephalus, and hormonal changes
IV. Primary brain tumors are categorized by their cell type; metastatic brain tumors are of the cell type of the primary tumor (Table 7-5)

Clinical Presentation
I. Subjective
   A. Headache
      1. Occurs at night after retiring
      2. Present and worse on awakening
      3. May be relieved by midmorning
   B. Visual changes
II. Objective
   A. Seizures: new onset
   B. Personality changes
   C. Vomiting without preceding nausea
      1. More common in morning
   D. Papilledema
   E. Change in LOC
   F. Hormonal changes if pituitary involved
   G. Specific to affected area of brain (Table 7-6)
III. Diagnostic
   A. Hormone levels: may be abnormal if pituitary tumor
   B. Chest X-ray: may show primary tumor of lung
   C. Skull X-ray: may show shift of pineal gland
   D. EEG: aids in identification of seizure activity
   E. Brain scan: identifies the tumor
   F. Bone scan: may show bone cancer
   G. CT: identifies the tumor
   H. MRI: identifies the tumor and effect on surrounding tissue
   I. Angiography: may show vascular shifts due to tumor or may show vascularity of tumor
   J. Biopsy: classifies tumor cell type

Nursing Diagnoses
I. Decreased Adaptive Capacity: Intracranial related to failure of normal intracranial compensatory mechanisms
II. Alteration in Cerebral Tissue Perfusion related to intracranial hypertension
III. Pain related to intracranial hypertension, stretching of dura at tumor site
IV. Ineffective Airway Clearance related to increased secretions, diminished LOC, inadequate protective reflexes

Table 7-5 Types of Brain Tumors	
Type	**Comments**
Gliomas • Astrocytomas (initially benign but prone to become malignant) • Oligodendrogliomas (usually benign but may become malignant) • Ependymomas (usually benign but may become malignant) • Medulloblastomas (highly malignant) • Glioblastoma multiforme (highly malignant)	• Most in cerebrum but medulloblastoma in cerebellum and ependymomas in ventricular system • Most grow rapidly but medulloblastoma is rapidly invasive • Most nonencapsulated; cannot be incised completely
Meningioma	• Benign, slow growing • Usually encapsulated; surgical cure possible • Recurrence possible
Pituitary adenoma	• Usually benign • Surgical approach usually successful
Acoustic neuroma	• Benign or low-grade malignancy • Arise from sheath of Schwann cells found on eighth cranial nerve • Will regrow if not completely excised • Surgical resection often difficult due to location
Metastatic tumor	• Malignant • Cancer cells spread to the brain via the circulatory system, usually lung, breast, or prostate cancer • Surgical resection difficult and prognosis poor

V. Risk for Fluid Volume Deficit related to decreased fluid intake, increased fluid loss, diabetes insipidus

VI. Risk for Fluid Volume Excess related to fluid resuscitation, SIADH

VII. Risk for Infection related to invasive procedures, traumatic wounds, surgical wounds

VIII. Potential for Injury related to seizure activity, inadequate protective reflexes

IX. Altered Nutrition: less than body requirements related to decreased protein/calorie intake, hypermetabolism

X. Impaired Verbal Communication related to dysphasia, aphasia, intubation

XI. Impaired Physical Mobility related to injury, paresis or plegia, bed rest, altered LOC

XII. Sensory/Perceptual Alterations related to altered LOC

XIII. Self-Care Deficits related to decreased motor function due to tumor growth and pressure

XIV. Ineffective Individual Coping related to situational crisis, powerlessness, change in role

XV. Anticipatory Grieving related to diagnosis of cancer

XVI. Ineffective Family Coping related to critically ill family member

Collaborative Management

I. Prevent/monitor for clinical indications and treat intracranial hypertension (see Intracranial Hypertension section in Chapter 6); glucocorticoids are often used to reduce cerebral edema

II. Maintain airway, oxygenation, ventilation
  A. Maintain airway
    1. Oropharyngeal or nasopharyngeal airway may be needed to hold tongue away from hypopharynx in obtunded patient
    2. Endotracheal intubation may be needed in patients without airway protective reflexes
  B. Maintain oxygenation and ventilation
    1. Administer oxygen as needed to maintain SpO_2 95% or greater unless contraindicated
    2. Initiate mechanical ventilation as needed for hypoventilation
  C. Prevent aspiration
    1. Position patient on side
    2. Have suction equipment available

III. Prepare patient for surgery, radiation, and/or chemotherapy
  A. Surgery
    1. Purposes of craniotomy for brain tumor
      a) Debulk tumor to relieve pressure
      b) Resect and remove tumor (usually followed by radiation)
      c) Insert shunt for hydrocephalus
    2. Postcraniotomy care (see Craniotomy section)
  B. Radiation: after surgery for incompletely excised tumor or for nonsurgically accessible tumor
    1. Whole-brain radiation therapy in high doses or superfractionated therapy
    2. Brachytherapy or interstitial irradiation: placement of a radioactive source in contact with or implanted into the brain tumor

Table 7-6	Clinical Manifestations of Tumors Specific to Affected Area of Brain
Area	**Clinical Manifestations**
Frontal lobe	• Personality changes • Inappropriate behavior: loss of social behavior • Inappropriate affect: quiet, flat • Inattentiveness, inability to concentrate • Emotional lability • Recent memory loss • Decreased intellectual ability • Motor changes: hemiparesis, hemiplegia • Seizure activity possible • If dominant hemisphere: expressive aphasia
Parietal lobe	• Sensory changes: hyperesthesia, paresthesia, loss of two-point discrimination • Constructional apraxia • Loss of right-left discrimination • Homonymous hemianopsia • Seizure activity possible
Temporal lobe	• Poor judgment • Irritability • Regressive behavior • Auditory disturbances • Olfactory, visual, gustatory hallucinations • Psychomotor seizures • If dominant hemisphere: receptive aphasia
Occipital lobe	• Visual disturbances: visual field defects • Visual hallucinations • Seizure activity possible: visual aura
Pituitary or hypothalamus	• Visual disturbances • Hormone imbalance: hypopituitarism or hyperpituitarism • Temperature regulation problems • Changes in sleep patterns
Brainstem	• Dysphagia • Vomiting • Ataxia • Nystagmus • Vomiting: with or without nausea • Decreased corneal reflex • Ventilatory pattern changes
Cerebellum	• Ataxia • Nystagmus • Unsteady gait • Decreased coordination • Vomiting: with or without nausea • Intentional tremors • Seizure activity possible

C. Radiosurgery: closed-skull destruction of an intracranial target with ionizing beams of radiation; an intracranial guiding device aids in focusing the beams of radiation
  1. Bragg peak proton beam

  2. Linear accelerator radiosurgery
  3. Gamma knife therapy
D. Chemotherapy
  1. Used after debulking in combination with radiotherapy, after irradiation, or for tumor recurrence
  2. Antineoplastic agent determined by tumor type; more than one agent may be used
IV. Monitor for complications
  A. Cerebral ischemia
  B. Hydrocephalus
  C. Cerebral edema
  D. Seizures
  E. Herniation

Status Epilepticus

Definitions

I. Seizure: sudden, paroxysmal episode of exaggerated activity or abnormal behavior caused by excessive discharge of cerebral neurons; Table 7-7 describes types of seizures
II. Status epilepticus: seizure activity of 30 minutes or more duration caused by a single seizure or a series of seizures in which consciousness does not return between seizures

Etiology

I. Withdrawal from anticonvulsant medications
II. Acute alcohol withdrawal
III. Acute withdrawal from chronically used drugs that have sedative or depressant effects
IV. Toxic levels of drugs: theophylline; lidocaine
V. CNS infection: meningitis; encephalitis: abscess
VI. Stroke: ischemic or hemorrhagic
VII. Brain tumors
VIII. Cerebral edema or trauma
IX. Metabolic disorders
  A. Hypoglycemia
  B. Hepatic failure
  C. Electrolyte imbalance
    1. Hyponatremia
    2. Hypocalcemia
    3. Hypomagnesemia
  D. Uremia

Pathophysiology

I. Prolonged grand mal seizures may deplete the brain of oxygen and glucose, which may produce hypoxia and neuronal death
II. Early: hypersympathetic phase
  A. Cerebral blood flow increases
  B. Tachycardia, hypertension
  C. Blood pH falls, Pao_2 falls, $Paco_2$ rises
  D. Glucose and potassium rise
III. Late: after 25 to 30 minutes of seizure activity
  A. Cerebral blood flow is unable to keep up with cerebral metabolic demands
  B. Bradycardia, hypotension, dysrhythmias, hypoglycemia
  C. Marked elevations of CK and potassium

Table 7-7	Types of Seizures		
Type	**Features**		**Duration**
	Generalized: Loss of Consciousness		
Absence (petit mal)	• Momentary loss of consciousness • Blank stare, cessation of activity • Eye blinking, lip smacking may occur • May lose muscle tone		Seconds
Tonic-clonic (grand mal)	• May be preceded by an aura and a cry from forced expiration • Loss of consciousness • Symmetrical tonic-clonic extremity movements • May experience apnea with cyanosis until tonic phase ends • May bite tongue, may be incontinent • Postictal fatigue, muscle soreness, confusion, lethargy, and/or headache		3-5 minutes
Myoclonic	• Short, abrupt muscle contractions of arms, legs, and torso • Contractions may be symmetrical or asymmetrical		Seconds
Clonic	• Muscle contraction and relaxation but slower than with myoclonic seizure		Several minutes
Tonic	• Abrupt increase in muscle tone of torso and face • Flexion of arms; extension of legs		Seconds
Atonic	• Abrupt loss of muscle tone • May cause falling and injuries related to fall		Seconds
	Partial: Focal at Onset but May Evolve into a Generalized Seizure		
Simple partial	• Consciousness not impaired • Abnormal unilateral movement of arm, leg, or both • Patient may sense abnormal smell, sound, or sensation, such as numbness, tingling, burning • Tachycardia or bradycardia, tachypnea, skin flushing, epigastric discomfort		Seconds to minutes
Complex partial	• Loss of consciousness but eyes may be open • Lip smacking, chewing, picking at clothing • Mumbling, speaking in repetitive phrases • Posturing or jerking movements • Postictal confusion, amnesia common		Minutes

D. Ventricular fibrillation may occur
E. Rhabdomyolysis-induced renal failure may occur

Clinical Presentation

I. Subjective
   A. History may include precipitating event or condition
     1. History of epilepsy
     2. History of noncompliance in taking anticonvulsant drugs
     3. History of chronic drug or alcohol use
II. Objective
   A. Alteration in LOC
   B. Tonic and/or clonic body movements
   C. Incontinence of urine or stool
   D. Involuntary motor activities: lip smacking, swallowing, chewing
III. Diagnostic
   A. Serum
     1. Electrolytes: hyperkalemia
     2. Glucose: increased early, decreased late
     3. CK: increased
     4. Lactic acid: increased
     5. Alcohol: may be positive for presence and quantity of alcohol

     6. Anticonvulsant drug levels: may show subtherapeutic or therapeutic drug levels
   B. Urine: may show myoglobinuria
   C. Skull X-rays: may show cause
   D. EEG: will show seizure activity
   E. CT: may indicate pathologic conditions (e.g., mass lesions)
   F. LP: may show meningitis as cause

Nursing Diagnoses

I. Decreased Adaptive Capacity: Intracranial related to failure of normal intracranial compensatory mechanisms
II. Alteration in Cerebral Tissue Perfusion related to intracranial hypertension
III. Ineffective Airway Clearance related to increased secretions, diminished LOC, inadequate protective reflexes
IV. Ineffective Breathing Patterns related to obstruction of airway by tongue
V. Risk for Infection related to invasive procedures, traumatic wounds, surgical wounds
VI. Hyperthermia related to seizure activity
VII. Risk for Injury related to seizure activity, inadequate protective reflexes

VIII. Pain related to meningeal irritation if CNS infection
IX. Hyperthermia related to infection
X. Sensory/Perceptual Alterations related to altered LOC
XI. Ineffective Individual Coping related to situational crisis, powerlessness, change in role
XII. Ineffective Family Coping related to critically ill family member

Collaborative Management

I. Establish and maintain airway and adequate ventilation
   A. Insert artificial airway if ventilation and oxygenation are inadequate
      1. Utilize nasopharyngeal airway or nasotracheal intubation if mouth cannot be opened; do not try to force mouth open
      2. Monitor ABGs and pulse oximetry
   B. Maintain oxygenation and ventilation
      1. Administer oxygen as needed to maintain Spo_2 95% or greater unless contraindicated
      2. Initiate mechanical ventilation as needed for hypoventilation
   C. Prevent aspiration
      1. Position on side: do not just turn head to side; turn body on side
      2. Have suction equipment available; suction as indicated
II. Assess causes or contributing factors
   A. Analyze blood for glucose, sodium, potassium, calcium, phosphorus, magnesium, BUN
   B. Screen for drugs
      1. Barbiturates
      2. Tricyclic antidepressants
      3. Alcohol
   C. Obtain anticonvulsant drug levels
   D. Obtain blood cultures if patient is hyperthermic
III. Protect patient from injury
   A. Call for help
   B. Do not leave patient
   C. Loosen constrictive clothing
   D. Remove pillow from under head
   E. Do not restrain, but gentle guiding of extremities is acceptable
   F. Pad siderails with blankets or pillows
   G. Maintain privacy
   H. Assess for injury
IV. Stop seizure activity
   A. Initiate IV
   B. Administer 100 mg thiamine and 50 ml of $D_{50}W$ as prescribed if alcohol ingestion or hypoglycemia is suspected (thiamine is given with the dextrose to prevent Wernicke's encephalopathy, especially if the patient has chronic malnutrition)
   C. Administer benzodiazepine or other drugs if seizures persist after dextrose and thiamine
      1. Diazepam (Valium) (see Table 7-8)
      2. Lorazepam (Ativan) (see Table 7-8)
      3. Phenytoin (Dilantin) (see Table 7-8)
      4. Phenobarbital (see Table 7-8)
      5. Neuromuscular blockade may be initiated
      6. General anesthesia may be needed on rare occasion
   D. Prepare patient for surgical procedures, which may be required for removal of tumor, hematoma, abscess
V. Monitor and assess condition closely to prevent complications
   A. Insert nasogastric tube to prevent vomiting and aspiration
   B. Initiate IV for medications
   C. Monitor cardiac rate and rhythm and BP
   D. Have cardiovascular drugs available
   E. Assess neurologic status frequently
   F. Treat hyperthermia with antipyretics or hypothermia blanket
VI. Monitor and document duration of seizure activity, patient's LOC, drugs
   A. Aura: presence or absence; nature if present
   B. Cry: presence or absence
   C. Onset: site of initial body movements, deviation of head and eyes, chewing and salivation, posture of body, sensory changes
   D. Tonic and clonic phases: movement of body during progression, skin color and airway, pupillary changes, incontinence, duration of each phase
   E. Relaxation phase: duration and behavior
   F. Postictal phase: duration, ability to remember anything about the seizure, orientation, pupillary changes, headache, injuries
   G. Duration: from aura to relaxation
   H. Drugs administered
VII. Maintain fluid and electrolyte balance
   A. Assess electrolytes, calcium and magnesium, renal and hepatic function
   B. Monitor for indications of myoglobinuria (e.g., tea- or cola-colored urine); administer treatment for myoglobinuria as prescribed (fluids and osmotic diuretics [e.g., mannitol])
VIII. Provide reassurance and comfort during postictal period
   A. Elevate head of bed 30 degrees
   B. Reassure and reorient patient as he or she awakens
   C. Provide privacy and calm environment
   D. Discretely clean patient if incontinent
   E. Allow the patient to sleep
IX. Monitor for complications
   A. Injury during seizure
   B. Acute respiratory failure
   C. Aspiration
   D. Acid-base imbalance, electrolyte imbalance
      1. Respiratory or metabolic acidosis
      2. Hyperkalemia
   E. Hypoglycemia
   F. Hyperthermia
   G. Renal failure related to myoglobinuria
   H. Permanent neurologic damage

Table 7-8	Anticonvulsant Drugs		
Drug	**IV Dosage**	**Onset/ Duration of Action**	**Adverse Effects**
Diazepam (Valium)	0.15-0.25 mg/kg at a rate of no faster than 2 mg/min	1-3 minutes/15-30 minutes	• Respiratory depression • Tachycardia • Hypotension • Dysrhythmias
Lorazepam (Ativan)	0.1-0.2 mg/kg (not to exceed 8 mg/kg) at a rate no faster than 2 mg/min	6-10 minutes/12-24 minutes	• Respiratory depression • Tachycardia • Hypotension • Dysrhythmias
Phenytoin sodium (Dilantin)	10-20 mg/kg at a rate no faster than 50 mg/min; must be mixed in saline	10-30 minutes/24 hours	• Hypotension • Dysrhythmias • Hepatitis • Nephritis • Blood dyscrasias
Fosphenytoin (Cerebyx)	10-20 phenytoin equivalent (PE) mg/kg at a rate no faster than 150 mg/min	10-30 minutes/24 hours	• Hypotension • Dysrhythmias • Nephritis • Blood dyscrasias
Phenobarbital (Phenobarbital Sodium, Luminal)	20 mg/kg at a rate no faster than 60 mg/min	20-30 minutes/48 hours	• Respiratory depression • Hypotension • Angioedema • Thrombophlebitis

CNS Infections

Definitions

I. Meningitis: acute inflammation of the brain and spinal cord that may involve all meningeal membranes; may be bacterial, fungal, or viral

II. Encephalitis: acute inflammation of the parenchyma of the brain and meninges

III. Brain abscess: accumulation of pus within the brain tissue; surrounded by inflamed tissue

Etiology

I. Meningitis

A. Bacterial

  1. Associated factors

    a) Otitis media

    b) Sinusitis, upper respiratory infection, or pneumonia

    c) Penetrating head injury

    d) Basal skull fracture

    e) Intracranial surgery

    f) ICP monitoring

    g) Septicemia, septic embolus

  2. Organisms

    a) *Haemophilus influenzae*

    b) *Neisseria meningitidis* (meningococcal)

    c) *Diplococcus pneumoniae* (pneumococcal)

    d) *Streptococcus pneumoniae*

    e) *Escherichia coli*

    f) *Enterobacter*

    g) *Klebsiella*

    h) *Pseudomonas*

    i) *Serratia*

    j) *Salmonella*

    k) Gonococcus

B. Fungal

  1. Associated factors

    a) Immunosuppression

      (1) AIDS

      (2) Histoplasmosis

      (3) Postorgan transplantation

      (4) Steroid therapy

      (5) Cancer

    b) Contaminated needles or syringes from drug abuse

  2. Organisms

    a) Cryptococcosis

    b) Coccidioidomycosis

    c) Mucormycosis

    d) Candidiasis

    e) Aspergillosis

C. Viral

  1. Associated factors

    a) Immunosuppression

  2. Organisms

    a) Coxsackievirus

    b) Echovirus

    c) Adenovirus

    d) Arbovirus

    e) Poliovirus

    f) Herpes simplex virus

    g) Myxovirus (e.g., influenza, mumps, measles)

    h) Western equine

D. Parasitic

  1. *Plasmodium* (malaria)

  2. *Toxoplasma gondii*

II. Encephalitis (almost always viral)

A. Associated factors

  1. Mosquito or tick bite (arbovirus)

2. Recent viral infection
3. Recent vaccination: measles, mumps, rubella
B. Organisms
   1. Arbovirus
   2. Herpes simplex
   3. Rubella
   4. Rubeola
   5. Mumps
   6. Mononucleosis
III. Brain abscess
   A. Associated factors
      1. Middle-ear and mastoid infection
      2. Sinus infection
      3. Penetrating head injuries
      4. Compound fractures
      5. Osteomyelitis of the skull
      6. Metastatic abscess
   B. Organisms
      1. *Streptococci*
      2. *Staphylococci*
      3. *Pneumococci*

Pathophysiology

I. Meningitis
   A. Pathologic organisms gain access to subarachnoid space and meninges
   B. Exudate forms in subarachnoid space and inflammation of meninges occurs
   C. Congestion of tissues and blood vessels
   D. Hyperemia of meningeal vessels
   E. Intracranial hypertension may result from hydrocephalus or cerebral edema
II. Encephalitis: virus acts as an intracellular parasite, damaging the nervous system by destroying selected neuronal cells
III. Brain abscess
   A. Bacteria is introduced into the brain tissue
   B. Local edema, hyperemia, infiltration by leukocytes, and softening of the parenchyma occurs
   C. Surrounding brain tissue becomes necrotic and edematous
   D. Central liquefaction occurs and becomes encapsulated
   E. The abscess acts as a mass lesion and may cause intracranial hypertension

Clinical Presentation

I. Meningitis
   A. Subjective
      1. History of precipitating event or condition
      2. Headache that gets progressively worse
      3. Chills
      4. Nausea, vomiting
      5. Photophobia, pain when moving eyes
   B. Objective
      1. Infectious signs
         a) Fever
         b) Tachycardia
         c) Chills
         d) Skin rash: most likely with meningococcal meningitis

2. Meningeal irritation
   a) Headache
   b) Nuchal rigidity
   c) Brudzinski's sign
   d) Kernig's sign
3. Neurologic abnormalities
   a) Change in LOC
   b) Cranial nerve involvement (e.g., pupil changes)
   c) Focal neurologic signs
   d) Seizures
C. Diagnostic
   1. Serum
      a) Blood cultures: may be positive for causative organism
      b) WBC: elevated
   2. LP
      a) Elevated CSF pressure (normal LP 80-180 mm/H_2O, measured at lumbar level, with patient in side-lying position)
      b) Increased WBCs in CSF
      c) Elevated protein in CSF in most cases
      d) Decreased glucose content in CSF in bacterial meningitis (glucose in CSF is normally 60% of serum glucose)
      e) CSF is cloudy in bacterial meningitis
      f) Glucose content in CSF is normal and CSF is clear in viral meningitis
      g) Culture: may identify organism
      h) CT: normal
II. Encephalitis
   A. Subjective
      1. History may include precipitating event or condition
      2. Headache
      3. Blurred vision, diplopia
      4. Weakness
      5. Dysphagia
   B. Objective
      1. Change in level of consciousness
      2. Fever
      3. Nuchal rigidity
      4. Dysphasia, aphasia
      5. Hemiparesis
      6. Nystagmus
      7. Facial muscle weakness
      8. Seizures
   C. Diagnostic
      1. Lumbar puncture
         a) Elevated or normal pressure
         b) Elevated protein
         c) Increased WBC
         d) Normal or low glucose
         e) Culture: may identify organism
      2. Brain biopsy: required for diagnosis of herpes simplex encephalitis
      3. EEG: may show seizure activity
      4. CT: normal early in course; low-density lesions may be seen later
      5. MRI: may be more definitive than CT scan

III. Brain abscess
  A. Subjective
    1. History may include precipitating event or condition
    2. Headache: constant and severe; increased with straining
    3. Malaise
    4. Irritability
    5. Chills
    6. Nausea, vomiting
    7. Muscle weakness
    8. Symptoms vary according to location of brain
  B. Objective
    1. Change in LOC
    2. Confusion
    3. Hemiplegia
    4. Fever
    5. Nuchal rigidity may be present
    6. Dysphasia/aphasia
    7. Seizures
    8. Signs vary according to location of brain
  C. Diagnostic
    1. CT scan: may show localized changes in brain density
    2. EEG: may show electrical silence at abscess location
    3. Lumbar puncture
      a) Increased pressure
      b) Increased WBC
      c) Elevated protein
      d) Normal glucose
    4. Brain biopsy: may identify organism
    5. Brain scan: locates abscess more than 1 cm in size
    6. Angiogram: locate temporal lobe and cerebellar abscesses

Nursing Diagnoses

  I. Decreased Adaptive Capacity: Intracranial related to failure of normal intracranial compensatory mechanisms
  II. Alteration in Cerebral Tissue Perfusion related to intracranial hypertension
  III. Pain related to meningeal irritation
  IV. Ineffective Airway Clearance related to increased secretions, diminished LOC, inadequate protective reflexes
  V. Risk for Fluid Volume Deficit related to decreased fluid intake, increased fluid loss, diabetes insipidus
  VI. Risk for Fluid Volume Excess related to fluid resuscitation, SIADH
  VII. Risk for Infection related to invasive procedures, traumatic wounds, surgical wounds
  VIII. Risk for Injury related to seizure activity, inadequate protective reflexes
  IX. Ineffective Individual Coping related to situational crisis, powerlessness, change in role
  X. Ineffective Family Coping related to critically ill family member

Collaborative Management

  I. Maintain airway, ventilation, and oxygenation
    A. Maintain airway
      1. Oropharyngeal or nasopharyngeal airway may be needed to hold tongue away from hypopharynx in obtunded patient
      2. Endotracheal intubation may be needed in patients without airway protective reflexes
    B. Maintain oxygenation and ventilation
      1. Administer oxygen as needed to maintain SpO_2 95% or greater unless contraindicated
      2. Initiate mechanical ventilation as needed for hypoventilation
    C. Prevent aspiration
      1. Position patient on side
      2. Have suction equipment available
  II. Treat infection
    A. Administer antibiotics (need to be fat-soluble to cross blood–brain barrier) as prescribed (e.g., usually penicillin IV or chloramphenicol IV)
    B. Administer antivirals to treat herpes simplex encephalitis as prescribed
    C. Prepare patient for surgical excision and drainage of brain abscess
  III. Prevent/monitor for clinical indications and treat intracranial hypertension (see Intracranial Hypertension section in Chapter 6); steroids may be prescribed to decrease inflammation after antibiotics are started
  IV. Maintain fluid and electrolyte balance; monitor for overhydration, diabetes insipidus
  V. Control body temperature to less than 38° C (100.4° F)
    A. Administer antipyretics
    B. Utilize hypothermia blanket
    C. Utilize meperidine (Demerol) as prescribed to control shivering
  VI. Prevent, monitor for, and control seizures
    A. Institute seizure precautions
    B. Administer anticonvulsant therapy as prescribed
  VII. Treat headache with nonsedating analgesics (e.g., codeine)
  VIII. Prevent transmission of disease; respiratory isolation is required only for meningococcal meningitis
  IX. Monitor for complications
    A. Seizures
    B. Disseminated intravascular coagulation (DIC)
    C. SIADH
    D. Cerebral edema and intracranial hypertension
    E. Subdural effusions
    F. Hydrocephalus
    G. Cranial nerve deficits
    H. Waterhouse-Friderichsen syndrome
      1. A major complication of meningococcal meningitis
      2. Overwhelming bacteremia with massive bilateral adrenal hemorrhage
      3. Causes acute adrenal crisis and potentially death
    I. Persistent neurologic deficits

LEARNING ACTIVITIES

1. **DIRECTIONS:** Match the following signs or symptoms with the neurologic conditions with which they are associated.

    ____brainstem lesion
    ____chronic subdural hematoma
    ____subarachnoid hemorrhage
    ____status epilepticus
    ____dural tear
    ____postcraniotomy
    ____upper motor neuron lesion
    ____meningeal irritation
    ____intracranial hypertension
    ____basal skull fracture

    a. Kernig's sign
    b. Babinski's reflex
    c. absence of doll's eyes (oculocephalic reflex)
    d. change in LOC, pupillary changes, respiratory pattern changes, Cushing's triad
    e. periorbital edema
    f. Battle's sign
    g. rhinorrhea
    h. personality change
    i. "worst headache of my life"
    j. myoglobinuria

2. **DIRECTIONS:** Your patient has had a hemorrhagic stroke. She has nuchal rigidity and decerebrate posturing. She does not vocalize at all and will not open her eyes even to pain. What is her Glasgow Coma Score? What grade bleed is this on the Hunt and Hess aneurysm grading scale?

3. **DIRECTIONS:** Identify the following factors as being associated with which complication of subarachnoid hemorrhage: vasospasm or rebleed.

	Vasospasm	Rebleed
Occurs most often immediately after the bleed or between 7 and 10 days after the bleed		
Caused by calcium influx into the vessel		
Occurs anytime after 3 days		
Treated by hypervolemic hemodilution and calcium channel blockers		
Caused by lysis of the protective clot		
Prevented by early clipping if the patient is stable enough		

4. **DIRECTIONS:** Describe CSF changes in the following conditions.

Bacterial meningitis	
Viral meningitis	
Subarachnoid hemorrhage	

5. **DIRECTIONS:** Describe the following types of spinal cord injuries.

Type of Injury	Motor Changes Below the Injury	Sensory Changes Below the Injury
Complete lesion		
Central cord syndrome		
Brown-Séquard syndrome		
Anterior cord syndrome		

6. **DIRECTIONS:** Identify five clinical indications of spinal shock.

    1. _____
    2. _____
    3. _____
    4. _____
    5. _____

7. **DIRECTIONS:** Complete the following table about autonomic dysreflexia.

Clinical Presentation	Collaborative Management

8. **DIRECTIONS:** List observations to make and interventions to perform during a seizure.

Observations to Make	Interventions

9. **Directions:** Complete the following crossword puzzle dealing with neurologic assessment, conditions, and treatment.

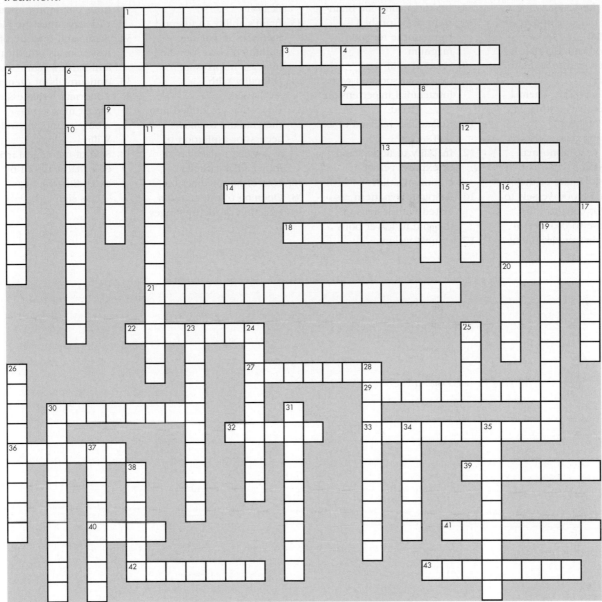

Across

1. Class of drugs used initially in status epilepticus
3. Abnormal sensitivity to light
5. Steroid often used for neurologic conditions (generic)
7. Loss of sensation
10. Testing for this reflex is also referred to as caloric testing
13. Diabetes _____ is a complication of craniotomy that causes polyuria
14. Type of asphasia that is also referred to as sensory aphasia
15. Unsteady or staggering gait
18. CSF drainage from the ear
19. Severe injury to the brain that causes prolonged unconsciousness, brainstem dysfunction, and profound residual deficits (abbrev.)
20. Side-to-side herniation
21. Temporary method to constrict cerebral vessels and decrease intracranial pressure
22. Type of paralysis seen with lower motor neuron lesion
27. Type of paralysis seen with upper motor neuron lesion
29. CSF drainage from the nose
30. Osmotic diuretic (generic)
32. Type of fracture associated with raccoon eyes and Battle's sign
33. Calcium channel blocker often used for cerebral artery spasm (generic)
36. Type of fracture that may interrupt major vascular channels and cause epidural hematoma
39. Complication of cerebral aneurysm that often occurs about 7 to 10 days after the bleed
40. Focal cerebral ischemic event that lasts longer than 24 hours (abbrev.)
41. Basal skull fractures involving this fossa may cause rhinorrhea and injury to the olfactory nerve
42. Scoring system used to standardize observation of responsiveness in neurologic patients
43. Pathologic reflex that indicates upper motor neuron lesion

Down

1. Respiratory pattern associated with lesions of the lower pons or upper medulla: ____'s
2. Type of asphasia that is also referred to as motor aphasia
4. Focal cerebral ischemia that resolves within 24 hours (abbrev.)
5. Posturing that is also referred to as abnormal extension
6. Intrinsic ability of the cerebral blood vessels to dilate or constrict in response to changes in the brain's environment

8. Herniation with downward shift of the brain, causing the brainstem to be pushed through the foramen magnum
9. Triad of vital sign changes associated with intracranial hypertension: ____'s triad
11. Reflex also referred to as doll's eyes
12. Inability to understand or express verbal communication
16. Respiratory pattern associated with lesions of the mid to lower pons
17. Double vision

19. Posturing that is also referred to as abnormal flexion
23. Brain's ability to tolerate increases in volume without a corresponding increase in pressure
24. Difficulty with swallowing
25. Holes that are drilled into the cranium to allow access for aspiration of a clot or to place an intracranial catheter
26. Loss of motor function
28. Opening of the cranium
30. Infection of the meninges

31. Complication of cerebral aneurysm that occurs most commonly about 3 to 5 days after the bleed
34. Basal skull fracture of this fossa causes otorrhea and Battle's sign
35. Anticonvulsant (generic)
37. Abnormal weakness of artery; most commonly occurs in circle of Willis
38. Sign of meningeal irritation that is tested by extending the leg: ____'s sign

LEARNING ACTIVITIES ANSWERS

1.

_c_ brainstem lesion	a.	Kernig's sign
_h_ chronic subdural hematoma	b.	Babinski's reflex
_i_ subarachnoid hemorrhage	c.	absence of doll's eyes (oculocephalic reflex)
_j_ status epilepticus	d.	change in LOC, pupillary changes, respiratory pattern changes, Cushing's triad
_g_ dural tear	e.	periorbital edema
_e_ postcraniotomy	f.	Battle's sign
_b_ upper motor neuron lesion	g.	rhinorrhea
_a_ meningeal irritation	h.	personality change
_d_ intracranial hypertension	i.	"worst headache of my life"
_f_ basal skull fracture	j.	myoglobinuria

2. GCS: 4

Hunt and Hess aneurysm grade: V

3.

	Vasospasm	Rebleed
Occurs either immediately after the bleed or between 7 and 10 days after the bleed		✔
Caused by calcium influx into the vessel	✔	
Occurs anytime after 3 days	✔	
Treated by hypervolemic hemodilution and calcium channel blockers	✔	
Caused by lysis of the protective clot		✔
Prevented by early clipping if the patient is stable enough		✔

4.

Bacterial meningitis	• Elevated pressure • Increased WBC • Normal or elevated protein • Decreased glucose • Cloudy appearance
Viral meningitis	• Elevated pressure • Normal or increased WBC • Normal or elevated protein • Clear appearance
Subarachnoid hemorrhage	• Elevated protein • Bloody appearance if acute • Dark amber (xanthochromic) if >5 days old

5.

Type of Injury	Motor Changes Below the Injury	Sensory Changes Below the Injury
Complete lesion	Complete loss	Complete loss
Central cord syndrome	Greater loss in upper extremities than in lower extremities	Varies
Brown-Séquard syndrome	Ipsilateral loss	Iipsilateral loss of position and vibratory sense Contralateral loss of pain and temperature
Anterior cord syndrome	Complete loss	Loss of pain and temperature

6. 1. Flaccid paralysis and areflexia below the level of the injury
2. Bradycardia
3. Hypotension
4. Paralytic ileus
5. Urinary retention

7.

Clinical Presentation	Collaborative Management
Throbbing headache Blurred vision Nasal congestion Flushing of the face and neck Anxiety Hypertension Bradycardia Sweating above the lesion	Place patient in sitting position or elevate the head of bed 30-45 degrees Identify cause: check bladder, check rectum, check skin Eliminate cause: irrigate or change indwelling bladder catheter, insert straight urinary catheter, disimpact the rectum using Nupercainal ointment Administer antihypertensive agents

8.

Observations to Make	Interventions
Preceding events: Was there an aura?	• Do not leave patient; provide privacy
Onset: • Body movements • Deviation of head and eyes • Chewing and salivation • Posture of body • Sensory changes	• Loosen clothing • Open airway but do not try to pry mouth open; nasopharyngeal or nasotracheal airways may be used if necessary • Turn patient to side • Administer oxygen • Do not restrain; gentle guiding of extremities is acceptable
Tonic and clonic phases: • Progression of movements of the body • Skin color and airway • Pupillary changes • Incontinence • Duration of each phase	• Pad siderails with blankets or pillows • Administer anticonvulsants (e.g., diazepam, phenytoin) • Reorient patient after seizure • Clean patient if incontinence has occurred • Allow patient to sleep
Level of consciousness during seizure	
Postictal phase • Duration • General behavior • Memory of events • Orientation • Pupillary changes • Headache • Aphasia • Injuries	
Duration of entire seizure	
Medications given and response	

9.

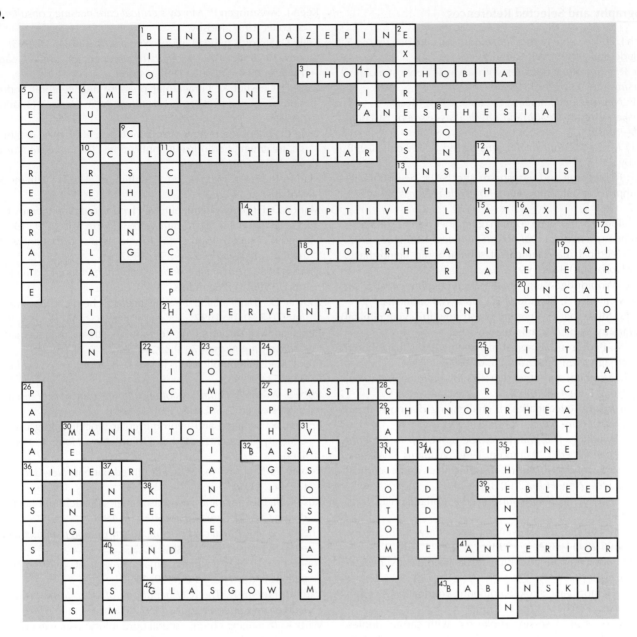

Across / Down crossword grid:

1. BENZODIAZEPINE
3. PHOTOPHOBIA
5. DEXAMETHASONE
7. ANESTHESIA
10. OCULOVESTIBULAR
13. INSIPIDUS
14. RECEPTIVE
15. ATAXIC
18. OTORRHEA
19. DAI
20. UNCAL
21. HYPERVENTILATION
22. FLACCID
27. SPASTIC
29. RHINORRHEA
30. MANNITOL
32. BASAL
33. NIMODIPINE
36. LINEAR
39. REBLEED
40. RIND
41. ANTERIOR
42. GLASGOW
43. BABINSKI

Down:
1. BIO
2. EXR
4. TORSSION
6. BUTREGULATION
8. HON
9. CSHING
11. OULOCEPHAIC
12. AHH
16. PNEA
17. DP
23. COMPLIANCE
24. DYGIAS
25. BURR
26. PARALYSIS
27. SPHGIA
28. CRATOMY
31. VSOSPASM
34. MIDDLE
35. PHNY
37. ANEURYSM
38. KERNIG

Bibliography and Selected References

Alspach J, editor: *Core curriculum for critical care nursing,* ed 5, Philadelphia, 1998, WB Saunders.

Arbour R: Controlling seizures with a vagal nerve stimulator, *Nursing97* 27 (6):32cc1, 1997.

Baker E: *Neuroscience nursing,* St Louis, 1994, Mosby.

Barkauskas V et al: *Health and physical assessment,* St Louis, 1994, Mosby.

Beare P, Myers J: *Adult health nursing,* ed 3, St Louis, 1998, Mosby.

Bleck T: Rebleeding and vasospasm after SAH: new strategies for improving outcome, *Journal of Critical Illness* 12(9):572, 1997.

Bleck T: Today's approach to managing aneurysmal subarachnoid hemorrhage, *Journal of Critical Illness* 12(6):347, 1997.

Bleck T: Medical management of subarachnoid hemorrhage, *New Horiz* 5 (4):387, 1997.

Boggs R, Wooldridge-King M: *AACN procedure manual for critical care,* ed 3, Philadelphia, 1993, WB Saunders.

Bouma G, Muizelaar P: Cerebral blood flow in severe clinical head injury, *New Horiz* 3 (3):384, 1995.

Brisman M, Bederson J: Surgical management of subarachnoid hemorrhage, *New Horiz* 5 (4):376, 1997.

Bullock R: Mannitol and other diuretics in severe neurotrauma, *New Horiz* 3 (3):448, 1995.

Campbell J: Viral encephalitis: a challenging diagnosis in an ICU, *Critical Care Nurse* 18 (3):58, 1998.

Chernow B, editor: *The pharmacologic approach to the critically ill patient,* ed 3, Baltimore, 1994, Williams & Wilkins.

Chestnut R: Secondary brain results after head injury: clinical perspectives, *New Horiz* 3 (3):366 1995.

Clochesy J et al: *Critical care nursing,* ed 2, Philadelphia, 1996, WB Saunders.

Cunning S, Houdek D: Preventing secondary brain injury, *Nursing98* 28 (11):32cc1, 1998.

Davies P: Caring for patients with diabetes insipidus, *Nursing96* 26 (5):62, 1996.

Franges E: Hemorrhagic stroke: promoting your patient's recovery, *Nursing98* 28 (6):32hn1, 1998.

French-Sherry et al: Assessing stroke risk with carotid duplex ultrasound scanning, *Journal of Critical Illness* 13 (7):448, 1998.

Gahart B, Nazareno A: *1999 intravenous medications,* St Louis, 1999, Mosby.

Gawlinski A, Hamwi D: *Acute care nurse practitioner clinical curriculum and certification review,* Philadelphia, 1999, WB Saunders.

Keen J, Swearingen P: *Mosby's critical care nursing consultant,* St Louis, 1997, Mosby.

Kelly D: Steroids in head injury, *New Horiz* 3 (3):453, 1995.

Kinney M et al: *AACN clinical reference for critical care nursing,* ed 4, St Louis, 1998, Mosby.

Lang E, Chesnut R: Intracranial pressure and cerebral perfusion pressure in severe head injury, *New Horiz* 3 (3):400, 1995.

Long L: Epilepsy: a review of seizure types, etiologies, diagnosis, treatment, and nursing implications, *Critical Care Nurse* 16 (4):83, 1996.

Marino P: *The ICU book,* ed 2, Baltimore, 1998, Williams & Wilkins.

Marion D, Firlik A, McLaughlin M: Hyperventilation therapy for severe traumatic brain injury, *New Horiz* 3 (3):439, 1995.

McNew C, Hunt S, Warner L: How to help your patient with epilepsy, *Nursing97* 27 (9):57, 1997.

Mims B et al: *Critical care skills: a clinical handbook,* Philadelphia, 1996, WB Saunders.

Mower D: Brain attack: treating acute ischemic CVA, *Nursing97* 27 (3):35, 1997.

Petterson M: Thrombolytic therapy in stroke management, *Critical Care Nurse* 17 (5):89, 1997.

Piek J: Medical complications in severe head injury, *New Horiz* 3 (3):534, 1995.

Price S, Wilson L: *Pathophysiology: clinical concepts of disease processes,* ed 5, St Louis, 1997, Mosby.

Prielipp R; Sedative and neuromuscular blocking drug use in critically ill patients with head injury, *New Horiz* 3 (3):456, 1995.

Roberts P: Nutrition in the head-injured patient, *New Horiz* 3 (3):506, 1995.

Rusy K: Rebleeding and vasospasm after subarachnoid hemorrhage, *Critical Care Nurse* 16 (1):41, 1996.

Thelan L et al: *Critical care nursing: diagnosis and management,* ed 3, St Louis, 1998, Mosby.

Tonneson A: Hemodynamic management of brain-injured patients, *New Horiz* 3 (3):499, 1995.

Varon J, Fromm R: *The ICU handbook of facts, formulas, and laboratory values,* St Louis, 1997, Mosby.

Wirtz K: Managing chronic spinal cord injury: issues in critical care, *Critical Care Nurse* 16 (4):24, 1996.

Zhuang J et al: Colloid infusion after brain injury: effect on intracranial pressure, cerebral blood flow, and oxygen delivery, *Crit Care Med* 23 (1):140, 1995.

Zornow M, Prough D: Fluid management in patients with traumatic brain injury, *New Horiz* 3 (3):488, 1995.

Gastrointestinal System

Selected Concepts in Anatomy and Physiology

General Information About the Gastrointestinal System

I. Functions of the gastrointestinal system
   A. Digestion and absorption of nutrients
   B. Elimination of waste material
   C. Detoxification and elimination of bacteria, viruses, chemical toxins, and drugs

II. Process of the gastrointestinal system (Fig. 8-1)
   A. Ingestion
   B. Digestion
   C. Absorption
   D. Elimination

III. Structures of the gastrointestinal system (Fig. 8-2)
   A. Alimentary canal: from the mouth to the anus
      1. Oropharynx
      2. Esophagus
      3. Stomach
      4. Small intestine: divided into duodenum, jejunum, and ileum
      5. Large intestine: divided into cecum, ascending colon, transverse colon, descending colon, sigmoid colon, and rectum
   B. Accessory organs of digestions
      1. Liver
      2. Gallbladder
      3. Pancreas

IV. Cell layers (Fig. 8-3)
   A. All areas of the gastrointestinal tract have the same cell layers (external to internal)
      1. Serosa: outermost layer that is often continuous with the peritoneum
      2. Muscularis
      3. Submucosa
      4. Mucosa: innermost layer that is exposed to dietary nutrients

V. Peritoneum
   A. The abdominal viscera is covered by the peritoneum
      1. The parietal layer lines the abdominal cavity wall
      2. The visceral layer covers the abdominal organs
      3. The peritoneal cavity is a potential space between the parietal and visceral layers
   B. The peritoneum has two folds
      1. The mesentery contains blood and lymph vessels and attaches the small intestine and part of the large intestine to the posterior abdominal wall
      2. The omentum contains fat and lymph nodes
         a) Lesser omentum from lesser curvature of stomach and upper duodenum to the liver
         b) Greater omentum from stomach over the intestines

Alimentary Canal

I. Oropharynx
   A. Location: mouth to esophagus
   B. Description
      1. Oral cavity
         a) Lips
         b) Cheeks
         c) Palate
         d) Teeth
         e) Tongue
            (1) Mucus glands
            (2) Serous glands
         f) Salivary glands
            (1) Parotid glands (2)
            (2) Submandibular glands (2)
            (3) Sublingual glands (2)
      2. Muscles of mastication
      3. Pharynx
         a) Nasopharynx
         b) Oropharynx
         c) Laryngopharynx
   C. Secretions: saliva (Table 8-1)
      1. Stimulated by the thought, sight, smell, or taste of food
      2. Consists of:
         a) Ptyalin (amylase): begins the breakdown

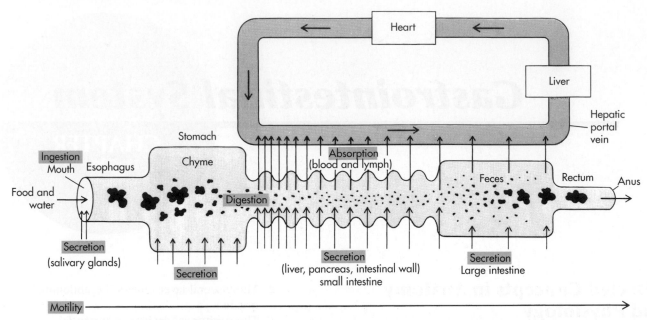

Figure 8-1 Summary of processes of the gastrointestinal system. (From Kinney MR, Packa DR, Dunbar SB: *AACN's clinical reference for critical-care nursing,* ed 4, St Louis, 1998, Mosby.)

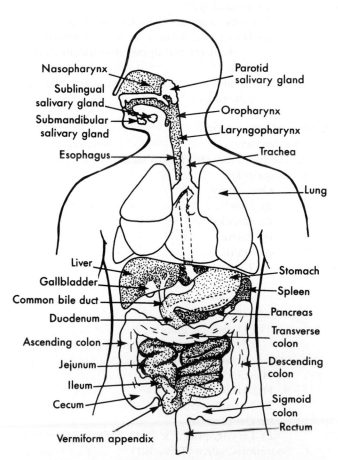

Figure 8-2 Structures of the gastrointestinal system. (From Kinney MR, Packa DR, Dunbar SB: *AACN's clinical reference for critical-care nursing,* ed 4, St Louis, 1998, Mosby.)

of polysaccharides (starches) to disaccharides
b) Mucus: provides lubricant
3. Volume: 1,500 ml/day
D. Process
1. The teeth break up the food into smaller pieces to increase surface area for digestive enzymes to act upon
2. The masseter muscles are innervated by cranial nerve V (trigeminal)
3. The tongue moves the food around in the mouth for better chewing and moves the food to the back of the throat to begin the process of swallowing
4. Swallowing (deglutination) (Fig. 8-4) consists of three stages; only stage one occurs in the mouth
a) Voluntary: the tongue forces the bolus of food into the pharynx
b) Pharyngeal: the bolus of food passes from the pharynx to the esophagus; the epiglottis closes to protect the larynx
c) Esophageal: the bolus of food passes from the esophagus to the gastroesophageal sphincter
E. Functions: Table 8-2
II. Esophagus
A. Location
1. Lies behind the trachea
2. Passes through the thoracic cavity and the diaphragm; passes through the diaphragm at the diaphragmatic hiatus

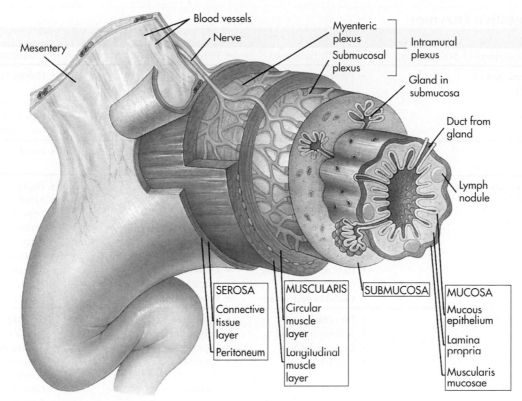

Figure 8-3 Cell layers of the gastrointestinal tract. (From Doughty DB, Jackson DB: *Gastrointestinal disorders: Mosby's clinical nursing series,* St Louis, 1993, Mosby.)

B. Description: hollow tube from the pharynx to the stomach; approximately 25 cm in length and 2 cm in diameter

C. Structure (Fig. 8-5)
1. Cell layers (external to internal)
   a) Does not have a serosa layer
   b) Muscularis
      (1) Type of muscle
         (a) Upper one third: skeletal muscle
         (b) Lower two thirds: smooth muscle
      (2) Direction of muscle
         (a) Inner: circular
         (b) Outer: longitudinal
   c) Submucosa
   d) Mucosa: lined with mucous membrane that secretes a protective mucoid substance
2. Sphincters
   a) Hypopharyngeal
      (1) Also referred to as the *upper esophageal sphincter* (UES)
      (2) Made of cricopharyngeal muscle
   b) Gastroesophageal
      (1) Also referred to as the *lower esophageal sphincter* (LES)
      (2) A physiologic rather than anatomic sphincter: consists of the last 2 to 4 cm of the esophagus

D. Secretions: mucus

E. Process: final phase of swallowing (involuntary)
1. When a bolus of food enters the esophagus, the hypopharyngeal sphincter opens
2. Food is moved through the esophagus by gravity and peristaltic action; peristalsis is the alternating contraction and relaxation of muscle fibers, which propels the substance in a wavelike motion through the esophagus, stomach, and intestines
3. The gastroesophageal sphincter opens and food enters the stomach
4. The process takes 5 to 10 seconds

F. Functions: Table 8-2

III. Stomach (Fig. 8-6)
A. Location: inferior to the diaphragm, with approximately 80% to 85% of the organ to the left of midline
B. Description
1. Largest dilation of the GI tract
2. Approximately 25 to 30 cm in length and 10 to 15 cm at maximal diameter
3. Relatively little muscle tone, which permits increased distention
C. Structure
1. Anatomic divisions
   a) Cardia: portion of stomach that immediately adjoins the esophagus
   b) Fundus: dome-shaped portion of stomach that extends left of the cardia

Table 8-1 **Digestive Enzymes**

Source	Enzyme	What it Acts On	What is Produced
Salivary glands (saliva) (1,500 ml/day)	• Ptyalin (amylase)	• Polysaccharides (starches)	• Disaccharides
Stomach (gastric juice) (2,500 ml/day)	• Pepsin	• Proteins	• Polypeptides
	• Gastric lipase	• Emulsified fats	• Fatty acids • Glycerol
	• Rennin	• Soluble milk protein	• Insoluble form
Liver (bile) (500 ml/day)	• None	• Nonemulsified fats	• Emulsified fats
Pancreas (pancreatic juice) (1,500 ml/day)	• Trypsin	• Denatured proteins • Polypeptides	• Peptides • Amino acids
	• Chymotrypsin	• Proteins • Polypeptides	• Peptides • Amino acids
	• Pancreatic lipase	• Emulsified fats	• Fatty acids • Glycerol
	• Pancreatic amylase	• Disaccharides	• Monosaccharides
	• Nucleases	• Nucleic acids	• Nucleotides
	• Carboxypeptidase	• Polypeptides	• Smaller polypeptides
Small intestine (1,000 ml/day)	• Enterokinase	• Trypsinogen	• Trypsin
	• Aminopeptidase	• Polypeptides	• Smaller polypeptides
	• Dipeptidase	• Dipeptides	• Amino acids
	• Sucrase	• Sucrose	• Glucose • Fructose
	• Lactase	• Lactose	• Glucose • Galactose
	• Maltase	• Maltose	• Glucose
	• Nucleotidase	• Nucleotides	• Nucleosides • Phosphoric acid
	• Nucleosidase	• Nucleosides	• Purine • Pentose
	• Intestinal lipase	• Fat	• Glycerides • Fatty acids • Glycerol

c) Greater curvature: lateral, convex side
d) Body: major area (belly) of stomach
e) Lesser curvature: medial, concave side
f) Antrum: lower portion close to pylorus
2. Sphincters
  a) Cardiac: between esophagus and stomach
  b) Pyloric: between stomach and duodenum
3. Layers of stomach wall (external to internal)
  a) Serosa: continuous with the peritoneum
  b) Muscularis
    (1) Outer: longitudinal muscle fibers
    (2) Middle: circular muscle fibers
    (3) Inner: transverse muscle fibers
  c) Submucosa
    (1) Blood vessels
    (2) Lymph vessels
    (3) Connective tissue
    (4) Fibrous tissues
  d) Mucosa: contains rugae, which are thick folds on the interior of the stomach; rugae do all of the following:
    (1) Increase surface area for exposure
    (2) Allow for distention

    (3) Contain the openings of the gastric glands
  e) Gastric glands
    (1) Cardiac glands: just distal to the gastroesophageal junction; secrete pepsinogen, mucus
    (2) Oxyntic glands: fundic area
      (a) Mucous neck cells secrete mucus
      (b) Chief cells secrete pepsinogen
      (c) Oxyntic (also referred to as *parietal*) cells secrete:
        (i) Hydrochloric acid
        (ii) Intrinsic factor
      (d) Enterochromaffin (endocrine) cells secrete serotonin
    (3) Pyloric glands: antral area
      (a) Gastrin secreted by G-cells
      (b) Serotonin secreted by enterochromaffin cells
D. Secretions: Table 8-1
  1. Gastric secretions are clear and contain water, salts, enzymes, hydrochloric acid

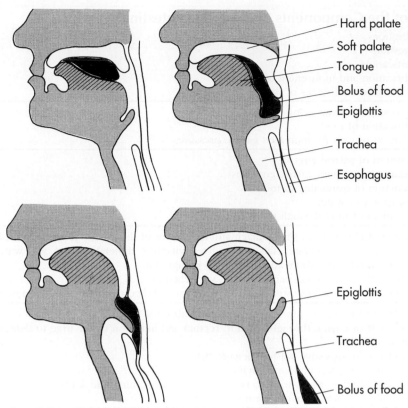

Hard palate
Soft palate
Tongue
Bolus of food
Epiglottis
Trachea
Esophagus

Epiglottis
Trachea
Bolus of food

Figure 8-4   The swallowing mechanism. (From Abels LF: *Critical care nursing,* St Louis, 1986, Mosby.)

2. Gastric secretions are stimulated when a bolus of food enters the upper portion of the stomach
3. Gastric secretions contain the following:
   a) Hydrochloric acid
      (1) Stimulated by: histamine, acetylcholine, gastrin
      (2) Functions include the following:
         (a) Denatures protein and break intermolecular bonds
         (b) Activates a number of enzymes secreted by stomach
         (c) Kills bacteria
   b) Pepsinogen
      (1) Pepsinogen is activated by hydrochloric acid to form pepsin
      (2) Pepsin catalyzes splitting of bonds between particular types of amino acids in protein chains
   c) Intrinsic factor: mucoprotein necessary for intestinal absorption of vitamin B_{12} in the ileum; deficiency of vitamin B_{12} causes pernicious anemia
   d) Mucus: contributes to the maintenance of the gastric mucosal barrier
4. Control of gastric secretions
   a) Cephalic phase
      (1) Mediated by parasympathetic nervous system (PNS)
      (2) Release of hydrochloric acid (HCl) when stimulated by thought, sight, smell, or taste of food
   b) Gastric phase
      (1) Enhances acid secretion
      (2) Stimulated by distention of stomach and digestion products of food
   c) Intestinal phase
      (1) Continuation of gastric acid secretion but in lesser amounts
      (2) Stimulated by distention, hypertonic solution, acid, and fat within duodenum
E. Process
   1. As food moves toward the pyloric sphincter at the distal end of the stomach, peristaltic waves increase in force and intensity
   2. The food bolus becomes a substance known as *chyme*
   3. Gastric motility is affected and controlled by various factors
      a) Affected by the following:
         (1) Quantity and pH of contents
         (2) Degree of mixing

Table 8-2	Functions of the Components of the Gastrointestinal System
Oropharynx	• Salivation • Ingestion • Mastication • Lubrication and moistening of food • First and second stages of swallowing
Esophagus	• Third stage of swallowing • Lubrication of food • Provision of vent for increased gastric pressures
Stomach	• Secretion of gastric enzymes • Mixing of food with gastric enzymes • Reduction of osmolality of food • Absorption of water • Movement of food through the pylorus
Small intestine	• Receipt of chyme from the stomach and movement of the chyme forward to facilitate proper absorption of proteins, carbohydrates, fats, electrolytes, vitamins, minerals, drugs, and water • Receipt of bile and pancreatic fluid to aid in digestion • Movement of chyme via peristalsis and segmentation • Bacteria in the small intestine help break down and digest protein and, to some degree, fat
Large intestine	• Secretion of mucus to lubricate and protect intestinal lining • Movement of chyme through colon to rectum and initiation of the urge to defecate • Storage of feces • Elimination of digestive wastes (defecation) • Absorption of water and electrolytes • Synthesis of vitamins (folic acid, riboflavin, vitamin K, nicotinic acid) • Metabolism of blood urea to ammonia
Liver	• Secretion of bilirubin, bile salts, cholesterol, fatty acids, calcium, and other electrolytes into bile • Storage of amino acids, glucose, vitamins, minerals (copper, iron), and blood • Vitamins: riboflavin, nicotinic acid, pyridoxine, vitamins A, D, E, K, B_{12} • Conversion of complex sugars to simple sugars • Conversion of carbohydrates to fats • Conversion of stored glucose (glycogen) to glucose (process is called *glycogenolysis*) • Conversion of amino acids and fats to glucose (process is called *gluconeogenesis*) • Conversion of amino acids to fatty acids and triglycerides • Formation of phospholipids and cholesterol • Formation of lipoproteins from triglycerides and peptides • Conversion of amino acids to plasma proteins (e.g., albumin, fibrinogen, globulins) • Phagocytosis of old RBCs • Formation of clotting factors and heparin • Conversion of ammonia to urea • Conversion of creatine to creatinine • Conversion of vitamin D_3 to 25-hydroxycholecalciferol • Detoxification of bacteria • Biotransformation of drugs to active and/or inactive metabolites • Deactivation of certain hormones
Gallbladder	• Collection, concentration, and storage of bile • Passageway for bile from liver to intestine • Regulation of bile flow • Release of bile

Pancreas	• Exocrine function
	  • Secretion of pancreatic juice for digestion of carbohydrates, proteins, and fats
	  • Secretion of bicarbonate to neutralize chyme
	• Endocrine function
	  • Secretion of insulin and glucagon

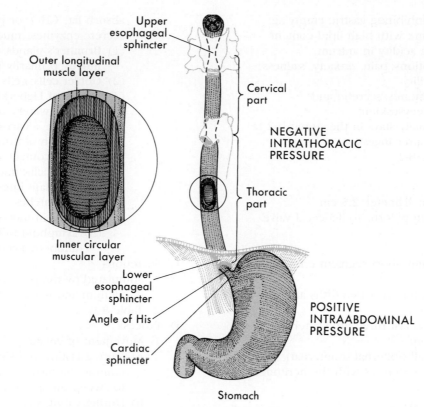

Figure 8-5   Anatomy of the esophagus. (From Beare PG, Myers JL: *Principles and practice of adult health nursing,* ed 2, St Louis, 1994, Mosby.)

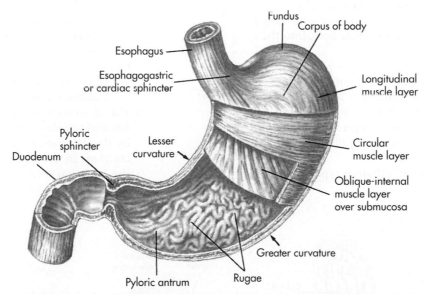

Figure 8-6   Anatomy of the stomach. (From Thompson JM et al: *Mosby's clinical nursing,* ed 3, St Louis, 1993, Mosby.)

(3) Peristalsis
(4) Ability of the duodenum to accept the chyme
b) Controlled by the following:
  (1) Sympathetic and parasympathetic nervous systems
  (2) Reflexes
  (3) Gastric hormones
4. Chyme is pumped through the pyloric sphincter into the duodenum

5. The stomach empties as chyme moves through the pyloric channel
  a) Rate of gastric emptying proportional to the volume of the stomach's contents
  b) Regulation of gastric emptying affected by the following:
    (1) Consistency of the fluid chyme; liquids selectively move through the pylorus before solids
    (2) Receptiveness of the duodenum

c) Factors inhibiting gastric emptying:
   (1) Chyme with high lipid content
   (2) High acidity in antrum
   (3) Emotions: pain, anxiety, sadness, hostility
   (4) Hormones: secretin and cholecystokinin
d) Food usually stays in the stomach 2 to 6 hours after ingestion

F. Function: Table 8-2

IV. Small intestine
  A. Description
    1. Length: 7 m; diameter: 2.5 cm
    2. Extends from pylorus to ileocecal valve
  B. Structure
    1. Divisions
      a) Duodenum: short segment only 30 cm long
      b) Jejunum: the next two fifths after the duodenum
      c) Ileum: the last three fifths after the duodenum
    2. Layers of wall (external to internal)
      a) Serosa: continuous with the peritoneum
      b) Muscular
      c) Submucosal
      d) Mucosal
    3. Sphincters
      a) Pylorus: from stomach to duodenum
      b) Ileocecal: controls flow of contents into large intestine and prevents reflux from the large intestine back into the ileum
    4. Villi (Fig. 8-7)
      a) Fingerlike projections of mucosa and submucosa prominent in duodenum and jejunum increase surface area
      b) Contain a single lymph vessel called a *lateal* and a dense capillary bed to aid in absorption
      c) Contain many different types of cells to absorb fat, CHO, or protein and/or to secrete enzymes, mucus
      (1) Brunner's glands: cells that secrete mucus; primarily in duodenum
      (2) Goblet cells: cells that secrete mucus
      (3) Crypts of Lieberkühn: cells that produce watery mucus called *succus entericus*, a carrier substance for absorption of nutrients when the villi come in contact with the chyme
      (4) Paneth's cells: uncertain function but may regulate intestinal flora
      (5) Peyer's patches
        (a) Cells in mucosa and submucosa
        (b) Lymphoid follicles that carry out antibody synthesis

  C. Secretions
    1. Stimulated by the presence of chyme in the duodenum and release of gastric hormones
    2. Table 8-1
  D. Process
    1. Movement of chyme
      a) During fasting and sleeping states: muscle contraction moves from antrum to ileum to sweep the gut of contents
      b) During eating state
        (1) Concentric, segmenting contractions take place in the jejunum; help to mix secretions of the small intestines with the chyme particles
        (2) Slow, propulsive contractions (peristalsis) slowly push the chyme in the direction of the large intestine
        (3) Continuous shortening and lengthening of the villi constantly stirs the intestinal contents
      c) The movement of chyme from the small intestine to the large intestine is regulated by the gastroileal reflex; increased contractions in the ileum as the chyme nears the large intestine

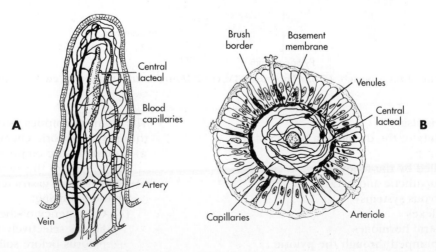

Figure 8-7   Villi. **A,** Longitudinal. **B,** Cross section. (From Abels LF: *Critical care nursing,* St Louis, 1986, Mosby.)

d) Movement of chyme through the small intestine takes approximately 3 to 10 hours

E. Function: Table 8-2

V. Large intestine

A. Description: length: 90 to 150 cm; diameter: 4 to 6 cm extending from ileum to anus

B. Structure
  1. Divisions (Fig. 8-8)
     a) Cecum
     b) Colon
        (1) Ascending colon
        (2) Transverse colon
        (3) Descending colon
        (4) Sigmoid colon
     c) Rectum
  2. Flexures
     a) Hepatic: bend at the liver; in the RUQ
     b) Splenic: bend at the spleen; in the LUQ
  3. Sphincters
     a) Ileocecal: from small intestine to cecum
     b) Anal: internal and external anal sphincters
  4. Layers of large intestinal wall
     a) Serosa: continuous with the peritoneum
     b) Muscularis
     c) Submucosa
     d) Mucosa

C. Process
  1. Movement of intestinal contents
     a) Haustral shuttling
        (1) Periodic uncoordinated tonic contractions or segmentations of both the longitudinal and circular muscles
        (2) Contents displaced short distances
        (3) Weak peristaltic contractions that move the contents through the large intestine

b) Phasic, random, nonpropulsive contractions
   (1) Last 30 seconds to 2 minutes
   (2) Contents displaced short distances in both directions
   (3) Mixes the contents and helps in the absorption of liquid contents without advancement toward the anus
c) Spontaneous mass movements
   (1) Fecal contents are pushed forward by mass movements that typically occur only a few times each day
   (2) Mass movements are stimulated by gastrocolic reflexes initiated when food enters the duodenum from the stomach, especially after the first meal of the day
   (3) These movements move feces into the rectum
   (4) The defecation reflex occurs when feces enters the rectum; peristaltic waves in the rectum and relaxation of the internal and external anal sphincters occurs
   (5) Afferent impulses are transmitted to the sacral segment of the spinal cord, from which reflex impulses are transmitted back to the colon and rectum, initiating relaxation of the internal anal sphincter
   (6) Evacuation of the colon may be facilitated by Valsalva maneuver

2. Factors that enhance colonic motility
   a) High-residue diets
   b) Fluids
   c) Irritation of colon (e.g., spicy foods)
   d) Irritant laxatives
3. Factors that inhibit colonic motility
   a) Low-residue diet
   b) Anticholinergic drugs
   c) Opiates
4. Movement of fecal contents through the small intestine takes approximately 12 hours

D. Function: Table 8-2

Accessory Organs of Digestion (Fig. 8-9)

I. Liver

A. Location: in RUQ, fitting snugly against right inferior diaphragm

B. Description
  1. Largest organ in the body: 1.5 kg
  2. Attached to the abdominal wall by the falciform ligament, which also divides the left and right lobes
  3. Four main lobes
     a) Right: larger than left
     b) Left
     c) Caudate
     d) Quadrate
  4. Covered by a thick capsule of connective

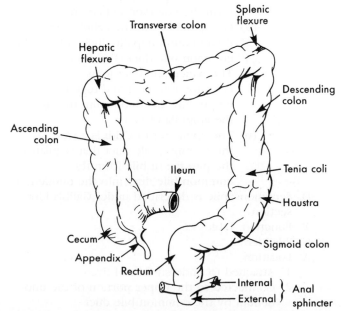

Figure 8-8 Anatomy of the colon. (From Kinney MR, Packa DR, Dunbar SB: *AACN's clinical reference for critical-care nursing,* ed 4, St Louis, 1998, Mosby.)

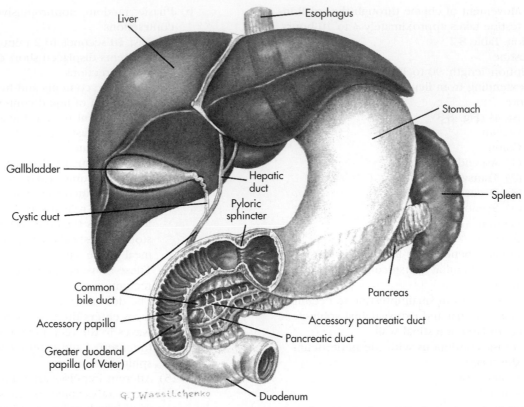

Figure 8-9   Accessory organs of the gastrointestinal system. (From Doughty DB, Jackson DB: *Gastrointestinal disorders: Mosby's clinical nursing series,* St Louis, 1993, Mosby.)

tissue (called *Glisson's capsule*); contains blood vessels, lymphatics
5. Capsule covered by a layer of serosa continuous with the peritoneum
C. Structure (Fig. 8-10)
   1. Lobes are divided into more than 1 million lobules
   2. Lobules are the functioning unit of the liver
      a) Hepatic cells (hepatocytes) are arranged in chains around a central vein
      b) Blood flows through sinusoids, which separate the hepatic chains
      c) The sinusoids receive oxygenated blood from branches of the hepatic artery and nutrient-rich blood from branches of the hepatic portal vein; the hepatic cells remove oxygen, nutrients, and toxins from the blood
      d) Each lobule has its own hepatic artery, portal vein, and bile duct, collectively called the *portal triad*
      e) The lobule consists of branching plates of liver cells radiating from center to periphery
      f) Kupffer cells, which are responsible for phagocytosis, line the sinusoids; Kupffer cells are a part of the reticuloendothelium system; they destroy old or defective red blood cells and remove bacteria and foreign particles from the blood

g) Ducts
   (1) Bile canaliculi are located between the hepatic cells and empty bile into the small bile ducts
   (2) Small bile ducts join to form the right and left hepatic ducts
   (3) Left and right hepatic ducts merge to form the common hepatic duct
   (4) Cystic duct from the gallbladder joins the common hepatic duct to form the common bile duct (Fig. 8-11)
   (5) The pancreatic duct joins the common bile duct and together empty into the duodenum through the ampulla of Vater
   (6) The sphincter of Oddi is a valve in the common bile duct that regulates the passage of bile from the common bile duct into the duodenum
D. Secretions: bile is described under Gallbladder section
E. Function: Table 8-2
II. Gallbladder
   A. Location
      1. Attached to undersurface of liver
      2. Connected to the upper portion of the duodenum by the common bile duct
   B. Description
      1. Saclike organ about 7 to 10 cm in length and 3 cm in diameter

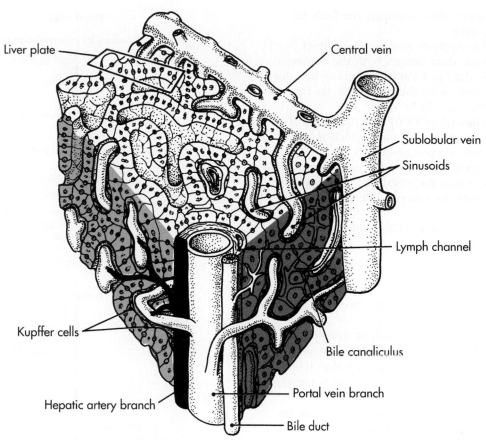

Figure 8-10   Microscopic structure of the liver lobule. (From Lewis SM, Collier IC: *Medical-surgical nursing,* ed 3, St Louis, 1992, Mosby.)

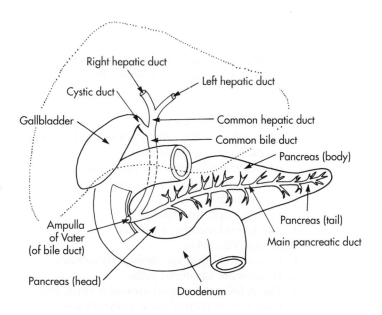

Figure 8-11   Ductal systems of the gastrointestinal tract. (From Kinney MR, Packa DR, Dunbar SB: *AACN's clinical reference for critical-care nursing,* ed 4, St Louis, 1998, Mosby.)

2. Storage capacity of 50 to 70 ml
3. Layers (exterior to interior)
   a) Serous layer: continuous with the peritoneum
   b) Smooth muscle layer
   c) Mucous membrane layer (has rugae that allow an increase in gallbladder size)

C. Structure
   1. The gallbladder has four anatomic divisions
      a) Fundus: distal portion of the body that forms a blind sac
      b) Body: connects the fundus to the infundibulum

c) Infundibulum: connects the body to the neck

d) Neck: narrows into the cystic duct

2. The cystic duct merges with the common hepatic duct to form the common bile duct, which joins with the pancreatic duct to form the ampulla of Vater

3. The sphincter of Oddi is at the terminal end of the common bile duct, which is located at the entrance into the duodenum

 a) Regulates the flow of bile and pancreatic juices into the intestine

 b) Inhibits the entry of bile into the pancreatic duct

 c) Prevents reflux of intestinal contents into the duct

D. Secretions

 1. Table 8-1

 2. Bile

 a) Bile is produced by the liver and stored in the gallbladder

 b) The gallbladder contracts in response to the hormone cholecystokinin when food is present in the small intestine; release is stimulated when fatty food is present in the small intestine

 c) Bile assists in the absorption of fats by emulsifying the fat and breaking down large fat droplets into small droplets

 d) Bile consists of the following:

 (1) Water

 (2) Bile pigments

 (3) Bile salts

 (4) High concentration of cholesterol

 (5) Some neutral fat, phospholipid, and inorganic salts

 e) The major bile pigment is bilirubin, a breakdown product of hemoglobin

 (1) Metabolism (Fig. 8-12)

 (a) The heme portion of the hemoglobin molecule is converted to bilirubin by reticuloendothelial cells, released into the bloodstream, and binds to albumin as fat-soluble unconjugated bilirubin (indirect)

 (b) In the liver, indirect bilirubin bonds to glucuronic acid to form water-soluble conjugated (direct) bilirubin, which is excreted into the hepatic ducts

E. Process

 1. Contraction of the gallbladder is stimulated by the hormone cholecystokinin

F. Function: Table 8-2

III. Pancreas

A. Location: lies in the posterior curvature of the stomach; lies behind the duodenum and the spleen

B. Description

 1. Length: 15 to 20 cm; diameter: 5 cm

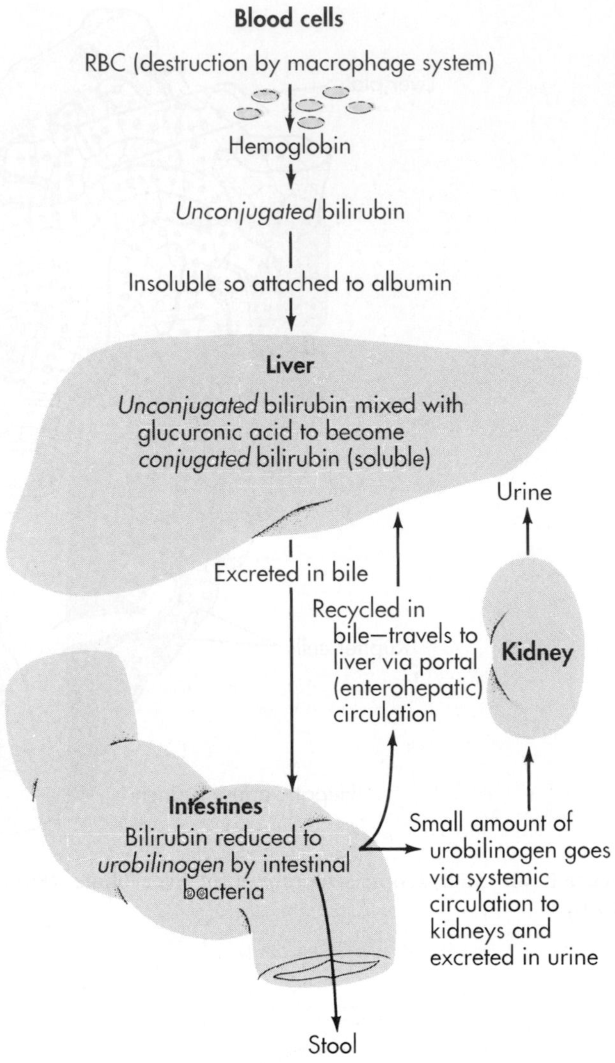

Figure 8-12 Bilirubin metabolism. (From Lewis SM, Collier IC: *Medical-surgical nursing,* ed 3, St Louis, 1992, Mosby.)

2. Anatomic divisions

 a) Head: over the vena cava in the C-shaped curve of the duodenum

 b) Body: lies behind the duodenum and extends across the abdomen behind the stomach

 c) Tail: under the spleen

3. Not surrounded by a capsule

C. Structure (Fig. 8-13)

 1. Connected lobes are formed by lobules

 2. Lobules are clustered cells

 3. The acini are arranged around a small central lumen; they secrete their enzymes into the central lumen

 4. These central lumina are drained into ductules

 5. Ductules drain into intralobular ducts, which drain into interlobular ducts, which empty into the pancreatic duct (also called the *duct of Wirsung*)

 6. The pancreatic duct runs from the tail to the head of the pancreas and unites with the

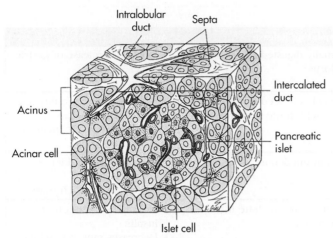

Figure 8-13   Pancreatic acini and ducts. (From Doughty DB, Jackson DB: *Gastrointestinal disorders: Mosby's clinical nursing series,* St Louis, 1993, Mosby.)

common bile duct to form the ampulla of Vater, which empties into the duodenum
   7. Cells have exocrine and endocrine functions
      a) Acinar cells have exocrine (through a duct) functions
      b) Alpha and beta cells of the islets of Langerhans have endocrine (ductless) functions
         (1) Alpha cells secrete glucagon
         (2) Beta cells secrete insulin
         (3) Delta cells secrete somatostatin
   D. Secretions: Table 8-1
      1. Pancreatic secretions are triggered by the presence of undigested food in the small intestine
      2. Acinar cells secrete a high concentration of sodium bicarbonate, water, sodium, potassium and digestive enzymes (lipase, amylase, trypsin, ribonuclease, deoxyribonuclease)
         a) Trypsinogen: secreted in inactive form; activated by contact with bile salts
         b) Chymotrypsinogen: secreted in inactive form; activated by contact with bile salts
      3. Secretions are controlled by the following:
         a) Vagus nerve and parasympathetic nervous system
         b) Hormonal: secretin and cholecystokinin
   E. Functions: Table 8-2

Gastrointestinal Hormones (Table 8-3)
Blood Supply (Fig. 8-14)
I. Arterial: aorta, aortic arch, thoracic arch, abdominal aorta
   A. Celiac artery: the following branches of the celiac artery supply the specified organs:
      1. Left gastric: supplies stomach, esophagus
      2. Hepatic to right gastric: supplies stomach
      3. Gastroduodenal: supplies stomach, duodenum
      4. Cystic: supplies gallbladder
      5. Splenic: supplies stomach, pancreas, spleen

   B. Superior mesenteric arteries supply the following:
      1. Jejunum
      2. Ileum
      3. Cecum
      4. Ascending colon
      5. Part of transverse colon
   C. Inferior mesenteric arteries supply the following:
      1. Transverse, descending, and sigmoid colon
      2. Rectum
   D. Hepatic artery and portal vein supply the liver
II. Venous
   A. Portal vein collects and delivers blood from entire venous drainage of GI tract to liver; branches include: gastric, splenic, superior mesenteric, inferior mesenteric
   B. Portal vein subdivides into liver sinusoids, which then unite with branches from hepatic artery to form hepatic vein, which empties into the inferior vena cava
   C. Partially metabolized digestive products are brought to liver sinusoids, where hepatocytes complete the next stage of metabolism

Nervous Innervation
I. Extrinsic
   A. Parasympathetic nervous system (PNS): increases the activity of the GI tract; innervated via the vagus nerve
   B. Sympathetic nervous system (SNS): decreases the activity of the GI tract; innervated via SNS fibers, which parallel the major blood vessels of the GI tract
II. Intrinsic
   A. Located inside the wall of the GI tract
   B. Consists of extensions from extrinsic nerves of the autonomic nervous system (ANS)
   C. Forms two major and three minor networks of plexuses

Functions of the Gastrointestinal System
I. Ingestion
   A. Ingestion begins with the sensation of hunger, controlled by the feeding center of the hypothalamus
   B. Ingestion ends with the sensation of satisfaction provided by the satiety center also in the hypothalamus
   C. Food and liquids enter the alimentary tract at the mouth
II. Secretion: Table 8-1
III. Digestion
   A. Carbohydrates: 4 kcal/g
      1. Digestion begins in the mouth where polysaccharides (starch) are broken down into disaccharides (e.g., sucrose, lactose, maltose) by the action of ptyalin (amylase)
      2. The process continues when the disaccharides are broken down into monosaccharides (e.g., glucose, galactose, fructose) by the

Table 8-3	Gastrointestinal Hormones		
Hormone	**Source**	**Stimulus for Release**	**Action**
Gastrin	Gastric mucosa of the antrum of the stomach and the pylorus	Partially digested proteins in pylorus	• Stimulates release of gastric juices
Secretin	Duodenal mucosa	Partially digested proteins, fats, acid in the intestine	• Inhibits gastric motility and acid secretions • Causes pancreatic bicarbonate secretion
Cholecystokinin	Duodenal mucosa	Fats in duodenum	• Increases gallbladder contraction • Decreases stomach tone
Gastric inhibitory peptide	Small intestine mucosa	Fat and carbohydrate in duodenum	• Stimulates secretion of insulin • Decreases motor activity of the stomach • Slows emptying of gastric contents into the small intestine
Vasoactive intestinal peptide	Small intestine mucosa	Acid in the duodenum	• Stimulates intestinal juice • Inhibits gastric secretion
Enterogastrone	Small intestine mucosa	Partially digested proteins, fats, and acids in intestine	• Inhibits gastric secretion and motility • Causes relaxation of sphincter of Oddi and contraction of gallbladder
Villikinin	Small intestine mucosa	Chyme in intestine	• Stimulates movement of intestinal villi
Pancreozymin	Duodenal mucosa	Partially digested proteins, fats, and acids in duodenum	• Stimulates pancreatic juice

action of pancreatic amylase and intestinal enzymes (e.g., sucrase, lactase, maltase)

B. Proteins: 4 kcal/g

1. Digestion begins in the stomach where pepsin breaks down proteins into polypeptides

2. The process continues when the polypeptides are broken down into peptides and amino acids in the small intestine by the action of trypsin, chymotrypsin, and carboxypeptides from the pancreas and aminopeptidases and dipeptidase from the intestinal villi

C. Fats: 9 kcal/g

1. Digestion of fats that are already emulsified (e.g., cream and butter) begins in the stomach by lipase

2. Digestion of nonemulsified fat occurs in the small intestine with emulsification of the fat by bile and pancreatic lipase

3. Fat is broken down into glycerol and fatty acids

IV. Absorption

A. Basic absorption mechanisms

1. Active transport requires an energy source (e.g., ATP) to move substances into and out of the cell; substances absorbed by active transport include proteins, glucose, sodium, and potassium

2. Passive diffusion is passive movement from an area of high-solute concentration to an area of low-solute concentration; substances absorbed by passive diffusion include free fatty acids and water

3. Facilitated diffusion is movement that requires a carrier that moves into the cell but does not require energy; a substance absorbed by facilitated diffusion is fructose

4. Nonionic transport is movement of solutes freely into and out of the cell; substances absorbed by nonionic transport include unconjugated bile salts, drugs

5. Solvent drag is flow of water to higher osmotic concentration; it contributes to absorption and reduction in osmolality that occurs in the jejunum

B. Specific absorption in small intestine

1. Electrolyte absorption: active transport from all areas of intestine

2. Water absorption: small and large intestine

a) Approximately 2 L of fluid are ingested daily

b) Approximately 7 L of fluid are secreted by the GI tract daily

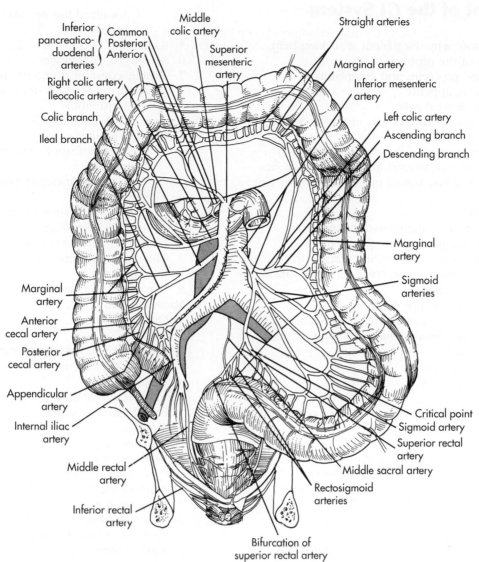

Inferior pancreatico-duodenal arteries
Common
Posterior
Anterior
Right colic artery
Ileocolic artery
Colic branch
Ileal branch
Middle colic artery
Superior mesenteric artery
Straight arteries
Marginal artery
Inferior mesenteric artery
Left colic artery
Ascending branch
Descending branch
Marginal artery
Marginal artery
Anterior cecal artery
Posterior cecal artery
Appendicular artery
Internal iliac artery
Middle rectal artery
Inferior rectal artery
Sigmoid arteries
Critical point
Sigmoid artery
Superior rectal artery
Middle sacral artery
Rectosigmoid arteries
Bifurcation of superior rectal artery

Figure 8-14 Arterial blood supply of the gastrointestinal system. (From Society of Gastroenterology Nurses and Associates SGNA: *Gastroenterology nursing: a core curriculum,* St Louis, 1993, Mosby.)

c) Of these 9 L, 7,500 ml are reabsorbed with only 1,500 ml reaching the cecum
d) Additional fluid is reabsorbed in the large intestine, but only 200 ml is lost in the stool
3. CHO absorption
   a) Fructose by facilitated diffusion
   b) Glucose and galactose by active transport
4. Protein absorption: amino acids absorbed by active transport in the ileum and the jejunum (**Note:** there are 22 basic amino acids; 9 are generally considered essential amino acids)
5. Fat absorption
   a) Micellar solubilization of fatty acid with bile salt to form micelle
   b) Diffusion of micelle into jejunal cell
   c) Delivery of fatty acids to circulation via lymphatic system
6. Water-soluble vitamin absorption: all areas of small intestine by passive diffusion (absorption of B_{12} requires intrinsic factor)

7. Fat-soluble vitamins absorption: absorbed in jejunum (bile salts required)
8. Calcium absorption: mainly in duodenum (vitamin D required)
9. Iron absorption: all areas of the intestine (especially in duodenum) by active transport; stored as protein-bound iron
V. Synthesis
   A. Bacteria in the large intestine produce vitamin K
   B. Peyer's patches in the small intestine play a role in antibody synthesis
VI. Effect on fluid and electrolyte balance
   A. Gastric losses are acidic; increased gastric losses (e.g., nasogastric suction, vomiting) cause metabolic alkalosis, hypokalemia, hyponatremia, hypovolemia
   B. Intestinal losses are alkaline: increased intestinal losses (e.g., biliary losses, pancreatic fistula, intestinal suction, diarrhea) cause metabolic acidosis, hypokalemia, hyponatremia, hypovolemia

Assessment of the GI System

Interview

I. Chief complaint: why the patient is seeking help and duration of the problem
  A. Nonspecific problems and complaints
    1. Change in appetite
    2. Fatigue or weakness
    3. Unintentional weight loss or weight gain
    4. Fever, chills
  B. Abdominal pain: describe PQRST (Table 8-4)
    1. Provocation: relationship to food, drugs, activity, position, bowel movements, breathing, stress
    2. Palliation
      a) Effective or ineffective treatments
      b) Alleviating factors (e.g., position)
    3. Quality: sharp, dull, tearing, cramping, burning, gnawing, stabbing, aching, colicky
      a) Visceral pain
        (1) Dull, poorly localized
        (2) May be caused by organic lesions or functional disturbance within the GI tract
      b) Somatic pain
        (1) Sharp, well localized
        (2) May be caused by inflammation of abdominal organs, which causes peritoneal irritation
    4. Region: location
      a) May be poorly localized
      b) May be referred pain (Fig. 8-15)
        (1) Pain may be felt in a remote area that is supplied by the same nerve as the diseased or damaged organ
        (2) Referred pain is usually sharp and localized but not over the area of injury
    5. Radiation
    6. Severity: 0 to 10 scale
    7. Timing: constant or intermittent; duration; relationship to food, alcohol, activity, position
  C. Abdominal distention
  D. Change in bowel elimination
    1. Change in color of stools
      a) Clay-colored stools indicate biliary obstruction
      b) Tarry stools (melena) indicate upper GI bleeding
      c) Bloody stools (hematochezia) indicate lower GI bleeding
    2. Change in consistency of stools
    3. Change in frequency of stools
    4. Excessive flatus
    5. Use of laxative, enemas
  E. Nausea/vomiting
    1. Onset, duration
    2. Frequency
    3. Character and color; presence of blood in vomitus (hematemesis)
    4. Palliation
      a) Effective or ineffective treatment
      b) Alleviating factors
    5. Timing
      a) Time of day
      b) Relationship to food, odors, drugs, alcohol, activity, bowel movements
    6. Aggravating factors
    7. Associated pain
  F. Abdominal trauma
    1. Gunshot entrance and exit wound
    2. Knife wounds

Table 8-4	Differentiation of Abdominal Pain		
Condition	**Location of Pain**	**Quality of Pain**	**Associated Symptoms**
Gastritis	• Epigastric or slightly left of midline	• May be described as indigestion	• Nausea and vomiting • May have hematemesis • Abdominal tenderness
Peptic ulcer	• Epigastric or RUQ	• Gnawing, burning	• Abdominal tenderness • Hematemesis (gastric) or melena (duodenal)
Pancreatitis	• Epigastric or LUQ • May radiate to back, flanks, or left shoulder	• Boring • Worsened by lying down	• Nausea and vomiting • Mild fever • Abdominal tenderness
Cholecystitis	• Epigastric or RUQ • May be referred to below right scapula	• Cramping	• Nausea and vomiting • Abdominal tenderness in RUQ
Appendicitis	• Epigastric or periumbilical pain; later localizes to RLQ	• Dull to sharp	• Anorexia, nausea, vomiting • Fever • Diarrhea • Rebound tenderness • Leukocytosis
Intestinal obstruction	• Epigastric or umbilical	• Spastic to dull	• Change in bowel habits • Melena or hematochezia • Hyperactive to hypoactive bowel sounds

3. Burns or abrasions
4. Ecchymotic areas associated with blunt trauma

G. Dentition problems
1. Caries
2. Gingivitis
3. Poor fitting dentures

H. Painful swallowing
I. Dysphagia
J. Dyspepsia
K. Eructation
L. Flatulence
M. Edema
N. Abnormal bruising or bleeding
O. Jaundice
P. Change in color of urine: dark brown or orange urine may indicate biliary obstruction
Q. Pruritus
R. Fecal incontinence
S. Rectal bleeding
T. Anal discomfort

II. History of present illness: use PQRST format
III. Past medical history
A. Past illnesses
1. Jaundice
2. Anemia
3. Obesity: use of liquid diets, gastrointestinal bypass, gastric balloon, etc.
4. Eating disorders (e.g., bulimia, anorexia nervosa)
5. Alcoholism
6. Peptic ulcer disease
7. GI hemorrhage
8. Cholclithiasis
9. Hepatic disease
   a) Cirrhosis
   b) Hepatitis
   c) History of blood transfusion
10. Pancreatitis
11. Cancer

12. Irritable bowel syndrome
13. Inflammatory bowel disease (e.g., ulcerative colitis, Crohn's disease)
14. Diverticulitis
15. Polyps
16. Hemorrhoids
17. Renal disease
18. Cardiovascular disease
19. Diabetes mellitus
20. COPD (high incidence of peptic ulcer disease)

B. Past injury: abdominal trauma
C. Past surgical procedures
D. Past diagnostic studies (e.g., endoscopy, X-rays, stool exam for occult blood)
E. Food intolerances or allergies; type of reaction if allergy

IV. Family history
A. Eating disorder (e.g., obesity, anorexia nervosa, bulimia)
B. Obesity
C. Anemia
D. Peptic ulcer disease
E. Pancreatic disease (e.g., pancreatitis, pancreatic cancer)
F. Diabetes mellitus
G. Liver disease (e.g., cirrhosis, hepatitis)
H. Malabsorption syndrome
I. Inflammatory bowel disease (e.g., ulcerative colitis, Crohn's disease)
J. Irritable bowel syndrome
K. Alcoholism
L. Cancer

V. Social history
A. Relationship with spouse or significant other; family structure
B. Occupation
C. Educational level
D. Stress level and usual coping mechanisms
E. Recreational habits

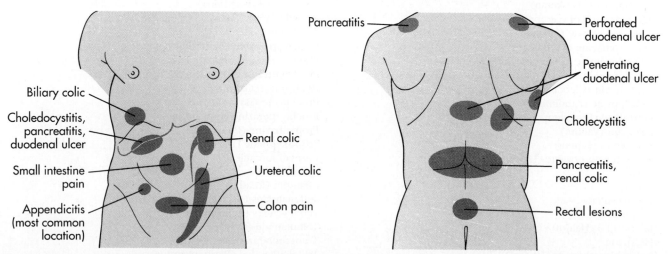

Figure 8-15   Common areas of referred abdominal pain. (Beare PG, Myers JL: *Principles and practice of adult health nursing,* ed 2, St Louis, 1994, Mosby.)

F. Exercise habits
G. Dietary habits
  1. Appetite
  2. Usual foods
  3. Number and time of meals, snacks
  4. Fluid intake
  5. Food restrictions
    a) Intolerances
    b) Prescribed restrictions
    c) Religious restrictions
  6. Change in eating habits
H. Usual bowel habits
I. Caffeine intake
J. Tobacco use: record as pack-years (number of packs per day times the number of years he or she has been smoking)
K. Alcohol use: record as alcoholic beverages consumed per month, week, or day
L. Exposure to toxins or infectious disease
M. Travel
VI. Medication history
A. Prescribed drug, dosage, frequency, time of last dose
B. Nonprescribed drugs
  1. Over-the-counter drugs, including vitamins and herbs
  2. Substance abuse
C. Patient understanding of drug actions, side effects

D. Drugs causing potential problems for patients with gastrointestinal problems
  1. Antibiotics
  2. Aspirin
  3. Nonsteroidal antiinflammatory drugs (e.g., ibuprofen [Motrin])
  4. Corticosteroids
  5. Acetaminophen (Tylenol)
  6. Many drugs have anorexia, nausea, vomiting as side effects
  7. Many drugs are hepatotoxic (Box 8-1)
E. Drugs often used for gastrointestinal problems
  1. Antacids
  2. Stool softeners
  3. Laxatives
  4. Cathartics
  5. Anticholinergics
  6. Corticosteroids
  7. Antidiarrheals
  8. Antiemetics
  9. Tranquilizers
  10. Sedatives
  11. Barbiturates

Vital Signs

I. BP: sitting; lying; standing especially in hemorrhaging patient; systolic BP less than 100 mm Hg and

---

BOX 8-1   Hepatotoxic Agents

6-Mercaptopurine (Purinethol)
Acetaminophen (Tylenol)
Acetylsalicylic acid (ASA)
Allopurinol (Zyloprim)
Amiodarone (Cordarone)
Amitriptyline (Elavil)
Ampicillin (Polycillin)
Carbamazepine (Tegretol)
Carbon tetrachloride
Chlorambucil (Leukeran)
Chloramphenicol (Geopen)
Chlordiazepoxide (Librium)
Chlorpromazine (Thorazine)
Chlorpropamide (Diabinese)
Cimetidine (Tagamet)
Clindamycin (Cleocin)
Cyclosporine (Sandimmune)
Dantrolene (Dantrium)
Diazepam (Valium)
Doxepin (Sinequan)
Erythromycin estolate (Ilosone)
Ethanol
Ethrane
Ferrous sulfate
Fluothane
Haloperidol (Haldol)
Halothane
Hydrochlorothiazide (HydroDIURIL)
Imipramine (Tofranil)

Indomethacin (Indocin)
Isoniazid (Isoniazid)
Ketoconazole (Miconazole)
Meprobamate (Equanil)
Methotrexate (Methotrexate)
Methyldopa (Aldomet)
Monoamine oxidase (MAO) inhibitors
Nicotinic acid
Oral contraceptives
Oxacillin (Prostaphlin)
Penicillin (Pen Vee K)
Penthrane
Phenazopyridine (Pyridium)
Phenobarbital (Luminal)
Phenylbutazone (Butazolidin)
Phenytoin (Dilantin)
Probenecid (Benemid)
Prochlorperazine (Compazine)
Promethazine (Phenergan)
Propoxyphene (Darvon)
Propylthiouracil (PTU)
Quinidine
Rifampin (Rifadin)
Sulfonamides (Bactrim, Septra, Gantrisin)
Tetracyclines (Achromycin)
Tolbutamide (Orinase)
Trimethobenzamide (Tigan)
Tripelennamine (Pyribenzamine)

HR greater than 100/min often indicates a blood loss of at least 20% reduction in blood volume
II. HR
III. Respiratory rate
IV. Temperature
V. Height
VI. Weight

Inspection

I. Landmarks (Fig. 8-16)
   A. Xiphoid
   B. Costal margin
   C. Midline
   D. Umbilicus
   E. Anterior superior iliac crest
   F. Symphysis pubis
   G. The abdomen may be divided into:
      1. Four quadrants (Fig. 8-17): horizontal and vertical lines intersect at the umbilicus
      2. Nine regions (Fig. 8-18)
II. General survey
   A. Apparent health status
   B. Apparent age relative to chronologic age
   C. Level of consciousness
   D. Gross deformity
   E. Nutritional status
   F. Stature/posture
      1. Patient flexing his or her knees to relieve abdominal tension is often seen in peritonitis
      2. Patient leaning forward to relieve abdominal pain is often seen in pancreatitis
   G. Gait
III. Mouth
   A. Lips: color, texture, lesions, swelling, symmetry
   B. Gums: inflammation, retraction, hypertrophy, bleeding, lesions
   C. Teeth: caries, state of repair, occlusion, dentures: fit, gum ulceration caused by ill-fitting dentures
   D. Tongue: swelling, laceration, lesions, coating
   E. Mucosa: moisture, lesions, color
   F. Odor
      1. Fetor hepaticus: sweet fecal odor caused by hepatic failure
      2. Feculent breath: foul fecal odor caused by reverse peristalsis with small bowel obstruction
      3. Severe halitosis: foul odor may be caused by poor dental hygiene, neoplasms of esophagus or stomach
IV. Skin
   A. Color: should be homogenous over the entire abdomen
      1. Pallor: anemia
      2. Jaundice: occurs when bilirubin is greater than 3.0 mg/dl; associated with any of the following:
         a) Liver disease
         b) Biliary obstruction
         c) Excessive hemolysis

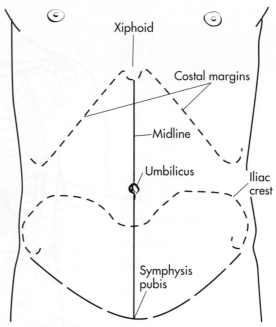

Figure 8-16   Landmarks of the abdomen.

      3. Bluish: due to infiltration of the abdominal wall with blood
         a) Location
            (1) Grey Turner's sign: ecchymosis to flanks indicative of retroperitoneal bleeding (e.g., from pancreas, duodenum, kidneys, vena cava, aorta)
            (2) Cullen's sign: ecchymosis around umbilicus indicative of intraperitoneal bleeding (e.g., liver or spleen)
         b) Causes
            (1) Hemorrhagic pancreatitis
            (2) Infarcted bowel
            (3) Ruptured ectopic pregnancy
   B. Lesions or discoloration
      1. Scars: trauma; surgical procedures
      2. Striae
         a) Usually vertical
         b) Initially pinkish or bluish, become silvery with time
         c) May be caused by pregnancy, obesity, ascites
         d) Purplish striae may be caused by Cushing's syndrome
      3. Rash
      4. Ecchymosis
      5. Abrasions
      6. Spider angioma: may be associated with elevated estrogen levels (e.g., pregnancy, liver disease)
      7. Palmar erythema: seen in cirrhosis, hepatic failure
   C. Shiny, edematous abdomen
      1. Ascites: intraperitoneal fluid often associated with cirrhosis or intraabdominal malignancy (e.g., liver, ovarian)

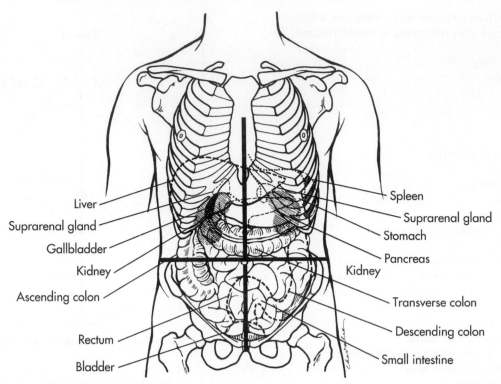

Figure 8-17   The abdomen divided into four quadrants. (From Abels LF: *Critical care nursing,* St Louis, 1986, Mosby.)

2. Anasarca: entire body edema that may be seen in end-stage heart failure or renal failure
D. Superficial vascularity
   1. May be caused by obstruction of inferior vena cava or portal vein
   2. Caput medusae: pronounced dilation of the periumbilical veins radiating from the umbilicus; seen in severe portal venous hypertension
E. Stoma: location, color, drainage, condition of peristomal skin
F. Draining wounds: location, drainage, condition of surrounding skin
G. Fistula: location, drainage, condition of surrounding skin
V. Contour of abdomen
   A. Profile
      1. Normal: flat from xiphoid process to pubic symphysis
      2. Scaffold: concave abdomen seen in malnutrition
      3. Distention or protuberance
         a) Diffuse and symmetrical
            (1) Fat
            (2) Flatus
            (3) Fetus (i.e., pregnancy)
            (4) Feces (i.e., obstruction)
            (5) Fluid (i.e., ascites)
            (6) Fatal growths (i.e., malignancy)
            (7) Fibroids
         b) Distention in upper quadrants: gastric dilation, pancreatic cyst, malignancy

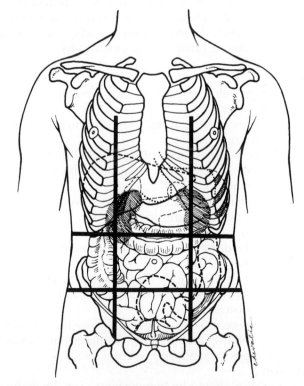

Figure 8-18   The abdomen divided into nine regions. (From Abels LF: *Critical care nursing,* St Louis, 1986, Mosby.)

         c) Distention in lower quadrants: pregnancy, uterine fibroid, distended bladder, ovarian tumor
         d) Distention in one quadrant: hernia, tumor, cyst, obstruction, organomegaly

VI. Abdominal girth
   A. Measure abdominal girth at largest area
   B. Mark on either side of tape measure so that measurements are consistently at same location
   C. One inch increase is equal to an increase in intraabdominal volume of 500 to 1000 ml

VII. Weakness of abdominal wall
   A. Diastasis recti abdominis: abnormal separation of the two abdominal rectus muscles when the patient tenses abdominal muscles by raising his or her head from the bed
   B. Hernia: abdominal, umbilical, or inguinal

VIII. Movement of abdomen
   A. Breathing: normal
      1. Women generally breathe thoracically when upright
      2. Both men and women generally breathe abdominally when supine
   B. Peristalsis: abnormal to see waves of peristalsis across the abdomen: generally associated with intestinal obstruction
   C. Aortic pulsation: normally visible at the end of expiration in a supine patient, especially if patient is thin; pulsatile swelling in the epigastrium suggests an abdominal aortic aneurysm or an epigastric solid tumor overlying the aorta

IX. Umbilicus
   A. Color
      1. Bluish (Cullen's sign): due to infiltration of the abdominal wall with blood
      2. Inflammation: may be seen with poor hygiene
   B. Contour
      1. Deeply inverted: obesity
      2. Everted: pregnancy or ascites
      3. Nodular (Sister Mary Joseph's nodule): may indicate intraabdominal carcinoma (especially stomach) with metastasis to the navel

Auscultation

I. Auscultation is done prior to percussion or palpation to prevent "stirring up" the abdomen; order for physical assessment of the abdomen, therefore, is inspection, auscultation, percussion, palpation

II. Preparation: may be helpful to put pillow under knees to relax abdominal muscles

III. Bowel sounds
   A. Method
      1. Use diaphragm with light pressure for 1 minute in each of the four abdominal quadrants
      2. Disconnect nasogastric suction for auscultation
      3. If bowel sounds are hypoactive, 5 minutes of auscultation without audible bowel sounds is required before documenting the absence of bowel sounds
   B. Normal bowel sounds: bubbling or soft gurgling noises heard every 5 to 20 seconds in an irregular pattern; heard in all quadrants

   C. Abnormal bowel sounds
      1. Very infrequent or absent bowel sounds
         a) Functional obstruction: paralytic ileus
         b) Advanced mechanical intestinal obstruction
      2. Loud, hyperactive bowel sounds (may be called *borborygmi*): hyperperistalsis (e.g., diarrhea, catharsis caused by GI bleeding)
      3. High-pitched "rushing" bowel sounds: early mechanical small intestinal obstruction
      4. Low-pitched "rushing" bowel sounds: early mechanical large intestinal obstruction
      5. Succussion splash: splashing sound audible when rolling the patient side to side; indicative of pyloric obstruction

IV. Vascular sounds
   A. Method: use bell over specified areas
   B. Bruits
      1. Listen over midline and renal and femoral arteries
      2. If bruit is noted, check circulation to extremities; if decreased blood flow is noted, aneurysm should be suspected
         a) Notify physician
         b) Keep patient quiet
         c) Do not palpate abdomen
   C. Venous hum: hum of medium tone created by blood flow in a large, engorged vascular organ such as liver or spleen

V. Peritoneal friction rub: scratchy sound heard over inflamed spleen or neoplastic liver

Percussion

I. Percussion tones normally heard over abdomen
   A. Dull: liver, full sigmoid colon, full bladder
   B. Flat: bone
   C. Tympany: gastric bubble, bowel

II. Tests for ascites
   A. Fluid wave: tap one side of the abdomen and feel for the fluid wave to hit the hand on the other side of the abdomen; have a colleague or the patient place the ulnar surface of his or her hand at the abdomen's midline to stop skin transmission
   B. Shifting dullness: percuss dullness indicating fluid at flanks while patient supine, mark fluid level, turn patient on one side and note shift of dullness line (Fig. 8-19)
   C. Midline dullness: dullness at midline with the patient leaning forward in a standing position indicates intraabdominal fluid

III. Organ borders
   A. Liver (dullness between right lung resonance and bowel tympany)
      1. Normal span 6 to 12 cm in the right midclavicular line
      2. Enlarged and tender in RVF, hepatitis, mononucleosis
      3. May be large or small in cirrhosis
      4. Absence of liver dullness: may indicate free air in peritoneum from bowel perforation

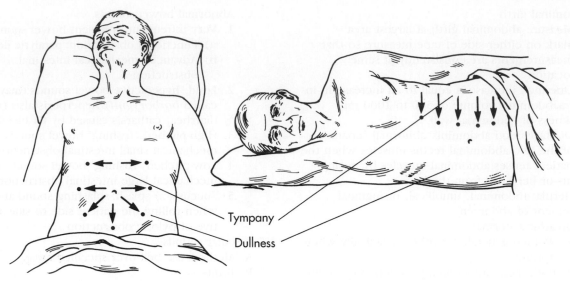

Figure 8-19 Test for ascites: shifting dullness. (Beare PG, Myers JL: *Principles and practice of adult health nursing*, ed 2, St Louis, 1994, Mosby.)

B. Spleen (dullness under left diaphragm): if percussible should be less than 7 cm at the left midaxillary line
C. Stomach (tympany under left costal margin)
D. Bladder (dullness above symphysis pubis): percussible only if enlarged
E. Intestine (tympany over abdomen): may percuss dullness over LLQ if sigmoid colon is full

Palpation
I. Method
  A. Warm hands
  B. Examine each quadrant
  C. Always palpate tender areas last
  D. Carry on conversation with patient to keep him or her (and abdominal muscles) relaxed; place a pillow under the knees and a pillow under the head
II. Light palpation: use fingertips to depress 1 to 2 cm; note the following:
  A. Temperature
  B. Moisture
  C. Superficial skin reflexes: movement of the umbilicus toward the quadrant that is stroked
  D. Voluntary guarding
    1. Patient may voluntarily splint abdominal muscles, especially when sensitive spot is touched; watch for nonverbal indicators of pain during palpation
  E. Involuntary guarding or rigidity
    1. Diffuse rigidity suggests an infectious, neoplastic, or inflammatory process in the peritoneal cavity
    2. Rigid, boardlike abdomen is associated with acute perforation of a viscus with spillage of air or GI contents into the peritoneal cavity
  F. Tender areas

G. Large masses
  1. If mass is pulsatile, refrain from additional abdominal palpation because it may be an abdominal aortic aneurysm
  2. If mass is not pulsatile, describe the following:
    a) Size
    b) Location
    c) Consistency
    d) Contour
    e) Tenderness
    f) Mobility
III. Deep palpation: use one hand on top of the other to depress 4 to 5 cm
  A. Do not use deep palpation in the following situations:
    1. Polycystic kidneys
    2. After renal transplant
    3. Malignant tumor: may cause seeding
    4. Recent surgery
  B. Note the following:
    1. Direct tenderness
      a) Associated with local inflammation of the abdominal wall, the peritoneum, or a viscus
    2. Rebound (or indirect) tenderness (also referred to as *Blumberg's sign*)
      a) Performed by pressing into the tender area and then letting go
      b) If the pain is exacerbated when pressure is released, rebound tenderness is present and peritoneal inflammation is suspected
      c) Rebound tenderness is especially significant when it occurs at a site away from the area of direct tenderness
    3. Organ size
      a) Liver edge: may be palpable
        (1) Ask the patient to take a deep breath

and move your hand in and up to check for tenderness, smoothness of edge

 (a) Tenderness is often caused by hepatitis or liver engorgement caused by right ventricular failure

 (b) Hard, lumpy liver is associated with cancer or cirrhosis

(2) A normal-size liver may be palpable, especially in patients with COPD due to hyperinflation of lungs; hepatomegaly exists only if the liver span by percussion is more than 12 cm at MCL

 b) Gallbladder: palpable only if enlarged with stones; if palpable, located under liver edge in right upper quadrant

4. Splenic tenderness

 a) Palpate left side of abdomen with patient supine and taking a deep breath

 b) Note any tenderness

 c) Spleen is palpable only if significantly enlarged (e.g., injury, leukemia, mononucleosis, portal hypertension)

5. Aortic pulsation: check for lateral expansion, which may indicate an aneurysm

IV. Ballottement

 A. Gentle repetitive bouncing of tissues against the hand

 B. May be used to evaluate organ enlargement

Diagnostic Studies

I. Serum chemistries

 A. Sodium: normal 136 to 145 mEq/L; elevated in dehydration from severe diarrhea or intestinal obstruction

 B. Potassium: normal 3.5 to 5.0 mEq/L; decreased in GI losses from upper or lower GI tract

 C. Chloride: normal 96 to 106 mEq/L
  1. Elevated in dehydration
  2. Decreased in vomiting, diarrhea, or intestinal obstruction

 D. Calcium: normal 8.5 to 10.5 mg/dl; decreased in acute pancreatitis

 E. Phosphorus: normal 3.0 to 4.5 mg/dl
  1. Elevated in intestinal obstruction
  2. Decreased in malnutrition or malabsorption syndromes

 F. Magnesium: normal 1.5 to 2.5 mEq/L; decreased in chronic diarrhea

 G. Glucose: normal 70 to 110 mg/dl; elevated in diabetes mellitus, pancreatitis

 H. BUN: normal 5 to 20 mg/dl

 I. Creatinine: normal 0.7 to 1.5 mg/dl

 J. Gastrin: normal less than 200 ng/L; elevated in Zollinger-Ellison syndrome (gastrin-producing pancreatic tumor) or G-cell hyperplasia, which may cause peptic ulcer disease

 K. Ammonia: normal 15 to 110 µg/dl; elevated in hepatic failure, renal failure, heart failure

 L. Iron: normal 50 to 150 µg/dl

 M. Iron-binding capacity: 250 to 410 µg/dl

 N. Lactate: negative

 O. Carcinoembryonic antigen (CEA): normal less than 2 ng/ml; elevated in cancer of the colon, lung, pancreas, stomach, breast, head, neck, prostate

 P. Bilirubin
  1. Total: normal 0.3 to 1.3 mg/dl; elevated in hepatic disease, biliary obstruction, or excessive hemolysis
  2. Direct: normal 0.1 to 0.3 mg/dl; elevated in biliary obstruction
  3. Indirect: normal 0.1 to 1.0 mg/dl; elevated in hepatic disease or excessive hemolysis

 Q. Serum proteins
  1. Total protein: normal 6 to 8 g/dl
  2. Albumin: normal 3.5 to 4.5 g/dl; half-life is 19 to 20 days, so poor indicator of acute changes in nutritional status
  3. Prealbumin: normal 15 to 32 mg/dl; half-life is only 2 to 3 days, so indicates changes in nutritional status better than albumin
  4. Transferrin: normal 250 to 300 mg/dl; half-life is only 8 to 10 days, so indicates changes in nutritional status better than albumin
  5. Globulin: normal 1.5 to 3 g/dl
  6. Albumin/globulin ratio (A/G): normal 1.5/1 to 2.5/1; reverse in chronic hepatitis, chronic liver disease
  7. Fibrinogen: normal 200 to 400 mg/dl

 R. Serum lipids
  1. Cholesterol: normal 150 to 200 mg/dl
  2. Triglycerides: normal 40 to 150 mg/dl

 S. Pepsinogen: normal 200 to 425 U/ml
  1. Elevated in hemoconcentration
  2. Decreased in malnutrition or hemorrhage

 T. Enzymes
  1. Alkaline phosphatase: normal 30 to 85 IU/L; elevated in cirrhosis, rheumatoid arthritis, biliary obstruction, liver tumor, hyperparathyroidism
  2. Amylase: normal 56 to 190 IU/L; elevated in acute pancreatitis, pancreatic cancer, pancreatic pseudocysts, perforated peptic ulcer, mesenteric thrombosis, ectopic pregnancy, renal failure, mumps
  3. Lipase: normal up to 1.5 U/ml; elevated in acute or chronic pancreatitis, duodenal ulcer, biliary obstruction, cirrhosis, hepatitis; stays elevated longer than amylase in pancreatitis
  4. Alanine aminotransferase (ALT): normal 5 to 36 U/ml
   a) Formerly called *SGPT*
   b) Elevated in hepatitis, cirrhosis, liver tumor, hepatotoxic drugs, cholestasis, infectious mononucleosis

5. Aspartate aminotransferase (AST): normal
   15 to 45 U/ml
   a) Formerly called *SGOT*
   b) Elevated in hepatitis, cirrhosis, acute
      pancreatitis, skeletal muscle disease or
      trauma, liver tumor
6. Gamma-glutamyl transferase (GGT): normal
   5 to 38 IU/L; elevated in hepatitis, cirrhosis,
   liver tumor, cholestasis, alcohol ingestion,
   myocardial infarction
7. Lactate dehydrogenase (LDH): normal 90 to
   200 IU/L; elevated in hepatitis, hemolytic
   anemia, pancreatitis, muscular dystrophy, pulmonary infarction, myocardial infarction, pernicious anemia, renal disease
U. Serology for viral hepatitis

II. Hematology
A. Hematocrit: normal 40% to 52% for males; 35%
   to 47% for females
B. Hemoglobin: normal 13 to 18 g/dl for males;
   12 to 16 g/dl for females
C. White blood cells (WBC): normal 3,500 to
   11,000 mm^3
   1. Differential: shift to left (increase in bands)
      indicates acute infection
D. Erythrocyte sedimentation rate: normal up to
   15 mm/hr for males; up to 20 mm/hr for
   females
E. Total lymphocyte count: normal 1,000 to
   4,000/mm^3 or 20% to 40% of WBC count

III. Clotting profile: may be abnormal in liver disease
A. Prothrombin time (PT): normal 12 to 15
   seconds; therapeutic 1.5 to 2.5 times normal
B. Activated partial thromboplastin time (aPTT):
   normal 25 to 38 seconds; therapeutic 1.5 to
   2.5 times normal
C. Activated clotting time (ACT): normal 70 to
   120 seconds; therapeutic 150 to 190 seconds
D. Thrombin time: normal 10 to 15 seconds
E. Bleeding time: normal 1 to 9.5 minutes
F. International Normalized Ratio (INR): normal
   less than 2.0
G. Platelets: normal 150,000 to 400,000/mm^3

IV. Urine
A. Glucose: normal negative
B. Ketones: normal negative
C. Amylase: normal negative
D. Bilirubin: normal negative
E. Bilinogen: normal 0.3 to 3.5 mg/dl
   1. Elevated in hepatocellular disease
   2. Decreased in complete biliary obstruction
F. Specific gravity: 1.005 to 1.030
G. Osmolality: 50 to 1200 mOsm/L

V. Gastric contents
A. Gastric analysis with a nasogastric tube
   1. Histamine or insulin is administered prior
      to collection of a sample of gastric contents
   2. Gastric contents are analyzed for the pres-
      ence of hydrochloric acid
   3. Have antihistamine (e.g., diphenhydramine
      [Benadryl]) or 50% dextrose available

B. pH determination
   1. Method
      a) Flush nasogastric tube with 20 ml of tap
         water and then clear tube with air
         before aspirating
      b) Do not use the same syringe used to
         give antacids to obtain the sample for
         pH testing
   2. Used for the following:
      a) To determine tube placement: stomach
         pH 1 to 3, intestine pH 6.5 or greater
      b) To determine effectiveness of H$_2$-
         receptor antagonist and/or antacid
         therapy: pH of 3.5 to 5.0 is desirable

VI. Stool
A. Fecal occult blood test: normal negative
B. Ova, parasites, blood (OPB): normal negative;
   specimen must be warm
C. Fecal fat: normal 5 g/24 hr
   1. Elevated in cystic fibrosis, Crohn's disease,
      biliary tract obstruction, pancreatic duct
      obstruction
   2. Specimen must be sent to laboratory in a
      wax-free container
D. Urobilinogen: normal 0 to 4 mg/day
   1. Decreased in biliary obstruction
   2. Specimen must be sent to laboratory in a
      light-resistant container
E. Culture: normal intestinal flora
F. Assay for *Clostridium difficile* toxin A or B:
   positive if diarrhea is caused by *C. difficile,* an
   opportunistic infection caused primarily by
   suppression of normal flora by antibiotic
   therapy

VII. Measurement of intraabdominal pressure (IAP)
A. Catheter inserted into peritoneal cavity and
   attached to transducer
B. Normal mean IAP is 0-subatmospheric; after
   abdominal surgery, the normal range may be
   slightly higher, averaging 3 to 15 mm Hg
   1. IAP may be increased with ascites, postop-
      erative bleeding, intestinal obstruction,
      ruptured abdominal aortic aneurysm
   2. Pressures greater than 30 to 40 mm Hg are
      associated with intraabdominal hyperten-
      sion and, potentially, abdominal com-
      partment syndrome

VIII. Other diagnostic studies (Table 8-5)

Malnutrition

Definition: Dietary intake of essential
nutrients is insufficient to meet the metabolic
demands of the body
I. Macronutrients: carbohydrate (CHO), protein, fat
II. Micronutrients: vitamins, minerals, water

Etiology
I. Decreased nutrient intake
A. Recent weight loss

Table 8-5 DIAGNOSTIC STUDIES

Study	Evaluates	Comments
Barium enema (also called *lower GI series*) **Note:** meglumine diatrizoate (Gastrografin) may be used, especially if bowel perforation is suspected	• Visualizes the movement, position, and filling of various segments of the colon after installation of barium by enema • Diagnoses colorectal lesions, diverticulitis, inflammatory bowel disease, strictures, fistulas • Evaluates colon size, length, and patency	• Low-fiber diet for 1-3 days prior to the study • Bowel preparation with bowel irrigation (e.g., GoLYTELY) and cathartics • NPO for 8-12 hours prior to study • Cathartics must be given after study • Contraindicated if bowel perforation or obstruction exists
Barium swallow, upper GI series, and small bowel follow-through **Note:** ordered according to which area or areas need to be evaluated (e.g., upper GI with small bowel follow-through means stomach, pylorus, duodenum; barium swallow with upper GI means esophagus, stomach, pylorus) **Note:** meglumine diatrizoate (Gastrografin) may be used, especially if bowel perforation is suspected	• Visualizes the position, shape, and activity of the esophagus, stomach, duodenum, and jejunum • Diagnoses esophageal lesions, varices, or esophageal motility disorders, hiatal hernia, gastric ulcers and tumors, small bowel obstruction, small bowel lesions, Crohn's disease • Evaluates gastric and small bowel motility	• Bowel preparation with bowel irrigation (e.g., GoLYTELY) and cathartics • NPO for 8-12 hours prior to study • Cathartics must be given after study • Contraindicated if bowel perforation or obstruction exists

Celiac or mesenteric angiography	• Evaluates portal vasculature
	• Diagnoses source of gastrointestinal bleeding
	• Evaluates cirrhosis, portal hypertension, vascular damage resulting from trauma, intestinal ischemia, tumors
	• May be used to treat GI bleeding using vasopressin
		• Bowel preparation (e.g., cathartics) as prescribed
		• NPO for 8 hours prior to the study
		• Sedative is usually prescribed prior to the procedure
		• Contrast media used
		  • Check for allergy to iodine prior to the study
		  • Monitor for allergic reaction following procedure
		  • Ensure hydration following procedure
		Postprocedure
		• Keep extremity in which catheter was placed immobilized in a straight position for 6-12 hours
		• Monitor arterial puncture point for hemorrhage or hematoma
		• Monitor neurovascular status of affected limb
		• Monitor for indications of systemic emboli

Cholecystography (oral, intravenous, percutaneous transhepatic, or common bile duct)	• Assesses gallbladder function, patency of the biliary system, and presence of gallstones • Diagnoses extrahepatic or intrahepatic jaundice, biliary calculi, biliary obstruction, common bile duct injury	• Percutaneous transhepatic cholangiography is contraindicated in patients with bleeding disorders • Fatty meal the day before the study, but the evening meal is fat free • Enema may be given the evening prior to the study • NPO 8-12 hours prior to the study • Contrast medium is administered orally the evening prior to the study, administered intravenous immediately prior to the study, injected percutaneously into the bile duct, or injected directly into the common bile duct during surgery • Check for allergy to iodine prior to the study

Continued

Table 8-5	DIAGNOSTIC STUDIES—cont'd	
Study	**Evaluates**	**Comments**
		• Monitor for allergic reaction following procedure • Ensure hydration following procedure • Monitor for clinical indications of bile leakage, hemorrhage, or peritonitis after percutaneous transhepatic cholangiography

Computed tomographic (CT) scan of abdomen	• Diagnoses tumors, pancreatic cancer or cysts, pancreatitis, biliary tract disorders, obstructive versus nonobstructive jaundice, cirrhosis, liver metastases, ascites, lymph node metastases, aneurysm
	• Evaluates vasculature and focal points found on nuclear scans
	• Used to direct biopsy of tumors or aspiration of abscess
		• No special preparation required
		• Contrast medium may be used; if used:
		  • Check for allergy to iodine prior to the study
		  • Monitor for allergic reaction following procedure
		  • Ensure hydration following procedure

Endoscopic retrograde cholangiopancreatography (ERCP)	• Diagnoses biliary stones, ductal stricture, ductal compression, neoplasms of the pancreas and biliary system • Evaluates patency of biliary and pancreatic ducts, jaundice, pancreatitis, cholecystitis, hepatitis	• Same as for esophagogastroduodenoscopy • Contraindicated if patient is uncooperative or if bilirubin is >3.5 mg/dl • Monitor for clinical indications of pancreatitis (most common complication) after study • Monitor for clinical indications of sepsis
Endoscopy • Esophagogastroduodenoscopy • Colonoscopy • Proctosigmoidoscopy	• Directly visualizes mucosa of areas of the GI tract • Esophagogastroduodenoscopy can be extended to visualize the pancreas and gallbladder • Esophagogastroduodenoscopy is used to diagnose esophagitis, esophageal ulcers, esophageal strictures, esophageal varices, hiatal hernia, gastritis, gastric ulcers, pyloric obstruction, pernicious anemia, foreign bodies, duodenal inflammation or ulcers and evaluates esophageal or gastric motility, bleeding, lesions, status of surgical anastomoses • Esophagoscopy, gastroscopy may also be used therapeutically for sclerosis of varices • Proctosigmoidoscopy is used to diagnose rectosigmoid cancer, strictures, polyps, inflammatory processes, hemorrhoids and to evaluate bleeding from rectosigmoid, surgical anastomoses • Colonoscopy is used to diagnose diverticular disease, obstruction, strictures, radiation injury, polyps, neoplasms, bleeding, ischemia • Colonoscopy or sigmoidoscopy may be used therapeutically for removal of polyps • Biopsies may be taken during any endoscopy	• Sedation may be prescribed especially for colonoscopy • Bowel preparation with gastric irrigation (e.g., GoLYTELY) and cathartics required before lower GI endoscopy • NPO 4-8 hours prior to study • Keep NPO until gag reflex returns if sedation used • Monitor closely after procedure for clinical indications of perforation, hemorrhage
Flat plate of abdomen	• Diagnoses perforated viscus, paralytic ileus, mechanical obstruction, intraabdominal mass • Evaluates the distribution of visceral gas (and identifies free air in the peritoneum indicative of bowel perforation) • Evaluates organ size	• No preparation required

Table 8-5	DIAGNOSTIC STUDIES—cont'd	
Study	**Evaluates**	**Comments**

Liver biopsy	• Obtains tissue specimen for microscopic evaluation
	• Diagnoses liver disease or malignancy
		• May be performed open or closed
		  • Open is done in surgery
		  • Closed biopsy may be done at bedside
		• Clotting profile is evaluated preprocedure
		  • Closed biopsy is contraindicated if platelet count is <100,000/mm^3
		• Patient must be cooperative because he or she must take a deep breath and hold for closed biopsy
		• Type and crossmatch for two units of blood preprocedure
		• NPO for 4-8 hours before study
		Postprocedure
		• Position patient on right side for 2 hours
		• Pressure dressing is applied, and the patient is on bed rest for 24 hours
		• Observe for:
		  • Hemorrhage: hypotension, dyspnea (subphrenic hematoma)
		  • Pneumothorax: dyspnea; chest pain; diminished breath sounds on right; hypoxemia
		  • Sepsis: fever; leukocytosis; rebound tenderness

Liver scan	• Diagnoses cirrhosis, hepatitis, tumors, abscesses, cysts, tuberculosis	• No preparation required
Magnetic resonance imaging (MRI)	• Evaluates liver, biliary tree, pancreas, spleen • Differentiation between cyst and solid mass • Diagnoses hepatic metastasis • Evaluates abscesses, fistulas, source of GI bleeding • Used for staging of colorectal cancer	• Cannot be used in patients with any implanted metallic device, including pacemakers • No special preparation required • Cannot be done on a patient being mechanically ventilated
Paracentesis	• Analysis of fluid removed during peritoneal tap • Diagnoses intraperitoneal bleeding with diagnostic peritoneal lavage	• Monitor for peritoneal leakage after tap • Monitor for clinical indications of infection or peritonitis after tap
Percutaneous transhepatic portography	• Diagnoses esophageal varices and visualizes portal venous circulation	• As for angiogram
Radionuclide imaging (hepatobiliary scintigraphy) • HIDA scan • PIPIDA scan	• Diagnoses hepatocellular disease, hepatic metastasis, biliary disease, lower GI bleeding, gastric reflux	• NPO 2 hours prior to study
Schilling's test	• Evaluates ileal absorption of vitamin B_{12} • Diagnoses pernicious anemia caused by intrinsic factor and inadequate ilial absorption of intrinsic factor-vitamin B_{12} complex	• IM vitamin B_{12} and oral radioactive B_{12} are given, and 24-hour urine specimen is collected
Ultrasound of abdomen	• Evaluates the pancreas, biliary ducts, gallbladder, liver • Identifies tumor, abdominal abscesses, hepatocellular disease, splenomegaly, pancreatic or splenic cysts • Differentiates obstructive from nonobstructive jaundice	• All barium must have been cleared from the GI tract prior to ultrasonography • NPO for 8 hours prior to study • If for evaluation of gallbladder: fat-free meal the evening prior to study

B. Recent change in diet; fad or limited diet
C. Eating disorder (e.g., obesity, bulimia, anorexia nervosa); **Note:** obesity is not overnourishment; many obese patients are protein malnourished
D. Anorexia
E. Nausea
F. Difficulty chewing or swallowing
G. Depression
H. Alcoholism or drug addiction
I. Social history of poverty, disability, living alone
J. Loss of the sense of taste or smell
K. Use of drugs known to alter dietary intake or food utilization (e.g., antacids, antibiotics, laxatives, antineoplastics)

II. Increased nutrient losses
A. Recurrent vomiting, diarrhea
B. GI disease such as peritonitis, inflammatory bowel disease

III. Increased nutrient requirements
A. Recent surgery or trauma
B. Chronic illnesses such as malignancy or renal, liver, lung, or heart disease or diabetes mellitus
C. Prolonged hypercatabolic state (e.g., multiple trauma, major surgery, sepsis, burns)

Pathophysiology

I. Inadequate calories causes glycogenolysis and gluconeogenesis
II. Stress of critical illness causes hypermetabolism, increased glucose utilization, gluconeogenesis with increased protein and fatty acid utilization, insulin resistance, and depletion of lean body tissue
III. Malnutrition causes immunodeficiency, poor wound healing, or eventual organ failure

Clinical Presentation

I. Subjective
A. Anorexia
B. Diarrhea
C. Fatigue, apathy
D. Irritability
E. Headache

II. Objective
A. Brittle hair
B. Pale, dry skin
C. Poor skin turgor
D. Fissures at corners of lips (cheilosis)
E. Hyperemic tongue; papillae may be hypertrophic or atrophic
F. Gum and teeth problems: loss of teeth; dental caries; bleeding or receding gums
G. Muscle wasting
H. Peripheral edema
I. Ascites
J. Hepatomegaly
K. Integumentary changes (e.g., poor wound healing)
L. Weight loss
1. Degrees of loss: 10% loss significant; 20% loss indicates malnutrition
2. Loss of more than 1 kg/wk associated with primarily protein loss

3. Body mass index (BMI)
a) Formula: Weight (kg)/Ht (m) × Ht (m)
b) Optimal: 20 to 25
c) Obesity: more than 25
d) Underweight: less than 20
M. Diminished skinfold and arm circumference measurement
1. Triceps skinfold
a) Measurement of skinfold thickness with calipers
b) Reflects measurement of the subcutaneous fat reserves of the body; normal 7.5 to 16.5 mm; less than 3 mm indicates severely depleted fat stores
2. Midarm muscle circumference
a) Measurement of middle of upper nondominant arm
b) Reflects measurement of body's muscle stores
N. Calculation of nutritional requirements
1. Protein: basal requirements 0.8 g/kg/day of body weight; critical illness requirements 1.5 to 2.5 g/kg/day
2. Calories: 25 to 80 kcal/kg/day
a) Basal or minimal illness: 25 kcal/kg/day
b) Moderate illness: 35 kcal/kg/day
c) Sepsis or extensive trauma: 45 kcal/kg/day
d) Burns: 80 kcal/kg/day
3. Fluids: 25 to 35 ml/kg/day

III. Diagnostics
A. Visceral protein measurements
1. Albumin: decreased; half-life 10 to 20 days
2. Transferrin: decreased; half-life 8 to 10 days
3. Prealbumin: decreased; half-life 2 to 3 days; better tool to evaluate visceral protein loss
4. Retinol-binding protein: decreased; half-life 10 hours; decreases with even minor stress; significance not fully understood
5. Hemoglobin/Hematocrit: may be decreased
6. Tests for immunocompetence
a) Total lymphocyte count: decreased
b) Cell-mediated immunity: skin tests for the following:
(1) *Candida albicans*
(2) Mumps
(3) Purified protein derivative (PPD) of tuberculin
B. Somatic (skeletal) protein measurements
1. Midarm muscle circumference
2. 24-hour urine specimen for creatinine
C. Nitrogen balance study (24-hour dietary record to evaluate nitrogen intake and urine collection to measure urine urea nitrogen and evaluate nitrogen loss): may show negative nitrogen balance

Nursing Diagnoses

I. Altered Nutrition: Less than Body Requirements related to inability to ingest, digest, absorb, or utilize nutrients, hypermetabolism
II. Risk for Infection related to anergy, immunocompromise, placement of central venous catheter

III. Risk for Aspiration related to enteral feeding, poor airway protective mechanisms, delayed gastric emptying, gastroesophageal incompetence with nasogastric and nasointestinal tubes

IV. Risk for Fluid Volume Deficit related to hyperosmolar feedings, hyperglycemia

V. Diarrhea related to bolus feeding, lactose intolerance, hyperosmolality, medications, contaminated formula, low-fiber formula, *Clostridium difficile*

VI. Impaired Tissue Integrity related to mechanical irritation of enteral tube, central venous catheter

Collaborative Management

I. Prevent/detect negative nitrogen balance and malnutrition
  A. Weigh daily at same time, on same scale
  B. Assess for changes in bowel sounds
  C. Monitor diagnostic studies reflective of visceral protein stores (e.g., albumin, transferrin, prealbumin)

II. Ensure delivery of adequate and appropriate nutrients
  A. Provide nutritional support for patients required to be NPO for more than 5 days or if patient unable to meet nutritional needs with oral feedings
    1. One liter of 5% dextrose provides only 170 kcal/L; while this provides fluids and delays gluconeogenesis for a short period, catabolism occurs after approximately 5 days at basal metabolic rate and earlier in a hypermetabolic patient
  B. Provide appropriate distribution of nutrients
    1. CHO: 50% to 60%
    2. Protein: 15% to 20%
    3. Fats: 25% to 30%
    4. New concepts in nutritional support (Table 8-6)
  C. Administer enteral nutritional support (Table 8-7) to patients with a functioning GI tract requiring nutritional support

D. Administer parenteral nutritional support (Table 8-8) to patients without a functioning GI tract requiring nutritional support; may also be used with oral or enteral nutrition to increase the amount of nutrients provided in hypermetabolic patients

GI Hemorrhage

Peptic Ulcer: May be gastric or duodenal

I. Definition: a sharply defined erosion in mucosa, which may involve the submucosa and muscular layers of the esophagus, stomach, and duodenum

II. Etiology
  A. *Helicobacter pylori:* a bacterial infection that has now been identified as a common cause of recurrent ulcer disease
  B. Other predisposing factors
    1. Genetic predisposition
    2. Smoking
    3. Diet
      a) Coffee or tea
      b) Carbonated beverages
      c) Beer
    4. Drugs and therapies
      a) Antineoplastics
      b) Radiation therapy
      c) Drugs that alter the mucosal barrier
        (1) Alcohol
        (2) Nonsteroidal antiinflammatory drugs: ASA, ibuprofen, indomethacin
      d) Drugs that decrease gastric mucosal renewal: corticosteroid, phenylbutazone
      e) Drugs that increase acid stimulation
        (1) Coffee (because of peptides, not caffeine)
        (2) Nicotine
        (3) Reserpine
      f) Hormones (e.g., estrogen)
    5. High emotional stress (e.g., Type A personality)

Table 8-6	**New Concepts in Nutritional Support**
Glutamine	• Nonessential neutral amino acid that plays an important role in maintaining normal intestinal structure and function • May be "conditionally" essential in critical illness, so providing glutamine to stressed patients may support the integrity of the gut, decrease the susceptibility to bacterial translocation and sepsis, and decrease the rate of protein catabolism
Arginine	• Semiessential amino acid that promotes nitrogen retention, improves protein turnover, improves wound healing, and enhances immune function • Arginine supplementation reduces the risk of infection and sepsis and promotes wound healing
Branched-chain amino acids	• Leucine, isoleucine, valine • Have beneficial effects on nitrogen balance in patients under stress • May be especially helpful in patients with hepatic failure or encephalopathy
Medium-chain triglycerides (MCT)	• Less irritating and more easily absorbed by the small bowel mucosa • Better than long-chain triglycerides (LCT) for patients with compromised GI function
Essential polyunsaturated fatty acids (PUFAs)	• Omega-6 (e.g., linoleic acid) and omega-3 (e.g., α-linolenic acid) fatty acids • Balance between these fatty acids aids in efficient functioning of the immune system

Table 8-7	**Enteral Nutritional Support**
Indications	• Patient has functioning GI tract but is unable or unwilling to consume nutrients
Advantages	• Preferred route for patients with functional GI tract • Fewer complications than parenteral route • Less expensive • Use of GI tract reduces incidence of sepsis by prevention of translocation of GI bacteria into blood or lymph • Use of GI tract maintains absorptive ability of GI tract

Types (Fig. 8-20) and choice of tubes	• Nasogastric
	• Nasoduodenal
	• Nasojejunal
	• Esophagostomy
	• Gastrostomy (including percutaneous endoscopic gastrostomy [PEG])
	• Jejunostomy (including needle jejunostomy, which may be done at the conclusion of a laparotomy)
	Choice
	• Small-gauge tube or tube that is placed below the gastroesophageal sphincter (such as PEG tube or jejunostomy tube) is preferred
	• Short-term (<6 weeks)
	  • Nasogastric
	  • Nasointestinal tube
	  • Needle jejunostomy
	• Long-term (>6 weeks)
	  • Gastrostomy
	  • Jejunostomy

Types of formulas	• Oligomeric (or *elemental*) and peptide enteral diets (e.g., Vivonex, Vivonex HN, Criticare HN, Vital HN, Travasorb NH, Impact, Stresstein): required when feeding is delivered distal to presence of digestive enzymes (distal jejunum)
	• Polymeric formulas require a functional GI system
	  • Intact protein and lactose-free enteral diets (e.g., Sustacal, Ensure, Enrich, Osmolite)
	  • Intact protein, lactose-free, high-density enteral diets (e.g., Magnacal, Isocal HCN, Sustacal HC, Ensure Plus, Ensure Plus HN)
	  • Blenderized meat-based enteral diets (e.g., Vitaneed, Compleat B)
	  • Specialized enteral diets
	    • Trauma (e.g., Traumacal, Traum-Aid HBC, Vivonex TEN)
	    • Hepatic (e.g., Travasorb Hepatic, Hepatic-Aid): increased branched-chain amino acids
	    • Pulmonary (e.g., Pulmocare): higher proportion of fats, less CHO to reduce CO_2 production
	    • Renal (e.g., Travasorb Renal, Amin-Aid): essential amino acids
	    • Diabetic (e.g., Glucerna, Suplena)
	    • Fiber-containing formulas (e.g., Ensure with fiber, Jevity, Sustacal with fiber)
	• Modular
	  • CHO (e.g., Polycose, Nutrisource Modular System [carbohydrate])
	  • Protein (e.g., Promod, Nutrisource Modular System [protein])
	  • Lipid-Medium Chain Triglycerides (e.g., MCT oil, Nutrisource Modular System [lipid])
	  • Lipid-Long Chain Triglycerides (e.g., Nutrisource Modular System [lipid LCT])
	• Note calorie concentration (most 1 kcal/ml but some critical care formulas have 2 kcal/ml)
	• Note osmolality (isotonic is 250-350 mOsm/L, hypertonicity contributes to dehydration and diarrhea)

Pattern of delivery	• Intermittent (cannot be used below the pylorus) • Continuously • Cyclic: feeding may be occasionally discontinued during the 24-hour period (e.g., turned off at night)

Monitor	• Placement and positioning of the feeding tube
	  • X-ray if mercury-weighted tube
	  • Injection of air with auscultation over stomach
	  • Check pH of gastric aspirate: pH 1-3 in stomach without pH-altering drugs, 3-5 in stomach with pH-altering drugs, >7 in small intestine
	• Intake and output totaled every 8-12 hours
	• Weight daily
	• Bedside glucose testing by fingerstick every 6 hours; serum glucose by laboratory daily
	• Electrolytes daily initially
	• BUN daily initially
	• Proteins, trace elements, liver function studies weekly

Table 8-7	**Enteral Nutritional Support—cont'd**
General guidelines	• Use an infusion pump for continuous infusion • Check for residual volume every 4 hours or before next intermittent feeding; if residual greater than 100-150 ml, delay feeding for at least 1 hour and then check again; patients with persistent retention benefit from having the tube advanced into the intestine (intestinal motility usually not affected by same factors as gastric motility) • Administer room-temperature fluids to prevent cramping and nausea • Begin with ¼-½ strength at slow rate; increase gradually • Administer free water in volume of 1 ml/kcal to prevent hyperosmolality • Keep head of bed elevated at least 30 degrees during and after intermittent feeding; continuously for continuous feeding
Complications of enteral alimentation	• Nausea/vomiting 　• Slow feeding 　• Allow feeding to come to room temperature before infusion 　• Decrease amount of fat in feeding 　• Administer lactose-free formula • Endotracheal aspiration of tube feeding 　• Elevate head of bed at all times if feeding is continuous; during and for 60 minutes after intermittent feeding 　• Keep cuff inflated during feeding if patient intubated or has tracheostomy 　• Check for residual volume in stomach every 4 hours • Hyperosmolar, hyperglycemic, nonketotic dehydration 　• Monitor serum glucose every 6 hours by fingerstick; administer insulin as prescribed to keep scrum glucose between 100-200 mg/dl • Diarrhea; caused by any of the following: 　• Decreased plasma colloidal oncotic pressure (COP) due to low serum proteins 　• Bacterial contamination: do not allow solutions to hang at room temperature for more than 8 hours; avoid antidiarrheals, which slow peristalsis and increase the risk of sepsis 　• Hypertonicity: use isotonic solutions if possible; administer adequate amounts of free water 　• Alteration in normal flora from antibiotics and proliferation of *Clostridium difficile*; administer metronidazole (Flagyl) or vancomycin; yogurt (with active cultures) or *Lactobacillus acidophilus* may be used to rcstore normal flora • Constipation 　• Add fiber 　• Increase free water

6. High physiologic strcss situation
   a) COPD
   b) Multiple trauma
   c) Major surgery
   d) Myocardial infarction
   e) Hepatic failure
   f) Renal failure
   g) Burns: referred to as *Curling's ulcer*
   h) Cerebral trauma: referred to as *Cushing's ulcer*
   i) Acute respiratory distress syndrome
   j) Mechanical ventilation for more than 5 days
   k) Coagulopathy
   l) Sepsis
   m) Shock

III. Pathophysiology
   A. Injury caused by one or more of the following factors:
      1. Presence of *Helicobacter pylori* bacteria
      2. Increased acid production or inability to buffer acid
      3. Impaired mucosal barrier to acid
      4. Impaired gastric motility

5. Stress
   a) Acid hypersecretion related at least in part to increased endogenous (or exogenous) glucocorticoids
   b) Decreased mucosal pH
   c) Ischemia
   d) Altered mucosal defense mechanisms

B. Ulceration occurs when mucosa is injured, allowing acid to diffuse back through the broken barrier

C. Hemorrhage, perforation, or scarring with obstruction indicate the need for immediate treatment
   1. Gastric ulcers are more likely to present with hematemesis or perforation
   2. Duodenal ulcers are more likely to present with melena, perforation, or scarring with obstruction

IV. Clinical presentation
   A. Subjective
      1. History: epigastric pain, previous ulcer, previous GI bleeding, alcoholism, liver disease
      2. Epigastric pain
      3. Fatigue, weakness

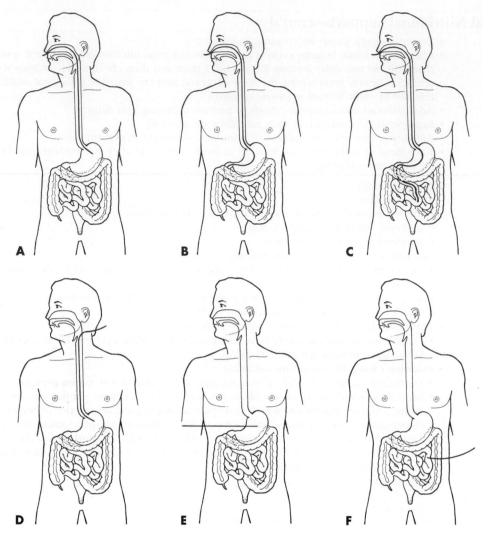

Figure 8-20 Enteral nutrition routes. **A,** Nasogastric. **B,** Nasoduodenal. **C,** Nasojejunal. **D,** Esophagostomy. **E,** Gastrostomy. **F,** Jejunostomy. (From Flynn JBM, Bruce NP: *Introduction to critical care skills,* St Louis, 1993, Mosby.)

4. Thirst
5. Anxiety
B. Objective
1. Blood or coffee-ground material appears in vomitus if gastric ulcer; black stools if duodenal; may have bloody stools in duodenal ulcer and hyperperistalsis
2. If bleeding is gradual, faintness, fatigue, and pallor may be only indications
3. Patient may have signs of acute abdomen if ulcer perforated (Box 8-2); other terms for an acute abdomen include *surgical abdomen* or *"hot belly"*
C. Diagnostic
1. Serum
   a) Chemistry
      (1) Gastrin level: may be elevated in gastric ulcer
      (2) Amylase: elevated if perforation causes penetration into the pancreas and causes acute pancreatitis
      (3) Total proteins, albumin, transferrin:

may be decreased because many of these patients are malnourished
      b) Hematology: Hgb, Hct may be decreased but changes take approximately 4 to 6 hours after acute bleed
      c) Clotting studies: PT, aPTT, prolonged if liver is affected
2. Gastric analysis: may show hyperacidity; may show blood in the gastric secretions
3. Stools for occult blood: positive
4. ECG: may show indications of ischemia (e.g., ST-T-wave changes)
5. Flat plate of abdomen: may show free air under diaphragm indicates perforation
6. Gastroscopy: important in differentiating cause of upper GI bleeding; can determine ulcer presence, location, and stage of healing
7. Upper GI series: may show anatomic deformity created by ulcer crater; may show delayed gastric emptying if edema or scarring is present

Table 8-8	**Parenteral Nutritional Support**

Indication	• When the enteral route is contraindicated (GI disorders)
	  • Bowel resection or other abdominal surgery
	  • Bowel obstruction
	  • Mesenteric ischemia
	  • Ileus
	  • Short-bowel syndrome
	  • Severe malabsorption
	• When the enteral route is ineffective (high caloric needs or shock)

Routes	• Central vein: referred to as *total parenteral nutrition* (TPN)
	  • Allows the administration of hypertonic glucose solutions because of rapid dilution by blood as the solution enters the great vessel
	  • Subclavian or internal jugular usually used
	• Peripheral vein: referred to as *peripheral parenteral nutrition* (PPN)
	  • Used for patients who cannot take in sufficient nutrition enterally for 5-7 days but who are not hypermetabolic
	  • Not usually adequate to provide sufficient calories for critically ill patient because of osmolality (and therefore calorie) limitations

Type of catheter	• Short term: peripheral or central venous catheter; multilumen catheter usually used to provide lumen for parenteral nutrition, lumen for blood and/or fluids, lumen for parenteral drugs • Long term: Hickman (Fig. 8-21), Broviac, or Groshong catheter; Infuse-a-Port; Port-a-Cath

Solution: 1 L of standard TPN formula (25% dextrose and 8.5% amino acids) provides ~1,000 kcal (1 kcal/ml)	• CHO: hypertonic dextrose (peripheral 10%; central usually 25% but may be as high as 35%)
	  • CHO and fats provide enough calories for maximal protein-sparing effect
	  • Dextrose provides 3.4 calories/g
	• Protein: crystalline amino acids 2.5%-8.5%; includes essential and nonessential amino acids
	  • Amino acids provide 4.3 calories/g
	  • Specialized formulas are available for specific diseases
	    • Hepatic failure (e.g., HepatAmine, Branch Amin): branched-chain amino acids
	    • Renal failure (e.g., RenAmin, NephrAmine): essential amino acids
	• Fats: 30% of nonprotein calories are supplied by fats; linoleic acid, the only essential fatty acid, should provide 4% of the total calorie intake to prevent deficiency of essential fatty acid
	  • 10% lipids provide 1 kcal/ml
	  • 20% lipids provide 2 kcal/ml
	• Electrolytes: sodium chloride, potassium, calcium, magnesium, phosphate
	• Buffer: acetate or bicarbonate
	• Minerals: iron, zinc, copper, manganese, cobalt, iodine, chromium, selenium
	• Vitamins: multivitamins 1 ampule/day
	  • Vitamin K (10-20 mg) should be administered every week; may be given IM or SC or added to TPN solution as phytonadione (AquaMephyton)

Possible additives	• Regular insulin (sliding-scale insulin will still be administered as needed) • Heparin • H_2-receptor antagonists • Metoclopramide (Reglan) • **Note:** All additives should be added under laminar hood (in pharmacy department) rather than on nursing unit
Monitor	• Vital signs and infusion rate at least every 4 hours (depending on the acuity of the patient) • Intake and output totaled every 8-12 hours • Weight daily • Bedside glucose testing by fingerstick every 6 hours; serum glucose by laboratory daily • Electrolytes daily • BUN daily • CBC, proteins, trace elements, liver function studies, triglycerides, cholesterol, platelet count, prothrombin time weekly • Catheter site
General guidelines	• Utilize strict sterile technique during catheter insertion and management • Assess patient for central venous catheter insertion complications (pneumothorax, hemothorax, chylothorax, arterial puncture); request chest X-ray after insertion of central venous catheter; do not initiate fluids at a rate faster than KVO until chest X-ray confirms placement • Do not use a catheter (or lumen of a multilumen catheter) that has been previously used for CVP measurements or for the prolonged administration of crystalloid solution or blood products • Do not use the catheter (or lumen) for drawing blood samples or infusing any other fluids

Table 8-8	**Parenteral Nutritional Support—cont'd**

	• Do not hang cloudy solutions
	• Monitor closely for emulsion crack if hanging 3-in-1 solution (also called *total nutrient admixture* [TNA]); do not hang solution if a layer of fat is seen separated at top of bag
	• Utilize an inline filter; 0.22 micron if lipids are piggybacked in distal to filter; 1.2 micron if TNA used as smaller filter will not allow lipids to flow through
	• Initiate at 1,200-2,400 cal/day and increase to desired caloric intake as prescribed
	• Remove from refrigerator 30 minutes prior to infusing
	• Keep rate constant (volumetric pump required)
	• Change dressing every 48 hours or according to hospital policy or anytime that the dressing becomes soiled
	  • Gauze and tape or semipermeable transparent dressing (e.g., Op-Site, Tegaderm)
	    • Semipermeable transparent dressings have been associated with a higher rate of catheter-related infection and sepsis than standard gauze and tape probably because of inadequate permeability and infrequency of dressing change; they should not be used in patients with oily skin or acne near catheter insertion site
	• Change tubing every 24-72 hours or according to hospital policy; lipid tubing (including TNA tubing) should be changed every 24 hours

Complications	• Allergic reaction (especially to lipids)
	  • Note fever, chills, shivering, chest or back pain
	  • Stop infusion
	• Infection and sepsis
	  • Utilize meticulous aseptic technique with all aspects of catheter care; change dressing every 48 hours or whenever soiled; change tubing every 24-72 hours; minimize number of entries into the system
	  • Monitor for clinical indications of catheter-related sepsis: fever, leukocytosis, glucose intolerance, redness, swelling, tenderness, and purulent drainage at insertion site
	  • Obtain blood cultures (not through this catheter), remove catheter and culture tip
	• Hyperglycemia
	  • Monitor serum glucose levels
	  • Administer insulin therapy; usually administered as insulin drip if serum glucose >500 mg/dl
	• Hyperglycemic/hyperosmolar nonketotic (HHNK) dehydration
	  • Monitor serum glucose levels
	  • Administer insulin therapy; usually administered as insulin drip if serum glucose >500 mg/dl
	  • Administer hypotonic saline (¼ or ½) or D_5W (depending on patient's serum osmolality) to correct free water deficit
	  • Discontinue TPN until patient stable as prescribed
	• Hypoglycemia
	  • Prevent interruption of TPN infusion (e.g., catheter occlusion or accidental removal)
	  • Use infusion pump (mandatory)
	  • Never discontinue TPN abruptly unless for HHNK
	• Electrolyte imbalances: hyperchloremic metabolic acidosis; hyponatremia; hypokalemia; hypocalcemia; hypomagnesemia; hypophosphatemia
	  • Adjust TPN solution concentration and/or alter infusion rate as prescribed
	• Refeeding syndrome: fluid imbalance; hypokalemia; hypophosphatemia; hypoglycemia or hyperglycemia
	  • Monitor fluid, electrolyte, glucose levels especially during the first 24-48 hours after TPN initiated
	  • Adjust TPN solution concentration and/or alteration of infusion rate as prescribed
	• Increased CO_2 production
	  • Monitor closely for clinical indications of hypercapnia; request ABGs as indicated
	  • Decrease the percentage of calories supplied by CHO and increase percentage of calories supplied by fats if hypercapnia occurs or during weaning
	• Air embolus
	  • Prevent air embolus by the following:
	    • Asking patient to hold breath or Valsalva during catheter insertion, tubing changes, and catheter removal
	    • Purge all air from tubings before attachment to catheter
	    • Use air-eliminating filters on central line tubings
	    • Use Luer-Lok connections
	  • Note dyspnea, hypotension, churning murmur over precordium, confusion
	  • If clinical indications occur: place patient in Trendelenburg position on left side and aspirate air with a syringe attached to the central venous catheter; administer oxygen
	• Subclavian thrombosis (rare)
	  • Monitor for swelling of involved arm, face, neck, erythema, fever
	  • Remove catheter
	  • Administer thrombolytic or anticoagulation therapy as prescribed

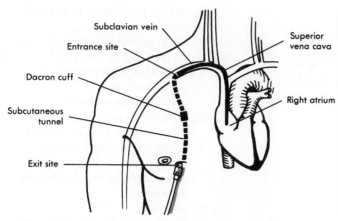

Figure 8-21 Hickman catheter for administration of TPN. (From Long BC, Phipps WJ, Cassmeyer VL: *Medical-surgical nursing: a nursing process approach,* ed 3, St Louis, 1993, Mosby.)

BOX

8-2   Clinical Indications of an Acute Abdomen

- Abdominal pain
- Abdominal distention
- Rigid, boardlike abdomen
- Rebound tenderness
- Diminished or absent bowel sounds
- Nausea, vomiting
- Fever
- Leukocytosis

---

8. Biopsy: may be done to rule out gastric cancer or malignant gastric ulcer
9. Angiography: may reveal bleeding site or sites; may include the placement of a catheter for administration of vasopressors (e.g., vasopressin)

V. Nursing Diagnoses

A. Alteration in Fluid Volume: Deficit related to hemorrhage, fluid shifts
B. Decreased Cardiac Output related to decreased preload
C. Altered Tissue Perfusion: Cerebral, Cardiopulmonary, Renal, Gastrointestinal, Peripheral related to anemia, hypovolemia, vasopressin therapy
D. Risk for Aspiration related to hematemesis
E. Potential for Impaired Gas Exchange related to anemia, aspiration
F. Alteration in Nutrition: Less than Body Requirements related to poor intake and altered food metabolism
G. Ineffective Individual Coping related to situational crisis, powerlessness, change in role
H. Ineffective Family Coping related to critically ill family member
I. Knowledge Deficit related to required lifestyle changes

VI. Collaborative management

A. Ensure airway, oxygenation, ventilation
 1. Elevate head of bed 30 to 45 degrees for optimal ventilation
 2. Administer oxygen as necessary to maintain SpO_2 95% unless contraindicated; in patients with COPD, administer oxygen to achieve an SpO_2 of ~90%
B. Restore circulating blood volume and control bleeding
 1. Insert at least two short (1¼ inch) large-gauge (16-18) peripheral intravenous catheters; draw labs and type and crossmatch for 6 units of blood
 2. Insert indwelling urinary catheter to evaluate hourly urine output
 3. Assist with insertion of arterial catheter and pulmonary artery catheter in patients with severe hemorrhage
 4. Administer crystalloids and colloids as prescribed
  a) Maintain urine output of 0.5 to 1 ml/kg/hr
  b) Maintain PAOP of ~12 to 15 mm Hg
  c) Avoid lactated Ringer's in patients with liver disease
 5. Administer blood and blood products as prescribed
  a) Packed red cells should be given early if significant blood loss is suspected to prevent tissue hypoxia
   (1) Fresh blood is preferred because it is lower in ammonia than banked blood
   (2) Hematocrit should be kept greater than 30% if possible
  b) After multiple transfusions, consideration should be given to replacement of clotting factors, platelets, and calcium
 6. Administer vasopressin intravenous as prescribed; vasopressin slows blood loss by constricting the splanchnic arteriolar bed and decreasing portal venous pressure
  a) Administer through a central line at a dose of 0.2 to 0.6 U/min for up to 36 hours; the dose is then slowly decreased
  b) Monitor for adverse effects of vasopressin: bradycardia, hypertension, water retention causing hyponatremia (SIADH), chest pain, dysrhythmias, abdominal cramping and pain, oliguria
   (1) Because vasopressin may cause constriction of coronary arteries, nitroglycerin infusion may be used concurrently to prevent chest pain
   (2) Close monitoring of the blood pressure is essential because hypertension may increase bleeding
  c) May also be infused directly into the superior mesenteric artery by a catheter placed during angiography
 7. Insert large-bore NG tube to perform gastric lavage to monitor bleeding and remove ni-

trogenous materials from the GI tract; Ewald tube may be used to aid in evacuation of large amounts of blood or clots

a) This procedure does not truly aid in clotting as previously believed and may dislodge clots; it is performed to monitor bleeding and to remove nitrogenous materials (blood) out of the gut so that they will not be converted to ammonia

b) Use room-temperature saline for lavage

(1) Iced lavage may cause:

(a) Hydrochloric acid to diffuse back into submucosa and cause more bleeding

(b) Prolongation of clotting times

(c) Hypothermia

(i) Causing a shift of the oxyhemoglobin dissociation curve to the left, decreasing tissue delivery of oxygen

(ii) Causing the patient to shiver, increasing oxygen consumption

c) Administer osmotic laxatives (e.g., sorbitol) as prescribed

d) Administer magnesium sulfate and saline enemas as ordered to evacuate the colon of bloody material

8. Assist with diagnostic/therapeutic endoscopy

a) Diagnostic: to identify the specific cause of the bleeding

b) Therapeutic

(1) Endoscopic thermal therapy uses heat to cauterize the bleeding vessel

(2) Endoscopic injection therapy uses hypertonic saline, epinephrine, or dehydrated alcohol to cause localized vasoconstriction of the bleeding vessel

9. Prepare patient for surgery if necessary to control bleeding

a) Indications for surgery

(1) Continuation of bleeding despite treatment

(2) Administration of more than 8 U of blood over 24 hours

(3) Hemorrhage to the point of hypotension or shock

(4) Rebleeding after hemostasis achieved

b) Surgical interventions

(1) Oversewing of bleeding point

(2) Pyloroplasty: revision of the pyloric valve

(3) Antrectomy: removal of the antrum; decreases acidity by removing antrum and decreasing gastric acid secretion

(4) Vagotomy: dividing the vagus nerve along the esophagus

(a) Decreases acid secretion in the stomach

(b) If ulcer is prepyloric, vagotomy should be performed to prevent obstruction

(5) Gastrectomy: partial or total

(a) Types (Fig. 8-22)

(i) Billroth I: antrectomy, vagotomy, and gastroduodenostomy

(ii) Billroth II: antrectomy, vagotomy, and gastrojejunostomy

(iii) Total gastrectomy: gastrectomy with anastomosis of esophagus to the duodenum or jejunum

(b) Monitor for:

(i) Early dumping syndrome (hyperosmolality effect related to a hyperosmolar bolus of food being "dumped" into the duodenum because of absence of pyloric valve and normal, more gradual gastric emptying): occurs within 30 minutes after eating; causes dizziness, weakness, tachycardia, and cool, clammy skin

(ii) Late dumping syndrome (hyperinsulinism effect related to an increase in insulin production by the pancreas in response to a large bolus of food, causing an increase in blood glucose): occurs 2 hours after meal; causes dizziness, weakness, restlessness, tachycardia, malabsorption, and cool, clammy skin

(iii) Pernicious anemia: related to removal of parietal cells, which make intrinsic factor necessary for the absorption of B_{12} in the ileum

C. Increase intragastric pH

1. Maintain pH 3.5 to 5.0 (normal pH of gastric secretions 1 to 3)

a) Administer agents that decrease gastric acidity and/or protect gastric mucosa (Table 8-9)

(1) Discussion of major disadvantage of reducing the acidity of the stomach

(a) Hydrochloric acid normally kills bacteria

(b) By neutralizing this effect, bacteria is allowed to proliferate in the stomach

(c) Bacteria may colonize into the esophagus, where it may migrate into the tracheobronchial tree

(d) Patient may aspirate gastric content (containing live bacteria) into the tracheobronchial tree

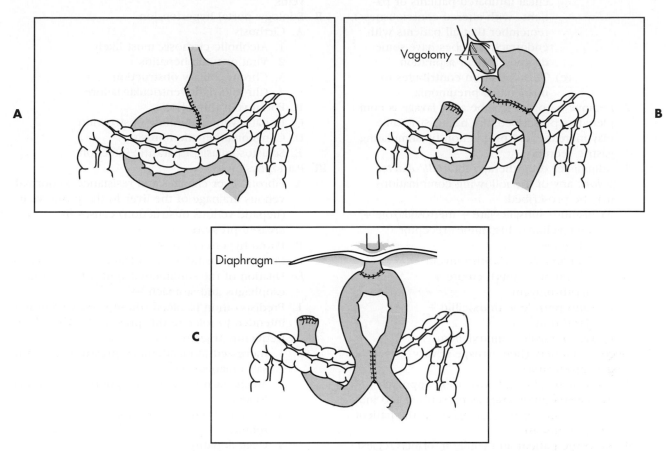

Figure 8-22   Gastric resection procedures. **A,** Billroth I. **B,** Billroth II. **C,** Total gastrectomy.

Table 8-9	Agents That Decrease Gastric Acidity and/or Protect Gastric Mucosa	
Category	**Examples**	**Actions**
Antacids	• Aluminum-magnesium complex (Riopan) • Magnesium hydroxide and aluminum hydroxide (Maalox, Mylanta) • Calcium carbonate (Tums)	• Buffers gastric acid • Increase in pH decreases the activity of pepsin
Histamine (H_2) receptor antagonists	• Cimetidine (Tagamet) • Ranitidine (Zantac) • Famotidine (Pepcid) • Nizatidine (Axid)	• Blocks the action of histamine on parietal cells to inhibit volume and concentration of gastric secretions
Proton pump inhibitors	• Omeprazole (Prilosec) • Lansoprazole (Prevacid) • Rabeprazole sodium (AcipHex)	• Inactivates hydrogen pump, causing prevention of the formation of hydrochloric acid by parietal cells
Mucosal protectant (prostaglandin E_1-analog)	• Misoprostol (Cytotec)	• Enhances the body's normal gastric mucosal protective mechanisms • Increases mucosal blood flow • Decreases gastric acid secretion
Mucosal protectant (aluminum hydroxide, sulfated sucrose)	• Sucralfate (Carafate)	• Combines with gastric acid and forms an adhesive protective coating over an ulcer crater • Adsorbs pepsin

in patients with poor protective mechanisms (e.g., endotracheal intubated patients or patients with altered consciousness); remember that all patients with endotracheal tubes have some degree of silent aspiration

    (e) This condition contributes to nosocomial pneumonia

2. Remove nasogastric tube after lavage is completed as prescribed; the nasogastric tube may increase acid production by stimulating gastric secretion

3. Administer drug therapy for *Helicobacter pylori;* any of the following combinations may be prescribed:

    a) Bismuth subsalicylate + metronidazole + tetracycline + histamine$_2$ receptor antagonist

    b) Omeprazole + clarithromycin

    c) Ranitidine bismuth citrate + clarithromycin

    d) Lansoprazole + amoxicillin + clarithromycin

    e) Lansoprazole + amoxicillin

D. Decrease anxiety (hemorrhage is very anxiety-producing)

1. Maintain a calm and reassuring approach

2. Administer anxiolytics as prescribed and indicated; avoid hepatotoxic agents if the patient has liver disease

3. Keep the patient and family informed regarding patient status

4. Encourage discussion of fears and concerns

E. Maintain fluid and electrolyte balance: evaluate sodium, potassium, calcium, magnesium and replace as prescribed

F. Maintain nutritional status by administering nutrients when appropriate

1. Provide bland proteins and fats in small, frequent meals

2. Avoid stimulants of gastric secretions (e.g., coffee, tea, cola, spicy foods, alcohol)

3. Progress to full diet as soon as possible

G. Monitor for complications

1. Aspiration pneumonitis

2. Recurrent bleeding, hemorrhage

3. Perforation

4. Peritonitis

5. Penetration into surrounding tissues (e.g., acute pancreatitis)

6. Obstruction due to ulcer scarring at the pylorus

7. Myocardial infarction

8. Cerebral infarction

9. Disseminated intravascular coagulation (DIC)

10. Sepsis

11. Shock: hypovolemia or septic

Esophageal Varices

I. Definition: dilation of the submucosal esophageal veins

II. Etiology: portal hypertension

A. Cirrhosis

1. Alcoholic cirrhosis: most likely

2. Viral or toxic hepatitis

3. Chronic biliary obstruction

4. Chronic right ventricular failure

B. Portal vein thrombosis

C. Hepatic venous outflow obstruction

D. Congenital hepatic fibrosis

E. Schistosomiasis: a parasitic infection

III. Pathophysiology

A. Fibrotic liver changes and resistance to normal venous drainage of the liver to the portal vein (hepatic venous obstruction) causes increased pressure →

B. Portal hypertension →

C. Pressure transmitted to collateral circulation →

D. Dilation of the submucosal veins of the distal esophagus and stomach →

E. Predisposition to bleed (these vessels were not intended to tolerate this pressure) → bleeding frequently triggered by:

1. Increased intraabdominal pressure (e.g., Valsalva maneuver)

2. Mechanical trauma (e.g., poorly chewed hard foods)

3. Chemical trauma (e.g., gastroesophageal reflux)

4. Coagulopathy

F. Massive bleeding from mouth (note that these patients do not truly vomit; they simply open their mouth and massive amounts of blood are emitted)

IV. Clinical presentation

A. Subjective

1. History of precipitating causes (e.g., excessive, chronic alcohol intake)

2. Report of sudden, painless hemorrhage orally

B. Objective

1. Bright, red blood gushing from mouth

2. Jaundice

3. Abdominal distention

4. Hyperactive bowel sounds

5. Melena

6. Hepatomegaly

7. Splenomegaly

8. Clinical indications of hypoperfusion: tachycardia, tachypnea, hypotension, cool clammy skin, decreased urine output, agitation, confusion

C. Diagnostic

1. Serum

    a) Chemistry

      (1) BUN: elevated

      (2) Bilirubin: may be elevated

      (3) Albumin: decreased because of liver disease

(4) AST, ALT, LDH: elevated due to liver disease

b) Hematology: Hgb, Hct decreased

c) Clotting studies: PT, aPTT prolonged because of liver disease

d) Arterial blood gases: may reveal metabolic acidosis related to shock and hypoperfusion

2. Stool: positive for occult blood

3. ECG: may show indications of ischemia (e.g., ST-T-wave changes)

4. Barium swallow: reveals the presence of esophageal varices

5. Esophagogastroduodenoscopy: reveals the presence of esophageal varices

6. Percutaneous transhepatic portography: reveals esophageal varices and measures pressure in the portal circulation

7. Angiography: may reveal bleeding site or sites; may include the placement of a catheter for administration of vasopressors (e.g., vasopressin)

V. Nursing Diagnoses

A. Alteration in Fluid Volume: Deficit related to hemorrhage, fluid shifts

B. Decreased Cardiac Output related to decreased preload

C. Altered Tissue Perfusion: Cerebral, Cardiopulmonary, Renal, Gastrointestinal, Peripheral related to anemia, hypovolemia, vasopressin therapy

D. Risk for Aspiration related to hematemesis

E. Ineffective Airway Clearance related to displacement of esophageal balloon in balloon tamponade

F. Alteration in Nutrition: Less than Body Requirements related to poor intake and altered food metabolism

G. Impaired Gas Exchange related to anemia, aspiration, airway compromise from balloon tamponade

H. Potential for Injury related to coagulopathy, esophageal varices, altered consciousness

I. Ineffective Individual Coping related to situational crisis, powerlessness, change in role

J. Ineffective Family Coping related to critically ill family member

K. Knowledge Deficit related to required lifestyle changes

VI. Collaborative management

A. Ensure airway, oxygenation, ventilation

1. Elevate head of bed 30 to 45 degrees for optimal ventilation

2. Administer oxygen as necessary to maintain SpO_2 95% unless contraindicated; in patients with COPD, administer oxygen to achieve an SpO_2 ~90%

3. Assist with endotracheal intubation as requested prior to endoscopy or balloon tamponade

B. Restore circulating blood volume and control bleeding

1. Insert at least two short (1¼ inch) large-gauge (16-18) peripheral intravenous catheters; draw labs and type and crossmatch for 6 units of blood

2. Insert indwelling urinary catheter to evaluate hourly urine output

3. Assist with insertion of arterial catheter and pulmonary artery catheter in patients with severe hemorrhage

4. Administer crystalloids and colloids as prescribed

a) Maintain urine output of 0.5 to 1 ml/kg/hr

b) Maintain PAOP of ~12 to 15 mm Hg

c) Avoid lactated ringers in patients with liver disease

5. Administer blood and blood products as prescribed

a) Packed red cells should be given early if significant blood loss is suspected to prevent tissue hypoxia

(1) Fresh blood is preferred because it is lower in ammonia than banked blood

(2) Hematocrit should be kept greater than 30% if possible

b) After multiple transfusions, consideration should be given to replacement of clotting factors, platelets, and calcium

6. Insert large-bore NG tube to perform gastric lavage to ensure adequate visualization and to remove nitrogenous material from the GI tract (**Note:** Studies have not shown that insertion of NG tube is associated with trauma to varices and increase in bleeding)

7. Assist with diagnostic/therapeutic endoscopy

a) Diagnostic: to identify the specific cause of the bleeding

b) Therapeutic

(1) Sclerotherapy

(a) Sclerosing agent (ethanolamine oleate [Ethamolin], morrhuate sodium [Scleromate], sodium tetradecyl [Sotradecol]) is injected into the varix and surrounding tissue; the sclerosing agent causes variceal inflammation, venous thrombosis, and eventually scar tissue; repeated injections may be necessary to completely decompress the bleeding varix and to decrease the risk of recurrent hemorrhage

(b) Varices are categorized as I to IV by their size; class III and IV are

at high risk to bleed if not
already bleeding
(c) Monitor for complications of
sclerotherapy
(i) Retrosternal pain
(ii) Transient fever
(iii) Transient dysphagia
(iv) Local ulceration
(v) Pulmonary symptoms, including diminished breath
sounds
(vi) Bleeding
(vii) Stricture
(viii) Perforation
(ix) Sepsis
(d) Sclerosing is repeated in 4 to 7
days and every 6 to 8 months
thereafter
(2) Esophageal variceal ligation: rubber-
bands or O-rings are placed on the
target vessels at gastroesophageal
junction
8. Administer vasopressin intravenously as prescribed; vasopressin slows blood flow by
constricting the splanchnic arteriolar bed
and decreasing portal venous pressure
a) Administer through a central line:
loading dose of 20 U in 50 to 100 ml
D_5W over 20 minutes followed by a dose
of 0.1 to 0.6 U/min for up to 36 hours;
the dose is then slowly decreased
b) Monitor for adverse effects of vasopressin: bradycardia, hypertension, water retention causing hyponatremia (SIADH),
chest pain, dysrhythmias, abdominal
cramping and pain, oliguria
(1) Because vasopressin may cause constriction of coronary arteries, nitroglycerin infusion may be used
concurrently to prevent chest pain
(2) Close monitoring of the blood pressure is essential because hypertension may increase bleeding
c) May also be infused directly into the superior mesenteric artery by a catheter
placed during angiography
9. Administer octreotide acetate (Sandostatin)
as prescribed; octreotide reduces splanchnic
blood flow, gastric acid secretion, GI mobility, and pancreatic exocrine function
a) Administer IV or SC 50 μg/hr for 24
hours or until TIPS or portosystemic
shunt is completed
b) Monitor for adverse effects of octreotide:
pain or burning at injection site, abdominal pain, diarrhea
10. Remove nitrogenous materials from the GI
tract
a) Perform gastric lavage with room-
temperature saline

b) Administer osmotic laxatives (e.g., sorbitol) as prescribed
c) Administer magnesium sulfate and saline
enemas as ordered
11. Stop bleeding through measures that lower
venous pressure
a) Administer beta-blockers (e.g., propranolol) as prescribed
b) Assist in placement of a multilumen tube
for balloon tamponade (Fig. 8-23 and
Table 8-10)
12. Prepare patient for surgery if necessary to
control bleeding
a) Indications for surgery
(1) Continuation of bleeding despite
treatment
(2) Administration of more than 8 U of
blood over 24 hours
(3) Hemorrhage to the point of hypotension or shock
(4) Rebleeding after hemostasis achieved
b) Portal-systemic shunt: portacaval, meso-
caval, or splenorenal
(1) Lowers portal pressure by diverting
blood flow
(2) Associated with a higher incidence
of hepatic encephalopathy and
avoided if possible
c) Transjugular intrahepatic portosystemic
shunt (TIPS)
(1) Invasive angiographic method; less
invasive than surgical shunt
(2) Shunts blood between the portal and
systemic venous systems entirely
within the liver; connection is made
between the hepatic and portal
veins and a stent is placed in the
tract
(3) Complications: hemorrhage, renal
failure, septic shock, shunt stenosis,
hepatic encephalopathy
C. Increase intragastric pH
1. Maintain pH 3.5 to 5.0 (normal pH of
gastric secretions 1 to 3)
2. Remove nasogastric tube after lavage completed; the nasogastric tube may increase
acid production by stimulating gastric
secretion
3. Administer agents that decrease gastric
acidity and/or protect gastric mucosa
(Table 8-10)
D. Decrease anxiety because hemorrhage is very
anxiety-producing
1. Maintain a calm and reassuring approach
2. Administer anxiolytics as prescribed and indicated; avoid hepatotoxic agents if the
patient has liver disease
3. Keep the patient and family informed regarding patient status
4. Encourage discussion of fears and concerns

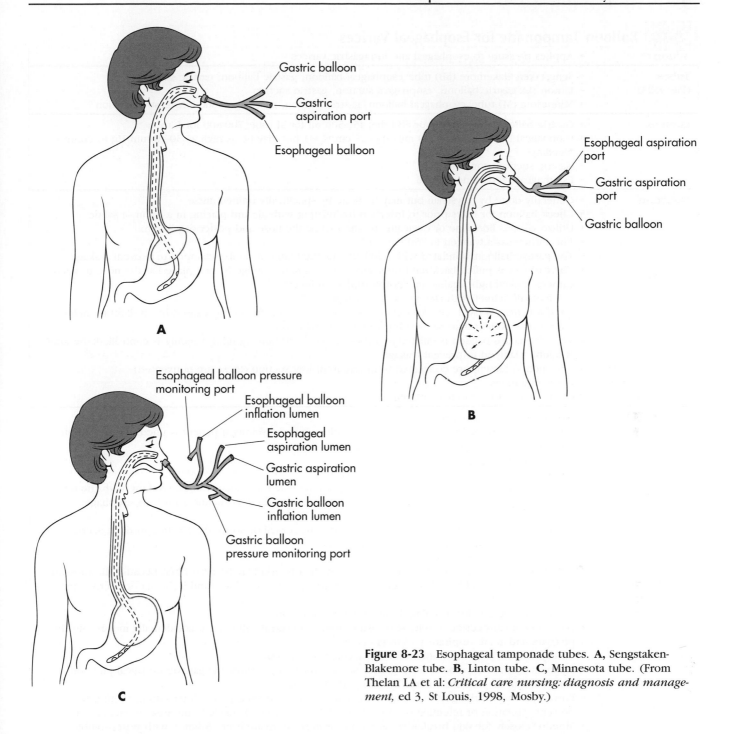

Gastric balloon

Gastric aspiration port

Esophageal balloon

A

Esophageal aspiration port

Gastric aspiration port

Gastric balloon

B

Esophageal balloon pressure monitoring port

Esophageal balloon inflation lumen

Esophageal aspiration lumen

Gastric aspiration lumen

Gastric balloon inflation lumen

Gastric balloon pressure monitoring port

C

Figure 8-23 Esophageal tamponade tubes. **A,** Sengstaken-Blakemore tube. **B,** Linton tube. **C,** Minnesota tube. (From Thelan LA et al: *Critical care nursing: diagnosis and management,* ed 3, St Louis, 1998, Mosby.)

E. Maintain fluid and electrolyte balance; evaluate sodium, potassium, calcium, magnesium and replace as prescribed

F. Correct coagulopathy
    1. Administer vitamin K IV or IM as prescribed
    2. Monitor closely for bleeding
    3. Monitor clotting studies
    4. Avoid invasive procedures and injections

G. Maintain nutritional status by administering appropriate nutrients when appropriate
    1. Give clear liquids initially; progress diet as indicated

2. Avoid alcohol-containing mouthwash, drugs

3. Encourage thorough chewing of foods, especially hard, sharp foods like crackers because they may mechanically injure varices, causing recurrence of bleeding

H. Assess for alcohol withdrawal syndrome (Table 8-11)
    1. If present, administer CNS depressants (e.g., diazepam [Valium], chlordiazepoxide [Librium]) as prescribed; most drugs used for this purpose, including diazepam [Valium] and chlordiazepoxide (Librium), have potential for liver toxicity; dosage is

Table 8-10	**Balloon Tamponade for Esophageal Varices**
Action	• Applies pressure to esophageal and intragastric varices
Tubes (Fig. 8-23)	• Sengstaken-Blakemore (SB) tube: esophageal balloon, gastric balloon, gastric suction • Linton (L): gastric balloon, esophageal suction, gastric suction • Minnesota (M) tube: esophageal balloon, gastric balloon, esophageal suction, gastric suction
Lumens	• Gastric balloon: 200-500 ml for SB tube; 450-500 ml for M tube; 700-800 for L tube • Esophageal balloon: usually 20 mm Hg (25 cm H_2O); but may be as high as 30-40 mm Hg to control bleeding • Gastric suction: nonvented • Esophageal suction: nonvented

Insertion	• Generally done by physician but may be done by specifically trained nurse
	• Check balloon for leaks prior to insertion by inflating with air and placing in a basin of saline
	• Utilize viscous lidocaine or Cetacaine to anesthetize the nose and posterior pharynx
	• The catheter is advanced to ~50 cm mark
	• The gastric balloon is inflated with ~200-300 ml; the lumen is double-clamped to prevent leakage
	• The catheter is pulled back until resistance is met; a nasal sponge is then placed at the nose to keep catheter pulled tight against the gastroesophageal junction
	  • A football helmet with face mask may also be used
	    • If a helmet is used, check fit closely; skin breakdown is frequently caused by an ill-fitting helmet
	  • 0.5-1.0 kg weight may be used hung over the end of the bed
	• The esophageal balloon is inflated to a pressure of 20-40 mm Hg until bleeding is controlled; the lumen is double-clamped to prevent leakage
	• The suction lumens are connected to intermittent low suction (these are nonvented)
	• Label all lumens
	• Obtain chest X-ray to check placement

Management	• Monitor and maintain airway
	  • Elevate head of bed to 45 degrees unless patient is unconscious; if patient is unconscious, elevate head of bed 15 degrees and position patient on left side
	  • Have suction equipment available
	  • Intubation is desirable but not absolutely required
	  • Suction the oropharynx and nasopharynx often because the patient cannot swallow with the tube in
	    • Not as much of an issue with Minnesota tube because there is suction above the esophageal balloon
	    • A small nasogastric tube may be inserted into the nostril opposite the SB tube to drain secretions that collect above the esophageal balloon
	• Maintain pressures at prescribed levels
	  • Periodic deflation at specific intervals (e.g., every 4 hours) may be prescribed because the pressures required to control bleeding exceed the pressure of capillary filling, and ischemia or necrosis may occur
	    • Monitor closely for bleeding during any time of deflation
	• Have scissors at bedside to release pressure from esophageal balloon if it accidentally moves into the pharynx and acute respiratory distress occurs
	  • Keep second tube in the room for replacement if necessary
	• Maintain traction on tube to keep gastric balloon pulled up against the gastroesophageal junction
	• Note amount of pressure/volume in each part of the tube
	• Ensure patency of the gastric suction lumen and keep connected to low intermittent suction to prevent aspiration or retention of blood in the GI tract, which is likely to increase ammonia levels
	• Monitor closely for skin breakdown at mouth or nose; lubricate every 8 hours with water-soluble lubricant
	• Deflation of the esophageal balloon is usually done at 24 hours; deflation of the gastric balloon is usually done at 48 hours; monitor closely for recurrent bleeding when balloons are deflated

Complications	• Airway obstruction • Aspiration • Perforation of esophagus: sudden epigastric or substernal pain, respiratory distress, increased bleeding, shock • Dysrhythmias • Chest pain • Bronchopneumonia • Laceration, ulceration of stomach • Pressure necrosis of hypopharynx, esophagus, or upper stomach • Hiccoughs

adjusted and liver function studies are monitored

I. Monitor for complications
   1. Aspiration pneumonitis
   2. Recurrent bleeding, hemorrhage
   3. Myocardial infarction
   4. Cerebral infarction
   5. Disseminated intravascular coagulation (DIC)
   6. Sepsis
   7. Shock: hypovolemia or septic

Other Possible Causes of Upper GI Hemorrhage

I. Mallory-Weiss tear
   A. Definition: acute longitudinal tear of the esophagus caused by forceful retching
   B. Etiology: caused by forceful retching and vomiting (e.g., alcoholism, bulimia)
   C. Pathophysiology: tear causes arterial bleeding
   D. Collaborative management: usually self-limiting

Table 8-11	Alcohol Withdrawal Syndrome	
Early	**Late**
Mild tachycardia	Marked tachycardia
Mild hypertension	Marked hypertension
Nausea, vomiting	Hyperthermia
Diaphoresis	Dehydration
Pruritus	Delirium
Visual disturbances	Delusions
Time disorientation	Illusions
Tremors	Hallucinations
Anxiety, agitation	Tonic clonic seizures
Sleep disturbances	

II. Gastritis
   A. Definition: a generalized inflammation of the gastric mucosa
   B. Etiology
      1. Dietary intolerances, especially milk intolerance
      2. Alcohol
      3. Drugs such as aspirin, steroids, NSAIDs
      4. Uremia
      5. Certain systemic diseases such as hepatitis
      6. Ingestion of strong acids or alkalis (referred to as *corrosive gastritis*)
   C. Pathophysiology: irritants cause inflammation of the gastric mucosa and oozing of blood
   D. Collaborative management: removal of irritant; similar to management of peptic ulcers
III. Vascular gastric tumors

Hepatic Failure/Encephalopathy
Definitions

I. Hepatic failure: inability of the liver to perform organ functions
II. Hepatic encephalopathy: neurologic failure as a result of hepatic failure

Etiology

I. Acute liver failure
   A. Viruses
      1. Fulminant viral hepatitis (Table 8-12)
      2. Herpes simplex
      3. Cytomegalovirus
   B. Hepatotoxic drugs (Box 8-1) (e.g., acetaminophen, halothane, methyldopa, isoniazid [INH]) or toxins (*Amanita* mushrooms, carbon tetrachloride)

Table 8-12	Types of Viral Hepatitis				
Type	**Route**	**Incubation Period**	**Onset/Chronicity**	**Comments**
A (HAV; infectious hepatitis)	Fecal-oral	2-6 weeks	Acute onset Chronicity does not develop	99% resolves but 1% becomes fulminant
B (HBV; serum hepatitis)	Parenteral Sexual	4-24 weeks	Insidious onset Chronicity develops in <5%	1% becomes fulminant 15%-25% develop liver cancer
C (HCV; non-A, non-B hepatitis; posttransfusion hepatitis)	Parenteral Sexual	2-20 weeks	Insidious onset Chronicity develops in 50%-60%	20%-50% develop cirrhosis 20% develop liver cancer 20% develop liver failure
D (HDV; Delta virus)	Superinfection or coinfection in patient with chronic hepatitis B	4-24 weeks	Acute onset Chronicity common with superinfection	Up to 30% become fulminant Most have worsening active hepatitis
E (HEV; enteric non-A, non-B hepatitis)	Fecal-oral	2-8 weeks	Acute onset Chronicity does not develop	10%-20% mortality in pregnant women

C. Ischemia (e.g., shock and multiple organ dysfunction syndrome [MODS])

D. Trauma

E. Reye's syndrome

F. Acute fatty liver of pregnancy

G. Acute hepatic vein occlusion

II. Chronic liver failure

A. Cirrhosis

B. Wilson's disease

C. Primary or metastatic tumors of the liver

Pathophysiology

I. Cirrhosis

A. Liver parenchymal cells are progressively destroyed and replaced with fibrotic tissue, resulting in impaired hepatic function; three quarters of the liver can be destroyed before symptoms appear

B. Distortion, twisting, and constriction of central sections cause impedance of portal blood flow and portal hypertension

II. Fulminant hepatitis: liver cells fail to regenerate and necrosis occurs

III. Portal hypertension and impaired hepatic function

A. Esophageal varices may develop (see Esophageal Varices section)

B. Splenomegaly may occur, causing thrombocytopenia: thrombocytopenia and vitamin K deficiency cause clotting abnormalities

C. Inability of the liver to produce adequate amounts of bile and impairment in protein, carbohydrate, and fat metabolism

1. Serum bilirubin levels become elevated because the liver is unable to conjugate the bilirubin and make bile

2. Deficiency of fat-soluble vitamins may occur because bile salts are required for absorption

3. Hypoglycemia may occur

D. Inability of the liver to manufacture plasma proteins and inactivate hormones (e.g., aldosterone, estrogen)

1. Causes decreased capillary oncotic pressure and shifting of fluid into the "third space," causing peripheral edema, ascites, pleural effusion

2. Causes increased circulating amounts of aldosterone and continuing retention of sodium and water by the kidney along with increased excretion of potassium

3. Ascites may develop

E. Inability of the liver to detoxify toxins and drugs and remove bacteria

1. Drug or toxin intoxication may occur

2. Hepatic encephalopathy may eventually occur

a) Ammonia is a byproduct of protein metabolism

b) The diseased liver is unable to convert ammonia to urea

c) Neurologic toxic effects result from elevation in blood ammonia

3. Bacteria is not removed from the circulating blood, which increases risk of infection and sepsis

F. Inability to store vitamins and manufacture clotting factors

1. Vitamin deficiencies may occur

2. Clotting abnormalities may occur

Clinical Presentation

I. Subjective

A. History of precipitating event

B. Irritability

C. Personality change

D. Disorientation

E. Weakness, fatigue

F. Anorexia, nausea, vomiting

G. Right upper quadrant dull abdominal pain

H. Abdominal fullness

I. Change in bowel habits

J. Weight loss

II. Objective

A. General: emaciation, cachectic appearance

B. Cardiovascular

1. Tachycardia, dysrhythmias

2. Bounding pulses

3. Hypertension or hypotension

4. Flushed skin

5. Spider angioma on upper trunk, face, neck, arms

6. Jugular venous distention

7. Distended superficial vessels on abdomen (caput medusae)

C. Pulmonary

1. Tachypnea or hyperpnea

2. Decreased respiratory excursion

D. Neurologic

1. Peripheral neuropathy

2. Slow, slurred speech

3. Asterixis

4. Hyperactive reflexes

5. Seizures

6. Positive Babinski reflex in encephalopathy

7. Extreme lethargy or coma in encephalopathy

E. Gastrointestinal

1. Fetor hepaticus

2. Ascites

3. Hematemesis

4. Hepatomegaly early; liver is small late

5. Splenomegaly

6. Ascites

7. Bowel sounds: diminished

8. Clay-colored (pale) stools if biliary obstruction

9. Steatorrhea (excessive fat in stool)

10. Esophageal varices and/or hemorrhoids

F. Renal

1. Oliguria

2. Dark amber urine

G. Hematologic/Immunologic

1. Abnormal bruising, bleeding

2. Susceptibility to infection
3. Poor wound healing
H. Integumentary
  1. Jaundice
  2. Palmar erythema
  3. Petechiae
  4. Bruises
  5. Edema
  6. Pruritus
  7. Spider angioma
I. Endocrine changes
  1. Hypogonadism: testicular atrophy and reduced testosterone levels in men
  2. Gynecomastia in men
  3. Altered hair distribution
III. Diagnostic
  A. Serum
    1. Chemistry
      a) Sodium: may be decreased or normal
      b) Potassium: may be decreased
      c) Calcium: may be decreased
      d) Magnesium: may be decreased
      e) BUN: may be elevated due to dehydration, hepatorenal syndrome, or GI bleeding
      f) Glucose: may be elevated or decreased
      g) Creatinine: may be elevated due to hepatorenal syndrome
      h) Cholesterol: elevated
      i) ALT, AST, LDH: elevated
        (1) AST/ALT ratio more than 1 suggests chronic liver failure or tumor
        (2) AST/ALT ratio less than 1 suggests hepatitis
      j) Alkaline phosphatase: elevated
      k) Bilirubin: elevated
      l) Ammonia: elevated in encephalopathy
      m) Total protein, serum albumin, fibrinogen: decreased
    2. Hematology
      a) Hgb, Hct: may be decreased if hemorrhage or hypersplenism
      b) WBC: decreased; if normal or elevated, infection may be present
      c) Platelets: decreased in splenomegaly
    3. Clotting studies: PT, aPTT prolonged
    4. Arterial blood gases
      a) Respiratory alkalosis
      b) Hypoxemia may be seen
  B. Urine
    1. Sodium: decreased
    2. Bilirubin: elevated in biliary obstruction
    3. Urobilinogen
      a) Elevated in hepatocellular disease
      b) Decreased in complete biliary obstruction
  C. Chest X-ray: may show pleural effusion or atelectasis
  D. Flat plate of abdomen: may reveal hepatosplenomegaly; abdominal haziness may be seen if ascites is present
  E. Abdominal ultrasound: may reveal intraabdominal fluid if ascites is present

F. Barium swallow or esophagogastroduodenoscopy: may be done to identify presence of esophageal varices
G. Liver scan: may show diffuse changes of cirrhosis
H. Liver biopsy: may show fatty infiltration (early) or severe degeneration and scarring (advanced)
I. Endoscopic retrograde cholecystopancreatography: may identify biliary obstruction
J. Paracentesis: cytologic examination may be done to rule out malignancy; ascites fluid has low specific gravity, low protein concentration, and cell counts
K. EEG: shows abnormal and generalized slowing in patients with encephalopathy
L. Lumbar puncture: may be done to rule out neurologic cause of altered consciousness; CSF shows increase in glutamine
IV. Stages of encephalopathy (Table 8-13)

Nursing Diagnoses
I. Impaired Gas Exchange related to ventilation/perfusion mismatching, intrapulmonary shunting, diminished diaphragmatic excursion
II. Fluid Volume Deficit related to fluid sequestration (e.g., ascites, peripheral edema, pleural effusion), hypoalbuminemia, diuretic therapy
III. Decreased Cardiac Output related to decreased preload
IV. Fluid Volume Excess related to altered regulatory mechanisms
V. Sensory/Perceptual Alterations related to elevated ammonia levels
VI. Pain related to liver enlargement ascites
VII. Alteration in Nutrition: Less than Body Requirements related to anorexia, nausea, malabsorption
VIII. Potential for Injury related to coagulopathy, altered consciousness, seizures
IX. Impairment in Skin Integrity related to skin fragility, pruritus
X. Impaired Physical Mobility related to fatigue, ascites, hepatic encephalopathy
XI. Alteration in Bowel Elimination related to diarrhea
XII. Ineffective Individual Coping related to situational crisis, powerlessness, change in role
XIII. Ineffective Family Coping related to critically ill family member
XIV. Knowledge Deficit related to required lifestyle changes

Collaborative Management
I. Identify and treat cause of hepatic failure
  A. Avoid hepatotoxic drugs
  B. Avoid alcohol-containing mouthwash or medications
  C. Monitor liver function studies
II. Maintain airway, oxygenation, ventilation
  A. Elevate head of bed 30 to 45 degrees, especially if ascites restricts diaphragmatic excursion
  B. Administer oxygen as necessary to maintain

Table 8-13	**Stages of Encephalopathy**
Stage I	• Mild confusion • Decreased attention span • Decreased response time • Forgetfulness • Mood changes • Slurred speech • Personality changes • Irritability • Change in sleep patterns • EEG normal
Stage II	• Lethargy • Confusion • Apathy • Aberrant behavior • Asterixis (liver flap) • Inability to reproduce simple designs (constructional apraxia) • EEG normal
Stage III	• Severe confusion and incoherence • Somnolent with diminished responsiveness to verbal stimuli • Speech incomprehensible • Asterixis • Hyperactive deep tendon reflexes • Hyperventilation • EEG abnormal
Stage IV	• No response to stimuli • Abnormal posturing: decorticate (abnormal flexion) or decerebrate (abnormal extension) • Areflexia except for pathologic reflexes • Positive Babinski's reflex • Fetor hepaticus • EEG abnormal

Spo$_2$ 95% unless contraindicated; in patients with COPD, administer oxygen to achieve an Spo$_2$ of ~90%

C. Artificial airways may be necessary in patients with altered consciousness and airway protective mechanisms (e.g., gag reflex)

D. Monitor for and prevent aspiration

E. Assist in management of ascites, which causes decreased diaphragmatic excursion and ventilation difficulties
1. Assist with paracentesis as necessary; patient may need paracentesis if extremely dyspneic, which occurs with severe ascites
2. Administer aldosterone-antagonists (also referred to as *potassium-sparing diuretics*) (e.g., spirolactone [Aldactone]) as prescribed; loop diuretics may also be required because aldosterone-antagonists tend to lose their effectiveness
3. Restrict sodium to 500 mg/day as prescribed
4. Restrict fluids to 1,500 ml/day as prescribed; be alert to clinical indications of hypovolemia

5. LeVeen or Denver shunt may be performed when patient is stable
   a) Surgical procedures that shunt ascites fluid into the superior vena cava
   b) LeVeen uses positive abdominal pressure caused by diaphragm descent during inspiration to open an intraperitoneal valve and shunt fluid from the peritoneum to the superior vena cava
   c) Denver shunt adds a subcutaneous pump that can be compressed manually to irrigate the intraperitoneal tubing

III. Maintain adequate circulating volume and fluid and electrolyte balance
   A. Colloids may be used to restore circulating blood volume (crystalloids are more likely to leave the vascular space, increasing edema)
      1. Avoid lactated Ringer's solution because the liver is responsible for converting lactate to bicarbonate
      2. Avoid protein-containing colloids (e.g., albumin) in hepatic encephalopathy
      3. Monitor for hepatorenal syndrome: cause is not completely understood but results from decreased albumin and portal hypertension; urine output decreases and serum creatinine increases
         a) Observe urine output closely
         b) Avoid thiazide diuretics and other hepatotoxic agents
         c) Hemodialysis may be indicated if liver status may improve
   B. Administer histamine$_2$-receptor antagonists and/or antacids as prescribed to maintain pH 3.5 to 5.0 to reduce the risk of GI bleeding
   C. Administer electrolyte replacement as prescribed
      1. Potassium: excessive (because of inadequate detoxification by the liver) aldosterone causes excessive elimination of potassium; loss accentuated by potassium-losing diuretics
      2. Magnesium: deficiency often related to malnutrition and diuretics
   D. Measure abdominal girth daily for patients with ascites
   E. Weigh daily at same time on same scales

IV. Empty bowel of nitrogen-containing materials
   A. Stop nitrogen-containing drugs: ammonium chloride, urea
   B. Administer neomycin orally or via NG tube as prescribed to kill bacteria that convert nitrogenous wastes to ammonia because the liver cannot further metabolize the ammonia; monitor for auditory or renal toxicity because small amounts of neomycin are absorbed
   C. Administer lactulose (osmotic laxative) orally or via NG tube as prescribed
      1. Acts as a chelating (bonds with) agent of ammonia by changing gut pH, resulting in ammonia excretion

2. Changes gut flora to foster growth of nonammonia-forming bacteria
3. Acts as an osmotic laxative; dose is usually adjusted for two semi-formed stools/day
   D. Administer magnesium citrate orally and/or tap water enemas as prescribed to remove nitrogenous wastes from the GI tract
   E. Prevent constipation with fiber, stool softeners, enemas
V. Identify and monitor stages of encephalopathy
   A. Perform frequent neurologic checks
   B. Avoid any hepatotoxic agents (Box 8-1)
   C. Avoid sedatives and analgesics and/or reduce dosage if necessary; diphenhydramine (Benadryl) or oxazepam (Serax) may be used for restlessness because they can safely be eliminated
   D. Maintain safety: seizure precautions
VI. Decrease portal hypertension: beta-blockers may be prescribed
VII. Administer appropriate nutritional support considering restrictions
   A. Administer $D_{10}W$ to prevent tissue catabolism and hypoglycemia initially
   B. Increase dietary protein (0.6-1.0 g/kg/day) for patients with cirrhosis and hepatic failure but restrict dietary protein (to less than 0.5 g/kg/day) in hepatic encephalopathy
      1. Give adequate CHO to prevent muscle (protein) catabolism and muscle wasting (caloric requirements 35-40 kcal/kg/day)
      2. Add protein in 20-g increments during recovery from encephalopathy
   C. Use appropriate route for nutritional support
      1. Oral: administer antiemetics as prescribed and indicated to prevent nausea (nausea is a significant impairment to oral nutritional intake in these patients); treat prior to each meal and whenever indicated
      2. Enteral: necessary in patients with altered consciousness
      3. Parenteral: branched-chain amino acid formulas may be used in encephalopathy; dextrose and lipids are needed to prevent the metabolism of parenteral amino acids or somatic protein (i.e., catabolism) for energy requirements
   D. Administer vitamins and minerals
      1. Fat-soluble vitamins: A, D, E, K
      2. Thiamine and other B vitamins
VIII. Prevent, assess for, and treat intracranial hypertension
   A. Avoid activities that increase ICP; decrease stimuli
   B. Teach the patient to avoid Valsalva maneuver and other activities that increase intraabdominal or intrathoracic pressure
   C. Administer mannitol as prescribed for cerebral edema
IX. Prevent and monitor for bleeding
   A. Administer vitamin K and fresh frozen plasma as prescribed
   B. Avoid injections if possible
X. Provide adequate rest; maintain bed rest in hepatic encephalopathy
XI. Prevent and monitor for infection
XII. Prevent and monitor for skin breakdown
   A. Alleviate pruritus: cornstarch baths, skin lubricating lotions, calamine lotion
   B. Apply cotton gloves to prevent scratching while sleeping
   C. Administer cholestyramine (Questran) as prescribed to reduce bile pigment accumulation in skin
XIII. Assess for clinical indications of alcohol withdrawal syndrome (Table 8-11)
   A. If present, administer sedatives as prescribed; most of these agents, including chlordiazepoxide (Librium) and diazepam (Valium), are hepatotoxic; doses are adjusted and liver enzymes are monitored
   B. Avoid alcohol-containing mouthwash or medications
XIV. Register patient for liver transplant if appropriate
XV. Monitor for complications
   A. Malnutrition results in:
      1. Immunosuppression
      2. Poor wound healing
      3. Edema, ascites
   B. Hemorrhage may be due to:
      1. Esophageal varices
      2. Coagulopathy
      3. Disseminated intravascular coagulation (DIC)
   C. Hypoglycemia
   D. Electrolyte imbalance
   E. Acute respiratory failure related to intrapulmonary shunt or noncardiac pulmonary edema
   F. Peritonitis
   G. Sepsis
   H. Hepatorenal syndrome
      1. Type of renal failure where loss of function is gradual but no signs of tissue damage are present
      2. Associated with cirrhosis of the liver and hepatitis but exact cause is unknown
      3. Clinical indications include oliguria with low urinary sodium
      4. Management may include dialysis but usually unresponsive to treatment
   I. Acute renal failure related to hepatorenal syndrome, acute tubular necrosis, or hypovolemia
   J. Cerebral edema

Acute Pancreatitis

Definition: Acute inflammation of the pancreas; forms include the following:

I. Interstitial pancreatitis: edematous pancreas with little necrosis damage; hypovolemia may occur as a result of fluid leak into peritoneal cavity
II. Hemorrhagic pancreatitis: extensive necrosis of pancreas and peripancreatic tissue and fat; erosion into blood vessels; hemorrhage occurs; SIRS often occurs

Etiology

I. Alcoholism: most common cause
  A. Chronic alcohol intake leads to secretory and structural changes in the pancreas, contributing to duct obstruction
  B. Alcohol increases the amount of trypsinogen

II. Obstruction of common bile duct: second most common cause
  A. Cholelithiasis
  B. Postendoscopic retrograde cholangiopancreatography (ERCP)

III. Hypertriglyceridemia

IV. Drugs
  A. Thiazide diuretics
  B. Furosemide
  C. Estrogen
  D. Procainamide
  E. Tetracycline
  F. Sulfonamides
  G. Corticosteroids
  H. Azathioprine (Imuran)
  I. Opiates

V. Peptic ulcer with perforation

VI. Cancer, especially tumors of pancreas or lung

VII. Injury to pancreas
  A. Trauma
  B. Surgical
    1. Gastric
    2. Biliary
    3. Duodenal
  C. Iatrogenic

VIII. Radiation injury

IX. Pregnancy: third trimester, ectopic pregnancy

X. Ovarian cyst

XI. Hypercalcemia

XII. Lupus erythematosus

XIII. Infections
  A. Mumps
  B. Coxsackievirus B
  C. Mycoplasma
  D. Infectious mononucleosis
  E. Viral hepatitis
  F. Human immunodeficiency virus (HIV)

XIV. Ischemia (e.g., shock and multiple organ dysfunction syndrome)

XV. Postcardiopulmonary bypass

XVI. Infection, sepsis

XVII. Hereditary factors

XVIII. Idiopathic (20% of cases)

Pathophysiology

I. Etiologic factor triggers activation of pancreatic enzymes and pancreatic cell injury

II. Autodigestion of pancreas caused by the escape of prematurely activated proteolytic enzymes from the acinar space or cells into the periacinal tissue
  A. Trypsin causes edema, necrosis, and hemorrhage
  B. Elastase causes hemorrhage
  C. Phospholipase A causes fat necrosis and damages the pulmonary capillary endothelium; may lead to ARDS
  D. Kallikrein causes edema, vascular permeability, smooth muscle contraction, shock

III. Damage to the acinar cells

IV. Erosion into vessels may cause hemorrhage

V. Inflammatory process causes necrosis of fat in pancreas and exudates with high albumin content, leading to hypoalbuminemia and ascites; fat necrosis results in precipitation of calcium, leading to hypocalcemia

VI. Release of necrotic toxins may cause sepsis and/or systemic inflammatory response syndrome (SIRS)

Clinical Presentation

I. Subjective
  A. Abdominal pain
    1. Precipitation: may occur after a heavy meal or a drinking binge
    2. Palliation: may be eased by leaning forward or by assuming fetal position
    3. Quality: "boring"
    4. Region: left upper quadrant or epigastrium
    5. Radiation: to back or flanks
    6. Severity: severe
    7. Timing: sudden onset, constant
  B. Associated symptoms
    1. Abdominal tenderness, guarding
    2. Nausea, vomiting, retching
    3. Dyspepsia
    4. Flatulence
    5. Weight loss
    6. Weakness

II. Objective
  A. Tachycardia
  B. Hypotension may be seen because of:
    1. Decreased circulating volume due to effusion or hemorrhage
    2. Septic shock
  C. Fever: usually low-grade (e.g., 37.8 to 39° C [~100° F])
  D. Jaundice possible
  E. Vomiting
  F. Hematemesis
  G. Grey Turner's signs or Cullen's sign may be seen in hemorrhagic pancreatitis
  H. Abdominal distention
  I. Guarding during palpation of the abdomen
  J. Epigastric mass may be palpable
  K. Ascites may be present
  L. Decreased bowel sound
  M. Steatorrhea (bulky, pale, foul-smelling, floating)
  N. Breath sound changes: may be diminished due to atelectasis, pleural effusion, or ARDS; crackles may also be heard
  O. Chvostek's or Trousseau's signs may be positive in hypocalcemia

III. Diagnostic
  A. Serum
    1. Chemistry
      a) Potassium: decreased

b) Calcium: decreased

c) Magnesium: decreased

d) Glucose: elevated if endocrine function of the pancreas is compromised

e) Triglycerides: may be elevated

f) Amylase: elevated; peaks at 4 to 24 hours after onset of symptoms; usually returns to normal within 4 days

g) Lipase: elevated, stays elevated longer than amylase

h) Albumin: decreased

i) BUN: may be elevated due to hypovolemia

j) AST, ALT, LDH, alkaline phosphatase, bilirubin: elevated in liver or biliary disease

2. Hematology

a) Hct: decreased with hemorrhage; increased with hemoconcentration due to third-spacing

b) WBC: usually elevated

3. Arterial blood gases

a) Metabolic acidosis

b) Respiratory complications may cause respiratory acidosis and hypoxemia

B. Urine: amylase usually elevated

C. Stool: increase in fecal fat

D. ECG: may suggest MI (e.g., ST-T-wave elevations)

E. Chest X-ray

1. May show left pleural effusion, elevated left hemidiaphragm, left atelectasis

2. May show pulmonary complications of pancreatitis (e.g., atelectasis, pneumonia, ARDS, pleural effusion)

F. Flat plate of abdomen

1. May show cause (e.g., cholelithiasis)

2. May show ileus and bowel dilation

G. Upper GI

1. May show delayed gastric emptying

2. May show enlargement of duodenum

3. May show presence of dilated loop of smooth bowel adjacent to the pancreas

H. Abdominal ultrasound: may show pancreatic swelling, edema, gallstone, pseudocyst, or peripancreatic fluid collections

I. CT scan

1. May show enlargement, edema, or necrosis of the pancreas

2. May show complications of pancreatitis (e.g., pancreatic pseudocyst or abscess)

J. MRI: shows inflammatory changes within the pancreas

K. Endoscopic retrograde choleangiopancreatography (ERCP)

1. Contraindicated in acute pancreatitis

a) Remember that pancreatitis is a complication of this study

b) Used more often in chronic pancreatitis; identifies ductal changes or calculi

L. HIDA scan: may identify hepatocellular disease from biliary obstruction as cause of pancreatitis

M. Peritoneal lavage: positive for blood in hemorrhagic pancreatitis

Nursing Diagnoses

I. Pain related to pancreatic inflammation, peritoneal inflammation

II. Fluid Volume Deficit related to vomiting, nasogastric suction, hemorrhage, fluid sequestration within peritoneum

III. Decreased Cardiac Output related to decreased preload

IV. Impaired Gas Exchange related to diminished lung expansion, anemia, atelectasis, ARDS

V. Alteration in Nutrition: Less than Body Requirements related to poor intake, impaired digestion, NPO or dietary restrictions, hypermetabolism

VI. Risk for Infection related to peritonitis, abscess

VII. Altered Protection related to electrolyte imbalance

VIII. Ineffective Individual Coping related to situational crisis, powerlessness, change in role

IX. Ineffective Family Coping related to critically ill family member

X. Knowledge Deficit related to required lifestyle changes

Collaborative Management

I. Maintain airway, oxygenation, ventilation

A. Elevate head of bed 30 to 45 degrees, especially if ascites restricts diaphragmatic excursion

B. Administer oxygen as necessary to maintain Spo_2 95% unless contraindicated; in patients with COPD, administer oxygen to achieve an Spo_2 of ~90%

C. Monitor Spo_2 closely and evaluate work of breathing in detection of development of atelectasis and/or ARDS

II. Maintain adequate circulating volume and fluid and electrolyte balance

A. Administer crystalloids and colloids as prescribed to restore circulating blood volume

B. Monitor sodium, calcium, potassium, magnesium, and phosphate

1. Administer calcium replacement orally or intravenous as prescribed

2. Administer potassium replacement as prescribed

3. Restrict sodium to 500 to 1000 mg/day for patients with ascites

C. Measure abdominal girth daily for patients with ascites

D. Weigh daily at same time on same scale

III. Decrease release of and destruction by pancreatic enzymes

A. NPO

B. Keep environment free of food odors

C. Perform mouth care with water or normal

saline only; do not use alcohol-containing or flavored mouthwash or toothpaste

D. Insert nasogastric tube and maintain suction to keep stomach decompressed and inhibit secretion of pancreatic juices

E. Administer octreotide acetate (Sandostatin) IV or SC as prescribed to suppress pancreatic secretions

F. Perform peritoneal lavage as prescribed: used for acute fulminant pancreatitis
   1. Performed percutaneous or via laparotomy
   2. Intraperitoneal space is rinsed with lavage fluid to remove toxic substances released from the pancreas
   3. May be done for 2 to 3 days
   4. Technique is the same as for peritoneal dialysis for renal failure (see Peritoneal Dialysis section in Chapter 9)

IV. Increase intragastric pH to prevent stress ulcer
   A. Maintain pH 3.5 to 5.0 (normal pH of gastric secretions 1 to 3)
   B. Administer agents that decrease gastric acidity and/or protect gastric mucosa (Table 8-9)

V. Prevent and treat pain and discomfort
   A. Maintain bed rest; knee-to-chest positioning may be helpful in relief of pain
   B. Maintain quiet environment, comfortable temperature, dim lighting
   C. Administer analgesics
      1. Opiates preferably administered via patient-controlled analgesia (PCA)
         a) **Note:** although meperidine (Demerol) has long been considered the analgesic of choice in acute pancreatitis, recent studies show no significant difference between morphine and meperidine in the degree of spasm of the sphincter of Oddi
      2. Octreotide acetate (Sandostatin) IV or SC to suppress pancreatic secretions for pain relieved by opioids
      3. Neurolytic block of the celiac plexus for severe persistent pain
   D. Encourage knee flexing while in supine position to relax abdominal muscles
   E. Utilize nonpharmacologic pain relief methods (e.g., imagery, distraction)
   F. Treat nausea with prescribed antiemetics
   G. After NG tube removal: perform mouth care after emesis should it occur

VI. Administer appropriate nutritional support considering restrictions
   A. Administer nutritional support during acute phase of illness
      1. Parenteral nutrition
      2. Enteral nutrition below the duodenum (**Note:** Enteral feeding has traditionally been thought to be contraindicated in acute pancreatitis, but recent studies indicate that enteral feeding may be safely administered

if the tube is below the duodenum [e.g., jejunostomy tube])

B. Clear liquids or elemental diet (e.g., Vivonex) may be used after inflammation subsides (pain subsides, serum amylase normal), progressing to low-fat, full liquids and eventually progressing to a regular diet

C. Avoid alcohol and food high in fat

D. Administer fat-soluble vitamins, thiamine, folic acid as prescribed

E. Monitor serum glucose levels closely and administer glucose or insulin as indicated

VII. Provide adequate rest

VIII. Prevent and monitor for infection
   A. Prophylactic antibiotics are contraindicated (they mask pancreatic sepsis); antibiotics are prescribed if infection exists
   B. Monitor for clinical indications of abscess formation
      1. Increase in abdominal pain
      2. Vomiting
      3. Fever
      4. Leukocytosis

IX. Assess for clinical indications of alcohol withdrawal syndrome (Table 8-12)
   A. If present, administer sedatives as prescribed; most of these agents, including chlordiazepoxide (Librium) and diazepam (Valium), are hepatotoxic; doses are adjusted and liver enzymes are monitored
   B. Avoid alcohol-containing mouthwash or medications

X. Prepare patient for surgical measures for relief of pancreatitis if necessary (during acute phase, surgery is performed only if absolutely necessary)
   A. Cholecystectomy if bile reflux is the cause of pancreatitis
   B. Drainage and removal of abscess or pseudocysts
   C. Pancreatic resection/total pancreatectomy
      1. Used if pancreas and/or other organs are necrotic
      2. Total pancreatectomy; results in diabetes and other metabolic difficulties
         a) Islet cell autotransplantation is sometimes performed
         b) Segmental pancreatic autotransplantation is sometimes performed: part of viable pancreatic tissue reimplanted following total pancreatectomy

XI. Monitor for complications
   A. Hypoglycemia or hyperglycemia
   B. Hypocalcemia
   C. Pseudocysts
      1. Caused by collection of inflammatory debris, pancreatic secretions, and necrotic tissue in the pancreatic tissue; may cause compression of portal vein or bile duct or rupture and peritonitis and sepsis
      2. Clinical presentation includes epigastric

pain, persistent nausea and vomiting, weight loss, jaundice, low-grade fever
3. Collaborative management includes surgical drainage
D. Pancreatic abscess
1. Caused by accumulation of pancreatic enzyme-rich fluid in the peritoneal cavity
2. Clinical presentation includes fever, palpable mass, abdominal tenderness, nausea, vomiting, leukocytosis
3. Collaborative management includes surgical drainage
E. Pancreatic fistula
1. Caused by a communication between the pancreas and the skin
2. Clinical presentation includes drainage of extremely alkaline pancreatic secretions onto the skin and severe excoriation
3. Collaborative management includes fluid and electrolyte replacement; octreotide acetate (Sandostatin) may be used
F. Hypovolemic shock
1. Caused by exudate of protein-rich fluid into retroperitoneal space or by erosion into the vascular bed and hemorrhage
2. Clinical presentation includes tachycardia, hypotension, oliguria, and other indications of hypoperfusion
3. Collaborative management includes volume resuscitation, including crystalloids, colloids, blood administration for hemorrhagic pancreatitis
G. Systemic inflammatory response syndrome (SIRS)
H. Acute respiratory distress syndrome
I. Disseminated intravascular coagulation (DIC)
J. Sepsis
K. Acute renal failure
L. Perforation

Intestinal Infarction/Obstruction/Perforation

Definitions
I. Intestinal infarction: necrosis of the intestinal wall resulting from ischemia
II. Intestinal obstruction: failure of the intestinal contents to progress forward through the lumen of the bowel
A. Functional obstruction: caused by loss of peristalsis; usually referred to as *paralytic ileus*
B. Mechanical obstruction: caused by factors that occlude the bowel lumen
1. Simple: luminal obstruction without compromise of blood supply
2. Strangulated: luminal obstruction with compromise of blood supply
III. Intestinal perforation: penetration of the lumen of the intestine with resultant spillage of intestinal contents into the peritoneal cavity

Etiology
I. Infarction
A. Arteriosclerosis
B. Vasculitis
C. Mural thrombus, emboli: post-MI, atrial fibrillation, ventricular aneurysm, endocarditis
D. Hypercoagulability (e.g., polycythemia, postsplenectomy)
E. Surgical procedures involving aortic clamping (e.g., abdominal aortic aneurysm repair)
F. Vasopressors
1. Endogenous due to sympathetic nervous system stimulation (e.g., shock)
2. Exogenous (e.g., norepinephrine, high-dose dopamine)
G. Strangulated intestinal obstruction
H. Intraabdominal infection
I. Cirrhosis
II. Obstruction
A. Functional (paralytic ileus)
1. Abdominal surgery
2. Hypokalemia
3. Intestinal distention
4. Peritonitis
5. Intestinal ischemia
6. Severe trauma
7. Spinal cord injury
8. Ureteral distention
9. Pneumonia
10. Pleuritis
11. Subphrenic abscess
12. Pancreatitis
13. Acute cholecystitis
14. Pelvic abscess
15. Narcotics (e.g., morphine)
16. Sepsis
B. Small bowel
1. Adhesions: most common
2. Incarcerated hernia
3. Volvulus
4. Foreign body
5. Neoplasm
C. Large bowel
1. Neoplasm: most common
2. Stricture
3. Intussusception
4. Diverticulitis
5. Fecal or barium impaction
III. Perforation
A. Peptic ulcer
B. Bowel obstruction
C. Appendicitis
D. Penetrating wound

Pathophysiology
I. Infarction
A. Decrease in blood flow to major mesenteric vessels causes vasoconstriction, vasospasm
B. Prolonged ischemia →
C. Edema of intestinal wall →
D. Full thickness necrosis →

E. Perforation →

F. Peritonitis

II. Obstruction

  A. Obstruction of bowel prevents adequate movement of bowel contents →

  B. Intestinal fluid accumulation above the obstruction →

    1. Fluid and electrolyte imbalance; fluid and electrolyte imbalance is more severe in small bowel obstruction

    2. Distention of the bowel eventually causes perforation

III. Perforation

  A. Leakage of gastrointestinal content into peritoneal cavity →

    1. Leakage of bacteria (especially *E. coli*) causes infection

    2. Chemical irritation causes inflammation

  B. Peritonitis and potentially sepsis

Clinical Presentation

I. Infarction

  A. Subjective

    1. May have history of precipitating event

    2. Anorexia

    3. Pallor

    4. Abdominal pain: severe cramping periumbilical or nonspecific diffuse

    5. Abdominal tenderness

    6. Urgent bowel movements

  B. Objective

    1. Tachycardia

    2. Hypotension

    3. Tachypnea

    4. Fever

    5. Clinical indications of dehydration

    6. Vomiting: persistent, may be bloody

    7. Abdominal distention

    8. Abdominal guarding and rigidity

    9. Urgent and bloody diarrhea

    10. Hypoactive or absent bowel sounds

    11. Weight loss

  C. Diagnostic

    1. Serum

      a) BUN: elevated due to dehydration

      b) Alkaline phosphatase: elevated

      c) Amylase: elevated

      d) Hematocrit: elevated

      e) WBC: elevated

      f) Arterial blood gases: metabolic acidosis

    2. Stool: guaiac positive

    3. Angiography: shows occlusion of the arterial supply

    4. Sigmoidoscopy: shows dusky, ischemic bowel

II. Obstruction

  A. Small bowel

    1. Subjective

      a) May have history of precipitating event

      b) Severe, sharp episodic pain

    2. Objective

      a) Vomiting early: may be projectile and/or fecal

      b) Clinical indications of dehydration

      c) Bowel sounds: high-pitched

        (1) Increased early

        (2) Decreased late

    3. Diagnostic

      a) Serum

        (1) Sodium: decreased

        (2) Potassium: decreased

        (3) Chloride: decreased

        (4) BUN: elevated due to dehydration

        (5) Hct: elevated

        (6) WBC: elevated

        (7) Arterial blood gases: usually metabolic acidosis, but metabolic alkalosis may be seen with proximal obstruction and gastric losses

      b) Upper GI: may show point of obstruction

      c) Flat plate of abdomen: shows dilated loops of gas-filled bowel

  B. Large bowel

    1. Subjective

      a) May have history of precipitating event

      b) Dull pain

      c) Change in bowel habits

      d) Decrease in flatus

    2. Objective

      a) Vomiting late

      b) Abdominal distention

      c) Bowel sounds: low-pitched

        (1) Increased early

        (2) Decreased late

    3. Diagnostic

      a) Serum

        (1) Sodium: decreased

        (2) Potassium: decreased

        (3) Chloride: decreased

        (4) BUN: elevated due to dehydration

        (5) CEA: elevated if due to cancer

        (6) Hematocrit: may be elevated due to dehydration or decreased due to hemorrhage; large bowel tumor often causes slow bleed

        (7) WBC: elevated

        (8) Arterial blood gases: metabolic acidosis

      b) Stools: may be positive for occult blood

      c) Flat plate of abdomen: shows dilated loops of gas-filled bowel

      d) Barium enema: may show point of obstruction

      e) Endoscopy: obstruction may be visible on sigmoidscopy or colonoscopy

III. Perforation

  A. Subjective

    1. Abdominal pain

    2. Abdominal tenderness

    3. Anorexia

    4. Nausea

  B. Objective

    1. Tachycardia

    2. Tachypnea

    3. Fever

4. Vomiting
5. Rigid, "boardlike" abdomen
6. Rebound tenderness
7. Absence of liver dullness due to free air in peritoneum
8. Bowel sounds: diminished or absent

C. Diagnostic
1. Serum: WBC elevated
2. Flat plate of abdomen: free air in peritoneum may be seen
3. Upper GI: contraindicated

Nursing Diagnoses

I. Pain related to bowel ischemia, perforation, peritonitis
II. Fluid Volume Deficit related to vomiting, fluid shifts
III. Impaired Gas Exchange related to diminished lung expansion
IV. High Risk for Infection related to bowel ischemia, perforation
V. Alteration in Nutrition: Less than Body Requirements related to poor intake and altered food metabolism
VI. Alteration in Bowel Elimination related to impaired bowel motility
VII. Ineffective Individual Coping related to situational crisis, powerlessness, change in role
VIII. Ineffective Family Coping related to critically ill family member
IX. Knowledge Deficit related to required lifestyle changes

Collaborative Management

I. Maintain airway, oxygenation, ventilation
   A. Elevate head of bed 30 to 45 degrees
   B. Administer oxygen as necessary to maintain SpO_2 95% unless contraindicated; in patients with COPD, administer oxygen to achieve an SpO_2 of ~90%
II. Maintain adequate circulating volume and fluid and electrolyte balance
   A. Administer crystalloids and colloids as prescribed to restore circulating blood volume
   B. Administer blood and blood products as prescribed; whole blood or packed cells should be given early if significant bleeding suspected; after multiple transfusions, consideration should be given to replacement of clotting factors, platelets, and calcium
   C. Monitor sodium, calcium, potassium, and phosphate; administer electrolyte replacement as indicated
   D. Discontinue vasopressors if cause of ischemia
   E. Weigh daily at same time on same scale
III. Prevent and treat pain and discomfort
   A. Maintain bed rest
   B. Maintain quiet environment, comfortable temperature, dim lighting
   C. Administer analgesics (e.g., morphine) (**Note:** analgesics are sometimes withheld until the diagnosis is made)

D. Encourage knee flexing while in supine position to relax abdominal muscles
E. Utilize nonpharmacologic pain relief methods (e.g., imagery, distraction)
F. Treat nausea with prescribed antiemetics
G. Perform mouth care after emesis

IV. Prevent perforation of bowel if obstruction present
   A. Assist in insertion of nasointestinal tube (e.g., Miller-Abbott or Cantor tube) for proximal decompression of the bowel
      1. Do not tape at nose because these tubes move through the GI tract by peristalsis
      2. Elevate head of bed 30 degrees and turn the patient every 1 to 2 hours to encourage movement of the tube; these tubes usually move 4 to 5 cm/hr
      3. Use pH of aspirate to assess movement of the tube through the pylorus: acidic pH in stomach, alkaline pH in intestine
      4. Get flat plate of abdomen as requested to assess final position, then tape tube in place
      5. Provide frequent nose and mouth care while tube is in place
   B. Do not give cathartics or enemas to patients with complete obstruction

V. Prevent and monitor for infection
   A. If perforation has occurred:
      1. Keep the patient immobilized to reduce the chemical irritation to the peritoneum
      2. Antibiotics are given preoperatively
      3. Antibiotic lavage may be done during surgery
      4. Antibiotics are given postoperatively
   B. Postoperatively clean around drains aseptically and protect skin around drains

VI. Administer appropriate nutritional support considering restrictions
   A. Administer nutritional support parenterally in the acute phase
   B. Provide oral feedings and advance diet when condition is surgically resolved
   C. Administer vitamin and mineral supplements

VII. Provide adequate rest

VIII. Prepare patient for surgical measures if necessary
   A. Bowel preparation with cathartics, enemas, and sterilization prior to surgery
      1. Nonabsorbable aminoglycoside (e.g., neomycin) is usually used for bowel sterilization
      2. Do not give cathartics or enemas for patients who have complete obstruction
   B. Procedures
      1. Infarction
         a) Revascularization techniques (e.g., bypass, embolectomy)
         b) Bowel resection with debridement of necrotic tissue; usually with end-to-end anastomosis, although temporary bowel diversion may be performed to allow anastomosis to heal

2. Obstruction
   a) Correction of cause
      (1) Lysis of adhesion
      (2) Herniorrhaphy
      (3) Reduction of volvulus or intussusception
   b) Bowel resection with debridement of necrotic tissue
      (1) With end-to-end anastomosis
      (2) With temporary diversion (e.g., colostomy)
      (3) With abdominoperineal resection with permanent colostomy; especially for rectal malignancy
3. Perforation
   a) Repair of perforation may require bowel resection; a temporary bowel diversion may be performed to allow the anastomosis to heal
   b) Antibiotic lavage may be done during surgery
IX. Prepare patient for other therapies (e.g., radiation, antineoplastic agents) if malignancy
X. Monitor for complications
   A. Fluid and electrolyte imbalance
   B. Hemorrhage
   C. Sepsis
   D. Peritonitis
   E. Respiratory distress secondary to abdominal distention
   F. Shock: hypovolemic or septic
   G. Abscess
   H. Perforation

Abdominal Trauma

Definition: Trauma that occurs between the nipple line to mid-thigh

Etiology

I. Penetrating trauma (e.g., motor vehicle collision, assault, sharp instruments [e.g., knife, gunshot wound, impalement])
II. Blunt trauma (e.g., motor vehicle collision, assault, fall, sport injury)
III. Iatrogenic trauma
   A. Peritoneal tap
   B. Endoscopy
   C. Biopsy
   D. Cardiopulmonary resuscitation

Pathophysiology

I. Seldom a single organ injury
II. High-velocity penetrating trauma
   A. Extensive destruction of contact tissue
   B. Severe associated blast effect on the surrounding tissues
   C. Liver most often affected by penetrating trauma
III. Blunt trauma
   A. Due to direct injury, crushing force between two objects, acceleration/deceleration, shearing, twisting
   B. Pressure injury
   C. Spleen most often affected by blunt trauma
      1. Pancreas is often injured with spleen

Clinical Presentation

I. Subjective
   A. Abdominal pain: may be poorly localized or referred
      1. Kehr's sign: left shoulder pain indicative of splenic rupture caused by blood below diaphragm that irritates the phrenic nerve
   B. Abdominal tenderness
II. Objective
   A. Seatbelt marks
   B. Hematoma: note location
      1. Hematoma in flank area may be seen in renal injury
   C. Entrance and exit wounds
   D. Grey Turner's or Cullen's sign: may be seen
   E. Coopernail sign (ecchymosis of scrotum or labia): indicative of fractured pelvis
   F. Rigid abdomen: may indicate intraabdominal bleeding
   G. Ballance's sign (resonance over right flank with patient on left side): indicative of ruptured spleen
   H. Diminished femoral pulses: may be seen in vascular injury
   I. Loss of liver dullness: indicates perforation with free air in peritoneum
   J. Bowel sounds: diminished or absent
   K. Clinical indications of hypoperfusion or shock
   L. Clinical indications of perforation
   M. Specifics related to organ injured (Table 8-14)
III. Diagnostic
   A. Serum
      1. Glucose: elevated due to stress
      2. Amylase: may be elevated if injury to pancreas or bowel
      3. ALT, AST, LDH: may be elevated if liver injury
      4. Hgb, Hct: decreased with hemorrhage
      5. WBC: may be elevated if infection is present or if spleen is ruptured
      6. Platelets: elevated if spleen is injured
      7. PT, aPTT: may be prolonged
      8. Drug and alcohol screens: may be positive
   B. Urine
      1. May show hematuria if renal trauma
      2. May show myoglobinuria if crush injury has occurred
   C. Stool: may be positive for occult blood
   D. Chest X-ray: rule out concurrent thoracic injury; identify free air under diaphragm
   E. Flat plate of abdomen: may show free air in peritoneum if bowel is perforated
   F. IVP: if hematuria is present to look for renal trauma
   G. Angiography: may show vascular injury
   H. CT scan or MRI: to identify areas of injury

Table 8-14	Clinical Indications of Organ Injury
Organ	**Clinical Indications of Injury**
Liver	• Local sign of injury (RUQ) • RUQ pain and guarding • Lower right rib fracture • Abdominal tenderness • Abdominal distention • Increased pain on inspiration • Leukocytosis • Elevated ALT, AST, LDH • Positive peritoneal lavage
Spleen	• Local sign of injury (LUQ) • LUQ pain • Lower left rib fracture • Abdominal tenderness • Increased abdominal girth • Kehr's sign • Ballance's sign • Increased pain on inspiration • Positive peritoneal lavage • Shock
Pancreas	• Epigastric or back pain • Abdominal tenderness • Abdominal distention • Increased abdominal girth • Diminished bowel sounds • Hyperglycemia • Elevated amylase • Positive peritoneal lavage • Shock
Intestine	• Local sign of injury (e.g., ecchymosis, abrasion) • Nausea, vomiting • Abdominal pain: may be referred or rebound • Absent bowel sounds • Leukocytosis • Positive peritoneal lavage
Abdominal vessels	• Abdominal distention • Increased abdominal girth • Diminished femoral pulses • Mottled lower extremities • Shock

I. Diagnostic peritoneal lavage: may be done to assess for intraabdominal bleeding
  1. Technique
    a) Placement of peritoneal catheter
      (1) If gross blood is obtained with catheter insertion, immediate exploratory laparotomy is indicated
    b) Instillation of 1 L of normal saline over 15 to 20 minutes
    c) Move the patient side to side after fluid instillation to distribute the lavage fluid
    d) Drain
  2. Considered positive if lavage fluid is grossly bloody or contains:
    a) RBC greater than 100,000 mm^3
    b) WBC greater than 500 mm^3
    c) Amylase greater than 175 U/dl

    d) Bile, bacteria, intestinal content
    e) Newsprint sign: newsprint cannot be read through the lavage fluid
  3. Limitation: does not detect diaphragmatic or retroperitoneal injuries

Nursing Diagnoses
I. Fluid Volume Deficit related to hemorrhage or blood sequestration, sepsis
II. Pain related to trauma, surgery
III. Alteration in Nutrition: Less than Body Requirements related to altered food metabolism, hypermetabolism
IV. Impaired Gas Exchange related to diminished lung expansion, splinting
V. Risk for Infection related to peritonitis
VI. Impairment in Skin Integrity related to trauma, surgery
VII. Ineffective Individual Coping related to situational crisis, powerlessness, change in role
VIII. Ineffective Family Coping related to critically ill family member
IX. Knowledge Deficit related to required lifestyle changes

Collaborative Management
I. Maintain airway, oxygenation, ventilation
  A. Stabilize the cervical spine
  B. Elevate head of bed 30 to 45 degrees to allow for optimal diaphragmatic excursion
  C. Administer oxygen as necessary to maintain Spo_2 95% unless contraindicated; in patients with COPD, administer oxygen to achieve an SpO_2 of 90% by pulse oximetry
II. Detect bleeding and maintain adequate circulating volume
  A. Detect bleeding by performing head-to-toe assessment and assisting with peritoneal lavage, which is especially important in an unconscious patient since subjective report of tenderness, pain is absent
  B. Insert indwelling urinary catheter to evaluate hourly urine output
  C. Assist with insertion of arterial catheter and pulmonary artery catheter in patient with hemodynamic instability
  D. Insert two short (1¼ inch) large-gauge (16-18) peripheral intravenous catheters; draw labs and type and crossmatch for blood
  E. Administer crystalloids and colloids as prescribed to restore circulating blood volume
  F. Administer blood and blood products as prescribed; whole blood or packed cells should be given early if significant bleeding suspected; after multiple transfusions, consideration should be given to replacement of clotting factors, platelets, and calcium
  G. Control bleeding
    1. Pressure can be applied to overt bleeding site

2. Prepare patient for exploratory laparotomy as indicated
   a) Penetrating injury invading the peritoneum
   b) Clinical indications of perforation (e.g., acute abdomen)
   c) Free air in peritoneum on X-ray
   d) Shock
   e) GI hemorrhage
   f) Massive hematuria
   g) Evisceration
   h) Positive peritoneal lavage
   i) Surgical indications on CT scan or angiography

III. Maintain fluid and electrolyte balance
   A. Insert indwelling urinary catheter to monitor hourly urine output
   B. Monitor sodium, calcium, potassium, and phosphate
      1. Administer electrolyte replacement as indicated

IV. Prevent and treat pain and discomfort
   A. Maintain bed rest
   B. Maintain quiet environment, comfortable temperature, dim lighting
   C. Administer analgesics (e.g., morphine); may be contraindicated until diagnoses are made
   D. Encourage knee flexing while in supine position to relax abdominal muscles in patients with peritoneal irritation
   E. Utilize nonpharmacologic pain relief methods (e.g., imagery, distraction)

V. Decompress GI tract
   A. Insert nasogastric tube
   B. Monitor NG output for color, amount, and odor of drainage

VI. Administer appropriate nutritional support considering restrictions
   A. Administer nutritional support parenterally acutely
   B. Provide oral feeding and advance diet when condition is surgically resolved
   C. Administer vitamin and mineral supplements

VII. Prevent and monitor for infection
   A. Observe for signs of peritonitis
   B. Monitor abdominal girth
   C. Maintain asepsis of drains
   D. Monitor bowel sounds
   E. Evaluate tetanus immunization status and administer tetanus toxoid as prescribed and indicated by penetrating trauma, abrasion, cuts, etc.

VIII. Monitor for complications
   A. Obstruction
   B. Perforation
   C. Peritonitis
   D. Pancreatitis
   E. Abscess
   F. Sepsis
   G. Hemorrhage
      1. Retroperitoneal
      2. Intraperitoneal
   H. Shock: hypovolemic or septic
   I. DIC
   J. Pneumonia
   K. Atelectasis
   L. Organ failure

LEARNING ACTIVITIES

1. **DIRECTIONS:** Complete the following crossword puzzle related to gastrointestinal anatomy and physiology.

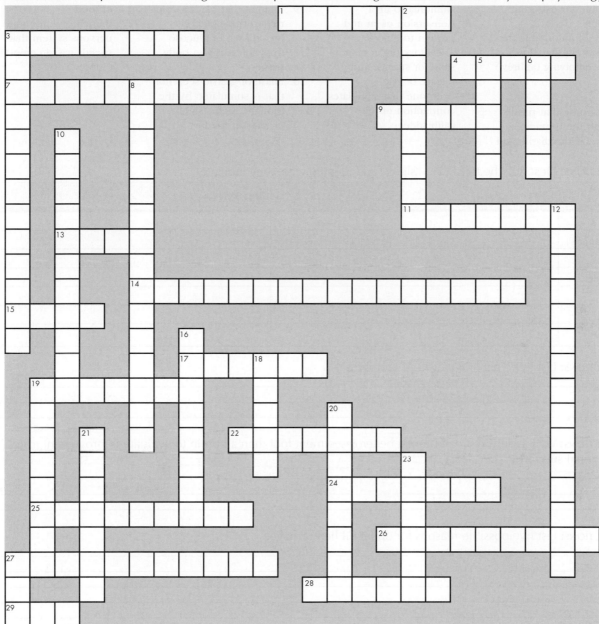

Across

1. Cells that line the sinusoids of the liver that are responsible for phagocytosis
3. Shortest segment of the small intestine
4. Fingerlike projections of mucosa and submucosa in the duodenum and jejunum that increase surface area
7. Breakdown of stored carbohydrate
9. Viscous, semifluid stomach contents that moves through the pylorus into the small intestine
11. Flexure of the large intestine that is in the LUQ
13. Fluid produced by the liver and stored in the gallbladder
14. Also referred to as the lower esophageal sphincter
15. Sphincter of _____ is a valve in the common bile duct that regulates the passage of bile from the common bile duct into the duodenum
17. Lower portion of the stomach, close to the pylorus
19. Enzyme that breaks down protein into amino acids
22. One of these lymph vessels is located in each villus
24. Flexure of the large intestine that is in the RUQ
25. This factor is necessary for the intestinal absorption of vitamin B_{12}
26. Major bile pigment

27. Alternate contraction and relaxation of muscle fibers that propels food and chyme through the GI tract
28. Cells in the pancreas responsible for exocrine function
29. Branch of autonomic nervous system that slows gastric emptying (abbrev.)

Down
2. Hollow tube that passes through the thoracic cavity and the diaphragm

3. Another term for swallowing
5. Last section of the small intestine
6. Accessory organ responsible for conversion of ammonia to urea
8. Conversion of fat and protein to glucose
10. Accessory organ responsible for storage and release of bile
12. Hormone that stimulates contraction of the gallbladder

16. Accessory organ with endocrine and exocrine functions
18. Thick folds on interior of stomach that increase surface area
19. Vitamin that plays a chief role in the metabolic breakdown of glucose to yield energy in body tissues
20. Phase of gastric secretion that is stimulated by the thought, sight, smell, or taste of food

21. Hormone responsible for the secretion of hydrochloric acid
23. Oral secretion stimulated by the thought, sight, smell, or taste of food
27. Branch of autonomic nervous system that speeds gastric emptying (abbrev.)

2. **DIRECTIONS:** Describe the following "signs" and identify what they indicate.

Sign	Description	Indicates
Ballance's		
Grey Turner's		
Cullen's		
Coopernail		
Kehr's		
Chvostek		
Trousseau's		

3. **DIRECTIONS:** List three general causes of jaundice.
1. _____
2. _____
3. _____

4. **DIRECTIONS:** Why is serum prealbumin a better assessment tool than albumin to evaluate improvement from nutritional support?

_____
_____
_____

5. **DIRECTIONS:** List five possible reasons for upper GI hemorrhage.
1. _____
2. _____
3. _____
4. _____
5. _____

6. **DIRECTIONS:** List five methods to control bleeding in esophageal varices.
1. _____
2. _____
3. _____
4. _____
5. _____

7. **DIRECTIONS:** List four classifications of drugs that are used to prevent ulcers and an example of each one.

Type	Example
1.	
2.	
3.	
4.	

8.   DIRECTIONS: List one classification of diuretic that is indicated and one type of diuretic that is contraindicated for ascites in hepatic failure.

Indicated	Contraindicated

9.   DIRECTIONS: List five common causes of paralytic ileus.

1. _____
2. _____
3. _____
4. _____
5. _____

10.   DIRECTIONS: List five classic indications of an "acute abdomen" seen in intestinal perforation.

1. _____
2. _____
3. _____
4. _____
5. _____

11.   DIRECTIONS: Calculate the caloric intake for a patient receiving total parenteral nutrition (TPN) with daily intake of 42 grams of protein, 250 grams of carbohydrate, and 140 grams of fat.

_____
_____
_____

12.   DIRECTIONS: Complete the following table. You may include more than one condition for each but include only conditions discussed in this chapter.

Clinical Finding	Condition
Elevated lipase, amylase	
Sudden, painless hematemesis	
Decreased protein	
Rebound tenderness	
Jaundice	
Hypocalcemia	
Bleeding tendencies	
Elevated ammonia	
Bloody diarrhea	
Hyperbilirubinemia	
Fetor hepaticus	
High-pitched rushing bowel sounds	
Succussion splash	

Management	Condition
Irrigate NG tube until clear	
Neomycin and lactulose	
Sclerosis during endoscopy	
Aldosterone-antagonist diuretics	
NPO status	
Sengstaken-Blakemore tube	
Volume and blood replacement	
Billroth I or II	

13. **DIRECTIONS:** Complete the following crossword puzzle related to gastrointestinal assessment, conditions, and treatments.

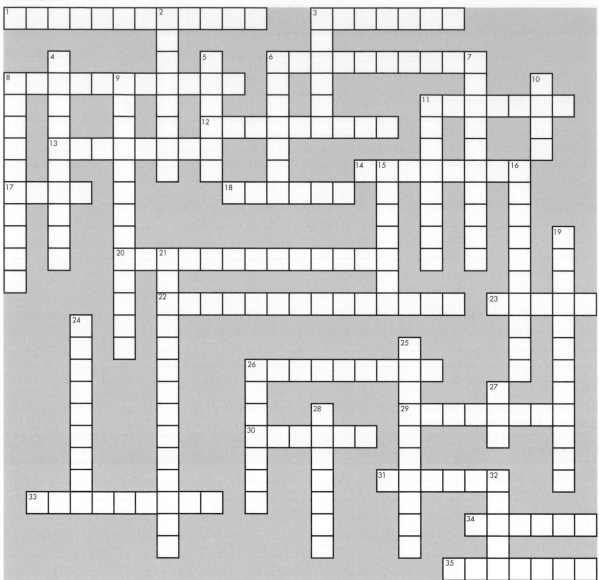

Across

1. Nutrient source that is broken down to glucose, fructose, and galactose
3. Obstruction here is manifested by a succussion splash
6. Anemia caused by deficiency of intrinsic factor
8. Location of pain in acute pancreatitis
11. Abnormal accumulation of fluid in the peritoneal cavity
12. Osmotic laxative often used in hepatic encephalopathy (generic)
13. Vitamin deficiency commonly seen in alcoholism

14. Maneuver that facilitates evacuation of the colon
17. Serious pulmonary complication of acute pancreatitis (abbrev.)
18. Mercury-weighted intestinal tube used to decompress the intestine
20. Drug often used for suicide gesture that may cause hepatic failure (generic)
22. Second most common cause of acute pancreatitis
23. Form of fluid replacement indicated in acute hemorrhage

26. Adverse effect of cimetidine seen often in elderly patients
29. _____'s sign is indicative of splenic rupture
30. Shunt used for ascites
31. *Helicobacter* _____ is a bacterium associated with peptic ulcer
33. Manifested by coffee-ground gastric aspirate; oozing noted on gastroscopy
34. Type of ulcer that causes an erosion in mucosa of the esophagus, stomach, or duodenum
35. _____'s is a stress ulcer associated with cerebral trauma

Down

2. Type of drug often given to patients with ascites
3. Hypertension of this circulation system is seen in cirrhosis
4. Histamine$_2$-receptor antagonist (generic)
5. _____'s sign is a bluish discoloration around the umbilicus; indicative of intraabdominal bleeding
6. Nutrient source that is broken down to amino acids
7. Mucosal barrier used to protect the gastric mucosa (generic)
8. Belching

9. Complication of hernia that may cause bowel ischemia or infarction
10. ____'s sign is caused by phrenic nerve irritation by subphrenic blood
11. Generalized, massive edema

15. Elevated levels of ____ are the cause of the neurologic changes seen in hepatic encephalopathy
16. Most common cause of acute pancreatitis
19. Electrolyte imbalance seen in acute pancreatitis

21. Abnormal function of the brain
24. Also referred to as liver flap
25. Loud, hyperactive bowel sounds
26. ____'s is a stress ulcer associated with burns

27. Nutrient source that is broken down to fatty acids
28. Tenderness that hurts more on release than with pressure
32. Functional obstruction of the bowel

LEARNING ACTIVITIES ANSWERS

1.

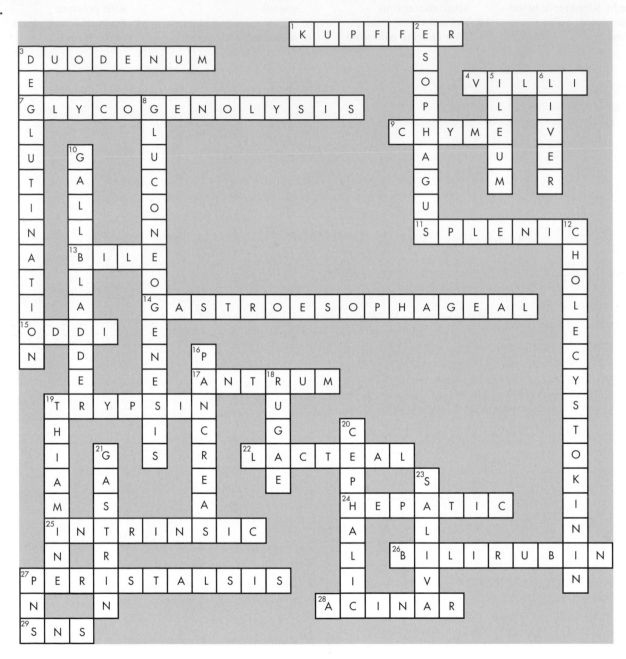

Across:
1. KUPFFER
3. DUODENUM
4. VILLI
7. GLYCOGENOLYSIS
9. CHYME
11. SPLENIC
13. BILE
14. GASTROESOPHAGEAL
15. ODDI
17. ANTRUM
19. TRYPSIN
22. LACTEAL
24. HEPATIC
25. INTRINSIC
26. BILIRUBIN
27. PERISTALSIS
28. ACINAR
29. SNS

Down:
2. ESOPHAGUS
5. LLVLUME
6. LIVER
8. GLUCONEOGENE
10. GALLBLADDER
12. CHOLECYSTOKININ
16. PUGRE
18. RUGE
20. CEPHALIV
21. GAS
23. SL

2.

Sign	Description	Indicates
Ballance's	Dullness over right flank with patient on left side	Ruptured spleen
Grey Turner's	Ecchymosis to flank	Retroperitoneal bleeding
Cullen's	Ecchymosis around umbilicus	Intraperitoneal bleeding
Coopernail	Ecchymosis of scrotum or labia	Pelvic fracture
Kehr's	Left shoulder pain	Splenic rupture
Chvostek	Spasm of the facial muscles elicited by tapping on the facial nerve	Hypocalcemia
Trousseau's	Carpal spasm induced by inflating a BP cuff on the upper arm to a pressure exceeding systolic blood pressure	Hypocalcemia

3.
1. Liver disease (e.g., cirrhosis, hepatitis)
2. Biliary obstruction (e.g., cholelithiasis)
3. Excessive hemolysis (e.g., hemolytic blood transfusion reaction)

4. The half-life of serum prealbumin is 2 to 3 days versus albumin with a half-life of 10 to 20 days; therefore, serum transferrin will show improvement or decline more quickly.

5.
1. Peptic ulcer
2. Esophageal varices
3. Mallory-Weiss tear
4. Gastritis
5. Vascular tumor

6.
1. Sclerotherapy of varices
2. Variceal ligation
3. Intrahepatic or portosystemic shunt
4. Balloon tamponade
5. Vasopressin or octreotide acetate (Sandostatin)

7.

Type	Example
Antacids	• Maalox • Mylanta
Histamine (H$_2$) receptor antagonists	• Cimctidine (Tagamet) • Ranitidine (Zantac) • Famotidine (Pepcid) • Nizatidine (Axid)
Proton pump inhibitors	• Omeprazole (Prilosec) • Lansoprazole (Prevacid) • Rabeprazole (Acipttex)
Mucosal barrier	• Sucralfate (Carafate)

8.

Indicated	Contraindicated
Aldosterone-antagonist (potassium-sparing)	Thiazide

9. Any five of the following:
- Abdominal surgery
- Hypokalemia
- Intestinal distention
- Peritonitis
- Intestinal ischemia
- Severe trauma
- Spinal cord injury
- Ureteral distention
- Pneumonia
- Pleuritis
- Subphrenic abscess
- Pancreatitis
- Acute cholecystitis
- Pelvic abscess
- Narcotics (e.g., morphine)
- Sepsis

10.
1. Abdominal pain
2. Rebound tenderness
3. Abdominal distention
4. Rigid "boardlike" abdomen
5. Diminished bowel sounds
6. Fever
7. Leukocytosis
8. Nausea, vomiting

11. 2,428 calories

12.

Clinical Finding	Condition
Elevated lipase, amylase	Acute pancreatitis
Sudden, painless hematemesis	Esophageal varices
Decreased protein	Acute pancreatitis, liver disease, malnutrition
Rebound tenderness	Peritonitis
Jaundice	Liver disease, biliary obstruction, hemolysis
Hypocalcemia	Acute pancreatitis
Bleeding tendencies	Liver disease
Elevated ammonia	Hepatic failure, hepatic encephalopathy
Bloody diarrhea	Intestinal infarction
Hyperbilirubinemia	Liver disease, biliary obstruction, hemolysis
Fetor hepaticus	Hepatic failure
High-pitched rushing bowel sounds	Small bowel obstruction
Succussion splash	Pyloric obstruction
Management	**Condition**
Irrigate NG tube until clear	Upper GI bleed
Neomycin and lactulose	Hepatic failure; hepatic encephalopathy
Sclerosis during endoscopy	Esophageal varices
Aldosterone-antagonist diuretics	Hepatic failure; hepatic encephalopathy
NPO status	Pancreatitis; intestinal infarction, obstruction, or perforation
Sengstaken-Blakemore tube	Esophageal varices
Volume and blood replacement	GI bleed
Billroth I or II	Gastric ulcer

13.

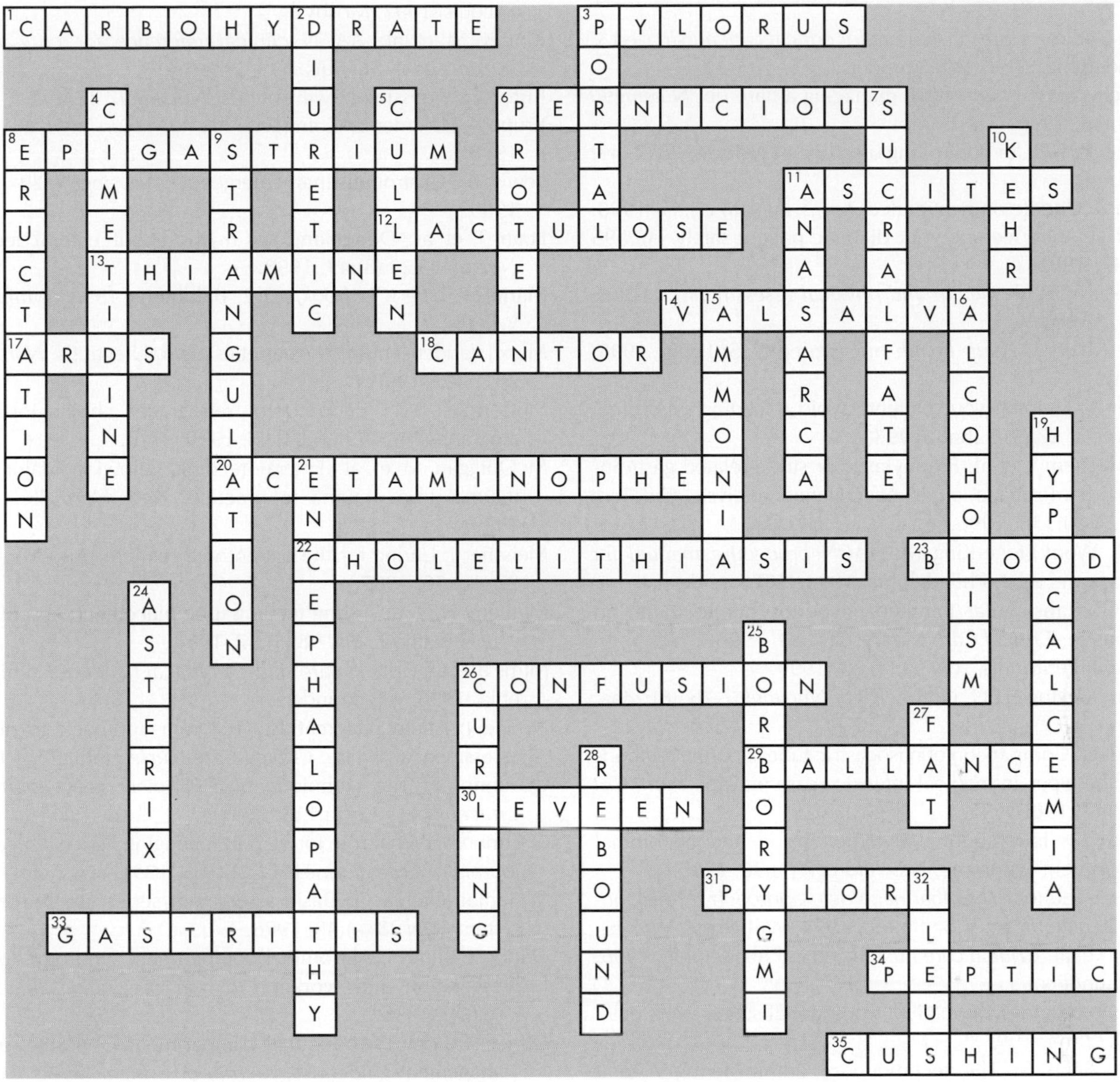
Across:
1 CARBOHYDRATE
3 PYLORUS
6 PERNICIOUS
8 EPIGASTRIUM
11 ASCITES
12 LACTULOSE
13 THIAMINE
14 VALSALVA
17 ARDS
18 CANTOR
20 ACETAMINOPHEN
22 CHOLELITHIASIS
23 BLOOD
26 CONFUSION
29 BALLANCE
30 LEVEEN
31 PYLORI
33 GASTRITIS
34 PEPTIC
35 CUSHING
Down:
2 DIURETIC
3 PORTAL
4 CIMETIDINE
5 CULLEN
6 PROTEIN
7 SUCRALFATE
8 ERUCTATION
9 STRANGULATION
10 KEHR
11 ANASARCA
15 AMMONIA
16 ALCOHOLISM
19 HYPOCALCEMIA
21 ENCEPHALOPATHY
24 ASTERIXIS
25 BORBORYGMI
27 FAT
28 REBOUND
32 ILEUS

Bibliography and Selected References

Alspach J, editor: *Core curriculum for critical care nursing,* ed 5, Philadelphia, 1998, WB Saunders.

Ambrose M et al: Pancreatitis: managing a flare-up, *Nursing96* 26 (4):33, 1996.

Angelucci P: TIPS for controlling bleeding, *Nursing95* 25 (7):43, 1995.

Aronson B: Update on peptic ulcer drugs, *AJN* 98 (1):41, 1998.

Bak L et al: Tube feeding your diabetic patient safely, *AJN* 96 (12):47, 1996.

Barkauskas V et al: *Health and physical assessment,* St Louis, 1994, Mosby.

Beare P, Myers J: *Adult health nursing,* ed 3, St Louis, 1998, Mosby.

Belcaster A: Helping your patients avoid refeeding syndrome, *Nursing97* 27 (9):32hn8, 1997.

Ben-menachem T et al: Prophylaxis for stress-related gastrointestinal hemorrhage: a cost effectiveness analysis, *Crit Care Med* 24 (2):338, 1996.

Boggs R, Wooldridge-King M: *AACN procedure manual for critical care,* ed 3, Philadelphia, 1993, WB Saunders.

Bouley G: Transjugular intrahepatic portosystemic shunt: an alternative, *Critical Care Nurse* 16 (1):23, 1996.

Breitfeller J: Peritonitis, *AJN* 99 (4):33, 1999.

Brown L: Giving TPN in the ICU, *Nursing96* 26 (8):24aa, 1996.

Burns S et al: Comparison of nasogastric tube securing methods and tube types in medical intensive care patients, *Am J Crit Care* 4 (3):198, 1995.

Cheatham M: Intra-abdominal hypertension and abdominal compartment syndrome, *New Horiz* 7 (1):96, 1999.

Chernow B, editor: *The pharmacologic approach to the critically ill patient,* ed 3, Baltimore, 1994, Williams & Wilkins.

Clochesy J et al: *Critical care nursing,* ed 2, Philadelphia, 1996, WB Saunders.

Cobb M: Improving your patient's nutritional status, *Nursing97* 27 (6):32hn4, 1997.

Dove D, Sahn S: The technique of administering enteral nutrition, *Journal of Critical Illness* 10 (12):881, 1995.

Eckler J: Preventing hepatitis, *Nursing99* 29 (8):66, 1999.

Fischer J: Does your patient need an albumin infusion? *Nursing98* 28 (11):32cc10, 1998.

Forloines-Lynn S: How to smooth the way for cyclic tube feedings, *Nursing96* 26 (3):57, 1996.

Forloines-Lynn S: Knowing how to manage complications of tube feeding, *Nursing96* 26 (3):32M, 1996.

Gahart B, Nazareno A: *1999 intravenous medications,* St Louis, 1999, Mosby.

Gallagher TJ: *Postoperative care of the critically ill patient,* Baltimore, 1995, Williams & Wilkins.

Gawlinski A, Hamwi D: *Acute care nurse practitioner clinical curriculum and certification review,* Philadelphia, 1999, WB Saunders.

Heslin J: Peptic ulcer disease: making a case against the prime suspect, *Nursing97* 27 (1):34, 1997.

Kamen B: Battling lower GI bleeding, *Nursing99* 29 (8):32hn1, 1999.

Kamen B: Combating upper GI bleeding, *Nursing99* 29 (7):32hn1, 1999.

Keen J, Searingen P: *Mosby's critical care nursing consultant,* St Louis, 1997, Mosby.

Kinney M et al: *AACN clinical reference for critical care nursing,* ed 4, St Louis, 1998, Mosby.

Kirton C: Assessing bowel sounds, *Nursing97* 27 (3):64, 1997.

Krupp K, Heximer B: Going with the flow, *Nursing98* 28 (4):54, 1998.

Lewis A: Gastrointestinal emergency! *Nursing99* 29 (4):52, 1999.

Loan T et al: Debunking six myths about enteral feeding, *Nursing98* 28 (8):43, 1998.

Marino P: *The ICU book,* ed 2, Baltimore, 1998, Williams & Wilkins.

Marx J: Understanding the varieties of viral hepatitis, *Nursing98* 28 (7):43, 1998.

McCormick M: Endoscopic retrograde cholangiopancreatography, *AJN* 99 (2):24HH, 1999.

McQuiggan M et al: Enteral feeding following major torso trauma: from trauma to practice, *New Horiz* 7 (1):131, 1999.

Meissner J: Caring for the patient with pancreatitis, *Nursing97* 27 (10):50, 1997.

Metheny N et al: Testing feeding tube placement: auscultation vs. pH method, *AJN* 98 (5):37, 1998.

Mims B et al: *Critical care skills: a clinical handbook,* Philadelphia, 1996, WB Saunders.

Noone J: Acute pancreatitis: an Orem approach to nursing assessment and care, *Critical Care Nurse* 15 (8):27, 1995.

O'Connor F: The technique of TIPS placement, *Journal of Critical Illness* 12 (2):113, 1997.

O'Connor F: What role for TIPS in managing variceal bleeding, *Journal of Critical Illness* 12 (2):103, 1997.

O'Hanlon-Nichols T: Basic assessment series: gastrointestinal system, *AJN* 98 (4):48, 1998.

Offner P, Burch J: Abdominal compartment syndrome, part 1: presentation and workup, *Journal of Critical Illness* 13 (10):639, 1998.

Offner P, Burch J: Abdominal compartment syndrome, part 2: management guidelines, *Journal of Critical Illness* 13 (10):634, 1998.

Price S, Wilson L: *Pathophysiology: clinical concepts of disease processes,* ed 5, St Louis, 1997, Mosby.

Salavec L: Splenic injury, *AJN* 99 (9):32, 1999.

Sheff B: Minimizing the threat of *C. difficile, Nursing99* 29 (2):35, 1999.

Siconolfi L: Clarifying the complexity of liver function tests, *Nursing95* 25 (5):39, 1995.

Teran J et al: A three-step nutritional approach to patients with hepatic encephalopathy, *Journal of Critical Illness* 10 (5):309, 1995.

Thelan L et al: *Critical care nursing: diagnosis and management,* ed 3, St Louis, 1998, Mosby.

Town J: Bringing acute abdomen into focus, *Nursing97* 27 (5):52, 1997.

Trujillo E et al: Nutritional assessment in the critically ill, *Critical Care Nurse* 19 (1):67, 1999.

Varon J, Fromm R: *The ICU handbook of facts, formulas, and laboratory values,* St Louis, 1997, Mosby.

Viall C: Taking the mystery out of TPN, part one, *Nursing95* 25 (4):34, 1995.

Viall C: Taking the mystery out of TPN, part two, *Nursing95* 25 (5):57, 1995.

Warmkessel J: Caring for the patient with colon cancer, *Nursing97* 27 (4):34, 1997.

Weigelt J, Lewis F: *Surgical critical care*, Philadelphia, 1996, WB Saunders.

Younossi Z, Canuto P: Hepatitic C update: implications of the blood transfusion "lookback," *Cleve Clin J Med* 65 (8):412, 1998.

Zakko W, Van Dam J: Techniques for nutritional assessment, *The Journal of Critical Illness* 11 (6):405, 1996.

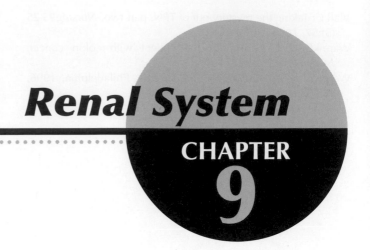

Renal System

CHAPTER 9

Selected Concepts in Anatomy and Physiology
General Information
I. Functions of the renal system
  A. Regulation of homeostasis and the body's internal environment
    1. Regulation of extracellular fluid volume
    2. Regulation of extracellular fluid osmolality
    3. Regulation of electrolyte balance
    4. Excretion of metabolic wastes
    5. Regulation of acid-base balance (in conjunction with the pulmonary system)
  B. Production and release of hormones
    1. Regulation of blood pressure influenced by aldosterone and antidiuretic hormone (ADH)
    2. Stimulation of RBC production via erythropoietin
    3. Synthesis and release of prostaglandins
  C. Bone mineralization
II. Components of the renal system (Fig. 9-1)
  A. Two kidneys
  B. Two ureters
  C. Urinary bladder
  D. Urethra

Functional Anatomy
I. General characteristics of the kidney
  A. Location of kidney
    1. Posterior abdominal wall behind peritoneum
    2. Opposite last thoracic and first three lumbar vertebrae on each side of spine
    3. Right kidney slightly lower than left as a result of liver location
  B. Size, shape, weight of the kidney
    1. Size: approximately 10 × 5 × 2.5 cm or approximately fist-sized
    2. Shape: beanlike with convex lateral border, convex and concave medial border; long axis approximately vertical
    3. Weight: 120 to 170 g each kidney

II. Extrarenal structures
  A. Renal capsule
    1. Thin, smooth layer of fibrous membrane that surrounds each kidney
    2. Acts as a protective layer
    3. Prevents kidney swelling
    4. Contains pain receptors
  B. Perirenal fat and renal fascia
    1. Support and protect the kidney
    2. Hold kidney in place
  C. Adrenal gland (also referred to as the *suprarenal gland*): rests on top of each kidney
  D. Hilum
    1. Concave notch of medial aspect of kidney
    2. Entry site for renal artery and nerves
    3. Exit site for renal vein and ureter
  E. Ureters
    1. Fibromuscular tubes located behind peritoneum; extend from kidney to posterior part of bladder floor
    2. Ureter walls composed of smooth muscle with mucosa lining and fibrous outer coat
    3. Collect urine from the renal pelvis and propel it to the bladder by peristaltic waves
    4. Ureters enter the superior, posterior bladder at an oblique angle; this angle and the peristaltic action of the ureters prevent reflux of urine
  F. Bladder
    1. Located behind symphysis pubis, below peritoneum
    2. Collapsible bag of smooth muscle
    3. Acts as a reservoir for urine until a sufficient amount accumulates for elimination; expels urine from body via the urethra
      a) Adults void approximately 5 to 9 times/day
      b) Volume of each voiding usually 100 to 300 ml but may be as much as 1 L
  G. Urethra
    1. Located behind symphysis pubis, anterior to

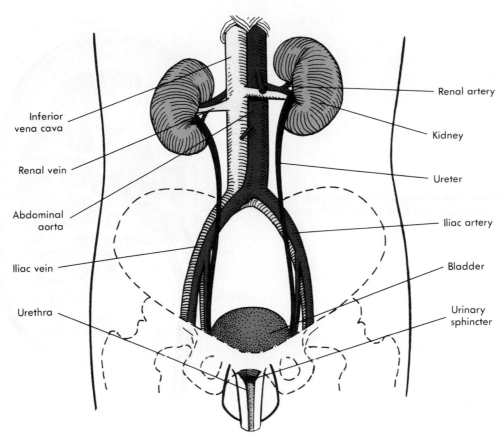

Figure 9-1 The kidneys and other structures of the urinary tract. (From Long BC, Phipps WJ, Cassmeyer VL: *Medical-surgical nursing: a nursing process approach*, ed 3, St Louis, 1993, Mosby.)

the vagina in females; extends through the prostate gland and penis in males
2. Acts as passageway for expulsion of urine from the urinary bladder to the urinary meatus, where it is expelled from the body

III. Renal structures (Fig. 9-2)
 A. Renal parenchyma
   1. Cortex
     a) Approximately 1 cm wide, pale and granular appearance
     b) Metabolically active portion of kidney where aerobic metabolism occurs and ammonia and glucose are formed
     c) Site of glomerulus, proximal and distal tubules
   2. Medulla
     a) Approximately 5 cm wide, darker than cortex and striated
     b) Consists of 6 to 10 pyramids formed by collecting tubules and ducts
       (1) Pyramids are triangular wedges of medullary tissue and are composed of collecting tubules
       (2) Columns are inward extensions of cortical tissue between the pyramids; much of the kidney's blood vessels and nerves are in these columns

       (3) Renal lobe consists of a pyramid and surrounding cortical tissue
     c) Site of deepest part of loop of Henle
 B. Renal sinus: spacious cavity filled with adipose tissue, the renal pelvis, minor and major calyces, and the origin of the ureter
   1. Calyces
     a) Calyces are cuplike structures that drain the papillae
     b) Eight to twelve minor calyces open into two to three major calyces that form the renal pelvis
   2. Renal pelvis
     a) Papillae are at the apices of the renal pyramids; collecting tubules drain into minor calyces at papillae
     b) Renal pelvis is like a small funnel tapering into the ureter; formed by the union of several calyces
     c) Urine flows from collecting duct to renal pelvis and into the ureter
 C. Nephron: microscopic functional unit of kidney (Fig. 9-3)
   1. Approximately 1 million in each kidney
   2. Able to compensate for significant degree of nephron destruction by:
     a) Filtering a greater solute (dissolved substances) load

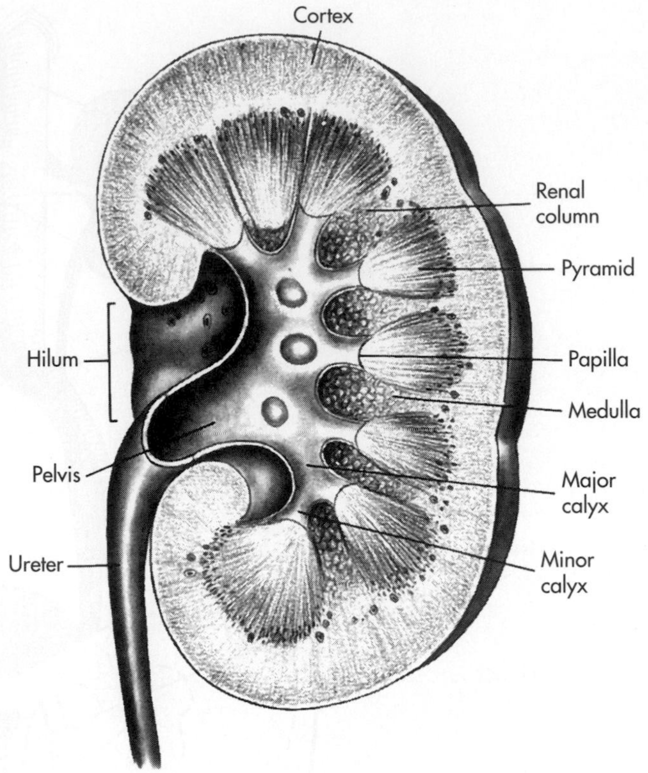

Figure 9-2   The kidney parenchyma. (From Thompson JM et al: *Mosby's clinical nursing,* ed 4, St Louis, 1997, Mosby.)

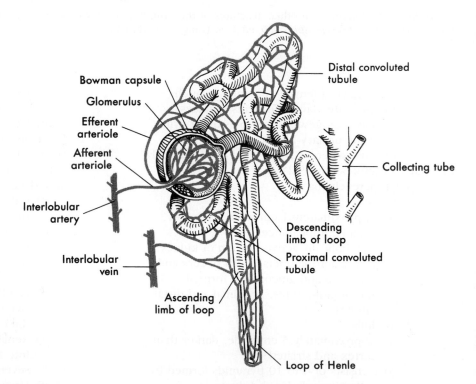

Figure 9-3   The nephron. (From Long BC, Phipps WJ, Cassmeyer VL: *Medical-surgical nursing: a nursing process approach,* ed 3, St Louis, 1993, Mosby.)

b) Hypertrophy of remaining functional nephrons
3. Types of nephrons
  a) Cortical (85% of nephrons)
    (1) The glomerulus is located in the outer cortex

(2) Cortical nephrons contain short loops of Henle, which dip into the outer edge of the medulla
b) Juxtamedullary (15% of nephrons)
  (1) The glomerulus is located in the inner cortex

(2) Juxtamedullary nephrons contain long loops of Henle that penetrate deep into the medulla

(3) These nephrons are important in the kidney's ability to concentrate the urine

4. Functional segments
   a) Renal corpuscle: consists of Bowman's capsule and glomerulus
      (1) The glomerulus is a cluster of tightly coiled capillaries that produces an ultrafiltrate; a portion of this ultrafiltrate eventually becomes urine
      (2) Bowman's capsule is the funnel-shaped upper end of the proximal tubule
   b) Renal tubules
      (1) Segmentally divided into proximal convoluted tubule, loop of Henle, distal convoluted tubule
      (2) Responsible for reabsorption and secretion, which alter the volume and composition of the ultrafiltration to form the final urine volume and composition
   c) Collecting duct
      (1) Several nephrons converge into a collecting duct
      (2) The collecting duct relays the urine from the tubules to the minor calyx

D. Renal vasculature
   1. Pathway of blood supply
      a) Renal arteries branch from the aorta
      b) The renal arteries branch into interlobar arteries → arcuate arteries → interlobular arteries
      c) The interlobular arteries become the afferent arteriole, which forms the glomerulus
      d) The efferent arteriole leads out of the glomerulus and forms the peritubular capillary network
      e) The efferent arteriole from the juxtamedullary nephron forms a different capillary network called the *vasa recta*
         (1) The vasa recta is a complex of long straight capillary loops that run parallel to the ascending and descending loop of Henle
         (2) It plays an important role in concentrating interstitial fluid found in the medulla
         (3) Blood flow through the vasa recta is sluggish
      f) The peritubular capillary network leads to the interlobular vein, which leads to the arcuate vein
      g) The arcuate vein leads to the interlobar vein, which leads to the renal vein
      h) The renal vein empties into the inferior vena cava

2. Renal blood flow
   a) The kidneys receive 20% to 25% of the cardiac output, or approximately 1,200 ml/min (600 ml/min for each kidney)
   b) Autoregulation maintains constancy in glomerular filtration rate (GFR)
      (1) Systemic mean arterial pressure (MAP) between 80 to 180 mm Hg prevents large changes in GFR because of the afferent arteriole's ability to constrict or dilate
         (a) Increases in MAP cause constriction of the afferent arteriole, which prevents the increased arterial pressure from raising the pressure in the glomerulus
         (b) Decreases in MAP cause dilation of the afferent arteriole, so more blood is allowed to flow into the glomerulus
      (2) Filtration ceases at MAP of 40 to 60 mm Hg or less

3. Juxtaglomerular apparatus consists of the macula densa and the juxtaglomerular cells
   a) The macula densa is a part of the distal tubule that lies close to the afferent and efferent arterioles
   b) Juxtaglomerular cells produce and store the enzyme renin, which is secreted in response to renal hyperfusion

E. Lymphatics
   1. The supply of lymphatic to the kidney is abundant
   2. Lymphatics from the kidney drain into the thoracic duct

F. Nervous innervation
   1. The autonomic nervous system (ANS) supplies the primary innervation of the kidney and the urinary tract
   2. The renal plexus is formed by the superior and inferior splanchnic nerves and enters the kidney at the hilum; the bladder, ureters, and urethra are supplied by the inferior mesenteric plexus, the hypogastric plexus, and the pudic nerve from the sacral region
   3. Both the sympathetic nervous system (SNS) and the parasympathetic nervous system (PNS) innervate the kidney, but the SNS has the prominent effect on the kidney; SNS fiber endings are found in the afferent and efferent arterioles and in all sections of the tubule; effects on the kidney include the following:
      a) Low level: increased sodium reabsorption within the proximal tubule
      b) Moderate level: constriction of afferent and efferent arterioles to decrease renal blood flow and glomerular filtration rate
      c) High level: predominant effect of afferent arteriole constriction; extreme reduction in renal blood flow and potential cessation of glomerular filtration rate

Physiology

I. Formation of urine involves three processes: filtration, reabsorption, and secretion (Fig. 9-4); major functions of each portion of the nephron (Fig. 9-5)

A. Glomerular filtration: the pressure of the blood within the glomerular capillaries causes fluid to be filtered into Bowman's capsule, where it begins to pass down to the tubule

1. Filtration is the transfer of water and dissolved substances through a permeable membrane from a region of high pressure to low pressure

2. Filtration depends on hydrostatic pressure, which may be affected by the following:

a) Diminished renal perfusion from hypovolemia

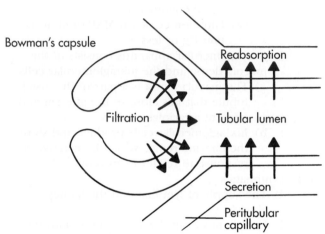

Figure 9-4   Processes of filtration, secretion, and reabsorption in the formation of urine. (From Richard C: *Comprehensive nephrology nursing,* Boston, 1987, Little Brown.)

b) Occlusion of the glomeruli from diabetic neuropathy

c) Alteration in the plasma protein concentration from hypoproteinemia

d) Alterations in the basement membrane from an autoimmune disorder

e) Arteriolar constriction from SNS stimulation or vasopressors

3. Glomerular filtration rate (GFR) is clinically measured by creatinine clearance

a) Formula for $GFR = \dfrac{Ux \times v}{Px}$

where:

x = substance freely filtered through glomerulus and not secreted or absorbed by tubules (e.g., creatinine)

U = urine concentration of x (e.g., creatinine)

v = urine flow rate/min

P = plasma concentration of x (e.g., creatinine)

b) Creatinine clearance is a calculation of GFR by comparing serum creatinine with the amount of creatinine excreted in the urine over a 24-hour period

c) GFR must be maintained at a constant rate, and autoregulation ensures this constant rate; systemic arterial pressure must be maintained between 80 to 180 mm Hg to maintain autoregulation

4. The glomerular membrane is porous but semipermeable

a) Glomerular filtrate (also called *ultrafiltrate*) is similar in composition to blood except that it lacks blood cells, platelets, and large plasma proteins; water, sodium, glucose, potassium, chloride,

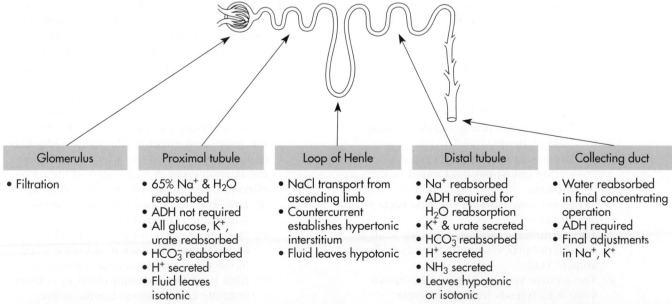

Glomerulus	Proximal tubule	Loop of Henle	Distal tubule	Collecting duct
• Filtration	• 65% Na⁺ & H₂O reabsorbed • ADH not required • All glucose, K⁺, urate reabsorbed • HCO₃⁻ reabsorbed • H⁺ secreted • Fluid leaves isotonic	• NaCl transport from ascending limb • Countercurrent establishes hypertonic interstitium • Fluid leaves hypotonic	• Na⁺ reabsorbed • ADH required for H₂O reabsorption • K⁺ & urate secreted • HCO₃⁻ reabsorbed • H⁺ secreted • NH₃ secreted • Leaves hypotonic or isotonic	• Water reabsorbed in final concentrating operation • ADH required • Final adjustments in Na⁺, K⁺

Figure 9-5   Major functions of each portion of the nephron. (Redrawn with permission from Llach F: *Papper's clinical nephrology,* ed 3, Boston, 1993, Little Brown.)

phosphate, urea, uric acid, creatinine, ammonia, phenol, calcium, and magnesium pass through the glomerular membrane

b) Glomerular filtrate volume is usually 120 ml/min, but 99% of this volume is reabsorbed in the renal tubule

B. Reabsorption: passage of a substance that the body needs from the lumen of the tubules through the tubular cells and into the capillaries
1. Processes
   a) Active transport
      (1) The force used when the cell membranes must move molecules "uphill" against a concentration gradient
      (2) Requires the use of energy and a carrier substance; the substance combines with a "carrier" and diffuses through the tubular membrane where they reenter the bloodstream
      (3) Substances moved by active transport include glucose, protein, amino acids, phosphate
   b) Passive transport: processes of osmosis and diffusion
      (1) Diffusion: the passive movement of solute from an area of higher concentration to an area of lower concentration; urea, electrolytes are moved by diffusion
      (2) Osmosis: the passive movement of water from an area of lower solute concentration to an area of higher solute concentration
2. Maximal tubular transport capacity: maximum amount of a substance that can be completely reabsorbed in 1 minute and that reflects the renal threshold of a substance; if this threshold is exceeded, the substance appears in the urine (e.g., glucosuria)

C. Tubular secretion: passage of a substance not needed by the body from the capillaries through the tubular cells into the lumen of the tubule

D. Countercurrent mechanism
1. Utilizes the juxtamedullary nephrons with their long loops of Henle and occurs within the renal medullary interstitium
2. Countercurrent *multiplication* is the mechanism that enables the body to excrete urine with an osmolality higher than the osmolality of serum
   a) Sodium chloride is transported out of the filtrate as it moves up the ascending limb of the loop of Henle, but water is not able to follow because this limb is impermeable to water
   b) Some sodium chloride enters the peritubular capillaries and is removed from the kidney, but some reenters the descending limb of the loop of Henle, making the filtrate more concentrated than the blood from which it was derived
   c) This process increases the osmotic pressure in the capillaries and tubules of the papillary region of the kidney until it is four times stronger than that of the blood in the afferent arteriole
3. Countercurrent *exchange* is the maintenance component of the countercurrent mechanism
   a) The vasa recta minimizes the loss of solute from the interstitium by passive diffusion, maintaining the osmotic gradient necessary for the countercurrent multiplication process

E. Total of 99% of the glomerular filtrate is reabsorbed from the tubules (especially the proximal limb); the remaining 1% is excreted as urine output
1. Normal urine output is approximately 1,500 ml/day
2. Urine composition
   a) Water
   b) Nitrogenous wastes: urea, uric acid, creatinine, ammonia
   c) Ions: potassium, sodium, calcium, chloride, bicarbonate, hydrogen, phosphate, sulfate
   d) Hormones and their breakdown products
   e) Vitamins: particularly water-soluble B vitamins and vitamin C
   f) Toxins
   g) Drugs
3. Abnormal constituents: glucose, albumin, RBCs, calculi, casts

II. Excretion of metabolic waste products
A. Urea
1. Protein (either ingested or catabolized from protein stores) is broken down into amino acids and nitrogenous wastes
2. Urea nitrogen is the end product of protein metabolism; it circulates in the bloodstream and is excreted in the urine
3. Blood urea nitrogen (BUN) varies with protein intake and hydration status so it provides an unreliable evaluation of renal function

B. Creatinine
1. Creatinine is a waste product of muscle metabolism
2. The normal kidney excretes creatinine at a rate equal to the kidney's blood flow or GFR
3. Serum creatinine is a better test for evaluation of renal function than BUN; urine creatinine clearance, which provides a comparison of serum creatinine and

24-hour urine creatinine, is an even better evaluation of renal function

III. Renal regulation of acid-base balance (for more on acid-base balance see Chapter 4)
   A. Tubular excretion of H^+ ions in exchange for sodium reabsorption
   B. Bicarbonate reabsorption into the circulation or excretion into the urine
   C. Excretion of H^+ ions in the urine as: NH_4Cl, H_2PO_4, H_2O
   D. Renal response to acidosis
      1. Increased hydrogen ion secretion
      2. Increased bicarbonate reabsorption
      3. Production of ammonia to accommodate hydrogen ion excretion
   E. Renal response to alkalosis
      1. Decreased hydrogen ion secretion
      2. Increased bicarbonate excretion
      3. Decreased production of ammonia

IV. Fluid balance
   A. Body fluids are dilute solutions of water and solutes
   B. Measurement methods
      1. Milliliter (ml): the unit of measure for fluid volume
      2. Milliequivalent (mEq): the unit of measure for chemical-combining activity of an electrolyte
      3. Milliosmols (mOsm): the unit of measure for osmotic pressure based on the number of dissolved particles in solution
         a) Osmolality: number of osmoles per kg of solution; expressed as mOsm/kg
         b) Osmolarity: number of osmoles per liter of solution
            (1) Isotonic: the tonicity of body fluids; osmolarity of 280 to 295 mOsm/L
            (2) Hypotonic: lower tonicity than body fluids
            (3) Hypertonic: higher tonicity than body fluids
         c) Osmolality and osmolarity: often used interchangeably, although most calculations of body fluids are based on osmolarity
   C. The human body is mostly water
      1. Volume
         a) Adult males: 60% of total body weight in adult males is water
         b) Adult females: slightly less water at 55% of total body weight due to higher percentage of body fat
         c) Older adults: less water at 45% to 55% of total body weight
         d) Obesity: body water decreases with increasing body fat
      2. Distribution (Fig. 9-6)
         a) Intracellular
            (1) Fluid contained within the cells
            (2) Accounts for 40% of total body weight

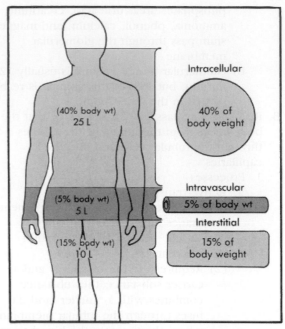

Figure 9-6 Distribution of body fluids. (From Thelan LA et al: *Critical care nursing: diagnosis and management*, ed 3, St Louis, 1998, Mosby.)

         b) Extracellular
            (1) Fluid outside the cells
            (2) Accounts for 20% of total body weight
            (3) Distribution
               (a) Interstitial
                  (i) Fluid surrounding the cells
                  (ii) Accounts for 15% of total body weight
               (b) Intravascular
                  (i) Fluid contained within the blood vessels
                  (ii) Accounts for approximately 4% of total body weight
               (c) Transcellular
                  (i) Fluid contained within specialized cavities of the body (e.g., cerebrospinal, pericardial, pleural, synovial, intraocular, digestive fluids)
                  (ii) Accounts for approximately 1% of total body weight
   D. Homeostasis is the state of internal equilibrium within the body; fluid, electrolyte, and acid-base are in balance
      1. Water and solutes are in constant movement and are exchanged continuously
         a) Most of the membranes of the body are semipermeable, allowing free movement of water and many nonelectrolytes and selective movement of electrolytes according to concentration gradients
         b) Movement of fluids, electrolytes, and

other solutes occurs by the following processes:

(1) Diffusion: solutes move from an area of higher solute concentration to an area of lower solute concentration

(2) Osmosis: solutions move from an area of lower solute concentration to an area of higher solute concentration

(3) Active transport: use of an energy source to move solutes from an area of lower solute concentration to an area of higher solution concentration

(4) Filtration: use of the pushing pressure of hydrostatic pressure to move water and selective solutes through a semipermeable membrane

c) Movement into and out of the cell occurs by diffusion, osmosis, and active transport

(1) Hydrostatic pressures push

(a) Capillary hydrostatic pressure pushes fluid out of capillary and into interstitium

(b) Interstitial hydrostatic pressure pushes fluid out of interstitium and into the capillary

(2) Colloidal oncotic pressures pull

(a) Capillary colloidal oncotic pressure pulls and holds fluid in the capillary

(b) Interstitial colloidal oncotic pressure pulls and holds fluid in the interstitium

(3) Starling's law of the capillaries describes the movement of fluid into and out of the capillaries (for more on capillary dynamics, see Chapter 2)

(a) Pressure differences at the venous and arterial ends of the capillaries influence the direction and rate of water and solute movement

(b) Pressures pushing fluid out of the capillary dominate at the arterial end; pressures pushing fluid back into the capillary dominate at the venous end

d) Pathology

(1) Third spacing: fluid accumulation in any space that is not intravascular or intracellular (e.g., interstitial edema, ascites, pleural effusion, pericardial effusion, into the lumen of the intestine)

(a) HF: peripheral edema is caused by venous congestion and excessive hydrostatic pressure at the venous end

(b) Malnutrition: decrease in plasma proteins decreases capillary colloidal oncotic pressure and allows excessive fluid to leak out of the capillary

(c) Fluid resuscitation with hypotonic solutions (e.g., D_5W): fluids with osmolality less than serum causes movement of fluid out of the vascular bed into the interstitium

2. Normal functioning of cells requires constancy of the body's compartments; imbalances disrupt homeostasis

E. Water exchanges occur continuously

1. Loss of water: total ~2,500 ml/24 hr

a) Lungs (400 ml)
b) Skin (400 ml)
c) Kidneys (1,500 ml)
d) Intestines (200 ml)
e) Losses are increased by any of the following:

(1) Increased respiratory rate
(2) Fever
(3) Hot, dry environment
(4) Injury to the skin (e.g., burns)

2. Gains of water: total ~2,500 ml/24 hr

a) Liquids (1,000 ml)
b) Food (1,200 ml)
c) Oxidation of food and body tissues (300 ml)

F. Body fluid is regulated by the following mechanisms:

1. Thirst

a) Thirst mechanism is located in the anterior hypothalamus; osmoreceptor cells sense changes in serum osmolality and initiate impulses to produce the thirst sensation and the release of ADH

b) The mechanism is stimulated by any of the following:

(1) Intracellular dehydration
(2) Hypertonic body fluids
(3) Extracellular fluid loss
(4) Hypotension or decreased cardiac output
(5) Angiotensin
(6) Dry mouth

c) The effect of thirst is the conscious desire to drink fluids (**Note:** Thirst is unreliable in the elderly or confused patient)

2. Antidiuretic hormone

a) ADH is produced by the hypothalamus, stored in and released by the posterior pituitary gland; release may be altered by intracranial processes (e.g., head injury, tumors, craniotomy) and extracranial processes (e.g., mechanical ventilation, tuberculosis)

b) ADH is stimulated by any of the following:
   (1) Hyperosmolality of extracellular fluid
   (2) Decrease in extracellular fluid volume
   (3) Hyperthermia
c) Effects of ADH include the following:
   (1) Acts on distal and collecting tubules, causing more water to be pulled from the tubule back into the blood
   (2) Increases total volume of body fluid by decreasing urine volume

3. Renin-angiotensin-aldosterone (RAA) system (Figure 2-21)
   a) RAA system is stimulated by any of the following:
      (1) Decreased blood pressure stimulating stretch receptors in juxtaglomerular cells
      (2) Sympathetic nervous system stimulation
      (3) Hyponatremia, hyperkalemia
      (4) Increased adrenocorticotropin hormone (ACTH) levels
   b) Effects of the RAA system include the following:
      (1) Angiotensin II causes vasoconstriction and secretion of aldosterone, a mineralocorticoid produced by the adrenal cortex
      (2) Aldosterone stimulates the renal tubules to reabsorb more sodium and water, which causes sodium retention, water retention, and decreased urine volume
      (3) Vasoconstriction and sodium and water retention increases blood pressure, which decreases renin secretion

4. Atrial natriuretic peptide (ANP)
   a) ANP is a hormonelike substance that is synthesized and stored by specialized atrial muscle cells
   b) ANP secretion is stimulated by the following:
      (1) Volume expansion
      (2) Elevated cardiac filling pressures
   c) Effects of ANP include the following:
      (1) Increased excretion of sodium and water by the kidney
      (2) Decreased synthesis of renin and decreased release of aldosterone

5. Countercurrent mechanism of kidney: mechanism for concentration and dilution of urine

V. Electrolyte balance
   A. Solutes are substances dissolved in a solution; they may be electrolytes or nonelectrolytes
      1. Nonelectrolytes (e.g., glucose, proteins, lipids, oxygen, carbon dioxide, urea, creatinine, bilirubin) are solutes without an electrical charge; they stay intact in solution
      2. Electrolytes are solutes that dissociate into positive or negative ions when in solution and generate an electrical charge when in solution
         a) Electrical charge
            (1) Cations are positive-charged ions
               (a) Major intracellular cation is potassium (K^+)
               (b) Major extracellular cation is sodium (Na^+)
               (c) Other cations: Ca^{++}, Mg^{++}, H^+
            (2) Anions are negative-charged electrolytes
               (a) Major intracellular anion is chloride (Cl^-)
               (b) Major extracellular anion is phosphate (PO_4^{3-})
               (c) Other anions: HCO_3^-
            (3) In each fluid compartment, the various cations and anions balance each other to achieve electrical neutrality; no net charge exists within a fluid compartment (Fig. 9-7)
   B. Summary of electrolyte normal values, roles, regulation, and food sources (Table 9-1)

VI. Renal role in regulation of blood pressure
   A. Juxtaglomerular apparatus is a combination of specialized cells located near the glomerulus at the junction of the afferent and efferent arterioles; juxtaglomerular cells contain granules of inactive renin
   B. The process of the juxtaglomerular apparatus is as follows:
      1. Renin is released in response to decreased arterial blood pressure, renal ischemia, hypovolemia, increased urinary sodium concentration, and norepinephrine
      2. Renin-angiotensin-aldosterone system is depicted in Figure 2-21

VII. Red blood cell synthesis and maturation
   A. Erythropoietin secretion
      1. Stimulates production of RBCs in bone marrow
      2. Prolongs life of RBC
   B. Postulated methods of erythropoietin synthesis and stimulus for secretion
      1. Normal kidneys either produce erythropoietin or synthesize an enzyme that catalyzes its formation
      2. Stimulation for formation is believed to be decreased Pao_2 in renal blood
   C. Interference in this process causes anemia in patients with chronic renal failure

VIII. Prostaglandin synthesis
   A. Process occurs primarily in the medulla
   B. Types of prostaglandins are as follows:
      1. Vasodilators: PGE_2, PGD_2, PGI_2
      2. Vasoconstrictors: PGA_2

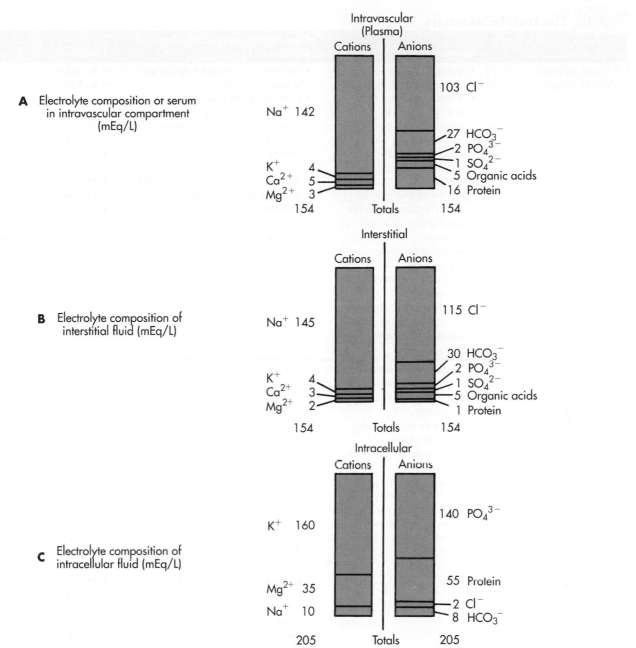

Figure 9-7   Electrolyte content of fluid compartments. **A,** Electrolyte composition of serum in intravascular compartment (mEq/L). **B,** Electrolyte composition of interstitial fluid (mEq/L). **C,** Electrolyte composition of intracellular fluid (mEq/L). (From Lewis SM, Collier IC: *Medical-surgical nursing,* ed 3, St Louis, 1992, Mosby.)

C. Release is stimulated by vasoactive substances (e.g., angiotensin, norepinephrine, bradykinins)

D. Effects of prostaglandins include the following:

1. Modulate the vasoconstrictive effects of angiotensin and norepinephrine; interference with this process may be one factor contributing to hypertension in patients with renal failure

2. Increase renal blood flow, which results in arterial vasodilation, inhibition of the distal tubule's response to ADH, and promotion of sodium and water excretion

IX. Renal role in bone mineralization

A. Vitamin D is metabolized by the kidney from an inactive form to an active metabolite called 1,25-dihydroxycholecalciferol necessary for the absorption of calcium and phosphorus from the intestine

B. Interference in this process causes osteodystrophy in patients with chronic renal failure

Table 9-1	Electrolyte Summary		

Electrolyte	Functions	Regulation and Factors Affecting Serum Level	Food Sources
Sodium: normal 136-145 mEq/L	• Maintains extracellular osmolality and volume • Maintains active transport mechanism in conjunction with potassium • Influences the kidney's regulation of the body's water and electrolyte status • Promotes the irritability of nerve tissue and the conduction of nerve impulses • Facilitates muscle contraction • Aids in some enzyme activities • Combines with bicarbonate and chloride to help regulate acid-base balance	• Aldosterone: causes sodium and water retention • Glomerular filtration rate: sodium excretion is increased when GFR is high; decreased when GFR is low • "Third factor": promotes sodium excretion by inhibiting sodium reabsorption; suppression of this factor ensures sodium reabsorption • Increase in sodium concentration stimulates water retention by ADH release, diluting sodium back to normal level • Some excretion through skin in perspiration	• Bouillon • Celery • Cheeses • Dried fruits • Frozen, canned, or packaged foods • Monosodium gluconate (MSG) • Mustard • Olives • Pickles • Preserved meat • Salad dressings and prepared sauces • Sauerkraut • Snack foods • Soy sauce
Potassium: normal 3.5-5.0 mEq/L	• Promotes transmission of nerve impulses • Maintains intracellular osmolality • Activates several enzymatic reactions • Helps regulate acid-base balance • Influences kidney function and structure • Promotes myocardial, skeletal, and smooth muscle contractility	• Aldosterone: increase in intracellular potassium or decrease in serum sodium causes aldosterone release and potassium excretion • GFR: potassium excretion is directly related to GFR in a normal kidney • Obligatory loss: the kidneys are unable to conserve potassium; it may be flushed out by diuresis even in the presence of a body deficit; 40-50 mEq lost each day • Renal failure: if kidneys fail to excrete potassium normally from the body (e.g., renal failure), toxic levels can occur • pH: potassium shifts into the cell in alkalosis (causing hypokalemia) and out of the cell in acidosis (causing hyperkalemia)	• Apricots • Artichokes • Avocado • Banana • Cantaloupe • Carrots • Cauliflower • Chocolate • Dried beans, peas • Dried fruit • Mushrooms • Nuts • Oranges, orange juice • Peanuts • Potatoes • Prune juice • Pumpkin • Spinach • Sweet potatoes • Swiss chard • Tomatoes, tomato juice, tomato sauce
Calcium: normal 8.5-10.5 mg/dl or 4.5-5.8 mEq/L (**Note:** Calcium is affected by albumin levels; to correct calcium, add 0.8 mg/dl for each 1 g/dl decrease in albumin)	• Hardens and strengthens bones and teeth • Aids in blood coagulation • Transmits neuromuscular impulses • Maintains cellular permeability • Serves essential role in cardiac contractility	• PTH: stimulated by a decrease in serum calcium; promotes calcium transfer from bone to plasma and aids in renal and intestinal absorption • Phosphorus: inhibits calcium absorption; calcium and phosphorus have an inverse relationship; if calcium goes up, phosphorus goes down and vice versa • Vitamin D: necessary for GI absorption; promotes calcium absorption • Calcitonin: aids transfer of calcium from plasma to bone, which directly lowers serum calcium	• Brazil nuts • Broccoli • Cheese • Collard, mustard, turnip greens • Cottage cheese • Eggnog • Ice cream • Milk and cream • Milk chocolate • Molasses • Oat flakes • Rhubarb • Seafood, especially sardines with bones • Sesame seeds • Soy flour • Spinach • Yogurt

Table 9-1	Electrolyte Summary—cont'd		
Electrolyte	**Functions**	**Regulation and Factors Affecting Serum Level**	**Food Sources**
Calcium—cont'd: normal 8.5-10.5 mg/dl or 4.5-5.8 mEq/L (**Note:** Calcium is affected by albumin levels; to correct calcium, add 0.8 mg/dl for each 1 g/dl decrease in albumin)		• Albumin: 50% of serum calcium is bound to serum albumin; therefore, a decrease in serum albumin lowers the total calcium level but not the ionized calcium level and the patient will not have symptoms of hypocalcemia • pH: alkalosis increases binding between albumin and calcium so that the patient will exhibit clinical indications of hypocalcemia though total body calcium is normal; acidosis decreases binding between albumin and calcium, so that the patient may exhibit clinical indications of hypercalcemia • Corticosteroids: contribute to demineralization of the bone and calcium loss; large doses decrease calcium absorption in GI tract • Diuretic effect: calcium is lost along with potassium and magnesium in patient on diuretics	
Phosphorus: normal 3.0-4.5 mg/dl	• Aids in structure of cellular membrane • Essential for glucose metabolism in red cells; produces 2,3-diphosphoglyceric acid (2,3-DPG) as an end product • Regulates the delivery of oxygen to the tissues; 2,3-DPG encourages unloading between hemoglobin and oxygen • Essential for ATP or high-energy phosphate formation • May be connected with DNA, RNA, genetic coding • Helps maintain bone hardness • Aids in enzyme regulation (ATPase) • Used by kidney to buffer hydrogen ions (PO_4)	• PTH: inhibits renal reabsorption of phosphates; calcium and phosphorus have an inverse relationship; if calcium goes up, phosphorus goes down and vice versa • Alterations in GFR affect phosphate excretion; increased GFR decreases reabsorption of phosphorus; decreased GFR increases reabsorption of phosphorus	• Dried beans and peas • Eggs and egg products • Fish, poultry • Meats, especially organ meats • Milk and milk products • Nuts • Seeds • Whole grains

Continued

Assessment of Fluid, Electrolyte, and Renal Status

Interview

I. Chief complaint: common symptoms of fluid, electrolyte, or renal conditions

   A. Flank or costovertebral angle pain

      1. Unilateral or bilateral

      2. Constant or intermittent

      3. Aggravated by costovertebral angle percussion

      4. Dull ache to stabbing or throbbing pain

      5. Relieved only by analgesics or treatment of underlying disease

      6. Accompanying findings: hematuria, pyuria, change in urine volume

Table 9-1	Electrolyte Summary—cont'd		
Electrolyte	Functions	Regulation and Factors Affecting Serum Level	Food Sources
Magnesium: normal 1.5-2.5 mEq/L	• Aids in neuromuscular transmission • Aids in cardiac contractility • Activates enzymes for cellular metabolism of CHO and proteins • Aids in maintaining the active transport mechanism at the cellular level • Aids in the transmission of hereditary information to offspring	• Not completely understood • Factors that influence calcium and potassium balance also affect magnesium • Deficiencies of these electrolytes usually occur together (e.g., diuretics cause the loss of all three) • Availability of sodium: sodium is necessary for the absorption of magnesium • Diuretics: cause the loss of excessive magnesium • PTH: affects magnesium reabsorption as it does calcium	• Bananas • Chocolate • Coconut • Grapefruit • Green, leafy vegetables • Legumes • Milk • Molasses • Nuts and seeds • Oranges • Refined sugar • Seafood • Soy flour • Wheat bran
Chloride: normal 96-106 mEq/L	• Maintains serum osmolality (along with sodium) • Combines with major cations to form important compounds (e.g., NaCl, HCl, KCl, CaCl) • Helps maintain acid-base balance through HCl production	• Indirectly affected by aldosterone • Changes almost always linked to sodium • pH: acidosis causes bicarbonate to be reabsorbed while chloride is excreted; alkalosis causes bicarbonate to be excreted while chloride is reabsorbed	• Bananas • Celery • Cheese • Dates • Eggs • Fish • Milk • Spinach • Table salt • Turkey

7. Possible causes: renal calculi, bladder cancer, bacterial cystitis, acute glomerulonephritis, obstructive uropathy, perirenal abscess, polycystic kidney disease, acute pyelonephritis, renal infarction, renal cancer, renal trauma, renal vein thrombosis, acute pancreatitis

B. Changes in pattern of urination
1. Frequency: frequent voiding
2. Nocturia: getting up at night to void (more than twice)
3. Dysuria: painful urination
4. Urgency: a feeling of the need to void immediately
5. Hesitancy: difficulty starting the flow of urine
6. Change in stream
7. Retention: incomplete emptying of the bladder
8. Incontinence: inability to control urination
9. Enuresis: incontinence of urine in bed at night

C. Change in urine output: increased or decreased amount

D. Change in appearance of urine
1. Dilute: clear to light yellow
2. Concentrated: dark, amber
3. Pyuria: cloudy
4. Hematuria: pink to red
5. Bilirubinemia: orange to brown
6. Myoglobinuria: tea or cola-colored
7. Hemoglobinuria: wine-colored

E. Neurologic
1. Visual changes: may be associated with uremia, fluid overload, or electrolyte imbalance
2. Paresthesias: may be associated with hypocalcemia
3. Headaches: may be associated with fluid overload or uremia
4. Seizures: may be associated with uremia, electrolyte imbalances, fluid overload
5. Decreased ability to concentrate: may be associated with uremia, electrolyte imbalance, or fluid overload
6. Apathy: may be associated with uremia

F. Cardiovascular
1. Palpitations: may be seen with dysrhythmias in electrolyte imbalance
2. Chest pain: may be seen with uremia or electrolyte imbalance
3. Edema: may be associated with uremia, fluid overload, or hypoproteinemia

G. Pulmonary
1. Dyspnea: may be seen in renal failure patients as a result of left ventricular failure or pleural effusion
2. Hemoptysis: seen in Goodpasture's syndrome

H. Gastrointestinal
1. Halitosis: foul odor to breath; urinelike odor to breath may be associated with uremia; metallic taste in mouth
2. Anorexia: may be associated with uremia
3. Nausea, vomiting: may be associated with

uremia, electrolyte imbalance, or fluid overload

   4. Constipation or diarrhea: may be related to fluid electrolyte imbalance
 I. Musculoskeletal
   1. Joint pain: may be associated with uremia, fluid imbalance, electrolyte imbalance
   2. Muscle weakness: may be associated with fluid electrolyte imbalance
   3. Muscle pain or cramps: may be associated with uremia or electrolyte imbalance
 J. Dermatologic
   1. Pruritus: may be associated with uremia
   2. Bruising: may be associated with uremia
   3. Delayed healing: may be associated with uremia
 K. Sexual
   1. Impotence: may be related to uremia
   2. Diminished libido: may be related to uremia
   3. Infertility: may be related to uremia
 L. Other general symptoms
   1. Fatigue: may be associated with uremia
   2. Fever: may be associated with infection or dehydration
   3. Thirst: may be associated with fluid imbalance
   4. Change in body weight: may be associated with uremia or fluid imbalance
II. History of present illness
 A. PQRST
 B. Accompanying symptoms
III. Past medical history
 A. Renal/urinary tract
   1. Urinary tract infection
   2. Calculi
   3. Renal insufficiency/failure
     a) Dialysis
     b) Renal transplantation
   4. Surgical procedures
 B. Cardiovascular
   1. Hypertension
   2. Arteriosclerosis/atherosclerosis
   3. Heart failure
   4. Bacterial endocarditis
 C. Pulmonary
   1. Goodpasture's syndrome: hemoptysis with glomerulonephritis
   2. Tuberculosis
 D. Endocrine/metabolic
   1. Diabetes mellitus
   2. Gout
 E. Immunologic/hematologic
   1. Connective tissue disorders
     a) Lupus erythematosus
     b) Scleroderma
   2. Hemophilia
   3. Disseminated intravascular coagulation
   4. Sickle-cell disease
   5. Malignancy
   6. Blood transfusion
 F. Gynecologic: toxemia of pregnancy

 G. Infection
   1. Recent beta-hemolytic streptococcal infection
   2. Urinary tract infection
IV. Family history
 A. Renal
   1. Inherited glomerulonephritis
   2. Polycystic disease
   3. Inherited nephritis (Alport's syndrome)
   4. Amyloidosis
   5. Malignancy
 B. Cardiovascular
   1. Hypertension
   2. Coronary artery disease
 C. Immunologic/hematologic
   1. Hemophilia
   2. Sickle cell disease
 D. Endocrine: diabetes mellitus
V. Social history
 A. Occupational exposure to toxins: lead, mercury, pesticides, methanol, radiation, carbon tetrachloride, phenol
 B. Exercise habits (strenuous exercise in an unconditioned person may cause rhabdomyolysis and myoglobinuria)
 C. Fluid intake: type of fluids
 D. Smoking (increased incidence of bladder cancer)
 E. Use of saccharine (increased incidence of bladder cancer)
VI. Medication history
 A. Potentially nephrotoxic agents
   1. Antibiotics/antiinfectives
     a) Aminoglycosides
     b) Cephalosporins
     c) Sulfonamides
     d) Amphotericin B
     e) Bacitracin
     f) Rifampin
   2. Nonsteroidal antiinflammatory agents (e.g., ibuprofen, indomethacin, aspirin)
   3. ACE inhibitors (e.g., captopril)
   4. Antineoplastics (e.g., cisplatin, methotrexate)
   5. Analgesics containing phenacetin
   6. Cyclosporin A
   7. Methanol, ethylene glycol
   8. Carbon tetrachloride
   9. Contrast media
   10. Heavy metals (e.g., lead, arsenic, mercury, uranium)
   11. Insecticides and fungicides
   12. Phencyclidine (PCP) and other street drugs
 B. Diuretics
 C. Antihypertensives
 D. Anticoagulants
 E. Electrolyte replacement therapy
 F. Immunosuppressives
   1. Corticosteroids
   2. Azathioprine (Imuran)
   3. Cyclophosphamide (Cytoxan)

Vital Signs

I. Blood pressure
  A. Increased: seen in fluid overload, renal disease, hypertension
  B. Decreased: must be fluid loss of 15% to 25% before systolic blood pressure falls
  C. Postural drop (tilt positive): decrease of 15 mm Hg in systolic pressure when patient sits or stands may be earlier change of hypovolemia
II. Pulse
  A. Increased: seen in SNS stimulation because may be seen in fluid overload or dehydration; response blunted or eliminated by beta-blockers
  B. Postural: increases of pulse by 20 BPM when the patient sits or stands may be earlier change of hypovolemia
III. Respiratory rate and rhythm
  A. Tachypnea: seen in sympathetic nervous system stimulation as may be seen in fluid overload or dehydration
  B. Kussmaul's: rapid, deep, gasping breaths seen in metabolic acidosis
IV. Temperature: hyperthermia may be seen in dehydration
V. Weight changes
  A. Change of 1 lb is equal to 500 ml; change of 1 kg is equal to 1 L
  B. Evaluate weight before and after hemodialysis; evaluate weight after drainage of dialysate in patients on peritoneal dialysis
  C. Weight loss resulting from generalized debilitation may be seen in renal failure

Inspection and Palpation

I. Skin
  A. Color
    1. Yellowish-gray cast is seen in renal failure
    2. Pallor may indicate anemia
    3. Petechiae, bruising may be seen in renal failure as a result of platelet dysfunction
  B. Skin texture
    1. Rough, dry skin is seen in renal failure
    2. Uremic frost, a filmy coating over the skin, is seen in untreated uremia
  C. Lesions: scratch marks may be seen as a result of pruritus in renal failure
  D. Skin turgor
    1. Recoil should be immediate; decrease in skin turgor indicates interstitial dehydration but is not an early sign
    2. Evaluation of skin turgor to determine hydration status is not reliable in elderly patients because of poor elasticity
  E. Edema
    1. Late change of overhydration since patient may gain 3 to 4 kg before edema is noticeable
    2. Location
      a) Edema related to renal disease is often facial initially
      b) Anasarca (generalized, massive edema

and does not pit) may be seen in end-stage renal disease
II. Mouth
  A. Halitosis: uremic fetor (urinelike odor to the breath) noted in renal failure
  B. Mucous membranes: stickiness of the oral mucous membranes and tongue is the preferred indicator of dehydration in the elderly; use a tongue blade to evaluate stickiness
III. Eyes
  A. Periorbital edema seen in nephrotic syndrome and other forms of renal disease
  B. Cataract formation common in renal failure
IV. Ears: nerve deafness common in renal failure
V. Neurologic status
  A. Change in level of consciousness may indicate azotemia or electrolyte imbalance
  B. Confusion may be indicative of uremia
  C. Seizures may indicate hyponatremia, cerebral edema
  D. Neuromuscular irritability and changes in muscle strength may reflect electrolyte imbalance
VI. Cardiovascular
  A. Dysrhythmias are common in electrolyte imbalance
  B. Jugular venous distention (see Figure 2-26 for illustration)
    1. To evaluate JVD
      a) Place patient in a 45-degree angle
      b) Identify the angle of Louis: raised notch that is created where the manubrium and the body of the sternum join; also called *manubriosternal junction* or *sternal angle*
      c) Measure height of neck vein distention
      d) Normal height of neck vein distention is 1 to 2 cm above the angle of Louis; neck vein distention of greater than 2 cm above the angle of Louis may be indicative of hypervolemia
VII. Abdomen
  A. Generalized edema and/or ascites: may be seen in renal failure
  B. Kidney
    1. The kidney may be palpated by "capture" technique; put one hand under the patient below the costal margin and the other hand on the abdomen below the costal margin; ask the patient to take a deep breath and move hands together to try to "capture" the kidney
    2. The lower pole of a normal right kidney may be palpable because it is lower than the right (pushed down by the liver)
    3. A normal left kidney is not palpable
    4. If kidney is palpable, evaluate the following:
      a) Size: normal size is 10 × 5 × 2.5 cm or about the size of a fist
        (1) Increased size may be seen in acute

renal disease, polycystic disease, obstructive uropathy, pyelonephritis, renal abscess or tumor
 (2) Decreased size may be seen in advanced chronic renal failure
 b) Discomfort: pain or discomfort during palpation may indicate infection, calculi, tumor, hydronephrosis, glomerulonephritis
C. Bladder
 1. The bladder is palpable in suprapubic area only when full
 2. If palpable, the bladder should be felt as a smooth, round, firm organ that is sensitive to palpation
VIII. Extremities
 A. Asterixis: a hand-flapping tremor induced by extending the arm and dorsiflexing the wrist; indicative of increased ammonia levels; seen in renal failure and hepatic encephalopathy
 B. Vascular access (e.g., fistula, AV graft, shunt)
  1. Thrill over access indicates patency
  2. Visible blood in tubing (e.g., shunt) should be bright red

Percussion
I. Thorax: flatness at lung bases may indicate pleural effusion, which is often seen in renal failure
II. Abdomen
 A. Elicitation of a fluid wave: indicative of ascites, which is often seen in end-stage renal failure
 B. Costovertebral angle (CVA) (Fig. 9-8): tap over costovertebral angle with ulnar surface of hand
  1. CVA tenderness may be seen in pyelonephritis, renal calculi, renal abscess or tumor, glomerulonephritis, or intermittent hydronephrosis
  2. Bruising over CVA may indicate renal trauma
 C. Bladder
  1. The bladder is percussible in suprapubic area only when it contains at least 150 ml
  2. Dullness is audible above the symphysis pubis if the bladder is full of urine
  3. Pain during percussion may indicate cystitis

Auscultation
I. Vascular sounds
 A. Renal bruit: may be audible to the left or right of midline in periumbilical region in renal vascular disease or renal vascular trauma
 B. Vascular access (e.g., fistula, AV graft, shunt) bruit: indicates patency
II. Heart sounds
 A. Rate and rhythm: dysrhythmias may be seen in electrolyte imbalance
 B. S_3: indicates heart failure
 C. Flow murmur: mitral regurgitation murmur (systolic murmur heard best at apex with diaphragm) may be heard with fluid overload
 D. Pericardial friction rub: may indicate pericarditis, a common complication of renal failure

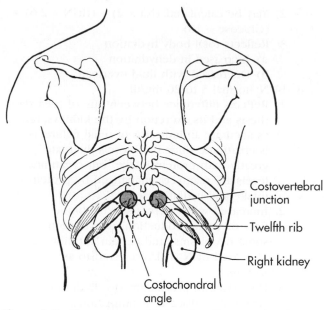

Figure 9-8 The costovertebral angle. (From Barkauskas VH et al: *Health and physical assessment,* St Louis, 1994, Mosby.)

III. Breath sounds: crackles may indicate fluid overload, heard initially at bases
IV. Bowel sounds: changes may indicate electrolyte imbalance
 A. Hypoactive bowel sounds in hypokalemia
 B. Hyperactive bowel sounds in hyperkalemia

Urine Output
I. Important indicator of GFR
II. Decreased with diminished cardiac output or dehydration
III. Increased in overhydration
IV. Volume parameters
 A. Normal output = 1,500 ml/24 hr or at least 0.5 ml/kg/hr
 B. Polyuria: greater than 2,500 ml/24 hr
 C. Oliguria: 100 to 400 ml/24 hr
 D. Anuria: 0 to 100 ml/24 hr

Hemodynamic Monitoring
I. Right atrial pressure (RAP) (from proximal port of pulmonary artery catheter) or central venous pressure (CVP) (from catheter in superior vena cava): normal 2 to 6 mm Hg
 A. Increased in hypervolemia
 B. Decreased in hypovolemia
II. Pulmonary artery occlusive pressure (PAOP): normal 6 to 12 mm Hg
 A. Increased in hypervolemia
 B. Decreased in hypovolemia

Diagnostic Studies
I. Serum
 A. Osmolarity: normal 280 to 295 mOsm/L
  1. Measures particles exerting osmotic pull per U of water

2. May be calculated: $(Na \times 2) + (BUN \div 2.6) + (Glucose \div 18)$

3. Reflects total body hydration
   a) Increased in dehydration
   b) Decreased with fluid overload

B. BUN: normal 5 to 20 mg/dl
   1. Reflects difference between rate of urea synthesis and its excretion by the kidneys; not as accurate an indicator of renal failure as is creatinine since BUN levels fluctuate greatly with protein intake, but creatinine levels are relatively unchanged by protein intake and hydration level
   2. Increased with decreased renal blood flow or urine production, dehydration, some neoplasms, and certain antibiotics; increased BUN is also referred to as *uremia*
   3. Decreased in pregnancy, overhydration, severe liver disease, malnutrition
   4. Normal BUN:creatinine ratio is 10:1
      a) When BUN is elevated disproportionately to the creatinine (e.g., BUN:creatinine ratio 20:1), consider an extrarenal cause such as one of the following:
         (1) Volume depletion
            (a) Insufficient fluid intake
            (b) Excessive fluid loss
               (i) Diuresis
               (ii) Vomiting
         (2) Poor renal perfusion
            (a) Shock
            (b) Sepsis
            (c) Decreased cardiac output
            (d) Renovascular disease
         (3) Protein catabolism
            (a) Starvation
            (b) Blood in the GI tract
            (c) Corticosteroids
      b) When BUN and creatinine are elevated maintaining the normal 10:1 ratio, consider a renal cause such as acute or chronic renal failure

C. Creatinine: normal 0.7 to 1.5 mg/dl
   1. Measures products of muscle metabolism
   2. More accurate than BUN in evaluating renal function because creatinine is normally filtered by the glomerulus and not reabsorbed by the tubule; unaffected by diet and fluid intake
   3. Elevated when 50% or more of the nephrons are destroyed
   4. Decreased in muscular dystrophy

D. Electrolytes
   1. Sodium: normal 136 to 145 mEq/L
   2. Potassium: normal 3.5 to 5.0 mEq/L
   3. Chloride: normal 96 to 106 mEq/L
   4. Calcium: normal 8.5 to 10.5 mg/dl
   5. Phosphorus: normal 3.0 to 4.5 mg/dl
   6. Magnesium: normal 1.5 to 2.5 mEq/L

Table 9-2	Anion Gap
Calculation of Anion Gap	$(Na + K) - (Cl + HCO_3^-)$
Normal value	5-15
Causes of Metabolic Acidosis with normal anion gap: bicarbonate loss	Intestinal loss of bicarbonate • Diarrhea • Pancreatic fistula • Ureterosigmoidostomy Renal loss of bicarbonate • Carbonic anhydrase inhibitors (e.g., acetazolamide [Diamox]) • Aldosterone-antagonists (also referred to as *potassium-sparing diuretics*) (e.g., triamterene [Dyrenium], spironolactone [Aldactone]) • Renal tubular acidosis • Adrenal insufficiency • Primary hypoaldosteronism Excessive gain of chloride • Large quantities of normal saline • Ammonium chloride • Arginine hydrochloride
Causes of Metabolic Acidosis with increased anion gap: metabolic acid gain	Renal failure Lactic acidosis • Shock • Hypoxemia/hypoxia • Severe anemia • Status epilepticus • Cyanide poisoning Ketoacidosis • Diabetic ketoacidosis • Starvation • Alcohol Drugs and toxins • Salicylates • Methanol • Ethylene glycol • Paraldehyde • High-dose carbenicillin Rhabdomyolysis

E. Anion gap: a calculated parameter (Table 9-2)
   1. Calculated by subtracting the anion from the cations
      a) (Sodium + Potassium) − (Chloride + bicarbonate)
      b) Normal: 5 to 15
   2. Helpful in determining cause of metabolic acidosis
      a) A normal anion gap indicates that the reason for the metabolic acidosis is bicarbonate loss
      b) An elevated anion gap indicates that the reason for the metabolic acidosis is an acid gain (e.g., lactic acid, ketoacid, toxins)

F. Glucose: normal 70 to 110 mEq/L

G. Arterial blood gases
  1. pH: normal 7.35 to 7.45
  2. $Paco_2$: normal 35 to 45 mm Hg
  3. HCO_3^-: normal 22 to 26 mEq/L
  4. Pao_2: normal 80 to 100 mm Hg
H. Hematology
  1. Hematocrit: normal 40% to 52% for males; 35% to 47% for females
     a) Measures portion of blood volume occupied by RBCs
     b) Increased in dehydration or polycythemia
     c) Decreased with low RBCs or with normal hemoglobin and water overload
  2. Hemoglobin: normal 13 to 18 g/dl for males; 12 to 16 g/dl for females
  3. White blood cells (WBC): 3,500 to 11,000 mm^3
I. Clotting profile
  1. Prothrombin time (PT): normal 12 to 15 seconds
  2. Activated partial thromboplastin time (aPTT): normal 25 to 38 seconds
  3. Thrombin time: normal 10 to 15 seconds
  4. Bleeding time: normal 1 to 9.5 minutes
  5. Platelets: normal 150,000 to 400,000/mm^3
J. Serum proteins
  1. Total protein: normal 6 to 8 g/dl
  2. Albumin: normal 3.5 to 4.5 g/dl
K. Serum lipids
  1. Cholesterol: 150 to 200 mg/dl
  2. Triglycerides: 40 to 150 mg/dl
II. Urine
A. Visual examination: clear, yellow
B. Glucose: normal negative; glycosuria occurs when renal threshold for glucose is exceeded; renal threshold is variable and patient-specific, so no accurate method is available to predict serum glucose
C. Ketones: normal negative; ketonuria is seen in catabolism (e.g., starvation or diabetic ketoacidosis)
D. Protein: normal 0 to 18 mg/dl
  1. Proteinuria may occur after ingestion of a high-protein meal or can accompany renal changes of pregnancy
  2. Consistent proteinuria suggests compromise of the glomerular membrane (e.g., nephrotic syndrome, glomerulonephritis)
E. Bilirubin: normal negative; urobilinogen indicates biliary obstruction or liver disease
F. Specific gravity: 1.005 to 1.030
  1. Increased with any condition causing hypoperfusion of kidneys leading to oliguria (e.g., shock, severe dehydration, proteinuria, glycosuria, contrast media)
  2. Decreased in diabetes insipidus, over-hydration, and when renal tubules lose their ability to reabsorb water and concentrate urine as in early pyelonephritis

G. Osmolality: 50 to 1,200 mOsm/L
  1. Measures number of particles per unit of water in urine
  2. Depends on the circulating titer of ADH and the rate of urinary solute excretion; should be 1.5 times that of serum osmolality
  3. Increased in fluid volume deficit resulting from retention of fluid by the body
  4. Decreased in fluid volume excess resulting from fluid being excreted by the kidney
H. Creatinine clearance
  1. Estimate of GFR
  2. Urine specimen for 24-hour period and a serum creatinine required
  3. Normal: 85 to 135 ml/min
I. Culture and sensitivity: normal, no bacteria present; if bacteria are present, appropriate antibiotic therapy is identified
J. pH: normal 4.0 to 8.0 with average of 6.0
  1. Increased urinary acidity indicates that the body is retaining bicarbonate
  2. Decreased urinary acidity (more alkaline) indicates that the kidney is retaining sodium and acids
     a) Alkaline urine may be associated with urinary tract infection
     b) Alkaline urine and serum acidosis is associated with renal tubular acidosis
K. Spot urine electrolytes
  1. Evaluates the kidney's ability to conserve sodium and concentrate urine
  2. Measures sodium, potassium, and chloride concentrations in the urine
     a) Sodium: normal 40 to 220 mEq/L/24 hr
     b) Potassium: normal 25 to 120 mEq/L/24 hr
     c) Chloride: normal 110 to 250 mEq/24 hr
L. Sediment
  1. Casts: precipitation from the kidney that takes the shape of the tubule where it was formed; normally none or occasional hyaline casts
     a) Hyaline casts: small amounts normal but if large amounts indicative of significant proteinuria
     b) Erythrocyte casts: indicative of glomerulonephritis or vasculitis
     c) Leukocyte casts: indicative of infectious process
     d) Granular casts: indicative of acute tubular necrosis, interstitial nephritis, acute or chronic glomerulonephritis, chronic renal failure
     e) Fatty casts: indicative of lipoid nephrosis or nephrotic syndrome
     f) Renal tubular casts: indicative of acute renal failure
  2. Bacteria: abnormal in catheterized specimen
  3. Erythrocytes: small numbers normal; large numbers indicative of glomerulonephritis,

interstitial nephritis, malignancy, infection, calculi, cystitis, or trauma
4. Leukocytes: small numbers normal; large numbers indicative of infection, interstitial nephritis
5. Renal epithelial cells: indicative of acute tubular necrosis, glomerulonephritis, interstitial nephritis
6. Crystals: indicative of stone formation
7. Eosinophils: indicative of allergic reaction in kidney
III. Other diagnostic studies (Table 9-3)

Fluid and Electrolyte Imbalances
Hypovolemia
I. Etiology
  A. Insufficient intake
  B. Inadequate replacement following excess fluid loss
  C. Excessive fluid losses
    1. Hemorrhage
    2. GI losses
      a) Nasogastric or intestinal suction
      b) Vomiting
      c) Diarrhea
      d) Fistula
    3. Renal losses
      a) Diuretics
      b) Aldosterone insufficiency
      c) Diuretic phase of acute renal failure
      d) Osmotic diuresis resulting from hyperglycemia or osmotic dyes
    4. Increased insensible losses
      a) Diaphoresis
      b) Tachypnea
    5. Draining wounds
  D. Intravascular to extravascular shift (also called *third-spacing*)
    1. Ascites
    2. Intestinal obstruction
    3. Hypoproteinemia
    4. Burns
II. Clinical presentation
  A. Tachycardia
  B. Orthostatic hypotension
  C. Decreased CVP, RAP, PAOP, CO/CI
  D. Increased SVR
  E. Weight loss more than 5% of body weight
  F. Flat jugular veins with head of bed elevated at 45° angle
  G. Weakness
  H. Anorexia, nausea, vomiting, constipation
  I. Flushed skin (fluid loss) or cool, clammy skin (blood loss)
  J. Dry, sticky tongue and mucous membranes
  K. Poor skin turgor
  L. Thirst
  M. Low-grade fever
  N. Syncope
  O. Lethargy, disorientation, coma

  P. Oliguria
  Q. Urine specific gravity more than 1.030 if ADH osmoreceptor mechanism is intact
  R. Increased BUN; normal creatinine
  S. Increased hematocrit and serum osmolality if fluid lost; decreased hematocrit if blood lost
III. Nursing diagnoses
  A. Fluid Volume Deficit related to excessive fluid losses, inadequate intake or replacement, third-spacing
  B. Decreased Cardiac Output related to decreased preload
  C. Altered Tissue Perfusion related to decreased hemoglobin, cardiac output
IV. Collaborative management
  A. Monitor urine output, I & O, daily weight, laboratory studies
  B. Treat the cause of hypovolemia (e.g., antidiarrheals for diarrhea, control of hemorrhage)
  C. Replace fluids carefully to prevent hypervolemia
    1. Oral fluids for mild deficits
    2. Parenteral fluids for moderate or severe deficits; replace fluids lost with similar fluids (e.g., blood for hemorrhage, normal saline with electrolytes for excessive diuresis)
  D. Provide frequent oral and skin care

Water Loss Syndromes: Serum osmolality more than 295 mOsm/L (may be referred to as *hyperosmolar hypernatremia*)
I. Etiology: water loss without sodium loss
  A. Inadequate water intake
  B. Hypertonic fluids or feedings (e.g., TPN, hyperosmolar enteral feedings)
  C. Diabetes insipidus
  D. Diabetes mellitus
  E. Watery diarrhea
II. Clinical presentation
  A. Tachycardia
  B. Hypotension
  C. Flushed skin
  D. Dry, sticky tongue and mucous membranes
  E. Poor skin turgor
  F. Thirst
  G. Low-grade fever
  H. Mental irritability, confusion
  I. Oliguria to anuria (except diabetes insipidus)
  J. Elevated hematocrit, serum osmolality, serum sodium
III. Nursing diagnoses
  A. Fluid Volume Deficit related to excessive fluid losses, inadequate intake or replacement, third-spacing
  B. Decreased Cardiac Output related to decreased preload
  C. Altered Tissue Perfusion related to decreased hemoglobin, cardiac output
IV. Collaborative management
  A. Monitor urine output, I & O, daily weight, laboratory studies

Table 9-3	DIAGNOSTIC STUDIES	
Study	**Purposes**	**Comments**
Computed tomographic (CT) scan	• Provides a view of kidneys, retroperitoneal space, bladder, prostate • Evaluates kidney size • Evaluates the kidney for tumors, abscesses, and obstruction	• No special preparation required • Can be safely used in patients with renal failure • Contrast medium may be used
Cystometrogram	• Evaluates the pressure exerted against the wall of the bladder to evaluate bladder tone	• No special preparation required • Urinary catheter inserted and saline instilled into bladder • Postprocedure monitor for clinical indications of urinary tract infection
Cystoscopy	• Visualizes bladder and urethra for identification pathology	Preprocedure • NPO after midnight if general anesthesia is to be used • Administer sedative if prescribed • No special preparation required Postprocedure • Pink-tinged urine is normal but gross hematuria is abnormal; monitor urine output • Encourage fluids

Intravenous pyelogram (IVP)	• Evaluates position, size, shape, and location of kidneys
	• Provides visualization of internal kidney (parenchyma, calyces, pelvis)
	• Evaluates filling of renal pelvis
	• Outlines ureters and bladder
	• Identifies presence of cysts and tumors
	• Identifies obstruction, congenital abnormality
		• Also called *excretory urogram*
		• Contraindicated in renal insufficiency, multiple myeloma, pregnancy, HF, sickle cell disease
		• Bowel preparation (e.g., cathartics as prescribed)
		• NPO for 8 hours prior to the test
		• Contrast media used
		  • Check for allergy to iodine prior to the study
		  • Monitor for allergic reaction postprocedure
		  • Ensure hydration postprocedure

Kidneys, ureters, and bladder (KUB)	• Outlines kidneys, ureters, bladder • Evaluates size, shape, and position of kidneys • Identifies location of calculi	• Also called *flat plate of abdomen* • Bowel preparation (e.g., cathartics) may be prescribed if to be followed by IVP
Magnetic resonance imaging (MRI)	• Differentiates between cyst and solid mass • Identifies infarction, trauma, obstruction	• More specific than renal ultrasonography or CT scan because it shows subtle density changes • Cannot be used in patients with any implanted metallic device, including pacemakers • No special preparation required

Nephrotomogram	• Evaluates segments of the kidney at different levels
	• Differentiates between cysts and solid mass
		• Bowel preparation (e.g., cathartics) as prescribed
		• NPO for 8 hours prior to the test
		• Contrast media used
		  • Check for allergy to iodine prior to the study
		  • Monitor for allergic reaction postprocedure
		  • Ensure hydration postprocedure

Renal angiography	• Evaluates renal vasculature • Identifies renal artery stenosis • Identifies cysts, tumors, infarction, trauma	• Bowel preparation (e.g., cathartics) as prescribed • NPO for 8 hours prior to the test • Sedative is usually prescribed prior to the procedure

Continued

Table 9-3 | **DIAGNOSTIC STUDIES—cont'd**

Study	Purposes	Comments

Renal angiography—cont'd		• Contrast media used
		  • Check for allergy to iodine prior to the study
		  • Monitor for allergic reaction postprocedure
		  • Ensure hydration postprocedure
		Postprocedure
		• Keep extremity in which catheter was placed immobilized in a straight position for 6-12 hours
		• Monitor arterial puncture point for hemorrhage or hematoma
		• Monitor neurovascular status of affected limb
		• Monitor for indications of systemic emboli

Renal biopsy	• Obtains tissue specimen for microscopic evaluation	• May be performed open or closed • Clotting profile is evaluated preprocedure • Type and crossmatch for two units of blood preprocedure • Usually not preformed if patient has only one functioning kidney (unless being done to evaluate possible transplant rejection) • Closed biopsy contraindicated in bleeding abnormalities, polycystic disease, hydronephrosis, neoplasm, urinary tract infection, and uncooperative patient Postprocedure • Pressure dressing is applied, and the patient is on bed rest for 24 hours • Observe for hematuria, flank pain, or hypotension
Renal radionuclide scan (renogram)	• Evaluates position, size, shape, and location of kidneys • Identifies obstruction, abscesses, cysts, tumors • Evaluates renal perfusion • Evaluates glomerular filtration, tubular function, and excretion • Assesses status of renal transplant	• Assure patient that the amount of radioactive material is minimal • Do not schedule within 24 hours after IVP • Ask patient to void prior to scan • Encourage fluids after the procedure

Retrograde pyelogram	• Evaluates position, size, shape, and location of kidneys
	• Outlines ureters and bladder
	• Identifies presence of cysts and tumors
	• Identifies presence of obstruction
		• Does not require the kidney to excrete the dye, so may be used in patients with renal insufficiency
		• Bowel preparation (e.g., cathartics) as prescribed
		• NPO for 8 hours prior to the test
		• Contrast media used
		  • Check for allergy to iodine prior to the study
		  • Monitor for allergic reaction postprocedure
		  • Ensure hydration postprocedure
		• Monitor patient for clinical indications of urinary tract infection or sepsis

Ultrasonography	• Evaluates fluid versus solid mass • Identifies obstructions • Identifies cysts, abscesses, tumors, polycystic kidney disease • Identifies hemorrhage • Identifies urinary tract obstruction and leaks	• No special preparation required • Can be safely used in patients with renal failure • Contrast media may be used
Voiding cystourethrography	• Identifies abnormalities of lower urinary tract to determine presence of reflux and residual urine	• No special preparation required • Encourage fluids postprocedure

B. Treat the cause
  1. Vasopressin for central diabetes insipidus; chlorpropamide (Diabinese) for nephrogenic diabetes insipidus
  2. Insulin for diabetes mellitus, hyperglycemia
  3. Antidiarrheals for diarrhea
C. Provide appropriate volume replacement and normalize serum osmolality: administer water in excess of sodium (e.g., D_5W or ½NS)
D. Maintain adequate urine output with adequate volume replacement and dopamine at renal dosages (1-2 µg/kg/min) as prescribed
E. Provide frequent oral and skin care

Hypervolemia

I. Etiology
  A. Excessive fluid intake
    1. Excessive oral or parenteral fluids
    2. Excessive use of saline enemas
  B. Retention of sodium and water
    1. Steroid therapy
    2. Heart failure
    3. Liver disease (e.g., cirrhosis)
    4. Stress response via ADH secretion, renin-angiotensin-aldosterone system
    5. Nephrotic syndrome
    6. Acute or chronic renal failure
  C. Interstitial to intravascular shift
    1. Remobilization of fluids after treatment of burns
    2. Administration of hypertonic or hyperosmolar solutions (e.g., albumin, 3% saline)
II. Clinical presentation
  A. Tachycardia
  B. Increased BP
  C. Increased CVP, RAP, PAOP
  D. Weight gain more than 5% of body weight
  E. Jugular venous distention
  F. Tachypnea, dyspnea, crackles
  G. Peripheral edema
  H. Ascites
  I. Increased urine output
  J. Urine specific gravity less than 1.010 if ADH osmoreceptor mechanism is intact
  K. Muscle weakness
  L. Lethargy, apathy, disorientation, coma
  M. Clinical indications of pulmonary or cerebral edema
  N. Decreased hematocrit
  O. Decreased BUN
  P. Chest X-ray: may show pulmonary vascular congestion
III. Nursing diagnoses
  A. Fluid Volume Excess related to decreased fluid elimination, excessive fluid intake or replacement
  B. Impaired Gas Exchange related to intraalveolar fluid
  C. Decreased Adaptive Capacity: Intracranial related to cerebral edema
IV. Collaborative management

A. Monitor urine output, I & O, daily weight, laboratory studies
B. Prevent hypervolemia by closely monitoring IV fluids; volumetric or controller pumps should be used for patients predisposed to hypervolemia
C. Decrease excess volume
  1. Restrict fluids and/or sodium
  2. Administer diuretics as prescribed
  3. Hemodialysis or continuous renal replacement therapy may be utilized, especially if renal insufficiency is present
D. Provide frequent oral and skin care

Water Excess Syndromes: Serum osmolality less than 280 mOsm/L (may be referred to as *hypoosmolar hyponatremia*)

I. Etiology: water increased in excess of sodium
  A. Replacement of isotonic body fluids with hypotonic solution (e.g., D_5W)
  B. Use of tap water enemas
  C. Psychogenic polydipsia
  D. GI or GU irrigation with hypotonic fluids (e.g., tap water or distilled water)
  E. Excessive ice chips
  F. Syndrome of inappropriate antidiuretic hormone (SIADH)
  G. Administration of oral hypoglycemic agents, tricyclic antidepressants
II. Clinical presentation
  A. Anorexia, nausea, vomiting
  B. Abdominal and muscle cramps
  C. Headache, confusion
  D. Weakness
  E. Edema
  F. Lethargy
  G. Muscle twitching, seizures
  H. Decreased hematocrit, serum osmolality, serum sodium
III. Nursing diagnoses
  A. Fluid Volume Excess related to decreased fluid elimination, excessive fluid intake or replacement
  B. Impaired Gas Exchange related to intraalveolar fluid
  C. Decreased Adaptive Capacity: Intracranial related to cerebral edema, seizures
IV. Collaborative management
  A. Monitor urine output, I & O, daily weight, laboratory studies
  B. Decrease water and normalize osmolality
    1. Restrict fluids
    2. Administer diuretics as prescribed
    3. Administer hypertonic (3%) saline as prescribed for severe hyponatremia
      a) Usually 250-500 ml administered over several hours at rate of 1-2 ml/kg/hr for serum sodium less than 115 mEq/L or if patient is having seizures
      b) Monitor closely for clinical indications of

fluid overload since it pulls fluid into the vascular space

    4. Initiate CRRT as prescribed

    5. Administer demeclocycline or lithium as prescribed for nephrogenic SIADH

C. Provide frequent oral and skin care

D. Monitor for clinical indications of cerebral edema: institute seizure precautions

E. Monitor for clinical indications of pulmonary edema

Hyponatremia: Sodium less than 136 mEq/L with normal serum osmolality

I. Etiology: both sodium and water decreased
    A. Decreased sodium intake
        1. Sodium-restricted diet
        2. Alcoholism
    B. Increased sodium excretion
        1. Skin losses
            a) Diaphoresis
            b) Burns
        2. GI losses
            a) GI suctioning
            b) Vomiting
            c) Diarrhea
            d) Draining wound or fistula
            e) Laxative abuse
        3. Renal losses
            a) Diuretics: thiazide, loop
            b) Adrenal insufficiency
II. Clinical presentation
    A. Tachycardia
    B. Postural hypotension
    C. Anorexia, nausea, vomiting, abdominal cramps
    D. Diarrhea
    E. Weight loss
    F. Decreased skin turgor
    G. "Fingerprinting" over sternum
    H. Apprehension
    I. Headache
    J. Weakness, fatigue
    K. Personality changes
    L. Lethargy progressing to coma
    M. Mental confusion, disorientation
    N. Muscle cramps, muscle twitching, increased deep tendon reflexes (DTR)
    O. Tremors, seizures
    P. Oliguria
III. Nursing diagnoses
    A. Fluid Volume Deficit related to excessive fluid and sodium losses, inadequate intake or replacement
    B. Decreased Cardiac Output related to decreased preload
IV. Collaborative management
    A. Monitor urine output, I & O, daily weight, laboratory studies
    B. Restore normal serum electrolyte levels
        1. Encourage sodium in diet in mild deficiency

    2. Administer sodium parenterally for moderate or severe deficiency
        a) Normal saline as prescribed
        b) Hypertonic (3%) saline as prescribed for severe hyponatremia
            (1) Usually 250-500 ml administered over several hours at rate of 1-2 ml/kg/hr for serum sodium; less than 115 mEq/L or if patient is having seizures
            (2) Monitor closely for clinical indications of fluid overload since it pulls fluid into the vascular space
    3. Potassium replacement may also be needed
C. Monitor for neurologic changes; institute seizure precautions
D. Provide frequent oral and skin care

Hypernatremia: Sodium more than 145 mEq/L with normal serum osmolality

I. Etiology: both sodium and water are increased
    A. Excessive salt (sodium chloride) consumption
    B. Excessive administration of normal saline or hypertonic saline solution
    C. Administration of sodium-containing drugs (e.g., sodium bicarbonate, sodium polystyrene sulfonate [Kayexalate])
    D. Heart failure
    E. Renal failure
    F. Cirrhosis
    G. Steroid therapy
    H. Cushing's syndrome
    I. Primary hyperaldosteronism
    J. Salt water near-drowning, ingestion of salt water
II. Clinical presentation
    A. Tachycardia
    B. Hypertension
    C. Weight gain
    D. Edema
    E. Thirst
    F. Low-grade fever
    G. Dry, sticky tongue and mucous membranes
    H. Flushed, dry skin
    I. Muscle rigidity and weakness
    J. CNS irritability: restlessness, agitation
    K. Mental confusion, disorientation
    L. Muscle cramps, muscle twitching, increased deep tendon reflexes (DTR)
    M. Tremors, seizures
    N. Oliguria
III. Nursing diagnoses
    A. Risk for Fluid Volume Excess related to decreased fluid elimination, excessive fluid intake or replacement
    B. Risk for Injury related to potential seizures
IV. Collaborative management
    A. Monitor urine output, I & O, daily weight, laboratory studies
    B. Treat the cause

C. Restore normal serum electrolyte levels
  1. Restrict sodium
  2. Administer diuretics as prescribed
D. Provide frequent oral and skin care
E. Monitor for change in neurologic status; institute seizure precautions

Hypokalemia: Potassium less than 3.5 mEq/L

I. Etiology
  A. Poor potassium intake
    1. Starvation
    2. Alcoholism
    3. Administration of potassium-deficient parenteral fluids or nutrition
    4. Use of low potassium dialysate
  B. Increased GI losses
    1. GI surgery
    2. Gastric or intestinal suction
    3. Vomiting
    4. Fistula
    5. Diarrhea
    6. Chronic malabsorption syndrome
    7. Laxative abuse
  C. Increased renal losses
    1. Diuretics: thiazide, loop
    2. Polyuria
    3. Renal tubular acidosis
    4. Sodium restriction
    5. Hypomagnesemia
    6. Hyperaldosteronism; licorice excess (increases aldosterone effect)
    7. Heart failure
    8. Steroid therapy or Cushing's syndrome
    9. Cirrhosis
    10. Stress via renin-angiotensin-aldosterone system and release of corticosteroids
    11. Burns (as fluid shifts back into intravascular space 48 to 72 hours after fluid resuscitation)
  D. Skin losses: diaphoresis
  E. Extracellular to intracellular shift
    1. Alkalosis
    2. Insulin
    3. Treatment of diabetic ketoacidosis
II. Clinical presentation
  A. Orthostatic hypotension
  B. Anorexia, nausea, vomiting
  C. Decreased GI motility and bowel sounds, paralytic ileus, constipation, abdominal distention
  D. Malaise, fatigue
  E. Muscle cramps, muscle weakness, possibly flaccid paralysis
  F. Decreased DTR
  G. Dizziness
  H. Apathy, mental confusion, drowsiness to coma
  I. Respiratory muscle weakness causing shallow respirations, dyspnea progressing to respiratory paralysis and respiratory arrest
  J. Polyuria, polydipsia
  K. Enhanced digitalis effect

  L. ECG changes
    1. Flat T-waves and prominent U-waves
    2. Depressed ST segment
    3. Prolonged QT and PR intervals
    4. Dysrhythmias (e.g., PVCs, ventricular tachycardia, ventricular fibrillation)
  M. Cardiac arrest
III. Nursing diagnoses
  A. Decreased Cardiac Output related to dysrhythmias
  B. Ineffective Breathing Pattern related to respiratory muscle weakness
  C. Constipation related to decreased GI motility
IV. Collaborative management
  A. Monitor urine output, I & O, daily weight, laboratory studies
  B. Treat the cause
  C. Restore normal serum electrolyte levels
    1. Increase dietary potassium for mild hyperkalemia; encourage use of potassium chloride salt substitute
    2. Administer potassium supplements orally as prescribed
    3. Administer potassium parenterally as prescribed for severe hypokalemia
      a) Add potassium to IV solution
      b) Administer potassium "runs" IV usually via minibag (usual safe maximum 10 mEq/100 ml over 1 hour but may be administered at 20 mEq/hr if serum potassium is less than 2.5 mEq/L)
        (1) Administer at no greater concentration than 10 mEq/100 ml if given via peripheral catheter or 20 mEq/100 ml if given via a central venous catheter
        (2) **Note:** It takes 100 to 200 mEq of potassium to increase serum potassium by 1 mEq/L
    4. Correct alkalosis
    5. Correct hypomagnesemia and/or hypocalcemia; hypokalemia that is refractory to treatment is often accompanied by hypomagnesemia and/or hypocalcemia
  D. Monitor for clinical indications of digitalis toxicity if patient receiving digitalis preparation
  E. Teach patient about adequate potassium replacement if receiving diuretics; potassium-sparing diuretics may be used

Hyperkalemia: Potassium more than 5.0 mEq/L

I. Etiology
  A. Increased potassium intake
    1. Excessive administration/ingestion of potassium: oral or parenteral
    2. Excessive or too rapid potassium replacement
    3. Excessive use of KCl salt substitute
    4. Transfusion of banked blood; the longer the blood has been stored, the higher the extracellular potassium content

B. Decreased potassium excretion
1. Acute and chronic renal disease
2. Adrenal insufficiency (Addison's disease)
3. Potassium-sparing diuretics
4. Angiotensin-converting enzyme (ACE) inhibitors
C. Cellular disruption with leak of intracellular potassium
1. Crush injuries
2. Rhabdomyolysis
3. Hemolysis (e.g., blood transfusion reaction, fresh water near-drowning)
4. Early burns
5. Trauma
6. Catabolism
7. Lysis of tumor cells from chemotherapy
D. Intracellular to extracellular shift
1. Acidosis
2. Hypertonic glucose with insulin deficiency
3. Massive digitalis overdosage
4. Muscle-paralyzing agents (e.g., succinylcholine)

II. Clinical presentation
A. Initially tachycardia progressing to bradycardia and cardiac arrest
B. Decreased contractility, decreased cardiac output, hypotension
C. Nausea, vomiting, intestinal colic, diarrhea
D. Muscle weakness progressing to flaccid paralysis
E. Numbness, paresthesia of extremities
F. Respiratory muscle weakness may cause hypopnea, dyspnea, respiratory distress
G. Increased deep tendon reflexes
H. Fatigue, lethargy, apathy, mental confusion
I. Oliguria
J. ECG changes
1. Tall, narrow, peaked T-waves
2. Wide QRS complex
3. Prolonged PR interval
4. Flattened to absent P-wave
5. Dysrhythmias (e.g., bradycardia, idioventricular rhythm, asystole)

III. Nursing diagnoses
A. Decreased Cardiac Output related to decreased contractility, dysrhythmias
B. Ineffective Breathing Pattern related to respiratory muscle weakness
C. Diarrhea related to increased GI motility

IV. Collaborative management
A. Monitor urine output, I & O, daily weight, laboratory studies
B. Treat the cause
C. Restore normal serum electrolyte levels
1. Limit potassium intake
a) Make sure that IV solution or TPN do not contain potassium
b) Check medications for potassium content
2. Check BUN, creatinine levels for data about renal function
3. If potassium more than 6.5 or dysrhythmias present: administer dextrose and insulin as prescribed; this treatment moves potassium

back into the cell and the effect lasts about 4 to 6 hours; sodium polystyrene sulfonate (Kayexalate) should be given during this time
a) Usual dosage is 50 ml of 50% dextrose and 10 U insulin
b) Patients with chronic renal failure may tolerate high levels of potassium and not be symptomatic until 7.0 mEq/L or greater
4. Administer sodium polystyrene sulfonate (Kayexalate), an exchange resin, orally or by retention enema; this drug exchanges sodium for potassium and moves potassium out of the body via the GI tract
a) Usual dosage is 30 g in 50 ml of 20% sorbitol orally or 50 g in 200 ml of dextrose as retention enema (**Note:** Sorbitol, an osmotic laxative, produces a cathartic effect only when given orally and may contribute to intestinal necrosis when given by enema)
5. Administer bicarbonate as prescribed to correct acidosis; this effect lasts 1 to 2 hours; monitor for hypernatremia and hyperosmolality
6. Initiate dialysis if due to renal failure
D. Monitor for and prevent cardiac effects of hyperkalemia
1. Administer calcium IV (usually 10 ml of 10% calcium gluconate) as prescribed for serum potassium levels of more than 6.5 mEq/L to block the neuromuscular and cardiac effects; contraindicated if patient is receiving digitalis

Hypocalcemia: Calcium less than 8.5 mg/dl (<4.5 mEq/L)

I. Etiology
A. Decreased calcium intake or absorption
1. Chronic insufficient dietary calcium intake
2. Hypoparathyroidism
3. Hypomagnesemia
4. Acute and chronic renal failure
5. Vitamin D deficiency or resistance
6. Liver disease
7. Postgastrectomy
8. Chronic malabsorption syndrome
9. Alcoholism
10. Cushing's syndrome
11. Steroid therapy
B. Increased calcium excretion
1. Diuretic therapy: loop, osmotic, potassium-sparing, carbonic anhydrase inhibitors
2. Chronic diarrhea
3. Hyperphosphatemia
4. Diuretic phase of acute renal failure
C. Increased calcium binding, decreased ionized calcium
1. Citrated blood administration
2. Alkalosis
3. Acute pancreatitis
4. Drugs (e.g., aminoglycosides, cimetidine, heparin, theophylline)

II. Clinical presentation
   A. Abdominal cramps, biliary colic
   B. Paresthesia of fingertips, circumoral area
   C. Chvostek's sign: facial twitching in response to tapping on the facial nerve
   D. Trousseau's sign: carpal spasm after 3 minutes of inflation of a blood pressure cuff to a level above systolic pressure
   E. Muscle cramps, tremors
   F. Increased deep tendon reflexes (DTRs), carpopedal spasm
   G. Irritability, confusion, psychosis
   H. Memory loss
   I. Laryngospasm, stridor
   J. Tetany (characterized by cramps, twitching of the muscles, sharp flexion of the wrist and ankle joints, seizures)
   K. Seizures
   L. Hyperphosphatemia
   M. Decreased contractility, cardiac output
   N. Oliguria, anuria if renal calculi obstructive
   O. Bruising, bleeding
   P. ECG changes
      1. Prolonged QT interval
      2. Dysrhythmias (e.g., torsades de pointes)

III. Nursing diagnoses
   A. Potential Ineffective Breathing Patterns related to laryngospasm
   B. Potential for Decreased Cardiac Output related to altered conductivity, contractility
   C. Risk for Injury related to seizures

IV. Collaborative management
   A. Monitor airway patency and ventilation: cricothyroidotomy may be necessary for severe laryngospasm
   B. Monitor urine output, I & O, daily weight, laboratory studies
   C. Treat the cause
   D. Restore normal serum electrolyte levels
      1. Encourage a high-calcium, low-phosphorus diet
      2. Administer oral calcium with vitamin D supplements as prescribed for mild hypocalcemia
      3. Administer calcium gluconate or calcium chloride IV as prescribed
         a) Administer slowly: 10 ml of calcium gluconate contains 4.5 mEq of calcium, whereas 10 ml of calcium chloride contains 13.6 mEq of calcium; administer both no more rapidly than 1 ml/min
         b) Administer through central venous catheter if possible; if administered through a peripheral catheter, prevent extravasation, which may cause necrosis and sloughing
      4. Administer phosphate-binding antacids as prescribed for hyperphosphatemia
      5. Administer magnesium as prescribed (hypocalcemia unresponsive to treatment may indicate concurrent hypomagnesemia)
   E. Monitor for and prevent neurologic complications; institute seizure precautions

Hypercalcemia: Calcium more than 10.5 mg/dl (>5.8 mEq/L)

I. Etiology
   A. Increased calcium intake
      1. Excessive intake of calcium supplements or calcium antacids
      2. Milk-alkali syndrome related to milk and antacid intake
   B. Increased calcium absorption: hypophosphatemia
   C. Increased mobilization of calcium from bone
      1. Hyperparathyroidism
      2. Vitamin D excess
      3. Immobility
      4. Osteolytic lesions
      5. Malignancy, especially breast, lung, lymphoma, multiple myeloma
      6. Paget's disease
      7. Granulomatous disease (e.g., sarcoidosis, TB, histoplasmosis)
      8. Thyrotoxicosis
   D. Decreased calcium excretion
      1. Thiazide diuretics
      2. Adrenal insufficiency (Addison's disease)
      3. Renal tubular acidosis
      4. Hyperparathyroidism
      5. Oliguric phase of acute renal failure
   E. Increased ionized calcium: acidosis

II. Clinical presentation
   A. Anorexia, nausea, vomiting, abdominal pain, decreased bowel sounds, constipation, paralytic ileus
   B. Bone and/or flank pain; pathologic fractures may occur
   C. Malaise, fatigue
   D. Neuromuscular weakness to flaccidity; decreased deep tendon reflexes (DTR)
   E. Confusion
   F. Depression, lethargy, stupor, coma
   G. Subtle personality changes progressing to psychosis
   H. Renal calculi
   I. Polyuria, polydipsia
   J. Azotemia
   K. Hypophosphatemia
   L. Enhanced digitalis effect
   M. Dysrhythmias and/or blocks
   N. ECG change: shortened QT interval
   O. X-ray: osteoporosis

III. Nursing diagnoses
   A. Decreased Cardiac Output related to dysrhythmias
   B. Risk for Injury related to neurosensory changes
   C. Altered Urinary Elimination related to renal calculi
   D. Constipation related to decreased bowel motility

IV. Collaborative management
   A. Monitor urine output, I & O, daily weight, laboratory studies
   B. Treat the cause (e.g., discontinuance of thiazide

diuretics, surgery, radiation, antineoplastics for malignancy, partial parathyroidectomy for hyperparathyroidism)
- C. Restore normal serum electrolyte levels
  1. Decrease calcium absorption
     a) Low-calcium, high-phosphorus diet
     b) Corticosteroids
  2. Increase calcium excretion
     a) Oral fluids, parenteral NS as prescribed
     b) Any of the following as prescribed:
        (1) Loop diuretics (e.g., furosemide [Lasix])
        (2) Phosphorus
        (3) Corticosteroids
        (4) Calcitonin
        (5) EDTA (disodium salt)
  3. Decrease bone resorption of calcium
     a) Weight-bearing activities
     b) Any of the following as prescribed:
        (1) Pamidronate (Aredia)
        (2) Plicamycin (formerly known as *mithramycin*) (Mithracin)
        (3) Gallium nitrate
        (4) Calcitonin
- D. Monitor for and prevent cardiac effects of hypercalcemia: calcium channel blockers as prescribed
- E. Prevent renal calculi while correcting hypercalcemia: agents to acidification urine may be used because acidification of urine increases solubility of calcium
- F. Monitor for clinical indications of digitalis toxicity

Hypophosphatemia: Phosphorus less than 3.0 mg/dl
- I. Etiology
  - A. Inadequate intake of phosphorus
    1. Malnutrition
    2. Alcoholism
    3. Severe, prolonged vomiting
    4. Prolonged low-phosphorus or phosphate-free IV therapy or total parenteral nutrition therapy
  - B. Decreased GI absorption or increased intestinal loss
    1. Excessive use of phosphate-binding gels such as aluminum hydroxide (Amphojel)
    2. Prolonged vomiting, gastric suction, sucralfate (Carafate)
    3. Chronic diarrhea
    4. Chronic malabsorption syndrome
    5. Vitamin D deficiency
  - C. Increased renal excretion of phosphorus
    1. Thiazide diuretics
    2. Hypomagnesemia
    3. Hypokalemia
    4. Hyperglycemia
    5. Hyperparathyroidism
    6. Fanconi's syndrome

- D. Extracellular to intracellular shifts
  1. Parenteral glucose or insulin administration
  2. Respiratory alkalosis
  3. Large amounts of carbohydrate (refeeding syndrome)
  4. Diabetic ketoacidosis (with treatment)
- II. Clinical presentation
  - A. Tachycardia, hypotension
  - B. Anorexia, nausea, vomiting
  - C. Malaise, fatigue
  - D. Paresthesia, tremors
  - E. Nystagmus, anisocoria
  - F. Uncoordination, ataxia
  - G. Mental confusion, lethargy, coma
  - H. Seizures
  - I. Memory loss
  - J. Muscle weakness, especially respiratory muscles
  - K. Bone pain
  - L. Chest pain
  - M. Hypercalcemia
  - N. Heart failure: dyspnea, crackles
  - O. Weight loss
  - P. Hemolytic anemia
  - Q. Indications of platelet dysfunction (e.g., petechiae)
  - R. Dysrhythmias
  - S. X-ray: skeletal abnormalities
- III. Nursing diagnoses
  - A. Potential Ineffective Breathing Patterns related to laryngospasm
  - B. Potential for Decreased Cardiac Output related to altered conductivity, contractility
  - C. Ineffective Breathing Patterns related to decreased respiratory muscle strength
  - D. Impaired Gas Exchange related to decreased 2,3-DPG levels
  - E. Risk for Injury related to seizures
- IV. Collaborative Management
  - A. Monitor urine output, I & O, daily weight, laboratory studies
  - B. Treat the cause (e.g., discontinuance of phosphate-binding gels, correction of hypercalcemia if cause of hypophosphatemia)
  - C. Restore normal serum electrolyte levels
    1. High-phosphorus, low-calcium diet
    2. Oral phosphate supplements (e.g., Neutra-Phos [sodium and potassium phosphate], Phospho-Soda [sodium phosphate], K-Phos (potassium phosphate) as ordered and monitor for signs of hypocalcemia when giving supplements
    3. Parenteral sodium phosphate or potassium phosphate IV as ordered and monitor for signs of hypocalcemia
       a) If phosphate less than 1 mg/dl without adverse effects: usual dose is 0.6 mg/kg/hr
       b) If phosphate less than 2 mg/dl with adverse effects: usual dose is 0.9 mg/kg/hr

c) Infuse through central venous catheter if possible
D. Monitor for cardiovascular, pulmonary, neurologic effects of hypophosphatemia

Hyperphosphatemia: Phosphate more than 4.5 mg/dl

I. Etiology
A. Increased phosphorus intake
1. Cathartic abuse with phosphate-containing laxatives and enemas
2. Excessive vitamin D
B. Decreased phosphorus excretion
1. Acute or chronic renal failure
2. Hypoparathyroidism
3. Extracellular shifts
4. Diabetic ketoacidosis (before treatment)
5. Respiratory acidosis
C. Cellular destruction
1. Neoplastic disease treated with chemotherapy
2. Catabolism
3. Rhabdomyolysis
II. Clinical presentation: same as hypocalcemia
III. Nursing diagnosis
A. Potential Ineffective Breathing Patterns related to laryngospasm
B. Potential for Decreased Cardiac Output related to altered conductivity, contractility
C. Risk for Injury related to seizures
IV. Collaborative management
A. Monitor airway patency; cricothyroidotomy may be necessary for severe laryngospasm
B. Monitor urine output, I & O, daily weight, laboratory studies
C. Treat the cause (e.g., correct hypocalcemia)
D. Restore normal serum electrolyte levels
1. Low-phosphorus, high-calcium diet
2. Sucralfate (Carafate) or aluminum antacids to bind with phosphate in the GI tract as prescribed
3. Dialysis if renal failure is cause
E. Monitor for and prevent neurologic complications; institute seizure precautions

Hypomagnesemia: Magnesium less than 1.5 mEq/L

I. Etiology
A. Decreased magnesium intake or absorption
1. Protein-calorie malnutrition
2. Starvation
3. Alcoholism
4. Prolonged low-magnesium or magnesium-free IV therapy or total parenteral nutrition therapy
B. Impaired absorption
1. Alcoholism
2. Intestinal malabsorption syndrome
3. Acute pancreatitis
C. Increased magnesium loss
1. Diuretics
2. Alcoholism
3. Diuretic phase of acute renal failure
4. Vomiting, gastric suction, fistula
5. Chronic diarrhea (e.g., ulcerative colitis; laxative abuse)
6. Hyperparathyroidism
7. Hyperaldosteronism
8. Steroids
9. Diabetic ketoacidosis
10. Heart failure
D. Increased magnesium binding: citrated blood administration
E. Extracellular to intracellular shift
1. Concentrated glucose solutions
2. Amino acid solutions
3. Insulin
4. Acute myocardial infarction
II. Clinical presentation
A. Tachycardia, hypotension
B. Anorexia, nausea, vomiting, abdominal distention
C. Paresthesia of fingertips, circumoral area
D. Chvostek's and Trousseau's signs
E. Muscle cramps, tremors
F. Increased DTRs, carpopedal spasm
G. Confusion, psychosis
H. Memory loss
I. Laryngospasm, stridor
J. Tetany
K. Seizures
L. Concurrent hypocalcemia, hypokalemia
M. Decreased contractility, cardiac output
N. Increased digitalis effect
O. ECG changes
1. Prolonged QT interval
2. Dysrhythmias, especially torsades de pointes
III. Nursing diagnoses
A. Potential Ineffective Breathing Patterns related to laryngospasm
B. Potential for Decreased Cardiac Output related to altered conductivity, contractility
C. Risk for Injury related to seizures
IV. Collaborative Management
A. Monitor airway patency; cricothyroidotomy may be necessary for severe laryngospasm
B. Monitor urine output, I & O, daily weight, laboratory studies
C. Treat the cause (e.g., improve nutrition, use potassium-sparing diuretics if diuretics are needed because they spare magnesium)
D. Restore normal serum electrolyte levels
1. High-magnesium diet
2. Oral magnesium supplements in the form of magnesium antacids as prescribed
3. Magnesium sulfate IV as prescribed
a) Usually administered in 1 to 2 g in 100 ml over 1 to 2 hours
b) May be diluted in 10 ml and given over 1 to 2 minutes when life-threatening dysrhythmias (e.g., torsades de pointes) occur

    c) Monitor calcium levels during magnesium replacement; increase dietary calcium or administer IV calcium as prescribed

  E. Monitor for and prevent neurologic complications; institute seizure precautions

  F. Monitor for clinical indications of digitalis toxicity

Hypermagnesemia: Magnesium more than 2.5 mEq/L

I. Etiology
- A. Increased magnesium intake
  1. Magnesium antacids
  2. Magnesium sulfate IV
  3. Magnesium-containing laxatives, enemas
- B. Decreased magnesium excretion
  1. Acute/chronic renal failure
  2. Hypoparathyroidism
  3. Hypoaldosteronism
  4. Hypothyroidism
- C. Intracellular to extracellular shift
  1. Untreated ketoacidosis
  2. Burns
  3. Rhabdomyolysis

II. Clinical presentation
- A. Bradycardia, hypotension
- B. Facial flushing
- C. Muscle weakness progressing to paralysis
- D. Decreased DTRs: loss of patellar reflex occurs at levels greater than 8 mEq/L
- E. Respiratory muscle weakness may cause hypoventilation and dyspnea
- F. Respiratory muscle paralysis and apnea may occur with levels greater than 10 mEq/L
- G. Confusion, lethargy, coma
- H. Cardiopulmonary arrest

III. Nursing diagnoses
- A. Potential Ineffective Breathing Patterns related to respiratory muscle weakness
- B. Potential for Decreased Cardiac Output related to altered conductivity, contractility
- C. Risk for Injury related to seizures

IV. Collaborative management
- A. Monitor and maintain airway and ventilation; intubation and mechanical ventilation may be necessary
- B. Monitor urine output, I & O, daily weight, laboratory studies
- C. Treat the cause
- D. Restore normal serum electrolyte levels
  1. Low-magnesium diet
  2. Discontinuance of magnesium-containing antacids or laxatives, IV magnesium
  3. NS or ½NS and diuretics as prescribed if normal renal function
  4. Dialysis if renal failure is cause of hypermagnesemia
- E. Monitor for and prevent neuromuscular, pulmonary, cardiovascular complications
  1. Parenteral calcium as prescribed

Acute Renal Failure

Definition: Any sudden severe impairment or cessation of kidney function; characterized by accumulation of nitrogenous wastes and fluid and electrolyte imbalances

Etiology and Pathophysiology (Fig. 9-9 and Table 9-4)

Clinical Presentation

I. Subjective
- A. Flank pain may be present
- B. Uremic syndrome
  1. Irritability
  2. Insomnia
  3. Inability to concentrate
  4. Anorexia, nausea, vomiting
  5. Metallic taste
  6. Fatigue, weakness
  7. Anxiety
- C. Dyspnea if pulmonary edema is present
- D. Headache
- E. Pruritus
- F. Decreased libido
- G. Weight loss or weight gain

II. Objective
- A. Genitourinary
  1. Decrease in urine volume
     a) Nonoliguria: dilute urine output more than 400 ml/24 hr
     b) Oliguria: urine output less than 400 ml/24 hr
     c) Anuria: urine output less than 100 ml/24 hr
        (1) Rare but may be seen in complete obstruction (postrenal)
  2. Altered excretion of drugs; toxic drug levels
  3. Bladder distention may be noted with postrenal failure
- B. Neurologic
  1. Change in behavior
  2. Confusion
  3. Change in level of consciousness
  4. Tremors, twitching
  5. Asterixis
  6. Seizures
- C. Gastrointestinal
  1. Bleeding gums
  2. Uremic breath
  3. Abdominal distention
  4. GI bleeding, melena
  5. Constipation or diarrhea
  6. May have paralytic ileus
- D. Respiratory
  1. Deep, rapid breathing (Kussmaul's)
  2. Pulmonary edema
     a) Bilateral crackles
  3. Hemoptysis may be seen along with acute renal failure in Goodpasture's syndrome
- E. Cardiovascular

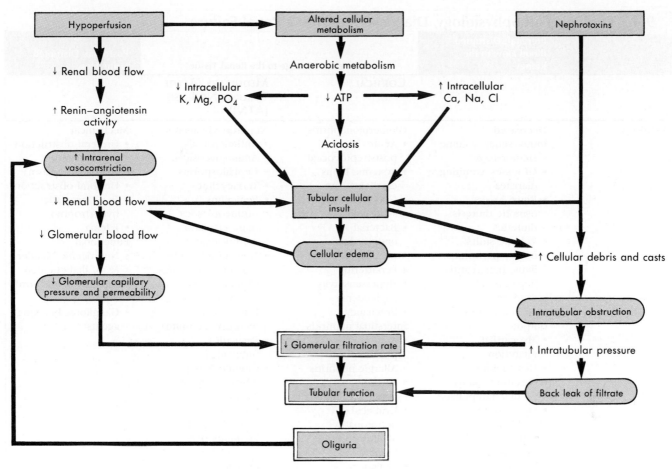

Figure 9-9 Pathophysiology of acute renal failure. (From Kinney MR, Packa DR, Dunbar SB: *AACN's clinical reference for critical-care nursing,* ed 4, St Louis, 1998, Mosby.)

1. Tachycardia
2. Dysrhythmias
3. Uremic pericarditis
   a) Pericardial friction rub
4. Hypertension
5. Vascular access
   a) Bruit
   b) Thrill
   c) Color of blood in tubing if visible (e.g., shunt)
   d) Neurovascular assessment of limb
F. Musculoskeletal
   1. Impaired mobility
   2. Muscle weakness
G. Integument
   1. Dry skin
   2. Pruritus
   3. Edema
   4. Bruising
   5. Pallor
   6. Uremic frost (end-stage)
H. Hematologic/Immunologic
   1. Increased susceptibility to infection
   2. Bleeding tendency
III. Diagnostic
   A. Serum
      1. Elevated BUN, creatinine
      2. Hyperkalemia

3. Hyperphosphatemia
4. Hypocalcemia
5. Hypermagnesemia
6. Sodium level is dependent on water balance; normal or dilutional hyponatremia
7. Arterial blood gases: metabolic acidosis with increased anion gap
8. Hematocrit, hemoglobin usually decreased; may be increased in prerenal failure caused by dehydration
9. Platelets: decreased
10. Clotting Profile: bleeding time may be increased
11. For other specifics, see Table 9-4
B. Urine
   1. Varies dependent on type of acute renal failure (Table 9-4)
   2. Decreased creatinine clearance
C. Radiologic
   1. KUB, IVP may indicate cause of postrenal failure
   2. Chest X-ray may show:
      a) Pericardial effusion
      b) Pleural effusion
      c) Pulmonary edema
D. Renal biopsy: most definitive diagnostic test, especially for glomerulonephritis
IV. Stages of acute renal failure (Table 9-5)

Table 9-4	Etiology, Pathophysiology, Diagnostics of Acute Renal Failure			
	Prerenal: Disrupted Blood Flow to the Kidney	**Intrarenal: Damage to the Renal Tissue**		**Postrenal: Disrupted Urine Flow**
		CORTICAL	**MEDULLARY (ACUTE TUBULAR NECROSIS [ATN])**	
Etiology	Decreased intravascular volume • Hemorrhage • GI losses: vomiting; diarrhea • Renal losses: osmotic diuresis, diuretics • Volume shifts: burns, peritonitis, ileus, pancreatitis, hepatorenal syndrome Decreased cardiac output • Myocardial infarction • Heart failure • Cardiomyopathy • Cardiac tamponade • Dysrhythmias Vasodilation • Sepsis • Anaphylaxis • Vasodilators Renovascular disease • Renovascular obstruction	Glomerulonephritis • Acute poststreptococcal • Systemic lupus erythematosus • Goodpasture's syndrome • Bacterial endocarditis Vasculitis • Periarteritis • Hypersensitivity angioedema • Pregnancy Interstitial nephritis • Acute pyelonephritis • Allergic nephritis • Severe hypercalcemia • Uric acid nephropathy • Myeloma of the kidney • Malignant hypertension	Nephrotoxic agents • Antimicrobials • Aminoglycosides • Cephalosporins • Tetracyclines • Penicillins • Antineoplastics (e.g., cisplatin, methotrexate) • Nonsteroidal anti-inflammatory drugs • Contrast dyes • Heavy metals (e.g., lead, arsenic, mercury, uranium) • Pesticides, fungicides • Chemicals (e.g., ethylene glycol, carbon tetrachloride) • Multiple myeloma • Pigments (e.g., hemoglobin, myoglobin) Prolonged ischemic injury • MAP <60 mm Hg for 40 minutes or more • Aortic cross-clamping • Bilateral emboli to both kidneys causing renal infarction • Vasoconstriction • Vasopressors (e.g., norepinephrine [Levophed], high-dose dopamine) Any cause of pre-renal failure that is prolonged	Mechanical • Ureteral obstruction (e.g., strictures, calculi, neoplasm) • Urethral obstruction (e.g., prostatic hypertrophy) • Edema Functional • Neurogenic bladder (e.g., diabetic neu-ropathy, spinal cord injury) • Ganglionic-blocking agents
Pathophysiology	• Decreased pressure to renal artery • Decreased afferent arterial pressure • Diminished glomer-ular filtration rate • Oliguria • Usually reversible if nephrons are intact	• Renal capillary swelling • Cellular proliferation • Obstruction of glo-merulus or tubular structures by edema or cellular debris • Oliguria	• Prolonged ischemia destroys tubular basement membrane • Nephrotoxic injury affects epithelial cellular layer	• Obstruction to urinary flow at or below the collect-ing ducts • Backpressure causes increased renal in-terstitial pressure • Decreased GFR • Oliguria

Table 9-4 | Etiology, Pathophysiology, Diagnostics of Acute Renal Failure—cont'd

	Prerenal: Disrupted Blood Flow to the Kidney	Intrarenal: Damage to the Renal Tissue		Postrenal: Disrupted Urine Flow
		Cortical	Medullary	
Diagnostics	• Oliguria • Urinary sodium <20 mEq/L • Increased BUN with BUN:creatinine ratio >10:1 (usually 20:1) • Urine specific gravity >1.020 • Urine osmolality increased except with metabolic acidosis or diuretics • Urine pH <6.0 • No protein in urine or only minimal amount of protein in urine • Sediment in urine: hyaline casts, finely granular casts	• Urine output may be normal (nonoliguria), oliguria, or polyuria • Urine sodium <20 mEq/L • BUN:creatinine increased with 10:1 ratio • Urine specific gravity varies • Urine pH >6.0 • Moderate to heavy proteinuria • Sediment in urine: RBCs, WBCs, casts	• Urine output may be normal (nonoliguria), oliguria, or polyuria • Urine sodium >20 mEq/L • Urine specific gravity 1.010 • BUN:creatinine elevated with 10:1 ratio • Urine pH >6.0 • Minimal to moderate proteinuria • Sediment in urine: tubular epithelial cells, tubular casts, rare RBC	• Oliguria with partial obstruction; anuria with complete obstruction • Urine sodium >20 mEq/L/day • BUN:creatinine elevated with 10:1 ratio • Urine specific gravity 1.010-1.015 • Urine pH >6.0 • Sediment in urine: RBCs, WBCs, calculi, uric acid crystals, hyaline casts • KUB, IVP may show obstruction and/or ureteral dilatation • May have positive culture for bacteria

Table 9-5 | Stages of Acute Renal Failure

	Onset	Oliguric-anuric	Diuretic	Recovery
Definition	Period of time from the precipitating event to the beginning of oliguria or anuria	Period of time when urine output is <400 ml/24 hr	Period of time between urine output is >400 ml/24 hr until laboratory values stabilize	Period of time between when the laboratory values stabilize until they are normal
Duration	Hours to days	1-2 weeks	1-2 weeks	3-12 months
BUN/creatinine	Normal or slight increase	Increased	Begins to decrease	Almost normal
Urine output	Decreased; about 20% of normal	<400 ml/24 hr; about 5% of normal	May exceed 3 L/24 hr; about 150-200% of normal	Back to 100% of normal
Mortality	5%	50%-60%	25%	10%-15%
Other characteristics		• Metabolic acidosis • Water gain with dilutional hyponatremia • Hyperkalemia • Hypocalcemia • Hyperphosphatemia • Hypermagnesemia • Azotemia	• Metabolic acidosis • Sodium may be normal or decreased • Hyperkalemia continues	• Uremia, acid-base imbalances, and electrolyte imbalances gradually resolve

Note: Some patients (especially when acute renal failure is related to nephrotoxins) go through only three phases: onset, nonoliguric, recovery

Nursing Diagnoses

I. Risk for Fluid Volume Excess related to inability of kidney to eliminate fluid during the oliguric phase

II. Risk for Fluid Volume Deficit related to diuresis during the diuretic phase

III. Altered Renal Tissue Perfusion related to hypovolemia, pump failure, vasodilation

IV. Risk for Injury related to uremia, electrolyte imbalance, metabolic acidosis, diminished drug metabolism and excretion

V. Risk for Infection related to suppressed immune response associated with uremia, malnutrition, invasive devices

VI. Activity Intolerance related to uremia, anemia

VII. Alteration in Nutrition: less than body requirements related to uremia, anorexia, dietary restrictions

VIII. Impairment in Skin Integrity related to pruritus and scratching, needle puncture sites at fistula

IX. Body Image Disturbance related to arteriovenous access, peritoneal access, dependency on life-sustaining technology

X. Anxiety related to change in health status

XI. Knowledge Deficit related to required lifestyle changes

XII. Ineffective Individual Coping related to situational crisis, powerlessness, change in role

XIII. Ineffective Family Coping related to critically ill family member

Collaborative Management

I. Improve renal perfusion
   A. Support renal perfusion and improve glomerular filtration rate
      1. Volume to improve preload in patients with hypovolemia as evidenced by decreased RAP, PAOP
      2. Inotropes to improve contractility in patients with decreased contractility as evidenced by decreased RVSWI, LVSWI
      3. Vasopressors to increase afterload in patients with massive vasodilation as evidenced by decreased SVR
      4. Dopamine may be prescribed at renal doses (e.g., 1-2 µg/kg/min) although it has shown no evidence of benefit when used in patients with acute oliguric renal failure, and it can predispose the patient to bowel ischemia through splanchnic vasoconstriction (no longer recommended for the management of acute oliguric renal failure)
      5. Fenoldopam (Corlopam) may be prescribed to increase renal blood flow
   B. Administer diuretic challenge as prescribed if patient is not anuric (Table 9-6)
      1. Furosemide (Lasix)
      2. Bumetanide (Bumex)
      3. Mannitol (Osmitrol): contraindicated in HF, pulmonary edema

II. Maintain fluid, electrolyte, acid-base balance
   A. Fluid
      1. Monitor for clinical indications of fluid overload
      2. Maintain sodium and water restriction and encourage the patient to remain within prescribed restrictions
         a) Restrict fluid: 24-hour restriction usually determined by adding 500 ml (for insensible loss) to the previous day's urine output

         b) Space fluid allowances over the entire 24-hour period
         c) Treat thirst by offering ice chips (must be included as intake), wet washcloths, misting the mouth, and providing mouth care
         d) Restrict sodium (usually 1-2 g/day)
   B. Potassium
      1. Monitor for clinical indications of hyperkalemia
      2. Maintain potassium restriction (usually 40 mEq/day); do not allow salt substitute (KCl) on dietary trays
   C. Phosphorus
      1. Monitor for clinical indications of hyperphosphatemia
      2. Maintain phosphorus restrictions
      3. Administer phosphate-binding agents (e.g., Basaljel, Amphojel)
         a) These aluminum-containing phosphate-binding agents may contribute to dialysis encephalopathy due to accumulation of aluminum; calcium carbonate (Caltrate) or calcium acetate (PhosLo) may be prescribed instead
   D. Magnesium
      1. Monitor for clinical indications of hypermagnesemia
      2. Maintain dietary magnesium restrictions
      3. Do not administer magnesium-containing medications (e.g., Maalox, magnesium sulfate, magnesium citrate)
   E. Monitor arterial blood gases for acid-base imbalance
      1. Initiate dialysis as prescribed to eliminate nitrogenous wastes and correct metabolic acidosis
      2. Administer sodium bicarbonate or Carbicarb as prescribed
         a) Generally used only for severe metabolic acidosis (pH <7.0)
         b) Monitor for hypernatremia
         c) Monitor for hypocalcemia

III. Diminish the accumulation of nitrogenous wastes
   A. Maintain protein restriction; usually 0.6 g/kg/day initially but may be as high as 1.0 to 1.5 g/kg/day if on hemodialysis and 1.5 to 2 g/kg/day if on peritoneal dialysis
   B. Provide adequate caloric intake to prevent catabolism and utilization of dietary protein for energy needs: usually approximately 35 to 40 kcal/kg/day
   C. Initiate dialysis as indicated and prescribed; indications for dialysis in the patient with acute renal failure generally include the following:
      1. Volume overload (especially with pulmonary edema)
      2. Uncontrollable hyperkalemia
      3. Uncontrollable hyperphosphatemia
      4. Uncontrollable acidosis

Table **9-6** | **Diuretic Summary**

Classification	Examples	Mechanism of Action	Potential Adverse Effects
Thiazide diuretics	• Hydrochlorothiazide (HydroDIURIL)	• Inhibit sodium reabsorption in the ascending loop of Henle and the early distal tubule • Decrease water reabsorption	• Hyponatremia • Hypokalemia • Hypercalcemia • Hypomagnesemia • Hypovolemia • Hyperglycemia • Hyperuricemia • Increased BUN • Hepatitis • Anemia, thrombocytopenia, neutropenia
Loop diuretics	• Furosemide (Lasix) • Ethacrynic acid (Edecrin) • Bumetanide (Bumex)	• Inhibit sodium reabsorption in the ascending loop of Henle • Decrease water reabsorption	• Hyponatremia • Hypokalemia • Hypocalcemia • Hypomagnesemia • Hypochloremic alkalosis • Hypovolemia • Hyperglycemia • Hyperuricemia • Increased BUN • Hearing loss • Thrombocytopenia, agranulocytosis, leukopenia, anemia
Osmotic diuretics	• Mannitol (Osmitrol)	• Expand intravascular volume and increase GFR • Increase osmolality of the tubular fluid, leading to decreased absorption of sodium and water	• Hyponatremia • Hypokalemia • Hypocalcemia • Hypomagnesemia • Initial intravascular hypervolemia followed by hypovolemia • Increased intravascular volume may cause pulmonary edema in patients with poor cardiac function • Hyperglycemia • Hyperuricemia • Increased BUN • Confusion
Potassium-sparing diuretics	• Spironolactone (Aldactone) • Triamterene (Dyrenium) • Amiloride (Midamor)	• Act as an aldosterone-antagonist • Block sodium and potassium exchange mechanism in the distal tubule, causing loss of sodium and water and retention of potassium	• Hyponatremia • Hyperkalemia • Hypocalcemia • Hypomagnesemia • Hypovolemia • Hyperchloremic metabolic acidosis
Carbonic anhydrase inhibitors	• Acetazolamide (Diamox)	• Block the action of carbonic anhydrase in the proximal tubule, preventing bicarbonate and sodium reabsorption • Cause increased water loss and a decrease in serum pH	• Hyponatremia • Hypokalemia • Hypocalcemia • Hypomagnesemia • Hypovolemia • Hyperchloremic metabolic acidosis • Thrombocytopenia, agranulocytosis, leukopenia, anemia

5. Symptomatic uremia (e.g., neurologic changes)
6. Pericarditis
7. Seizures or coma
8. BUN 80 to 100 mg/dl or greater but may be initiated at BUN more than 50 to 60 mg/dl
9. Serum creatinine 10 mg/dl or greater

IV. Prevent further damage to the kidney by nephrotoxic agents
   A. Note that dosages of drugs eliminated by the kidney are decreased and the interval between doses is increased
   B. Monitor peak/trough serum drug levels
   C. Monitor urine creatinine clearance when patient is receiving nephrotoxic agents

V. Provide adequate nutrition while maintaining dietary restrictions
   A. Provide high biologic protein (i.e., proteins containing all essential amino acids) within protein restriction
   B. Provide enough calories to prevent catabolism of somatic protein stores
   C. Increase dietary calcium
   D. Decrease dietary sodium, potassium, phosphorus

VI. Prevent fluid volume deficit during the diuretic phase
   A. Monitor for clinical indication of fluid volume deficit
   B. Volume may be replaced hourly during this phase by replacing the last hour's urine output during the following hour

VII. Prevent infection: initiate dialysis as prescribed when BUN level more than 80 to 100 mg/dl because BUN values above this level are associated with increased risk of infection

VIII. Prevent injury: initiate dialysis as prescribed when BUN level more than 80 to 100 mg/dl because BUN values above this level are associated with neurologic changes

IX. Maintain patency of vascular access (if present)
   A. Palpate shunt, fistula, AV graft for thrill; auscultate for bruit; note any change in bright red color in tubing if shunt; palpate pulses and check capillary refill distal to access
   B. Do not allow venipuncture, IV cannulation, injections, blood pressure measurements in limb with shunt, fistula, AV graft
   C. Monitor for constrictive clothing or dressing in limb with shunt, fistula, AV graft
   D. Monitor for bleeding; use pressure dressing or clamp on tubing if shunt to stop bleeding
   E. Note any redness, induration, or purulent drainage around access; culture any purulent drainage; change dressing as for central venous catheter
   F. Instruct patient not to disturb scabs at puncture sites at fistula, AV graft for hemodialysis

X. Prevent infection and maintain patency of peritoneal access
   A. Note any redness, induration, or purulent drainage around access; culture any purulent drainage
   B. Provide aseptic catheter care
      1. Wash with antibacterial soap
      2. Dress with light gauze dressing
      3. Aseptic catheter manipulation
   C. Culture peritoneal dialysate outflow fluid periodically or as indicated

XI. Promote comfort
   A. Administer antipruritics as prescribed
   B. Utilize emollient or cornstarch baths

XII. Monitor for and treat anemia
   A. Monitor hemoglobin, hematocrit, RBCs
   B. Monitor for bleeding: gums, NG aspirate or vomitus, stools, hematuria
   C. Administer folic acid, iron, vitamin B_{12} as prescribed
   D. Administer packed RBCs as prescribed; blood is usually only prescribed if the patient is symptomatic of anemia (e.g., dyspnea, chest pain, syncope, hypotension)
   E. Administer recombinant erythropoietin (Epogen) as prescribed

XIII. Monitor for complications
   A. Renal: chronic renal failure will develop in 25% to 30% of patients with acute renal failure
   B. Cardiovascular
      1. Dysrhythmias
      2. Hypertension
      3. Pericarditis, cardiac tamponade
      4. Pulmonary edema
   C. Neurologic
      1. Coma
      2. Seizures
   D. Metabolic
      1. Electrolyte imbalances
         a) Hyperkalemia
         b) Hyperphosphatemia
         c) Hypermagnesemia
         d) Hypocalcemia
      2. Acid-base imbalance: metabolic acidosis
   E. Gastrointestinal
      1. Peptic ulcer disease
      2. GI hemorrhage
   F. Hematologic
      1. Anemia
      2. Uremic coagulopathies
   G. Infection
      1. Increased susceptibility to pneumonias
      2. Septicemias
      3. Urinary tract and wound infections
   H. Miscellaneous: drug toxicity

Renal Replacement Therapy
Dialysis

I. Definition: separation of solutes by differential diffusion through a semipermeable membrane that is placed between the two solutions (Fig. 9-10)

II. Purposes
   A. Eliminate excess body fluids
   B. Maintain or restore electrolyte balance
   C. Maintain or restore acid-base balance
   D. Eliminate nitrogenous wastes and toxins from the blood
III. Indications
   A. Acute or chronic renal failure
   B. Severe water intoxication

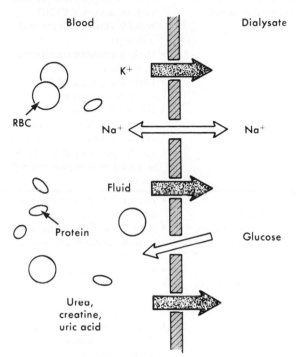

Figure 9-10   Osmosis and diffusion in dialysis. Net movement of major particles and fluid is illustrated. (From Long BC, Phipps WJ, Cassmeyer VL: *Medical-surgical nursing: a nursing process approach,* ed 3, St Louis, 1993, Mosby.)

C. Severe electrolyte imbalance
D. Drug intoxication (drug must be dialyzable [e.g., alcohol, aspirin, barbiturates, some poisons])
E. Hepatic encephalopathy/coma
IV. Components
   A. Dialysate: solution of water, electrolytes (sodium, chloride, magnesium, bicarbonate), nonelectrolytes (glucose), buffer (acetate)
      1. Electrolyte concentration in the dialysate is adjusted to the patient's needs
   B. Semipermeable membrane: peritoneum, extracorpeal membrane
   C. Patient's blood in contact with the membrane
V. Principles (Fig. 9-11)
   A. Osmosis: a hypertonic solution is used as the dialysate to move water across the semipermeable membrane
   B. Diffusion: the dialysate solution contains a concentration of selected solutes lower than the blood so that these solutes will move across the semipermeable membrane and into the dialysate solution
   C. Filtration: in some forms of dialysis, a pressure difference exists between the sides of the semipermeable membrane, with the highest pressure on the forward side of the membrane to act as a hydrostatic force pushing against the membrane to provide a filtration effect
   D. Convection (in continuous renal replacement therapy [CRRT]): the transfer of solutes and solutions simultaneously moving across the semipermeable membrane
VI. Variables affecting efficiency
   A. Size and number of the pores in the semipermeable membrane

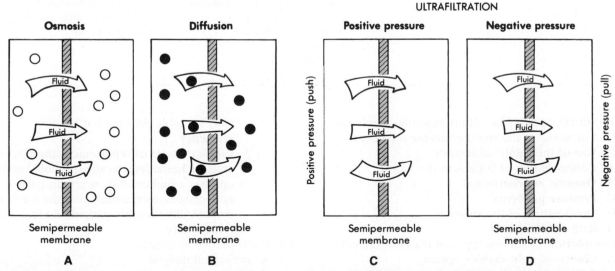

Figure 9-11   Dialysis is based on the following principles. **A,** osmosis. **B,** diffusion and ultrafiltration. Ultrafiltration occurs when either positive pressure **C** or negative pressure **D** is placed on the system. Ultrafiltration is maximized by exerting both positive and negative pressure on the system simultaneously. (From Long BC, Phipps WJ, Cassmeyer VL: *Medical-surgical nursing: a nursing process approach,* ed 3, St Louis, 1993, Mosby.)

<table>
Table 9-7 | Types of Dialysis
</table>

	Hemodialysis	Intermittent Peritoneal Dialysis	Continuous Renal Replacement Therapies (SCUF, CAVH, CAVHD, CVVHD)
Principles	• Osmosis • Diffusion • Filtration	• Osmosis • Diffusion • Filtration	• Osmosis • Diffusion • Filtration • Convection
Treatment requirements	• Membrane: extracorpeal membrane • Blood pump • Dialyzer • Dialysate • Vascular access • Anticoagulation	• Membrane: peritoneum • Dialysate: 1.5%, 2.5%, 4.25% • Access: peritoneal catheter	• Vascular access (SCUF, CAVH, CAVHD require arterial and venous access; CVVHD require venous access and a pump) • High-coefficient membrane hemofilter • Dialysate (usually 1.5% without potassium) • Systolic BP of at least 60 mm Hg; **Note:** continuous venous-venous hemodialysis can be performed if a pump is added to serve as arterial pressure
Specific indications	• Need for rapid treatment • Fluid overload unresponsive to diuretics • Electrolyte imbalance • Acute or chronic renal failure • Drug overdosage or poison intoxication with dialyzable agent • Pulmonary edema refractory to diuretics	• Fluid overload • Electrolyte imbalance • Acute or chronic renal failure • Drug overdosage or poison intoxication with dialyzable agent • Lack of availability of vascular access for hemodialysis • Inability to anticoagulate • Hemodynamic instability	• Fluid overload unresponsive to diuretics • Acute or chronic renal failure in hemodynamically unstable patient • Electrolyte imbalance • Drug overdosage or poison intoxication with dialyzable agent • Inability to tolerate hemodialysis or therapeutic anticoagulation
Contraindications	• Hemodynamic instability • Hypovolemia • Inadequate vascular access • Coagulopathy	• Rapid treatment required • Acute peritonitis • Recent abdominal surgery • Known abdominal adhesions • Abdominal trauma • Intraperitoneal hematoma • Recent vascular anastomosis of abdominal vessels • Respiratory distress • Sepsis • Extreme obesity • Coagulopathy	• Rapid treatment required • Systolic blood pressure <60 mm Hg for CAVH, CAVHD • Lack of arterial access for SCUF, CAVH, CAVHD • Hematocrit >45% • Inability to tolerate high volumes of fluid exchange • Coagulopathy

B. Surface area of the semipermeable membrane
C. Thickness of the semipermeable membrane
D. Size of the solute molecules
E. Concentration of solutes in the blood
F. Osmotic concentration
G. Pressure gradients
H. Temperature of the solution
I. Rate of blood flow
VII. Comparison of various types of dialysis (Table 9-7)
  A. Choice of right dialysis option
    1. Intermittent hemodialysis: therapy of choice for most patients; use is limited when patient is hemodynamically unstable
    2. Peritoneal dialysis: suited for hemodynami-cally unstable patients but has low efficiency
    3. Continuous renal replacement therapy: suitable for hemodynamically unstable patient and has a higher efficiency than peritoneal dialysis; increasingly popular for hemodynamically unstable patients with acute renal failure
VIII. Collaborative management
  A. Peritoneal dialysis
    1. Preparation
      a) Prepare patient for insertion of peritoneal catheter (Fig. 9-12)
        (1) Explain procedure to patient

Table 9-7	Types of Dialysis—cont'd		
	Hemodialysis	**Intermittent Peritoneal Dialysis**	**Continuous Renal Replacement Therapies (SCUF, CAVH, CAVHD, CVVHD)**
Advantages	• Rapid and efficient; only 4-6 hours per session (usually 3 times weekly) • Very efficient, corrects biochemical disturbances quickly	• Equipment is easily and readily assembled • Fairly simple, requiring less staff and patient education • Relatively inexpensive • Minimal danger of acute electrolyte imbalance or hemorrhage • Dialysate can be easily individualized • Anticoagulation not required	• Removes solutes gradually • Decreased risk of hemodynamic instability • Provides flexibility in fluid administration • Requires only minimal heparinization • Relatively inexpensive • Fairly simple, requiring less staff education • Can be used for physiologically unstable patients
Disadvantages	• Complex procedure requiring extensive staff training • Equipment expensive • Machine availability may be limited • Requires anticoagulation • Vascular access necessary	• Relatively slow to alter biochemical imbalances, usually requiring 36 hours for therapeutic effect • May cause protein loss • May be difficult to gain and maintain peritoneal access	• Not very efficient • Patient must be in bed during entire treatment • Requires anticoagulation • Vascular access necessary

Complications	• Access complications: bleeding, clotting, infection
	• Acute fluid and electrolyte imbalances
	• Hemorrhage
	• Hypovolemia
	• Air embolus
	• Disequilibrium syndrome caused by too-rapid removal of waste products
	• Allergic reaction to membrane
	• Hepatitis
	• Dialysis encephalopathy (related to accumulation of aluminum from water used to prepare dialysate)
	• Infection
	• Dysrhythmias
		• Access complications: infection, dialysate leak, bleeding, peritonitis
		• Too-rapid fluid removal causing:
		  • Hypovolemia
		  • Hypernatremia
		• Hypervolemia caused by dialysate retention
		• Hypokalemia caused by potassium-free dialysate usage
		• Alkalosis caused by alkaline dialysate usage
		• Disequilibrium syndrome caused by too rapid removal of waste products
		• Hyperglycemia caused by high glucose concentration of dialysate
		• Protein loss
		• Respiratory distress
			• Access complications: bleeding, clotting, infection
			• Depletion syndrome: loss of vitamins, amino acids, etc.
			• Acid-base imbalances
			• Fluid, electrolyte imbalances, especially fluid volume deficit if volume not adequately replaced
			• Hemorrhage related to:
			  • Anticoagulation
			  • Disruption of filter or tubing
			• Infection
			• Blood clotting in extracorpeal system
			• Loss of vascular access

(2) Ask patient to void or insert urinary catheter prior to abdominal puncture

b) Weigh patient before treatment, weigh patient daily after draining dialysate

2. Procedure (Fig. 9-13)
   a) Warm dialysate to body temperature
   b) Add prescribed medications to dialysate; possible additives include: heparin, potassium chloride, antibiotics, lidocaine
   c) Instill between 1 to 3 L of dialysate (usually 2 L) (inflow phase); this volume is usually infused at a rate of 2 L in 10 to 20 minutes
   d) Allow to dwell in intraperitoneal space for 20 to 30 minutes (**Note:** If first exchange, do not allow dialysate to dwell, drain immediately to ensure catheter patency and placement)
   e) Drain and measure dialysate (outflow phase)
   f) Assess appearance of dialysate
      (1) Normal: clear, pale yellow or straw-colored
      (2) Cloudy: suspect infection; culture and sensitivity is indicated
      (3) Bloody: if occurs after the first four exchanges, suspect intraabdominal bleeding or coagulopathy
      (4) Amber: suspect bladder perforation
      (5) Brownish: suspect bowel perforation

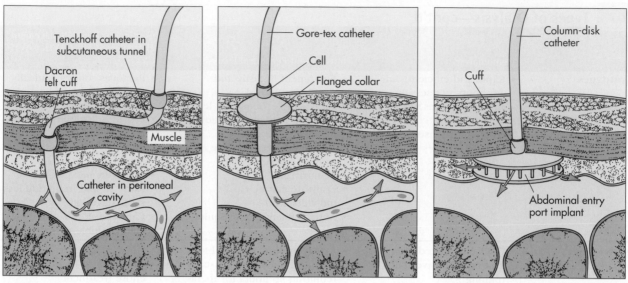

Figure 9-12   Three types of peritoneal dialysis catheters. **A,** Tenckhoff catheter has two Dacron felt cuffs that hold the catheter in place and prevent dialysate leakage and bacterial invasion. Subcutaneous tunnel also helps prevent infection. **B,** Gore-tex catheter with Dacron cuff above flanged collar. **C,** Column-disk catheter has cuff and large abdominal entry port implant. (From Beare P, Myers J: *Adult health nursing,* ed 3, St Louis, 1998, Mosby.)

Figure 9-13   Patient receiving peritoneal dialysis. Dialysate fluid is instilled into the peritoneal cavity, allowed to dwell for a given period of time, and then drained. (From Long BC, Phipps WJ, Cassmeyer VL: *Medical-surgical nursing: a nursing process approach,* ed 3, St Louis, 1993, Mosby.)

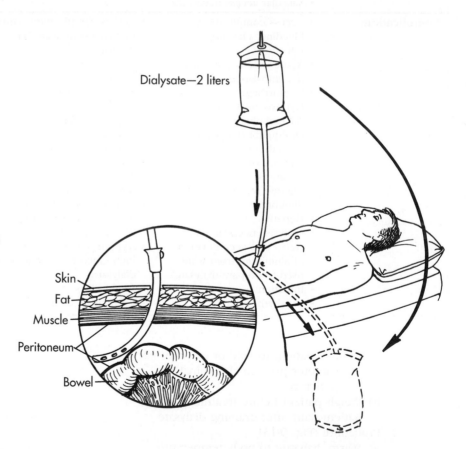

g) If the amount drained is less than the amount instilled, do the following:
   (1) Turn patient side to side
   (2) Apply gentle pressure to the abdomen
3. Keep meticulous cumulative intake and output records (e.g., if drain is 300 ml less than the amount instilled [+300 ml] during one exchange but the next exchange yields a drain volume of 400 ml more than the amount instilled [−400 ml], the cumulative volume is −100 ml)
4. Monitor for hypotension, respiratory distress, especially during inflow phase

Table 9-8	Forms of Vascular Accesses for Dialysis			
Access	**Advantages**	**Disadvantages**	**Management**
Double-lumen vascular catheter inserted into subclavian, jugular, or femoral vein	• Easy insertion • Immediate use • High flow rates are achieved • No venipuncture required for access	• Externally located • Can be easily dislodged • Prone to infection, thrombosis • Femoral catheters are associated with a higher incidence of infection	• Monitor site daily and provide site care • Restrict use of this catheter to dialysis only • Administer heparin into catheter if prescribed
Shunt (rarely used today; replaced by double-lumen vascular catheter)	• Immediate use • No venipuncture required for access	• Externally located (tubing in artery and tubing in vein connected with a T-connector; bright red blood is seen in tubing) • Can be easily dislodged or disconnected causing hemorrhage • Prone to infection, thrombosis • Short lifespan • Creates body image alteration	• Monitor site daily and provide site care • Keep clamps available in case of accidental disconnect; usually "bulldog" clamps attached to dressing • Do not use limb for BP, venipuncture, IV cannulation • Listen for bruit, feel for thrill: indicate patency • Assess color: bright red indicates patency • Assess neurovascular status of affected limb often • Administer heparin into shunt if prescribed
Fistula	• Located internally • Greater longevity • Lower clotting and infection rates than external devices • No danger of disconnect	• Requires 4-6 weeks to mature before use • Requires venipuncture for access • May result in ischemia to affected limb (referred to as *vascular steal syndrome*) • May thrombose	• Do not use limb for BP, venipuncture • Listen for bruit, feel for thrill: indicate patency • Assess neurovascular status of affected limb often • Teach patient exercises to increase blood flow in fistula (e.g., squeezing a ball) • Warn patient not to wear constrictive clothing
AV Graft	• As for fistula • May be used for patients with vessels inadequate for fistula formation • Can be used earlier than traditional fistula	• As for fistula • Infection is more serious than with traditional fistula due to risk of disintegration and hemorrhage • May cause aneurysm formation	• As for fistula • Rotating puncture sites and applying pressure on needle removal aids in prevention of aneurysm and pseudoaneurysm

5. Monitor vital signs during outflow phase
6. Monitor blood glucose levels in all patients; hyperglycemia is likely to occur in diabetic patients or when 4.25% dialysate is used
7. Provide peritoneal catheter exit site care

B. Hemodialysis
 1. Preparation
   a) Patient must have vascular access (Table 9-8 and Fig. 9-14)
   b) Weigh patient prior to hemodialysis
   c) Do not administer drugs that may cause hypotension prior to hemodialysis
     (1) Antihypertensives
     (2) Antiemetics
     (3) Narcotics
     (4) Beta-blockers
     (5) Calcium channel blockers
   d) Do not administer dialyzable drugs immediately prior to hemodialysis
 2. Procedure (usually performed by specially trained hemodialysis nurse rather than critical care staff) (Fig. 9-15)
   a) Vascular access is cannulated and/or connected to the dialyzer
   b) Anticoagulation is maintained
   c) Blood chemistries are monitored throughout the treatment
   d) Vital signs are monitored often for evaluation of hemodynamic stability and tolerance

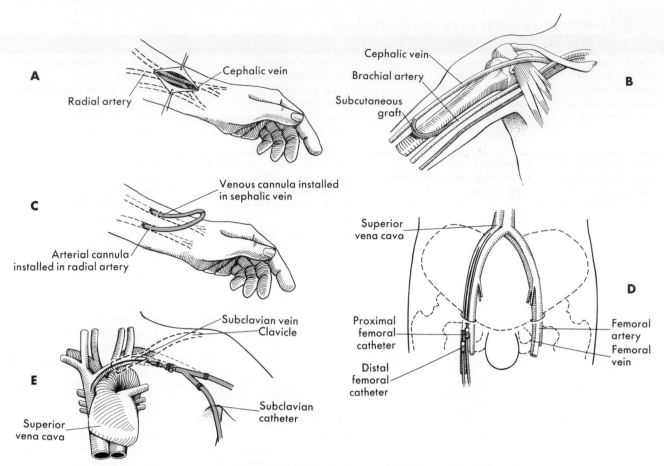

Figure 9-14   Vascular accesses for hemodialysis. **A,** Arteriovenous fistula. **B,** Arteriovenous graft. **C,** External arteriovenous shunt. **D,** Femoral vein catheter. **E,** Subclavian vein catheter. (From Long BC, Phipps WJ, Cassmeyer VL: *Medical-surgical nursing: a nursing process approach,* ed 3, St Louis, 1993, Mosby.)

e) Monitor the vascular access and the hemofilter for indications of clotting

C. Selected complications
1. Disequilibrium syndrome
   a) Caused by toxins (e.g., urea) being rapidly removed from the blood but not as rapidly removed from the cerebro-spinal fluid
   b) The higher concentration of toxins in the brain cells may cause a shift of fluid into brain cells and cerebral edema
   c) Clinical indications may include nausea, vomiting, headache, hallucinations, and seizures
   d) Collaborative management
      (1) Use a smaller dialyzer
      (2) Reduce blood pump speed
      (3) Shorten dialysis time and dialyze more often
      (4) Administer diazepam and phenytoin as prescribed for seizures
2. Muscle cramps
   a) Caused by rapid water removal and sodium shifts

b) Collaborative management
   (1) Administer quinine as prescribed prior to dialysis
   (2) Administer hypertonic saline during dialysis as prescribed

D. Continuous renal replacement therapy (Table 9-9 and Fig. 9-16)
1. Preparation
   a) Patient must have vascular access
   b) Heparin is usually administered after baseline clotting studies are obtained
2. Procedure
   a) Prepare hemofilter with dialysate solution
   b) Connect vascular access to hemofilter
   c) Fluid replacement is calculated according to the ultrafiltration rate
   d) Change the filter when the rate slows or if the filter ruptures or is clogged

Renal Transplant

I. Renal replacement therapy for patients with chronic renal failure
II. See Chapter 11

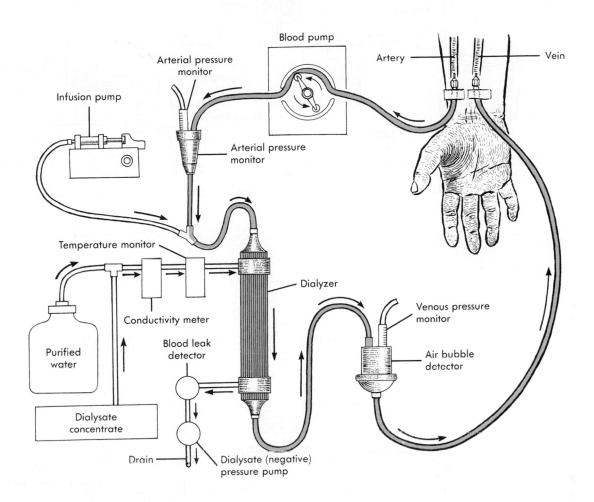

Figure 9-15   Components of a hemodialysis system. (From Thelan LS, Davie JK, Urden LD: *Critical care nursing: diagnosis and management,* ed 3, St Louis, 1998, Mosby.)

Table 9-9	**Continuous Renal Replacement Therapy (CRRT)**		
Type		**Ultrafiltration Rate**	**Function**
SCUF (Slow continuous ultrafiltration)		100-300 ml/hr	Fluid removal
CAVH (Continuous arteriovenous hemofiltration)		500-800 ml/hr	Fluid removal Moderate solute removal
CAVHD (Continuous arteriovenous hemodialysis) or CVVHD (Continuous venovenous hemodialysis)		500-800 ml/hr	Fluid removal Maximal solute removal

Modified from Price CA: *AACN clinical issues* 3 (3):597, 1992.

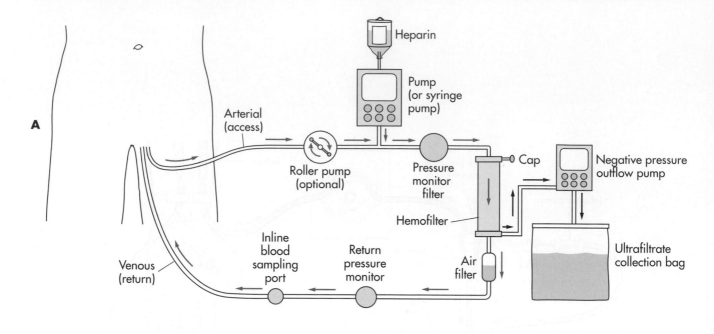

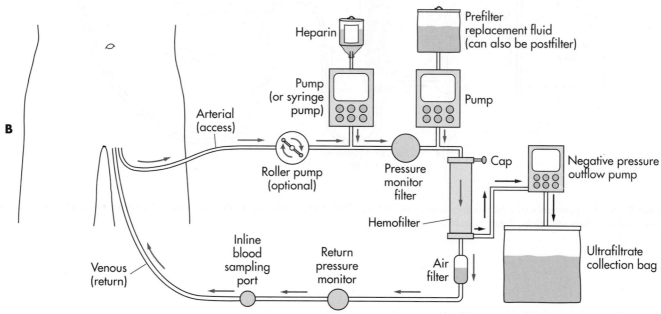

Figure 9-16   Continuous renal replacement therapy systems. **A,** SCUF setup. **B,** CAVH setup. Note that the systems are similar but vary in complexity, depending on what function is to be performed. For example, the CAVH setup differs from the SCUF setup in that it contains prefilter replacement fluid and a pump so that significant blood volume can be removed. (From Thelan LS, Davie JK, Urden LD: *Critical care nursing: diagnosis and management,* ed 3, St Louis, 1998, Mosby.)

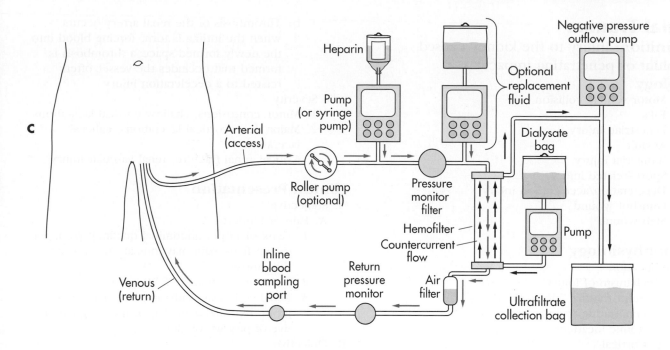

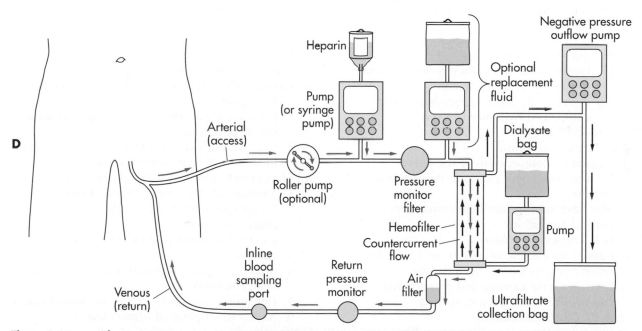

Figure 9-16, cont'd   C, CAVHD setup. **D,** CVVHD setup. Note that the CAVHD and CVVHD setup differ from the SCUF setup and CAVH setup in that they have additional countercurrent flow. (From Thelan LS, Davie JK, Urden LD: *Critical care nursing: diagnosis and management,* ed 3, St Louis, 1998, Mosby.)

Renal Trauma
Definition: Injury to the kidney caused by blunt or penetrating impact

Etiology
I. Motor vehicle collision
II. Falls
III. Pedestrian injury
IV. Assault
V. Industrial injury
VI. Sports-related injury
VII. Deceleration/acceleration injury
VIII. Gunshot wound
IX. Stab wound

Pathophysiology
I. Classification
 A. Mechanism of injury
  1. Blunt trauma: 70% to 80%
  2. Penetrating trauma: 20% to 30%
 B. Anatomic location
  1. Cortical
  2. Pedicle: vascular
  3. Collecting system
  4. Anatomic issues
   a) The right kidney is more vulnerable to injury than the left because it is lower
   b) Fracture of ribs 11, 12 may cause kidney penetration
   c) Renal trauma is almost always accompanied by other system problems
    (1) Injury to the left kidney is often accompanied by injury to spleen
    (2) Injury to the right kidney is often accompanied by injury to liver
 C. Classification (Fig. 9-17)
  1. Class I: renal contusion
   a) Caused by compression of the kidney between the lower ribs and the vertebral column
   b) May have subcapsular hematoma, minor cortical lacerations
  2. Class II: cortical laceration
   a) Caused by fracture of ribs 10 to 12 or the transverse process of the vertebrae
   b) Damages renal capsule and parenchyma; can involve the collecting system
  3. Class III: caliceal laceration
   a) Involves a larger laceration or multiple lacerations extending into the renal collection system
  4. Class IV: renal fracture (also referred to as *shattered kidney*)
   a) Involves extensive lacerations at various sites in the renal parenchyma; involves the collecting system
  5. Class V: vascular pedicle injury or renal artery thrombosis
   a) Vascular pedicle injury involves a tear or laceration to the renal vasculature; often caused by penetrating trauma

   b) Thrombosis of the renal artery occurs when the intima is torn, forcing blood into the newly formed space; a thrombosis is formed that occludes the vessel; often related to a deceleration injury
 D. Severity
  1. Minor: contusions, shallow cortical lacerations
  2. Major: deep cortical lacerations, caliceal laceration
  3. Critical: renal fracture, renal vascular injury

Clinical Presentation
I. Subjective
 A. Pain or tenderness
  1. Flank or upper abdominal quadrant pain; persistent flank pain may indicate renal artery thrombosis
  2. Costovertebral angle (CVA) pain
  3. Renal colic: pain radiating from flank into groin, external genitalia, or into thigh: indicative of passage of clots
II. Objective
 A. Hematuria: gross or microscopic
 B. Oliguria
 C. Hematoma over posterior aspect of rib 11 or 12 or in flank area
 D. Entrance/exit wound if penetrating trauma
 E. Flank swelling or mass
 F. Abdominal distention
 G. Abdominal bruit if renal artery thrombosis
 H. External genitalia: note any ecchymosis
 I. Urethral meatus: note any bleeding
 J. Clinical indications of retroperitoneal bleeding
  1. Back pain
  2. Clinical indications of hemorrhage: tachycardia, hypotension
  3. Grey Turner's sign: ecchymosis over the flank indicative of retroperitoneal bleeding
 K. Clinical indications of extravasated urine
  1. Midline bulging (overdistended bladder)
  2. Lower quadrant, flank or thigh distention (fluid collection)
  3. Lower abdominal pain or mass (bladder rupture)
  4. Abdominal pain, rebound tenderness (peritoneal irritation)
  5. Hematuria (trauma to kidney or urinary tract)
  6. Anuria (disruption of urinary tract)
III. Diagnostic
 A. Laboratory
  1. Serum
   a) BUN and creatinine: may be elevated if renal damage
   b) Hemoglobin and hematocrit: may be decreased if hemorrhage
   c) Potassium: may be elevated
  2. Urine: may be positive for blood or protein
 B. Chest X-ray: may show fractured ribs (11 to 12) on affected side
 C. KUB: may show any of the following:
  1. Rib fracture over kidney

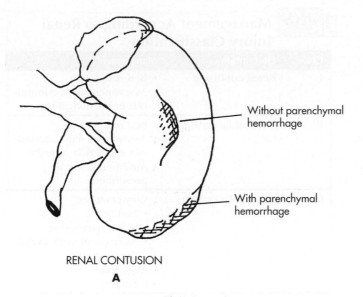

Without parenchymal hemorrhage

With parenchymal hemorrhage

RENAL CONTUSION
A

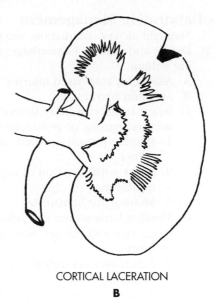

CORTICAL LACERATION
B

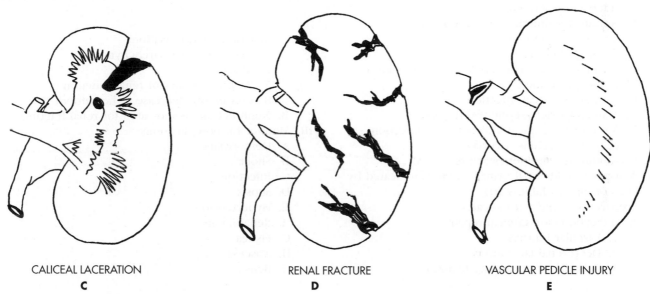

CALICEAL LACERATION
C

RENAL FRACTURE
D

VASCULAR PEDICLE INJURY
E

Figure 9-17   Renal trauma. **A,** Renal contusion. **B,** Cortical laceration. **C,** Caliceal laceration. **D,** Renal fracture. **E,** Vascular pedicle injury. (Drawing by Ann M. Walthall.)

2. Displacement of bowel
3. Obliteration of renal shadow
D. IVP may show any of the following:
   1. Delayed excretion of dye
   2. Renal outline enlargement
   3. Decreased concentration of contrast media in renal parenchyma
E. Ultrasonography: may show renal parenchymal injury
F. Renal scan: may show renal parenchymal injury and/or defect in renal blood flow

G. CT and/or MRI: may show extent of injury
H. Angiogram: may show vascular disruption, renal infarction, hematoma

Nursing Diagnoses

I. Altered Pattern of Urinary Elimination related to mechanical trauma, extravasation of urine
II. Risk for Fluid Volume Deficit related to hemorrhage
III. Risk for Infection related to bacterial contamination of urinary tract, invasive procedures
IV. Pain related to trauma, surgery

Collaborative Management

I. Maintain airway, ventilation, oxygenation
II. Detect and control hemorrhage; replace circulating volume
   A. Assess for associated injuries
   B. Maintain bed rest
   C. Insert urinary catheter unless blood noted at urethral meatus or resistance is met
      1. Prepare patient for urethrogram if resistance is met
      2. Assist with insertion of suprapubic catheter if indicated
      3. Monitor for hematuria
   D. Monitor hemoglobin and hematocrit
   E. Insert two large-gauge, short intravenous catheters
      1. Administer crystalloids or colloids as prescribed
      2. Type and crossmatch for blood; administer blood as prescribed
   F. Encourage fluids orally if injury is minor
III. Administer fluid and drug therapy to maintain urine output
   A. Administer appropriate fluid replacement
   B. Administer low-dose (1 to 2 µg/kg/mm) dopamine as prescribed
   C. Administer diuretics as prescribed
      1. Osmotic diuretics
      2. Loop diuretics
IV. Control pain: administer analgesics (e.g., morphine) as prescribed
V. Prevent and/or treat infection
   A. Maintain strict aseptic techniques
   B. Monitor for clinical indications of infection (e.g., fever, chills, pyuria)
   C. Administer antibiotics as prescribed
VI. Assist with additional management as indicated by class of injury (Table 9-10)
VII. Prepare for surgery if indicated
   A. Indications for surgical repair
      1. Vascular injuries
      2. Deep renal lacerations
      3. Pulsatile or expanding hematoma
      4. Urinary extravasation
      5. Necrotic renal parenchyma
      6. Abscess
      7. Progressive loss of renal function
      8. Continuing decrease in hematocrit
   B. Nephrectomy is indicated for renal fracture
VIII. Monitor for complications
   A. Hemorrhage
   B. Shock
   C. Infection
   D. Sepsis
   E. Hypertension
   F. Renal failure
   G. Fistula
   H. Abscess
   I. Ileus

Table 9-10 **Management According to Renal Injury Classification**

Class	Description	Management
I	Renal contusion	• Bed rest • Assessment with continuous evaluation of urine
II	Cortical laceration	• Bed rest • Assessment with continuous evaluation of urine • Antibiotics may be prescribed
III	Caliceal laceration	• Conservation • Bed rest • Blood transfusion • Assessment with evaluation of urine • Aggressive • Surgery
IV	Renal fracture	• Exploratory laparotomy and nephrectomy
V	Vascular pedicle injury or renal artery thrombosis	• Emergency surgical exploration with vascular repair • Blood transfusion

LEARNING ACTIVITIES

1. DIRECTIONS: Complete the following crossword puzzle related to renal anatomy and physiology.

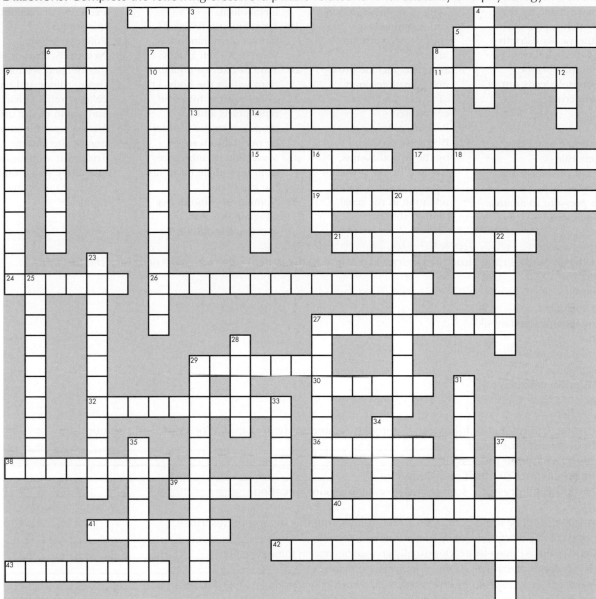

Across

2. Movement of solutes from an area of high solute concentration to an area of low solute concentration
5. Vitamin D is necessary for the absorption of this electrolyte
9. Loop of ____
10. Another term for glomerular filtrate
11. Passageway for expulsion of urine from the bladder to the urinary meatus
13. Hormone of the adrenal cortex that causes retention of sodium and water and excretion of potassium
15. Composed of 6 to 10 pyramids
17. Passage of a substance from the capillary into the tubule
19. Hormone that stimulates the release of RBCs from the bone marrow
21. Cluster of tightly coiled capillaries in the nephron
24. Site of the glomerulus, proximal and distal tubules
26. Process that maintains constancy in GFR
27. Waste product of muscle metabolism
29. Collapsible bag of smooth muscle
30. Small funnel tapering into the ureter
32. Includes the renal cortex and medulla
36. Positively charged ion
38. Ion whose concentration determines pH
39. Inward extension of cortical tissue between the pyramids

40. Capillary network that runs parallel to the ascending and descending loop of Henle (2 words)
41. Also referred to as the suprarenal gland
42. Substance made by the kidney that modulates the vasoconstrictive effects of angiotensin and norepinephrine
43. This arteriole leads out of the glomerulus

Down
1. This arteriole leads into the glomerulus
3. Movement of solutes and solutions from an area of high pressure to an area of low pressure

4. Human body is composed mostly of this substance
6. Type of fluid loss (or gains) that cannot be measured
7. Type of nephron important in the kidney's ability to concentrate urine
8. Segments include proximal convolute, loop of Henle, and distal convoluted
9. Pushing pressure
12. Hormone produced by the hypothalamus, released by the posterior pituitary; causes water retention in the renal tubule (abbrev.)

14. Movement of solution from an area of low solute concentration to an area of high solute concentration
16. End product of protein metabolism
18. Thin, smooth layer of fibrous membrane that surrounds each kidney
20. State of internal equilibrium within the body
22. Collects urine from the renal pelvis and propels it to the bladder by peristaltic waves
23. Movement of substances from the tubule back into the capillaries
25. Number of osmoles per kilogram of solution; expressed as mOsm/kg

27. Consists of Bowman's capsule and glomerulus
28. Cuplike structures that drain the papillae
29. Kidney aids in acid-base regulation, primarily by excreting or retaining this solute
31. Pulling pressure
33. Negatively charged ion
34. Cavity filled with adipose tissue, minor and major calices, renal pelvis, and origin of the ureter
35. Microscopic functional unit of the kidney
37. Triangular wedges of medullary tissue; composed of collecting tubules

2. **DIRECTIONS:** Number the structures below according to the order of their involvement in urine formation.
_____ Ureters
_____ Glomerulus
_____ Loop of Henle
_____ Proximal convoluted tubule
_____ Bladder
_____ Bowman's capsule
_____ Collecting ducts
_____ Distal convoluted tubule
_____ Urethra

3. **DIRECTIONS:** Complete the following statements related to the movement of solutes and solutions.
Water moves by the process of_____ .
Electrolytes move by the process of_____ .
The sodium-potassium pump is an example of_____ .
The use of a pushing pressure, such as hydrostatic pressure, is called_____ .

4. **DIRECTIONS:** Identify the electrolyte or electrolytes that the statement describes.
a. Serum levels of this electrolyte go up in acidosis and down in alkalosis._____
b. Imbalances of these three electrolytes usually go together and in same direction._____
c. Serum levels of this electrolyte go down in hypoalbuminemia._____
d. These two electrolytes have an inverse relationship: when one goes down, the other goes up._____
e. These two electrolytes are often deficient in malnourished patients._____
f. Loss of either of these two electrolytes causes hydrogen ions to move into the cell, resulting in metabolic alkalosis._____

5. **DIRECTIONS:** Specify whether the following causes of metabolic acidosis would have a normal anion gap or an increased anion gap.

Condition	Normal Anion Gap	Increased Anion Gap
Shock		
Renal failure		
Diarrhea		
Diabetic ketoacidosis		
Salicylate overdose		
Renal tubular acidosis		
Rhabdomyolysis		
Carbonic anhydrase inhibitors		

6. **DIRECTIONS:** Identify three major reasons for the BUN to be elevated in a patient with a normal creatinine.

1. _____
2. _____
3. _____

7. **DIRECTIONS:** Indicate whether these signs and symptoms are indicative of electrolyte deficit or excess.

Sign or Symptom	Excess (Hyper)	Deficit (Hypo)
Sodium		
Weight gain		
Abdominal cramps		
Flushed, dry skin		
Postural hypotension		
Headache		
Hypertension		
Potassium		
Flat T-waves, prominent U-waves		
Decreased GI motility, paralytic ileus		
Intestinal colic, diarrhea		
Muscle cramps to flaccid paralysis		
Decreased cardiac contractility		
Tall, peaked T-waves, widened QRS complex		
Calcium		
Tetany		
Decreased deep tendon reflexes		
Neuromuscular weakness, flaccidity		
Seizures		
Bone or flank pain		
Laryngospasm		
Phosphorus		
Tetany		
Fatigue		
Chest pain		
Dyspnea		
Increased deep tendon reflexes		
Abdominal cramps		
Magnesium		
Decreased deep tendon reflexes		
Anorexia, nausea, vomiting		
Cardiopulmonary arrest		
Lethargy		
Dysrhythmias, especially torsades de pointes		
Facial flushing		

8. **Directions:** Identify three electrolyte imbalances that enhance digitalis effect and increase the chance of digitalis toxicity.

1. _____
2. _____
3. _____

9. **Directions:** What fluid, electrolyte, or acid-base imbalances would these patients be predisposed to:

a. A patient receiving regular doses of furosemide.

1. _____
2. _____
3. _____
4. _____
5. _____
6. _____

b. A patient with persistent vomiting.

1. _____
2. _____
3. _____
4. _____

c. A patient with acute renal failure (oliguric phase).

1. _____
2. _____
3. _____
4. _____
5. _____
6. _____
7. _____

d. A patient with diabetic ketoacidosis (before treatment).

1. _____
2. _____
3. _____
4. _____

e. A patient receiving multiple units of banked blood.

1. _____
2. _____
3. _____

10. **Directions:** List three indications for dialysis in a patient with acute renal failure.

1._____
2._____
3._____

11. **DIRECTIONS:** Categorize the following causes of acute renal failure as prerenal, intrarenal, or postrenal:

Condition	Prerenal	Intrarenal	Postrenal
Acute pyelonephritis			
Benign prostatic hypertrophy			
Contrast dyes			
Diuretics			
Gentamycin			
Glomerulonephritis			
Goodpasture's syndrome			
Hemorrhage			
Hepatorenal syndrome			
Hypersensitivity reactions			
Intraabdominal tumor			
Malignant hypertension			
Neurogenic bladder			
Prolonged hypotension			
Renal calculi			
Rhabdomyolysis with myoglobinuria			
Septic shock			

12. **DIRECTIONS:** Identify the following characteristics as occurring during the oliguric or diuretic phase of acute renal failure or both.

Characteristic	Oliguric Phase	Diuretic Phase	Both
Elevated BUN			
Hyperkalemia			
Metabolic acidosis			
Volume deficit			
Volume excess			

13. **DIRECTIONS:** List three indications of extravasation of urine into the peritoneal cavity.

1. _____
2. _____
3. _____

14. **DIRECTIONS:** Complete the following crossword related to renal assessment, conditions, and treatments.

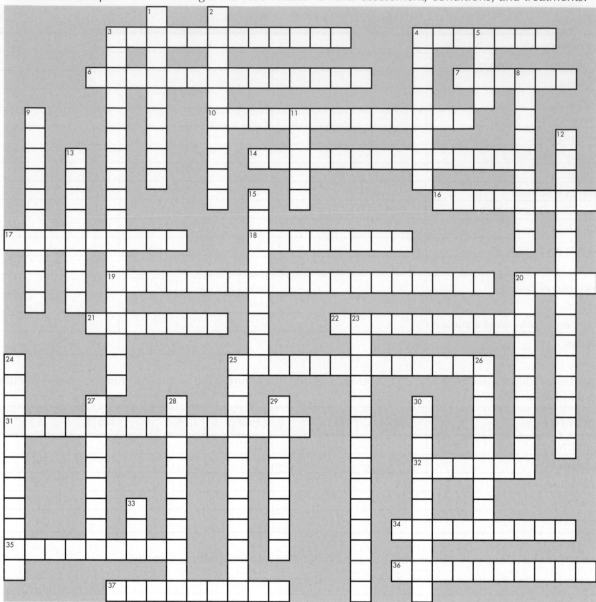

Across

3. Syndrome characterized by basement membrane damage and manifested by renal failure and hemoptysis (possessive)
4. Deficiency of this electrolyte may cause paresthesia, tetany, laryngospasm, seizures
6. Tenderness at this angle may indicate pyelonephritis
7. Increased levels of urea in the blood
10. Carbonic anhydrase inhibitor; often used to treat metabolic alkalosis (generic)

14. Potassium-sparing diuretic (generic)
16. Osmotic diuretic (generic)
17. Categorization of acute renal failure that is caused by disrupted renal flow; renal stone is an example of a cause of this type of renal failure
18. Phase of acute renal failure that is heralded by a dramatic increase in urine output
19. Thiazide diuretic (generic)

20. Precipitation from the kidney that takes the shape of the tubule where it was formed
21. Long-term vascular access consisting of an internal artery-vein anastomosis
22. Potentially permanent renal replacement therapy for patients with chronic renal failure
25. Electrolyte imbalance that occurs with osteolytic lesions
31. Calcium may be given for hypocalcemia, hyperkalemia, ____
32. Levels of this electrolyte are greatly affected by water balance

34. Significant change in serum levels of this electrolyte causes dysrhythmias
35. Presence of this substance in the urine is the result of the breakdown of skeletal muscle; may cause renal failure
36. Loop diuretic (generic)
37. Solution of glucose and electrolytes used on one side of the semipermeable membrane to pull fluid and electrolytes across the semipermeable membrane in dialysis

Down

1. Type of renal injury that is caused by compression of the kidney between the lower ribs and the vertebral column

2. Ion exchange agent used to decrease serum potassium (trade)

3. Infection of the kidney associated with beta-hemolytic streptococcal infection

4. Type of intrarenal failure that is caused by infectious processes

5. Renal replacement therapy that may be used in patients who cannot tolerate hemodialysis (abbrev.)

8. High levels of this electrolyte may cause respiratory paralysis and cardiopulmonary arrest

9. Presence of this substance in the urine is the result of massive hemolysis; may cause renal failure

11. Calculation of this gap differentiates metabolic acidosis caused by acid gain from metabolic acidosis caused by bicarbonate loss

12. Electrolyte imbalance that occurs in refeeding syndrome

13. Renal injury that involves multiple lacerations extending into the renal collection system

15. Type of intrarenal failure that is caused by nephrotoxic agents or prolonged ischemic injury

20. Breakdown of lean body tissue

23. Condition characterized by the breakdown of skeletal muscle

24. Surgical procedure performed for renal fracture

25. Electrolyte imbalance that occurs with crush injury, renal failure, hemolysis

26. Hand-flapping tremor seen in uremia

27. Categorization of acute renal failure that is caused by disrupted blood flow to the kidney; shock is an example of a cause of this type of renal failure

28. Categorization of acute renal failure that is caused by damage to renal tissue; acute tubular necrosis is an example of a cause of this type of renal failure

29. Separation of solutes by differential diffusion through a semipermeable membrane that is placed between the two solutions

30. High levels of this electrolyte occur in renal failure; low levels occur in malnutrition

33. Another term for this X-ray is "flat plate of abdomen" (abbrev.)

LEARNING ACTIVITIES ANSWERS

1.

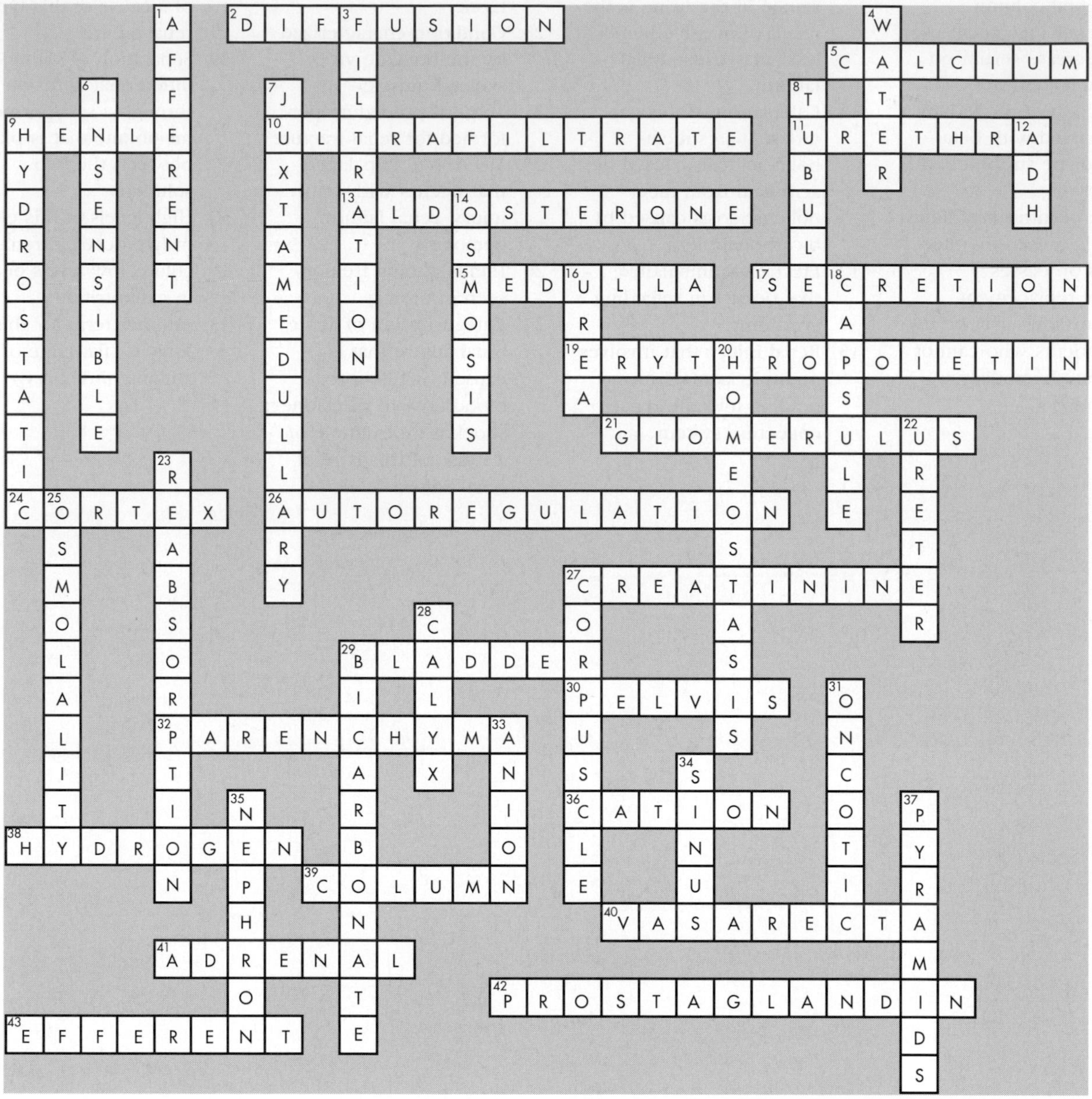

Crossword puzzle answers:

Across:
- 2 DIFFUSION
- 5 CALCIUM
- 9 HENLE
- 10 ULTRAFILTRATE
- 11 URETHRA
- 13 ALDOSTERONE
- 15 MEDULLA
- 17 SECRETION
- 19 ERYTHROPOIETIN
- 21 GLOMERULUS
- 24 CORTEX
- 26 AUTOREGULATION
- 27 CREATININE
- 29 BLADDER
- 30 PELVIS
- 32 PARENCHYMA
- 36 CATION
- 38 HYDROGEN
- 39 COLUMN
- 40 VASARECTA
- 41 ADRENAL
- 42 PROSTAGLANDIN
- 43 EFFERENT

Down:
- 1 AFFERENT
- 3 FILLTRATION
- 4 WATER
- 6 INSENSIBLE
- 7 JUXTAMEDULLARY
- 8 TUBULE
- 12 ADH
- 14 OSMOSIS
- 16 URORASIS
- 18 CABASTER
- 20 HOS
- 22 URETER
- 23 RABSORY
- 25 OSMOLALIT
- 27 CORS
- 28 CILL
- 30 PUSS
- 31 ONCOTIC
- 33 ANION
- 34 S
- 35 NEPHRON
- 37 PYRAMIDS

2.

_7_ Ureters
_1_ Glomerulus
_4_ Loop of Henle
_3_ Proximal convoluted tubule
_8_ Bladder
_2_ Bowman's capsule
_6_ Collecting ducts
_5_ Distal convoluted tubule
_9_ Urethra

3. Water moves by the process of <u>osmosis</u>.
   Electrolytes move by the process of <u>diffusion</u>.
   The sodium-potassium pump is an example of <u>active transport</u>.
   The use of a pushing pressure, such as hydrostatic pressure, is called <u>filtration</u>.

4.   a. Potassium
     b. Potassium, calcium, magnesium
     c. Calcium
     d. Calcium, phosphorus
     e. Magnesium, phosphorus
     f. Potassium, chloride

5.

Condition	Normal Anion Gap	Increased Anion Gap
Shock		✔
Renal failure		✔
Diarrhea	✔	
Diabetic ketoacidosis		✔
Salicylate overdose		✔
Renal tubular acidosis	✔	
Rhabdomyolysis		✔
Carbonic anhydrase inhibitors	✔	

6.   1. Volume depletion
     2. Catabolism including starvation, GI bleed
     3. Hypoperfusion

7.

Sign or Symptom	Excess (Hyper)	Deficit (Hypo)
Sodium		
Weight gain	✔	
Abdominal cramps		✔
Flushed, dry skin	✔	
Postural hypotension		✔
Headache		✔
Hypertension	✔	
Potassium		
Flat T-waves, prominent U-waves		✔
Decreased GI motility, paralytic ileus		✔
Intestinal colic, diarrhea	✔	
Muscle cramps to flaccid paralysis		✔
Decreased cardiac contractility	✔	
Tall, peaked T-waves, widened QRS complex	✔	
Calcium		
Tetany		✔
Decreased deep tendon reflexes	✔	
Neuromuscular weakness, flaccidity	✔	
Seizures		✔
Bone or flank pain	✔	
Laryngospasm		✔
Phosphorus		
Tetany	✔	
Fatigue		✔
Chest pain		✔
Dyspnea		✔
Increased deep tendon reflexes	✔	
Abdominal cramps	✔	
Magnesium		
Decreased deep tendon reflexes	✔	
Anorexia, nausea, vomiting		✔
Cardiopulmonary arrest	✔	
Lethargy	✔	
Dysrhythmias, especially torsades de pointes		✔
Facial flushing	✔	

8. 1. Hypercalcemia
   2. Hypokalemia
   3. Hypomagnesemia

9. a. A patient receiving regular doses of furosemide.
   1. Hypovolemia
   2. Hyponatremia
   3. Hypokalemia
   4. Hypocalcemia
   5. Hypomagnesemia
   6. Metabolic alkalosis (caused by hypochloremia and hypokalemia)

   b. A patient with persistent vomiting.
   1. Hypovolemia
   2. Hyponatremia

3. Hypokalemia
4. Metabolic alkalosis (caused by hypochloremia and hypokalemia)

c. A patient with acute renal failure (oliguric phase).
1. Hypervolemia
2. Hyponatremia
3. Hyperkalemia
4. Hypocalcemia
5. Hyperphosphatemia
6. Hypermagnesemia
7. Metabolic acidosis

d. A patient with diabetic ketoacidosis (before treatment).
1. Hyperkalemia
2. Hypophosphatemia
3. Hypermagnesemia
4. Metabolic acidosis

e. A patient receiving multiple units of banked blood.
1. Hyperkalemia
2. Hypocalcemia
3. Hypomagnesemia

10. a. BUN >100 mg/dl
b. Volume overload, especially with pulmonary edema
c. Uncontrollable hyperkalemia
d. Uncontrollable hyperphosphatemia
e. Uncontrollable acidosis
f. Pericarditis
g. Seizures or coma
h. Symptomatic uremia

11.

Condition	Prerenal	Intrarenal	Postrenal
Acute pyelonephritis		✔	
Benign prostatic hypertrophy			✔
Contrast dyes		✔	
Diuretics	✔		
Gentamycin		✔	
Glomerulonephritis		✔	
Goodpasture's syndrome		✔	
Hemorrhage	✔		
Hepatorenal syndrome	✔		
Hypersensitivity reactions		✔	
Intraabdominal tumor			✔
Malignant hypertension		✔	
Neurogenic bladder			✔
Prolonged hypotension		✔	
Renal calculi			✔
Rhabdomyolysis with myoglobinuria		✔	
Septic shock	✔		

12.

Characteristic	Oliguric Phase	Diuretic Phase	Both
Elevated BUN			✔
Hyperkalemia			✔
Metabolic acidosis			✔
Volume deficit		✔	
Volume excess	✔		

13. a. Midline bulging
   b. Lower quadrant, flank or thigh distention
   c. Lower abdominal pain or mass
   d. Abdominal pain, rebound tenderness
   e. Hematuria
   f. Anuria

14.

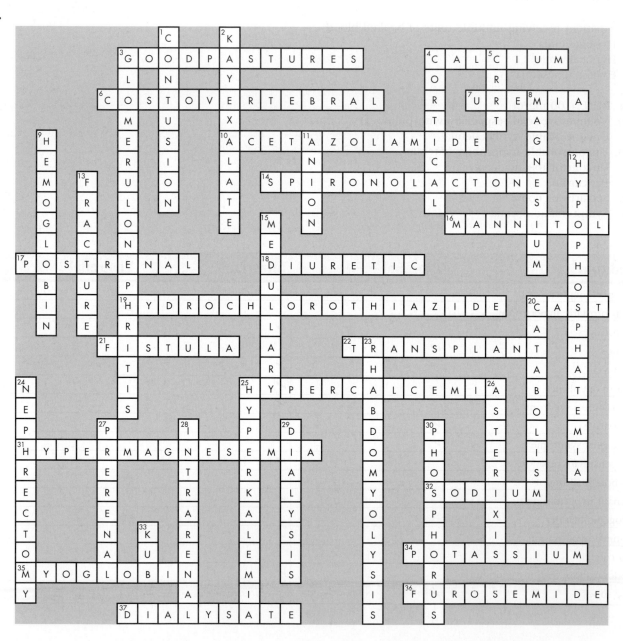

Bibliography and Selected References

Alspach J, editor: *Core curriculum for critical care nursing,* ed 5, Philadelphia, 1998, WB Saunders.

Barkauskas V et al: *Health and physical assessment,* St Louis, 1994, Mosby.

Beare P, Myers J: *Adult health nursing,* ed 3, St Louis, 1998, Mosby.

Bhatla B, Nolph K, Khanna R: Choosing the right dialysis option for your critically ill patient, *Journal of Critical Illness* 11 (1):21, 1996.

Boggs R, Wooldridge-King M: *AACN procedure manual for critical care,* ed 3, Philadelphia, 1993, WB Saunders.

Brar R, Hollenberg S: The technique of fluid resuscitation, *Journal of Critical Illness* 11 (8):550, 1996.

Brar R, Hollenberg S: Administering fluid resuscitation effectively for traumatic shock, *Journal of Critical Illness* 11 (10):672, 1996.

Bräxmeyer D: The pathophysiology of potassium balance, *Critical Care Nurse* 16 (5):59, 1996.

Chernow B, editor: *The pharmacologic approach to the critically ill patient,* ed 3, Baltimore, 1994, Williams & Wilkins.

Cirolia B: Understanding edema, *Nursing96* 26 (2), 66, 1996.

Clayton K: Cancer-related hypercalcemia, *AJN* 97 (5):42, 1997.

Clochesy J et al: *Critical care nursing,* ed 2, Philadelphia, 1996, WB Saunders.

DeJong M: Hyponatremia, *AJN* 98 (12):36, 1998.

Gahart B, Nazareno A: *1999 intravenous medications,* St Louis, 1999, Mosby.

Giuliano K, Pysznik F: Renal replacement therapy in critical care: implementation of a unit-based continuous venovenous hemodialysis program, *Critical Care Nurse* 18 (1):40, 1998.

Higley R: Continuous arteriovenous hemofiltration: a case study, *Critical Care Nurse* 16 (5):37, 1996.

Keen J, Searingen P: *Mosby's critical care nursing consultant,* St Louis, 1997, Mosby.

Kinney M et al: *AACN clinical reference for critical care nursing,* ed 4, St Louis, 1998, Mosby.

Laskowski-Jones L: Managing hemorrhage: taking the right steps to protect your patient, *Nursing97* 27 (9):36, 1997.

Marino P: *The ICU book,* ed 2, Baltimore, 1998, Williams & Wilkins.

Metheny N: Focusing on the dangers of D_5W, *AJN* 97 (10):55, 1997.

Mims B et al: *Critical care skills: a clinical handbook,* Philadelphia, 1996, WB Saunders.

O'Donnell M: Assessing fluid and electrolyte balance in elders, *AJN* 95 (11):41, 1995.

Price S, Wilson L: *Pathophysiology: clinical concepts of disease processes,* ed 5, St Louis, 1997, Mosby.

Roper M: Back to basics: assessing orthostatic vital signs, *AJN* 96 (8):43, 1996.

Rosen G et al: Intravenous phosphate repletion regimen for critically ill patients with moderate hypophosphatemia, *Crit Care Med* 23 (7):1204, 1995.

Rutecki G, Whittier F: Life-threatening phosphate imbalance: when to suspect, how to treat, *Journal of Critical Illness* 12 (11):699, 1997.

Rutecki G, Whittier F: Decision points in hypocalcemia: is emergent therapy required? *Journal of Critical Illness* 13 (2):84, 1998.

Sandrock J: Managing hypovolemia, *Nursing97* 27 (2):32aa, 1997.

Sandrock J: Treating traumatic hypovolemia: which fluid to choose?, *Nursing98* 28 (1):32cc1, 1998.

Stark J: Dialysis choices: turning the tide in acute renal failure, *Nursing97* 27 (2):41, 1997.

Thelan L et al: *Critical care nursing: diagnosis and management,* ed 3, St Louis, 1998, Mosby.

Varon J, Fromm R: *The ICU handbook of facts, formulas, and laboratory values,* St Louis, 1997, Mosby.

Wood J, Bosley C: Acute postrenal failure: reversing the problem, *Nursing95* 25 (3):48, 1995.

Young J: A closer look at IV fluids, *Nursing98* 28 (10):52, 1998.

Endocrine System

CHAPTER 10

Selected Concepts in Anatomy and Physiology

Functions: The endocrine system regulates secretion of hormones that alter metabolic body functions, including all of the following:

I. Chemical reactions and transport of chemicals across cell membranes
II. Growth and development
III. Metabolism
IV. Fluid and electrolyte balance
V. Acid-base balance
VI. Adaptation
VII. Reproduction

Components

I. Glands or glandular tissue that synthesize, store, and secrete hormones
   A. An endocrine gland is ductless but highly vascular
   B. The locations of the endocrine glands are depicted in Fig. 10-1
II. Hormones
   A. Definition: complex chemical substances produced in one part or organ of the body that initiate or regulate the activity of an organ or a group of cells in another part of the body
      1. Hormones are released by endocrine glands in response to specific signals (e.g., low target gland hormone levels)
      2. Hormones are released directly into the bloodstream to be distributed throughout the body and to the target gland or target organ to initiate a response
   B. Types include the following:
      1. Amines (e.g., epinephrine, dopamine, thyroid hormones)
      2. Peptides (e.g., growth hormone, follicle-stimulating hormone)
      3. Steroids (e.g., androgens, aldosterone, cortisol)
   C. Endocrine glands and hormones significant in the care of critically ill patients are summarized in Table 10-1; hormones are also secreted by the following organs, although these organs are not normally considered part of the endocrine system
      1. Gastrointestinal tract (e.g., gastrin, cholecystokinin, somatostatin)
      2. Heart (e.g., atrial natriuretic hormone)
      3. Kidney (e.g., erythropoietin, renin, calcitriol)
III. Receptor cells: located in an organ or a group of cells in another part of the body

Process of Hormone Synthesis, Secretion, Effect, Suppression (Fig. 10-2)
Regulation of Hormones

I. The hypothalamus
   A. The hypothalamus regulates the secretion of hormones through other stimulating hormones called *releasing factors*
   B. Releasing factors are keyed to cause the release of hormone from the target gland
II. Neurotransmitters
   A. Sympathetic nervous system: epinephrine, norepinephrine
   B. Parasympathetic nervous system: acetylcholine
III. Feedback regulation
   A. Allows self-regulation
   B. Based on the concentration of the hormone present in the circulation
   C. Also influenced by electrolyte levels, metabolites, osmolality, fluid status, and other hormones

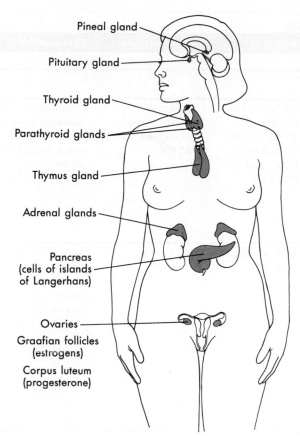

Pineal gland

Pituitary gland

Thyroid gland

Parathyroid glands

Thymus gland

Adrenal glands

Pancreas
(cells of islands
of Langerhans)

Ovaries
Graafian follicles
(estrogens)
Corpus luteum
(progesterone)

Figure 10-1   Location of endocrine glands. (From Beare PG, Myer JL: *Principles and practice of adult health nursing,* ed 2, St Louis, 1994, Mosby.)

D. Positive feedback: low hormone levels stimulate release of the releasing factor
E. Negative feedback: high hormone levels inhibit the release of the releasing factor (Fig. 10-3)

Endocrine Dysfunction
I. Classification
  A. Based on level of hormone activity
    1. Hyperfunction: increased hormonal activity
    2. Hypofunction: decreased hormonal activity
  B. Based on location of dysfunctional gland or response
    1. Primary disorders: disorder of the target gland (e.g., adrenal or thyroid gland)
    2. Secondary disorder: disorder of the stimulating gland (e.g., hypothalamus or pituitary)
  C. Based on acuity
    1. Acute: beginning abruptly with marked intensity
    2. Chronic: developing slowly and persisting for a long period, often for the remainder of the individual's lifetime
II. Causes of endocrine dysfunction
  A. Dysfunction of a particular gland
  B. Altered secretion of the stimulating hormones for that gland
  C. Altered response to the hormone at the target cell

Assessment of the Endocrine System
Interview
I. Chief complaint: why is the patient seeking help and the duration of the problem; because hormones affect every body tissue, numerous symptoms may indicate endocrine dysfunction
  A. General
    1. Easy fatigability, lethargy
    2. Sleep disorders
    3. Cold or heat intolerance
    4. Weight loss or gain, or rapid fluctuations in weight
    5. Increase in size of head, hands, feet
  B. Dermatologic
    1. Pruritus
    2. Hair loss
    3. Changes in hair distribution
    4. Changes in quality of hair
    5. Changes in skin color or pigmentation
    6. Striae
    7. Changes in skin moisture
  C. Eyes: visual changes
  D. Neck
    1. Jugular neck vein distention
    2. Enlargement or nodules
  E. Cardiovascular
    1. Palpitations
    2. Syncope
  F. Pulmonary: dyspnea
  G. Neurologic
    1. Voice changes
    2. Tremors
    3. Nervousness
    4. Loss of the sense of smell
    5. Headache
    6. Sensory changes
    7. Memory loss
    8. Personality changes
    9. Confusion, agitation
    10. Delusions, paranoia, depression
    11. Muscle twitching
    12. Seizures
  H. Gastrointestinal
    1. Change in appetite
    2. Nausea, vomiting
    3. Abdominal pain
    4. Constipation or diarrhea
    5. Incontinence
    6. Polyphagia
    7. Polydipsia
  I. Genitourinary
    1. Polyuria, oliguria, nocturia
    2. Incontinence
    3. Decreased libido
    4. Menstrual irregularities
  J. Musculoskeletal
    1. Muscle or joint pain or aching
    2. Muscle weakness
    3. Muscle cramping

Table 10-1 Hormones Significant in Critical Care Nursing

Hormone	Actions	Releasing Factors	Target	Hypersecretion	Hyposecretion
PITUITARY (HYPOPHYSIS)					
ANTERIOR PITUITARY (ADENOHYPOPHYSIS)					
Growth hormone (somatotropin)	• Stimulates protein anabolism • Mobilizes fatty acids • Conserves carbohydrates • Stimulates bone and cartilage growth	Growth hormone releasing hormone (GHRH) from hypothalamus in response to exercise, starvation, decreased amino acid levels, stress, hypoglycemia	All body cells capable of growth, especially muscle, bone, and cartilage cells	Giantism in children; acromegaly in adults	Dwarfism in children; possible decrease in organ weight in adults
Adrenocorticotropic hormone	• Stimulates growth and function of adrenal gland • Controls production and release of glucocorticoid hormones • Stimulates mineralocorticoid production • Stimulates androgen production	Corticotropin releasing hormone (CRH) from hypothalamus in response to hypoglycemia, decrease in cortisol levels, hypoxia, trauma, surgery, physical and/or psychologic stress	Cells of adrenal cortex	Cushing's disease	Adrenal insufficiency (chronic) and/or adrenal crisis (acute)
Thyroid-stimulating hormone (thyrotropin)	• Increases size and growth of thyroid cells • Increases synthesis of thyroid hormones • Releases stored thyroid hormones	Thyrotropin releasing hormone (TRH) from the hypothalamus in response to cold temperature or a decrease in thyroid hormone levels	Cells of the thyroid gland	Hyperthyroidism	Hypothyroidism
POSTERIOR PITUITARY (NEUROHYPOPHYSIS)					
Antidiuretic hormone (vasopressin)	• Increases water reabsorption (inhibits diuresis) by kidney tubules and collecting ducts • Causes vasoconstriction of arterioles • Causes abdominal cramping	Increase in serum osmolality, hypernatremia, hypovolemia, hypoxia, hypotension, pain, trauma, stress, nausea, pharmacologic agents	Distal renal tubules and collecting ducts; smooth muscle of arterioles and GI tract	Syndrome of inappropriate antidiuretic hormone (SIADH)	Diabetes insipidus (DI)
THYROID GLAND					
Triiodothyronine (T_3) and thyroxine (T_4) **Note:** T_3 is more biologically active	• Stimulates metabolic rate • Increases protein synthesis • Increases carbohydrate and fat metabolism • Increases bone growth • Increases oxygen consumption • Increases metabolism and clearance of drugs	Thyroid stimulating hormone (TSH) from anterior pituitary; TRH from hypothalamus; cold temperature	Most body cells	Hyperthyroidism (chronic); thyroid storm or crisis (acute)	Hypothyroidism (chronic); myxedema coma (acute)

Table 10-1	Hormones Significant in Critical Care Nursing—cont'd				
Hormone	**Actions**	**Releasing Factors**	**Target**	**Hypersecretion**	**Hyposecretion**
Thyrocalcitonin (calcitonin)	• Reduces plasma calcium levels by inhibiting bone lysis and decreasing calcium resorption by the kidney	Increase in serum calcium, magnesium, or glucagon	Bone cells, kidney cells	Not significant	Not significant
PARATHYROID GLAND					
Parathyroid hormone (parathormone)	• Increases serum calcium by accelerating bone breakdown with release of calcium into the blood, increasing calcium reabsorption from intestine and decreasing kidney tubule reabsorption of calcium • Decreases blood phosphate levels by increasing phosphate loss in urine • Increases reabsorption of magnesium by the renal tubules	Low serum calcium; high serum magnesium or phosphate level; catecholamines; cortisol	Bone cells, cells of GI tract and kidney	Hypercalcemia and hypophosphatemia; possibly renal calculi	Hypocalcemia and bone decalcification, hyperphosphatemia
ADRENAL CORTEX					
Glucocorticoids (i.e., cortisol)	• Increases blood glucose by stimulating gluconeogenesis in the liver • Inhibits glucose utilization by the cell • Inhibits protein anabolism • Promotes fatty acid mobilization • Inhibits inflammatory response	CRH from hypothalamus; ACTH from anterior pituitary	Most body cells	Cushing's syndrome	Addison's disease (chronic); adrenal crisis (acute)
Mineralocorticoids (i.e., aldosterone)	• Increases sodium and water reabsorption and potassium excretion	ACTH from anterior pituitary (minor effect); primary stimulus is renin-angiotensin system; decrease in serum sodium; increase in serum potassium	Distal and collecting tubules of kidney; sweat glands; salivary glands; intestines	Hyperaldosteronism	Addison's disease (chronic); adrenal crisis (acute)

Continued

Table 10-1 Hormones Significant in Critical Care Nursing—cont'd

Hormone	Actions	Releasing Factors	Target	Hypersecretion	Hyposecretion
ADRENAL MEDULLA					
Catecholamines (i.e., epinephrine, norepinephrine)	• Dilates pupils • Increases heart rate and contractility • Dilates blood vessels to heart, brain, and skeletal muscle • Constricts blood vessels to nonessential organs (i.e., skin, kidney, GI tract) • Bronchodilation • Increases respiratory rate and depth • Increases perspiration, peristalsis and secretion in GI tract • Increases blood sugar	Sympathetic nervous system innervation: insulin, histamine, anxiety, fear, pain, trauma, exercise, temperature extremes, hypoxia, hypotension, hypovolemia, excess thyroid hormone	Most body cells, vascular beds, smooth muscle	Exaggeration or prolongation of normal effects; may be caused by adrenal medulla tumor called *pheochromocytoma*	May have decrease in stress response or no noticeable effect
PANCREAS					
Glucagon (from alpha cells)	• Stimulates glycogenolysis and gluconeogenesis to increase blood glucose • Inhibits glycolysis • Increases lipolysis	Decrease in blood glucose; elevated blood amino acid; catecholamines; exercise; starvation	Most body cells, especially liver cells	Hyperglycemia	Hypoglycemia
Insulin (from beta cells)	• Enables glucose to move into the cell • Aids in muscle and tissue oxidation of glucose • Enhances storage of glycogen • Increases protein synthesis • Inhibits lipolysis	Increase in blood glucose; gastrin; increase in growth hormone; ACTH; glucagon	Most body cells, especially liver cells	Hypoglycemia	Hyperglycemia (diabetes mellitus [DM])

4. Muscle wasting
5. Twitching
6. Fractures

II. History of present illness: use PQRST format
III. Past medical history: past illnesses or pathologic conditions that may result in endocrine dysfunction
   A. Trauma
   B. Ischemia or infarction
   C. Neoplasm
   D. Inflammation, infection
   E. Autoimmune conditions
   F. Acquired immunodeficiency syndrome (AIDS)
   G. Irradiation, antineoplastic drugs
   H. Surgical removal of an endocrine gland

   I. Interruption of prescribed pharmaceutical agent for treatment of a preexisting chronic endocrine dysfunction
IV. Family history
   A. Diabetes mellitus (DM)
   B. Cardiovascular disease
   C. Cerebrovascular disease
   D. Cancer
V. Social history
   A. Relationship with spouse or significant other, family structure
   B. Occupation
   C. Educational level
   D. Stress level and usual coping mechanisms

E. Recreational habits
F. Exercise habits
G. Dietary habits
   1. Usual diet
   2. Compliance with prescribed limitations
H. Fluid intake
I. Caffeine intake
J. Tobacco use: recorded as pack-years (number of packs per day times the number of years he or she has been smoking)
K. Alcohol use: recorded as alcoholic beverages consumed per month, week, or day

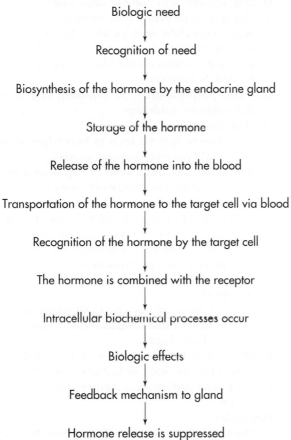

Figure 10-2   Process of hormone synthesis, secretion, effect, and suppression.

L. Toxin exposure
M. Travel
VI. Medication history
   A. Prescribed drug, dosage, frequency, time of last dose
   B. Nonprescribed drugs
      1. Over-the-counter drugs, supplements
      2. Substance abuse
   C. Patient understanding of drug actions, side effects, and sick day management
   D. Pharmacologic agents used to treat chronic endocrine dysfunction
      1. Hormone replacement
      2. Hormone suppressive agents
      3. Agents that trigger release of hormone or potentiate the effect of the hormone
      4. Vitamins or minerals necessary for body synthesis of hormones
   E. Evaluation of patient's compliance with prescribed therapy
   F. Pharmacologic agents that may alter endocrine function by either stimulating or inhibiting hormone release or that interfere with hormone action at the target tissue; pharmacologic agents that may cause endocrine dysfunction are listed under Etiology for each endocrine condition

Inspection and Palpation

I. Vital signs
   A. BP: lying, sitting, standing; orthostatic BP changes caused by hypovolemia may be seen in diabetes insipidus or diabetes mellitus
   B. Heart rate
      1. Bradycardia is often seen in hypothyroidism
      2. Tachycardia may be associated with hyperthyroidism, infection (which may be a cause of DKA or HHNK), hypovolemia (which may occur in DKA, HHNK, or DI), and hypervolemia (which may occur in SIADH)
   C. Respiratory rate
      1. Bradypnea is often seen in hypothyroidism
      2. Tachypnea may be associated with hyperthyroidism, infection (which may be a cause of

Target hormone level is low

Hypothalamus senses low level

Hypothalamus releases releasing factor

Releasing factor stimulates pituitary to secrete stimulating hormone

Stimulating hormone stimulates target gland to produce and/or release target hormone

Hypothalamus senses increase in circulating target hormone

Hypothalamus does not release releasing factor

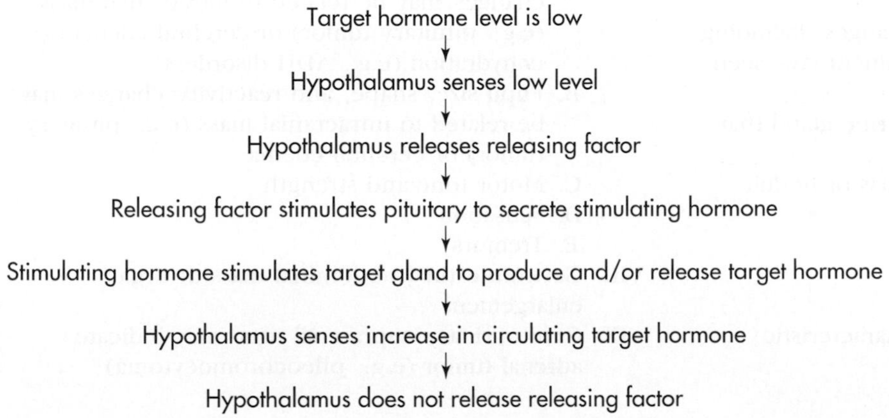

Figure 10-3   Negative feedback.

DKA or HHNK), hypovolemia (which may occur in DKA, HHNK, or DI), and hypervolemia (which may occur in SIADH)

D. Temperature
1. Hypothermia may be associated with hypothyroidism
2. Hyperthermia may be associated with hyperthyroidism with extreme hyperthermia during thyroid crisis
3. Hyperthermia may also indicate infection that may be a cause of DKA or HHNK

II. General survey
A. Apparent health status
B. Apparent age (consistency with chronologic age)
C. Gross deformity or asymmetry
D. Nutritional status
E. Stature and posture
F. Redistribution of body fat (e.g., Cushing's syndrome [hyperadrenocortical function] causes redistribution of fat with "buffalo hump," "moon face," thick trunk with thin arms and legs)
G. Gynecomastia in males: may be related to hypogonadism, hyperthyroidism, Cushing's syndrome
H. Mobility
I. Level of consciousness: changes in cerebral function may occur
J. Presence of Medic-Alert bracelet indicating chronic endocrine condition or steroid dependency

III. Head and neck
A. Eyes
1. Eyeballs
a) Protruding eyeballs (exophthalmos): often seen in hyperthyroidism; lid lag often seen in patients with exophthalmos
b) Sunken: may be seen in hypothyroidism or dehydration
2. Strabismus: may be seen with hyperthyroidism
B. Facial or periorbital edema: often seen in Cushing's syndrome; may also be seen in hypothyroidism
C. Changes in visual acuity and visual fields: may be related to pituitary tumor
D. Facial bone structure: facial changes, including protruding forehead and prominent jaw, seen in acromegaly
E. Thyroid gland (the only endocrine gland that can be palpated)
1. Enlargement or palpable mass or nodule
2. Tenderness
3. Presence of thrill

IV. Skin and appendages
A. Skin color changes
1. Addison's disease causes characteristic "bronzing" of the skin

2. Gray-brown pigmentation around neck and axillae may be seen in Cushing's syndrome
3. Yellowish skin discoloration may be seen in hypothyroidism

B. Skin temperature: skin temperature changes often seen in thyroid conditions
C. Skin moisture and turgor
1. Warm, moist, paper-thin skin may be seen in hyperthyroidism
2. Dry, scaly skin may be seen in hypothyroidism
3. Decreased skin turgor may be seen in dehydration, which may be seen in DI, DKA, HHNK
D. Skin lesions: acne, spider angiomata
E. Mucous membranes: note moisture
F. Scars (especially in neck area, which may indicate prior thyroid surgery)
G. Bruising: increased bruising may be seen in Cushing's syndrome
H. Striae: purplish striae on abdomen may be seen in Cushing's syndrome
I. Hair changes
1. Alopecia: may be seen in hyperthyroidism, hypothyroidism, hypopituitarism
2. Coarse hair: often seen in hypothyroidism
3. Thin, silky hair: frequently seen in hyperthyroidism
4. Increased body or facial hair: may be seen in acromegaly or Cushing's disease
J. Brittle nails: often seen in hypothyroidism
K. Enlargement and protrusion of tongue: may be seen in hypothyroidism or acromegaly

V. Cardiovascular
A. Point of maximal impulse (PMI) displacement: may indicate cardiomegaly, which may be seen in hypothyroidism
B. Heave: may be associated with heart failure, which may be seen in hyperthyroidism
C. Peripheral pulses: increased or decreased quality

VI. Pulmonary
A. Odor of breath: acetone (fruity) breath noted in DKA
B. Respiratory rate, depth, and rhythm

VII. Neurologic
A. Level of consciousness or mental status changes: may be related to intracranial mass (e.g., pituitary tumor) or cerebral edema or dehydration (e.g., ADH disorders)
B. Pupil size, shape, and reactivity: changes may be related to intracranial mass (e.g., pituitary tumor) or cerebral edema
C. Motor tone and strength
D. Sensation
E. Tremors

VIII. Gastrointestinal: abdominal mass or organ enlargement

IX. Genitourinary: suprarenal mass may indicate adrenal tumor (e.g., pheochromocytoma)

Percussion

I. Neurologic: changes in deep tendon reflexes (increased or decreased) may be related to serum sodium changes seen in DI or SIADH

Auscultation

I. Head and neck: thyroid gland bruits
II. Cardiovascular: heart sound changes
    A. S_3: indicative of HF, which may be seen in patients with hyperthyroidism
    B. Systolic murmur: often heard in high cardiac output states (e.g., hyperthyroidism)
III. Pulmonary: crackles noted with fluid overload and pulmonary edema, which may be seen in SIADH
IV. Gastrointestinal: bowel sounds changes (hyperactive or hypoactive)

Diagnostic Studies

I. Serum
    A. Sodium: normal 136 to 145 mEq/L
    B. Potassium: normal 3.5 to 5.0 mEq/L
    C. Chloride: normal 96 to 106 mEq/L
    D. Calcium: normal 8.5 to 10.5 mg/dl
    E. Phosphorus: normal 3.0 to 4.5 mg/dl
    F. Magnesium: normal 1.5 to 2.5 mEq/L
    G. Glucose: normal 70 to 110 mg/dl
    H. Glycosylated hemoglobin: normal 4% to 7%
    I. Osmolality: normal 280 to 295 mOsm/L
    J. BUN: normal 5 to 20 mg/dl
    K. Creatinine: normal 0.7 to 1.5 mg/dl
    L. Ketones: normal negative
    M. Hormone levels
        1. Thyroid-stimulating hormone (TSH): normal 2 to 10 mU/ml
        2. T_3: normal 0.2 to 0.3 µg/dl
        3. T_4: normal 6 to 12 µg/dl
        4. ACTH: normal 15 to 100 pg/ml in AM, less than 50 pg/ml in PM
        5. Cortisol: normal 6 to 28 µg/dl at 8 AM, 2 to 12 µg/dl at 4 PM
        6. ADH: normal 1 to 5 pg/ml
    N. Arterial blood gases
        1. pH: normal 7.35 to 7.45
        2. $Paco_2$: normal 35 to 45 mm Hg
        3. HCO_3: normal 22 to 26 mEq/L
        4. Pao_2: normal 80 to 100 mm Hg
    O. Hematocrit: normal 40% to 52% for males, 35% to 47% for females
    P. Hemoglobin: normal 13 to 18 g/dl for males, 12 to 16 g/dl for females
    Q. White blood cells (WBC): normal 3,500 to 11,000 mm^3
II. Urine
    A. Glucose: normal negative
    B. Ketones: normal negative
    C. Specific gravity: normal 1.005 to 1.030
    D. Osmolality: normal 50 to 1,200 mOsm/L
    E. 17-hydroxycorticosteroids: normal 4.5 to 10 mg/24 hr for males, 2.5 to 10 mg/24 hr for females

F. 17-ketosteroids: normal 8 to 15 mg/24 hr for males, 6 to 12 mg/24 hr for females
III. Radiologic studies
    A. Skull series
    B. Chest X-ray
    C. Flat plate of abdomen (KUB)
    D. CT (computed tomography) scan of head or abdomen
    E. Magnetic resonance imaging (MRI)
    F. Pancreatic scan
    G. Thyroid scan
    H. Thyroid ultrasound
    I. Fine-needle aspiration biopsy of thyroid gland
    J. Adrenal angiography
    K. Brain scan
IV. Other studies
    A. Electrocardiogram (ECG)
    B. Electroencephalogram (EEG)

Diabetes Insipidus (DI)

Definition: Clinical condition characterized by impaired renal conservation of water, resulting in polyuria, low urine specific gravity, dehydration, and hypernatremia; caused either by deficiency of ADH or decreased renal responsiveness to ADH

Etiology

I. Neurogenic (or central) DI: defect in release or synthesis of antidiuretic hormone (ADH)
    A. Congenital, idiopathic
    B. Intracranial tumors: especially hypothalamic or pituitary
    C. Extracranial neoplasm: leukemia, breast cancer
    D. CNS injury: especially basal skull fracture
    E. Postcraniotomy
    F. Intracerebral hemorrhage
    G. CNS infections (e.g., meningitis, encephalitis)
    H. Cerebral hypoxia and/or anoxic brain syndrome
    I. Granulomatous diseases
    J. Drugs that inhibit the secretion of ADH (Table 10-2)
        1. Ethanol
        2. Phenytoin (Dilantin)
        3. Chlorpromazine (Thorazine)
        4. Reserpine (Serpasil)
II. Nephrogenic DI: defect in renal tubular response to ADH; usually less severe than neurogenic DI
    A. Congenital
    B. Renal disease
    C. Drugs that block the effect of ADH on the renal tubules (Table 10-2)
        1. Lithium
        2. Demeclocycline (Declomycin), a tetracycline derivative
        3. α adrenergic agents (e.g., norepinephrine)
        4. Caffeine
        5. Amphotericin B

Table 10-2 Drugs Affecting the Action of ADH

Drugs That Decrease the Amount or Action of ADH (May Cause DI, Some May Be Used to Treat SIADH)	Drugs That Increase the Amount or Effect of ADH (May Cause SIADH, Some May Be Used to Treat DI)
• Ethanol alcohol • Phenytoin (Dilantin) • Chlorpromazine (Thorazine) • Reserpine (Serpasil) • Lithium • Demeclocycline (Declomycin), a tetracycline derivative • α adrenergic agents (e.g., norepinephrine) • Caffeine • Amphotericin B	• General anesthetics • Narcotics: morphine, meperidine • Barbiturates • Thiazide diuretics: hydrochlorothiazide (HydroDIURIL) • Tricyclic antidepressants: amitriptyline (Elavil) • Oral hypoglycemics: chlorpropamide (Diabinese) • Acetaminophen • Cytotoxic agents: vincristine (Oncovin); cyclophosphamide (Cytoxan) • Nicotine • Anticonvulsants: carbamazepine (Tegretol) • β adrenergic agents (e.g., isoproterenol) • Antihyperlipidemics: clofibrate (Atromid-S)

D. Result of electrolyte imbalance
 1. Hypokalemia
 2. Hypercalcemia
III. Psychogenic DI: result of psychogenic polydipsia

Pathophysiology (Fig. 10-4)
 I. Deficiency of ADH or inadequate renal tubule response to ADH, leading to inadequate antidiuresis
 II. Diuresis of large volumes of hypotonic urine
 III. Dehydration and hypernatremia
 IV. Potential shock and/or neurologic effects
 V. Permanent versus temporary
  A. Permanent DI follows hypophysectomy (removal of pituitary gland)
  B. Temporary DI usually resolves within 5 to 7 days

Clinical Presentation
 I. History of precipitating event: clinical indications may not occur for 1 to 3 days because of utilization of stored ADH
 II. Subjective
  A. Thirst, especially for cold liquids
  B. Fatigue, weakness
 III. Objective
  A. Polyuria: 5 to 15 L/24 hr; suspect DI if urine output is greater than 200 ml/hr for 2 consecutive hours
  B. Clinical indications of dehydration and volume depletion
   1. Weight loss
   2. Poor skin turgor
   3. Dry mucous membranes
   4. Sunken eyeballs
   5. Postural hypotension, tachycardia
   6. Decrease in CVP, RAP, PAP, PAOP, CO/CI
  C. Neurologic signs resulting from hyperosmolality and hypernatremia
   1. Restlessness, confusion, irritability
   2. Seizures
   3. Lethargy, coma

IV. Diagnostic
 A. Serum
  1. Sodium: elevated, usually greater than 145 mEq/L (hyperosmolar hypernatremia caused by water loss)
  2. BUN: elevated
  3. Increased serum osmolality: elevated, greater than 295 mOsm/L
  4. Hematocrit elevated
  5. Serum ADH level: decreased (<1 pg/ml)
 B. Urine
  1. Specific gravity: decreased, less than 1.005
  2. Osmolality: less than serum osmolality; less than 200 mOsm/L
 C. Water deprivation test may be performed (**Note:** Because of the risks of dehydration, this test is usually not performed on a critically ill patient)
  1. Prestudy weight, serum, urine osmolality, and urine specific gravity are measured
  2. Fluid intake is withheld
  3. Measurements are repeated hourly until one of the following occurs:
   a) Negative results: urine specific gravity exceeds 1.020, urine osmolality exceeds 800 mOsm/L
   b) Positive results: 5% of body weight is lost or urine specific gravity does not increase after 3 consecutive hours
  4. Discontinue if hypotension, tachycardia, or lethargy occur
  5. Inability to concentrate urine when fluid-deprived suggests diabetes insipidus, and a vasopressin test should be performed
 D. Vasopressin test
  1. Exogenous ADH (usually 5 U of aqueous vasopressin) is administered subcutaneously; urine specimens are collected every 30 minutes for 2 hours and evaluated for quantity and osmolality
   a) If neurogenic DI: urine output decreases and urine osmolality increases by more than 9%

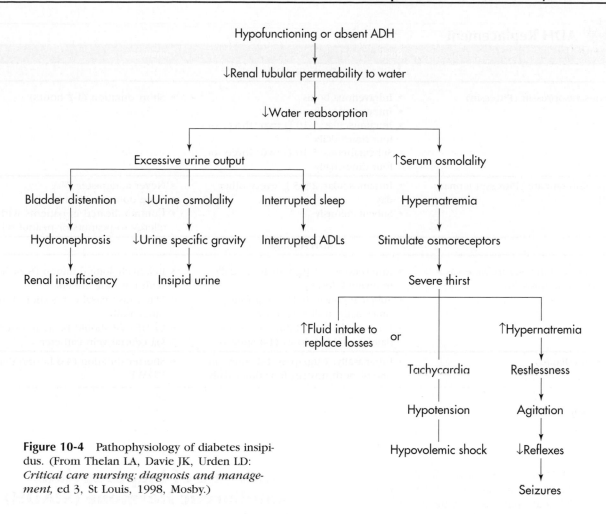

Figure 10-4   Pathophysiology of diabetes insipidus. (From Thelan LA, Davie JK, Urden LD: *Critical care nursing: diagnosis and management,* ed 3, St Louis, 1998, Mosby.)

b) If nephrogenic DI: no response to ADH will be seen

Nursing Diagnoses

I. Fluid Volume Deficit related to diuresis caused by ADH deficiency or decreased effect of ADH on renal tubule
II. Decreased Cardiac Output related to decreased preload
III. Risk for Injury related to altered consciousness, electrolyte imbalance
IV. Ineffective Individual Coping related to situational crisis, powerlessness, change in role
V. Ineffective Family Coping related to critically ill family member
VI. Knowledge Deficit related to health maintenance

Collaborative Management

I. Detect clinical indications of DI in high-risk patients
   A. Monitor urine output hourly; measure urine specific gravity if indicated by increase in urine output
   B. Monitor weight daily (1 kg = 1 L)
   C. Monitor serum sodium levels

D. Note or calculate serum osmolality
E. Monitor for clinical indications of hypovolemia, hypoperfusion
II. Correct fluid deficit
   A. Type of volume replacement: hypotonic solutions such as 0.45% sodium chloride solution or D_5W depending on degree of hyperosmolality; if patient very hyperosmolar, D_5W would be used; less hypersmolar, ½NS
   B. Rate of volume replacement: determined by volume of urine output and insensible losses (e.g., hourly urine output plus 50 ml/hr)
III. Treat the cause
   A. Administer exogenous ADH replacement as prescribed for neurogenic DI (Table 10-3)
      1. Side effects to monitor for: hypertension, chest pain, water intoxication, abdominal cramping
   B. Assist in preoperative preparation and postoperative management after hypophysectomy if pituitary tumor is the cause; usually done by transsphenoidal approach (see Fig. 7-2)
      1. Incision is made in the gingiva above the maxilla and then pituitary gland is removed through the sphenoid

Table 10-3 ADH Replacement

Drug	Route	Comments
Synthetic ADH		
Aqueous vasopressin (Pitressin)	• Intravenous bolus • Intravenous infusion • Intramuscular: 5-10 U two, three, or four times daily • Subcutaneous: 5-10 U two, three, or four times daily	• Short duration (1-2 hours)
Vasopressin tannate (Pitressin tannate in oil)	• Intramuscular: 2.5-5 U every other day • Subcutaneously	• Never administer IV • Long duration (72 hours) • Contraindicated in patients with allergy to peanuts or peanut oil
ADH Analogs		
DDAVP (1,deamino-8-D-arginine vaso-pressin) (Desmopressin)	• Intravenous: 2-4 μg four times daily in divided doses • Subcutaneously: 0.2-0.4 mg four times daily in divided doses • Intranasally: 0.1-0.4 mg four times daily in divided doses (1-4 sprays)	• Relatively long duration (8-24 hours) with few side effects • May cause nasal congestion if given intranasally • IV DDAVP should be administered via central vein catheter
Lypressin (Diapid)	• Intranasally: 7 μg/spray 1-2 sprays in one or both nostrils four times daily	• Shorter duration (4-6 hours) than DDAVP

2. Antibiotic-impregnated nasal packing is usually maintained for 48 to 72 hours
3. CSF leak may be seen during first 72 hours; mustache dressing is used to collect CSF
C. Administer ADH potentiator as prescribed for nephrogenic DI (Table 10-2)
   1. Chlorpropamide (Diabinese) used most often: stimulates the release of ADH from the pituitary gland and enhances its effect at the renal tubule; monitor for hypoglycemia
   2. Thiazide diuretics and sodium restriction may also be used: mild sodium depletion enhances water reabsorption
D. Administer pharmacologic agents as prescribed for obsessive compulsive behavior (e.g., serotonin reuptake inhibitors, tricyclic antidepressants, or monoamine oxidase inhibitors) for psychogenic polydipsia
IV. Correct electrolyte imbalance: potassium replacement usually required
V. Maintain patient safety
   A. Safe environment: siderails up, call light within reach
   B. Seizure precautions
   C. Frequent reorientation
VI. Monitor for complications
   A. Coma
   B. Hypovolemic shock
   C. Thromboembolism

Syndrome of Inappropriate Antidiuretic Hormone (SIADH)
Definition
I. Clinical condition characterized by impaired renal excretion of water, resulting in oliguria, high urine specific gravity, water intoxication, and hyponatremia
II. Caused either by excess of ADH or ADH-like substance or an increased renal responsiveness to ADH

Etiology
I. Neurogenic SIADH: increased production and/or release of ADH
   A. Pituitary tumor
   B. CNS trauma
   C. Stroke: thrombotic or hemorrhagic
   D. Intracranial hematoma
   E. CNS infection: encephalitis, meningitis
   F. CNS hemorrhage
   G. Guillain-Barré syndrome
   H. Cerebral infarction or atrophy
   I. Nonmalignant pulmonary disease
      1. Tuberculosis
      2. Pneumonia
      3. Lung abscess
      4. Chronic obstructive pulmonary disease
      5. Positive-pressure ventilation
II. Ectopic SIADH: production of a substance indistinguishable from ADH by tissue
   A. Oat-cell (small cell) cancer of the lung

B. Duodenal cancer
C. Pancreatic cancer
D. Prostatic cancer
E. Leukemia
F. Lymphoma: Hodgkin's and non-Hodgkin's
G. Thymoma
H. Lymphosarcoma

III. Nephrogenic SIADH: pharmacologic agents that increase ADH secretion or ADH effect (Table 10-2)
A. General anesthetics
B. Narcotics: morphine, meperidine
C. Barbiturates
D. Thiazide diuretics: hydrochlorothiazide (HydroDIURIL)
E. Tricyclic antidepressants: amitriptyline (Elavil)
F. Oral hypoglycemics: chlorpropamide (Diabinese)
G. Acetaminophen
H. Cytotoxic agents: vincristine (Oncovin), cyclophosphamide (Cytoxan)
I. Nicotine
J. Anticonvulsants: carbamazepine (Tegretol)
K. β adrenergic agents (e.g., isoproterenol)
L. Antihyperlipidemics: clofibrate (Atromid-S)

Pathophysiology (Fig. 10-5)

I. Increased secretion of ADH or ADH-like substance or increased renal responsiveness to ADH
II. Failure of negative feedback system: ADH secretion continues despite low serum osmolality
III. Renal reabsorption of water increases
IV. Water intoxication
V. Hyponatremia, hypoosmolality
VI. Potential cerebral edema and seizures

Clinical Presentation

I. Subjective
A. Anorexia
B. Nausea
C. Dyspnea may be reported if pulmonary edema develops
D. Headache
E. Inability to concentrate
F. Muscle weakness and/or cramps

II. Objective
A. Oliguria (<0.5 ml/kg/hr)
B. Clinical indications of fluid overload
1. Tachypnea
2. Hypertension
3. Weight gain without edema
4. Fever
5. Jugular venous distention (JVD)
6. Breath sound changes: crackles
7. Increased CVP, RAP, PAP, PAOP
C. GI
1. Vomiting
2. Diarrhea
3. Diminished bowel sounds
D. Neurologic
1. Personality changes

2. Altered level of consciousness: confusion, lethargy progressing to coma
3. Decreased deep tendon reflexes
4. Seizures related to hyponatremia

III. Diagnostic
A. Serum
1. Sodium: decreased; often less than 120 mEq/L (hypoosmolar hyponatremia caused by water retention)
2. Potassium: may be decreased
3. Calcium: may be decreased
4. BUN: decreased
5. Osmolality: decreased; less than 280 mOsm/L
6. Plasma ADH: more than 5 pg/ml
B. Urine
1. Specific gravity: elevated; more than 1.030
2. Osmolality: elevated; often greater than 1,200 mOsm/L
C. Water load test (**Note:** Because of the risks of fluid overload, this test is not usually performed in a critically ill patient)
1. Patient is given an oral or IV fluid load (usually 20 ml/kg)
2. Urine is collected over the next 5 to 6 hours
a) Normal (negative): excretion of 80% of amount of fluid administered
b) Positive: excretion of less than 40% of amount of fluid administered

Nursing Diagnoses

I. Fluid Volume Excess related to oliguria caused by excess ADH or effect of ADH
II. Risk for Decreased Adaptive Capacity related to hypervolemia, intracranial hypertension
III. Risk for Injury related to seizures, alteration in consciousness, electrolyte imbalance
IV. Ineffective Individual Coping related to situational crisis, powerlessness, change in role
V. Ineffective Family Coping related to critically ill family member
VI. Knowledge Deficit related to health maintenance

Collaborative Management

I. Detect clinical indications of SIADH in high-risk patients
A. Monitor urine output hourly; measure urine specific gravity if indicated by decrease in urine output
B. Monitor weight daily (1 kg = 1 L)
C. Monitor serum sodium levels
D. Note or calculate serum osmolality
E. Monitor for clinical indications of hypervolemia, pulmonary edema, intracranial hypertension
II. Treat the cause
A. Surgical intervention to remove malignant lesion if it is causative agent
B. Demeclocycline (Declomycin), phenytoin (Dilantin), or lithium may be used to inhibit the

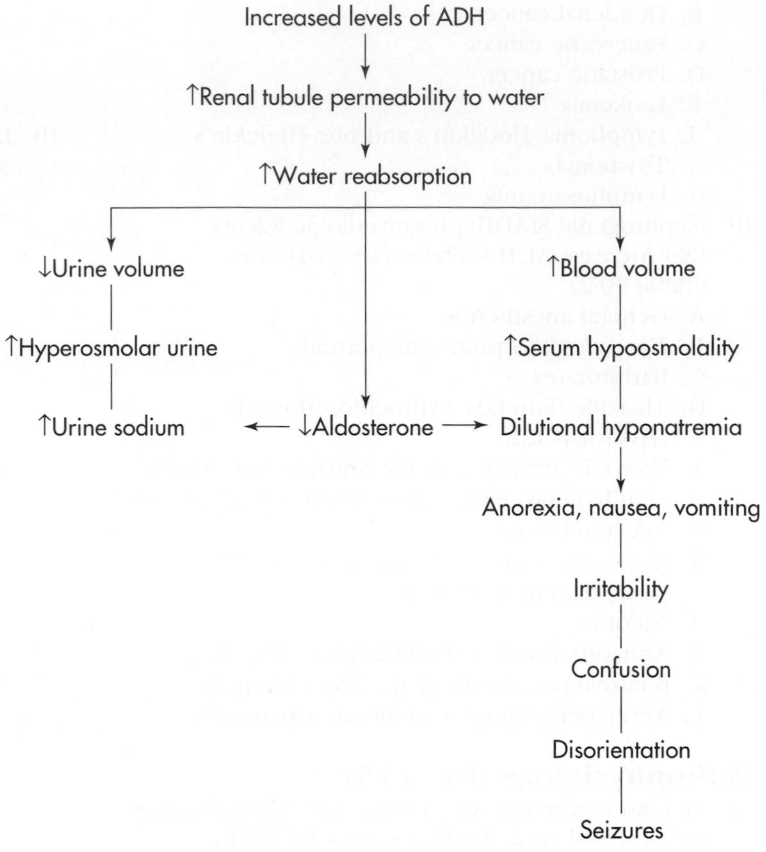

Increased levels of ADH
↓
↑Renal tubule permeability to water
↓
↑Water reabsorption

↓Urine volume   ↑Blood volume

↑Hyperosmolar urine   ↑Serum hypoosmolality

↑Urine sodium ←— ↓Aldosterone —→ Dilutional hyponatremia
↓
Anorexia, nausea, vomiting
↓
Irritability
↓
Confusion
↓
Disorientation
↓
Seizures

Figure 10-5 Pathophysiology of syndrome of inappropriate ADH secretion (SIADH). (From Thelan LA, Davie JK, Urden LD: *Critical care nursing: diagnosis and management,* ed 3, St Louis, 1998, Mosby.)

action of ADH on the renal tubules, especially with ectopic ADH
C. Discontinuance of causative drugs if possible
III. Correct fluid volume excess
A. Fluid restriction based on amounts lost in urine and insensible losses; usually restricted to 1,000 ml/day
B. Diuretics to promote water excretion: usually furosemide (Lasix) or mannitol (Osmitrol)
IV. Correct electrolyte imbalance
A. Dietary sodium should be encouraged
B. Hypertonic (3%) saline (usually 250-500 ml over several hours at rate of 1-2 ml/kg/hr) for serum sodium less than 115 mEq/L or if patient is having seizures
1. Hypertonic saline is usually discontinued when the serum sodium is 125 mEq/L
2. Monitor closely for clinical indications of pulmonary edema during and after hypertonic saline infusion
C. Potassium replacement may be needed
V. Provide for patient safety
A. Safe environment: siderails up, call light within reach
B. Seizure precautions
C. Frequent reorientation
VI. Monitor for complications
A. Intracranial hypertension
B. Seizures
C. Coma

Diabetic Ketoacidosis (DKA)
Definitions
I. Diabetes mellitus (DM): a group of metabolic diseases characterized by hyperglycemia (confirmed fasting serum glucose of greater than or equal to 126 mg/dl) that results from defects in insulin secretion, insulin action, or both
A. Type 1 diabetes is characterized by beta cell destruction, usually leading to absolute insulin deficiency; previously known as juvenile-onset, type I, insulin-dependent diabetes mellitus (IDDM)
B. Type 2 diabetes is characterized by insulin resistance and a relative (rather than absolute) insulin deficiency; previously known as age-onset, type II, non–insulin-dependent diabetes mellitus (NIDDM)
II. Hyperglycemic crises
A. Diabetic ketoacidosis: hyperglycemic crisis associated with metabolic acidosis and elevated serum ketones; the most serious metabolic disturbance of type 1 DM
B. Hyperglycemic hyperosmolar nonketotic condition: hyperglycemic crisis associated with the absence of ketone formation; most serious metabolic disturbance in type 2 DM

Etiology
I. Undiagnosed type 1 DM: 20% of patients with DKA
II. Causes in known type 1 DM
A. Illness or infection

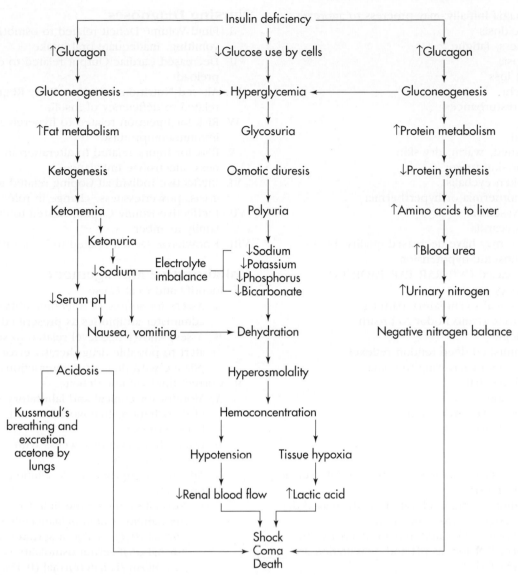

Figure 10-6 Pathophysiology of diabetic ketoacidosis. (From Thelan LA, Davie JK, Urden LD: *Critical care nursing: diagnosis and management,* ed 3, St Louis, 1998, Mosby.)

B. Omission of exogenous insulin
C. Trauma
D. Surgery
E. Noncompliance: too many calories
III. Causes in patients with or without diabetes
   A. Cushing's syndrome
   B. Hyperthyroidism
   C. Pancreatitis
   D. Pregnancy
   E. Drugs
      1. Glucocorticoids (e.g., prednisone)
      2. Thiazide diuretics (e.g., hydrochlorothiazide)
      3. Phenytoin (Dilantin)
      4. Sympathomimetics (e.g., epinephrine)
      5. Diazoxide (Hyperstat)

Pathophysiology (Fig. 10-6)

I. Insufficient insulin or cell's ability to use insulin
II. Without insulin, glucose cannot move into the cell and accumulates in the blood, causing hyperglycemia
III. Hyperglycemia causes an osmotic diuresis as the hypertonic solution goes through the renal tubules and pulls more water into the tubule; this diuresis causes glycosuria, dehydration, and electrolyte imbalance
IV. Breakdown of glycogen is activated and its synthesis inhibited; gluconeogenesis is stimulated to make new glucose from proteins and fats
V. Impaired glucose uptake by adipose tissue causes impaired triglyceride synthesis and liberation of free fatty acids (FFA) into blood
VI. Excessive fatty acids enter liver, leading to ketoacidosis

Clinical Presentation

I. Subjective
   A. Nausea
   B. Abdominal pain

C. Polyphagia initially; may progress to anorexia with acidosis

D. Weakness, fatigue

E. Polydipsia

F. Weight loss

G. Headache

H. Visual disturbances

II. Objective

A. General
  1. Flushed, warm, dry skin
  2. Poor skin turgor
  3. Sunken eyeballs
  4. Hypothermia or hyperthermia

B. Cardiovascular
  1. Tachycardia
  2. Pulse may have decreased quality: 1+/3+
  3. Orthostatic hypotension
  4. Decreased CVP, RAP, PAP, PAOP, CO

C. Pulmonary
  1. Kussmaul's ventilatory pattern
  2. Acetone (fruity) odor to breath

D. Neurologic
  1. Diminished deep tendon reflexes
  2. Lethargy progressing to coma

E. Gastrointestinal
  1. Vomiting
  2. Hypoactive bowel sounds

F. Renal: polyuria

III. Diagnostics

A. Serum
  1. Glucose: elevated 300 to 800 mg/dl; average 600 mg/dl
  2. Sodium: normal, elevated, or decreased depending on hydration status
  3. Potassium: elevated initially; decreases to normal or low as pH and dehydration are corrected
  4. Anion gap: elevated, more than 15
  5. Calcium: may be decreased
  6. Phosphorus: decreased
  7. Magnesium: elevated initially and then decreased
  8. Ketones: elevated, more than 3 mOsm/L
  9. BUN and creatinine elevated with BUN:creatinine ratio greater than 10:1
  10. Serum osmolality: elevated; usually 295 to 330 mOsm/L
  11. Lipids: may be elevated
  12. Arterial blood gases: metabolic acidosis often with some degree of respiratory compensation
      (1) pH less than 7.30
      (2) HCO_3 less than 15
      (3) $Paco_2$ less than 35 mm Hg
  13. Hematocrit: elevated
  14. WBC: elevated, unreliable indication of infection in DKA

B. Urine: positive for glucose and ketones

C. Electrocardiogram
  1. May show changes associated with potassium levels
  2. Sinus tachycardia is often seen

Nursing Diagnoses

I. Fluid Volume Deficit related to osmotic diuresis, vomiting, inadequate oral intake

II. Decreased Cardiac Output related to decreased preload

III. Altered Nutrition: Less than Body Requirements related to deficiency of insulin

IV. Risk for Infection related to hyperglycemia, immunocompromise

V. Risk for Injury related to alteration in consciousness, electrolyte imbalance

VI. Ineffective Individual Coping related to situational crisis, powerlessness, change in role

VII. Ineffective Family Coping related to critically ill family member

VIII. Knowledge Deficit related to health maintenance

Collaborative Management

I. Identify and treat cause

A. Assess for source of infection: obtain cultures; administer antibiotics as prescribed

B. Assess knowledge level related to self-care; be alert to possible drug therapy errors, noncompliance with diet, drug interactions

II. Correct fluid volume deficit

A. Monitor for clinical and laboratory indications of dehydration, hypovolemia, and hypoperfusion

B. Establish intravenous access with at least one large-gauge catheter

C. Administer appropriate IV solution as prescribed
  1. Normal saline for the first 1 to 2 L or until the patient is hemodynamically stable; then normal (0.9%) saline if serum sodium is normal or if serum osmolality is less than 320 mOsm/L; half-normal (0.45%) saline if hypernatremic or serum osmolality is greater than 320 mOsm/L
  2. Colloids such as albumin or plasma protein fraction may be needed, especially if the patient is hypotensive
  3. Dextrose 5% is added (e.g., D_5NS or $D_5\frac{1}{2}NS$) when serum glucose reaches 250 to 300 mg/dl
  4. Dextrose 10% may be used if serum glucose falls to 150 mg/dl or less

D. Administer IV fluid replacement at appropriate rate as prescribed
  1. First hour: 10 to 30 ml/kg for first hour
  2. After first hour: 500 to 1,000 ml/hr depending on cardiovascular status, volume deficit, and urine output
  3. Total volume deficit: usually 4 to 8 L

III. Normalize serum glucose level gradually

A. Administer IV regular insulin injection as prescribed: usually 10 to 20 U (or 0.15 U/kg) followed by infusion

B. Initiate IV regular insulin infusion as prescribed: usually 5 to 10 U/hr (or 0.1 U/kg/hr)
  1. Insulin is mixed in normal saline, and the IV tubing is flushed with 50 ml of insulin solu-

tion to saturate binding sites on the IV tubing before administration
2. Serum glucose should drop by no more than 75 to 100 mg/dl/hr to avoid hypoglycemia, hypokalemia, and cerebral edema
3. Insulin infusion is usually decreased to 3 to 5 U/hr when serum glucose is less than 250 mg/dl and usually discontinued 1 to 2 hours after subcutaneous insulin is started
C. Administer SC regular insulin as prescribed: usually administered by sliding scale when serum glucose is less than 250 mg/dl; pH greater than 7.2; bicarbonate greater than 18 mEq/L
IV. Correct electrolyte imbalance
A. Monitor for clinical and laboratory indications of hyperkalemia (initially) and hypokalemia, hypophosphatemia, and hypomagnesemia (with insulin therapy)
B. Replace potassium as prescribed
1. Potassium levels are monitored hourly initially
2. Usually total body potassium is severely depleted but serum levels show normal level or hyperkalemia because an intracellular to extracellular shift occurs because acidosis is present
3. Potassium replacement is started when potassium level is at upper limit of normal
   a) Usually in the form of KCl, but a portion may be given in the form of KPO_4 depending on phosphorus levels
4. Refractory hypokalemia suggests hypocalcemia and/or hypomagnesemia
C. Replace phosphorus as prescribed
1. Often low, especially with insulin therapy; replacement is indicated, especially if patient is anemic, has HF, pneumonia or any other cause of hypoxia (Remember that hypophosphatemia shifts the oxyhemoglobin curve to the left and impairs tissue oxygenation) or if serum phosphate level is less than 1 mg/dl
2. Two-thirds to one-half of potassium is replaced with KCl and one-third to one-half of potassium is replaced with KPO_4
3. To prevent hypocalcemia, phosphate administration should not exceed 1.5 mEq/kg/24 hr
D. Replace magnesium as prescribed; usually replaced as 1 to 2 g of 10% solution if renal function adequate
V. Correct acid-base imbalance
A. Provide adequate rehydration and insulin therapy
B. Administer sodium bicarbonate as prescribed; (**Note:** Sodium bicarbonate is only recommended today for severe acidosis [pH 7.0 or less] and should be discontinued as soon as pH is 7.2)

C. Monitor for hyperchloremic acidosis caused by NaCl and KCl administration
VI. Safety
A. Prevent aspiration resulting from paralytic ileus commonly seen in DKA
1. Keep head of bed elevated 30 degrees
2. Insert nasogastric tube as indicated
B. Maintain seizure precautions
C. Monitor serum glucose and electrolytes carefully
VII. Monitor for complications
A. Cardiovascular
1. Hypovolemic shock
2. Dysrhythmias
3. Thromboembolism
4. Myocardial infarction
5. Pulmonary edema
B. Neurologic
1. Cerebral edema
2. Seizures
3. Coma
C. Endocrine: hypoglycemia
D. Renal
1. Acute renal failure
2. Electrolyte imbalances: potassium, sodium, phosphorus, magnesium

Hyperglycemic Hyperosmolar Nonketotic Syndrome (HHNK)

Definition: Hyperglycemic crisis associated with the absence of ketone formation; most common severe metabolic disturbance in type 2 diabetes mellitus

Etiology: usually seen in patients over 50 years with glucose intolerance or type 2 diabetes mellitus; often iatrogenic, may be precipitated by any of the following:
I. Pancreatitis
II. Burns
III. Infection
IV. Hepatitis
V. Trauma
VI. Cushing's syndrome
VII. Hyperthyroidism
VIII. Renal disease
   A. Peritoneal dialysis
   B. Hemodialysis
IX. Hypertonic nutrition: enteral or parenteral
X. Alcohol
XI. Drugs
   A. Glucocorticoids (e.g., prednisone)
   B. Thiazide diuretics (e.g., hydrochlorothiazide)
   C. Loop diuretics (e.g., furosemide [Lasix])
   D. Phenytoin (Dilantin)
   E. Diazoxide (Hyperstat)
   F. Immunosuppressive drugs
   G. Beta-blockers (e.g., propranolol [Inderal])
   H. Chlorpromazine (Thorazine)

    I. Cimetidine (Tagamet)
    J. Calcium channel blockers
    K. Mannitol
    L. Sympathomimetics drugs (e.g., epinephrine)
    M. Thyroid preparations

Pathophysiology (Fig. 10-7)

I. Relative insulin deficiency
II. Without insulin, glucose cannot move into the cell and accumulates in the blood, causing hyperglycemia (hyperglycemia is severe)
III. Hyperglycemia causes an osmotic diuresis as the hypertonic solution goes through the renal tubules and pulls more water into the tubule; this diuresis causes glycosuria, dehydration, and electrolyte imbalance
IV. Sufficient insulin is present to inhibit gluconeogenesis; therefore breakdown of fat and protein with resultant ketoacidosis and muscle wasting does not occur
V. Osmotic diuresis causes serum hyperosmolality, cellular dehydration, and decreased glomerular filtration rate
VI. Thrombosis, renal failure, and neurologic changes may result

Clinical Presentation

I. Subjective: weakness, fatigue
II. Objective
  A. General
    1. Weight loss
    2. Flushed, warm, dry skin
    3. Poor skin turgor
    4. Polydipsia
    5. Fever common
  B. Cardiovascular
    1. Tachycardia
    2. Orthostatic hypotension
    3. Decreased CVP, RAP, PAP, PAOP, CO/CI
  C. Pulmonary: tachypnea
  D. Neurologic
    1. Sensory deficits: paresthesia
    2. Motor deficits: paresis, plegia
    3. Aphasia
    4. Decreased deep tendon reflexes
    5. Seizures
    6. Lethargy progressing to coma
  E. Renal: polyuria
III. Diagnostics
  A. Serum
    1. Glucose 600 to 2,000 mg/dl; average 1,100 mg/dl
    2. Sodium: normal or elevated
    3. Potassium: decreased
    4. Calcium: may be decreased
    5. Phosphorus: decreased
    6. Magnesium: decreased
    7. BUN and creatinine: elevated with BUN:creatinine ratio more than 10:1
    8. Serum osmolality elevated; often greater than 330; may be as high as 450 mOsm/L

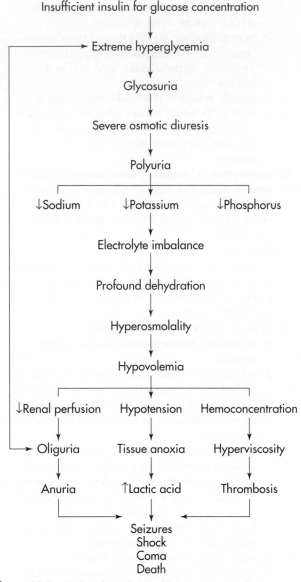

Figure 10-7 Pathophysiology of hyperglycemic hyperosmolar nonketotic syndrome. (From Thelan LA, Davie JK, Urden LD: *Critical care nursing: diagnosis and management,* ed 3, St Louis, 1998, Mosby.)

    9. Arterial blood gases: normal pH or only mildly acidotic; acidosis if present is lactic acidosis related to hypoperfusion instead of ketoacidosis
    10. Hematocrit: elevated
    11. WBC: elevated
  B. Urine
    1. Glucose: positive
    2. Ketones: negative
  C. Electrocardiogram
    1. May show changes associated with potassium levels
    2. May show sinus tachycardia

Nursing Diagnoses

I. Fluid Volume Deficit related to osmotic diuresis
II. Decreased Cardiac Output related to decreased preload

III. Altered Nutrition: Less than Body Requirements related to relative deficiency of insulin
IV. Risk for Infection related to hyperglycemia, immunocompromise
V. Risk for Injury related to alteration in consciousness, electrolyte imbalance
VI. Ineffective Individual Coping related to situational crisis, powerlessness, change in role
VII. Ineffective Family Coping related to critically ill family member
VIII. Knowledge Deficit related to health maintenance

Collaborative Management

I. Identify and treat cause
   A. Assess for source of infection: obtain cultures; administer antibiotics as prescribed
   B. Monitor serum glucose in patients on enteral and parenteral nutrition, glucocorticoids, dialysis, diuretics
   C. Assess knowledge level related to self-care; be alert to possible drug therapy errors, noncompliance with diet, drug interactions
II. Correct fluid volume deficit
   A. Monitor for clinical and laboratory indications of dehydration, hypovolemia, and hypoperfusion; hemodynamic monitoring is often necessary to guide fluid resuscitation because of the patient's age and health
   B. Establish intravenous access with at least one large-gauge catheter
   C. Administer appropriate IV solution as prescribed
      1. Normal saline usually used for the first 1 to 2 L or until the patient is hemodynamically stable; then normal (0.9%) saline if serum sodium normal or if serum osmolality is less than 320 mOsm/L; half-normal (0.45%) saline if hypernatremic or serum osmolality is greater than 320 mOsm/L
      2. Colloids such as albumin or plasma protein fraction may be needed, especially if the patient is hypotensive
      3. Dextrose 5% is added (e.g., D_5NS or $D_5\frac{1}{2}NS$) when serum glucose reaches 250 to 300 mg/dl
      4. Dextrose 10% may be used if serum glucose falls to 150 mg/dl or less
   D. Administer intravenous fluid replacement at appropriate rate
      1. First hour: 10 to 30 ml/kg for first hour
      2. After first hour: 500 to 1,000 ml/hr depending on cardiovascular status, volume deficit, and urine output
      3. Total volume deficit: usually 8 to 15 L
III. Normalize serum glucose level gradually (**Note:** Even though HHNK causes higher serum glucose levels, smaller amounts of insulin are needed to normalize serum glucose)
   A. Administer IV regular insulin injection as prescribed: usually 10 to 20 U (or 0.15-0.30 U/kg) followed by infusion

B. Initiate IV regular insulin infusion as prescribed: usually 5 to 10 U/hr (or 0.1 U/kg/hr)
   1. Insulin is mixed in normal saline, and the IV tubing is flushed with 50 ml of insulin solution to saturate binding sites on the IV tubing before administration
   2. Serum glucose should drop by no more than 75 to 100 mg/dl/hr to avoid hypoglycemia, hypokalemia, and cerebral edema
C. Administer SC regular insulin as prescribed
   1. Usually administered by sliding scale when serum glucose is less than 250 mg/dl; pH more than 7.2; bicarbonate more than 18 mEq/L
   2. IV insulin infusion usually discontinued when SC insulin is initiated; note that no overlap is usually required in HHNK
IV. Correct electrolyte imbalance
   A. Monitor for clinical and laboratory indications of hyperkalemia (initially) and hypokalemia, hypophosphatemia, and hypomagnesemia (with insulin therapy)
   B. Replace potassium as prescribed
      1. Potassium levels are monitored hourly initially
      2. Usually severely depleted; serum levels show severe hypokalemia since no intracellular to extracellular shift occurs because acidosis is not usually present
      3. Replacement usually in the form of KCl, but a portion may be in form of KPO_4 depending on phosphorus levels
   C. Replace phosphorus as prescribed
      1. Often low, especially with insulin therapy; replacement is indicated, especially if patient is anemic, has HF, pneumonia, or any other cause of hypoxia or if serum phosphate level is less than 1 mg/dl
      2. Two-thirds to one-half of potassium is replaced with KCl and one-third to one-half of potassium is replaced with KPO_4
      3. To prevent hypocalcemia, potassium phosphate administration should not exceed 1.5 mEq/kg/24 hr
   D. Replace magnesium as prescribed; usually replaced as 1 to 2 g of 10% solution if renal function adequate
V. Safety
   A. Prevent aspiration resulting from paralytic ileus commonly seen in DKA
      1. Keep head of bed elevated 30 degrees
      2. Insert nasogastric tube as indicated
   B. Maintain seizure precautions
   C. Monitor serum glucose and electrolytes carefully
VI. Monitor for complications
   A. Cardiovascular
      1. Hypovolemic shock
      2. Dysrhythmias
      3. Thromboembolism
      4. Myocardial infarction
      5. Pulmonary edema

B. Neurologic
1. Cerebral edema
2. Intracranial hypertension
3. Cerebral infarction
4. Coma
C. Endocrine: hypoglycemia
D. Renal
1. Acute renal failure
2. Electrolyte imbalances: potassium, sodium, phosphorus, magnesium

Hypoglycemia

Definition: Decrease in the amount of glucose in the blood; serum glucose level of 50 mg/dl or less or a sudden decrease in serum glucose even though the level is not less than 50 mg/dl

Etiology

I. Insufficient nutrient intake
   A. Missed or delayed meal
   B. Nausea, vomiting
   C. Interrupted enteral or parenteral nutrition
II. Excessive insulin dose
   A. Poor visual acuity causing dose inaccuracy
   B. Change from pork or beef insulin to human insulin (Humulin)
   C. Injection in area of improved absorption
III. Sulfonylurea therapy
   A. Renal insufficiency potentiates effects
   B. Hepatic insufficiency delays metabolism and excretion and impairs gluconeogenesis and glycogenolysis
   C. Potentiated by salicylates, sulfonamides, phenylbutazone, α-glucosidase inhibitors (e.g., acarbose [Precose], miglitol [Glyset])
IV. Inadequate production of glucose
   A. Strenuous physical exercise or stress with inadequate adjustment of food intake and/or insulin dosage
   B. Excessive alcohol intake ingested without adequate food intake
   C. Glucagon deficiency
V. Postgastrectomy
VI. Pancreatic islet cell necrosis: may occur with pentamidine therapy for *Pneumocystis carinii* infection; causes an acute increase in insulin release
VII. Pancreatic islet cell tumor (insulinoma)
VIII. Adrenal insufficiency
IX. Severe liver disease
X. Pregnancy

Pathophysiology

I. Too much insulin in relation to amount of glucose
II. Decrease in serum glucose levels to 50 mg/dl or below
III. Sympathetic nervous system (SNS) stimulation (**Note:** This stimulation and, therefore, the signs and symptoms are blocked by beta-blockers)
IV. Neuroglycopenic effects may cause neuronal damage: the brain must have a constant supply of glucose and cannot use any other substrates (e.g., protein, fat)
V. Rise in counterregulatory hormones: glucagon, epinephrine, cortisol, growth hormone with resultant rise in serum glucose

Clinical Presentation

I. Subjective
   A. Adrenergic (sympathetic) stimulation indicators
      1. Palpitations
      2. Irritability
      3. Anxiety
      4. Hunger
      5. Tingling
   B. Neuroglycopenic indicators
      1. Blurred vision, diplopia
      2. Headache
      3. Weakness
      4. Difficulty with concentration
      5. Fatigue
II. Objective
   A. Adrenergic (sympathetic) stimulation indicators
      1. Diaphoresis
      2. Pallor, cool skin
      3. Tremors
      4. Piloerection
      5. Tachycardia, tachypnea
   B. Neuroglycopenic indicators
      1. Vasomotor changes: hypotension
      2. Slurred speech
      3. Agitation
      4. Confusion
      5. Staggering gait
      6. Sensory changes: paresthesias
      7. Motor changes: paresis, hemiplegia, paraplegia
      8. Seizures
      9. Coma
   C. Nocturnal hypoglycemia
      1. Restless sleep
      2. Nightmares
      3. Early morning headache
III. Diagnostic
   A. Serum: glucose 50 mg/dl or less
      1. Glucose 20 to 40 mg/dl is associated with seizures
      2. Glucose less than 20 mg/dl is associated with coma
   B. Electrocardiogram: sinus tachycardia is seen

Nursing Diagnoses

I. Risk for Injury related to alteration in consciousness, seizures
II. Risk for Decreased Adaptive Capacity: Intracranial related to neuroglycopenic effects

Collaborative Management

I. Restore normal serum glucose level
   A. Measure serum glucose level immediately if clinical indications of hypoglycemia noted

B. Administer 10 to 15 g (40 to 60 cal) of carbohydrates for conscious patients (for examples see Box 10-1); glucose tablets or gel is required if the patient has been receiving an α-glucosidase inhibitor (e.g., acarbose [Precose], miglitol [Glyset])

C. Administer parenteral glucose if patient is unconscious
1. D$_{50}$W injection: usually 50 ml (25 g) over 3 to 5 minutes (**Note:** Thiamine 100 mg IV recommended prior to dextrose administration, especially in alcoholics to prevent Wernicke's encephalopathy)
2. D$_{10}$W or D$_5$W infusion as prescribed
3. Glucagon 1 mg IM: may be given to unconscious patients if unable to gain IV access

D. Provide longer acting carbohydrate source (milk, cheese, crackers) or regularly scheduled meal to avoid recurrence

E. Reassess serum glucose 15 minutes after treatment and every 15 minutes until serum glucose is within normal range

II. Prevent injury
A. Maintain airway if patient is unconscious
B. Monitor closely for seizures; maintain seizure precautions

III. Identify and treat cause of hypoglycemia
A. Assess serum glucose by laboratory or bedside glucose-monitoring device as indicated
B. Anticipate times when the patient is most likely to exhibit hypoglycemia
1. Be aware of peak times for administered insulin therapy (Table 10-4)
2. Be aware of missed or late meals or snacks, which predispose the patient to hypoglycemia
3. Be aware of excessive exertion, which may predispose the patient to hypoglycemia
4. Note any drugs that the patient is receiving, which may potentiate insulin
5. Be aware (and make patient and family aware) that beta-blockers block the SNS (early) symptoms of hypoglycemia; serum glucose testing should be done more often in patients on beta-blockers

C. Assess knowledge level related to self-care; be alert to possible drug therapy errors, noncompliance with diet, drug interactions
D. Assist with additional diagnostic studies if hypoglycemia is experienced by a patient who is not a known diabetic
E. Consider Somogyi phenomenon (insulin-induced posthypoglycemic hyperglycemia) as cause of early morning hyperglycemia

Table 10-4 Characteristics of Insulin Preparations

Insulin	Onset (hr)	Peak (hr)	Duration (hr)
Human regular (IV)	Immediate	¼-½	1-2
Human lispro (SC)	¼	½-1½	3-5
Human regular (SC)	½-1	2-3	5-7
Human NPH (SC)	2-4	4-10	14-18
Human Lente (SC)	3-4	4-12	16-20
Human Ultralente (SC)	6-10	14-24	20-36

1. The result of counterregulatory hormone secretion in response to hypoglycemia
2. Results in early morning hyperglycemia after nighttime hypoglycemia; needs to be differentiated from dawn phenomenon (hyperglycemia caused by nocturnal elevations in growth hormone)
3. Best documented by 3 AM serum glucose
4. Treated by a decrease in evening insulin dose and/or bedtime snack

IV. Monitor for complications
A. Myocardial ischemia or infarction
B. Seizures
C. Coma
D. Irreversible neurologic damage

LEARNING ACTIVITIES

1. **DIRECTIONS:** Complete the following crossword puzzle.

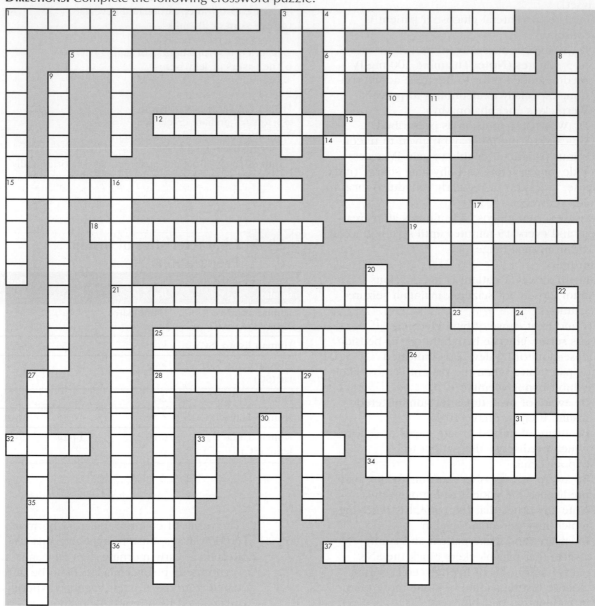

Across

1. Electrolyte imbalance noted initially in DKA
3. Hormone secreted by adrenal cortex, which causes the retention of sodium and water
5. Type of drug that blocks the early symptoms of hypoglycemia (2 words)
6. Caused by excessive secretion of growth hormone in an adult

10. Type of diabetes caused by ADH deficiency
12. Organ that produces glucagon and insulin
14. Hormone that enables glucose to move into the cell
15. Oral hypoglycemic that potentiates the action of ADH on the renal tubules (generic)

18. Type of DI caused by lack of responsiveness of the renal tubule to ADH
19. Type of regulation that controls the release or retention of hormone
21. Electrolyte imbalance that occurs in DKA with insulin therapy because glucose is able to move into the cell and increased amounts of ATP are produced

23. Hyperglycemic crisis that occurs in type 2 diabetics or patients with glucose intolerance (abbrev.)
25. Serum in SIADH becomes____
28. Change in urine output in DI, DKA, and HHNK
31. Hormone produced by the anterior pituitary gland and stored and released by the posterior pituitary gland (abbrev.)

32. Hormone produced by the anterior pituitary gland, which causes the production and release of hormones from the adrenal cortex (abbrev.)
33. Endocrine gland located in the neck, which produces hormones that control metabolic rate
34. Hormone released by adrenal cortex, which causes gluconeogenesis
35. Hormone produced by alpha cells of the pancreas, which causes glycogenolysis and gluco-neogenesis to increase serum glucose
36. Hyperglycemic crisis that occurs in type 1 diabetes (abbrev.)

37. Type of diabetes caused by insulin deficiency

Down
1. Result of insulin deficiency
2. This occurs in DKA but not in HHNK
3. Endocrine gland that produces sugar (cortisol), salt (aldosterone), and sex (androgens) and epinephrine and norepinephrine
4. Vasopressin replacement often used nasally in permanent DI (abbrev.)
7. Change in urine output in SIADH

8. ____'s syndrome is an excess of hormones from the adrenal cortex
9. Tetracycline derivative that may be used to treat SIADH
11. A serious complication of SIADH that results from hyponatremia
13. DKA causes an increase in this gap
16. Tumor of the adrenal medulla
17. Another term for the anterior pituitary
20. Type of DI that results from a decrease in the secretion of ADH from the posterior pituitary
22. Protruding eyeballs

24. Respiratory pattern seen in DKA
25. Serum in DI and HHNK becomes____
26. Another name for ADH
27. Type of DI that results from excessive water consumption
29. ____'s syndrome is a chronic deficiency of glucocorticoids and minerocorticoids
30. Color of the skin in a patient with Addison's disease
33. Hormone produced by the anterior pituitary, which stimulates the thyroid gland (abbrev.)

2. **Directions:** Identify whether these factors increase or decrease ADH release or action

Lithium	
Alcohol	
Chlorpropamide (Diabinese)	
Positive-pressure ventilation	
Chlorpromazine (Thorazine)	
Phenytoin (Dilantin)	
Hydrochlorothiazide (HydroDIURIL)	
Anesthetic agents	
Demeclocycline (Declomycin)	
Beta stimulants	
Morphine sulfate	

3. **Directions:** Identify whether these factors are increased or decreased in DI and SIADH.

	DI	SIADH
Serum ADH		
Urine output		
Urine specific gravity		
Urine osmolality		
Serum osmolality		
Serum sodium		
Right atrial/pulmonary artery occlusive pressures		

4.   **DIRECTIONS:** Complete this table.

	DKA	HHNK
Age		
Type of diabetes mellitus		
Serum glucose range		
Presence of ketosis		
pH		
Anion gap		
Respiratory pattern		
Breath odor		
Serum osmolality		
Serum sodium		
Serum potassium		
BUN		
Average fluid deficit		

5.   **DIRECTIONS:** Identify the following clinical indications as DKA, HHNK, or both.

Serum glucose >300 mg/dl	
Kussmaul's respirations	
pH <7.30	
Positive serum and urine ketones	
Abdominal pain	
Dehydration	
Lethargy progressing to coma	
Serum glucose >1,000 mg/dl	

6.   **DIRECTIONS:** Identify the following clinical indications as DKA, hypoglycemia, or both.

Headache	
Serum glucose >300 mg/dl	
Abdominal pain	
Cold, clammy skin	
Nervousness, tremors	
Polyuria	
Lethargy progressing to coma	
Seizures	
Glycosuria	
Tachycardia	
Agitation, inability to concentrate	
Weakness, fatigue	
Fruity breath	
Serum glucose <50 mg/dl	

7. **DIRECTIONS:** Match the following endocrine conditions with the appropriate pharmacologic therapy. More than one condition may be listed for each therapy and conditions may be listed more than once.

a. Neurogenic DI
b. Nephrogenic DI
c. SIADH
d. DKA
e. HHNK
f. Hypoglycemia

____ 50% dextrose
____ Chlorpropamide (Diabinese)
____ Parenteral fluids
____ Insulin
____ 3% saline
____ Thiazide diuretics
____ Loop diuretics
____ Demeclocycline (Declomycin)
____ Pitressin

LEARNING ACTIVITIES ANSWERS

1.

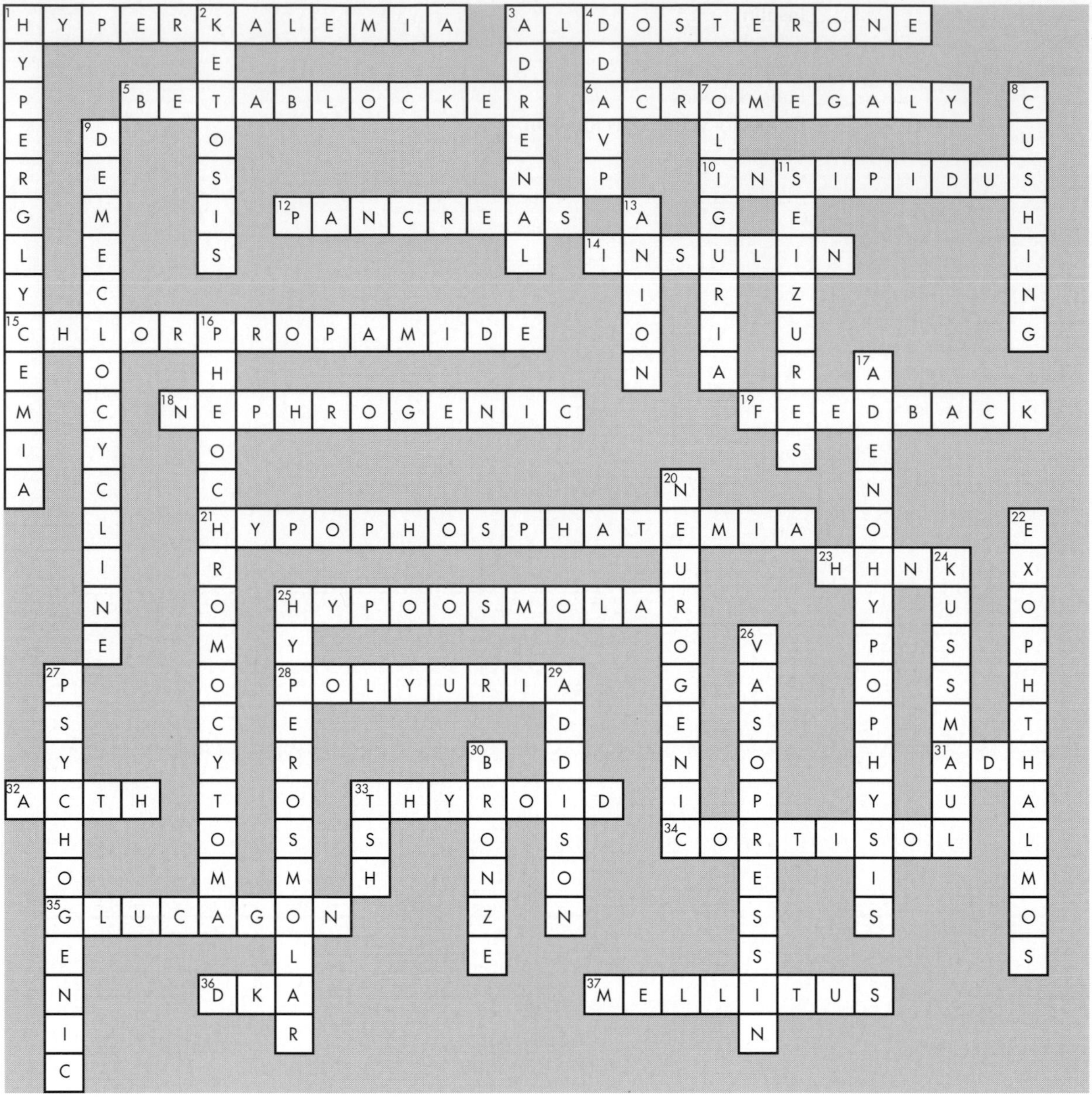

Across / filled answers in the crossword grid:

HYPERKALEMIA
ALDOSTERONE
BETABLOCKER
ACROMEGALY
INSIPIDUS
PANCREAS
INSULIN
CHLORPROPAMIDE
NEPHROGENIC
FEEDBACK
HYPOPHOSPHATEMIA
HHNK
HYPOOSMOLAR
POLYURIA
ADH
ACTH
THYROID
CORTISOL
GLUCAGON
DKA
MELLITUS

Down / intersecting answers:

HYPERGLYCEMIA
KETOSIS
ADRENAL
ADDISON
CUSHING
DEMECLOCYCLINE
BOSIS
PHCOC
AVP
ALIGN
SERIZUR
ANTIDIURETIC
ASCENSION
NONKETOGENIC
GLUCOGENESIS
VASOPRESSIN
KUSPMHYUL
EXOPHTHALMOS
PSYCHOGENIC
BSNZE
CORTISOL

2.

Lithium	Decrease
Alcohol	Decrease
Chlorpropamide (Diabinese)	Increase
Positive-pressure ventilation	Increase
Chlorpromazine (Thorazine)	Decrease
Phenytoin (Dilantin)	Decrease
Hydrochlorothiazide (HydroDIURIL)	Increase
Anesthetic agents	Increase
Demeclocycline (Declomycin)	Decrease
Beta stimulants	Increase
Morphine sulfate	Increase

3.

	DI	SIADH
Serum ADH	Decreased	Increased
Urine output	>200 ml/hr	<0.5 ml/kg/hr
Urine specific gravity	<1.005	>1.030
Urine osmolality	Low	High
Serum osmolality	>295 mOsm/L	<280 mOsm/L
Serum sodium	>145 mEq/L	<135 mEq/L
Right atrial/pulmonary artery occlusive pressures	RA <2 mm Hg; PAOP <6 mm Hg	RA >6 mm Hg; PAOP >12 mm Hg

4.

	DKA	HHNK
Age	Most often young	Most often old
Type of diabetes mellitus	1 (IDDM)	2 (NIDDM) or none
Average serum glucose	600 mg/dl	1,100 mg/dl
Presence of ketosis	Positive	Negative
pH	May be very acidotic	Normal or minimally acidotic
Anion gap	Increased	Normal
Respiratory pattern	Kussmaul's (rapid and deep)	Normal or tachypneic (rapid and shallow)
Breath odor	Acetone (fruity)	Normal
Serum osmolality	295-330 mOsm/L	330-450 mOsm/L
Serum sodium	Decreased, normal, or increased	Normal or increased
Serum potassium	Increased initially; drops with rehydration and correction of acidosis	Decreased
BUN	Mildly increased	Severely increased
Average fluid deficit	4-8 L	8-15 L

5.

Serum glucose >300 mg/dl	Both
Kussmaul's respirations	DKA
pH <7.30	DKA
Positive serum and urine ketones	DKA
Abdominal pain	DKA
Dehydration	Both
Lethargy progressing to coma	Both
Serum glucose >600 mg/dl	HHNK

6.

Headache	Hypoglycemia
Serum glucose >300 mg/dl	DKA
Abdominal pain	DKA
Cold, clammy skin	Hypoglycemia
Nervousness, tremors	Hypoglycemia
Polyuria	DKA
Lethargy progressing to coma	DKA
Seizures	Hypoglycemia
Glycosuria	DKA
Tachycardia	Both
Agitation, difficulty with concentration	Hypoglycemia
Weakness, fatigue	DKA
Fruity breath	DKA
Serum glucose <50 mg/dl	Hypoglycemia

7.

  __f__   50% dextrose
  __b__   Chlorpropamide (Diabinese)
__abde__ Parenteral fluids
 __de__ Insulin
  __c__   3% saline
  __b__   Thiazide diuretics
  __c__   Loop diuretics
  __c__   Demeclocycline (Declomycin)
  __a__   Pitressin

Bibliography and Selected References

Alspach J, editor: *Core curriculum for critical care nursing,* ed 5, Philadelphia, 1998, WB Saunders.

Barkauskas V et al: *Health and physical assessment,* St Louis, 1994, Mosby.

Beare P, Myers J: *Adult health nursing,* ed 3, St Louis, 1998, Mosby.

Boggs R, Wooldridge-King M: *AACN procedure manual for critical care,* ed 3, Philadelphia, 1993, WB Saunders.

Brar R, Hollenberg S: The technique of fluid resuscitation, *Journal of Critical Illness* 11 (8):550, 1996.

Brar R, Hollenberg S: Administering fluid resuscitation effectively for traumatic shock, *Journal of Critical Illness* 11 (10):672, 1996.

Chernow B, editor: *The pharmacologic approach to the critically ill patient,* ed 3, Baltimore, 1994, Williams & Wilkins.

Cirolia B: Understanding edema, *Nursing96* 26 (2), 66, 1996.

Clochesy J et al: *Critical care nursing,* ed 2, Philadelphia, 1996, WB Saunders.

Depree P: A short course on a quick performer: lispro insulin, *Nursing98* 28 (11):54, 1998.

Drass K, Peterson A: Type II diabetes: exploring treatment options, *AJN* 96 (11):45, 1996.

Fleming D: Challenging traditional insulin injection practices, *AJN* 99 (2):72, 1999.

Gahart B, Nazareno A: *1999 intravenous medications,* St Louis, 1999, Mosby.

Hernandez D: Microvascular complications of diabetes: nursing assessment and intervention, *AJN* 98 (6):26, 1998.

Keen J, Searingen P: *Mosby's critical care nursing consultant,* St Louis, 1997, Mosby.

Kinney M et al: *AACN clinical reference for critical care nursing,* ed 4, St Louis, 1998, Mosby.

Laskowski-Jones L: Managing hemorrhage: taking the right steps to protect your patient, *Nursing97* 27 (9):36, 1997.

Marino P: *The ICU book,* ed 2, Baltimore, 1998, Williams & Wilkins.

Matz R: Managing fluid abnormalities in uncontrolled diabetes mellitus, *Journal of Critical Illness* 12 (5):278, 1997.

Matz R: Coping with electrolyte imbalances in uncontrolled diabetes, *Journal of Critical Illness* 12 (6):341, 1997.

Mims B et al: *Critical care skills: a clinical handbook,* Philadelphia, 1996, WB Saunders.

Price S, Wilson L: *Pathophysiology: clinical concepts of disease processes,* ed 5, St Louis, 1997, Mosby.

Roper M: Back to basics: assessing orthostatic vital signs, *AJN* 96 (8):43, 1996.

Sandrock J: Managing hypovolemia, *Nursing97* 27 (2):32aa, 1997.

Sandrock J: Treating traumatic hypovolemia: which fluid to choose?, *Nursing98* 28 (1):32cc1, 1998.

Thelan L et al: *Critical care nursing: diagnosis and management,* ed 3, St Louis, 1998, Mosby.

Umpierrez G, Kitabchi A: Management strategies for diabetic ketoacidosis, *Journal of Critical Illness* 11 (7):437, 1996.

Umpierrez G, Kitabchi A: A rational approach to diagnosing diabetic ketoacidosis, *Journal of Critical Illness* 11 (7):428, 1996.

Varon J, Fromm R: *The ICU handbook of facts, formulas, and laboratory values,* St Louis, 1997, Mosby.

Hematologic and Immunologic Systems

CHAPTER 11

Selected Concepts in Anatomy and Physiology

Purposes of the Hematologic and Immunologic Systems

I. Hematologic
   A. Provides the medium for transportation of oxygen, carbon dioxide, and nutrients to the tissues
   B. Maintains hemostasis
   C. Maintains internal environment, including participation in regulation of temperature and acid-base balance
II. Immunologic: protects the internal environment from invading foreign material

Bone Marrow

I. Adults have 30 to 50 ml of bone marrow per kilogram of body weight
II. Most functioning bone marrow in adults is located in flat bones (vertebrae, skull, pelvic and shoulder girdles, clavicle, ribs, sternum) and proximal epiphysis of long bones
III. The functions of the bone marrow include the following:
   A. Production of the following:
      1. Erythrocytes (red blood cells)
      2. Leukocytes (white blood cells) including granulocytes, agranulocytes, and lymphocytes
      3. Thrombocytes (platelets)
   B. Recognition and removal of senescent cells
   C. Participation in cellular and humoral immunity

Spleen

I. White pulp: primarily concerned with humoral immunity; performs the following functions:
   A. Production of lymphocytes
   B. Stimulation of B-cell activity to produce immuno-globulins; therefore, splenectomized patients have a greatly increased risk of sepsis
II. Red pulp: contains reticuloendothelial tissue; performs the following functions:
   A. Storage and release of RBCs into the circulation
      1. Caused by contraction of smooth muscle in the capsule surrounding the spleen and in invaginations of the capsule, called *trabeculae*
      2. When stimulated by the SNS, as much as 100 ml of concentrated RBCs can be released into the circulation, raising the hematocrit by 1% to 2%
   B. Filtering and destruction (by the process of phagocytosis) of damaged or old erythrocytes (referred to as *culling*)
      1. Removes particles from intact RBCs without destroying them (referred to as *pitting*)
      2. Catabolizes hemoglobin released from RBCs that have been destroyed by the spleen; iron returned to the bone marrow for reuse
   C. Filtering and trapping foreign material, including bacteria and viruses
   D. Storage and release of platelets; destruction of damaged or senescent platelets

Liver: Performs the Following Functions:

I. Filtering of blood as it comes from the gastrointestinal tract
   A. Removal of foreign material, including microorganisms, damaged or old RBCs, and other degradation products by the Kupffer's cells lining the sinusoidal beds of the liver
   B. Destruction of RBCs produces bilirubin, which the liver converts to bile, necessary for fat digestion
II. Elimination of immune complexes (e.g., antigen-antibody complexes) from the blood

III. Detoxification of toxic substances that enter the blood
IV. Manufacture of some clotting factors and antithrombin
V. Storage of blood (e.g., in heart failure, the liver becomes engorged with blood)

Lymphatic System

I. Lymph: pale yellow fluid that transports lymphocytes
   A. Composition
      1. Contains lymphocytes, granulocytes, enzymes, and antibodies
      2. Deficient in platelets and fibrinogen, so it coagulates very slowly
   B. Function: returns proteins and fat from GI tract, certain hormones, and excess interstitial fluid to the blood
II. Lymph circulation
   A. Lymphatic capillaries are somewhat larger than blood capillaries and irregular in diameter
   B. Lymphatic vessels are formed by lymphatic capillaries
   C. Lymph ducts drain into subclavian veins
      1. The right lymphatic duct collects lymph from right side of head, neck, thorax, right arm, right lung, right side of heart, and right upper surface of diaphragm
      2. The thoracic duct collects lymph from all other parts of the body
   D. Lymph nodes are small, bean-shaped organs located along lymph vessels
      1. Spongy and multichanneled on inside
      2. Sites of B- and T-cell lymphocyte production and distribution
      3. Functions
         a) Lymph nodes filter and allow WBCs to phagocytosize bacteria and foreign material carried by lymph
         b) Granulocytes, macrophages, and lymphocytes pass through the lymph node to return to the blood
      4. Enlargement of lymph nodes
         a) This change occurs with infection or malignancy
         b) Enlarged superficial nodes can be palpated; enlarged deep nodes can only be visualized on X-ray
   E. Additional lymphoid tissue synthesizes IgA and IgE immunoglobulins and is located in the submucosa of the respiratory, intestinal, or genitourinary tracts
      1. Mucosal-associated lymphoid tissues (MALT): clusters of T and B lymphocytes and phagocytes dispersed in the mucosal linings of the respiratory, gastrointestinal, and genitourinary tracts
      2. Gut-associated lymphoid tissue (GALT): Peyer's patches in the intestinal tract

III. Thymus
   A. Location: anterosuperior mediastinum below the thyroid gland; each lobe packed with lymphocytes
   B. Function
      1. Site of maturation and distribution of T lymphocytes
      2. Secretes a hormone, thymosin, which is thought to stimulate immune function

Blood

I. Plasma constitutes 55% of total blood volume
   A. Composed of serum and plasma proteins, including albumin, serum globulins, fibrinogen, prothrombin, plasminogen
   B. Hematocrit expresses the percentage of red blood cells in the total blood volume
II. All blood cells originate from pluripotential stem cell
   A. Erythroid stem cells (pronormoblasts) develop into reticulocytes and finally into erythrocytes
   B. Myeloid stem cells (myeloblasts or monoblasts) develop into granulocytes and monocytes
   C. Lymphoid stem cells (lymphoblasts) develop into B and T lymphocytes
   D. Thrombocytic stem cells (megakaryoblasts) develop into thrombocytes
III. Erythrocytes are also referred to as *red blood cells* or *RBCs*
   A. Structure
      1. Erythrocytes are nonnucleated, round, biconcave cells
      2. The inner part of an RBC (referred to as *stoma*) is the location of hemoglobin attachment and contains the antigens that determine ABO and Rh blood type
   B. Function of RBCs
      1. Transport oxygen from lungs to tissues
      2. Participate in maintenance of acid-base balance
      3. Highly permeable to hydrogen, chloride, and bicarbonate ions and water
   C. Types of RBCs
      1. Reticulocytes: immature RBCs
         a) Useful in assessing erythrocyte production; elevated reticulocyte count means that production of new RBCs is greater than usual, such as may occur in acute hemorrhage
         b) Maturation to erythrocyte takes 1 to 4 days
      2. Erythrocytes: mature RBCs
         a) Lifespan is approximately 120 days
         b) The spleen acts as reservoir for RBCs; contains 1% to 2% of circulating RBCs
   D. Erythropoiesis
      1. Regulation
         a) Determined by relationship of cellular oxygen requirement and general metabolic activity
         b) Bone marrow stimulated to make more RBCs by the hormone erythropoietin;

erythropoietin is secreted by the kidney in response to hypoxemia

2. Nutritional requirements for RBC and hemoglobin production
   a) Iron
   b) Vitamin B_{12}
   c) Folic acid
3. Process
   a) Stem cell
   b) Erythroblast (has a nucleus)
   c) Expulsion of nucleus
   d) Erythrocyte
4. Hemoglobin (Hgb) synthesis
   a) Synthesis takes place in bone marrow
   b) Hemoglobin consists of four globins chains and four heme groups per hemoglobin molecule; each hemoglobin molecule has two different types of globin (e.g., normal adult hemoglobin [referred to as HbA]) and has two alpha chains and two beta chains

E. Destruction (hemolysis) of erythrocytes
   1. Destruction of old and immature RBCs occurs in the liver and spleen
   2. Destruction of immature RBCs occurs primarily because they are misshapen or damaged
   3. Presenescent RBCs are removed from the circulation by the spleen, liver, or bone marrow for any of the following reasons:
      a) RBC membrane abnormalities
      b) Hemoglobin abnormalities
      c) Abnormal metabolic functions
      d) Physical trauma to the RBC
      e) Antibodies
      f) Infectious agents and toxins
   4. Hgb and iron are returned to the bone marrow for reuse
   5. Erythrocyte destruction increases bilirubin production; bilirubin is transported to the liver attached to albumin
      a) Indirect bilirubin is unconjugated; this is before the liver has converted it to water-soluble; indirect bilirubin becomes elevated in hemolytic states that overwhelm the liver's ability to conjugate or in liver disease where the liver is unable to adequately conjugate
      b) Direct bilirubin is conjugated: this is after the liver has converted it to a water-soluble substance that will be excreted into the bile; direct bilirubin becomes elevated in biliary obstruction

IV. Leukocytes: phagocytic and immunologic systems
   A. Cytokines: protein hormones synthesized by the various leukocytes (Table 11-1)
      1. Act as chemical mediators of immunity and inflammation
      2. Important in regulation of normal immune and inflammatory responses
      3. Are causative factors in systemic inflam-

matory response syndrome (see Chapter 12)
      4. Types of cytokines
         a) Monokines are synthesized by mononuclear phagocytes
         b) Lymphokines are synthesized by lymphocytes
   B. Granulocytes: active phagocytes
      1. Neutrophils (also known as *polymorphonuclear leukocytes*); largest component of circulating WBC mass (40% to 80%)
         a) Function
            (1) Neutrophils leave the blood vessel, migrate through the tissues, and search for microorganisms or damaged or old body cells; they then engulf, kill, and digest them through the process of phagocytosis (Table 11-2 and Figure 11-1 describe some selected cellular processes of leukocytes, including phagocytosis)
               (a) Neutrophils are the most actively phagocytic of granulocytes
               (b) After phagocytosis, the neutrophil dies
               (c) Pus is the end product of neutrophil death
               (d) Neutrophils exhibit a burst of oxygen consumption during phagocytosis known as a *respiratory burst*; this burst produces superoxide, hydrogen peroxide, and hydroxyl radicals; these oxygen-derived radicals normally function in destruction of microorganisms but may be injurious to normal body tissue
            (2) Neutrophils contain cytoplasmic granules that include lysosomal enzymes, which aid in killing the microorganism
         b) Lifespan after maturation: half-life 4 to 10 hours
         c) Maturity
            (1) Bands are immature neutrophils
               (a) Phagocytic
               (b) Increase in bands seen in acute infection; often referred to as a *shift to the left*
            (2) Segmented neutrophils (referred to as *segs*) are mature neutrophils
               (a) Phagocytic
               (b) Increase in segs seen in liver disease and pernicious anemia; frequently referred to as a *shift to the right*
         d) Recruitment
            (1) Movement into the tissues is stimulated by microorganisms or antigen-antibody reactions

Table 11-1   Cytokines

Factor	Action
Chemotactic factors	• Attract macrophages and granulocytes to area of antigen
Granulocyte macrophage colony-stimulating factor (GM-CSF)	• Enhances production of neutrophils in the bone marrow
Interferon	• Inhibits viruses • Activates natural killer cells
Interleukin-1 (IL-1)	• Augments the immune response • Mediates the inflammatory response • Activates T-cells • Activates phagocytes • Promotes prostaglandin production • Induces fever
Interleukin-2 (IL-2)	• Induces T-cells to proliferate • Enhances activity of NK cells and cytotoxic T-cells
Interleukin-3 (IL-3)	• Regulates growth and differentiation of leukocytes in the bone marrow
Interleukin-4 (IL-4)	• Enhances antibody production through B-cell activation
Interleukin-5 (IL-5)	• Promotes growth and differentiation of B lymphocytes into IgA-secreting cells
Interleukin-6 (IL-6)	• Promotes the differentiation of B lymphocytes to plasma cells • Promotes hematopoiesis • Enhances the inflammatory process
Interleukin-7 (IL-7)	• Induces growth of immature T- and B-cells
Interleukin-8 (IL-8)	• Stimulates chemotaxis • Activates T lymphocytes and neutrophils
Interleukin-9 (IL-9)	• Induces growth of T-cells and mast cells
Interleukin-10 (IL-10)	• Inhibits proliferation of helper T-cells • Decreases production of some other cytokines (an antiinflammatory effect)
Lymphotoxin (LT)	• Cytotoxic: directly destroys the antigen
Macrophage activation factor (MAF)	• Enhances functioning of macrophages
Migration inhibition factor (MIF)	• Prevents migration of macrophages to area of antigen
Transfer factor (TF)	• Changes nonsensitized T lymphocytes to sensitized T lymphocytes
Transforming growth factor (TGF)	• Stimulates fibroblasts for wound healing • Inhibits the immune response
Tumor necrosis factor (TNF) (also called cachectin)	• Cytotoxic to tumor cells • Induces fever • In high concentrations (e.g., septic shock) causes endothelial cell damage and increases vascular permeability

(2) The bone marrow speeds maturation and release when more neutrophils are needed for phagocytosis

e) Destruction: lost from the blood via the GI tract, pulmonary or oral secretions, and urine and into the tissues

2. Eosinophils: constitute 0% to 5% of WBC mass

   a) Functions

      (1) Ingest immune complexes (antigen-antibody complexes) and inactive mediators of allergic response

      (2) Some phagocytic activity

      (3) Probably most important during parasitic infections and allergic reac-

tions; especially important in helminth infections because these parasitic worms are too large to be phagocytized and eosinophils secrete chemicals that destroy the surface of the helminth

b) Lifespan after maturation: half-life in circulation approximately 30 minutes; in tissues 12 days

c) Tissue eosinophils are present in large numbers on mucosal surfaces of the respiratory and gastrointestinal systems and the skin because these locations are common entry points for foreign material

Table 11-2	**Definitions of Selected Leukocyte Activities**
Opsonization	The process by which opsonins render bacteria more susceptible to phagocytosis by leukocytes; an opsonin is an antibody or complement split product that when attached to foreign material, a microorganism, or an antigen, enhances phagocytosis of the substances by leukocytes and other macrophages
Chemotaxis (Fig. 11-1)	The movement toward (positive) or away from (negative) a chemical stimulus; movement of neutrophils and monocytes toward an invading microorganism
Margination (Fig. 11-1)	The process of the white blood cell sticking to the capillary wall
Diapedesis (Fig. 11-1)	The passage of white blood cells through the walls of the vessels that contain them without damage to the vessels
Phagocytosis	The process by which certain cells engulf and destroy microorganisms and cellular debris; involves invagination, engulfment, internalization and formation of phagocyte vacuole, digestion of phagocytosed material by lysosomes and oxygen-derived radicals, and release of digested microbial products
Lysis	The destruction or dissolution of a cell through the action of a specific agent

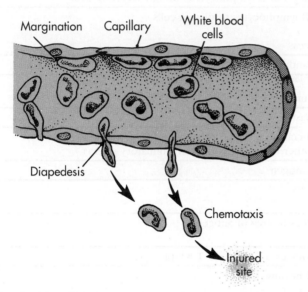

Figure 11-1 Illustration of margination, diapedesis, and chemotaxis. (From Lewis SM, Collier IC: *Medical-surgical nursing: assessment and management of clinical problems,* ed 3, St Louis, 1992, Mosby.)

3. Basophils: constitute 0% to 2% of WBC mass
  a) Function
    (1) Similar to mast cells, basophils contain heparin and histamine, which is released as they degranulate during acute local or systemic allergic reactions; mast cells stay in the tissue, whereas basophils stay in the circulatory system; if a basophil leaves the circulatory system to stay in the tissue, it becomes a mast cell
    (2) Basophils do not participate in phagocytic activity
  b) Lifespan after maturation: unknown

C. Agranulocytes
  1. Mononuclear phagocytes
    a) Monocytes: constitute 3% to 8% of WBC mass
      (1) Function
        (a) Some phagocytic activity
        (b) Differentiate into macrophages as they migrate into the tissues
      (2) Lifespan after maturation: circulating half-life 8 to 10 hours
    b) Macrophages (not measured in WBC count due to their location)
      (1) Function
        (a) Greater phagocytic ability than PMNs or monocytes; especially involved in removal of damaged or senescent cells, cellular debris, and mutant or cancer cells
        (b) Produce the cytokine interleukin-1 (IL-1), which increases proliferation of T-cells, stimulates the growth and development of B lymphocytes, causes fever, and stimulates the release of prostaglandin
        (c) Produce the cytokine alpha interferon, which is important in the body's defense against viruses and tumors
        (d) Also produce IL-6, IL-8, and tumor necrosis factor (TNF)
      (2) Fixed or mobile
        (a) Fixed (or tissue) macrophages: stay in one organ and phagocytize live and dead debris
          (i) Lung: alveolar macrophages
          (ii) Brain: microglia
          (iii) Liver: Kupffer cells
          (iv) Bone: osteoclast

(v) Peritoneum: peritoneal macrophages

(vi) Kidney: mesangial cells

(b) Mobile macrophages: found primarily at sites of inflammation and in peritoneal, pleural, and synovial spaces; migrate through the circulatory system as monocytes

(3) Lifespan: months or years

2. Lymphocytes: constitute 10% to 40% of WBC mass

a) T-cells: constitute approximately 70% to 80% of lymphocytes

(1) Develop in the bone marrow; mature and differentiate in the thymus

(2) Function: cellular immunity

(3) Types of T-cells

(a) Helper T-cells (also referred to as *CD4 T lymphocytes, T4 lymphocytes,* or T_H) detect foreign cells and produce lymphokines to stimulate the production or activation of other cells to fight infection; lymphokines are soluble proteins that function as chemical communicators to transmit instructions to macrophages, lymphocytes, and tissue cells

(b) Cytotoxic T-cells (also referred to as *killer cells* or T_c) emit chemicals that dissolve the foreign cell's membrane to kill the cell before the invader can use it as a base for multiplication

(c) Suppressor T-cells (also referred to as *CD8 T lymphocytes, T8 lymphocytes,* or T_S) modulate the overall immune system by signaling B-cells and T-cells to slow down or stop their activity

(d) Memory T-cells circulate in blood and lymph after the initial infection to allow a ready response to subsequent invasion by the same organism

(e) Helper T-cells typically carry the CD4 surface molecule, and suppressor and cytotoxic T-cells typically carry the CD8 surface molecule; normally twice as many CD4 cells as CD8 cells are present

b) B-cells: constitute approximately 10% to 20% of lymphocytes

(1) Develop and mature in the bone marrow (bursa)

(2) Function: production of immunoglobulins (humoral immunity)

(a) Once activated, B-cells become plasma cells

(i) Recognize specific foreign material

(ii) Develop specific immunoglobulins to that antigen

(b) Memory B-cells circulate in blood and lymph after the initial infection to allow a ready response to subsequent invasion by the same organism

c) Natural killer (NK) cells (also referred to as *null cells*): constitute approximately 10% of lymphocytes

(1) Large, granular cytotoxic lymphocytes that are neither T-cells nor B-cells (no surface marker exists on these lymphocytes)

(2) Function

(a) Kill nonspecifically and do not need prior exposure for activation

(b) Involved in surveillance against tumors, some parasites, and viruses

Inflammation

I. Sequential physiologic response the body makes to injuries, immunologic processes, or foreign substances in the body; may be acute or chronic

A. Occurs at sites of tissue damage irrespective of cause

B. May be local only or can become systemic; systemic response is now referred to as *systemic inflammatory response syndrome (SIRS)* (discussion of SIRS and multiple organ dysfunction syndrome (MODS) is in Chapter 12)

II. Process

A. Stage 1: vascular stage

1. Phases

a) Phase 1: immediate but temporary vasoconstriction caused by trauma to vascular smooth muscle

b) Phase 2

(1) Warmth, redness, swelling, pain, and loss of function are the five classic symptoms of the inflammatory response

(2) Injured tissues and cells secrete chemical mediators (Table 11-3); predominant effect is vasodilation and increase in capillary permeability, causing warmth, redness, and swelling

(a) Healing is enhanced by the increase in mobilization of nutrients to the area

(b) Tissue injury is decreased by diluting toxins or microorganisms that enter the area

(c) Pain is caused by tissue stretching and histamine and prostaglandin release

Table 11-3	**Chemical Mediators of the Inflammatory Process**
Chemical Mediator	**Action**
Bradykinin	• Vasodilation • Increased capillary permeability • Enhanced chemotaxis • Pain • Conversion of plasminogen to plasmin
Collagenase	• Clot degradation
Complement cascade	• Neutrophil aggregation • Increased capillary permeability • Activation of mast cells and basophils
Elastase	• Clot degradation
Endorphin	• Vasodilation • Analgesia
Fibrinolysin	• Digestion of fibrin
Histamine1 (H_1)	• Vasodilation • Increased capillary permeability • Smooth muscle contraction (bronchospasm)
Histamine2 (H_2)	• Vasodilation • Increased heart rate and contractility • Increased secretion of mucus and gastric acid • Inhibition of T-cells
Interleukin-1 (IL-1)	• Protein catabolism • Fever • Activation of lymphocytes • Stimulation of fibroblasts
Interleukin-2 (IL-2)	• Activation of B lymphocytes to make antibodies • Activation of macrophages
Leukotriene	• Vasoconstriction • Increased capillary permeability • Smooth muscle contraction (bronchospasm)
Lipase	• Fat degradation
Plasminogen	• Clot degradation (when activated to plasmin)
Prostacyclin	• Vasodilation • Platelet inhibition • Increased capillary permeability
Prostaglandin (PGD_2, PGF_{2a})	• Vasoconstriction • Bronchoconstriction
Prostaglandin (PGE_2, PGI_2)	• Vasodilation • Bronchodilation • Promotion of platelet aggregation • Increased capillary permeability • Activation of lysosomal enzymes • Potentiation of leukotriene • Pain
Serotonin	• Vasodilation • Increased capillary permeability • Pulmonary vasoconstriction • Smooth muscle contraction (bronchospasm)
Thromboxane	• Vasoconstriction • Pulmonary vasoconstriction • Platelet aggregation
Tumor necrosis factor (TNF)	• Necrosis of bacteria or tissue • Muscle breakdown • Induction of fever

(d) Loss of function is caused by tissue swelling and pain

2. The major leukocyte in this stage of inflammation is the tissue macrophage
   a) Response is immediate because the tissue macrophage is already in the tissue
   b) Colony-stimulating factor (G-CSF) is secreted by the macrophage to stimulate the bone marrow to speed up the maturation and release of leukocytes
   c) Cytokines secreted by the macrophage attract neutrophils to the area of injury or invasion

B. Stage II: cellular stage; major leukocyte in this stage of inflammation is the neutrophil, which attacks and destroys foreign material and removes necrotic tissue

C. Stage III: tissue repair and replacement
   1. Initiated at the time of injury
   2. Regeneration: replacement of lost cells with the same type of cells
   3. Repair: replacement of lost cells with connective tissue cells to form scar tissue; some loss of function occurs with the degree of loss, depending on the percentage of previously functional tissue replaced by scar tissue

Immunity

I. Definition: the protection of the body against pathogenic organisms or other foreign material; dependent on ability to recognize self from nonself
   A. Self is determined genetically; it is anything synthesized by a person's own particular DNA code
   B. Nonself describes anything that is different in its chromosome structure and that evokes a response from the immune system; antigens are chemical substances (almost always protein) that are viewed by the body as foreign (nonself)

II. Lines of defense
   A. First: skin and mucous membranes, acid secretions and enzymes, natural immunoglobulins
   B. Second: macrophages and neutrophils
   C. Third: cellular and humoral immunity

III. Innate immunity: body's inherent immune mechanisms; present at birth; do not require prior exposure to antigen for activation
   A. Anatomic: skin and mucous membranes
   B. Chemical
      1. Acid secretions in stomach, vagina, mouth
      2. Digestive enzymes in the GI tract
      3. Tears, perspiration
      4. Lysosomes
      5. Natural immunoglobulins
      6. Cytokines
      7. Pyrogen (produced by granulocytes to cause an increase in body temperature)
   C. Cellular
      1. Normal bacterial flora: GI tract, vagina, respiratory tract
      2. Tissue macrophages

3. Leukocytes and mobile macrophages
4. Inflammatory process

IV. Acquired immunity: immunity developed by the body through the creation of antibodies and formation of T and B memory cells in response to exposure to foreign material (antigen)
   A. Types
      1. Passive acquired immunity: produced by the injection of antibodies or sensitized lymphocytes
      2. Active acquired immunity: produced by natural exposure to an antigen (e.g., infection)
   B. Cell-mediated immunity
      1. Particularly effective against viruses, parasites, some fungi, and bacteria harbored inside of cells; responsible for delayed hypersensitivity, transplant rejection, and malignancy surveillance and, possibly, destruction
      2. Primarily mediated by T-cells
      3. Induced and regulated primarily through the production and activity of cytokines (Table 11-1)
      4. Process
         a) The macrophage is the first cell to detect most antigens
         b) The macrophage processes the antigen and "presents" it to both T- and B-cells
         c) T-cells recognize the antigen when it is on the macrophage cell membrane
         d) The antigen binds with an antigen receptor on the surface of the T-cell, sensitizing the T-cell
         e) Sensitized T-cells secrete lymphokines (Table 11-1), which regulate and coordinate the immune response to combat foreign cells, protect the body against mutant or cancer cells, and destroy foreign tissue; IL-8 is secreted by the macrophage and stimulates T-cell division
         f) T-cells are programmed to recognize the body's own tissue (self) from nonself (antigenic); autoimmune diseases are caused when the immune system cannot recognize self and the body is damaged by the immune system
         g) Natural killer cells also contribute to cellular immunity, especially in relation to cancer cell surveillance
   C. Humoral-mediated immunity
      1. Particularly effective against bacteria and viruses
      2. Primarily mediated by B-cells
      3. Process (Figure 11-2)
         a) Once activated, B-cells become plasma cells and recognize specific foreign cells or antigen
         b) Plasma cells make antibodies (also called *immunoglobulins*) (Table 11-4)
            (1) Immunoglobulins (antibodies) are

Figure 11-2 Primary and secondary immune responses. The introduction of antigen induces a response dominated by two classes of immunoglobulins, IgM and IgG. IgM predominates in the primary response, with some IgG appearing later. After the host's immune system is primed, another challenge with the same antigen induces the secondary response, in which some IgM and large amounts of IgG are produced. (From McCance KL, Huether SE: *Pathophysiology: the biological basis for diseases in adults and children,* ed 2, St Louis, 1994, Mosby.)

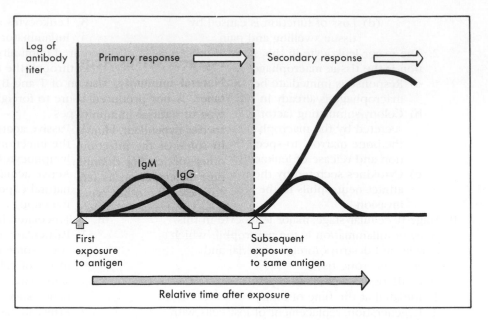

Table 11-4	Immunoglobulins (Ig)	
Ig	**Actions**	**Comments**
IgG	• Coats microorganisms (primarily bacteria and viruses) to enhance phagocytosis • Activates complement system	• Most abundant immunoglobulin (75%-80% of total) • Present in intravascular and extravascular spaces • Crosses the placental barrier and provides natural immunity
IgA	• Protects epithelial surfaces against antigen adhesion and invasion • Protects against entry via the respiratory, GU, GI tracts • Activates complement system	• Present in many body secretions (e.g., saliva, tears, sweat, mucus, breast milk) • 10% to 15% of total
IgM	• Kills bacteria in bloodstream • Activates complement system	• First responder to bacterial or viral invasion • Present mostly in intravascular space • 5% to 10% of total immunoglobulin
IgD	• Not well understood • May activate B-cells	• 1% of total immunoglobulins
IgE	• Attaches to mast cells and basophils and causes them to release their contents (e.g., histamine) in response to contact with specific antigens	• Present in serum, interstitial space, exocrine secretions, and on basophils and mast cells • Very small percentage (0.002%) of total immunoglobulins

serum proteins that bind to specific antigens; they begin the process that causes lysis or phagocytosis of an offending antigen

(2) One end of the immunoglobulin (Ig) molecule has a constant fragment with a fixed sequence of amino acids that is constant within the category of the immunoglobulin (e.g., IgG, IgM)

(3) The other end of the Ig has an antigen-binding fragment with an amino acid sequence specific to the antigen for which it was formed

c) The first exposure to an antigen is followed by a latent phase where no antibody levels are detected

d) Primary response follows as serum antibody levels rise rapidly; maximal antibody response takes 3 to 5 days

e) Levels plateau and finally decline

f) Subsequent exposure to the antigen results in more rapid production of antibodies to that antigen and higher concentrations of the antibody; this process is the basis for immunizations

g) Inflammation occurs because antigen-antibody complexes (referred to as

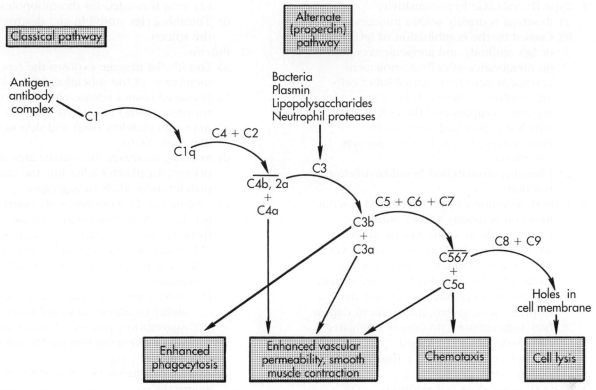

Figure 11-3   The complement cascade. (From Lewis SM, Collier IC: *Medical-surgical nursing: assessment and management of clinical problems,* ed 3, St Louis, 1992, Mosby.)

immune complexes) attract white blood cells
4. Immune complexes activate the complement cascade (Fig. 11-3)
   a) Complement is a group of blood proteins: more than 20 of these proteins exist, but 11 are considered the primary complement elements
      (1) These are labeled C1 to C9, with C1 having 3 subunits (C1q, C1r, C1s)
      (2) C1 is primarily synthesized by the intestinal epithelium
      (3) C2 and C4 are produced by macrophages
      (4) C3, C6, and C9 are synthesized by the liver
      (5) C5 and C8 are synthesized by the spleen
   b) When activated, they function as mediators to enhance various aspects of inflammatory response; they also do the following:
      (1) Attract and stimulate PMNs
      (2) Kill microorganisms by punching holes in their cell membranes, allowing intracellular fluid to leak out; mononuclear phagocytes and monocytes then clear the debris from the bloodstream
      (3) Agglutinate the bacteria
      (4) Activate basophils and mast cells

   c) They may be activated with or without previous exposure to the antigen
      (1) Anaphylactoid reaction: no previous exposure to the antigen; no true antigen-antibody interaction
      (2) Anaphylactic reaction: previous exposure to the antigen; involves antigen-antibody interaction
      (3) A more detailed description of anaphylactoid and anaphylactic reactions is given in Chapter 12
D. Hypersensitivity (allergic) reactions
   1. Type I: immediate hypersensitivity reactions ranging from mild reaction with localized response to a severe systemic reaction referred to as *anaphylaxis*
      a) Reaction occurs within minutes (usually 5 to 20 minutes) of exposure to even a minute amount of the antigen
      b) Caused by IgE specific to the antigen; the antigen binds to one end of IgE; IgE is bound to a mast cell or basophil; when the antigen attaches, the mast cell or basophil degranulates and histamine is released; slow-reacting substance of anaphylaxis (SRS-A) and eosinophil-chemotactic factor of anaphylaxis (ECF-A) are also released; eosinophils are recruited to the site
      c) Example: anaphylactic reaction to a penicillin, insect venom, foods, pollen

2. Type II: cytotoxic hypersensitivity
   a) Reaction is usually within minutes to days
   b) Caused by the combination of IgG, IgM, or IgA antibody and antigenic receptors on membranes of cells; complement cascade is activated; natural killer cells are involved in destruction of the immune complex and the cell to which it is attached, and macrophages may phagocytize the immune complexes
   c) Example: mismatched blood transfusion reaction
3. Type III: immune complex-mediated reaction
   a) Reaction is usually within hours
   b) Caused by large quantities of antigen-antibody (IgG, IgM, or IgA) complexes that cannot be quickly and efficiently cleared by the reticuloendothelial system; complement cascade is activated; neutrophils are activated at the site of deposition; inflammatory process is stimulated and mediators are released
   c) Example: environmental antigens (e.g., pollen, some drugs)
4. Type IV: delayed or cell-mediated hypersensitivity
   a) Reaction is within one or more days
   b) Cause is poorly understood but is presumed to be from cells that require time to migrate to the site; probably caused by previously sensitized lymphocytes and lymphokines that activate the inflammatory response at the site
   c) Example: skin testing for tuberculosis, contact dermatitis

Hemostasis

I. Definition: the termination of bleeding by a complex process that involves integrated interactions among blood vessels, platelets, clotting factors, and the fibrinolytic system
II. Hemostatic mechanisms
   A. Vascular response
      1. Disruption of vascular integrity causes a sympathetic nervous system response, resulting in vasospasm and blood vessel constriction in the injured vessel
      2. Thromboxane A_2, endothelin, the alpha-adrenergic system, and serotonin are thought to mediate this response
   B. Platelet aggregation
      1. Thrombocytes (platelets)
         a) Produced in bone marrow
         b) Lifespan is 9 to 12 days
         c) Thrombopoiesis
            (1) Thrombopoietin (a hormone like erythropoietin for RBCs) is postulated to stimulate the production and release of thrombocytes

(2) Iron is needed for thrombopoiesis
      d) Thrombocytes stored in and destroyed by the spleen
   2. Process
      a) Endothelial damage exposes the basement membrane of the subendothelial collagen
      b) Damaged tissues release chemicals (e.g., thromboplastin) to activate platelets
      c) Activated platelets swell and develop hair-like projections
      d) Swelling increases the surface area of the platelet for platelet adhesion and makes platelet more likely to aggregate
      e) Granules and components necessary for the clotting process are released from the platelets; adenosine diphosphate (ADP) released by degranulation of the platelet enhances adhesiveness and aggregation
         (1) Adhesiveness: stickiness that aids in ability to adhere to vessel walls
         (2) Aggregation: process of platelets adhering or clumping together to form the "platelet plug"
      f) Activated platelets become adhesive and aggregate
      g) Platelet aggregation becomes large enough to form a platelet plug (sometimes referred to as a *white clot*) that seals the damaged blood vessel
      h) During aggregation of the platelets, platelet factor III (PFIII), an important contributor in the intrinsic pathway, is released
      i) Platelets contain factor XIII (fibrin-stabilizing factor), which is essential to forming a stable fibrin clot
   3. Platelet function is affected by qualitative and quantitative factors
      a) Qualitative changes: drugs that decrease the ability of the platelets to aggregate
         (1) Alcohol
         (2) Aspirin (ASA)
         (3) Ticlopidine (Ticlid)
         (4) Clopidogrel (Plavix)
         (5) GP IIb/IIIa platelet receptor blockers (e.g., abciximab [ReoPro], eptifibatide [Integrilin], tirofiban HCl [Aggrastat])
         (6) Nonsteroidal antiinflammatory agents (e.g., phenylbutazone [Butazolidin], ibuprofen [Motrin])
         (7) Quinidine
         (8) Dextran 40 (low-molecular-weight dextran [LMD])
         (9) Heparin
      b) Quantitative changes
         (1) Thrombocytopenia
            (a) Significance
               (i) Platelet counts greater than 50,000/mm^3: surgery can generally be tolerated

(ii) Platelet counts 20,000 to 30,000/mm^3: spontaneous bleeding may occur

(iii) Platelet counts less than 10,000/mm^3: spontaneous intracranial hemorrhages likely

(b) Causes

(i) Decreased production (e.g., bone marrow depression, B$_{12}$ or folic acid deficiency)

(ii) Increased destruction (e.g., idiopathic thrombocytopenia purpura [ITP], disseminated intravascular coagulation [DIC], sepsis)

(iii) Hypersplenism (e.g., portal hypertension)

(iv) Heparin-induced thrombocytopenia and thrombosis (HITT): also called *heparin-associated thrombocytopenia and thrombosis (HATT)* or *white clot syndrome*; immune-mediated response caused by heparin

(v) Dilutional thrombocytopenia: caused by large volumes of fluids that do not contain platelets

(2) Thrombocytosis

(a) Significance: may cause excessive thrombosis or bleeding, depending on the quality of the platelets

(b) Causes

(i) Malignancy

(ii) Polycythemia vera

(iii) Leukemia

(iv) Postsplenectomy

(v) Rheumatoid arthritis

(vi) Trauma

C. Coagulation

1. Depends on presence of clotting factors and functioning of the pathways

2. Blood coagulation factors (Table 11-5)

a) Consist of proteins, lipoproteins, and calcium, which is critical in the intrinsic, extrinsic, and common pathways

b) Circulate as inactive; activated in a cascade fashion

3. Clotting pathways (Fig. 11-4)

a) Pathways are cascades where one action depends on a preceding action or interaction

b) A fibrin clot may be produced through activation of either the intrinsic or extrinsic pathway

(1) Intrinsic pathway

(a) Initiated by damage to red blood cells or platelets

(b) Time from activation through intrinsic pathway and common pathway to a clot: 2 to 6 minutes

(c) Tested by aPTT

(2) Extrinsic pathway

(a) Initiated by injured tissue

(b) Time from activation through extrinsic pathway and common pathway to a clot: as short as 15 to 20 seconds

(c) Tested by PT

c) Common pathway

(1) Platelet factor III and tissue thromboplastin combine to become a prothrombin activator

(2) Prothrombin is converted to thrombin

(3) Fibrinogen is converted to fibrin

(4) Fibrin clot is formed

(5) Pathway is tested by aPTT, PT, and thrombin time

4. Anticoagulants (Table 11-6)

D. Anticoagulant mechanisms in normal system

1. Fibrinolytic system (Fig. 11-5)

a) Activated clotting factors are cleared by the reticuloendothelial system

b) Clot-lysing activities maintain blood in fluid state

(1) Process of clot breakdown takes approximately 7 to 10 days

(2) Blood (intrinsic pathway) or tissue (extrinsic pathway) plasminogen activators activate plasminogen to plasmin; therefore, once a clot is developed, steps are initiated to eliminate it

(3) Plasmin works to lyse fibrin clots, producing fibrin split products (FSPs) (also referred to as *fibrin degradation products* [FDPs]; increased amounts of FSPs increase potential for patient to bleed

(4) Thrombolytics (or fibrinolytics) speed up this process by either directly providing tissue plasminogen activator (e.g., alteplase [Activase], reteplase [Retavase]) or by triggering the process by adding a complex to cause the activation of the fibrinolytic system (streptokinase [Streptase]) (discussion of these agents and implications is located in the MI section of Chapter 3)

c) Controls of fibrinolysis

(1) Plasminogen activator inhibitor type 1 inactivates tissue plasminogen activator

(2) Alpha$_2$-antiplasmin is an inhibitor of plasmin

2. Antithrombin system

a) Defends against excessive clotting

b) Release of antithrombin III from mast cells

c) Neutralizes the clotting capability of thrombin

Table 11-5   **Blood Coagulation Factors**

Factor	Name(s)	Comments
I	Fibrinogen	• Synthesized in liver • Precursor to fibrin (Ia)
Ia	Fibrin	• Activated fibrinogen (I) becomes fibrin (Ia)
II	Prothrombin	• Synthesized in liver • Vitamin K dependent • Precursor to thrombin (IIa)
IIa	Thrombin	• Activated prothrombin becomes thrombin
III	Tissue thromboplastin Tissue factor	• First factor of extrinsic pathway
IV	Calcium	• Acts as an enzyme cofactor for most of the activation steps in intrinsic, extrinsic, and common pathways
V	Proaccelerin Labile factor Ac globulin	• Synthesized in liver • Combines with Xa and phospholipid to accelerate conversion of prothrombin (II) to thrombin (IIa)
VI		No designated factor VI
VII	Proconvertin Stable factor	• Synthesized in liver • Vitamin K dependent • Part of extrinsic pathway • Complexes with tissue thromboplastin (III) to activate X
VIII	Antihemophiliac factor A	• Part of intrinsic pathway • Complexes with IXa and platelet phospholipid to activate X
IX	Plasma thromboplastin component (PTC) Christmas factor Antihemophiliac factor B	• Synthesized in liver • Vitamin K dependent • Associated with factors VIII, XI, XII in the intrinsic pathway
X	Stuart-Prower factor	• Synthesized in liver • Vitamin K dependent • Part of intrinsic and extrinsic pathways • Complexes with V and phospholipid to accelerate prothrombin (II) conversion
XI	Plasma thromboplastin antecedent (PTA)	• May be synthesized in liver • May be vitamin K dependent • Part of intrinsic pathway • Associated with factors VIII, IX, and XII in the intrinsic pathway
XII	Hageman factor Contact factor	• First factor in intrinsic factor • Indirectly activates plasmin and complement cascades
XIII	Fibrin-stabilizing factor Fibrinase Laki-Lorand factor	• May be synthesized in liver • Activated by thrombin (IIa) • Produces a stronger, insoluble clot; stabilizes clot formation

Note: "a" after the factor indicates an activated factor.

Blood Groups

I. Three systems describe the most important antigens on red blood cells, tissues, and other cells
 A. ABO system (Table 11-7)
  1. This system is concerned with antigens on the RBC, which are designated A and B; the presence of these antigens is genetically controlled
  2. Blood type is named for the antigen that is present on the RBC
  3. Antibodies are present in the plasma for the antigen or antigens that are not present (e.g., B antibodies are found in group A blood because B antigens are absent)
 4. Agglutination that occurs in mismatched blood is the basis for typing and crossmatching
  a) Blood typing detects the major antigens: A, B, Rh
  b) Crossmatching detects the presence of major or minor RBC antigens
 B. Rh system (Table 11-8)
  1. This system is concerned with a series of six common types of Rh antigens, each called an Rh factor
  2. Each person has one of each of three pairs, so they have three of these Rh factors designated c, C, d, D, e, E

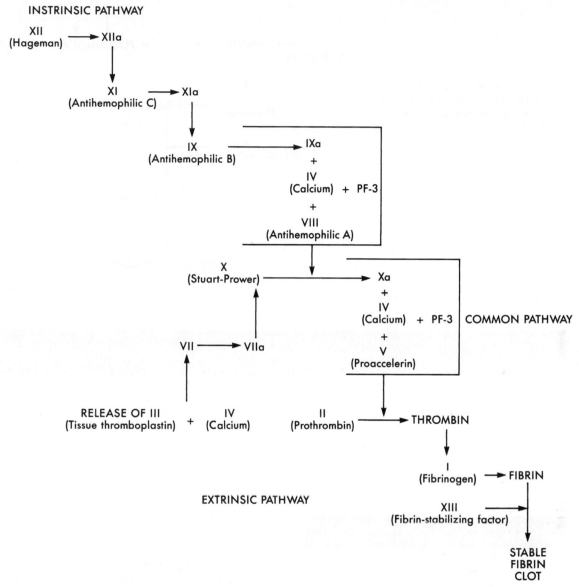

Figure 11-4 The clotting pathways: intrinsic, extrinsic, common. (From Kinney MR, Packa DR, Dunbar SB: *AACN's clinical reference for critical-care nursing,* ed 4, St Louis, 1998, Mosby.)

Table 11-6	**Anticoagulants**				
Drug	**Action**	**Location of Action**	**Duration**	**Desired Effect**	**Antidote**
Heparin	Prevents the conversion of prothrombin to thrombin and neutralizes the clotting capability of thrombin	Intrinsic and final common pathway	4 hours	aPTT 1.5-2.5 × laboratory control	Protamine sulfate
Warfarin (Coumadin)	Inhibits the synthesis of prothrombin	Extrinsic pathway	3-5 days	PT 1.5-2.0 × laboratory control	Vitamin K₁ (AquaMEPHYTON)

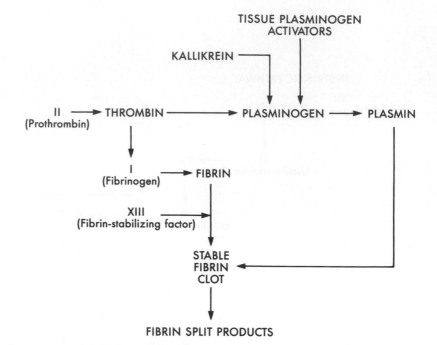

Figure 11-5 The fibrinolytic process. (From Kinney MR, Packa DR, Dunbar SB: *AACN's clinical reference for critical-care nursing,* ed 3, St Louis, 1993, Mosby.)

Table					

11-7 ABO Blood Groups

Patient's ABO Group	Percentage of Population	Antigen on RBC	Antibodies in Plasma	Compatible RBCs	Compatible Plasma
O	47%	None	Anti-A; Anti-B	O	O, A, B, AB
A	41%	A	Anti-B	O, A	A, AB
B	9%	B	Anti-A	O, B	B, AB
AB	3%	A and B	None	O, A, B, AB	AB

11-8 Rh Compatibility

Patient's Rh Type	RBC Rh Type for Transfusion	Plasma Rh Type for Transfusion
Positive	Positive or negative	Positive or negative
Negative	Negative	Positive or negative

3. Only C, D, E are antigenic enough to cause significant development of anti-Rh antibodies (and therefore to potentially cause blood transfusion reaction if nonmatched blood is administered)
4. If C, D, or E antigens are present, the person is Rh-positive; if none of these three antigens is present, the person is Rh-negative; most (85%) Americans are Rh-positive
5. Rh antibodies do not develop spontaneously; they only occur after exposure to Rh antigen (e.g., second exposure to non-Rh matched blood or Rh-negative mothers pregnant with the second Rh-positive fetus if anti-Rh globin [Rho-gam] was not given); delayed

transfusion reactions can occur even after the first exposure to Rh-positive blood and cause a mild transfusion reaction
C. Other red cell antigens
1. Cold agglutinins
a) These antibodies cause erythrocytes to coagulate when blood plasma temperature is below normal body temperature
b) Banked blood must be warmed to normal body temperature (37° C) before giving the blood to a patient who has cold agglutinins
2. Coombs' test: used to determine presence of hemolyzing antibodies
a) Direct: detects antibodies attached to red cells
b) Indirect: detects antibodies in serum
D. Uncrossmatched type O-negative packed red blood cells may be used in exsanguinating patient
1. Whole blood is avoided to decrease the risk of reaction caused by anti-A and anti-B antibodies in type O plasma
2. Blood antigen-antibody complexes may complicate later crossmatching and may cause

future blood transfusion reaction to own blood
type unless own blood type is O negative

3. Type-specific blood may be preferable, and
type matching takes only 5 to 15 minutes

E. Human leukocyte antigen (HLA)

1. Concerned with a group of antigenic substances found on many cell types (including
WBCs and platelets but not on erythrocytes)

2. Detected serologically by cytotoxicity assays;
HLA-A, HLA-B, HLA-C are found on all nucle-
ated cells but HLA-D and HLA-DR antigens
are only located on B lymphocytes, monocytes, and epidermal and endothelial cells

3. Very important in organ and tissue transplantation histocompatibility

Assessment of the Hematologic and Immunologic Systems

Interview

I. Chief complaint: why the patient is seeking help
and duration of the problem

A. Symptoms that may be related to hematologic
or immunologic conditions

1. General
   a) Fatigue
   b) Weakness
   c) Chills
   d) Fever
   e) Weight loss
   f) Night sweats
   g) Apathy
   h) Lethargy
   i) Malaise
   j) Abnormal bleeding, bruising, or swelling
   k) Chronic or recurrent infections
   l) Poor wound healing
   m) Enlarged and/or tender lymph nodes

2. Specific
   a) Skin
      (1) Dry, coarse skin
      (2) Bruising or bleeding
         (a) Prolonged bleeding
         (b) Petechiae
         (c) Bruising easily
      (3) Color changes
         (a) Jaundice
         (b) Pallor
         (c) Cyanosis
      (4) Rash
      (5) Pruritus
      (6) Lesions
      (7) Wounds: poor healing
      (8) Inflammation
   b) Eyes
      (1) Visual disturbances (e.g., blurring,
          diplopia)
      (2) Blindness related to retinal
          hemorrhage
      (3) Conjunctival pallor or inflammation

   c) Ears
      (1) Vertigo
      (2) Tinnitus
   d) Nasopharynx and mouth
      (1) Epistaxis
      (2) Dysphagia
      (3) Gingival bleeding
      (4) Painful lesions on mouth and lips
      (5) Sore tongue
      (6) Sore throat
      (7) Persistent hoarseness
   e) Neck: nuchal rigidity
   f) Lymph nodes
      (1) Swelling
      (2) Tenderness
   g) Cardiovascular
      (1) Chest pain
      (2) Sternal tenderness
      (3) Palpitations
      (4) Known murmurs
   h) Pulmonary
      (1) Exertional dyspnea
      (2) Cough
      (3) Sputum
      (4) Orthopnea
      (5) Respiratory tract infections, including
          Pneumocystis pneumonia, in immu-
          nodeficient patients
      (6) Hemoptysis
   i) Gastrointestinal
      (1) Anorexia
      (2) Abdominal pain and cramping
      (3) Abdominal fullness
      (4) Eructation
      (5) Bloody or black stools
      (6) Vomiting of blood or coffee ground
          material
      (7) Ulcers
      (8) Change in bowel habits
         (a) Diarrhea
         (b) Constipation
      (9) Rectal pain or bleeding
   j) Genitourinary
      (1) Hematuria
      (2) Pyuria
      (3) Menorrhagia
      (4) Amenorrhea
      (5) Incontinence, dysuria, hesitancy,
          frequency
      (6) Urinary retention
      (7) Pelvic or flank pain
   k) Neurologic
      (1) Change in level of consciousness
      (2) Confusion
      (3) Irritability
      (4) Memory loss
      (5) Headache
      (6) Ataxia
      (7) Sensory changes: paresthesia,
          anesthesia
      (8) Syncope, vertigo

l) Back and extremities
  (1) Pain and/or tenderness in joints, back, shoulder, or bone
  (2) Joint stiffness or swelling
  (3) Muscle weakness

II. Past medical history
  A. Surgical history
    1. Splenectomy
    2. Tumor removal
    3. Thymectomy
    4. Breast implants
    5. Organ or tissue transplant
    6. Prosthetic heart valves
    7. Tonsillectomy
    8. Surgical excision of duodenum
    9. Total or partial gastrectomy
    10. Response to dental extractions (e.g., excessive bleeding)
  B. Medical problems
    1. Recurrent infections
    2. Problems with wound healing
    3. Anemia
    4. Asthma
    5. Mononucleosis
    6. Malignancy, especially leukemia, lymphoma, multiple myeloma
    7. Autoimmune disease (e.g., lupus erythematosus)
    8. Radiation therapy
    9. Malabsorption syndrome
    10. Liver disease
    11. Renal failure
    12. Spleen disorders
    13. Diabetes mellitus
    14. Sexually transmitted disease
    15. HIV/AIDS
    16. Prolonged or excessive bleeding (e.g., after dental procedures, injury, or surgery)
    17. Deep vein thrombosis or pulmonary embolism
    18. Vitamin K deficiency
  C. Allergies
    1. Known allergies and type of reaction
      a) Inhalants
      b) Contactants
      c) Injectables
      d) Ingestibles
    2. Transfusion with blood or blood products
  D. Immunizations: types, dates, any adverse reactions

III. Family history
  A. Congenital immune deficiency
  B. Congenital bleeding disorder (e.g., hemophilia)
  C. Congenital RBC dyscrasias (e.g., sickle cell disease)
  D. Congenital anemia (e.g., Thalassemia)
  E. Asthma
  F. Allergies
  G. Anemia
  H. Jaundice
  I. Malignancies

J. Autoimmune disease (e.g., systemic lupus erythematosus [SLE], rheumatoid arthritis)

IV. Social history
  A. Relationship with spouse or significant other; family structure
  B. Occupation
    1. Occupational exposure to radiation
    2. Occupational exposure to chemicals (e.g., lead, benzene, ethylene oxide, insecticides, vinyl chloride)
    3. Military service; exposure to toxins
  C. Educational level
  D. Stress level and usual coping mechanisms; lifestyle changes
  E. Recreational habits
  F. Exercise habits
  G. Dietary habits; dietary deficiency: iron, folic acid, vitamin B_{12}
  H. Caffeine intake
  I. Tobacco use: record as pack-years (number of packs per day times the number of years he or she has been smoking)
  J. Alcohol use: record as alcoholic beverages consumed per month, week, or day
  K. Recent foreign travel
  L. Sexuality
    1. Safe sex practices
    2. Sexual preference: heterosexual, homosexual, bisexual
    3. Multiple sexual partners
    4. Sexual activity with prostitutes, homosexuals, or bisexuals

V. Medication history
  A. Agents used to treat existing hematologic conditions
    1. Drugs used for erythropoiesis: iron, vitamin B_{12}, pyridoxine, folic acid, recombinant human erythropoietin
    2. Drugs used for bleeding or clotting disorders: cryoprecipitate, anticoagulants
    3. Antineoplastic agents
    4. Antiviral, antibacterial, antifungal agents
    5. Drugs used to augment the immune system (e.g., interferon, interleukin-2, colony-stimulating factors)
  B. Agents that may exert a negative effect on hematologic/immunologic system
    1. Allergy medication
    2. Analgesics
      a) Acetaminophen: may decrease platelets; may cause hemolytic anemia
      b) Antiinflammatory agents
        (1) Antigout drugs (e.g., colchicine): may cause aplastic anemia
        (2) Aspirin: inhibits platelet aggregation; decreases macrophage activity
        (3) Corticosteroids (e.g., prednisone): suppress the immune/inflammatory process
        (4) Nonsteroidal (e.g., phenylbutazone [Butazolidin], ibuprofen [Motrin]):

inhibit platelet aggregation; depress bone marrow and may cause aplastic anemia; lyse T, B, and natural killer cells; inhibit interferon production; inhibits IL-1 and IL-2 production

  c) Narcotics
    (1) Heroin: may decrease platelets
    (2) Morphine sulfate: may decrease platelets

3. Antibiotics
  a) Oral antibiotics: may kill vitamin K–producing bacteria in the GI tract
  b) All antibiotics may cause opportunistic infections by altering normal flora in GI tract, mouth, vagina, etc.; *Clostridium difficile* is an example often seen in critical care units that causes severe diarrhea
  c) Tetracyclines: inhibit chemotaxis; inhibit activation of the lymphocytes
  d) Sulfonamides: inhibit chemotaxis; inhibit activation of the lymphocytes; may cause aplastic anemia; may decrease platelets
  e) Chloramphenicol: depresses WBC production; may cause aplastic anemia
  f) Penicillin: may decrease platelets
  g) Rifampicin: may decrease platelets

4. Anticonvulsants
  a) Phenytoin (Dilantin): inhibits the effects of corticosteroids; may cause lymph node hyperplasia; may cause anemia or thrombocytopenia
  b) Phenobarbital: may cause aplastic anemia

5. Antidysrhythmics
  a) Procainamide: may cause hemolytic anemia, thrombocytopenia; decreases production of WBCs
  b) Quinidine: may cause hemolytic anemia, thrombocytopenia
  c) Propranolol: inhibits platelet aggregation

6. Antifungals
  a) Amphotericin B: may cause anemia or thrombocytopenia

7. Antihypertensives
  a) Captopril (Capoten): may cause pancytopenia
  b) Methyldopa (Aldomet): may cause thrombocytopenia, anemia

8. Antituberculins (e.g., p-aminosalicylic acid [PAS], isoniazid [INH])

9. Diuretics
  a) Chlorothiazide (Diuril): may cause anemia or thrombocytopenia
  b) Furosemide (Lasix): may cause anemia or thrombocytopenia

10. Heparin: may decrease platelets

11. Histamine$_2$-receptor antagonists (e.g., cimetidine): may decrease platelets

12. Immunosuppressives

13. Oral contraceptives and diethylstilbestrol

14. Oral hypoglycemic agents (e.g., chlorpropamide) may cause anemia or thrombocytopenia

15. Sympathomimetics (e.g., epinephrine): decrease chemotaxis; decrease WBC production and response to antigens; alter antibody production

16. Anesthetic agents (e.g., halothane, nitrous oxide, cyclopropane): decrease phagocytosis and inhibit T-cell function

C. Nonprescribed drug use
1. Over-the-counter drugs
2. Vitamins, minerals, herbs
3. Substance abuse: injectable drug use, especially if needles are shared
  a) Intravenous drug use
  b) Intramuscular steroid use
  c) Intradermal "poppers"

Physical Examination

I. Vital signs
  A. Weight: weight loss
  B. Heart rate: tachycardia often seen with blood loss or infection
  C. Blood pressure: hypotension seen with blood loss
  D. Temperature: hyperthermia often seen with infection but less likely in elderly patients

II. Inspection
  A. Skin and appendages
    1. Color
      a) Pallor or flushing of mucous membranes and palmar creases
      b) Pallor of conjunctivae
      c) Cyanosis
      d) Jaundice
      e) Brownish skin discoloration
      f) Areas of hyperpigmentation
      g) Signs of inflammation
    2. Bleeding
      a) Petechiae
      b) Ecchymosis
      c) Purpura
      d) Mucous membrane bleeding
      e) Gingival bleeding
      f) Retinal hemorrhages
      g) Hemorrhage from orifices
    3. Moisture
      a) Dry, rough skin (xeroderma)
      b) Moisture-related skin breakdown may occur at skin folds (e.g., axillae, groin, perineal areas); fungal infections are common in these areas
    4. Lesions and wounds
      a) Rash
      b) Excoriated skin
      c) Leg ulcers
      d) Intravenous catheter insertion sites
      e) Chest tube insertion site
      f) Surgical or traumatic wounds

g) Orthopedic devices

h) Drains

5. Pitting edema of extremities

6. Hair: alopecia

7. Nail and nailbed

a) Pallor of nailbeds

b) Spoon nails

c) Clubbing

B. Mouth

1. Dryness of the mouth (xerostomia)

2. Gingival and mucosal ulceration

3. Swollen, reddened, bleeding gums

4. Smooth tongue texture

5. White coating on tongue (candidiasis, also called *thrush*)

6. White, irregular lesions on lateral surfaces of tongue (oral hairy leukoplakia often seen in HIV-positive patients)

7. Purplish lesions on tongue

8. Beefy red tongue

C. Gastrointestinal: nasogastric tube

D. Neuromuscular

1. Decreased level of consciousness

2. Pupil changes

3. Decreased sensation

4. Muscle weakness

III. Palpation

A. Enlargement or tenderness of superficial lymph nodes

B. Tenderness during sternal or rib palpation

C. Tenderness during abdominal palpation

D. Hepatomegaly

E. Splenomegaly

IV. Percussion

A. Decreased deep tendon reflexes

B. Diaphragmatic excursion

C. Hepatomegaly

D. Splenomegaly

V. Auscultation

A. Cardiovascular

1. Dysrhythmia

2. S_3

3. S_4

4. Murmur

5. Rub

6. Bruits over carotids, aorta

B. Pulmonary

1. Crackles

2. Pleural rub

C. Abdomen

1. Bowel sounds

2. Peritoneal friction rub

Diagnostic Studies

I. Blood

A. Hematology

1. Red blood cells (RBC): normal 4.4 to 5.9 $\times 10^6$/ml for males; 3.8 to 5.2 $\times 10^6$/ml for females

a) Elevated in dehydration, chronic hypoxemia, or high altitudes; may temporarily increase after a cold shower or with intense emotions

b) Decreased in hemorrhage, anemias, leukemias, or hypothyroidism

2. Reticulocyte count: normal 0.5% to 1.5% of RBC

a) Young RBCs

b) Assesses the responsiveness and potential of the bone marrow to respond to bleeding or hemolysis

3. Erythrocyte sedimentation rate (ESR or sed rate): normal 1 to 13 mm/hr for males, 1 to 20 mm/hr for females

a) Nonspecific test; measures the amount of RBCs that settle in 1 hour

b) Elevated in inflammatory processes (e.g., rheumatoid arthritis, malignancy, rheumatic fever, hemolytic anemia, thyroid disorders, autoimmune disorders, nephrotic syndrome)

c) Decreased in polycythemia vera, hypofibrinogenemia, sickle cell anemia, congestive heart failure

4. Hemoglobin: normal 13 to 18 g/dl for males; 12 to 16 g/dl for females

a) Elevated in polycythemia, which may occur in chronic hypoxia or high altitudes

b) Decreased in anemia, hemorrhage

5. Hematocrit: normal 40% to 52% for males; 35% to 47% for females

a) Elevated in dehydration or polycythemia

b) Decreased with anemia, leukemia, or with normal hemoglobin and water overload

6. Red cell indices

a) Mean corpuscular volume (MCV) (an average of size): normal 80 to 100 fl

b) Mean corpuscular hemoglobin (MCH) (an average of weight of hemoglobin in an RBC): normal 26.6 to 34.0 pg

c) Mean corpuscular hemoglobin concentration (MCHC): normal 31.4 to 36.3 g/dl

7. Peripheral smear: evaluation of blood cell size, shape, and composition

8. WBC: 3,500 to 11,000 mm^3

a) Elevated in infection, trauma, surgery, acute leukemia, stress

b) Decreased in bone marrow depression (e.g., aplastic anemia, agranulocytosis, chronic leukemia, sepsis, autoimmune disorders)

9. Differential

a) Neutrophils: normal 40% to 80%

(1) Elevated in infection, inflammatory processes, malignancy, trauma, hemorrhage, burns, tissue necrosis (e.g., myocardial infarction), ketoacidosis

(2) Decreased in overwhelming infection, bone marrow depression,

vitamin B$_{12}$ or folic acid deficiency, hypersplenism

b) Eosinophils: normal 0% to 5%
  (1) Elevated in:
    (a) Allergic conditions
      (i) Asthma
      (ii) Eczema
    (b) Leukemia
    (c) Autoimmune disorders
    (d) Parasitic infection, especially helminthic infections
  (2) Decreased in:
    (a) Adrenocortical stimulation
    (b) Stress
    (c) Cushing's syndrome
    (d) Systemic lupus erythematosus

c) Basophils: 0% to 2%
  (1) Elevated in allergic conditions, inflammatory processes, graft rejection, acute leukemia, recent splenectomy
  (2) Decreased in hyperthyroidism and long-term corticosteroid therapy

d) Monocytes: 3% to 8%
  (1) Elevated in chronic inflammatory conditions, anemia, malignancy, mononucleosis, acute HIV infection
  (2) Decreased in immunodeficiency disorders

e) Lymphocytes: 10% to 40%
  (1) Elevated in chronic lymphocytic leukemia, chronic infections: bacterial and viral, multiple myeloma, mononucleosis, Cushing's syndrome
  (2) Decreased in immunodeficiency disorders (e.g., AIDS, systemic lupus erythematosus, leukemia, antineoplastic drugs, steroids, sepsis)
  (3) Lymphocyte assays (Table 11-9)
    (a) T-cells
    (b) B-cells
    (c) Natural killer cells

f) Changes in differential
  (1) Shift to the left: increased percentage of bands; seen in infection
  (2) Shift to the right: increased percentage of segs; seen in pernicious anemia or hepatic disease
  (3) Regenerative shift: elevated WBC with increased percentage of bands; indicative of stimulation of bone marrow
  (4) Degenerative shift: decreased WBC with increased percentage of bands; indicative of bone marrow depression

10. Platelets: normal 150,000 to 400,000/mm^3; decreased in systemic lupus erythematosus, HIV infection, idiopathic thrombocytopenic purpura, DIC

Table 11-9 Lymphocyte Assays

Lymphocyte Type	Percentage of Lymphocytes
Total T-cells	70%-80%
CD4 (helper T-cells)	29%-60%
CD8 (suppressor T-cells)	18%-42%
CD4/CD8 (helper/suppressor ratio)	>1%
Total B-cells	10%-20%

B. Clotting profile
  1. Prothrombin time (PT): normal 12 to 15 seconds; assesses extrinsic coagulation pathway and the common pathway
  2. Activated partial thromboplastin time (aPTT): normal 25 to 38 seconds; assesses intrinsic coagulation pathway and the common pathway
  3. Thrombin time (TT): normal 10 to 15 seconds; assesses time for thrombin to convert fibrinogen to a fibrin clot
  4. Bleeding time: normal 1 to 4 minutes; assesses platelet function
  5. Lee White clotting time: normal 6 to 12 minutes; nonspecific test for clotting abnormalities
  6. Fibrinogen: normal 200 to 400 mg/dl
    a) Elevated in hypercoagulable states and inflammatory conditions
    b) Decreased in hypocoagulable states with propensity to bleed
  7. Fibrin split products (FSPs) (also referred to as *fibrin degradation products [FDPs]*): normal 0 to 10; elevated in excessive fibrinolysis (e.g., DIC)
  8. D-dimer: normal less than 250 ng/ml; elevated in DIC
  9. Specific factor assays: measure amounts of each factor in the blood

C. Serum proteins
  1. Total protein: normal 6 to 8 g/dl
  2. Albumin: normal 3.5 to 4.5 g/dl
  3. C-reactive protein: normal less than 0.8 mg/dl; nonspecific test for evaluating severity and course of inflammatory conditions
  4. Serum protein electrophoresis: immunoglobulin analysis (Table 11-10)
  5. Complement assay
    a) Components
      (1) Total complement: normal 41 to 90 hemolytic units
      (2) C1 esterase inhibitor: normal 16 to 33 mg/dl
      (3) C3: normal 88 to 252 mg/dl in men; 88 to 206 mg/dl in women
      (4) C4: normal 12 to 72 mg/dl in men; 13 to 75 mg/dl in women

Table 11-10 Immunoglobulin Analysis

Immunoglobulin	Increased	Decreased
IgG	• Infection • Hepatitis A • Glomerulonephritis • Rheumatoid arthritis • Systemic lupus erythematosus • AIDS • IgG myeloma	• Agammaglobulinemia • Chronic lymphocytic leukemia
IgM	• Hepatitis A and B • Chronic infections • SLE • Rheumatoid arthritis • Sjögren syndrome • AIDS	• Hypogammaglobulinemia • Chronic lymphocytic leukemia • IgG myeloma • IgA myeloma • Agammaglobulinemia
IgA	• SLE • Rheumatoid arthritis • IgA myeloma	• IgA deficiency • Acute and chronic lymphocytic leukemia • Agammaglobulinemia • IgG myeloma • Chronic infections
IgE	• Allergic rhinitis • Allergic asthma • Parasitic infection	• IgA deficiency • Intrinsic asthma
IgD	• Eczema • Skin disorders	• Unknown

b) Decreased total complement levels occur in the following:
  (1) Systemic lupus erythematosus (SLE)
  (2) Acute poststreptococcal glomerulonephritis
  (3) Acute serum sickness
  (4) Cirrhosis of the liver
  (5) Multiple myeloma
  (6) Severe immunodeficiency
  (7) Rapidly rejecting allografts
c) Elevated total complement levels occur in the following:
  (1) Obstructive jaundice
  (2) Thyroiditis
  (3) Acute rheumatic fever
  (4) Rheumatoid arthritis
  (5) Acute myocardial infarction
  (6) Ulcerative colitis
  (7) Diabetes mellitus
D. Chemistry
  1. Calcium: normal 8.5 to 10.5 mg/dl
  2. Bilirubin: normal total bilirubin 0.3 to 1.3 mg/dl
    a) Indirect (before being conjugated by liver): 0.1 to 1.0 mg/dl
    b) Direct (after being conjugated by liver): 0.1 to 0.3 mg/dl
  3. Iron: normal 50 to 150 µg/dl
  4. Total iron-binding capacity (TIBC): normal 250 to 410 µg/dl
E. Type and crossmatch
  1. Blood typing: determined by agglutination studies

2. Rh factor determination
3. Coombs' test: detects immune antibodies important in crossmatching
  a) Direct: normal negative; measures antibodies (IgG) attached to RBCs
  b) Indirect: normal negative; measures antibodies (IgG) in the serum
F. Human leukocyte antigens (HLA): evaluates tissue compatibility
  1. Tissue
    a) Complement-dependent cytotoxic assay
    b) Mixed lymphocyte culture
  2. Crossmatching
G. Immune profile
  1. CD4 cell count: normal 800 cells/mm^3; varies with age
    a) Measured helper T-cells
    b) Decreased in HIV infection and AIDS; assists in staging HIV infection
  2. T4/T8 (CD4/CD8) ratio
    a) Helper cells: suppressor/cytotoxic cells ratio: normal >1
    b) Normally more CD4 cells than CD8 cells
    c) Reverse ratio in HIV infection or AIDS
H. HIV antibody screening: normal negative
  1. Detects antibodies to HIV; present with exposure to HIV, but absence does not mean that the patient has not been exposed because time is required for development of antibodies
  2. Does not indicate immunity
  3. Types of tests
    a) Enzyme-linked immunosorbent assay

(ELISA): screening test subject to error; up to 10% false-positive results

    b) Western blot: more specific than ELISA

I. HIV virus screening (e.g., polymerase chain reaction [PCR]): normal negative

J. HIV viral load testing

    1. May range from imperceptible (<25 to 5,000 copies of HIV/ml) to 1 million or more copies/ml; consider that the higher the viral load, the more rapid the damage from HIV

    2. Used to evaluate the effectiveness of anti-retroviral therapy

II. Urine

    A. RBCs: normal 0 to 2/low-power field; RBCs in the urine may indicate trauma (e.g., renal calculi) or bleeding disorder (e.g., DIC)

    B. WBCs: normal 0 to 4/low-power field; WBCs in the catheterized urine specimen indicate urinary tract infection

    C. Bilirubin: normal none; urobilinogen indicates biliary obstruction or liver disease

III. Stool

    A. Blood: may be grossly bloody or guaiac positive in bleeding disorders

    B. Culture and/or toxins: may show opportunistic infections (e.g., *Clostridium difficile*) in immunodeficient patients

IV. Radiologic and radioisotope studies

    A. Chest X-ray

    B. Flat plate of abdomen

    C. Lymphangiography: visualizes the lymph system after injection of a dye; assists in node assessment

    D. Isotopic lymphangiography: uses technetium 99m and is less invasive than radiographic lymphangiography

    E. Scans: liver, spleen, or bone

    F. CT scan of abdomen for evaluation of liver, spleen, and lymph nodes

V. Biopsy

    A. Bone marrow

    B. Lymph node

        1. Open: direct visualization; performed in operating room

        2. Closed or needle: performed at bedside

    C. Synovial

    D. Biopsy of transplanted organs to look for indications of rejection

VI. Anergy panel testing

    A. Administration of antigen for observation of a delayed inflammatory skin reaction

        1. Tuberculosis, mumps, *Candida*, trichophytin are most often used

        2. Mumps antigen is contraindicated for patients allergic to chicken or eggs

    B. Normal response: a negative response to tuberculosis (unless the patient has been previously exposed to tuberculosis) and a positive reaction to several of the other antigens within 24 to 72 hours

C. Abnormal responses

    1. Anergy: failure to respond to any of the injections

    2. Immunodeficiency: induration of less than 5 mm in diameter

Blood and Blood Component Administration

Actions

I. Replacement of circulating volume, blood, or blood component

II. Improvement of oxygen-carrying capacity (RBCs, whole blood)

III. Replenishment of clotting factors (fresh frozen plasma, cryoprecipitate) and platelets (platelets)

IV. Replenishment of granulocytes (granulocytes)

Blood and Blood Products (Table 11-11)
Nursing Diagnoses

I. Fluid Volume Deficit related to blood loss

II. Impaired Tissue Perfusion related to inadequate hemoglobin

III. Altered Protection related to deficiency of clotting factors and/or platelets

IV. Risk for Fluid Volume Excess related to too rapid administration of blood

V. Risk for Injury related to transfusion reaction, blood-transmitted disease

Collaborative Management

I. Administer blood safely

    A. Insert or ensure patency of IV catheter; do not use a catheter (or lumen) smaller than 20 gauge

    B. Ensure that the type and crossmatch has been done and that blood or blood component is available

    C. Assess vital signs: notify physician if temperature is 37.8° C (100° F) or higher

    D. Request blood or blood component from blood bank when ready to administer it within 20 to 30 minutes; if you cannot begin the transfusion within 30 minutes after receiving it, return it to the blood bank

    E. Check all of the following before administration of blood or blood component

        1. Physician prescription for blood or blood product

        2. Consent form signed by the patient (if required by hospital policy)

        3. Confirm the following information with another registered nurse:

            a) Patient's name and hospital number on patient ID bracelet

            b) Type of blood component

            c) Patient's blood group and Rh type

            d) Donor's blood group and Rh type

            e) Unit number of blood or blood component

            f) Expiration date of the blood or blood component

Table 11-11 Blood And Blood Products

Product	Contents	Compatibility Required	Uses	Volume/Unit	Comments
Whole blood	RBCs, WBCs, platelets, plasma, and clotting factors	ABO, Rh-specific	Restores blood volume and oxygen-carrying capacity	Approximately 500 ml	• Must be fresh (<4 hours old) to preserve platelet function • Administer over 2-4 hours • Best for hemorrhagic shock
Packed red blood cells	RBCs and 20% plasma	ABO, Rh-specific preferred; ABO, Rh-compatible required	Restores oxygen-carrying capacity	Approximately 250 ml	• Increases hemoglobin by 1 gram/dl/unit and hematocrit by 2%-3%/U; this change takes approximately 4-6 hours • Administer over 2-4 hours
Washed red blood cells	RBCs and 20% plasma with fewer WBCs and platelets than packed RBCs	ABO, Rh-specific preferred; ABO, Rh-compatible required	Restores oxygen-carrying capacity for patients previously sensitized by transfusions	Approximately 250 ml	• As for packed RBCs
Platelets	Platelets, WBCs, plasma	ABO, Rh-specific or compatible	Corrects low platelet levels to aid in clotting	Approximately 50 ml	• Administer 1 U over 10 minutes • Will increase platelet count by 5,000-10,000/mm³ • Agitate often because platelets tend to settle
Fresh frozen plasma (FFP)	Water, plasma proteins, clotting factors	Rh-compatibility required; ABO-compatibility preferred	Expands blood volume Restores clotting factor deficiencies Contains no platelets	Approximately 250 ml	• Takes 20 minutes to thaw • Must be given within 6 hours of thawing • Administer 1 U over 1-2 hours or more rapidly if for hemorrhage
Granulocytes	WBCs, small amount of plasma	ABO, Rh-compatible; HLA (human leukocyte antigen) compatible if possible	Restores granulocytes in life-threatening granulocytopenia	Approximately 300 ml	• Administer rapidly • Chills, fever may occur; steroids and antihistamines may be given; meperidine may be used for shivering • Administer over 2-6 hours
Cryoprecipitate	VIII, XIII, fibrinogen, fibronectin	ABO-specific or compatible	Replaces clotting factors	Approximately 10 ml; usually 10 bags pooled	• Administer rapidly immediately after thawing • May administer 30 U at one time
Albumin	Albumin from plasma	No compatibility required	Provides volume expansion (no clotting factors)	5%: 200 or 500 ml 25%: 50 ml or 100 ml	• Administer 1 ml/min or more rapidly if patient is in shock • Chemically processed so no risk of hepatitis
Plasma protein fraction	Albumin and globulin in saline solution	No compatibility required	Provides volume expansion (no clotting factors)	5%: 200-500 ml	• Administer 10 ml/min • Chemically processed so no risk of hepatitis

F. Sign the transfusion record along with the RN who confirmed the above information

G. Prime the blood administration set with normal (0.9%) saline, allowing the normal saline to cover the filter; use only normal saline, do not use dextrose-containing solutions or lactated Ringer's solution

H. Warm the blood if indicated
   1. Blood may be warmed to avoid hypothermia in the patient receiving four or more units over 6 hours or in the patient who has tested positive for cold agglutinins
   2. Warm the blood to between 32° and 37° C using a blood-warming device in these situations

I. Clamp off the saline and start the blood or blood component

J. Adjust rate to administer slowly 25 to 50 ml within the first 15 minutes

K. Monitor for transfusion reaction (Table 11-12 and Box 11-1)
   1. Ask the patient to notify the nurse if he or she develops chills, low back pain, shortness of breath, nausea, sweating, itching, hives, or anxiety
   2. Assess for clinical indications of transfusion reaction (Table 11-12)
   3. Take appropriate action for transfusion reactions (Table 11-12 and Box 11-2) if they occur

L. Monitor vital signs every 15 minutes for the first hour and then every 30 minutes until transfusion complete or according to hospital policy

M. Adjust rate to infuse blood within 4 hours of initiating the infusion; FFP, platelet, granulocytes are administered more rapidly; if the blood slows, do the following:
   1. Ensure that the roller clamp is open
   2. Increase the height of the blood bag
   3. Gently squeeze the bag several times to agitate the blood cells
   4. Gently squeeze the tubing and flashbulb
   5. Remove dressing and check site
   6. Close the blood and open the saline to allow 50 to 100 ml to irrigate the line, then restart the blood

N. Flush administration set tubing with saline after transfusion complete

O. Disconnect the empty blood bag from the administration set and dispose of these items according to hospital policy

II. Monitor for adverse effects (Table 11-13) and complications
   A. Complications
      1. Hepatitis
         a) Hepatitis B transmission has been reduced by mandatory testing of all donor blood for hepatitis B surface antigen
         b) Non-A, non-B hepatitis (also referred to as *type C hepatitis*) accounts for 90% of transfusion-related hepatitis
      2. HIV: HIV transmission through blood transfusion has been greatly reduced by screening for HIV antibody started in 1985 and by careful history taking of potential donors for risk factors for HIV
      3. Cytomegalovirus (CMV)
         a) CMV is usually not a problem for immunocompetent patients but may be life-threatening in immunodeficient patients
         b) Clinical indications of CMV infection include mild fever, mild splenomegaly, and atypical serum lymphocytes
         c) CMV-negative blood products are indicated for immunodeficient patients
      4. Transfusion-related acute lung injury or ARDS

Disseminated Intravascular Coagulation
Definition
I. A syndrome characterized by thrombus formation and hemorrhage secondary to overstimulation of the normal coagulation process, with resultant decrease in clotting factors and platelets
II. DIC may be acute or chronic but this discussion is limited to acute DIC

Etiology: Always Secondary
I. Vascular disorders
   A. Shock
   B. Vasculitis
   C. Giant hemangioma
   D. Dissecting aneurysm
II. Infection and sepsis
   A. Bacterial
      1. Gram negative (e.g., *Escherichia coli,* meningococci)
      2. Gram positive (e.g., Staphylococcus, Streptococcus)
   B. Viral (e.g., influenza, herpes)
   C. Rickettsial (e.g., Rocky Mountain spotted fever)
   D. Protozoal (e.g., malaria)
   E. Fungal (e.g., aspergillosis)
III. Hematologic/immunologic
   A. Hemolytic blood transfusion reaction
   B. Massive blood transfusion
   C. Prolonged cardiopulmonary bypass
   D. Sickle cell crisis
   E. Thalassemia major
   F. Polycythemia vera
   G. Anaphylaxis
   H. Systemic lupus erythematosus
   I. Transplant rejection
IV. Trauma
   A. Multiple trauma
   B. Burns
   C. Acute anoxia
   D. Heat stroke
   E. Crush injury
   F. Head injury
   G. Surgery

Table 11-12
Types of Transfusion Reactions

Type of Reaction	Cause	Clinical Indications	Timing	Treatment
Febrile (nonhemolytic): most common type of transfusion reaction	Antigen-antibody reaction to WBCs, platelets, or plasma proteins in the blood product	• Fever (rise in temperature greater than 1° C) • Chills • Headache • Nausea, vomiting • Flushing • Anxiety • Muscle pain	Immediately or up to 6 hours after transfusion	• Stop transfusion • Keep vein open with saline • Notify physician and blood bank • Send blood specimens to blood bank • Administer antipyretics as indicated • Administer steroids as prescribed • Consider washed or leukocyte-poor blood for future transfusions
Mild allergic (Type I hypersensitivity reaction)	Allergic reaction to plasma-soluble antigen in blood product	• Flushing • Itching • Urticaria • Hives	During transfusion or up to 1 hour after transfusion	• If febrile, stop transfusion • If afebrile, slow transfusion to keep-vein-open rate until advised by physician • Notify physician and blood bank • Monitor vital signs • Administer antihistamines as prescribed
Anaphylaxis (Type I hypersensitivity reaction)	Allergic reaction in patients with IgA deficiency sensitized to IgA through previous transfusion or pregnancy	• Anxiety • Urticaria • Facial edema • Dysphagia • Abdominal cramps, diarrhea • Urinary incontinence • Dyspnea • Stridor • Wheezing • Cyanosis • Chest pain or pulmonary edema may occur • Shock may occur • Cardiopulmonary arrest may occur	Immediately; after transfusion of only a few mls of blood	• Stop transfusion • Keep vein open with saline • Notify physician and blood bank • Administer oxygen • Administer antihistamines, steroids, and/or epinephrine as prescribed • Establish emergency airway and/or CPR may be necessary • Consider washed or leukocyte-poor blood or blood from IgA-deficient donor for future transfusions
Acute hemolytic (Type II hypersensitivity reaction)	ABO group incompatibility; antibodies in recipient's plasma attach to antigens in transfused RBCs causing RBC destruction	• Burning sensation along vein • Lumbar pain • Chills • Fever • Flushing • Nausea, vomiting • Tachycardia, tachypnea • Hypotension (may be only sign in unconscious patient) **May even have:** • Dyspnea • Chest pain • Hemoglobinemia; hemoglobinuria • Anuria • Disseminated intravascular coagulation • Shock may occur • Cardiopulmonary arrest may occur	Usually within 15 minutes after initiation of transfusion but may occur any time during transfusion; may be delayed if Rh incompatibility	• Stop transfusion • Keep vein open with saline • Notify physician and blood bank • Send blood unit and blood sample from the patient to the blood bank immediately • Monitor vital signs and urine output • Administer fluids for shock as prescribed • Administer diuretics (usually mannitol) as prescribed (especially if hemoglobinuria occurs) • Monitor for acute renal failure and shock • Request new crossmatch

Table **11-12**	Types Of Transfusion Reactions—cont'd			
Type of Reaction	**Cause**	**Clinical Indications**	**Timing**	**Treatment**
Delayed hemolytic	Alloimmune response causes slow hemolysis	• Fever • Mild jaundice • Purpura • Anemia	Days to weeks after completion of transfusion	• Monitor urine output and hemoglobin and hematocrit levels
Noncardiac pulmonary edema	Donor antibodies react with recipient HLA antigen	• Fever, chills • Dyspnea • Cough • Crackles • Hypoxemia • Shock	During transfusion or shortly after the transfusion	• Stop transfusion • Administer oxygen • Assist with intubation and mechanical ventilation as necessary • Administer steroids as prescribed
Circulatory overload	Fluid administered faster than the cardiovascular system can accommodate	• Tachycardia • Hypertension • Headache • Jugular venous distension • Increased RAP, PAP, PAOP • Dyspnea • Cough • Crackles	During transfusion or shortly after the transfusion	• Administer RBCs no more rapidly than 4 ml/kg/hr unless severe hemorrhage occurring • Slow or stop transfusion • Continue IV saline slowly if transfusion discontinued • Position patient upright with legs over the side of bed • Administer oxygen as indicated • Administer diuretics or venous vasodilators as indicated
Sepsis	Transfusion of contaminated blood components (blood should be infused within 4 hours)	• Chills • Fever • Vomiting • Abdominal pain • Diarrhea (may be bloody) • Hypotension • Shock	During or after transfusion	• Stop the transfusion • Obtain cultures of patient's blood and send with remaining blood to blood bank • Administer antibiotics as prescribed • Administer fluids or steroids as prescribed • Administer vasopressors as needed
Graft versus host disease	Occurs in immunodeficient patients who receive lymphocytes; involves donor's lymphocytes mounting an attack against the recipient's tissues	• Fever • Rash • Stomatitis • Hepatitis • Severe diarrhea • Bone marrow suppression • Infection • Lymphadenopathy • Hepatosplenomegaly	Days to weeks after transfusion	• Administer steroids as prescribed • Administer methotrexate or azathioprine (Imuran) as prescribed

V. Neoplastic disorders
   A. Adenocarcinoma
      1. Pancreatic cancer
      2. Breast cancer
      3. Prostate cancer
      4. Ovarian cancer
      5. Lung cancer
      6. Colon cancer
      7. Stomach cancer
   B. Cancer of the urinary tract

BOX **11-1** **Clinical Indications of Blood Transfusion Reaction in an Unconscious or Sedated Patient**

Tachycardia or bradycardia
Hypotension
Fever
Visible signs of hemoglobin in urine (port-wine colored)
Oliguria or anuria
Bleeding

BOX

11-2 Nursing Actions for Suspected Transfusion Reaction

1. Stop transfusion
2. Maintain IV access with normal saline and new administration set
3. Reassure the patient; stay at the bedside
4. Notify physician and blood bank
5. Recheck blood numbers and type
6. Treat symptoms appropriately
7. Return unused portion of blood in blood bag and administration set to the blood bank
8. Collect and send blood and urine samples to the laboratory; send another urine specimen 24 hours after transfusion reaction
9. Document the transfusion reaction and treatment administered

    C. Sarcoma
    D. Leukemia
    E. Pheochromocytoma
  VI. Obstetric complications
    A. Abruptio placentae
    B. Retained dead fetus
    C. Retained placenta
    D. Septic abortion
    E. Hydatidiform mole
    F. Amniotic fluid embolism
    G. Acute fatty liver of pregnancy
    H. Toxemia
 VII. Embolism
    A. Pulmonary embolism
    B. Fat embolism
    C. Amniotic fluid embolism
VIII. Gastrointestinal and accessory organs
    A. Necrotizing enterocolitis
    B. Pancreatitis
    C. Obstructive jaundice
    D. Hepatitis
    E. Cirrhosis
    F. Acute hepatic failure
  IX. Pulmonary
    A. ARDS
    B. Pulmonary embolism
  X. Toxins
    A. Snake bites
    B. Aspirin poisoning
    C. Impure IV drugs
  XI. Prosthetic devices
    A. LeVeen or Denver shunt
    B. Intraaortic balloon pump

Pathophysiology (Fig. 11-6)

  I. The paradox of DIC: bleeding after clotting
 II. Triggered by:
    A. Intrinsic coagulation system activation: damage to vascular endothelium
    B. Extrinsic coagulation system activation: release of tissue thromboplastin
    C. Red cell or platelet injury

III. Clotting causes ischemia and tissue and organ necrosis; this process leads to multiple organ dysfunction syndrome
    A. Tissue damage releases thromboplastin into circulation
    B. Thromboplastin converts prothrombin into thrombin
    C. Abundant intravascular thrombin is produced that both converts fibrinogen to a fibrin clot and enhances platelet aggregation
    D. Excessive blood coagulation creates microvascular thrombi (referred to as *microclots*) in the microcirculation, causing ischemia
 IV. Bleeding causes loss of hemoglobin and oxygen-carrying capacity; leading to hypoxia and ischemia
    A. Excessive aggregation of platelets causes thrombocytopenia and excessive blood coagulation causes depletion of clotting factors (DIC is often referred to as a *consumptive coagulopathy*)
    B. A stable clot, therefore, cannot be formed at injury sites, predisposing patient to hemorrhage
  V. Fibrinolysis causes the destruction of once-stable clots and more bleeding
    A. Activation of plasminogen to plasmin causes lysis of preexisting clots and surface bleeding
    B. Naturally occurring antithrombins, which inhibit thrombin, are inactivated by plasmin
    C. Fibrinolysis causes production of fibrin split products (FSP), also referred to as *fibrin degradation products (FDP)*
    D. Fibrin split products are normally cleared by the reticuloendothelial system but overproduction overwhelms the system
    E. Fibrin split products act as an anticoagulant perpetuating bleeding
      1. FSPs coat the platelets and interfere with platelet function
      2. FSPs interfere with thrombin and disrupt coagulation
      3. FSPs attach to fibrinogen, which interferes with the polymerization process necessary to form a stable clot

Clinical Presentation

  I. Subjective
    A. History of predisposing factor
    B. Symptoms related to ischemia
      1. Chest pain
      2. Dyspnea
      3. Abdominal pain
 II. Objective
    A. Clinical indications of decreased perfusion (subjective included)
      1. Brain: change in level of consciousness, focal neurologic signs, seizures
      2. Heart: chest pain, ST segment elevation or depression, clinical indications of hypoperfusion
      3. Lung: dyspnea, chest pain, clinical indications of hypoxemia

Table 11-13 Potential Adverse Effects of Blood Transfusion

Complications	Clinical Indications	Prevention/Treatment

Citrate intoxication and hypocalcemia caused by binding of citrate with calcium	• Paresthesia of fingertips, circumoral area
	• Chvostek's sign
	• Trousseau's sign
	• Muscle cramps, tremors
	• Increased deep tendon reflexes (DTR), carpopedal spasm
	• Abdominal cramps, biliary colic
	• Confusion, psychosis
	• Memory loss
	• Laryngospasm, stridor
	• Tetany (characterized by cramps, twitching of the muscles, sharp flexion of the wrist and ankle joints, seizures)
	• ECG changes
	  • Prolonged QT interval
	  • Dysrhythmias
		• Monitor calcium in patients receiving multiple transfusions and/or patients with hepatic or renal disease
		• Administer 500 mg-1 g of calcium every 3-5 U of blood as prescribed

Hyperkalemia caused by hemolysis of stored blood and liberation of potassium
(**Note:** the older the blood, the higher the potassium in the blood)
	• Tachycardia progressing to bradycardia and cardiac arrest
	• Nausea, vomiting, intestinal colic, diarrhea
	• Muscle weakness progressing to flaccid paralysis
	• Numbness, tingling of extremities
	• Increased deep tendon reflexes
	• Fatigue
	• Lethargy, apathy, mental confusion
	• Respiratory muscle weakness may cause hypopnea, dyspnea
	• Respiratory distress
	• Oliguria
	• Decreased contractility, cardiac output
	• ECG changes
	  • Tall, peaked T-waves
	  • Wide QRS complex
	  • Prolonged PR interval
	  • Flattened to absent P-wave
	  • Bradycardia
	  • Dysrhythmias
		• Monitor potassium closely in patients receiving stored blood (especially patients with renal insufficiency)
		• Dextrose and insulin may be prescribed acutely for patients with cardiac effects of hyperkalemia

Loss of 2,3-DPG (2,3-DPG is a byproduct of glucose metabolism on the hemoglobin molecule, which encourages unloading between hemoglobin and oxygen; banked [refrigerated] blood is low in 2,3-DPG; decreased 2,3-DPG shifts the oxyhemoglobin dissociation curve to the left)	• Clinical indications of hypoxia (e.g., tachycardia, dysrhythmias, cyanosis, restlessness, confusion)	• Especially a problem if massive amounts (e.g., ~10 U) of banked blood are administered • Give fresh whole blood when possible for patients in need of multiple transfusions
Ammonia intoxication (**Note:** occurs in older blood; especially a problem for patients with hepatic disease)	• Decreased cardiac output: hypotension • Confusion • Altered level of consciousness • Elevated serum ammonia	• Avoid use of older blood, especially for massive transfusion • Monitor for ammonia intoxication in patients with hepatic disease
Dilutional coagulopathy	• Prolonged PT, aPTT • Bleeding from needle site, wound	• Administer 2 U FFP and/or platelets for every 10 U of packed RBCs as prescribed
Hypothermia	• Decrease in body temperature • Decrease in tissue delivery of oxygen caused by shift of the oxyhemoglobin dissociation curve to the left resulting in increased affinity between hemoglobin and oxygen	• Warm blood to 35-37° C if large quantities of blood are being administered

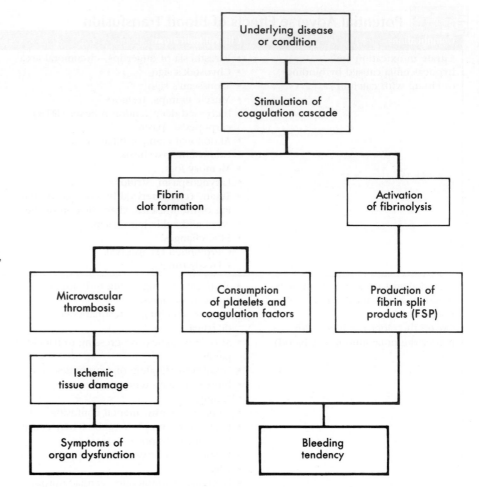

Figure 11-6 Brief schematic of pathophysiology of DIC. (From Kinney MR, Packa DR, Dunbar SB: *AACN's clinical reference for critical-care nursing,* ed 4, St Louis, 1998, Mosby.)

4. Kidney: decreased urine output, proteinuria, electrolyte imbalance
5. GI tract: abdominal pain, diarrhea (may be bloody)
6. Skin: acral cyanosis of toes, fingers, lips, nose, ears; mottling; coldness; necrosis
B. Clinical indications of platelet dysfunction
    1. Petechiae: often the first indication of DIC
    2. Ecchymoses
    3. Purpura
C. Clinical indications of hemorrhage
    1. Tachycardia: initially postural only then profound tachycardia
    2. Hypotension
        a) Initially narrowed pulse pressure
        b) Then postural hypotension
        c) Then profound hypotension
    3. Tachypnea
    4. Overt bleeding in a patient with no previous bleeding history
        a) Mucosal surfaces: gingival bleeding, epistaxis
        b) GU: hematuria
        c) GI: hematemesis, hematochezia, melena, guaiac-positive stool
        d) Pulmonary: hemoptysis
        e) Gynecologic: vaginal bleeding
        f) Skin: prolonged oozing from puncture points, IV sites, and wounds (referred to as *surface bleeding*), bruising

5. Occult bleeding
    a) Swollen joints, joint pain may indicate bleeding into the joint
    b) Abdominal distension, rebound tenderness may indicate intraperitoneal bleeding
    c) Back pain, leg numbness, hypotension may indicate retroperitoneal bleeding
    d) Headache, change in level of consciousness, pupillary changes may indicate intracerebral hemorrhage
    e) Visual changes (e.g., blurred vision, loss of visual fields) may indicate retinal hemorrhage
    f) Alterations in hemodynamic parameters: right atrial pressure, pulmonary artery occlusive pressure, cardiac output/cardiac index may be decreased
III. Diagnostic: all that bleeds is not DIC; diagnostic studies are definitive
    A. Serum
        1. Arterial blood gases: respiratory alkalosis initially progressing to metabolic acidosis due to lactic acidosis
        2. Platelet count: decreased ($<150,000/mm^3$)
        3. Prothrombin time (PT): prolonged (usually >40 seconds)
        4. Activated partial prothrombin time (aPTT): prolonged (usually >70 seconds)
        5. Thrombin time: prolonged (>15 seconds)

6. Fibrinogen level: decreased by 50% or more or less than 200 mg/dl
   a) Because fibrinogen is elevated in pregnancy, sepsis, and neoplastic conditions, a decrease of 50% is a more accurate indicator of DIC than an absolute value in these patients
7. Antithrombin III: decreased (usually <70% activity)
8. Fibrin split products (FSP) [also referred to as *fibrin degradation products (FDP)*]: elevated (usually >40 µg/ml)
   a) Measures the results of both fibrin and fibrinogen degradation
9. D-dimer (end-product of fibrin degradation): elevated (>250 ng/ml)
   a) Specific to the results of fibrin degradation
   b) More specific than FSP for diagnosis of DIC
10. Protamine sulfate test: strongly positive
    a) Protamine sulfate is added to plasma to scc if fibrin strands are formed
    b) A positive test reflects the formation of excessive amounts of thrombin
11. Clotting factor analysis: shows a decrease in factors I, V, VIII, and fibrinogen
12. Peripheral smear: shows presence of schistocytes, helmet cells, red cell fragments
13. Hemoglobin and hematocrit: may be decreased if blood loss is significant
B. Urine: may be positive for blood
C. Stool: may be positive for blood
D. Sputum: may be positive for blood

Nursing Diagnosis
I. Altered Peripheral, Cardiopulmonary, Cerebral, Renal Tissue Perfusion related to microclots and/or hemorrhage
II. Risk for Fluid Volume Deficit related to hemorrhage
III. Decreased Cardiac Output related to decreased preload
IV. Impaired Gas Exchange related to microclots in pulmonary circulation, shunting
V. Risk for Injury related to altered clotting, prescribed therapies
VI. Pain related to ischemia, necrosis
VII. Anxiety related to acute change in health status
VIII. Ineffective Individual Coping related to situational crisis, powerlessness, change in role
IX. Ineffective Family Coping related to critically ill family member

Collaborative Management
I. Detect DIC early and control causative factor
A. Identify and closely assess high-risk groups for clinical indications of DIC
   1. Monitor closely for thrombosis or bleeding
      a) Note petechiae, ecchymosis, acrocyanosis
      b) Test nasogastric aspirate or vomitus, stools, and urine for blood
      c) Monitor oral secretions, pulmonary secretions, and gums for bleeding
      d) Monitor peripheral pulses, capillary refill
   2. Monitor laboratory studies for diagnostic indications of DIC
   3. Monitor closely for clinical indications of hypoperfusion or intracranial hemorrhage
   4. Monitor hemodynamic parameters as indicated; insert indwelling urinary catheter to monitor hourly urine output
B. Control underlying causative factor
   1. Surgery
      a) Surgical debridement
      b) Abscess drainage
      c) Evacuation of the uterus
      d) Removal of tumor
   2. Antimicrobials for infection
   3. Antineoplastics for malignancy
II. Maintain airway, ventilation, and oxygenation
A. Administer oxygen to maintain PaO_2 of 80 mm Hg and SpO_2 of 95% unless contraindicated
B. Assist with intubation and mechanical ventilation as necessary
C. Suction only as necessary and with low suction to avoid trauma to the tracheobronchial mucosa
III. Correct hypovolemia, hypotension, hypoxia, and acidosis
A. Insert or ensure patency of peripheral intravenous catheter
B. Administer normal saline to replace volume until type and crossmatch are completed and blood is available
C. Administer volume replacement, inotropes, and/or vasopressors as prescribed to maintain MAP greater than 60 mm Hg
IV. Stop the microclotting to maintain perfusion and protect vital organ function
A. Administer intravenous heparin (usually 5 to 15 U/kg/hr) as prescribed; aPTT is not used to adjust dose because it is affected by the DIC
   1. Used primarily for patients with thrombosis who continue to bleed despite other rigorous treatment; often effective with underlying malignancy, acute promyelocytic leukemia, and purpura fulminans (may be seen in sepsis)
   2. Prevents further thrombosis in the microvasculature and prevents platelet aggregation; works with antithrombin III to neutralize circulating thrombin
   3. Continues to be controversial because it may potentiate or prolong bleeding, but thrombosis of small vessels has the greatest impact on morbidity and mortality in DIC, not hemorrhage
   4. Contraindicated in CNS or GI hemorrhage, DIC associated with hepatic failure, and

Table **11-14** **Treatments for DIC**

Treatment	Rationale	Controversy
Heparin	• Prevents further microclots and prevents platelet aggregation • Works with antithrombin III to neutralize circulating thrombin	• May perpetuate bleeding
Antithrombin III	• Works with heparin to neutralize circulating thrombin	• May perpetuate bleeding
Clotting factors • Fresh frozen plasma • Cryoprecipitate • Platelets	• Reestablishes normal hemostatic potential	• "Fuel to the fire" theory attests that until the clotting process is stopped, clotting factors increase the thrombosis and microclotting
Epsilon-aminocaproic acid (Amicar)	• Blocks the fibrinolytic system so that stable clots are not degraded • Decreases amount of FSPs, which have anti-coagulant effect	• Clearance of microclots from occluded vessels may be delayed • **Indicated only in primary fibrinolysis**

hemorrhagic obstetric causes (e.g., abruptio placentae)
   B. Administer antithrombin III as prescribed: antithrombin III inhibits the action of thrombin; may be administered if antithrombin levels are low
   C. Assist with plasmapheresis (may be utilized in severe cases)
   D. Note: Table 11-14 describes rationale and controversies regarding selected treatments
V. Stop the bleeding by supporting coagulation
   A. Administer blood products as prescribed to replace missing clotting factors
      1. Fresh frozen plasma (contains all clotting factors): used for bleeding patients with markedly prolonged PT and aPTT
      2. Cryoprecipitate (contains factors VIII, XIII, and fibrinogen): used to maintain fibrinogen levels above 100 mg/dl
      3. Platelets: used to maintain platelet count above 50,000/mm^3
      4. Packed red blood cells: may be needed if blood loss is significant
      5. May potentiate or prolong the clotting ("fuel to the fire" theory), so heparin may be given first
   B. Administer hemostatic cofactors as prescribed
      1. Vitamin K: needed for liver production of several clotting factors
      2. Folic acid: folic acid deficiency may cause thrombocytopenia
   C. Administer epsilon aminocaproic acid (Amicar) (antifibrinolytic agent) as prescribed for primary fibrinolysis; should be avoided in all other situations because it may enhance deposition of fibrin in the microcirculation and macrocirculation and lead to fatal DIC
   D. Apply thrombin-soaked gauze, pressure dressings, and/or ice packs to control bleeding sites
VI. Treat ischemic pain
   A. Administer analgesics as prescribed

   B. Apply cold compresses for pain caused by bleeding in joints and tissues
VII. Maintain skin integrity and minimize tissue trauma
   A. Provide meticulous skin cause
      1. Turn gently often and assess skin while repositioning
      2. Keep the skin moist with lubricating lotions
      3. Utilize specialized beds as needed
   B. Provide careful mouth care; use alcohol-free mouthwash and swabs
   C. Provide careful perianal care; avoid rectal temperatures, suppositories
   D. Alternate activity with rest; mobilize and ambulate patient progressively
   E. Use an electric rather than straight-edged razor
   F. Avoid tape if possible; use adhesive remover to remove tape
   G. Apply local pressure to any break in skin integrity
      1. Avoid intramuscular, subcutaneous infections
      2. Use arterial line or saline lock for blood sampling
         a) If venous puncture is necessary, apply pressure for 3 to 5 minutes after venous puncture
         b) If arterial puncture is necessary, apply pressure for 10 to 15 minutes after arterial punctures
   H. Reduce frequency of cuff BPs: an arterial line is ideal for pressure monitoring and obtaining blood specimens
   I. Do not give ASA or NSAID due to their effect on platelet aggregation
   J. Teach patient to avoid Valsalva maneuver
   K. Do not disturb any clot
VIII. Provide psychologic support and reassurance: reassure patient that treatment is being provided to stop the bleeding (hemorrhage causes extreme anxiety)

IX. Monitor for complications
   A. Intracerebral hemorrhage (a major cause of death)
   B. Hemorrhagic shock
   C. ARDS
   D. GI dysfunction
   E. Renal failure
   F. Infection

Immunodeficiency

Definition: A state of decreased responsiveness or unresponsiveness of the immune system, causing an impaired ability to defend the body against antigens

Etiology

I. Congenital immunodeficiency
II. Acquired immunodeficiency
   A. Acute and/or overwhelming infections
      1. Bacterial
      2. Viral
   B. Physical agents, chemicals, drugs
      1. Radiation
      2. Antibiotics
      3. Antineoplastic agents
      4. Steroids
      5. Antacids, histamine$_2$-receptor antagonists
      6. Immunosuppressive agents (e.g., for post-transplant patients)
      7. Anesthetic agents
      8. Alcohol
   C. Surgery
   D. Stress
      1. Physiologic
      2. Psychologic including noise
   E. Bone marrow depression
   F. Postsplenectomy
   G. Cancer, especially leukemia, lymphoma, multiple myeloma
   H. Chronic diseases (e.g., diabetes mellitus, inflammatory bowel disease, hepatic cirrhosis and/or failure, chronic renal failure, psychiatric illness)
   I. Malnutrition
      1. Protein-calorie malnutrition
      2. Zinc deficiency
   J. Alcohol or drug abuse
   K. Anaphylaxis
   L. Human immunodeficiency virus (HIV) disease or acquired immunodeficiency syndrome (AIDS)
   M. Aging (immunosenescence)
   N. Central nervous system depression

Pathophysiology

I. In addition to previously listed etiological factors, critically ill patients are likely to have:
   A. Altered skin barrier or mucous membranes caused by invasive catheters, nasogastric tubes, endotracheal tubes, chest tubes, indwelling urinary bladder catheter, trauma, burns, surgery, skin lesions
   B. Stress, which promotes catabolism, impairs healing, and causes immunodeficiency
   C. Multiple infections, which may overwhelm the immune system and bone marrow, causing a consumptive leukopenia
   D. Impaired gag, swallowing, and cough reflexes caused by impaired consciousness or tubes
   E. Increased gastric pH caused by antacids or histamine$_2$-receptor antagonists, which allows proliferation of bacteria in the stomach, which may migrate or be aspirated into the tracheobronchial tree and lungs
   F. Malnutrition caused by preexisting disease or inadequate nutritional replacement
   G. Altered perfusion of the intestinal tract, resulting in impaired integrity of the intestinal wall and translocation of microorganisms or their toxins from intestinal lumen into the blood
   H. Prolonged hospitalization increases risk of exposure to microorganisms in the hospital environment from contaminated objects, other patients, or transmitted by hospital personnel; the most common types of nosocomial infection are urinary tract infection, wound infection, respiratory tract infection, and septicemia
II. Reduction of resistance to infection resulting from decrease in number or effectiveness of leukocytes and lymphocytes and immune system suppression
III. Presence of opportunistic infection
   A. Chain of infection includes the following components:
      1. Source of infection
      2. Mechanism of spread
      3. Susceptible host
   B. Drug-resistance infections (e.g., methicillin-resistant *Staphylococcus aureus* [MRSA], vancomycin-resistant enterococcus [VRE]) are of increasing concern; factors that contribute to microbial resistance include the following:
      1. Increased use and misuse of antimicrobials
      2. Increased number of susceptible hosts
      3. Increased use of invasive procedures and devices
      4. Lack of diligence with infection control practices

Clinical Presentation

I. Subjective
   A. History of precipitating condition
   B. Increased susceptibility to infection
      1. Immunodeficiency is suspected when an individual experiences chronic recurrent infections that do not respond to therapy or do respond but recur
II. Objective
   A. Fever: greater than 101° F or 38.3° C
      1. Fever may be the only sign of infection in patients with leukopenia
      2. Not all patients can develop a fever since the

immune system (cytokines) is responsible for fever, so in immunodeficient patients temperature may be normal or below normal even in the presence of infection
B. Skin rash
C. Poor wound healing
D. Redness, swelling, induration at IV site, wounds, incisions
E. Recurrent abscess
F. Osteomyelitis
G. Hepatosplenomegaly
H. Presence of opportunistic infections (e.g., *Pneumocystis* pneumonia, oral candidiasis)
I. Presence of opportunistic malignancy (e.g., Kaposi's sarcoma)
J. Chronic diarrhea
K. Clinical indications of sepsis or septic shock may be seen

III. Diagnostic
A. Serum
1. WBC: total WBC may be decreased or one component of the differential may be decreased
2. T-cell count: may be decreased or T-cell count may be normal but T-cell function may be impaired
3. Albumin and total proteins: may be decreased if protein malnutrition is a causative factor
B. Cultures: may show causative organism(s)
C. Anergy profile: delayed or absent response to skin tests
D. Antibody titers: may be abnormal

Nursing Diagnosis

I. Risk for Infection related to immune system impairment
II. Impaired Skin Integrity related to invasive procedures and devices, edema, malnutrition, immunosuppression
III. Altered Nutrition related to anorexia, hypermetabolism
IV. Ineffective Individual Coping related to situational crisis, powerlessness, change in role
V. Ineffective Family Coping related to critically ill family member
VI. Knowledge Deficit related to health maintenance

Collaborative Management

I. Prevent and monitor for clinical indications of infection
A. Place in private room; limit number of visitors
B. Avoid contact with visitors or hospital staff who have any of the following:
1. Fever
2. Upper respiratory infection
3. Diarrhea
4. Open skin lesions
5. Exposure to contagious disease
C. Minimize potential of cross-contamination; do not assign this patient and a patient who has an infection to the same nurse

D. Institute and emphasize good handwashing
1. Handwashing should be for at least 10 seconds; friction is the most important aspect of effective handwashing
2. Hands should be washed at the following times:
a) Before and after patient contact
b) Before and after invasive procedures
c) After contact with soiled items
d) After toileting
e) After removal of gloves
E. Clean multiple patient equipment (e.g., stethoscope, BP cuff, IV pumps) with disinfectants between patients
F. Provide only food that is cooked, pasteurized, or sterilized; unpeeled fruit should be avoided
G. Sterile water may need to be used even for drinking
H. Minimize introduction of organisms
1. Avoid cut flowers, potted plants, and standing water
2. Damp-dust with disinfectant solution at least every 24 hours
I. Culture common sources of contamination (e.g., ventilator tubing)
J. Avoid intrusive procedures and invasive devices as much as possible
K. Teach and encourage necessary personal hygiene techniques
L. Assess oral mucosa daily and maintain oral hygiene
M. Decrease stress, noise, bright lights, and so on
N. Live vaccines should not be given
O. Encourage high-protein, high-calorie diet
P. Administer filgrastim (granulocyte-colony stimulating factor) (Neupogen) and sargramostim (granulocyte macrophage-colony stimulating factor) (Leukine, Prokine) as prescribed
1. These drugs stimulate proliferation and differentiation of hematopoietic cells, specifically neutrophils or neutrophils and monocytes
2. Indicated to decrease incidence of infection in patients with nonmyeloid malignancy receiving bone marrow suppressive antineoplastic agents and for ganciclovir-induced neutropenia in AIDS patients
II. Provide appropriate nutritional support
A. Enteral nutrition is preferred over parenteral nutrition because it helps to prevent translocation of gram-negative bacteria from the GI tract and helps to prevent stress ulcers
B. Nutritional support containing glutamine and arginine may also be helpful in preventing sepsis
III. Prevent breaks in skin integrity
IV. Maintain activity but provide for adequate rest
V. Assist in patient and family adjustment: provide appropriate reassurance that measures are being taken to prevent and treat infection

VI. Monitor for complications
    A. Poor wound healing
    B. Opportunistic infections
    C. Secondary infections
    D. Sepsis
    E. Septic shock

Acquired Immunodeficiency Syndrome

Definitions

I. Acquired immunodeficiency syndrome (AIDS) is a syndrome of immunodeficiency caused by the human immunodeficiency virus (HIV)

II. HIV is a retrovirus that invades cells that contain the CD4 molecule on their cell membranes; these cells include the helper T-cells, macrophages, glial cells, and dendritic cells
    A. A retrovirus is an RNA-containing virus with an enzyme (reverse transcriptase) that allows conversion of viral RNA to DNA
    B. The viral DNA then inserts itself into the infected host cell's DNA

Etiology

I. Exposure to the causative agent: human immunodeficiency virus (HIV), a CD4 cell retrovirus

II. High-risk groups
    A. Participants of high-risk sexual behavior; unprotected sex
        1. Anal: highest risk during unprotected intercourse
        2. Vaginal
        3. Oral
    B. Sex partners (heterosexual or homosexual) of infected persons
    C. Injectable drug users who share needles
        1. IV drug users
        2. IM steroid users (e.g., athletes)
        3. Users of "skin poppers"
    D. Recipients of blood products, especially prior to 1985; hemophiliacs significantly affected
    E. Newborns or breast-fed infants of infected mothers

Pathophysiology

I. Mode of transmission
    A. Sexual
        1. Semen
        2. Vaginal secretions
    B. Exposure to infected blood or blood products or other body fluids with high concentration of HIV (e.g., CSF of an infected person)
    C. Perinatally
    D. Breast milk

II. Course
    A. Exposure to seroconversion: approximately 6 weeks to 6 months; may take a year or longer in some persons; therefore, repeated testing necessary after suspected exposure

    B. Destruction of T4 cells and imbalance between T4 and T8 cells caused by HIV's use of the T4 cells' DNA for reproduction (Fig. 11-7)
    C. Decrease in cell-mediated immunity T-cells' ability to destroy foreign organisms that enter the body
    D. General decline in the immune system
    E. Presence of opportunistic infections and malignancies
    F. Incubation (exposure to symptoms) period: 6 months to 10 years; average 2 to 5 years

Clinical Presentation

I. Subjective
    A. High-risk group or activity by history
    B. Flulike symptoms initially
    C. Fatigue, lethargy
    D. Anorexia, nausea, vomiting
    E. Diarrhea
    F. Night sweats, chills
    G. Bruising, bleeding
    H. Dyspnea, cough
    I. Recurrent infections: upper respiratory infection, shingles

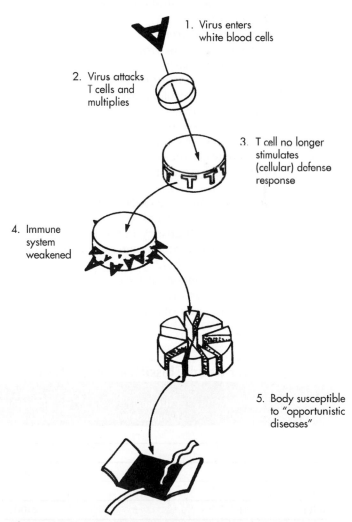

1. Virus enters white blood cells

2. Virus attacks T cells and multiplies

3. T cell no longer stimulates (cellular) defense response

4. Immune system weakened

5. Body susceptible to "opportunistic diseases"

Figure 11-7 Effect of the HIV retrovirus. (From Surgeon General's Report on Acquired Immune Deficiency Syndrome [United States Department of Health and Human Services].)

II. Objective
  A. Fever: recurrent
  B. Rash
  C. Weight loss: rapid, unplanned (may be referred to as *HIV wasting*)
  D. White spots or sores in mouth (hairy leukoplakia)
  E. Lymphadenopathy
  F. AIDS-defining illnesses
    1. Opportunistic infection: infection in the patient with HIV tend to be severe, disseminated, and recur
      a) Candidiasis: esophagus, trachea, bronchi, lungs
      b) Coccidioidomycosis: disseminated or extrapulmonary
      c) Cryptococcosis: extrapulmonary
      d) Cryptosporidia diarrhea for over 1 month
      e) Cytomegalovirus (CMV) disease or retinitis
      f) Encephalopathy: HIV-related
      g) Herpes simplex: skin ulcers for over 1 month, pneumonia, bronchitis, esophagitis
      h) Histoplasmosis: disseminated or extrapulmonary
      i) Isosporiasis: chronic diarrhea for over 1 month
      j) *Mycobacterium avium-intracellulare* or *Mycobacterium kansasii*: disseminated or extrapulmonary
      k) *Mycobacterium tuberculosis* (TB): pulmonary or extrapulmonary
      l) *Mycobacterium:* other species disseminated or extrapulmonary
      m) *Pneumocystis carinii* pneumonia (PCP)
      n) Pneumonia: recurrent
      o) Progressive multifocal leukoencephalopathy (PML)
      p) *Salmonella* septicemia: recurrent
      q) Toxoplasmic encephalitis
    2. Malignancy: malignancy in the patient with HIV tends to be more aggressive and respond more poorly to therapy
      a) Cervical cancer: invasive
      b) Kaposi's sarcoma (KS): in patients less than 60 years of age
      c) Lymphoma
        (1) Burkitt's
        (2) Immunoblastic
        (3) Primary lymphoma of the brain
    3. Wasting syndrome caused by HIV
III. Diagnostic
  A. Serum
    1. Tests for antibody to HIV
      a) ELISA
      b) Western blot: more definitive than ELISA
    2. Tests for HIV
      a) Cell culture
      b) Polymerase chain reaction (PCR)
    3. Hemoglobin and hematocrit: may be decreased
    4. White blood cells: may be decreased
    5. Platelets: may be decreased
    6. Lymphocyte count
      a) CD4 less than 500 cells/mm^3
      b) CD4 below 14%
      c) Ratio of CD4 to CD8 cells: less than 1.0
    7. Immune substances
      a) Acid-labile alpha interferon
      b) HLA-DR5
      c) Immunoglobulins: may be elevated in number but decreased in function
    8. Total protein, albumin, transferrin: decreased in protein malnutrition
  B. Skin tests: may be decreased or absent delayed hypersensitivity reactions to common antigens (e.g., *Candida*, mumps, PPD)
  C. Chest X-ray: may reveal pneumonia
  D. Bronchoscopy with lavage and/or biopsy: may be performed for diagnosis of PCP, KS, TB
IV. Walter Reed classification (Table 11-15)

Nursing Diagnoses
  I. Risk for Infection related to immunodeficiency
  II. Impaired Gas Exchange related to PCP
  III. Altered Nutrition: Less than Body Requirements related to HIV, drug adverse effects
  IV. Anticipatory Grieving related to diagnosis of disease with no known cure
  V. Diarrhea related to drug adverse effects, HIV
  VI. Anxiety related to acute change in health status

Table 11-15	**Walter Reed Classification System**					
Class	HIV Antibody Status	Chronic Lymphadenopathy	CD4 Count (in cm3)	Delayed Hypersensitivity	Oral Candidiasis	Opportunistic Infection/ Malignancy
WR0	−	−	>400	Normal	−	−
WR1	+	−	>400	Normal	−	−
WR2	+	+	>400	Normal	−	−
WR3	+	±	<400	Normal	−	−
WR4	+	±	<400	Partial Failure	−	−
WR5	+	±	<400	Partial or Complete Failure	±	−
WR6	+	±	<400	Complete Failure	±	+

VII. Ineffective Individual Coping related to situational crisis, powerlessness, change in role
VIII. Ineffective Family Coping related to critically ill family member
IX. Knowledge Deficit related to health maintenance

Collaborative Management

I. Minimize further immune system damage
  A. Administer antiretroviral agents (included in Table 11-16)
    1. Types include the following:
      a) Nucleoside analogs
        (1) First class of antiretroviral agents introduced
        (2) Prevent the viral enzyme reverse transcriptase from synthesizing DNA from viral RNA
        (3) Examples include zidovudine (Retrovir), didanosine (Videx), zalcitabine (Hivid), lamivudine (Epivir), stavudine (Zerit)
      b) Nonnucleoside reverse transcriptase inhibitors (NNRTI)
        (1) Interfere directly with reverse transcriptase
        (2) Resistance very common, so generally reserved for use in three-drug combinations
        (3) Examples include nevirapine, delavirdine, efavirenz
      c) Protease inhibitors
        (1) Prevent viral protein from being broken down into usable segments by the enzyme protease
        (2) Generally given in combination with two or more antiretroviral agents because of concern about HIV resistance
        (3) Combinations of two protease inhibitors are being used because of enhancement of effectiveness
        (4) Examples include ritonavir (Norvir), saquinavir (Invirase), indinavir (Crixivan), nelfinavir (Viracept)
    2. Multiple drug therapy is preferred because of the rapid development of resistance with monotherapy
      a) Recommendation is to use three or more drugs, including agents from two or more classes
      b) Common combinations include the following:
        (1) 2 nucleoside analogs + 1 or 2 protease inhibitors
        (2) 2 nucleoside analogs + 1 nonnucleoside reverse transcriptase inhibitors
    3. HIV viral load testing along with CD4 cell count are used to monitor the therapeutic effect of drugs
  B. Encourage adequate rest and nutrition
  C. Encourage avoidance of alcohol and nonprescribed drugs

II. Prevent infection
  A. Use good handwashing techniques
  B. Place patient in private room if possible to prevent transmission of infection to the patient
  C. Decrease number of visitors and do not permit visitors with infections (e.g., upper respiratory infection)

III. Identify and treat opportunistic infections and malignancy (Table 11-17)
  A. Monitor for complications of HIV and of drug therapy (Tables 11-16 and 11-17)
  B. Treat fever with antipyretics, tepid sponge baths, and fluid replacement
  C. Monitor for and treat PCP and acute respiratory failure
    1. Early symptoms include nonproductive cough, dyspnea, fever, chills, chest pain
    2. Diagnostic studies include chest X-ray (findings similar to ARDS), sputum culture (which often requires inducement with saline lavage), and/or bronchoscopy with bronchial lavage or brushing
    3. Collaborative management includes the following:
      a) Administer trimethoprim-sulfamethoxazole (TMP-SMX) orally or IV or pentamidine (Pentam) by inhalation or IV
        (1) TMP-SMX IV requires dilution in a large volume of fluid and may cause fluid overload
        (2) Pentamidine by inhalation may cause bronchospasm
        (3) Pentamidine IV may cause hypotension
      b) Administer oxygen for hypoxemia
      c) Initiate mechanical ventilation as prescribed for respiratory acidosis and fatigue
      d) Administered bronchodilators may be necessary for bronchospasm
      e) Provide appropriate rest periods
      f) Encourage fluids to liquefy secretions
      g) Encourage sustained inspiration and incentive spirometry; encourage the patient to cough; suction only if necessary
      h) Provide frequent oral and nasal care to prevent candidiasis

IV. Provide appropriate nutritional support
  A. Monitor nutritional status and electrolyte balance
  B. Monitor for and treat HIV wasting indicated by unexplained weight loss of more than 10% of body weight
    1. Provide diet that is high in protein and calories
      a) Discourage "empty calorie" foods
      b) Administer multivitamins as ordered
    2. Provide small, frequent meals with snacks as desired
    3. Provide the patient's favorite foods

Table **11-16** **Selected Antivirals and Anti-Infectives for HIV/AIDS**

Drug	Also Called	Indication	Adverse Effects
Abacavir (Ziagen)	1592/ABC	HIV: NRTI antiretroviral	• Systemic hypersensitivity reaction • Nausea, vomiting • Fever • Malaise
Acyclovir (Zovirax)		Viral infections • Herpes simplex 1 and 2 • Varicella-zoster	• Anorexia, nausea, vomiting, abdominal pain, diarrhea (PO) • Rash • Headache • Bone marrow depression (IV) • Nephrotoxicity (IV)

Amphotericin B (Fungizone)		Disseminated fungal infections	• Chills, fever
			• Anorexia, nausea, vomiting, diarrhea
			• Headache
			• Muscle and joint pain
			• Hypotension
			• Electrolyte imbalance
			  • Hypokalemia
			  • Hypomagnesemia
			• Bone marrow depression
			  • Leukopenia
			  • Thrombocytopenia
			  • Anemia
			• Hepatotoxicity
			• Nephrotoxicity
			• Seizures

Dapsone		*Pneumocystis carinii* pneumonia (PCP) prophylaxis	• Nausea, vomiting • Headache • Peripheral neuropathy • Anemia • Methemoglobinemia • Leukopenia • Hepatotoxicity • Nephrotoxicity • Visual changes
Delavirdine (Rescriptor)	DLV	HIV: NNRTI antiretroviral	• Nausea • Fever • Rash

Didanosine (Videx)	ddI	HIV: NRTI antiretroviral indicated for patients who cannot tolerate zidovudine (Retrovir) or who have become resistant to Retrovir	• Anorexia, nausea, vomiting, abdominal pain, diarrhea
			• Dry mouth
			• Headache
			• Peripheral neuropathy
			• Seizures
			• Pancreatitis
			• Elevated liver enzymes; hepatotoxicity
			• Bone marrow depression
			  • Leukopenia
			  • Thrombocytopenia
			  • Anemia

Efavirenz (Sustiva)	DMP 266	HIV: NNRTI antiretroviral	• Dizziness • Rash • Hepatitis
Fluconazole (Diflucan)		Fungal infections	• Nausea, vomiting, abdominal pain, diarrhea • Headache • Rash • Elevated liver enzymes

Table 11-16	Selected Antivirals and Anti-Infectives for HIV/AIDS—cont'd		
Drug	**Also Called**	**Indication**	**Adverse Effects**
Foscarnet (Foscavir)		Pulmonary cytomegalovirus	• Anorexia, nausea, vomiting, diarrhea • Dysrhythmias • Elevated liver enzymes • Nephrotoxicity • Electrolyte imbalance • Bone marrow depression • Bronchospasm • Myalgia • Seizures

Ganciclovir (Cytovene)		Cytomegalovirus (CMV)	• Chills, fever
			• Anorexia, nausea, vomiting, diarrhea
			• Rash
			• Bone marrow depression
			  • Leukopenia
			  • Thrombocytopenia
			  • Anemia
			• Elevated liver enzymes
			• Disorientation, confusion

Indinavir (Crixivan)	IND	HIV: protease inhibitor antiretroviral	• Diarrhea, abdominal pain, nausea, vomiting, anorexia • Headache • Renal stones • Hyperbilirubinemia • Elevated liver enzymes • Hyperglycemia

Lamivudine (Epivir)	3TC	HIV: NRTI antiretroviral	• Nausea, vomiting, anorexia, abdominal pain, diarrhea, dyspepsia
			• Headache
			• Pancreatitis
			• Photophobia
			• Rash
			• Renal stones
			• Myalgia, arthralgia
			• Bone marrow depression
			  • Leukopenia
			  • Thrombocytopenia
			  • Anemia

Nelfinavir (Viracept)	NFV	HIV: protease inhibitor antiretroviral	• Diarrhea • Elevated liver enzymes • Elevated cholesterol and triglycerides • Hyperglycemia
Nevirapine (Viramune)	NVP	HIV: NNRTI antiretroviral	• Nausea • Rash, Stevens-Johnson syndrome • Fever
Pentamidine (Pentam)		*Pneumocystis carinii* pneumonia (PCP)	• Nausea, vomiting • Metallic taste • Chills, facial flushing • Hypertension • Rash • Hypotension • Dysrhythmias • Hyperglycemia • Hyperkalemia • Nephrotoxicity • Elevated liver enzymes • Pancreatitis • Leukopenia • Thrombocytopenia

Continued

Table 11-16 Selected Antivirals and Anti-Infectives for HIV/AIDS—cont'd

Drug	Also Called	Indication	Adverse Effects
Ritonavir (Norvir)	RTV	HIV: protease inhibitor antiretroviral	• Anorexia, nausea, vomiting, abdominal pain, diarrhea • Buccal mucosa ulceration • Dry mouth, bitter taste • Headache • Paresthesia • Rash • Elevated cholesterol and triglycerides • Hyperglycemia
Saquinavir (originally Invirase, now Fortovase)	SQV	HIV: protease inhibitor antiretroviral	• Anorexia, nausea, vomiting, abdominal pain, diarrhea • Dry mouth • Headache • Somnolence • Rash
Stavudine (Zerit)	d4T	HIV: NRTI antiretroviral advanced HIV infection not responsive to other antiretrovirals	• Nausea, vomiting, anorexia, diarrhea, dyspepsia, stomatitis • Hepatotoxicity • Bone marrow depression: anemia • Peripheral neuropathy • Myalgia, arthralgia • Photosensitivity • Rash

Trimethoprim-sulfamethoxazole (TMP-SMX)	TMP-SMX	*Pneumocystis carinii* pneumonia (PCP)
		Isospora belli infection
		Salmonella infection
		Shigella infection
			• Rash
			• Fever
			• Nausea, vomiting
			• Peripheral neuritis
			• Bone marrow depression
			  • Leukopenia
			  • Thrombocytopenia
			• Headache
			• Elevated liver enzymes

Zalcitabine (Hivid)	ddC	HIV: NRTI antiretroviral combination treatment with zidovudine CD4 count of 300 cells/mm³ or less who have demonstrated clinical or immune system deterioration	• Anorexia, nausea, vomiting, abdominal pain, diarrhea, stomatitis
			• Rash, pruritus
			• Headache
			• Elevated liver enzymes
			• Bone marrow depression
			  • Leukopenia
			  • Thrombocytopenia
			• Peripheral neuropathy
			• Pancreatitis
			• Nephrotoxicity

Zidovudine (Retrovir)	AZT	HIV: NRTI antiretroviral CD4 count of 500/mm³ or lower even if asymptomatic	• Nausea, vomiting, abdominal pain, diarrhea
			• Taste changes
			• Rash, acne
			• Headache
			• Fatigue, malaise
			• Myalgia
			• Insomnia
			• Bone marrow depression
			  • Anemia
			  • Leukopenia
			  • Thrombocytopenia

Table 11-17 Opportunistic Infections and Malignancies Seen in AIDS and Treatment

BACTERIAL INFECTIONS

Infection	Treatment
Mycobacterium tuberculosis	• Isoniazid (INH) • Ethambutol (Myambutol) • Rifampin (Rifadin) • Pyrazinamide • Streptomycin • Para-amino-salicylic acid (PAS)
Mycobacterium avium-intracellulare	• Clarithromycin • Azithromycin (Zithromax) • Ethambutol (Myambutol) • Isoniazid (INH) • Rifampin (Rifadin) • Streptomycin • Amikacin (Amikin) • Ciprofloxacin (Cipro) • Clofazimine (Lamprene) • Rifabutin (Mycobutin) • Cycloserine (Seromycin)
Salmonella	• Chloramphenicol (Chloromycetin) • Ampicillin • Amoxicillin • Trimethoprim-sulfamethoxazole (TMP-SMX) • Ceftriaxone (Rocephin) • Ciprofloxacin (Cipro)
Shigella	• Trimethoprim-sulfamethoxazole (TMP-SMX) • Ciprofloxacin (Cipro) • Ampicillin • Nalidixic acid (NegGram) • Furazolidone
Treponema pallidum (syphilis)	• Penicillin
Neisseria gonorrhoeae	• Ceftriaxone sodium (Rocephin) • Cefixime (Suprax) • Ciprofloxacin (Cipro) • Ofloxacin (Floxin)

PROTOZOAL INFECTIONS

Infection	Treatment
Pneumocystis carinii	• Trimethoprim-sulfamethoxazole (TMP-SMX) • Pentamidine (Pentam) • Dapsone-trimethoprim
Cryptosporidium enteritidis	• Amphotericin B (Fungizone) • Spiramycin (Rovomycin)
Toxoplasma gondii	• Pyrimethamine (Daraprim) • Sulfadiazine • Pyrimethamine- sulfadiazine (Fansidar) • Clindamycin (Cleocin)
Isospora belli	• Trimethoprim-sulfamethoxazole (TMP-SMX)

VIRAL INFECTIONS

Infection	Treatment
Herpes (1 and 2)	• Acyclovir (Zovirax) • Foscarnet • Vidarabine (Vira-A)
Cytomegalovirus	• Ganciclovir (Cytovene) • Foscarnet sodium (Foscavir) for CMV retinitis
Varicella-zoster	• Acyclovir (Zovirax) • Foscarnet • Vidarabine (Vira-A)
Hepatitis A, B, or non-A/non-B	• Interferon alfa-2b for B and non-A/non-B

FUNGAL INFECTIONS

Infection	Treatment
Candida albicans	• Nystatin rinses (for oral candidiasis) • Clotrimazole (Mycelex) • Amphotericin B (Fungizone) • Fluconazole (Diflucan) • Ketoconazole (Nizoral) • Itraconazole (Sporanox)
Cryptococcus neoformans	• Amphotericin B (Fungizone) • Fluconazole (Diflucan) • Ketoconazole (Nizoral) • Itraconazole (Sporanox)
Histoplasma capsulatum	• Amphotericin B (Fungizone) • Fluconazole (Diflucan) • Ketoconazole (Nizoral) • Itraconazole (Sporanox)
Coccidioidomy-cosis	• Amphotericin B (Fungizone) • Fluconazole (Diflucan) • Itraconazole (Sporanox) • Ketoconazole (Nizoral)

MALIGNANCIES

Malignancy	Treatment
Kaposi's sarcoma	• Radiation • Surgical excision • Cryotherapy • Chemotherapy • Interferon alfa-2a • Doxorubicin (Adriamycin) • Bleomycin (Blenoxane) • Vinblastine (Velban) • Vincristine (Oncovin) • Methotrexate (Folex) • Cyclophosphamide (Cytoxan)
CNS lymphoma	• Radiation
Hodgkin's lymphoma	• Radiation • Chemotherapy
Non-Hodgkin's lymphoma	• Radiation • Steroids • Chemotherapy

C. Identify causes for and provide symptomatic relief of anorexia
   1. Possible causes of anorexia in the patient with HIV include medication adverse effects, altered taste, dysphagia, nausea, vomiting, weakness, lethargy
   2. Avoid providing fatty, spicy, or overly sweet foods
   3. Avoid metallic utensils and foods from metal cans
   4. Administer antiemetics as prescribed
   5. Administer other pharmacologic agents as prescribed to increase appetite and weight; these agents have less effect on lean body mass:
      a) Megestrol (Megace) is a synthetic progesterone derivative
      b) Dronabinol (Marinol) is an antiemetic and appetite stimulant
      c) Oxandrolone (Oxandrin) is an anabolic steroid
D. Provide symptomatic relief for stomatitis
   1. Provide a mixture of viscous lidocaine, diphenhydramine (Benadryl) elixir, and a magnesium or aluminum salt product such as Mylanta or sucralfate (Carafate) suspension before meals to reduce mouth pain while eating
   2. Provide meticulous mouth care
   3. Administer nystatin (Mycostatin) as prescribed for oral candidiasis
E. Provide symptomatic relief of diarrhea
   1. Replace fluids and electrolytes
      a) High-potassium foods
      b) Electrolyte-containing fluids (e.g., Gatorade) may be helpful
   2. Provide diet low in fat and lactose and high in soluble fiber (e.g., oatmeal, fruit)
   3. Avoid extreme temperature foods
   4. Avoid caffeine
   5. Administer antidiarrheal drugs as prescribed; acidophilus or Lactaid may also be helpful
F. Provide symptomatic relief of dysphagia
   1. Provide soft, bland, nutrient-dense foods and supplements; gelatin, yogurt, pudding are easy to swallow
   2. Provide small, frequent meals
G. Administer enteral or parenteral nutritional support as prescribed
   1. Assist with placement of an enteral feeding tube or vascular access
   2. Use medium chain triglycerides (MCTs) (e.g., Lipisorb or Peptamen) or elemental formulas (e.g., Vivonex TEN) as prescribed
V. Prevent transmission of HIV
   A. Consider all body secretions potentially infectious
   B. Use protective barriers when exposure to blood or body fluids is likely
      1. Gloves are worn when hands will come in contact with blood, body fluids, nonintact skin, or items or surfaces soiled with blood or body fluids
      2. Gown, mask, and goggles are worn whenever body fluids, especially blood, may be splattered
      3. Masks are worn whenever an airborne infection (e.g., tuberculosis) is present
      4. Mouthpieces and manual resuscitation bags are used for resuscitation
   C. Wash hands immediately after removing gloves and any time hands are contaminated with blood or other infectious substances
   D. Use caution with sharp instruments (e.g., needles, scalpels) and dispose of these objects safely
      1. Do not recap needles
      2. Place all sharps in puncture-resistant container
   E. Double-bag and label linens as infectious
   F. Decontaminate surfaces exposed to body fluids with 1:10 dilution of bleach solution
   G. Ensure that reusable equipment is washed and autoclaved
   H. Teach patient and significant others about transmission of HIV
      1. HIV is not transmitted by casual contact
      2. Saliva has not been shown to be a transmission medium, so eating utensils do not need to be disposable and should simply be washed after use
      3. HIV is transmitted via venereal fluids, blood, breast milk, and perinatally
         a) Toothbrushes, razors, needles, or other items that may be contaminated with blood should not be shared
         b) Sexual transmission should be prevented through the use of condoms with nonoxynol-9, which has been shown to kill HIV and to prevent other sexually transmitted diseases; this practice is considered safer than not using a condom but not safe
         c) HIV-positive women should not breast-feed infants; use of antiretrovirals perinatally have been shown to decrease transmission of the virus to the unborn child
         d) HIV-positive persons should not donate blood or expose anyone else to their blood
         e) HIV-positive persons should inform their dentist and other healthcare professionals of their HIV status
         f) Injectable drug users should safely discard or clean syringes and needles with a 1:10 dilution of bleach solution; syringes and needles should not be shared
VI. Provide compassionate emotional support and health counseling
   A. Be nonjudgmental and use scientific knowledge instead of prejudice in health counseling

B. Assess:
   1. The patient's level of knowledge about HIV and AIDS
   2. The patient's past experiences with others with HIV and AIDS
   3. The patient's perception of HIV and AIDS in light of his or her cultural and religious beliefs
C. Teach patient how to prevent transmission of HIV to others
D. Teach significant others what they can do to help and support patient and to protect themselves from HIV
E. Teach clinical indications of infection and what to do if they occur
F. Spend time listening to patient's fears and concerns; allow patient to express fear and grief

VII. Monitor for complications
   A. Acute respiratory failure: Pao_2 less than 50 to 60 mm Hg; $Paco_2$ greater than 50 mm Hg; pH less than 7.30
   B. Septic shock: tachycardia, tachypnea, hypotension, decreased systemic vascular resistance progressing to increased systemic vascular resistance, changes in sensorium, oliguria, elevated serum lactate
   C. Meningitis: headache, fever, nuchal rigidity, lethargy, confusion, seizures
   D. CNS lymphoma: headache, paresis or plegia, paresthesia, visual changes, ataxia, seizures
   E. HIV encephalopathy: personality changes, memory changes, paresis or plegia, aphasia, confusion
   F. Disseminated intravascular coagulation: surface bleeding from injection sites, lesions; peripheral mottling, cyanosis; bleeding from mucous membranes, orifices; prolonged PT, aPTT, bleeding times; decreased platelet counts; elevated fibrin split products
   G. CMV retinitis: progressive visual loss

Organ Transplantation
General Organ Recipient Criteria
   I. End-stage organ disease
   II. Positive psychosocial assessment factors
   III. Absence of the following:
       A. Infection or transmittable disease
       B. Malignancy
       C. Substance abuse
       D. Other organ system failure

General Organ Donor Criteria
   I. Requirements of cadaver donors (Note: live donors may be utilized for kidney, liver, or lung [one lobe] transplantation)
       A. Patient declared dead in either of the following ways:
           1. Irreversible cessation of circulatory and respiratory function

   a) Referred to as a non-heart-beating donor (NHBD)
   b) Constitutes only approximately 1% of cadaveric organ donors each year
   c) Potentially, kidneys are retrieved from NHBDs because this organ can generally withstand more anoxic damage than other organs
   2. Irreversible cessation of all functions of the entire brain, including the brainstem
       a) Recognizable cause of coma (e.g., severe head trauma, intracranial hemorrhage, anoxic encephalopathy following cardiac arrest, drowning, asphyxiation)
       b) Potentially reversible causes of coma (sedative drugs including alcohol, neuromuscular blocking agents, hypothermia, metabolic or endocrine disturbance) excluded
       c) No spontaneous ventilation when tested for a sufficient time; usually 3 to 5 minutes of $Paco_2$ of more than 60 mm Hg; apnea testing is performed by doing the following:
           (1) Disconnect the mechanical ventilator
           (2) Deliver 100% oxygen
           (3) Monitor for ventilatory effort
           (4) Measure arterial blood gases to confirm $Paco_2$ greater than 60 mm Hg
           (5) Reconnecting the ventilator
       d) No brainstem reflexes
           (1) No pupillary light reflex
           (2) No corneal reflex
           (3) No oculocephalic reflex (doll's eyes)
           (4) No oculovestibular reflex (caloric)
           (5) No gag reflex
       e) No motor response to central pain stimulation
       f) EEG: no electrical activity during a period of at least 30 minutes
       g) Cerebral angiography: no intracerebral filling in circle of Willis or at carotid bifurcation
       h) Cerebral blood flow scan: no uptake of radionuclide in brain parenchyma, indicating no cerebral blood flow
B. Organ function acceptable to transplant program
C. No prolonged hypotension or cardiopulmonary arrest
D. No active sepsis or cancer (except primary brain tumor)
E. Consent from next of kin or signed organ donation card
II. Exclusions
   A. General
       1. Untreated bacterial, fungal, or viral infection or sepsis
       2. Malignancy other than primary brain tumor or minor skin lesions
       3. Communicable disease (e.g., HIV, hepatitis B or C); although hepatitis type may be matched

to recipient (e.g., hepatitis B donor to hepatitis B recipient, etc.)
  B. Heart
     1. History of cardiac disease
     2. Suboptimal cardiac function after intervention
  C. Lungs
     1. Positive sputum Gram stain
     2. Pulmonary edema
     3. Pulmonary contusion
     4. Aspiration
  D. Liver: history of hepatitis B or C is generally an exclusion but the recipient may be given a choice of accepting a liver from a patient with hepatitis B or C; also may be acceptable if recipient has hepatitis
  E. Pancreas
     1. History of diabetes mellitus
  F. Kidneys
     1. History of hypertension: not absolute; biopsy may be done to determine viability
     2. History of diabetes mellitus: not absolute; biopsy may be done to determine viability

Preoperative Assessment of Recipient Patient

I. Diagnostic studies to evaluate current status of failing organ
  A. Heart
     1. ECG
     2. Echocardiogram
     3. Cardiac enzymes and isoenzymes
     4. Cardiac catheterization may be conducted
  B. Lung
     1. Chest X-ray
     2. Arterial blood gases
     3. Gram stain and culture of sputum
  C. Liver
     1. Liver function studies: ALT, AST, alkaline phosphatase, GGTP, LDH
     2. Bilirubin
     3. Hemoglobin, hematocrit
     4. PT, aPTT
     5. Total protein, albumin
  D. Pancreas
     1. Serum electrolytes
     2. BUN, creatinine
     3. Serum amylase
     4. Serum glucose
     5. Urine culture and urinalysis
  E. Kidney
     1. Serum electrolytes
     2. BUN, creatinine
     3. Urine culture and urinalysis
II. Tissue histocompatibility
  A. ABO compatibility: detects surface antigens on RBCs and other tissues
  B. Minor red cell antigen testing: detects surface antigens on RBCs
  C. Microlymphocytotoxicity testing: detects class I HLA antigens and match between donor and recipients

  D. Mixed leukocyte culture or mixed lymphocyte culture (MLC): detects class II HLA antigens (**Note:** takes too long to be used for cadaver organs; used for living kidney donors)
  E. White cell crossmatch: detects presence of preformed circulating cytotoxic antibodies in recipient to antigens on the lymphocytes of the donor
  F. Mixed lymphocyte crossmatch: detects presence of preformed circulating cytotoxic antibodies in recipient to antigens on the lymphocytes of the donor
III. Psychologic and emotional status
IV. Potential sources of postoperative infection

Collaborative Management of the Donor Pretransplant

I. Recognize the patient as a potential organ donor according to donor criteria and follow hospital protocol for notification of the local organ procurement organization
II. Collaborate with the physician and organ procurement coordinator in obtaining consent for organ donation from closest family member; if family is not available, look for signed organ donor card
  A. Offer the patient's family the option of organ donation as soon as brain death has been declared
  B. Ensure that the person who approaches the family is an expert regarding organ donation and has time to spend with the family
  C. Approach the family in a private, quiet location
  D. Allow time for the family to accept the death
  E. Use the word "dead" not "nearly dead," "almost dead," or "for all practical purposes dead"; avoid the term "brain dead" because families then tend to believe that there is something worse than brain dead and that the patient is being "kept alive" for organ retrieval; brain death is permanent and irreversible and when the brain is dead, the person is dead
  F. Use "recover," "retrieve," or "remove" organs; avoid the word "harvest"
  G. Use the patient's name and do not refer to the patient as "the donor"
  H. Believe in the benefit to the family of the donor as well as to the recipient
  I. Ensure confidentiality of the donor family and transplant recipients
III. Obtain necessary measurements and laboratory data
  A. Height and weight
  B. Serology screening for hepatitis antigen and antibody, human immunodeficiency virus (HIV), syphilis, cytomegalovirus (CMV)
  C. Blood type and crossmatch
  D. Tissue typing
  E. Diagnostic studies to evaluate organ status
IV. Maintain airway, oxygenation, and ventilation
  A. Ensure a patent airway

B. Administer oxygen to maintain Pao$_2$ of at least 80 mm Hg and Sao$_2$ greater than 95%

C. Provide mechanical ventilation to maintain Paco$_2$ 35 to 45 mm Hg

V. Maintain adequate organ perfusion and tissue oxygenation

A. Monitor vital signs, urine output, and hemodynamic parameters

B. Administer IV fluids, inotropes, and/or vasopressors as prescribed to maintain systolic BP of 100 mm Hg, MAP more than 70 mm Hg, and urine output more than 100 ml/hr; do not overhydrate

VI. Maintain adequate hydration and electrolyte balance

A. Monitor serum osmolality and electrolytes

B. Replace fluids and electrolytes as prescribed

C. Control diabetes insipidus with administration of aqueous vasopressin as prescribed

VII. Maintain normal body temperature

A. Utilize warm blankets, radiant heat lamps, warm inspired air by the ventilator, and/or warm IV fluids as indicated for hypothermia

B. Utilize antipyretics, tepid sponge baths as indicated for hyperthermia; ASA is preferred as an antipyretic because of potential adverse liver effects of acetaminophen

VIII. Prevent infection

A. Monitor for clinical indications of infection

B. Avoid intrusive procedures if possible

C. Use strict aseptic technique in IV, airway, tube management

D. Administer antibiotics as prescribed

IX. Transport the patient to the operating room when the organ procurement organization has found recipients for all of the organs that will be donated

Nursing Diagnoses for the Recipient Posttransplant

I. Risk for Infection related to immunosuppression

II. Risk for Fluid Volume Excess or Deficit related to heart failure, overhydration, hemorrhage, third-spacing

III. Impaired Gas Exchange related to heart failure, lung transplant

IV. Pain related to surgical procedure

V. Ineffective Individual Coping related to situational crisis, powerlessness, change in role

VI. Ineffective Family Coping related to critically ill family member

VII. Knowledge Deficit related to health maintenance

Collaborative Management of the Recipient Posttransplant

I. Relieve pain and anxiety

A. Administer narcotics (e.g., morphine) for pain relief

B. Administer anxiolytics (e.g., diazepam) as needed

C. Allow patient the opportunity to discuss feelings and concerns regarding the surgery and chances of success

II. Protect patient from infection

A. Monitor for clinical indications of infection; cytomegalovirus (CMV) is one common serious infection in immunodeficient patients

1. Clinical indications: fever; malaise; leukopenia, thrombocytopenia, or anemia; abnormal liver function studies; pneumonitis; hepatic or splenic enlargement; impaired graft function

2. Diagnosis by tissue biopsy (liver, bronchiole alveolar lavage, open lung)

B. Administer antimicrobials, antivirals as prescribed

III. Prevent and detect acute rejection of transplant (Table 11-18)

A. Administer antirejection agents (Table 11-19); corticosteroids and azathioprine (Imuran) or cyclosporine (Neoral) or tacrolimus (Prograf) are usually used for maintenance; other agents may be substituted or added for acute rejection

B. Monitor for clinical indications of acute rejection

1. General: fever, tachycardia, flulike symptoms

2. Organ-specific: usually pain around the transplanted organ (with exception of the heart because of denervation) and failure of the transplanted organ; organ biopsy is definitive for rejection

a) Heart

(1) Clinical indications of heart failure: S$_3$, dyspnea, crackles, peripheral edema, jugular venous distention, fatigue, ele-

Table 11-18 Forms of Rejection

Form	Time Frame	Mechanism	Response to Treatment
Hyperacute	Minutes to hours	Humoral response involving preexisting antibodies; causes infarction occurring before the end of the transplantation procedure or within a few hours after the surgical procedure	None Graft removal required
Accelerated	Within a few days	Humoral response	Poor
Acute	1 wk-1 yr	Cellular response	Good
Chronic	1-5 yr	Humoral response	Poor since progressive process

Table 11-19 | **Antirejection Agents**

Drug	Effects	Adverse Effects
Antithymocyte globulin (ATgam)	• Reduces number of circulating T-cells • Reduces the proliferative function of the T-cell	• Allergic reactions • Thrombocytopenia • Anaphylaxis • Increased incidence of malignancy • Decreased resistance to infection, especially viral infections (e.g., CMV, herpes)
Azathioprine (Imuran)	• Interferes with the purine synthesis necessary for the production of antibodies • Prevents synthesis of DNA/RNA in leukocytes • Prevents activation and rapid proliferation of T-cells responding to an antigen	• Stomatitis • Alopecia • Coagulopathy • Bone marrow depression: leukopenia, anemia, thrombocytopenia • Hepatotoxicity • Pancreatitis • Development of neoplasms • Decreased resistance to infection
Corticosteroids (e.g., prednisone)	• Inhibit inflammation by inhibiting production of prostaglandin • Impair the sensitivity of the T-cells to an antigen • Prevent proliferation of cytotoxic T-cells • Impair the production of interleukins • Decrease macrophage mobility	• Cushingoid appearance • GI irritation and/or hemorrhage • Sodium and water retention • Hypertension • Hyperglycemia • Mood swings • Protein catabolism • Delayed healing • Development of cataracts • Development of neoplasms • Aseptic bone necrosis • Decreased resistance to infection
Cyclosporine (Neoral)	• Interferes with the production and activity of cytotoxic and helper T-cells • Interferes with the secretion of interleukins by helper T-cells and the ability for cytotoxic T-cells to respond to interleukins • Interferes with the ability of macrophages to secrete interleukin	• Nausea • Gingival hyperplasia • Headache • Leg cramps • Hirsutism • Hypertension • Nephrotoxicity • Hepatotoxicity • Electrolyte imbalance: hyperkalemia, hypomagnesemia • Tremors, seizures • Lymphocytopenia • Development of neoplasms: lymphomas • Increased susceptibility to infection especially viral or fungal infections
Muromonab-CD3 (Orthoclone OKT3)	• Removes T-cells with the T3 surface antigen from the circulation • Alters T-cell function so that they are unable to recognize antigens	• Fever, chills • Nausea, vomiting, diarrhea • Malaise • Headache • Dyspnea • Chest pain • Wheezing • Tremors • Fluid retention • Thrombocytopenia • Leukopenia • Muscle and bone pain • Allergic reactions • Increased incidence of malignancy • Increased susceptibility to infections especially viral infections (e.g., CMV, herpes)

Table 11-19	Antirejection Agents—cont'd	
Drug	**Effects**	**Adverse Effects**
Mycophenolate mofetil (CellCept)	• Inhibits the proliferative responses of T and B lymphocytes • Blocks antibody formation • Blocks the generation of cytotoxic T-cell production	• Nausea • Diarrhea • Dyspnea • Hypertension • Thrombocytopenia • Leukopenia • Hematuria • Hypokalemia
Tacrolimus (Prograf), formerly referred to as FK 506	• Blocks production of IL-2 and other lymphokines that help activate T lymphocytes	• Anorexia, nausea, vomiting, abdominal pain, diarrhea • Headache • Circumoral numbness and tingling • Tremors • Headache • Hypertension • Flushing • Chest pain • Insomnia • Anemia • Edema • Elevated liver enzymes • Nephrotoxicity • Electrolyte imbalance: hyperkalemia, hypomagnesemia • Hypertension, rash if given with cyclosporine; *cyclosporine should be discontinued 24 hours before tacrolimus initiated* • Decreased resistance to infection

vated right atrial pressure, pulmonary artery occlusive pressure
(2) Dysrhythmias
(3) Decreased cardiac output/index with resultant clinical indicators of hypoperfusion (e.g., restlessness, cool skin, decreased bowel sounds, decreased urine output)
b) Lung
(1) Dyspnea, chest discomfort
(2) Oxygen desaturation with activity, progressive hypoxemia
(3) Breath sound changes: diminished breath sounds, crackles
(4) Abnormal pulmonary function studies (e.g., decreased forced expiratory volumes, vital capacity)
(5) Pulmonary infiltrates on chest X-ray
c) Liver
(1) Right upper quadrant pain
(2) Elevated bilirubin, liver enzymes; elevated ammonia may be seen
(3) Hepatomegaly
d) Pancreas
(1) Elevated serum glucose
(2) Decrease in urine amylase (in patient with exocrine urinary diversion)

e) Kidney
(1) Hypertension
(2) Swollen, tender kidneys; remember that transplanted kidneys are placed in the pelvis; therefore, pelvic rather than flank pain occurs (Fig. 11-8)
(3) Decreased urine volume
(4) Elevated BUN, creatinine
(5) Electrolyte imbalances
C. Teach patient about immunosuppressive drugs
1. Explain that they are the main defense against transplant rejection
2. Discuss the side effects of the prescribed medications
3. Stress that medications cannot be withdrawn suddenly
4. Teach the patient to notify the physician immediately of any indications of infection
5. Advise the patient to inform healthcare providers that he or she is receiving immunosuppressive drugs; the patient should not receive vaccination with live, attenuated organisms
6. Inform the patient that birds are not allowed and that other pets should be approved by the physician

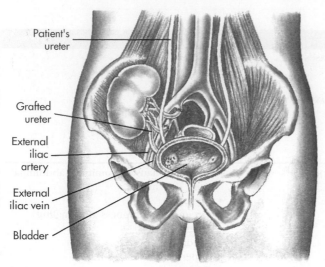

Patient's ureter

Grafted ureter

External iliac artery

External iliac vein

Bladder

Figure 11-8   Location of transplanted kidney. (From Thompson J, et al: *Mosby's clinical nursing,* ed 4, St Louis, 1997, Mosby.)

IV. Collaborative management specific to types of transplant
  A. Heart
    1. Monitor for and treat clinical indications of hypoperfusion
      a) Hemodynamic monitoring is indicated
      b) Inotropes are often required initially
        (1) Isoproterenol (Isuprel): increases heart rate, contractility, and decreases PVR
        (2) Dopamine or dobutamine: increases contractility
        (3) Temporary pacing: may be required to increase heart rate
    2. Monitor for and treat clinical indications of hypervolemia or hypovolemia: fluids, diuretics, or vasodilators may be required
    3. Monitor for and treat coagulopathy
      a) Protamine is given to reverse the heparin used while patient is on cardiopulmonary bypass
      b) Clotting factors, in the form of FFP, may be necessary
      c) Blood administration may be necessary
    4. Monitor for and treat dysrhythmias
    5. Monitor for and treat cardiac tamponade
  B. Lung
    1. Maintain airway, ventilation, oxygenation
      a) Monitor arterial blood gases closely
      b) Administer oxygen to maintain Spo$_2$ of at least 90%; mechanical ventilation may be necessary initially
      c) Ensure bronchial hygiene (secretions are thick and denervated lung does not have cough reflex): repositioning, deep breathing, incentive spirometry, postural drainage, coughing
    2. Monitor for and treat hypervolemia or hypovolemia

      a) Monitor hemodynamic parameters, chest tube drainage, and wound drainage
      b) Administer diuretics and/or venous vasodilators and utilize PEEP as prescribed to prevent or treat pulmonary edema
      c) Replace intravascular fluid volume cautiously
    3. Monitor for and treat dysrhythmias
    4. Monitor for and treat coagulopathy
      a) If the patient is put on cardiopulmonary bypass, protamine is given to reverse the heparin
      b) Blood administration is usually necessary; must be CMV-negative blood
    5. Monitor for clinical indications of anastomoses leak (e.g., subcutaneous emphysema, pneumothorax); although a bolus dose of corticosteroid is usually given in the OR, maintenance corticosteroids are generally not administered for 7 to 14 days after transplant since they decrease the healing of the tracheal and bronchial anastomoses
  C. Liver
    1. Avoid narcotics until the patient is awake and neurologic status can be assessed (patient may be bleeding and needs to be carefully assessed)
    2. Monitor for indications of biliary obstruction (e.g., decreased T-tube drainage, jaundice)
    3. Monitor for intraabdominal bleeding (e.g., increase in abdominal girth, increase in drainage from drains)
    4. Monitor for indications of coagulopathy (e.g., prolonged PT, aPTT, abnormal bleeding): administer FFP, platelets, vitamin K as prescribed
    5. Monitor for electrolyte imbalance, especially hypokalemia and hypocalcemia: replace electrolytes as prescribed
    6. Monitor for renal impairment
    7. Monitor for hypoglycemia
  D. Pancreas
    1. Monitor for indications of hypoglycemia or hyperglycemia; administer D$_{10}$W or insulin as indicated and prescribed
    2. Monitor for clinical indications of peritoneal irritation: abdominal pain, abdominal distention, absent bowel sounds, rebound tenderness
    3. Monitor for acidosis if exocrine drainage through bladder; sodium bicarbonate may be prescribed
  E. Renal
    1. Maintain patency of vascular access
    2. Monitor renal function
      a) Monitor hourly urine output
      b) Monitor BUN, creatinine
    3. Monitor for clinical indications of extravasation of urine (e.g., abdominal pain, rebound tenderness, diminished bowel sounds, abdominal distension)

LEARNING ACTIVITIES

1. **DIRECTIONS:** Complete the following crossword puzzle.

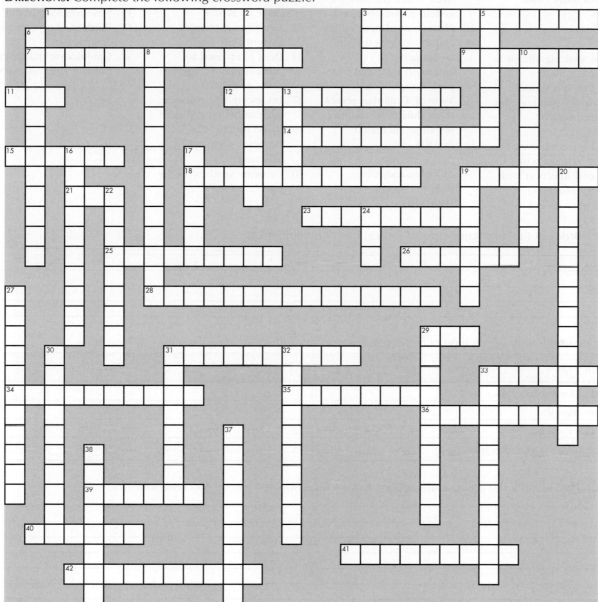

Across

1. Mature red blood cell
3. Most cellular immunity-specific immunosuppressive agent; used after organ transplantation
7. Process of erythrocyte production
9. Electrolyte that may decrease with administration of banked blood
11. Virus that causes AIDS (abbrev.)
12. Sequential physiologic response that the body makes to injury or invasion
14. Adherence of phagocytes to the vessel wall
15. Liquid portion of blood
18. Prevents excessive clotting
19. Parenteral anticoagulant (generic)
21. Type of pneumonia often seen in patients with AIDS (abbrev.)
23. Electrolyte that may increase with administration of banked blood
25. Clotting pathway initiated by tissue injury
26. Immunodeficient condition characterized by a lack of or diminished reaction to an antigen
28. Blood product administered to replace factor VIII in hemophiliacs
29. End result of fibrinolysis (abbrev.)
31. Cascade that can directly kill organisms
33. Site of T-cell distribution
34. Type of agranular leukocyte; T-cells and B-cells are examples
35. Type of immunity that is mediated by the T-cell
36. Clotting pathway that is initiated by endothelial injury
39. Site of B-cell distribution
40. Type of T-cell that is decreased in AIDS

41. Cell that can engulf and digest microorganisms and cellular debris
42. Movement of neutrophils and phagocytes through pores of small blood vessels

Down

2. Granulocyte significant in allergic reactions
3. Virus that is a serious problem for immunocompromised patients (abbrev.)
4. Fungal infection often seen in patients with AIDS; oral infection with this organism is referred to as *thrush*

5. Activated plasminogen; active agent in the fibrinolytic process
6. Immature reticulocyte
8. Infection that is more likely when the immune system is compromised
10. Movement of neutrophils and monocytes toward an antigen
13. Yellowish fluid that transports lymphocytes
16. Type of T-cell that serves to modulate the immune response; increased in AIDS
17. ____'s sarcoma is a type of malignancy often seen in patents with AIDS

19. Type of immunity mediated by B-cells; involves the development of antigen-specific antibodies
20. Synonym for antibody; made by B-cells
22. First sign of platelet dysfunction
24. Drug often used to prevent platelet aggregation (abbrev.)
27. Leukocyte that released granules when ruptured
29. Blood protein that becomes fibrin when activated
30. Cytokine synthesized by lymphocytes

31. Chemical mediators of immunity and inflammation
32. Agranulocyte that is the major phagocyte of the leukocytes
33. Synonym for platelet
37. Product of erythrocyte destruction
38. Granulocyte that releases heparin and histamine

---

2.   DIRECTIONS: List the five major clinical indications of inflammation.

1. _____
2. _____
3. _____
4. _____
5. _____

3.   DIRECTIONS: Identify which type of hypersensitivity reaction the following situations demonstrate.

Example	Type
Skin testing for tuberculosis	
Inhalation allergies	
Anaphylaxis to penicillin	
Hemolytic blood transfusion reaction	

4.   DIRECTIONS: Identify the appropriate actions to take for suspected transfusion reaction.

a. _____
b. _____
c. _____
d. _____
e. _____
f. _____
g. _____
h. _____
i. _____

5.   DIRECTIONS: Complete the following table.

	Platelet Plug	Intrinsic Pathway	Extrinsic Pathway	Common Pathway	Fibrinolytic System
Activation					
Laboratory Test					

6.   DIRECTIONS: Briefly describe the three major phases of DIC.

1.
2.
3.

7.   DIRECTIONS: Identify the direction of change of the following laboratory values in DIC.

Platelets	
PT	
aPTT	
Fibrin split products	
Factors V, VIII	
Fibrinogen	

8.   DIRECTIONS: Discuss the controversy of the following therapies in the treatment of DIC.

a. Heparin	
b. Clotting factors	

9.   DIRECTIONS: List five factors encountered in the critical care unit that affect the patient's immune response and may cause immunodeficiency.

1.
2.
3.
4.
5.

10.   DIRECTIONS: An HIV-positive patient admitted with PCP would be classified in what Walter Reed class.

WR_____

11.   DIRECTIONS: Identify three major adverse effects of the following antiretroviral agents.

Zidovudine (Retrovir)	1. 2. 3.
Didanosine (Videx)	1. 2. 3.
Zalcitabine (Hivid)	1. 2. 3.

12.   DIRECTIONS: Identify general and organ-specific indications of rejection after organ transplantation.

General:_____

Heart:_____

Lung:_____

Liver:_____

Pancreas:_____

Kidney:_____

13.   **DIRECTIONS:** Identify three major adverse effects of the following immunosuppressive agents.

Azathioprine (Imuran)	1. 2. 3.
Cyclosporine (Neoral)	1. 2. 3.
Orthoclone OKT3	1. 2. 3.
Prednisone	1. 2. 3.
Mycophenolate mofetil (CellCept)	1. 2. 3.
Tacrolimus (Prograf)	1. 2. 3.

LEARNING ACTIVITIES ANSWERS

1.

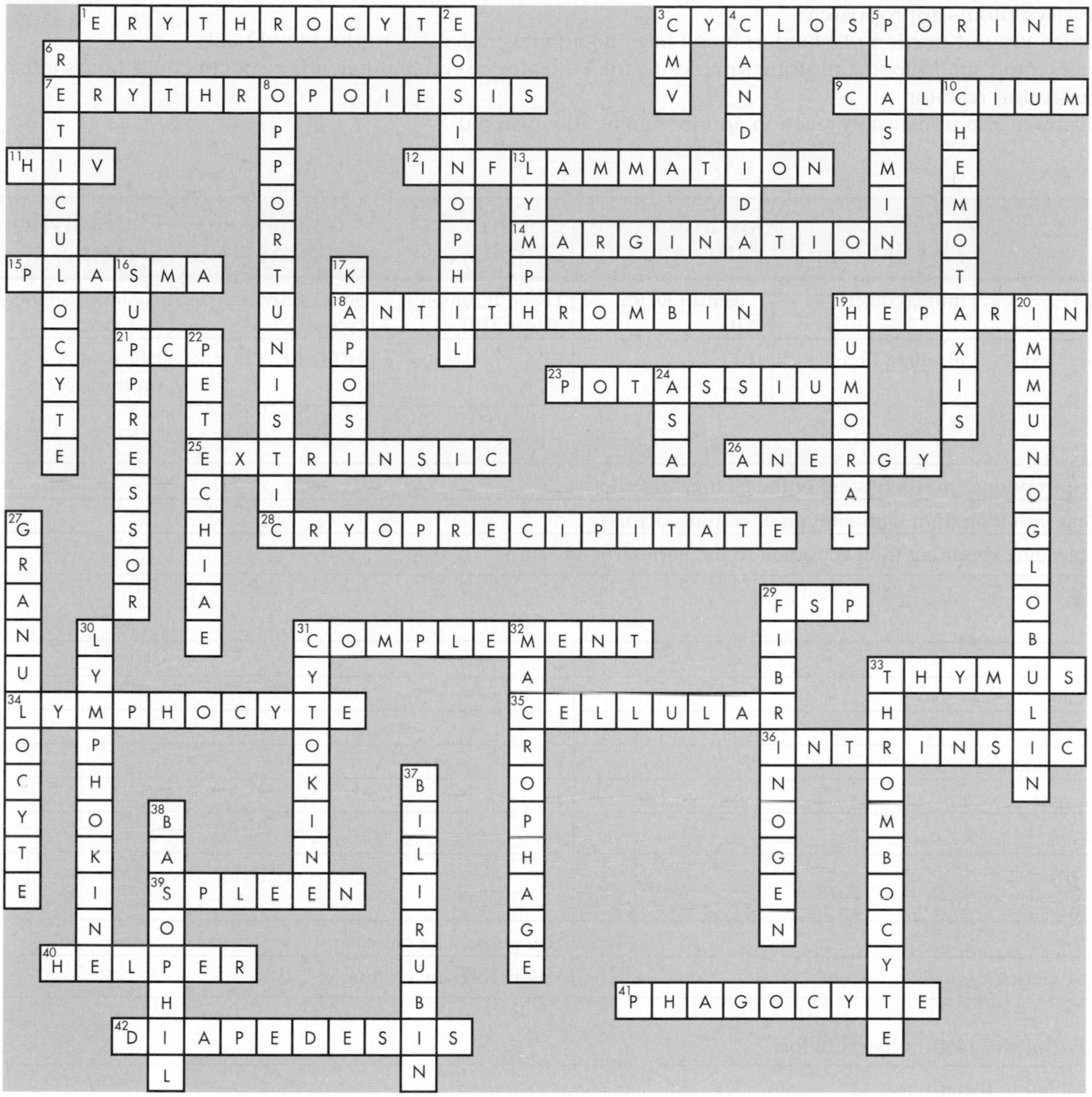

2.
1. Warmth
2. Redness
3. Swelling
4. Pain
5. Loss of function

3.

Example	Type
Skin testing for tuberculosis	IV
Inhalation allergies	III
Anaphylaxis to penicillin	I
Hemolytic blood transfusion reaction	II

4. a. Stop transfusion
   b. Maintain IV access with normal saline and new administration set
   c. Reassure the patient; stay at the bedside
   d. Notify physician and blood bank
   e. Recheck blood numbers and type
   f. Treat symptoms appropriately
   g. Return unused portion of blood in blood bag and administration set to the blood bank
   h. Collect and send blood and urine samples to the laboratory; send another urine specimen 24 hours after transfusion reaction
   i. Document the transfusion reaction and treatment administered

5.

	Platelet Plug	Intrinsic Pathway	Extrinsic Pathway	Common Pathway	Fibrinolytic System
Activation	Intimal defect	Hageman factor (XII)	Tissue thromboplastin (III)	Stuart-Prower factor (X)	Tissue plasminogen activator
Laboratory Test	Bleeding time	aPTT	PT	aPTT, PT, TT	Fibrin split products

6.

1. Clotting (resulting from activation of the clotting cascade[s])
2. Bleeding (resulting from consumption of clotting factors)
3. More bleeding (resulting from activation of the fibrinolytic system)

7.

Platelets	↓
PT	↑
aPTT	↑
Fibrin split products	↑
Factors V, VIII	↓
Fibrinogen	↓

8.

a. Heparin	May perpetuate bleeding
b. Clotting factors	May perpetuate clotting

9. Any five of the factors listed below.

Massive antibiotic therapy
Invasive procedures
Steroids
Stress
Antacids
Histamine$_2$-receptor antagonists
Anesthetic agents
Immunosuppressive agents
Malnutrition

10. WR6 (caused by presence of opportunistic infection)

11.

Zidovudine (Retrovir)	1. Bone marrow depression 2. GI symptoms 3. Headache or any of the adverse effects listed in Table 11-16
Didanosine (Videx)	1. Peripheral neuropathy 2. Pancreatitis 3. GI symptoms or any of the adverse effects listed in Table 11-16
Zalcitabine (Hivid)	1. Peripheral neuropathy 2. Bone marrow depression 3. GI symptoms or any of the adverse effects listed in Table 11-16

12.   General: flulike symptoms, fever, tachycardia
Heart: HF, dysrhythmias, decreased cardiac index with clinical indications of hypoperfusion
Lung: hypoxemia, especially with exertion; pulmonary infiltrates
Liver: right upper quadrant pain; elevated bilirubin, liver enzymes, ammonia; hepatomegaly
Pancreas: hyperglycemia, decrease in C-peptide level, decrease in urine amylase
Kidney: hypertension, swollen, tender kidneys, decrease in urine output, elevated BUN, creatinine

13.   Increased susceptibility to infection applies to all of these agents.

Azathioprine (Imuran)	1. Bone marrow depression 2. Hepatotoxicity 3. Pancreatitis or any of the adverse effects listed in Table 11-19
Cyclosporine (Neoral)	1. Nephrotoxicity 2. Hepatotoxicity 3. Hypertension or any of the adverse effects listed in Table 11-19
Muromonab-CD3 (Orthoclone OKT3)	1. Leukopenia 2. Thrombocytopenia 3. Allergic reactions or any of the adverse effects listed in Table 11-19
Prednisone	1. Sodium and water retention 2. Hypertension 3. Hyperglycemia or any of the adverse effects listed in Table 11-19
Mycophenolate mofetil (CellCept)	1. Nausea 2. Diarrhea 3. Hypertension or any of the adverse effects listed in Table 11-19
Tacrolimus (Prograf)	1. GI effects 2. Headache 3. Numbness and tingling or any of the adverse effects listed in Table 11-19

Bibliography and Selected References

Alcoser P, Burchett S: Bone marrow transplantation—immune system suppression and reconstitution, *AJN* 99 (6):26, 1999.

Alspach J, editor: *Core curriculum for critical care nursing,* ed 5, Philadelphia, 1998, WB Saunders.

Anastasi J, Sun V: Controlling diarrhea in the HIV patient, *AJN* 96 (8):35, 1996.

Barkauskas V, et al: *Health and physical assessment,* St Louis, 1994, Mosby.

Beare P, Myers J: *Adult health nursing,* ed 3, St Louis, 1998, Mosby.

Becker C, Petlin A: Heart transplantation, *AJN* 99 (5):8, 1999.

Bloom E, et al: Xenotransplantation: the potential and the challenges, *Critical Care Nurse* 19 (2):76, 1999.

Boggs R, Wooldridge-King M: *AACN procedure manual for critical care,* ed 3, Philadelphia, 1993, WB Saunders.

Bormann J, Kelly A: HIV & AIDS: are you biased? *AJN* 99 (9):38, 1999.

Borton D: Taking a commonsense approach to infection control, *Nursing98* 28 (5):32hn1, 1998.

Brar R, Hollenberg S: The technique of fluid resuscitation, *Journal of Critical Illness* 11 (8):550, 1996.

Brar R, Hollenberg S: Administering fluid resuscitation effectively for traumatic shock, *Journal of Critical Illness* 11 (10):672, 1996.

Calianno C, Pino T: Getting a reaction to anergy panel testing, *Nursing95* 25 (1):58, 1995.

Chabalewski F, Norris M: The gift of life: talking to families about organ and tissue donation, *AJN* 94 (6):28, 1994.

Chernow B, editor: *The pharmacologic approach to the critically ill patient,* ed 3, Baltimore, 1994, Williams & Wilkins.

Clochesy J, et al: *Critical care nursing,* ed 2, Philadelphia, 1996, WB Saunders.

Cohn S: Blood substitutes, *New Horizons* 7 (1):54, 1999.

Cook L: The value of lab values, *AJN* 99 (5):66, 1999.

Crone C: Psychiatric aspects of transplantation, I: evaluation and selection of candidates, *Critical Care Nurse* 19 (1):79, 1999.

Crone C: Psychiatric aspects of transplantation, II: preoperative issues, *Critical Care Nurse* 19 (3):51, 1999.

Crone C: Psychiatric aspects of transplantation, III: postoperative issues, *Critical Care Nurse* 19 (4):28, 1999.

Dikon A: Ways to prevent infection in patients with special needs, *Nursing98* 28 (5):32hn17, 1998.

Dressler D: Disseminated intravascular coagulation—coping with a paradoxical crisis, *Nursing96* 26 (11):32aa, 1996.

Ehrle R, Shafer T, Nelson K: Referral, request, and consent for organ donation: best practice—a blueprint for success, *Critical Care Nurse* 19 (2):21, 1999.

Evans B: Complementary therapy and HIV infection, *AJN* 99 (2):42, 1999.

Fitzpatrick L, Fitzpatrick T: Blood transfusion—keeping your patient safe, *Nursing97* 27 (8):34, 1997.

Fuss E: Managing antibiotic-resistant organisms, *Nursing97* 27 (9):70, 1997.

Gahart B, Nazareno A: *1999 intravenous medications,* St Louis, 1999, Mosby.

Giuliano K, Sims T: Transplant issues: bugs and drugs, *Nursing98* 28 (2):32cc1, 1998.

Hoffmann R, Reeder S: Mycophenolate mofetil (CellCept): the newest immunosuppressant, *Critical Care Nurse* 18 (3):50, 1998.

Holmquist M, et al: A critical pathway: guiding care for organ donors, *Critical Care Nurse* 19 (2):84, 1999.

Katzenstein D: Antiretroviral therapy for HIV: what to do in 1999, *Journal of Critical Illness* 14 (4):196, 1999.

Keen J, Searingen P: *Mosby's critical care nursing consultant,* St Louis, 1997, Mosby.

Kershaw D: Catching up with new AIDS drug treatment, *Nursing98* 28 (4):32hn1, 1998.

Kinney M, et al: *AACN clinical reference for critical care nursing,* ed 4, St Louis, 1998, Mosby.

Kirsten V: Treating HIV disease—hope on the horizon, *Nursing98* 28 (11):34, 1998.

Lewis D, Valerius W: Organs from non-heart-beating donors: an answer to the organ shortage, *Critical Care Nurse* 19 (2):70, 1999.

Lisanti P, Zwolski K: Understanding the devastation of AIDS, *AJN* 97 (7):26, 1997.

Marino P: *The ICU book,* ed 2, Baltimore, 1998, Williams & Wilkins.

McCoy J, Argue P: The role of critical care nurses in organ donation, *Critical Care Nurse* 19 (2):48, 1999.

Mims B, et al: *Critical care skills—a clinical handbook,* Philadelphia, 1996, WB Saunders.

Pelletier-Hibbert M: Coping strategies used by nurses to deal with the care of organ donors and their families, *Heart and Lung* 27 (4):230, 1998.

Price S, Wilson L: *Pathophysiology—clinical concepts of disease processes,* ed 5, St Louis, 1997, Mosby.

Ress B: Antiretroviral therapy for human immunodeficiency virus disease: implications for critical care nursing, *Critical Care Nurse* 18 (6):54, 1998.

Richards M, et al: Nosocomial infections in medical intensive care units in the United States, *Crit Care Med* 27 (5):887, 1999.

Riley L, Coolican M: Needs of families of organ donors: facing death and life, *Critical Care Nurse* 19 (2):53, 1999.

Russell B: Nosocomial infections, *AJN* 99 (6):24J, 1999.

Schroeter K, Taylor G: Ethical considerations in organ donation for critical care nurses, *Critical Care Nurse* 19 (2):60, 1999.

Sheff B: VRE & MRSA: putting bad bugs out of business, *Nursing98* 28 (3):40, 1998.

Sims H: Mechanisms of immune suppression in critically ill patients, *New Horizons* 7 (1):147, 1999.

Sullivan J, Seem D, Chabalewski F: Determining brain death, *Critical Care Nurse* 19 (2):37, 1999.

Tahan H: Patients waiting for heart transplantation, *Critical Care Nurse* 18 (4):40, 1998.

Tasota F, Fisher E, Coulson C, Hoffman L: Protecting ICU patients from nosocomial infections: practical measures for favorable outcomes, *Critical Care Nurse* 18 (1):54, 1998.

Thelan L, et al: *Critical care nursing: diagnosis and management,* ed 3, St Louis, 1998, Mosby.

Ungvarski P: Update on HIV infection, *AJN* 97 (1):44, 1997.

Varon J, Fromm R: *The ICU handbook of facts, formulas, and laboratory values,* St Louis, 1997, Mosby.

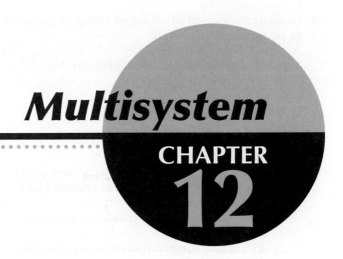

Multisystem

CHAPTER 12

Note: The blueprint includes cardiogenic shock and hypovolemic shock in cardiovascular, anaphylactic shock in hematology/immunology, and neurogenic shock in neurologic, but it is logical to discuss the similarities of all shock states together and then discuss their differences.

Shock

Definitions

I. Shock: condition of insufficient perfusion of cells and vital organs, causing tissue hypoxia; perfusion is inadequate to sustain life; results in cellular, metabolic, and hemodynamic derangements

II. Systemic inflammatory response syndrome (SIRS): the systemic response to a variety of insults that begin as local inflammation

III. Bacteremia: presence of viable bacteria in the blood

IV. Sepsis: SIRS caused by infection

V. Severe sepsis: sepsis with associated organ dysfunction

VI. Septic shock: sepsis with hypotension despite adequate fluid resuscitation and the presence of perfusion abnormalities

VII. Multiple organ dysfunction syndrome (MODS): failure of more than one organ in an acutely ill patient with SIRS to such an extent that homeostasis cannot be maintained without intervention

Classification by Etiology

I. Hypovolemic: caused by inadequate intravascular volume
   A. External losses
      1. Blood
         a) Gastrointestinal (e.g., esophageal varices, peptic ulcer, hemorrhoids)
         b) Genitourinary (e.g., antepartal or postpartum bleeding, hematuria)
         c) Amputations
         d) Major blood vessel disruption (may also be occult)
         e) Coagulopathy
            (1) Congenital coagulopathy (e.g., hemophilia)
            (2) Acquired coagulopathy (e.g., disseminated intravascular coagulation [DIC], excessive anticoagulation)
      2. Fluid
         a) Gastrointestinal (e.g., vomiting, diarrhea, nasogastric suction)
         b) Renal
            (1) DKA
            (2) HHNK
            (3) Diabetes insipidus
            (4) Hypoaldosteronism (Addison's disease)
            (5) Diuretics
            (6) Osmotic dyes
         c) Cutaneous
            (1) Burns
            (2) Exudative wounds
            (3) Excessive perspiration (e.g., heat exhaustion)
   B. Internal sequestration
      1. Blood
         a) Hemoperitoneum or retroperitoneal (e.g., hemorrhagic pancreatitis, ruptured spleen, lacerated liver)
         b) Thoracic trauma with hemothorax, hemomediastinum
         c) Dissecting aortic aneurysm
         d) Pelvic or long bone fractures
      2. Fluid
         a) Ascites: peritonitis, pancreatitis, cirrhosis, intraabdominal malignancies (e.g., liver, ovarian)
         b) Pleural effusion
         c) Internal obstruction

II. Cardiogenic: caused by impaired ability of the heart to pump blood effectively
  A. Decreased contractility
    1. MI (loss of 40% of left ventricular myocardium)
    2. Myocardial contusion
    3. Cardiomyopathy
    4. Myocarditis
    5. Severe HF
    6. Ventricular aneurysm
    7. Overdosage of myocardial depressant drugs (e.g., beta-blockers, calcium channel blockers, barbiturates)
    8. Stunned myocardium: transient cardiogenic shock
      a) Cardiac surgery: related to hypothermia, cardioplegic arrest, surgical incisions
      b) Reperfusion injury
      c) Post-CPR
      d) Hypoxemia
      e) Acidosis
      f) Hypoglycemia
      g) Electrolyte imbalance
  B. Impaired filling
    1. Dysrhythmias
    2. Cardiac tamponade
    3. Noncompliant ventricle (e.g., left ventricular hypertrophy, right ventricular hypertrophy)
  C. Impaired emptying (may be referred to as *obstructive*)
    1. Valvular dysfunction
      a) Chronic: stenosis or regurgitation
      b) Acute: papillary muscle rupture
    2. Ventricular septal rupture
    3. Intracardiac tumor
    4. Massive pulmonary embolism
    5. Tension pneumothorax
    6. Dissecting thoracic aortic aneurysm
III. Distributive or vasogenic: caused by massive vasodilation and a resultant relative hypovolemia
  A. Septic: resulting from massive vasodilation caused by release of mediators of the inflammatory process in response to overwhelming infection
    1. Factors that cause immunosuppression
      a) Extremes of age
      b) Malnutrition
      c) Alcoholism or drug abuse
      d) Debilitation
      e) Malignancy
      f) AIDS
      g) History of splenectomy
      h) Chronic health problems (diabetes mellitus, liver disease, heart disease [e.g., coronary artery disease or heart failure], renal failure)
      i) Bone marrow suppression
      j) Immunosuppressive therapies (e.g., immunosuppressive drugs, antineoplastic drugs, antibiotic therapy, corticosteroids)

    2. Factors that cause bacteremia, septicemia
      a) Invasive procedures and devices
      b) Pulmonary procedures
      c) Diagnostic procedures
      d) Surgical procedures or wounds
      e) Traumatic wounds or burns
      f) Genitourinary infection
      g) Untreated GI disease (cholelithiasis, intestinal obstruction, appendicitis, diverticulitis)
      h) Peritonitis
      i) Food poisoning
      j) Prolonged hospitalization
      k) Translocation of GI bacteria: NPO status, decreased peristalsis, and GI ischemia contribute to proliferation of gastrointestinal bacteria and translocation of these bacteria into blood or lymph
    3. Microorganisms
      a) Gram-negative bacteria (*indicates most likely)
        (1) *Escherichia coli**
        (2) *Klebsiella enterobacter**
        (3) *Pseudomonas aeruginosa**
        (4) *Proteus mirabilis*
        (5) *Enterococcus*
        (6) *Serratia marcescens*
        (7) *Bacteroides* organisms
        (8) *Haemophilus influenzae*
      b) Gram-positive organisms
        (1) *Staphylococcus aureus*
        (2) *Staphylococcus epidermidis*
        (3) *Streptococcus pneumoniae*
        (4) *Clostridium* organisms
        (5) *Pneumococcus*
      c) Less likely
        (1) Viruses
        (2) Fungi
        (3) Rickettsiae
        (4) Spirochaeta
        (5) Protozoa
        (6) Parasites
  B. Anaphylactic: resulting from massive vasodilation caused by release of histamine in response to a severe allergic reaction
    1. Foods, especially the following:
      a) Fish
      b) Shellfish
      c) Eggs
      d) Milk and milk products
      e) Wheat
      f) Strawberries
      g) Legumes (e.g., peanuts, soybeans)
      h) Nuts (e.g., walnuts, pecans)
      i) Chocolate
      j) Food coloring
      k) Preservatives
    2. Drugs
      a) Antibiotics, especially penicillin (penicillin

accounts for approximately one-quarter of all anaphylaxis)

   b) Aspirin

   c) Local anesthetics

   d) Narcotics

   e) Barbiturates

   f) Insulin: pork or beef

   g) Iodine-containing contrast media (e.g., Renografin)

   h) Chymopapain (enzyme used in chemical discectomy)

   i) Dextran

   j) Blood and blood products: blood transfusion incompatibilities

   k) Animal serums: antitoxins

   l) Allergic extracts in hyposensitization therapy

3. Bites or stings

   a) Venomous snakes

   b) Hymenoptera: wasps, hornets, bumble bees, yellow jackets

   c) Spiders

   d) Jellyfish

   e) Stingrays

   f) Deer flies

   g) Fire ants

4. Chemical

   a) Materials (e.g., latex)

   b) Hand lotions

   c) Soap

   d) Perfume

   e) Iodine-containing solutions (e.g., Betadine)

C. Neurogenic: resulting from massive vasodilation caused by suppression of the sympathetic nervous system

1. General anesthesia

2. Spinal anesthesia

3. Epidural block

4. Cervical spinal cord injury

5. Drugs

   a) Barbiturates

   b) Phenothiazines

   c) Sympathetic blocking agents (e.g., antihypertensives)

6. Head injury

7. Insulin shock

8. Exposure to unpleasant circumstances (e.g., fright, pain)

Pathophysiology

I. Stages of shock in general

  A. Initial stage is manifested by subclinical hypoperfusion caused by inadequate delivery or inadequate extraction of oxygen

    1. Shock is initiated by decreased tissue oxygenation caused by any of the following:

      a) Decrease in circulating blood volume (hypovolemic)

      b) Decrease in ability of the heart to pump blood (cardiogenic)

      c) Decrease in vascular tone (distributive, may also be referred to as *vasogenic*)

    2. Cardiac output and index are decreased but no clinical indications of hypoperfusion are present

  B. Compensatory stage is manifested by the attempts of the neuroendocrine systems to compensate and restore tissue perfusion to vital organs

    1. Clinical indications of sympathetic nervous system (SNS) stimulation are evident

      a) Baroreceptor reflex: decrease in blood pressure stimulates the baroreceptors, which then stimulate the vasomotor center in the medulla to activate the SNS

      b) SNS: epinephrine and norepinephrine released from adrenal medulla, causing the following physiologic responses:

        (1) Arterial vasoconstriction

          (a) Systemic response increases SVR and blood pressure

          (b) Constriction of afferent and efferent arterioles of kidneys decreases glomerular filtration rate (GFR) and urine output

        (2) Venous vasoconstriction

          (a) Widespread reflex venoconstriction increases venous return to the heart, which increases preload

          (b) Increased venous return and preload increases myocardial contractility by increasing myofibril stretch (Starling's Law of the Heart)

        (3) Heart rate and contractility increase

        (4) Blood is redistributed from nonessential (e.g., skin, bowel, kidney) to the essential (e.g., heart and brain) organs

      c) CNS ischemic response

        (1) Ischemia and elevated CO_2 cause the CNS ischemia response when MAP falls to less than 50 mm Hg

        (2) This response causes powerful stimulation of the SNS

    2. Hormonal compensation

      a) Activation of renin-angiotensin-aldosterone system (Fig. 2-21 in Chapter 2)

        (1) Vasoconstriction of arteries and arterioles

        (2) Increase in reabsorption of sodium and water by the renal tubule

      b) Release of glucocorticoids: stimulate glycogenolysis and gluconeogenesis to mobilize glucose for cellular energy

  C. Progressive stage is characterized by the inability of the compensatory mechanisms to maintain tissue perfusion

1. Clinical indications of decreased delivery or extraction of oxygen to the tissues now evident
2. Myocardial depression: caused by ischemia and myocardial depressant factor (MDF) released by the ischemic pancreas
3. Vasomotor center depression: caused by severe cerebral ischemia
   a) Increases capillary permeability
   b) Decreases circulating volume
   c) Results in decreased flow to vital organs
4. Deterioration of microcirculation
   a) Spasm of the precapillary sphincter and venules
   b) Continuing ischemia and local acidosis causes dilation of the precapillary sphincters, whereas the venules are more resistant to the effects of acidosis and remain constricted
   c) Blood enters capillaries and pools
   d) Stagnant blood increases capillary hydrostatic pressure and increases tissue edema
5. Thrombosis of small vessels
   a) Microcirculation is sluggish
   b) Microclots develop, which lead to organ ischemia, anoxia, and consumption of clotting factors, potentially leading to DIC
6. Cellular deterioration
   a) Reduced delivery of oxygen to tissues
   b) Change from aerobic to anaerobic metabolism (acidosis occurs because lactic acid is produced as a byproduct of anaerobic metabolism and accumulates in the blood)
   c) Depletion of cellular adenosine triphosphate (ATP) reserves (aerobic metabolism results in 18 times more ATP than the same amount of glucose metabolized anaerobically)
   d) Failure of sodium-potassium pump
   e) Cellular edema
   f) Organelle edema
      (1) Mitochondria can no longer use glucose and oxygen to make ATP
      (2) Lysosomes may rupture, releasing active enzymes into the cell
   g) Cellular destruction
   h) Organ failure
7. Massive ischemia of tissues, leading to the release of mediators of the inflammatory process and systemic inflammatory response syndrome (see next section on SIRS)
8. Effects of shock on specific organs and organ systems
   a) Heart
      (1) Dysrhythmias occur because of the failure of the sodium-potassium pump resulting from decreased ATP supplies, hypoxia, ischemia, and acidosis
      (2) Cardiac failure may occur because of ischemia, acidosis, and myocardial depressant factor (MDF)
   b) Lung
      (1) Endothelial damage in the capillary bed and precapillary arterioles and damage to the type II pneumocytes may cause acute respiratory distress syndrome (ARDS)
      (2) Hypoxemia causes hypoxemic vasoconstriction of pulmonary circulation and pulmonary hypertension
      (3) Ventilation-perfusion mismatch occurs because of disturbances in both ventilation and perfusion
      (4) Pulmonary edema may result from disruption of the alveolar-capillary membrane, ARDS, or from overaggressive fluid resuscitation
   c) Brain
      (1) Brain ischemia results when cerebral perfusion pressure is less than 50 mm Hg
      (2) Cerebral infarction may occur
   d) Kidney
      (1) Hypoperfusion of the kidney decreases glomerular filtration rate
      (2) Prolonged ischemia causes acute tubular necrosis and renal failure
      (3) Metabolic acids accumulate in the blood, worsens the metabolic acidosis caused by lactic acid production during anaerobic metabolism
   e) Liver
      (1) Hypoperfusion damages the reticuloendothelial cells, which causes recirculation of bacteria and cellular debris and predisposes to bacteremia and sepsis
      (2) Damage to the hepatocytes causes the liver to be unable to detoxify drugs, toxins, or hormones, or to conjugate bilirubin
      (3) Decreased ability to mobilize carbohydrate, protein, and fat stores results in hypoglycemia
   f) Pancreas
      (1) Pancreatic enzymes are released by the ischemic and damaged pancreas
      (2) Release of myocardial depressant factor (MDF) results in depression of cardiac contractility
   g) Gastrointestinal
      (1) Ischemia and increased gastric acid production caused by glucocorticoids increase risk of stress ulcer
      (2) Prolonged vasoconstriction and ischemia lead to the inability of the intestinal wall to act as intact barrier to prevent the migration of bacteria out of the gastrointestinal tract; this

change may allow translocation of bacteria from the GI tract into the lymphatic and vascular beds
   h) Hematologic/Immunologic
      (1) Sluggish blood flow, massive tissue trauma, and consumption of clotting factors may cause disseminated intravascular coagulation (DIC)
      (2) Bone marrow mobilizes the release of white blood cells, which causes leukocytosis early in shock; as depletion of WBCs in blood and in bone marrow occurs, leukopenia results
      (3) Massive tissue injury caused by widespread ischemia stimulates a systemic inflammatory response syndrome with massive release of mediators of the inflammatory process
II. Refractory stage is irreversible and refractory to conventional therapy
   A. Clinical indications of profound hypoperfusion and hypotension unresponsive to potent vasopressors
   B. Clinical indications of MODS
      1. ARDS
      2. DIC
      3. Hepatic dysfunction/failure
      4. ATN/renal failure
      5. Myocardial ischemia/infarction/failure
      6. Cerebral ischemia/infarction
III. Specific to hypovolemic (Fig. 12-1)
IV. Specific to cardiogenic (Fig. 12-2)
V. Specific to septic (Fig. 12-3)
VI. Specific to anaphylactic (Fig. 12-4)
   A. Anaphylactic reaction requires previous exposure to the antigen
      1. With first exposure to the antigen, specific IgE antibody is formed
      2. The antibody binds to the mast cells and basophils
      3. Repeat exposure triggers a response by the IgE antibodies
      4. Mast cells are triggered to degranulate
      5. Bioactive mediators are released
   B. Anaphylactoid reaction is clinically indistinguishable from anaphylactic reaction but does not require previous exposure to the antigen
      1. Non-IgE mediated
      2. Direct activation and degranulation of mast cells thought to be triggered by the complement system
VII. Specific to neurogenic (Fig. 12-5)

Clinical Presentation (Table 12-1)

I. Initial stage: no clinical indications; expert nurse may detect that "something is different" (referred to as *intuitive judgment* by Pat Benner)
II. Compensatory stage: SNS stimulation
   A. Subjective
      1. Anxiety, fear, feeling of impending doom
      2. Thirst

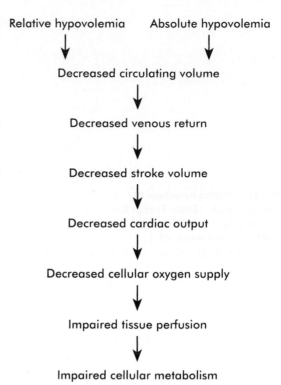

Figure 12-1 Pathophysiology of hypovolemic shock. (From Thelan L, et al: *Critical care nursing: diagnosis and management,* ed 3, St Louis, 1998, Mosby.)

   B. Objective
      1. Tachycardia
      2. Decreased pulse pressure: systolic BP increases or stays the same; diastolic BP increases
      3. Tachypnea
      4. Skin: cool, pale, clammy
      5. GI: decreased bowel sounds
      6. Renal: oliguria (<0.5 ml/kg/hr)
      7. CNS: irritability, restlessness, confusion
III. Progressive stage: hypoperfusion
   A. Subjective
      1. Anorexia, nausea
      2. Chest pain, palpitations may occur
      3. Dyspnea may occur
   B. Objective
      1. Tachycardia, dysrhythmias
      2. Hypotension
      3. Hypothermia (except early septic)
      4. Tachypnea
      5. Skin
         a) Bluish, mottled appearance
         b) Peripheral cyanosis
      6. GI: vomiting, absent bowel sounds
      7. Renal: anuria
      8. CNS: lethargy, coma
IV. Refractory stage: profound hypoperfusion and evidence of MODS
   A. ARDS: clinical indications of respiratory distress, crackles, decreased Pao_2, Sao_2, decreased pulmonary compliance, diffuse pulmonary infiltrates on chest X-ray

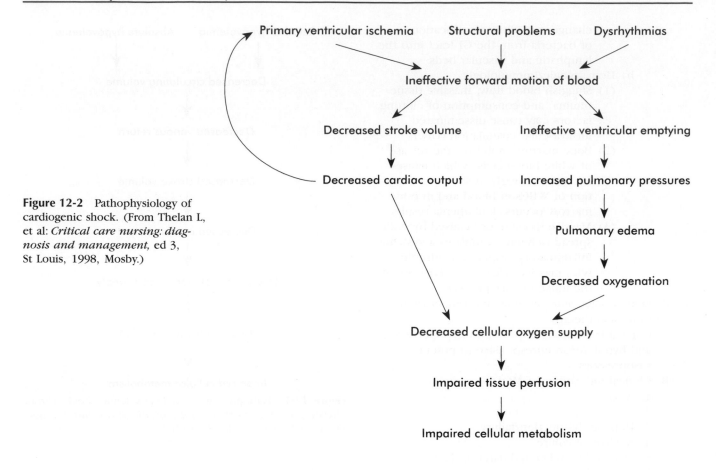

Figure 12-2   Pathophysiology of cardiogenic shock. (From Thelan L, et al: *Critical care nursing: diagnosis and management,* ed 3, St Louis, 1998, Mosby.)

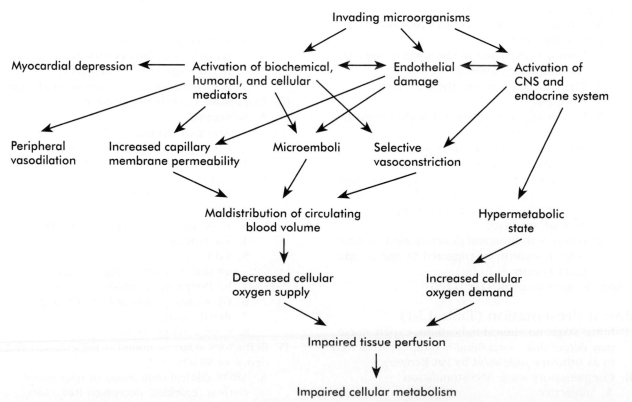

Figure 12-3   Pathophysiology of septic shock. (From Thelan L, et al: *Critical care nursing: diagnosis and management,* ed 3, St Louis, 1998, Mosby.)

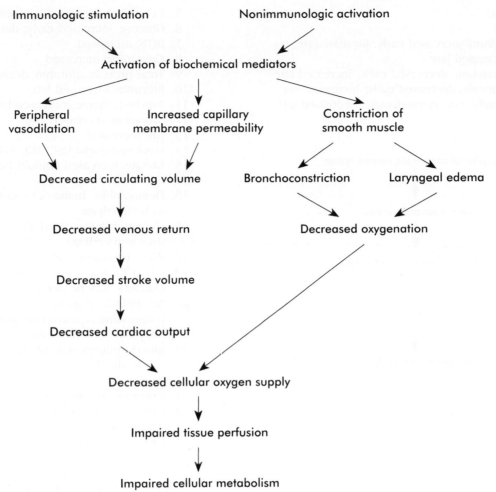

Figure 12-4   Pathophysiology of anaphylactic shock. (From Thelan L, et al: *Critical care nursing: diagnosis and management,* cd 3, St Louis, 1998, Mosby)

B. DIC: bleeding in a patient without a prior history of bleeding, petechiae, blood in sputum, vomitus, nasogastric aspirate, urine, stool, elevated PT, aPTT, decreased platelets, elevated FSP, positive D-dimer

C. Hepatic dysfunction/failure: jaundice, elevated bilirubin, elevated AST, ALT, LDH, hypoglycemia

D. Gastrointestinal: paralytic ileus, gastrointestinal bleeding

E. ATN/renal failure: oliguria or anuria, elevated BUN, creatinine, decreased urine creatinine clearance

F. Myocardial ischemia/infarction/failure: chest pain, ECG indicators of myocardial infarction, positive CK-MB and troponin, clinical indicators of left ventricular and/or right ventricular failure

G. Cerebral ischemia/infarction: change in level of consciousness, change in Glasgow Coma Score of 1 or more, focal signs (e.g., hemiparesis or hemiplegia, aphasia)

V. Hemodynamic parameters (Table 12-2)

A. Decreased oxygen delivery to the tissues (DO_2): common to all forms of shock

except early septic shock, in which DO_2 is increased but extraction and utilization are impaired

1. Oxygen delivery to the tissues
   a) Cao_2
      (1) Required to calculate DO_2 and DO_2I
      (2) Formula: $Hbg \times Sao_2 \times 1.34$
      (3) Normal: 18-20 ml/dl
   b) DO_2
      (1) Formula: $Cao_2 \times CO \times 10$ OR $Hgb \times Sao_2 \times 1.34 \times CO \times 10$
      (2) Normal: 900-1100 ml/min
   c) DO_2I
      (1) Formula: $Cao_2 \times Cl \times 10$
      (2) Normal: 550-650 ml/min/m^2

2. Oxygen consumption by the tissues
   a) VO_2
      (1) Formula: $CO \times Hgb \times 13.4 \times (Sao_2 - Svo_2)$
      (2) Normal: 200-300 ml/min
   b) VO_2I
      (1) Formula: $Cl \times Hgb \times 13.4 \times (Sao_2 - Svo_2)$
      (2) Normal: 110-160 ml/min/m^2

VI. Diagnostic
  A. Serum
    1. Sodium: increased early, increased or decreased late
    2. Potassium: decreased early, increased late
    3. Chloride: decreased early, increased late
    4. Bicarbonate: normal early, decreased late

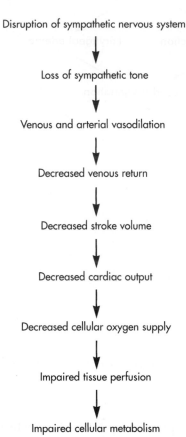

Figure 12-5 Pathophysiology of neurogenic shock. (From Thelan L, et al: *Critical care nursing: diagnosis and management,* ed 3, St Louis, 1998, Mosby.)

    5. CO₂: normal early, decreased late
    6. Glucose: increased early, decreased late
    7. BUN: increased
    8. Creatinine: increased
    9. Total protein, albumin: decreased
    10. Bilirubin: increased late
    11. Amylase, lipase: increased late
    12. Ammonia: increased late
    13. CK: increased
    14. Liver enzymes (AST, ALT, LDH): increased
    15. Lactate: increased (should be done on arterial blood)
    16. Hemoglobin, hematocrit: decreased if due to hemorrhage
    17. Hematocrit: increased if due to cause other than hemorrhage
    18. WBC: increased early, decreased late
    19. PT, aPTT: may be prolonged
    20. Platelets: may be decreased
    21. Arterial blood gases: respiratory alkalosis progressing to metabolic acidosis; Pao_2 and Sao_2 may be decreased
    22. Blood cultures: may identify organism if septic shock
  B. Urine
    1. Urine creatinine clearance: decreased
    2. Urine specific gravity: increased early, decreased late
    3. Urine osmolality: increased early, decreased late
    4. Urine sodium: decreased
  C. Other diagnostic studies may be done to evaluate the reason for shock
VII. Specific to hypovolemic shock
  A. Subjective: history of precipitating factor
  B. Objective
    1. Flat neck veins
    2. Parameters used for evaluation of severity of hemorrhagic shock (Table 12-3)
  C. Hemodynamics: Table 12-2

Table **12-1**	**Clinical Presentation of the Stages of Shock**		
Initial: Subclinical Hypoperfusion	**Compensatory: SNS**	**Progressive: Hypoperfusion**	**Refractory: Profound Hypoperfusion**
CI 2.2-2.5 L/min/m²	CI 2.0-2.2 L/min/m²	CI <2.0 L/min/m²	CI <1.8 L/min/m²
• No clinical indications of hypoperfusion but "something is different"	• Tachycardia • Narrowed pulse pressure • Tachypnea • Cool skin • Oliguria • Diminished bowel sounds • Restlessness to confusion	• Dysrhythmias • Hypotension • Tachypnea • Cold, clammy skin • Anuria • Absent bowel sounds • Lethargy to coma	• Life-threatening dysrhythmias • Hypotension despite potent vasopressors • ARDS • DIC • Hepatic dysfunction/failure • ATN • Mesenteric ischemia/infarction • Myocardial ischemia/infarction/failure • Cerebral ischemia/infarction

D. Diagnostic: hematocrit
   1. Elevated if due to dehydration
   2. Decreased if due to blood loss
VIII. Specific to cardiogenic shock
   A. Subjective
      1. History of precipitating factor
      2. Chest pain
      3. Dyspnea
      4. Thirst
      5. Anxiety, fear, feeling of impending doom
   B. Objectives
      1. Clinical indicators of LVF
         a) Tachycardia
         b) Dysrhythmias
         c) Pulsus alternans
         d) Tachypnea
         e) Heart sound changes: S_3
         f) Breath sound changes: crackles
      2. Clinical indicators of RVF
         a) Jugular venous distention
         b) Peripheral edema
         c) Hcpatosplenomegaly

C. Hemodynamics: Table 12-2; defining characteristics of cardiogenic shock
   1. CI: less than 2.0 L/min/m^2
   2. RAP/PAP/PAOP increased; PAOP usually more than 18 mm Hg
   3. SVR/SVRI increased; SVR usually more than 2000 dynes/sec/cm^{-5}
D. Diagnostic
   1. ECG
      a) May reveal acute or old myocardial infarction
      b) May reveal ventricular aneurysm
   2. Cardiac catheterization
      a) May reveal cause of cardiogenic shock
      b) May reveal abnormal intracardiac pressures
   3. Echocardiography: may reveal cause of cardiogenic shock
      a) Ventricular wall motion abnormality
      b) Valvular abnormality
      c) Cardiac tamponade
IX. Specific to septic shock (Table 12-4)
   A. Hemodynamics: Table 12-2

Table 12-2 Hemodynamic Alterations in Shock

	Hypovolemic	Cardiogenic	Early Septic	Late Septic	Anaphylactic	Neurogenic
HR	High	High	High	High	High	Nl or Low
BP	Nl → Low	Nl → Low	Nl → Low	Low	Nl → Low	Nl → Low
CO/CI	Low	Low	High	Low	Nl → Low	Nl → Low
RAP/PAOP	Low	High	Low	High but may be normal or low	Low	Low
SVR/SVRI	High	High	Low	High	Low	Low
SvO$_2$	Low	Low	High	Low	Low	Low

Table 12-3 Severity of Hemorrhagic Shock

Class	I	II	III	IV
Blood loss (% of blood volume)	<15%	15%-30%	30%-40%	>40%
Blood loss (ml)	<750 ml	750-1500 ml	1500-2000 ml	>2000 ml
Heart rate/min	<100	>100	>120	140 or >
Blood pressure	Normal	Normal	Decreased	Decreased
Pulse pressure	Widened or normal	Narrowed	Narrowed	Narrowed
Capillary refill	Normal	Delayed	Delayed	Delayed or absent
Respiratory rate/min	14-20	20-30	30-40	>35
Urine output (ml/hr)	30 or >	20-30	<20	Negligible
Skin appearance	Cool, pink	Cool, pale	Cold, moist, pale	Cold, clammy, cyanotic
Neurologic status	Slightly anxious	Mildly anxious	Anxious, confused	Confused, lethargy

Adapted from American College of Surgeons, Advanced Trauma Life Support program for physicians, Chicago, 1993.

Table 12-4	**Stages of Septic Shock**	
Early (Hyperdynamic)	**Late (Hypodynamic)**	
LOOKS LIKE INFECTION	**LOOKS LIKE SHOCK**	

Objective	
Tachycardia	Tachycardia
Pulses bounding	Pulses weak and thready
Blood pressure: normal or low	Hypotension
Wide pulse pressure	Narrow pulse pressure
Skin warm, flushed	Skin cool, pale
Hyperpnea	Bradypnea or tachypnea
Change in mental status (e.g., irritability, confusion)	Decreased level of consciousness (e.g., lethargy, coma)
Oliguria	Anuria
Hyperthermia	Hypothermia

Hemodynamic	
CO/CI increased	CO/CI decreased
RAP/PAP/PAOP decreased	RAP/PAP/PAOP usually increased but may be normal or decreased
SVR/SVRI decreased	SVR/SVRI increased
Svo_2 increased	Svo_2 decreased

Diagnostic	
ABGs: respiratory alkalosis with hypoxemia	ABGs: metabolic acidosis with hypoxemia
PT, aPTT increased	PT, aPTT increased
Platelets decreased	Platelets decreased
WBC increased	WBC decreased
Glucose increased	Glucose decreased
	BUN, creatinine increased
	Serum arterial lactate increased
	Amylase, lipase increased
	AST, ALT, LDH increased

Legend: *CO*, cardiac output; *CI*, cardiac index; *RAP*, right atrial pressure; *PAP*, pulmonary artery pressure; *PAOP*, pulmonary artery occlusive pressure; *SVR*, systemic vascular resistance; *SVRI*, systemic vascular resistance index; *Svo$_2$*, oxygen saturation of venous blood; *PT*, prothrombin time; *aPTT*, activated partial thromboplastin time; *WBC*, white blood cell; *BUN*, blood urea nitrogen; *AST*, aspartate aminotransferase (formerly called *SGOT*); *ALT*, alanine aminotransferase (formerly called *SGPT*); *LDH*, lactic dehydrogenase.

X. Specific to anaphylactic shock
  A. Subjective
    1. History of precipitating factor
    2. Vague uneasiness
    3. Warmth
    4. Nausea, abdominal cramping, abdominal pain
    5. Dyspnea
    6. Dizziness, vertigo
    7. Urticaria
    8. Feeling of a lump in throat
  B. Objective
    1. Cutaneous
      a) May be localized redness, swelling, and pruritus if due to bite or sting
      b) May be generalized
        (1) Angioedema (edema of membranous tissues). swelling of eyes, lips, tongue, hands, feet, and genitalia
        (2) Flushing
        (3) Warm to hot skin
        (4) Pruritus
        (5) Hives
        (6) Conjunctival injection, tearing
        (7) Watery rhinorrhea, sneezing
        (8) Erythema more in upper extremities
    2. Cardiovascular
      a) Tachycardia
      b) Hypotension
      c) Dysrhythmias
      d) ST-T-wave changes consistent with ischemia
      e) Cardiac arrest may occur
    3. Pulmonary
      a) Hoarseness
      b) Cough
      c) Prolonged expiration
      d) Breath sound changes: stridor, wheezing, crackles, rhonchi
      e) Respiratory arrest may occur
    4. Neurologic
      a) Restlessness
      b) Headache
      c) Paresthesia
      d) Change in level of consciousness
      e) Seizures

5. Genitourinary
   a) Urinary incontinence
   b) Urine output: may be decreased
   c) Vaginal bleeding
6. GI
   a) Dysphagia
   b) Vomiting
   c) Intestinal cramping, diarrhea
C. Hemodynamics: Table 12-2
D. Diagnostic: IgE levels may be used to confirm allergic origin
XI. Specific to neurogenic shock
   A. Subjective: history of precipitating factor
   B. Objective
      1. Bradycardia
      2. Hypotension
      3. Hypothermia
      4. Skin warm, dry, flushed
      5. Definite neurologic deficit
   C. Hemodynamics: Table 12-2

Nursing Diagnoses

I. Decreased Cardiac Output related to inadequate volume, inadequate cardiac contractility, inadequate vascular tone, dysrhythmias, ineffective timing of IABP
II. Fluid Volume Deficit related to blood or fluid loss
III. Ineffective Airway Clearance related to tracheobronchial obstruction due to laryngeal edema, laryngeal spasm, bronchospasm, increased secretions, artificial airways
IV. Ineffective Breathing Patterns related to immobility, analgesics
V. Impaired Gas Exchange related to alveolar-capillary membrane changes secondary to increased capillary permeability associated with histamine, acute respiratory distress syndrome, ventilation/perfusion mismatch
VI. Altered Cerebral Tissue Perfusion related to hypoxia, cerebral hypoperfusion
VII. Altered Peripheral Tissue Perfusion related to hypovolemia, fluid shifts, decreased blood flow secondary to IABP catheter position, vasopressors
VIII. Altered Nutrition: Less than Body Requirements related to hypermetabolism, paralytic ileus, decreased absorption
IX. Altered Urinary Elimination Pattern related to hypoperfusion, excretion of pigments (e.g., myoglobin, hemoglobin)
X. Impaired Skin Integrity due to urticaria, angioedema
XI. Risk for Infection related to invasive procedures, immunocompromise
XII. Pain related to invasive procedures
XIII. Risk for Injury related to intubation, invasive procedures, hemorrhage secondary to clotting abnormalities
XIV. Altered Protection related to electrolyte imbalance caused by fluid shifts and potential hemolysis
XV. Ineffective Individual and Family Coping related to sudden critical illness
XVI. Anxiety related to sudden critical illness, fear

of the unknown, fear of death, change in role relationships, change in self-concept

Collaborative Management

I. Maximize oxygen delivery to the tissues (Hgb, Sao_2, CO/CI)
   A. Maintain optimal hemoglobin and vascular volume: monitor and use CVP or PAOP when available
      1. Two intravenous catheters should be inserted immediately, especially in cases of hemorrhage; these catheters should be short and large-gauge
      2. Volume replacement for hypovolemic and vasogenic; may be necessary even in cardiogenic shock to achieve optimal PAOP
         a) Types of fluids used for fluid resuscitation (Table 12-5)
            (1) Crystalloids: solutions with dextrose or electrolytes; safe, effective, inexpensive and usually the initial fluid type
               (a) Isotonic solutions
                  (i) Have an osmolality close to blood osmolality (280-295 mOsm/L)
                  (ii) Tend to stay in the vascular space better than other crystalloids but still require replacement with 3 ml for every 1 ml lost since they do equilibrate across fluid compartments
                  (iii) Examples
                     [a] Normal (0.9%) saline: 154 mEq of sodium and 154 mEq of chloride, osmolality is 289 mOsm/L, pH is 5.7; large volumes may cause metabolic (hyperchloremic) acidosis
                     [b] Lactated Ringer's: 130 mEq/L, 109 mEq/L chloride, 4 mEq/L potassium, 3 mEq/L of calcium, osmolality is 273 mEq/L; pH 6.7; lactate is added as a buffer to make the solution less acidic (than without the lactate); lactate is converted to bicarbonate by the liver; large volumes may cause metabolic alkalosis; avoid in patients who have liver disease
               (b) Hypotonic solutions
                  (i) Have an osmolality less than blood

	Table 12-5	Types of Fluid Used for Fluid Resuscitation

Crystalloids	Colloids	Blood and Blood Products
Isotonic: NS; LR (D_5NS, D_5LR)	Albumin	Whole blood
Hypotonic: ½NS (D_5½NS, D_5W)	Plasma protein fraction (PPF)	Packed RBCs
Hypertonic: 3% saline; D_{10}W; TPN	Dextran 70/75	Fresh frozen plasma
	Hetastarch (Hespan)	

Key: *NS,* normal (0.9%) saline; *LR,* lactated Ringer's; *D_5NS,* 5% dextrose in normal saline; *D_5LR,* 5% dextrose in lactated Ringer's solution; *½NS,* 0.45% saline; *D_5½NS,* 5% dextrose in 0.45% saline; *D_5W,* 5% dextrose in water; *D_{10}W,* 10% dextrose in water; *TPN,* total parenteral nutrition (usually 25% dextrose)

Note: Dextrose solutions are in parentheses because even though 5% dextrose adds to osmolality in the bottle or bag, this small amount of dextrose is metabolized so quickly when in the body that it should not be considered in the osmolality of the solution. So consider D_5NS as NS, D_5½NS as ½NS, and D_5W as water. This last example is why D_5W is avoided except in extreme hyperosmolar condition. In significant volumes D_5W will dilute electrolytes, particularly sodium, and potentially cause neurologic changes including seizures.

(ii) Tend to leave the vascular space and replace the interstitial space better than the vascular space

(iii) Examples

[a] Half normal (0.45%) saline

[b] D_5W: 5% dextrose in water; although D_5W is isotonic in the bottle, the body quickly metabolizes the dextrose and free water is left; avoid this solution except in extremely hyperosmolar patients (e.g., HHNK, DI)

(c) Hypertonic solutions

(i) Have an osmolality greater than blood

(ii) Pull fluid from the interstitial space into the intravascular space; monitor closely for clinical indications of fluid overload when these solutions are administered

(iii) Examples

[a] Hypertonic (3%) saline

[b] D_{10}W (10% dextrose in water)

[c] D_{50}W (50% dextrose in water)

[d] Total parenteral nutrition solution (usually 10% is given via a peripheral vein, 25% is given via a central vein)

(2) Colloids: large molecule (protein or starch) solutions; considered when the patient's response to initial resuscitation efforts are insufficient

(a) Not only stay in the vascular space better than crystalloids but also contribute to intravascular colloidal oncotic pressure to pull more fluid into the vascular space

(b) May be used in hypovolemic shock (except early burns) or neurogenic shock; since septic and anaphylactic shock and early burn injury are associated with increased capillary permeability, they should be avoided at least initially

(c) Examples

(i) Albumin: plasma protein component, costly

(ii) Dextran: contains polymers of high-molecular-weight polysaccharides; may cause coagulopathy by decreasing platelet aggregation; causes allergic reactions; may cause acute tubular necrosis and renal failure, but this adverse effect is rare

(iii) Hetastarch: contains polymers of hydroxyethyl starch; may cause coagulopathy by decreasing platelet aggregation; may elevate serum amylase levels, but they return to normal at 5 to 7 days after hetastarch

(3) Blood and blood products: used only to achieve a specific physiologic goal, such as to increase oxygen delivery or clotting capability

(a) Contain plasma proteins that add to intravascular colloidal oncotic pressure; only solution that increases the CaO_2 (content of oxygen in arterial blood) since 97% of all oxygen is carried on the hemoglobin molecule

(b) Indicated when the patient has lost blood and clinical indications of hypoperfusion are present

(c) Hematocrit of 30% to 32% probably a reasonable goal since no significant increase in oxygen delivery is achieved and blood flow may become sluggish with a greater hematocrit

(d) Major disadvantages of blood and blood products: cost and risk of blood transfusion reaction or blood transmitted disease

(e) For more information on blood and blood products and administration of blood, see Chapter 11

b) Volume

(1) Typical fluid challenge is 250 to 500 ml of normal saline or lactated Ringer's solution over 5 minutes

(2) Continue to administer 200 ml every 5 minutes until an increase in BP is seen or until patient exhibits clinical indicators of fluid overload (e.g., dyspnea, jugular venous distention, S_3, systolic flow murmur, crackles)

3. Type and crossmatch immediately if patient is hemorrhaging; type-specific blood or O negative may be given in severe hemorrhage

4. Take care during fluid resuscitation to prevent hypothermia; fluids may need to be warmed if the patient's body temperature is low (35° C or less) at the initiation of fluid resuscitation or if multiple units of blood or multiple liters of IV fluids are needed

5. Administer venous vasodilators and/or diuretics as prescribed to decrease the preload (PAOP) in cardiogenic shock

B. Maintain optimal cardiac contractility and cardiac output

1. Monitor ECG, MAP, RAP, PAP, PAOP, CO/CI, LVSWI, RVSWI, neurologic status

2. Administer inotropes (e.g., dobutamine) as prescribed

3. Administer diuretics (e.g., furosemide) as prescribed

4. Administer vasoactive agents

a) Administer arterial vasodilators (e.g., nitroprusside [NTP]) to decrease afterload (SVR) and/or venous vasodilators (e.g., nitroglycerin [NTG]) to decrease preload (PAOP) as prescribed; these agents are typically needed in cardiogenic shock

b) Administer vasopressors (e.g., norepinephrine [Levophed], dopamine [Intropin]) as prescribed and in the lowest doses necessary to achieve desired effects

(1) Vasopressors are generally contraindicated in patients with cardiogenic shock because they increase afterload (SVR) and myocardial oxygen consumption

(2) Vasopressors are sometimes used in an effort to maintain MAP above 60 mm Hg to maintain perfusion pressure, but by constricting the vessels they may actually decrease blood flow to organs, even through the MAP is higher

5. Correct metabolic acidosis because it affects cardiac contractility

a) Improve oxygenation and perfusion by improving Hgb, Sao_2, Hgb

b) Administer sodium bicarbonate as prescribed; indicated only if pH 7.0 or less

6. Avoid overheating, which may cause vasodilation and decreased preload

C. Maintain optimal oxygen saturation

1. Monitor Spo_2, Svo_2, arterial blood gases

2. Ensure adequate airway; endotracheal intubation often necessary

3. Administer oxygen at 5 to 6 L/min initially

a) Higher concentrations may be necessary depending on Spo_2 and arterial blood gas values

b) CPAP or PEEP may be required for refractory hypoxemia

4. Initiate mechanical ventilation as prescribed for respiratory muscle fatigue, respiratory acidosis, and/or refractory hypoxemia

5. Monitor closely for changes in Spo_2, arterial blood gases, pulmonary vascular resistance, chest X-ray, and lung compliance indicative of ARDS

II. Minimize oxygen consumption of the tissues

A. Maintain bed rest and provide adequate rest periods

B. Control body temperature

1. Treat hyperthermia with cooling blankets as necessary: set at 1° below patient's temperature to avoid shivering and drift (continued decrease on temperature)

2. Avoid overheating, which may increase myocardial oxygen consumption

C. Monitor work of breathing; initiate mechanical ventilation as prescribed for respiratory fatigue

D. Treat pain and anxiety

1. Administer analgesics and/or anxiolytics as prescribed and indicated

2. Provide patient and family support

a) Keep patient and family informed

b) Encourage the patient and family to discuss fear, concerns

III. Prevent injury caused by decreased perfusion

A. Limit sedatives and other central nervous system (CNS) depressants

B. Administer drugs only IV because peripheral perfusion and drug absorption is impaired;

central venous catheter with multiple lumens is preferred

IV. Maintain or improve nutritional status

A. Provide enteral feedings unless absolutely contraindicated (e.g., paralytic ileus); glutamine, arginine, and omega-3 fatty acids may be important in the prevention and treatment of sepsis, septic shock, SIRS, and MODS

B. Provide parenteral feeding if enteral feedings are contraindicated or if parenteral supplementation of enteral feedings is needed to meet calorie and protein requirements

C. Monitor serum potassium, magnesium, and phosphate closely; replace or restrict as indicated

D. Add trace elements and vitamins as prescribed

V. Maintain renal perfusion and glomerular filtration rate (GFR)

A. Insert indwelling urinary catheter to monitor hourly urine output

B. Monitor BUN, creatinine, urine creatinine clearance, urine sodium

C. Replace volume as indicated by CVP or PAOP

D. Monitor closely for change in color of urine, which may indicate myoglobinuria, (tea-colored), hemoglobinuria (wine-colored)

E. Administer dopamine at 1 to 2 μg/kg/min as prescribed to improve renal and mesenteric blood flow

VI. Specific to hypovolemic

A. Treat the cause

1. Compression of any compressible vessels
2. Surgery may be necessary to control bleeding
3. Antidiarrheals for diarrhea
4. Insulin for hyperglycemia

B. Administer appropriate volume replacement

C. Utilize autotransfusion if appropriate; used primarily in chest trauma (or chest surgery) to decrease the risk of transfusion-transmitted disease (for more detailed discussion, see Chest Surgery and Chest Tubes section of Chapter 5)

VII. Specific to cardiogenic

A. Treat the cause

1. Pericardiocentesis for cardiac tamponade
2. Thrombolytics, anticoagulants for pulmonary embolism
3. Surgery for removal of intracardiac tumors, valve replacement, septal repair, etc.
4. Emergency decompression followed by chest tube for tension pneumothorax

B. Administer inotropes (e.g., dobutamine) to increase contractility

C. Administer diuretics (e.g., furosemide) or venous vasodilators (e.g., nitroglycerin [NTG]) to decrease preload (PAOP)

D. Administer arterial vasodilators (e.g., nitroprusside [NTP]) to decrease afterload

E. Administer antidysrhythmics as prescribed

F. Utilize mechanical supports (e.g., intraaortic balloon pump [IABP]) (Fig. 3-18, Fig. 3-19, and Table 3-16) or ventricular assist devices (Table 3-25); IABP is especially helpful in patients who have very high afterload that is refractory to arterial vasodilators or who are too hypotensive to utilize arterial vasodilators to reduce afterload

G. Prepare patient for emergency revascularization (e.g., percutaneous coronary intervention [PCI] or coronary artery bypass grafts [CABG])

H. Register patient for cardiac transplantation when available if appropriate

VIII. Specific to septic

A. Prevent infection and sepsis

1. Use good handwashing techniques and prevent cross-contamination
2. Avoid intrusive procedures if possible
3. Participate in early identification of focus of infection

   a) Monitor color, characteristics of sputum, urine, stools, wounds, etc.
   b) Culture secretions and wounds as indicated

4. Prepare patient for surgery as indicated for any of the following:

   a) Removal of all necrotic tissue
   b) Drainage of abscess
   c) Early debridement of burn eschar
   d) Prompt stabilization of fractures to minimize soft tissue damage, inflammation, infection

5. Perform meticulous oral and airway care; silent aspiration of oral, nasopharyngeal, sinus secretions around the endotracheal tube cuff occurs and is a cause of nosocomial pneumonia

6. Perform meticulous intravenous, intraarterial, pulmonary artery, and urinary catheter care according to Center for Disease Control (CDC) guidelines or hospital policy

7. Perform meticulous wound care as indicated by type and appearance of wound

8. Avoid NPO status to prevent translocation of enteric bacteria into the lymphatics and vascular bed

   a) Enteral feedings should be given if at all possible
   b) Selective gut decontamination (gut sterilization) with nonabsorbable antibiotics (e.g., neomycin) has been advocated for use with parenteral nutrition for patients that must be NPO; effectiveness has not been proven and cost may be prohibitive

9. Administer prophylactic antibiotic therapy as prescribed

   a) Controversial today as more microorganisms become resistant to available antibiotic therapy
   b) Many physicians prefer to have clinical indications of infection before prescribing antibiotic therapy

B. Treat infection and neutralize toxins
   1. Administer antibiotics as prescribed
   2. Use experimental therapies as prescribed; may only be available for compassionate use
      a) Monoclonal antibodies to endotoxin may neutralize endotoxins and prevent mediator release
      b) Plasmapheresis may be used to remove endotoxin and/or bacterial byproducts
C. Modify mediators (controversial because these mediators are important to the inflammatory process, but excess amounts may need to be modified or blocked)
   1. Antihistamines (e.g., diphenhydramine [Benadryl], ranitidine [Zantac]) to modify and/or block histamine
   2. Naloxone (Narcan) to modify and/or block endorphins
   3. Ibuprofen (Motrin) and indomethacin (Indocin) to modify and/or block prostaglandin
   4. Corticosteroids (e.g., hydrocortisone sodium succinate [Solu-Cortef]) may modify several mediators and stabilize the cell membrane
   5. Angiotensin-converting enzyme inhibitors (e.g., captopril [Capoten]) to decrease production of angiotensin II
   6. Anticoagulants (e.g., heparin) to modify the clotting cascade by blocking the conversion of prothrombin to thrombin
D. Control hyperthermia
   1. Monitor core body temperature
   2. Administer antipyretics as indicated
   3. Remove extra bed linens and utilize cooling blankets
E. Maintain MAP and tissue perfusion
   1. Administer volume and vasopressors as prescribed
   2. Administer inotropes as prescribed to maintain tissue perfusion; increasing cardiac output 50% or more above normal has been shown to improve survival; cardiac index greater than 4.5 L/min/m^2 may be used as a goal

IX. Specific to anaphylactic
A. Remove the offending agent or slow absorption of antigen
   1. Remove stinger if due to a sting and the stinger can be removed easily without squeezing
   2. Apply ice if due to sting or bite
   3. Discontinue infusion of dye, drug, or blood
   4. Lavage the stomach if an ingested antigen
   5. Flush skin with water if dermal contaminant
B. Maintain airway, oxygenation, and ventilation
   1. Ensure adequate airway
      a) Endotracheal tube may be needed
      b) Cricothyrotomy may be necessary because of laryngeal edema
   2. Administer oxygen at 5 to 6 L initially;

adjust to maintain Spo_2 at 95% unless contraindicated
   3. Initiate mechanical ventilation as prescribed
C. Modify or block the effects of biochemical mediators
   1. Administer sympathomimetic agents
      a) Epinephrine 0.3 to 0.5 ml of 1:1000 solution SC or 1 ml of 1:10,000 solution IV
      b) Glucagon 0.5 to 1.0 mg IV, especially if patient is receiving beta-blockers; can stimulate an increase in heart rate and contractility even with beta-blockade
   2. Administer antihistamines as prescribed to block histamine receptors
      a) Diphenhydramine (Benadryl) 25 to 50 mg IV
      b) Ranitidine (Zantac) 50 mg IV
   3. Administer bronchodilators as prescribed to reverse the bronchoconstriction caused by histamine, SRS-A, and bradykinin
      a) Epinephrine, an adrenergic agent, acts as a bronchodilator by stimulating beta$_2$-receptors
      b) Aminophyllin, a xanthine, acts as a bronchodilator by directing relaxing smooth muscle
   4. Administer steroids as prescribed to stabilize mast cells, decrease capillary permeability, prevent delayed reaction
      a) Hydrocortisone sodium succinate (Solu-Cortef)
      b) Methyl prednisolone sodium succinate (Solu-Medrol)
D. Maintain MAP and tissue perfusion: fluids, inotropes, and/or vasopressors may be necessary

X. Specific to neurogenic
A. Treat the cause: reverse anesthesia, etc.
B. Maintain MAP and tissue perfusion
   1. Maintain MAP more than 70 mm Hg
      a) Fluids: colloids are usually used because they are more likely to remain in vascular space and because increased capillary permeability is not a factor in neurogenic shock as it is in septic and anaphylactic shock; monitor closely for pulmonary or cerebral edema
      b) Inotropes and/or vasopressors may be necessary
   2. Maintain heart rate 60 to 100 bpm: atropine and/or pacemaker may be necessary
C. Prevent venous stasis and deep vein thrombosis: anticoagulants as prescribed

XI. Monitor for complications of shock
A. Dysrhythmias
B. GI ulceration
C. Mesenteric ischemia, infarction

XII. Monitor for indications of organ failure and multiple organ dysfunction syndrome (MODS)
A. Acute respiratory failure (ARDS)
B. Disseminated intravascular coagulation (DIC)
C. Hepatic failure

D. Renal failure

E. Myocardial infarction

F. Cerebral infarction

Systemic Inflammatory Response Syndrome (SIRS) and Multiple Organ Dysfunction Syndrome (MODS)

Definitions

I. Systemic inflammatory response syndrome (SIRS) (Fig. 12-6): "Widespread inflammation (or clinical response to that inflammation) that can occur in patients with such diverse disorders as infection, pancreatitis, ischemia, multiple trauma, shock, or immunologically mediated organ injury" (Bone R, Sprung C, Sibbald W, 1992)

II. Multiple organ dysfunction syndrome (MODS) (Fig. 12-7): "Presence of altered organ function in an acutely ill patient such that homeostasis cannot be maintained without intervention" (Bone R, Sprung C, Sibbald W, 1992)

A. "Primary multiple organ dysfunction syndrome occurs when there is a direct injury to the organ that becomes dysfunctional" (Bone R, Sprung C, Sibbald W, 1992)

B. "Secondary multiple organ dysfunction syndrome occurs as a consequence of trauma or infection in one part of the system that results in the systemic inflammatory response and dysfunction of organs elsewhere" (Bone R, Sprung C, Sibbald W, 1992)

Etiology

I. Mechanical tissue damage: trauma, burns, crush injuries, surgical procedures

II. Abscesses: intraabdominal, intracranial

III. Ischemic/necrotic tissue: prolonged shock, MI, pancreatitis, DIC

IV. Microbial invasion: immunosuppressed states, surgery/trauma, community exposure, nosocomial exposure

V. Endotoxin release: gram-negative sepsis, translocation of bacteria from gut (sepsis is the single most common etiologic factor, but 40% to 50% of MODS patients do not have positive blood cultures)

VI. Global perfusion deficits: shock, cardiopulmonary arrest

VII. Regional perfusion deficits: vascular injury, vascular repair procedures, thromboembolic events

Pathophysiology

I. May be triggered by infection or noninfective processes such as injury, ischemia, necrosis

II. Cascade of inflammation (Fig. 12-8): although the inflammatory process is necessary and helpful when localized, it may be destructive when generalized or systemic

III. Mediators (see Table 11-1 and Table 12-6)

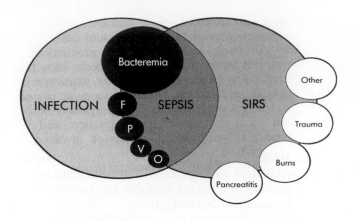

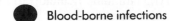

Blood-borne infections

F   Fungemia

P   Parasitemia

V   Viremia

O   Other

Figure 12-6 Interrelationships among systemic inflammatory response syndrome (SIRS), sepsis, and infection. (From American College of Chest Physicians/Society of Critical Care Medicine consensus conference committee, *Critical Care Medicine* 20 (6):865, 1992.)

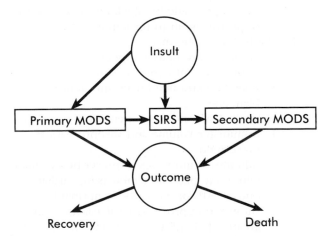

Figure 12-7 Different causes and results of primary and secondary multiple organ dysfunction syndrome (MODS). (From American College of Chest Physicians/Society of Critical Care Medicine consensus conference committee, *Critical Care Medicine* 20 (6):866, 1992.)

IV. Central nervous system, autonomic nervous system, endocrine system, and hematology and immunology systems respond as if an infection has occurred

V. MODS may occur due to hypoperfusion and generalized inflammatory process (Fig. 12-9)

Clinical Presentation

I. SIRS

A. Criteria (2 or more of the following) (Bone, 1991)

1. Tachycardia (>90/min)

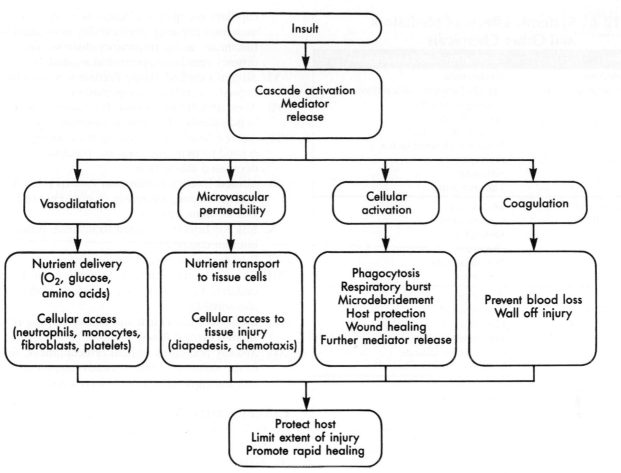

Figure 12-8 Cascade of inflammation. (From Huddleston SV: *Multiple organ dysfunction and failure,* ed 2, St Louis, 1996, Mosby.)

2. Hyperpnea (respiratory rate above 20/min or $Paco_2$ below 32 mm Hg)
3. Hyperthermia (temperature above 38° C or 100.4° F) or hypothermia (temperature below 36° C or 96.8° F) (hypothermia is more common in elderly patients)
4. WBC above 12,000 cells/mm³ or below 4,000 cells/mm³ or more than 10% bands

B. System assessment (Table 12-7)

II. MODS: dysfunction of one or more of the following organs:

A. Pulmonary (ARDS): absence of pulmonary embolism or bilateral pneumonia with the following:
1. Predisposing factor such as sepsis
2. Unexplained hypoxemia
3. Bilateral pulmonary infiltrates consistent with pulmonary edema
4. Pao_2/Fio_2 ratio less than 200
5. PAOP less than 18 mm Hg (to rule out cardiac pulmonary edema)

B. Hematologic (DIC): absence of liver failure, major hematoma, or anticoagulation therapy with the following:
1. Fibrin split products (FSP) more than 1:40 or D-dimer >200 ng/ml
2. Thrombocytopenia or a 25% drop from a previous value

3. Prolonged PT, aPTT
4. Clinical evidence of bleeding

C. Renal: absence of diuretic within 2 hours of urine analysis with the following:
1. Serum creatinine abnormal and urinary sodium is more than 40 mmol/L
2. If previous renal insufficiency, an increase in creatinine by 2.0 mg/dl not due to myoglobinuria

D. Hepatobiliary: absence of preexisting liver disease with the following:
1. Serum bilirubin more than 2.0 mg/dl
2. Alkaline phosphatase, ALT, AST, gamma-glutamyl transferase (GGT) over twice laboratory normal

E. Central nervous system: absence of sedation or paralyzing agents that would alter the patient's ability to respond with decrease in Glasgow Coma Score by one point

F. Degrees of organ dysfunction are described in Table 12-8

Nursing Diagnoses

I. Fluid Volume Deficit related to massive vasodilation and increased capillary permeability

II. Decreased Cardiac Output related to inadequate volume, inadequate cardiac contractility, inadequate vascular tone, dysrhythmias

Table 12-6	Systemic Effects of Mediators and Other Chemicals
Effect	**Chemical Mediators and Triggers**
Selective vasoconstriction	Angiotensin
	Catecholamines: epinephrine, norepinephrine
	Leukotrienes
	Oxygen-free radicals
	Platelet activating factor
	Prostaglandins
	Serotonin
	Thromboxane
Peripheral vasodilation	Bradykinin
	Complement
	Endorphins
	Histamine
	Prostaglandins
	Serotonin
Increased capillary permeability	Bradykinin
	Complement
	Histamine
	Leukotrienes
	Oxygen-free radicals
	Platelet activating factor
Coagulation	Complement
	Hageman factor
	Platelet aggregation
	Polymorphonuclear cell aggregation
	Tumor necrosis factor
Endothelial damage	Acidosis
	Complement
	Endotoxin
	Histamine
	Hypoxia
	Oxygen-free radicals
	Platelet activating factor
	Polymorphonuclear cell aggregation
	Tumor necrosis factor
	Interleukin-1
Depressed myocardial contractility	Complement
	Endorphins
	Histamine
	Impaired adrenergic response
	Lactic acid
	Myocardial depressant factor
Enhanced polymorphonuclear activity	Cellular debris
	Complement
	Elastase
	Kinins
	Interleukin-1
	Leukotrienes
	Platelet activating factor
	Platelet aggregation
	Prostaglandins
	Tumor necrosis factor

III. Ineffective Airway Clearance related to increased secretions, artificial airways
IV. Ineffective Breathing Patterns related to immobility, analgesics
V. Impaired Gas Exchange related to alveolar-capillary membrane changes secondary to increased capillary permeability associated with histamine, acute respiratory distress syndrome, ventilation/perfusion mismatch
VI. Altered Cerebral Tissue Perfusion related to hypoxia, cerebral hypoperfusion
VII. Altered Peripheral Tissue Perfusion related to hypovolemia, fluid shifts, vasopressors
VIII. Altered Nutrition: Less than Body Requirements related to hypermetabolism, paralytic ileus, decreased absorption
IX. Altered Urinary Elimination Pattern related to hypoperfusion, excretion of pigments (e.g., myoglobin, hemoglobin)
X. Risk for Infection related to invasive procedures, immunocompromise
XI. Pain related to invasive procedures
XII. Risk for Injury related to intubation, invasive procedures, hemorrhage secondary to clotting abnormalities
XIII. Ineffective Individual and Family Coping related to sudden critical illness
XIV. Anxiety related to sudden critical illness, fear of the unknown, fear of death, change in role relationships, change in self-concept

Collaborative Management

I. Prevent and treat infection (see Septic Shock section)
II. Maximize oxygen delivery to the tissues (see Shock section)
   A. Maintain cardiac index 4.5 L/min/m^2 or greater
      1. Administer fluids: crystalloids are used because capillary permeability is increased
      2. Administer inotropes (e.g., dobutamine) as prescribed
      3. Administer vasopressors (e.g., dopamine, norepinephrine) as prescribed when SVR is low
   B. Maintain hematocrit approximately 30% to 32%
      1. Administer blood and blood products as prescribed
      2. Correct coagulopathies; administer fresh frozen plasma, platelets, vitamin K as prescribed
   C. Maintain Spo$_2$, Sao$_2$: more than 95%
      1. Ensure adequate airway
      2. Administer oxygen as needed
      3. Initiate mechanical ventilation as needed; PEEP may also be necessary
   D. Monitor Svo$_2$
      1. Decreased Svo$_2$ to less than 60% indicates that oxygen delivery is impaired or oxygen consumption is increased
         a) Assess Sao$_2$
         b) Assess cardiac output/index
         c) Assess hemoglobin
         d) Assess for causes of increased consumption (e.g., shivering, fever, seizures)

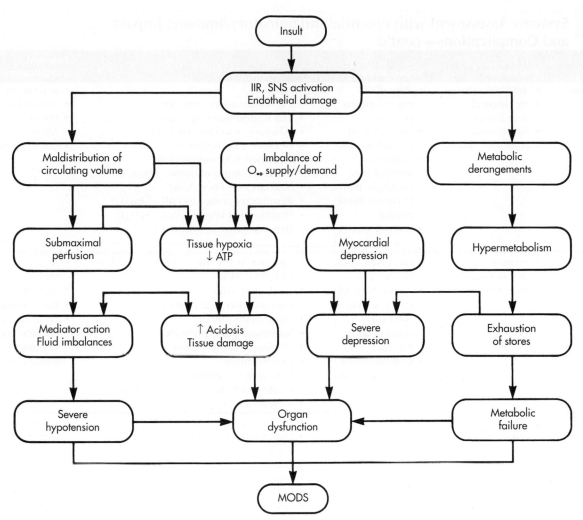

Figure 12-9   Pathophysiologic cascade mechanism of multiple organ dysfunction and failure. *IIR,* Inflammatory/immune response; *NE,* neuroendocrine; *PIRI,* postischemic reperfusion injury; *ATP,* adenosine triphosphate; *MSOF,* multisystem organ failure. (From Huddleston SV: *Multiple organ dysfunction and failure,* ed 2, St Louis, 1996, Mosby.)

Table 12-7	Systems Assessment with Potential Inflammatory/Immune Impact and Complications			
System	**Risk Factors**	**Impact on IIR**	**Assessment**	**Potential Complications**
CNS	• Invasive drains • ICP monitoring • Surgical incision • Cranial nerve involvement • Spinal cord injury	• Increased microbial access • IIR activation • Impaired natural defenses	• Decreased LOC, GCS • Decreased CCP • Inflammation at wound • Respiratory depression • Skin breakdown	• CNS infection • Aspiration • Corneal abrasions • Skin breakdown

Adapted from: Huddleston Secor V: *Multiple organ dysfunction and failure,* ed 2, St Louis, 1996, Mosby.
Legend: *IIR,* inflammatory/immune response; *CNS,* central nervous system; *ICP,* intracranial pressure; *LOC,* level of consciousness; *GCS,* Glasgow Coma Score; *CCP,* cerebral perfusion pressure; *FIo$_2$,* fraction of inspired oxygen; *Paco$_2$,* partial pressure of carbon dioxide in arterial blood; *Pao$_2$,* partial pressure of oxygen in arterial blood; *Spo$_2$,* oxygen saturation of hemoglobin by pulse oximetry; *Svo$_2$,* oxygen saturation of hemoglobin in venous blood; *Sao$_2$,* oxygen saturation of hemoglobin in arterial blood; *ARDS,* acute respiratory distress syndrome; *CV,* cardiovascular; *HR,* heart rate; *BP,* blood pressure; *CO/CI,* cardiac output/cardiac index; *PAP,* pulmonary artery pressure; *PAOP,* pulmonary artery occlusive pressure; *CVP/RAP,* central venous pressure/right atrial pressure; *SVR,* systemic vascular resistance; *GI,* gastrointestinal; *H$_2$,* histamine type 2 receptor; *GU,* genitourinary; *BUN,* blood urea nitrogen; *HCO$_3$,* bicarbonate

Continued

Table 12-7 Systems Assessment with Potential Inflammatory/Immune Impact and Complications—cont'd

System	Risk Factors	Impact on IIR	Assessment	Potential Complications
Pulmonary	• Artificial airway • Mechanical ventilation • Barotrauma • High FIo_2 levels	• Bypass of natural airway defenses • Increased microbial access • Activation of alveolar macrophages with toxic mediator release • Altered surfactant production	• Dyspnea • Use of accessory muscles • Thick, discolored sputum • Wheezes, crackles, rhonchi • Decreased compliance • Increased V/Q mismatching • Increased intrapulmonary shunt • Infiltrates on chest X-ray • Respiratory acidosis ($\downarrow$pH, $\uparrow$Paco$_2$) • Hypoxemia ($\downarrow$Pao$_2$, $\downarrow$Sao$_2$, Spo$_2$) • Hypoxia ($\downarrow$Svo$_2$, $\uparrow$ lactate)	• Aspiration • Atelectasis • Pneumonia • ARDS • Oxygen toxicity
CV	• Invasive monitoring • Poor perfusion	• Increased microbial access • Tissue ischemia to IIR activation with third spacing and edema • Cellular activation and mediator release	• Changes in HR, BP, CO/CI, PAP, PAOP, CVP/RAP, SVR • Cold, pale skin • Inflammation at access sites • Diminished pulses • Narrowed pulse pressure • Decreased urine output • Dysrhythmias • Myocardial ischemia or infarction • Positive cardiac isoenzymes, troponin • Increased lactate	• Reperfusion injury • Cellulitis • Bacteremia/Sepsis • Endothelial damage and clotting abnormalities
GI	• Nasogastric tube • Antacid therapy • H$_2$-Blocker therapy • Stress ulceration • Antibiotics • Ileus	• Increased gastric pH to bacterial colonization • IIR activation • Inhibition of normal flora's protective function • Inability to clear bacterial load	• Decreased bowel sounds • Upper or lower GI bleeding • Abdominal distention • Diarrhea • Constipation, impaction • Ileus • Stress • Ulceration/erosion • Guaiac + stool • Enteric organisms on blood culture • Jaundice • Ascites • Decreased drug clearance • Abnormal bleeding • Increased liver enzymes • Hypoglycemia • Increased ammonia • Decreased plasma proteins • Decreased clotting factors • Hepatomegaly/splenomegaly	• Colonization of esophagus and tracheobronchial tree • Pneumonia • Overgrowth of pathogenic organisms in the GI tract (e.g., *C. difficile*) • Translocation of bacteria to the lymph and blood
GU	• Bladder catheter • Antibiotics • Hyperglycemia	• Increased microbial access • Altered normal flora in vagina • Promotion of yeast growth	• Changes in urine output, malodorous urine, or vaginal discharge • Peripheral edema • Increased CVP/RAP, PAP, PAOP • Increased BUN and creatinine metabolic acidosis ($\downarrow$ pH, $\downarrow$ HCO$_3$)	• Urinary tract infection • Septicemia • *Candida* infections

Adapted from: Huddleston Secor V: *Multiple organ dysfunction and failure*, ed 2, St Louis, 1996, Mosby.

Legend: *IIR*, inflammatory/immune response; *CNS*, central nervous system; *ICP*, intracranial pressure; *LOC*, level of consciousness; *GCS*, Glasgow Coma Score; *CCP*, cerebral perfusion pressure; *FIo$_2$*, fraction of inspired oxygen; *Paco$_2$*, partial pressure of carbon dioxide in arterial blood; *Pao$_2$*, partial pressure of oxygen in arterial blood; *Spo$_2$*, oxygen saturation of hemoglobin by pulse oximetry; *Svo$_2$*, oxygen saturation of hemoglobin in venous blood; *Sao$_2$*, oxygen saturation of hemoglobin in arterial blood; *ARDS*, acute respiratory distress syndrome; *CV*, cardiovascular; *HR*, heart rate; *BP*, blood pressure; *CO/CI*, cardiac output/cardiac index; *PAP*, pulmonary artery pressure; *PAOP*, pulmonary artery occlusive pressure; *CVP/RAP*, central venous pressure/right atrial pressure; *SVR*, systemic vascular resistance; *GI*, gastrointestinal; *H$_2$*, histamine type 2 receptor; *GU*, genitourinary; *BUN*, blood urea nitrogen; *HCO$_3$*, bicarbonate

Table 12-8	**Definitions Degrees of Organ Dysfunction**					
				Organ Dysfunction		
Organ system	Parameter	Normal	Mild	Moderate	Severe	Extreme
CV	Systolic BP (mm Hg)	>90	<90 but fluid responsive	<90 not fluid responsive	<90 not fluid responsive	<90 not fluid responsive
	Arterial pH	≥7.3	≥7.3	≥7.3	<7.3	<7.2
Pulmonary	Pao_2/FIo_2 (mm Hg)	>400	301-400	201-300	101-200	<100
CNS	GCS	15	13-14	10-12	7-9	≥6
Coagulation	Platelet count (1,000/ml)	>120	81-102	51-80	21-50	≥20
Renal	Creatinine (mg/dl)	<1.5	1.5-1.9	2.0-3.4	3.5-4.9	≥5.0
Hepatic	Bilirubin (mg/dl)	<1.2	1.2-3.5	3.6-7.0	7.1-14.0	>14.0

Bone R: Managing sepsis: what treatments can we use today? *Journal of Critical Illness* 12 (1):15, 1997.

2. Increased Svo_2 to more than 80% indicates that oxygen extraction is impaired
III. Minimize oxygen consumption of the tissues (see Shock section)
IV. Maintain or improve nutritional status (see Shock section)
V. Use experimental therapies as prescribed; may only be available for compassionate use
   A. Modify cytokine response
     1. Antiendotoxin: monoclonal antibodies
     2. Antioxidants: allopurinol (Zyloprim), mannitol, vitamins C and E, superoxide dismutase (SOD)
     3. Antiprostaglandin: ibuprofen (Motrin)
     4. Antihistamines: diphenhydramine (Benadryl), ranitidine (Zantac)
     5. Opiate receptor blockers: naloxone (Narcan)
     6. Corticosteroids: block neutrophils, lysosomes, arachidonic acid and complement cascades, interleukins, and inflammation
   B. Utilize extracorporeal membrane oxygenation (ECMO) as prescribed: blood is removed from body, taken through a bubble oxygenator, and then returned to the body in an oxygenated state
VI. Monitor for complications
   A. Shock (if not caused by shock)
   B. Organ failure
   C. Death

Burns
Etiology
I. Thermal: contact with flames, hot liquids or steam (scald), hot objects, or flash (explosion of a flammable liquid)
   A. The severity of the burn is determined by temperature, duration, and location
   B. Scald is the most common of all burns; thicker liquids maintain contact for longer period and cause a more severe burn

II. Electrical: contact with an electrical power source, including lightning
   A. The severity of the burn is determined by the current and the electrical resistance of the body parts
   B. More injury occurs to the less resistant tissues, such as nerves, blood vessels, and muscle
III. Chemical: contact with a caustic chemical
   A. The severity of the injury is determined by the concentration of the chemical and the duration of the exposure
   B. Acids cause necrosis and loss of protein; alkali penetrate deeper into tissues and continue to produce tissue necrosis for several hours after contact
IV. Radiation: exposure to ionizing radiation
   A. The severity of the injury is determined by duration of the exposure and the distance from the source
   B. Alpha and beta radiation are the least dangerous; damage occurs primarily from gamma radiation or X-ray particles

Pathophysiology
I. Damage to skin or body tissue interferes with normal skin functions
   A. Compromises protection against infection
   B. Causes loss of body fluids
   C. Alters control of body temperature
   D. Interferes with vitamin D activation
   E. Alters sensory and excretory functions
   F. Alters body image
II. Zones of injury (Fig. 12-10 and Table 12-9) relate tissue changes to severity of injury and viability of tissue
III. The response to the injury follows a predictable sequence, but the magnitude of the response is proportional to the extent of the injury (Fig. 12-11)
   A. Cellular damage occurs at 45° C (113° F)
   B. Inflammatory process is initiated
     1. Cellular enzymes and mediators of the

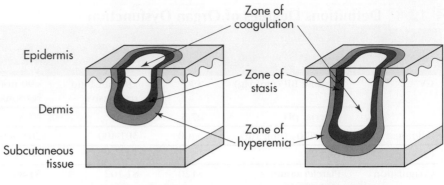

Figure 12-10 Zones of thermal injury. Thermal energy produces concentric zones of decreasingly severe tissue injury. (Modified from Jackson DM: *Br J Surg* 40:558, 1953.)

	Zone	Description
Table 12-9	**Zones of Thermal Injury**	
	Zone of coagulation	• Center of burn, which has the most contact with the heat source • Cells coagulate and necrosis occurs • White or gray without blanching
	Zone of stasis	• Area surrounding center • Injured cells suffer vascular damage • Edematous and red without blanching • May recover or go on to become necrotic
	Zone of hyperemia	• Area around injured zone • Red with blanching • Minimally injured; vascularity is maintained • No cell death • Recovers within approximately 5 days

inflammatory process are released; complement system is activated

2. Vasodilation and increased capillary permeability occur
3. Vessels become permeable to fluids, electrolytes, and proteins

C. Fluid shift from intravascular space to interstitial space
   1. Plasma proteins leak through injured capillary membranes, causing decreased capillary oncotic pressure and increased tissue oncotic pressure, leading to a fluid shift into interstitial space
   2. Lymph flow initially increases but then decreases due to blockage of lymph vessels by serum proteins leaking from the capillary

D. Decreased circulating blood volume and sympathetic nervous system innervation (causing an increase in SVR) lead to a low cardiac output and decreased tissue perfusion; hypovolemic shock may occur
   1. Stasis of blood and metabolic acidosis occurs
   2. Hyperkalemia occurs due to hemolysis and acidosis

E. Edema occurs around the burned area
   1. Edema may be generalized in burns with burn surface area (BSA) of more than 20% due to systemic inflammatory response and hypoproteinemia
   2. Large fluid resuscitation volumes may also contribute to edema
   3. Cellular edema occurs during extensive burns due to a shift of sodium and water into the cell

F. The primary barrier to microorganisms (the skin) is injured, and the immune system is compromised by the overwhelming inflammatory response; infection and sepsis may occur

G. Inflammatory mediators cause pulmonary hypertension; smoke inhalation causes damage to type II pneumocytes, causing a surfactant deficiency that leads to atelectasis and potentially acute respiratory distress syndrome; this pathophysiology leads to ventilation-perfusion mismatch, intrapulmonary shunt, and hypoxemia

H. Decreased renal perfusion and myoglobinuria or hemoglobinuria may cause acute tubular necrosis and acute renal failure
   1. When capillary membrane integrity is reestablished (at about 72 hours), diuresis occurs
   2. Lymphatics have also recovered enough to be able to return fluid to the vascular space about the same time, which contributes to diuresis

I. Hypovolemia and sympathetic nervous system redistribution of blood flow causes hypoperfusion of the gastrointestinal tract leading to paralytic ileus; ischemia and increased acidity caused by glucocorticoid release may cause stress ulcer (often referred to as *Curling's ulcer* in burn patients)

J. Massive tissue injury stimulates the extrinsic clotting pathway and may lead to disseminated intravascular coagulation (DIC)

K. Hypermetabolism occurs, which is probably stimulated by the sympathetic nervous system

L. Inhalation injury is the leading cause of death in the first 24 hours after a burn injury
   1. Burns that occur in enclosed areas or that

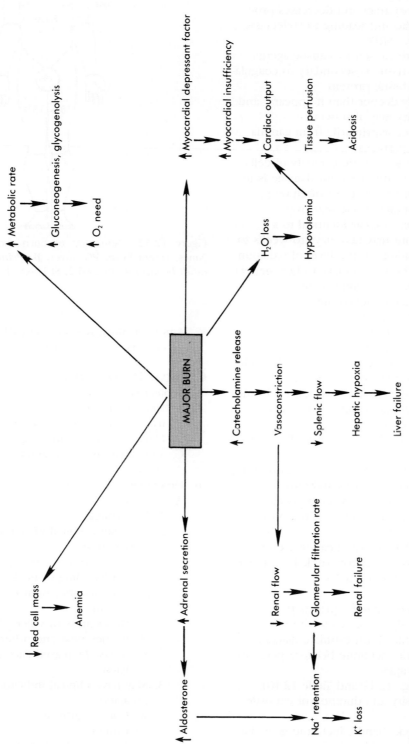

Figure 12-11 Pathophysiology of a major burn. (From Long BC, Phipps WJ, Cassmeyer VL: *Medical-surgical nursing: a nursing process approach*, ed 3, St Louis, 1993, Mosby.)

affect the head and neck are likely to be associated with inhalation injury
2. Inhalation of hot air and smoke causes cellular and capillary damage, leading to airway edema and potential airway obstruction
3. Inhalation of toxins destroys epithelial cells of the respiratory tract and decreases production of surfactant, leading to atelectasis and, potentially, ARDS

M. Chemical burns are caused by caustic agents
1. Destruction of tissue is secondary to coagulation or leak of tissue protein
2. Injury is usually deeper than it appears, and systemic toxicity may also occur

N. Radiation burns occur primarily from gamma radiation or X-ray particles
1. Radiation damages mitotic capacity of cells, leading to cell death; the most damage is to cells that are in mitosis most often (e.g., mucous membranes, bone marrow)
2. These burns may appear identical to a thermal burn but may take days to weeks to manifest depending on the level of radiation

O. Electrical burn occurs secondary to heat generation as current passes through tissue
1. Extent of damage depends on:
   a) Duration of contact
   b) Intensity of current
   c) Resistance of the system
   d) Course electrical current travels through body until it reaches the ground
2. Extent of damage caused by electrical burns is often greater than it initially appears (iceberg principle)
3. Dysrhythmias often occur, especially asystole or ventricular fibrillation
4. Sustained muscle contraction may cause long bone or vertebral fractures and muscle destruction, leading to myoglobinemia

IV. Factors that determine the severity of the burn
A. Size of the burned area
1. Rule of nines (Fig. 12-12): head 9%, each arm 9%, each leg 18%, anterior trunk 18%, posterior trunk 18%, perineum 1%
2. Rule of palms
   a) Size of patient's palm equal to 1%
   b) Especially helpful for scatter burns
3. Lund and Browder burn estimate diagram (Fig. 12-13): more accurate because percentages vary with ages

B. Depth of burn (Fig. 12-14 and Table 12-10): depends on intensity and duration of exposure

C. Location of burn
1. Face, head, neck, hands, feet, and genitalia create particular problems
2. Circumferential burns are also very serious

D. Age of patient: higher mortality rates in patients younger than 10 years of age and older than 50 years of age

E. Concomitant illness and injury (e.g., diabetes mellitus, multiple trauma)

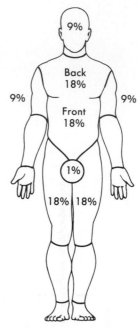

Figure 12-12 Estimation of burn surface area by Rule of Nines. (From Beare PG, Myer, JL: *Principles and practice of adult health nursing,* ed 2, St Louis, 1994, Mosby.)

V. American Burn Association (ABA) burn injury severity criteria (see Table 12-11)

Clinical Presentation

I. Subjective
A. History of exposure to fire, hot object, electricity, chemical, radiation, explosion
B. May have history of drug or alcohol intoxication
C. May have history of abuse and be related to abuse

II. Objective
A. Pulmonary
1. Tachypnea
2. May have clinical indications of airway obstruction
   a) Circumoral, pharyngeal, or neck burns
      (1) Swelling of neck
      (2) Inelastic, tight eschar of neck
   b) Stridor
   c) Hoarseness or voice change
   d) Restlessness and other signs of hypoxia
   e) ABGs: decreased PaO_2 and/or increased $PaCO_2$
3. May have clinical indications of smoke inhalation
   a) Chest tightness
   b) Cough
   c) Circumoral, pharyngeal, or neck burns
   d) Smoky-smelling breath
   e) Dusky to cyanotic mucous membranes
   f) Restlessness and other signs of hypoxia
   g) Hoarseness or voice change
   h) Singed nasal hairs
   i) Sooty sputum

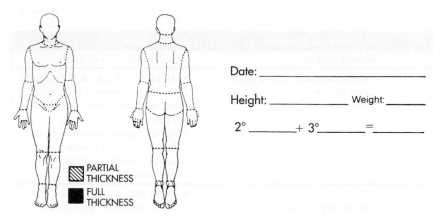

Date: _____

Height: _____ Weight: _____

2° _____ + 3° _____ = _____

PARTIAL THICKNESS

FULL THICKNESS

Percent Surface Area Burned
(Berkow Formula)

Area	0-1 YEAR	1-4 YEARS	5-9 YEARS	10-14 YEARS	15 YEARS	ADULT	2°	3°
Head	19	17	13	11	9	7		
Neck	2	2	2	2	2	2		
Ant. Trunk	13	13	13	13	13	13		
Post Trunk	13	13	13	13	13	13		
R. Buttock	2 1/2	2 1/2	2 1/2	2 1/2	2 1/2	2 1/2		
L. Buttock	2 1/2	2 1/2	2 1/2	2 1/2	2 1/2	2 1/2		
Genitalia	1	1	1	1	1	1		
R.U. Arm	4	4	4	4	4	4		
L.U. Arm	4	4	4	4	4	4		
R.L. Arm	3	3	3	3	3	3		
L.L. Arm	3	3	3	3	3	3		
R. Hand	2 1/2	2 1/2	2 1/2	2 1/2	2 1/2	2 1/2		
L. Hand	2 1/2	2 1/2	2 1/2	2 1/2	2 1/2	2 1/2		
R. Thigh	5 1/2	6 1/2	8	8 1/2	9	9 1/2		
L. Thigh	5 1/2	6 1/2	8	8 1/2	9	9 1/2		
R. Leg	5	5	5 1/2	6	6 1/2	7		
L. Leg	5	5	5 1/2	6	6 1/2	7		
R. Foot	3 1/2	3 1/2	3 1/2	3 1/2	3 1/2	3 1/2		
L. Foot	3 1/2	3 1/2	3 1/2	3 1/2	3 1/2	3 1/2		
TOTAL								

Figure 12-13   Estimation of burn surface area by Lund and Browder's burn estimate diagram. (From Cardona VD: *Trauma nursing from resuscitation through rehabilitation,* Philadelphia, 1995, WB Saunders.)

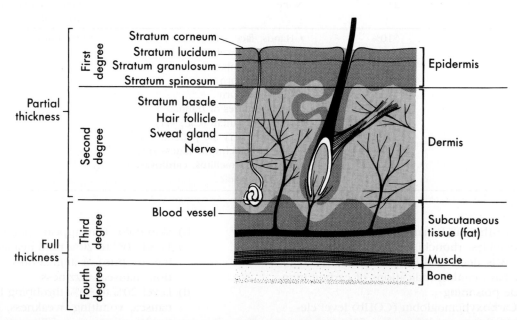

Figure 12-14   Diagram showing depth of burn. (From Beare PG, Myer, JL: *Principles and practice of adult health nursing,* ed 2, St Louis, 1994, Mosby.)

Table **12-10** Depth of Burn

	Superficial Partial Thickness	Deeper Partial Thickness	Full Thickness
Previously called	First degree	Second degree	Third and fourth degree
Depth	• Epidermis	• Epidermis and upper layers of the dermis	• All layers of skin and into subcutaneous tissue (3rd); may even be into muscle or bone (4th) • All skin appendages (e.g., hair follicles, sweat glands, sebaceous glands, etc.) are destroyed
Skin appearance	• Pink or red • Blanches on pressure • Little or no edema • Dry and intact • May be small blisters	• Red • Blanches on pressure • Edematous • Wet, weeping, shiny surface • Fluid-filled blisters	• Deep red, brown, black, or white leathery appearance • Edematous • Exposed subcutaneous layer may be visible • Does not blanch to pressure • Thrombosed blood vessels appear as brownish streaks • Sunken due to loss of underlying fat and/or muscle
Pain	• Painful at first but decreases with cooling; itches later	• Very painful • Extremely sensitive to touch, temperature, air currents	• Complete superficial anesthesia; deep pain (e.g., ischemia, inflammation) is intact
Healing time	• <1 week	• 1 week - 1 month	• > 1 month
Healing process	• Heals spontaneously without scarring	• May heal spontaneously • If converts to full-thickness burn, may require skin grafting	• If < 4 cm in diameter, granulation and migration of healthy epithelium from wound edges occur; grafting is required for wounds ≥ 4 cm

Table **12-11** American Burn Association (ABA) Burn Injury Severity Criteria

	Partial Thickness	Full Thickness	Complicating Factors	Recommended Treatment Facility
Minor	<15%	<2%	None	Outpatient facility (e.g., emergency department, clinic)
Moderate	15%-25%	2%-10%	None	General hospital; may be outpatients
Major	>25%	>10%	• Hands, face, eyes, ears, feet, or perineum involved • Inhalation injury • Electrical burn • Chemical burn • Other injuries or trauma • High-risk patient (e.g., very young or very old patient, patient has chronic illness such as diabetes mellitus, cardiovascular disease, etc.)	Burn unit or burn center

j) Breath sound changes: stridor, wheezing, crackles, rhonchi
k) ABGs: decreased Pao_2, increased $Paco_2$
4. May have clinical indications of carbon monoxide poisoning
   a) Carboxyhemoglobin (COHb) level elevated (normal is less than 5% for nonsmoker and less than 10% for smoker)
b) Skin color may appear cherry red
c) Level 10% to 20%: mild headache, flushing, dyspnea or angina on vigorous exertion, nausea, dizziness
d) Level 20% to 30%: throbbing headache, nausea, vomiting, weakness, dyspnea on moderate exertion, ST segment depression

e) Level 30% to 40%: severe headache, visual disturbances, syncope, vomiting

f) Level 40% to 50%: tachypnea, tachycardia, worsening syncope

g) Level 50% to 60%: chest pain, respiratory failure, shock, seizures, coma

h) Level 60% to 70%: respiratory failure, shock, coma, death

5. May have restrictive process due to tight eschar around chest

   a) Tachypnea

   b) Dyspnea

   c) Decrease in tidal volume, vital capacity

B. Cardiovascular

1. Clinical manifestations of hypovolemic shock (e.g., tachycardia, hypotension, decreased or absent peripheral pulses, pallor, thirst, decreased urine output)

2. Dysrhythmias, especially if electrical burn

C. Integumentary

1. Skin appearance changes depending on depth of burn (Table 12-10) (**Note:** true depth of burn may not be evident for several hours to days after burn injury)

2. Entrance and exit wounds are apparent in electrical burns

3. Lightning may cause linear and feathering burns on skin, especially at moist areas

D. Neuromuscular

1. Tingling, numbness in extremities, especially if circumferential burn

2. May have change in level of consciousness depending on cerebral perfusion

3. Visual disturbances, paralysis, twitching, seizures, coma may be seen in electrical burns

E. Renal

1. Oliguria

2. May have reddish (sometimes described as port wine colored) urine of hemoglobinuria or brownish (sometimes described as tea colored) urine of myoglobinuria

F. GI

1. Diminished or absent bowel sounds, especially during first 72 hours after burn

2. Anorexia, nausea, vomiting, diarrhea may be seen in radiation burns

G. Hematologic: purpura, hemorrhage, infection may be seen in radiation burns

III. Hemodynamics

A. RAP, PAP, PAOP decreased initially

B. CO/CI decreased initially and increases as fluid shifts back into vascular space

C. SVR increased

IV. Diagnostic

A. Serum

1. Potassium

   a) May be increased for first 24 to 48 hours secondary to hemolysis

   b) May be decreased after 48 hours secondary to diuresis that occurs with fluid shifting back into vascular space

2. Sodium: may be increased initially because of fluid resuscitation with lactated Ringer's or normal saline

3. Calcium: may be decreased initially

4. Phosphorus: may be decreased 3 to 9 days after burn

5. Bicarbonate: decreased in lactic acidosis, rhabdomyolysis

6. Glucose: may be increased

7. BUN: may be increased because of hypovolemia and dehydration (prerenal failure) or protein catabolism

8. Creatinine: may be increased if intrarenal failure (e.g., acute tubular necrosis because of myoglobinuria or hemoglobinuria or prolonged hypoperfusion of the kidney)

9. Total protein, albumin: may be decreased because of plasma protein leak into the interstitial space

10. Creatine kinase: may be increased because of muscle damage; especially helpful in evaluation of extent of electrical burns

11. Hemoglobin: may be decreased because of hemolysis

12. Hematocrit

   a) Increased for first 24 to 48 hours secondary to shift of fluid out of vascular space

   b) Decreased after 48 hours secondary to shift of fluid back into vascular space

13. White blood cell

   a) May be increased because of inflammatory response and/or infection

   b) May be decreased because of consumption late in burn sepsis

14. Clotting profile

   a) PT, aPTT: may be prolonged

   b) Platelet count: may be decreased

15. Arterial blood gases

   a) May show hypoxemia caused by smoke inhalation or ARDS

   b) May show metabolic acidosis caused by lactic acidosis from hypoperfusion or carbon monoxide poisoning

16. Toxicology

   a) Carboxyhemoglobin levels: elevated with smoke inhalation and carbon monoxide intoxication

   b) Toxicology screen: may reveal drugs or alcohol

17. Blood culture and sensitivity: may reveal infection

B. Urine

1. Urine specific gravity: increased

2. Proteinuria may be seen

3. Glycosuria may be seen

4. Myoglobinuria or hemoglobinuria may be seen

5. Toxicology screen: may reveal drugs or alcohol

C. Wound culture and sensitivity: may reveal infection
D. Chest X-ray: may reveal atelectasis, pulmonary edema, ARDS
E. Bronchoscopy: may be used to identify (and remove) carbonaceous material and to assess the condition of the tracheobronchial mucosa
F. Pulmonary function studies: tidal volume, vital capacity, maximal inspiratory force may be decreased
G. ECG: may show myocardial damage in electrical burn
H. MRI: may be used to assess extent of electrical burn

Nursing Diagnoses

I. Ineffective Airway Clearance related to tracheal edema, epidermal sloughing, smoke inhalation, impaired cough, artificial airway
II. Ineffective Breathing Patterns related to smoke inhalation, airway edema
III. Impaired Gas Exchange related to atelectasis, pneumonia, pulmonary edema, acute respiratory distress syndrome, carbon monoxide poisoning
IV. Fluid Volume Deficit related to increased capillary permeability, increased evaporation loss
V. Decreased Cardiac Output related to fluid shifts, dysrhythmias, diuresis
VI. Altered Cerebral Tissue Perfusion related to hypoxia, cerebral hypoperfusion
VII. Altered Peripheral Tissue Perfusion related to swelling, circumferential burns, thrombus formation, disseminated intravascular coagulation (DIC)
VIII. Hypothermia related to epithelial skin loss

IX. Alteration in Nutrition: Less than Body Requirements related to hypermetabolism, paralytic ileus, decreased absorption
X. Altered Urinary Elimination Pattern related to hypoperfusion, excretion of pigments (e.g., myoglobin, hemoglobin)
XI. Impaired Skin Integrity due to burns, invasive procedures
XII. Risk for Infection related to loss of normal body defenses (e.g., skin), invasive procedures, immunocompromise
XIII. Pain related to exposure of nerve endings, invasive procedures, inflammation
XIV. Risk for Injury related to impaired immunity, intubation, aspiration, invasive procedures, stress ulcer
XV. Altered Protection related to fluid shifts, potential hemolysis, electrolyte imbalance
XVI. Ineffective Individual and Family Coping related to sudden critical illness
XVII. Anxiety related to sudden critical illness, fear of the unknown, fear of death, fear of disfigurement, change in role relationships, change in self-concept, change in body image

Collaborative Management: Priorities vary during the three major treatment phases (Table 12-12)

I. Limit further injury
  A. Stop the burning process
    1. Thermal
      a) Remove clothing
      b) Remove rings, bracelets, jewelry, belts, or encircling, constricting objects before swelling begins

Table 12-12	Treatment Phases of Burn Injury			
Phase	**Time Period**	**Focus of Care**	**Major Complications**
Resuscitative (also called *emergent*) phase	• From injury until early inflammatory reaction and resultant fluid shifts are resolved • Lasts approximately 24 to 72 hours	• Prevent shock • Maintain organ function • Prevent infection and promote wound healing	• Shock • Respiratory failure
Acute phase	• From the initiation of diuresis until all wounds are closed • From day 3 up to several months	• Prevent infection • Promote wound healing • Support skin grafting	• Sepsis
Rehabilitation phase	• From the time wounds are closed until rehabilitation is complete • May last for several years	• Restore patient's functional abilities • Return patient to role in family, workplace, community • Support decisions related to cosmetic and/or reconstructive surgery	• Body image alteration • Self-concept alteration

c) Immerse area in cool water or normal saline initially to remove dirt, ash, soot, and other foreign material; use cool water to cool down tar, asphalt

d) Wrap uninvolved areas with warm blankets to prevent systemic hypothermia

2. Electrical

a) Turn off source of electricity

b) Do not touch the patient until source of electricity has been turned off

3. Chemical

a) Brush off any dry chemical first (protecting yourself from the chemical with gloves, gowns, goggles)

b) Dermal decontamination

(1) Remove and discard clothing

(2) Do not try to neutralize since neutralizing agents may produce heat as they interact with the chemical

(3) Flush skin gently with water for at least 15 to 30 minutes or until skin pH is normal if chemical was an acid or an alkali

(4) Cover areas with damp sterile dressings

4. Radiation

a) Remove the patient from the area

b) Protect the patient (and yourself) with lead-lined garment

II. Maintain airway, oxygenation, ventilation

A. Assess for clinical indications of airway obstruction or smoke inhalation

B. Assess for circumferential neck or chest burns with swelling and tight, inelastic eschar formation; escharotomy may be needed to relieve obstruction and constriction of chest

1. Escharotomy is incision through eschar of a burned trunk (or limb)

2. This procedure is usually done at the bedside

3. Cuts are made through the eschar to relieve constriction and to allow expansion, releasing constriction on chest excursion (or on arteries and nerves if a limb)

C. Monitor ABGs and pulse oximetry

1. Pulse oximetry may detect an inadequate signal in circumferential burn

2. Elevated carbon monoxide levels cause an inaccurate (falsely elevated) SpO_2

D. Elevate head of bed to 30 degrees to enhance respiratory excursion

E. Encourage deep breathing and incentive spirometry if appropriate; encourage coughing if rhonchi are audible; if rhonchi are audible and cough is inadequate, nasotracheal suctioning or suctioning via endotracheal tube is indicated

F. Assist with maintenance of airway

1. Endotracheal intubation may need to be performed early because swelling may hinder intubation attempts later

2. Cricothyrotomy may be needed for emergency opening of the airway if swelling is too severe to allow endotracheal intubation

G. Administer humidified oxygen

1. Adjust the oxygen concentration to maintain a SpO_2 of at least 95%

2. Utilize CPAP (or PEEP if patient is being mechanically ventilated) to increase the driving pressure of oxygen for refractory hypoxemia or ARDS

3. Treat carbon monoxide poisoning

a) Administer high concentrations (100%) of oxygen by a nonrebreathing mask; decreases COHb levels by one-half in 40 minutes

b) Utilize hyperbaric oxygen therapy for carboxyhemoglobin levels greater than 25%; burn patients are unable to significantly increase their PaO_2, so they may require hyperbaric oxygen therapy at 2 to 3 atmospheres

H. Initiate mechanical ventilation as necessary for respiratory failure

I. Administer pharmacologic agents as prescribed

1. Bronchodilators may be prescribed for bronchospasm

2. Steroids may be prescribed to decrease inflammation, but their use is controversial because they may increase the chance of sepsis

J. Prevent aspiration by inserting a nasogastric tube for gastric decompression; most patients with a burn surface area of more than 30% will have paralytic ileus

K. Assist with laryngoscopy and/or bronchoscopy; performed to determine state of mucosa in inhalation injuries and to determine the presence of carbonaceous material and remove it

III. Maintain circulation

A. Insert large-gauge intravenous catheter(s)

1. Number

a) If burn surface area is 15% to 40%: one

b) If burn surface area is more than 40%: two

2. Location: avoid inserting through burned skin if possible

B. Administer large volume of crystalloids (usually LR) during the first 24 to 48 hours

1. Utilize the American Burn Association (ABA) consensus formula of 2 to 4 ml/kg per percentage of burn surface area to calculate the approximate fluid requirements during the first 24 hours; one-half of the volume is given during the first 8 hours postburn (not postadmission), and the remainder is given during the next 16 hours; increase fluid requirements by approximately 25% to 50% if inhalation injury has occurred

a) Adjust rate of fluids according to clinical

indicators of adequate fluid resuscitation, including the following:
(1) Urine output of 1 ml/kg/hr
(2) PAOP approximately 15 mm Hg
(3) HR less than 120/min
(4) Systolic greater than 100 mm Hg; mean arterial pressure greater than 70 mm Hg
(5) Serum bicarbonate levels greater than 18 mEq/L
(6) Clear, lucid sensorium
  b) Avoid hypervolemia, which increases edema formation and predisposes the patient to heart failure, pulmonary edema, and acute respiratory distress syndrome
   (1) Monitor for clinical indications of volume overload (e.g., S_3, crackles, JVD)
   (2) Monitor hemodynamic parameters
 2. Avoid colloids until after the first 24 hours because of increased capillary permeability; colloids may be used the second 24 hours
  a) If percentage of total BSA is 30% to 50%, albumin at 0.3 ml/kg per percentage of total BSA
  b) If percentage of total BSA is 51% to 70%, albumin at 0.4 ml/kg per percentage of total BSA
  c) If percentage of total BSA is more than 70%, albumin at 0.5 ml/kg per percentage of total BSA
 3. Crystalloids during the second 24-hour period are usually at a rate of 25% to 50% that for the first 24 hours or whatever rate maintains urine output at 0.5 to 1.0 ml/kg/hr; dextrose is added during this time period, and the osmolality is determined by the patient's serum osmolality and serum sodium level (e.g., D_5W if very hyperosmolar, D_5NS if isotonic)
 4. Decrease infusion rates as spontaneous diuresis occurs (usually 72 to 96 hours postburn)
C. Administer inotropes as prescribed; they may be needed if cardiac output/index is inadequate even with adequate volume replacement (as evidenced by PAOP of approximately 15 mm Hg)
D. Administer blood as prescribed to decrease anemia, improve acid-base imbalance, improve capillary oncotic pressure and hypoproteinemia, improve oxygenation and hemodynamics, and decrease tissue edema; often needed by 4 to 5 days postburn due to hemolysis that has occurred
E. Monitor weight
 1. Weigh patient daily at same time and on same scale
 2. Remember that 1 kg is equal to 1 L fluid
IV. Assess for additional injuries

V. Relieve pain and discomfort
A. Assess degree of discomfort utilizing the following methods:
 1. Patient report using a 0 to 10 scale
 2. Nonverbal indicators of pain
  a) Tachycardia
  b) Hypertension or hypotension
  c) Tachypnea
  d) Pupil dilation
  e) Rigid muscle tone
  f) Immobility and guarded position
B. Administer IV narcotics; morphine sulfate is most often used either by IV titration, continuous infusion, or by patient-controlled analgesia pump when the patient is awake, alert, and able to participate in care
C. Administer intravenous sedative as indicated (after neurologic evaluation is complete)
D. Cover wounds to prevent stimulation of nerve endings
E. Position for comfort while still maintaining limbs in functional position
F. Teach relaxation techniques (e.g., imagery, diaphragmatic breathing)
G. Utilize music, white noise, or nature recordings to create a calming environment
H. Encourage diversionary activities (e.g., television, radio, reading, needlework)
I. Provide uninterrupted sleep and rest periods
VI. Prevent heat loss and hypothermia; maintain core body temperature at 35° to 38.3° C (95° to 101° F)
A. Initially wrap uninvolved areas with warm blankets to prevent systemic hypothermia
B. Avoid wet linens and dressings
C. Keep room between 85° to 90° F (29° to 32° C); prevent drafts
D. Use radiant heat lamps as necessary
E. Warm IV fluids as necessary
VII. Maintain renal function
A. Insert indwelling urinary catheter to monitor hourly urine assessment
B. Monitor urine output and color
C. Monitor urine for myoglobinuria, hemoglobinuria; if present, management may include the following:
 1. Fluids to maintain urine output greater than 1/ml/kg/hr
 2. Osmotic diuretics (e.g., mannitol) to "flush" the renal tubules; monitor closely for volume depletion if osmotic diuretics are used
 3. Sodium bicarbonate to alkalinize the urine
VIII. Replace electrolytes
A. Monitor potassium, calcium, magnesium, and phosphorus levels closely
B. Replace electrolytes as indicated; potassium replacement especially during diuresis (72 to 96 hours after burn)
IX. Maintain peripheral circulation
A. Keep burned extremities at or above heart level

B. Perform neurovascular assessment of burned limbs every hour
   1. Remember the 6 Ps of acute arterial occlusion: pain, pallor, pulselessness, paralysis, paresthesia, polar (cold)
   2. Check pulses with Doppler stethoscope if nonpalpable; pulses may be difficult to palpate due to severe edema; if present, they should be audible with a Doppler stethoscope
   3. Check capillary refill if there are no pulse points distal to burn; capillary refill is normally 2 to 3 seconds; report capillary refill greater than 4 seconds
C. Assist with escharotomy as necessary to relieve compression from swelling
   1. Indications of arterial and nerves compression include the following:
      a) Weak or absent peripheral pulses
      b) Progressive neurologic changes (e.g., paresthesia, paralysis)
      c) Cyanosis of distal unburned digits
   2. Incision is made along midlateral or midmedial line; if pulses do not return within 15 minutes, a second line is cut on the other side; fasciotomy, a deeper cut through the fascia, may be required if escharotomy does not restore peripheral perfusion

X. Prevent wound infection and promote wound healing
A. Administer adsorbed tetanus diphtheria (Td) toxoid 0.5 ml IM as prescribed if more than 5 years have elapsed since last tetanus booster to prevent *Clostridium tetani*; administer tetanus immune globulin 250 units IM if no prior immunization or last booster was more than 10 years ago
B. Prevent and monitor for wound infection and sepsis; sepsis and septic shock are the primary causes of death in burn injury
   1. Use sterile technique or aseptic technique as indicated; reverse isolation with a private room may be required, especially if open method of wound management being used
   2. Shave area around burn (do not shave eyebrows)
   3. Monitor closely for clinical indications of wound infection, including the following:
      a) Edema
      b) Erythema of unburned skin at wound edges
      c) Black or red hemorrhage areas in eschar
      d) Pus beneath eschar
      e) Unexpected rapid eschar separation
      f) Poor graft take
      g) Granulation tissue becomes pale and boggy
      h) Exudate that may be foul smelling
   4. Culture wound if appropriate
      a) Organism count more than 10^5/g of tissue indicates infection

b) Common causative organisms include *Pseudomonas aeruginosa*, *Klebsiella*, *Serratia*, *Escherichia coli*, *Enterobacter cloacae*
   5. Monitor closely for clinical indications of sepsis (e.g., fever, hyperglycemia, decreased urine output, altered LOC, increased CO/CI, decreased SVR, increased Svo_2)
   6. Administer antibiotics as prescribed for infection; prophylactic antibiotics are not indicated
C. Provide wound care
   1. Cleanse and irrigate wound
   2. Debride eschar and necrotic tissue
      a) Used to remove foreign material and cellular debris from the burn wound
         (1) Necrotic tissue acts as a physical barrier to epithelization and wound healing
         (2) Moist eschar is an excellent medium for bacteria
      b) Techniques
         (1) Autolytic: use of semipermeable transparent dressings (e.g., OpSite, Tegaderm); minor burns only
         (2) Mechanical
            (a) Cutting away loose tissue with forceps and scissors
            (b) Sponging wound surfaces during hydrotherapy
            (c) Wound irrigation
            (d) Wet-to-wet or wet-to-moist dressings
            (e) Wet-to-dry dressings: may cause damage to granulation tissue
         (3) Chemical: use of enzymatic ointments (e.g., Accuzyme, Collagenase, Elase)
         (4) Surgical: surgical excision of eschar and necrotic tissue to prepare the wound for grafting
            (a) Tangential excision: sequential shaving of the eschar until viable, bleeding tissue is reached
               (i) Only nonviable tissue is sacrificed, so better cosmetic result is achieved
               (ii) Blood loss can be high
            (b) Fascial excision: surgical removal of all eschar and tissue down to the level of the fascia
               (i) Used for very deep, extensive burns
               (ii) Less blood loss but fat and lymphatic tissues are sacrificed
               (iii) Cosmetic defect permanent and more pronounced than with tangential excision

c) Caution necessary in patients with thrombocytopenia and/or prolonged PT, aPTT

3. Provide hydrotherapy
   a) Used to prevent buildup of microorganisms on the wound surface and to loosen and remove dead tissue present on the wound
   b) Techniques of hydrotherapy
      (1) Immersing patient in Hubbard tank
          (a) May cause autocontamination from one burn area to another
          (b) May cause cross-contamination between patients; cleansing and monitoring of tank between patients is critical
      (2) Sitting or standing in a shower
      (3) Gently spraying burn areas while the patient is seated or lies on a stretcher

4. Utilize appropriate dressing techniques
   a) Open method: application of an antimicrobial cream to the burned areas and then leaving it exposed to air
      (1) Better detection of infection
      (2) Eliminates painful dressing changes
      (3) Less risk of diminishing circulation due to constrictiveness of dressings
   b) Semi-open method: application of an antimicrobial cream and a fine mesh gauze is then used to cover the burn area
   c) Closed method: application of an occlusive dressing to cover the burn
      (1) Less heat loss
      (2) Faster eschar separation
      (3) Barrier isolation is not required
      (4) Poor detection of infection
      (5) Risk of diminishing circulation due to constrictiveness of dressings
      (6) Dressings are changed two to three times daily, requiring significant nursing time
   d) If dressings are used, consider the following:
      (1) Burn wound surfaces must not be wrapped together
      (2) Bulky dressings decrease mobility, so keep dressings as light as appropriate
      (3) Wrap dressings from distal to proximal to decrease edema formation and promote venous return
      (4) Dependent areas are often Ace-wrapped to limit edema

5. Utilize topical antibiotics (Table 12-13) as prescribed

Table 12-13 Topical Antimicrobials Commonly Used for Burns

Agent	Application	Advantages	Disadvantages
Mafenide acetate (Sulfamylon)	Daily or twice daily	• Requires no dressing, thereby increasing mobility • Good penetration of eschar • Effective against most gram-positive and gram-negative organisms • Effective against anaerobes	• Causes burning for approximately 30 min • May cause metabolic acidosis • May cause allergic reaction
Silver nitrate (0.5% solution)	Change dressing 2-3 times/day; necessary to keep dressing soaked	• Low cost • Painless application • Effective against staphylococci, streptococci, and some strains of *Pseudomonas*	• Black staining • Poor penetration of eschar • Requires dressing, which decreases mobility • May cause hyponatremia, hypochloremia, hypokalemia • May cause methemoglobinemia
Silver sulfadiazine (Silvadene)	Daily or twice daily	• Painless application • Keeps eschar pliable • Requires no dressing, thereby increasing mobility • Nonstaining • Effective against most gram-positive and gram-negative organisms • Effective against fungi	• Intermediate penetration of eschar • May cause allergic reactions • May decrease granulocyte and lymphocyte formation
Clotrimazole cream (Lotrimin)	Twice daily with dressing changes	• Painless application • Effective against a broad spectrum of fungi	• Not effective against bacteria, so an antibacterial ointment must also be used • May cause skin irritation and blistering

D. Assist with sequential excision and grafting; often begins as early as 2 to 4 days after injury and continues at four- to five-day intervals
  1. Temporary wound coverings: temporary closure before autografting
    a) Biologic dressings: skin obtained from living or recently deceased animals or humans
      (1) Heterografts (xenografts): from other species
        (a) Bovine: cow
        (b) Porcine: pig
      (2) Homografts (allografts): from human cadavers
    b) Dermal replacements (e.g., Integra): synthetic dermal substitute that is covered with an ultrathin split-thickness autograft after the dermal component has become vascularized
    c) Biosynthetic dressings: combination of biologic and synthetic materials
      (1) Biobrane: nylon fabric that is partially embedded into a silicone film; may be used as covering for donor sites or autografts; requires a cover dressing until adherence of Biobrane to wound is achieved
      (2) Calcium alginate (e.g., Curasorb, Kalginate): naturally occurring polysaccharides found in seaweed; able to absorb many times its own weight in wound fluid while providing a moist environment for wound healing; requires a cover dressing
    d) Synthetic dressings
      (1) Thin-film dressings (e.g., OpSite, Tegaderm, Bioclusive); useful only for small, discrete partial-thickness wounds and donor sites
      (2) Composite dressings (e.g., LYOfoam, Curafoam): provide one layer to absorb and wick away exudate while another layer maintains a moist environment to facilitate healing; useful only for partial-thickness wounds
      (3) Hydrocolloid dressings (e.g., Derma-SORB, Wound Contact Layer): used for small, clean partial-thickness wounds or donor sites
      (4) Nonadherent fine-mesh gauze dressings (e.g., Scarlet Red ointment dressing, Xeroform, Aquaphor): used over donor site or autografts
  2. Autografts: permanent coverage of burn wounds
    a) Types
      (1) Full-thickness skin grafts: excision of entire thickness of the donor skin to the level of the subcutaneous tissue
        (a) Permits transfer of entire dermal layer with greater durability and less wound contracture than with split-thickness
        (b) Requires suture repair or split-thickness skin grafting to donor site
        (c) Useful only for repair of small burns
      (2) Split-thickness skin grafts: excision of a thin dermal layer of the donor skin; used as sheet grafts or meshed to provide expansion
        (a) Sheet grafts provide better functional and cosmetic result, but drainage beneath the graft may result in loss of graft; examine often for sub-graft hematoma or seroma formation
        (b) Mesh grafts cover a larger area but require a longer time for interstitial closure and have a greater propensity for scar formation
      (3) Cultured epithelial autograft (CEA): thin cultured skin that is attached to a fine-mesh gauze backing
        (a) Used when little unburned skin is available
        (b) Sample taken at time of admission; it takes 20 to 30 days for the culture to be ready for grafting
  3. Management and assessment of graft sites and donor site
    a) Immobilize the grafted area
      (1) Sheet and mesh grafts: 5 to 7 days
      (2) CEA: 2 weeks
    b) Elevate the grafted extremity to the level of, or slightly higher than, the heart to minimize edema
    c) Avoid pressure on or shearing of the graft area
    d) Monitor for bleeding, subgraft hematoma or seroma
    e) Monitor for clinical indications of infection (e.g., purulent drainage, poorly defined borders, foul odor)

XI. Maintain adequate nutrition
  A. Assess for clinical indications of paralytic ileus (e.g., absent bowel sounds, abdominal distention, abdominal tenderness); most patients with BSA of more than 20% have paralytic ileus initially
  B. Provide nutritional requirements: high-protein and high-calorie diet
    1. Protein recommendation is 1.5 to 2.0 g/kg/day
    2. Calorie recommendation is 25 kcal/kg/day plus 40 kcal/percentage of BSA
      a) Enough carbohydrates must be provided

so that the protein is used for anabolism and not for basal caloric requirements
   b) Calories required usually 3,500 to 7,000 kcal/day
3. Vitamin and mineral supplements are needed
   a) Vitamin B complex
   b) Vitamin C
   c) Zinc
   d) Fat-soluble vitamins: A, D, E, K
C. Utilize appropriate nutritional support methods
1. NPO initially with parenteral nutrition
2. Enteral feedings by small, frequent oral feedings with supplements or nasogastric, gastric, duodenal, or jejunal tube after paralytic ileus has resolved and GI tract is functional
   a) Early enteral feedings may decrease chance of sepsis; duodenal feedings may be initiated even when gastric suctioning is necessary
   b) TPN and Intralipid may be necessary even with enteral or oral feedings to meet caloric requirements
XII. Maintain GI integrity
A. Insert nasogastric tube and maintain nasogastric suction initially
B. Monitor for return of bowel sounds
C. Administer oral or nasogastric feedings when bowel sounds return; nasogastric suction and duodenal feeding may be utilized prior to return of bowel sounds
D. Monitor for and prevent stress ulcer
1. Utilize the enteral route for nutritional support; food in the stomach helps to reduce acidity
2. Administer antacids and/or histamine receptor antagonists (e.g., cimetidine [Tagamet]) as prescribed to maintain the gastric pH 3.5 or greater
3. Administer sucralfate (Carafate) as prescribed to adhere to any ulcer site
4. Check nasogastric aspirate and stools for blood
XIII. Maintain use of limbs
A. Provide range-of-motion (ROM) exercises at least every 4 hours
1. Often combined with hydrotherapy
2. Reinstitute ROM exercises on fifth postgraft day for newly grafted limbs
B. Apply splints as recommended by physical therapy to maintain functional position of limbs and to prevent contracture development
XIV. Assist in rehabilitation
A. Assist with effort to regain or compensate for functions lost as a result of the burn
B. Prepare patient for surgical procedures for scar contracture control and scar revision
C. Assist with body image adjustments
1. Assess the patient's perceptions and feelings

about the burn injury, changes in lifestyle, changes in relationships
2. Respect the patient's need to express anger; do not be judgmental or punitive
3. Provide information about cosmetic aids and use of concealment with clothing
4. Encourage attempts to enhance appearance (e.g., putting on lipstick)
D. Refer to local support groups for burned patients
XV. Monitor for complications
A. Cardiovascular
1. Hypovolemic shock
2. Heart failure
3. Acute arterial occlusion with resultant loss of limb
B. Pulmonary
1. Pneumonia
2. Atelectasis
3. Acute respiratory distress syndrome (ARDS)
4. Pulmonary embolism
5. Pulmonary fibrosis
C. Renal: acute renal failure
D. GI
1. Paralytic ileus
2. Curling's ulcer
3. Hepatic failure
4. Malnutrition
E. Hematologic/Immunologic
1. Wound infection
2. Sepsis and septic shock
3. Disseminated intravascular coagulation (DIC)
F. Musculoskeletal: contractures
G. Psychosocial
1. Drug dependency
2. Depression

Near-Drowning
Definitions
I. Drowning: suffocation from immersion in a liquid; death within 24 hours
II. Near-drowning: survival for more than 24 hours after asphyxia related to submersion
III. Secondary drowning: death that occurs after the initial injury and recovery
IV. Immersion syndrome: sudden death after submersion in extremely cold water; probably due to dysrhythmias
V. Hyperventilation submersion syndrome: death following hyperventilation and underwater swimming; the swimmer hyperventilates in an attempt to increase underwater time; this decreases $Paco_2$ but does not significantly increase Pao_2 or decrease oxygen requirements, so the patient may lose consciousness due to hypoxia and drowns before stimulated to breath again and to come up for air

Etiology: Immersion in a Liquid
I. Contributing factors
A. Overestimation of swimming capability

B. Alcohol or drug intoxication
C. Seizure
D. Spinal cord or head injury
E. Myocardial infarction
F. Dysrhythmia
G. Hypoglycemia
H. Air embolism (scuba diving)
I. Attempted suicide, homicide, or child abuse

Pathophysiology

I. Depends on the following:
   A. Temperature of water
      1. Water has a thermal conductive property that is 32 times that of air, so the body temperature rapidly changes toward the temperature of the water
      2. Cold water is water with a temperature of less than 20° C (68° F)
         a) Sometimes increases the period that a victim can remain submerged before rescue and recovery; survival rates are greater than for warm water because of the following:
            (1) Hypothermic mechanism: reduction of cerebral metabolic rate reduces cerebral oxygen requirements
            (2) Diving reflex: decreases the heart rate and shunts blood to the brain and heart; probably less of a factor in adults but is a significant reflex in children
         b) Adverse effects
            (1) May cause fatal dysrhythmias
            (2) May increase blood viscosity and slow circulation of blood through the coronary and cerebral arteries
            (3) Perpetuates hypoxia by shifting the oxyhemoglobin dissociation curve to the left, which increases the affinity between hemoglobin and oxygen and decreases oxygen unloading at the tissue level
            (4) May cause hyperventilation, hypocapnia, disorientation, and possible loss of consciousness leading to drowning
   B. Quantity of water
      1. Dry: accounts for 10% to 20% of near-drowning events
         a) Aspiration does not occur, but the patient becomes hypoxic from laryngospasm or breath holding
         b) Laryngospasm causes hypercapnia and respiratory acidosis and hypoxemia, hypoxia, and metabolic acidosis with eventual cerebral anoxia
      2. Wet: accounts for 80% to 90% of near-drowning events
         a) Aspiration of water or gastric contents into lungs occurs
         b) Aspiration of at least 22 ml/kg of fluid is required to cause significant changes in electrolytes, and aspiration of at least 11 ml/kg is required to cause changes in blood volume; only approximately 15% of drowning victims ever aspirate that much fluid
         c) Aspiration of acidic gastric contents may cause pneumonitis and acute respiratory distress syndrome; aspiration of solid gastric contents may cause airway obstruction or contribute to intrapulmonary shunt
   C. Type of water: fresh or salt water; presence of contaminants
      1. Because so few patients aspirate enough fluid into their lungs to cause fluid and electrolyte problems, the difference between salt and fresh water is more theoretic than clinically pertinent, but for those patients who do aspirate significant amounts of fluid into their lungs, the following physiologic changes occur:
         a) Salt water (hypertonic)
            (1) Fluid is drawn from the vascular space and interstitium into the alveoli
            (2) This leads to hemoconcentration and pulmonary edema
            (3) This causes intrapulmonary shunt and hypoxemia
            (4) Hypernatremia, hyperchloremia, and hypermagnesemia occur
         b) Fresh water (hypotonic)
            (1) Hemodilution, hypervolemia, and acute hemolysis along with damage to the type II pneumocytes occurs
            (2) This leads to a decrease in surfactant and resultant alveolar collapse and atelectasis
            (3) This results in intrapulmonary shunt and hypoxemia
            (4) Seizures may occur due to dilutional hyponatremia
      2. Particulate matter: sand, algae, weeds, mud, chloride, or bacteria
         a) Lung infection and even pulmonary fibrosis may occur
         b) Salt water is considered twice as lethal as fresh water per unit volume because of the degree of impurity
   D. Length of time submersed: the longest recorded survival time (approximately 40 minutes) was in cold fresh water; this is twice as long as the longest recorded survival rate for cold sea water and four times as long as the longest recorded survival rate for warm fresh water
II. Pulmonary consequences
   A. Aspiration causes laryngospasm, which causes asphyxia and loss of consciousness
   B. Glottic relaxation usually follows, which leads to additional aspiration of water into the lungs
   C. Aspirated fluid causes an inflammatory reaction in the alveolar-capillary membrane
   D. Pulmonary edema occurs as interstitial fluid moves into the alveolus

E. This fluid shift dilutes and inactivates the surfactant and causes atelectasis

F. Hypoxemic vasoconstriction occurs and pulmonary hypertension occurs

G. Ventilation/perfusion mismatch, intrapulmonary shunt, increased pathologic dead space, and decreased pulmonary compliance occur

H. Atelectasis, pneumonitis, and eventually ARDS occur

III. Cardiovascular consequences: hypothermia, hypoxemia, and acidosis may cause fatal dysrhythmias

IV. Neurologic consequences

A. Hypoxemia, hypercapnia, and decreased cerebral perfusion pressure cause cerebral hypoxia and intracranial hypertension

B. Permanent brain injury occurs as the period of cerebral hypoxia and anoxia continues

C. Fresh water drowning may cause hyponatremia and seizures

V. Renal consequences: hypoxia, hypoperfusion, myoglobinuria, hemoglobinuria may lead to acute tubular necrosis and intrarenal renal failure

A. Myoglobinuria may occur secondary to muscle trauma or seizures

B. Hemoglobinuria may occur secondary to hemolysis as occurs after the aspiration of significant amounts of fresh water

Clinical Presentation

I. Subjective

A. History of submersion

B. History of contributing event (e.g., alcohol or drug intoxication, MI, SCI)

C. Dyspnea

D. Substernal burning and/or pleuritic chest pain

II. Objective

A. Dysrhythmias or cardiopulmonary arrest

B. Hypotension

C. Tachypnea

D. Use of accessory muscles

E. Cough: may have pink, frothy sputum

F. Cyanosis

G. Chest dullness to percussion

H. Breath sound changes: crackles, rhonchi, wheezes

I. Abdominal distention may be present due to swallowing large volumes of water

J. Change in level of consciousness with signs of cerebral anoxia may be evident

K. Paralysis may be evident if a spinal cord injury has been sustained

L. Hyporeflexia or seizures may occur related to hyponatremia in fresh water near-drowning

M. Oliguria, proteinuria, and elevated BUN may be seen if acute tubular necrosis develops

N. Brownish (tea-colored) urine may be seen if myoglobinuria is present; reddish (port wine-colored) urine may be seen if hemoglobinuria is present

O. Temperature may be increased or decreased

1. May be hypothermic related to exposure in cold water

2. May have fever related to pulmonary infection

P. Signs of trauma may be evident

III. Diagnostic

A. Serum

1. Hematocrit: may be increased in salt water drowning and decreased in fresh water drowning

2. Hemoglobin: may be decreased along with later potassium and bilirubin increase if significant hemolysis occurs (must have aspiration of at least 11 ml/kg of fresh water)

3. Electrolytes

a) Sodium, chloride, potassium, and magnesium may be decreased in fresh water near-drowning and increased in salt water near-drowning

b) Potassium may be increased if any of the following occurs:

(1) Fresh water near-drowning with significant hemolysis

(2) Hypothermia

(3) Renal failure

4. White blood cells (WBC)

a) May be increased due to pulmonary infection

b) May be decreased in hypothermia due to cells being sequestered in the liver and spleen

5. Coagulation studies (e.g., PT, aPTT, platelet count, fibrin split products)

a) May be abnormal due to DIC

b) PT, aPTT may be prolonged and platelets may be decreased in hypothermia due to cells being sequestered in the liver and spleen

6. Arterial blood gases

a) Respiratory acidosis progressing to metabolic acidosis

b) Hypoxemia

7. Drug and alcohol levels may be indicated

B. Urine

1. May show hemoglobinuria

2. May show myoglobinuria

C. ECG: may show dysrhythmias

1. Bradycardia to asystole

2. Ventricular fibrillation

D. Chest X-ray

1. May show diffuse indistinct, nodular infiltrates

2. May show atelectasis, pneumonia, pulmonary edema, and/or acute respiratory distress syndrome (ARDS)

E. Spine X-rays: may be indicated to rule out spinal fracture

F. EEG: may indicate seizure activity

G. CT of head: may indicate head injury

Nursing Diagnoses

I. Ineffective Airway Clearance related to aspiration of water, gastric content, and/or particulate matter, accumulated secretions, artificial airway

II. Impaired Gas Exchange related to atelectasis, pneumonia, pulmonary edema and/or ARDS

III. Hypothermia related to submersion in cold water

IV. Decreased Cardiac Output related to dysrhythmias, hypoxia, hypotension, excessive PEEP, hypovolemia

V. Altered Cerebral Tissue Perfusion related to hypoxia, cerebral hypoperfusion, intracranial hypertension

VI. Risk for Injury related to seizures, intubation, invasive procedures, hemorrhage, electrolyte imbalance

VII. Risk for Fluid Volume Excess or Fluid Volume Deficit related to fluid shifts

VIII. Risk for Infection related to aspiration of contaminants in water

IX. Ineffective Individual and Family Coping related to sudden critical illness

Collaborative Management

I. Maintain airway, oxygenation, and ventilation

A. Provide basic and advanced life support at the scene and in the emergency department

1. Precautions should be taken to immobilize the cervical spine if cervical trauma is possible

2. If the patient is hypothermic and in ventricular fibrillation, consider the following:

a) Limit defibrillation to one series of three (200, 300, 360 joules)

b) If unsuccessful, continue CPR but do not defibrillate again until core body temperature is at least 30° C (86° F)

c) Do not use catecholamines (e.g., epinephrine) until the patient's temperature is at least 30° C (86° F); they are not generally effective in patients with severe hypothermia

B. Administer oxygen to all near-drowning patients to maintain SpO_2 more than 95%

1. Initially use 100% oxygen; decrease oxygen levels if possible

2. CPAP may be delivered by mask prior to the need for intubation if the patient is hypoxemic even on 100% oxygen but able to maintain normal $PaCO_2$ levels; do not administer CPAP by mask in an obtunded or unconscious patient due to risk of vomiting and aspiration

C. Assist with intubation and initiation of mechanical ventilation as necessary; PEEP is used to increase driving pressure of oxygen and to maintain acceptable PaO_2 with the lowest FIO_2, to decrease atelectasis and shunt, and to increase intraalveolar pressure to decrease movement in fluid into the alveolus

D. Administer bronchodilators as prescribed for bronchospasm: beta$_2$ stimulants and/or xanthines

E. Assist with bronchoscopy; may be performed for removal of aspirated foreign solid material

F. Administer blood as prescribed to improve tissue oxygen delivery if significant hemolysis

has occurred due to aspiration of large volumes of fresh water

II. Monitor fluid, electrolyte, and renal status

A. Perform hemodynamic monitoring to evaluate and monitor fluid status; fluid prescription will be determined by the patient's serum sodium and osmolality (e.g., NS if isotonic, ½NS if hypertonic)

B. Monitor serum electrolyte values closely

C. Monitor urine output, BUN, and creatinine closely

D. Administer fluids, diuretics (e.g., mannitol), and sodium bicarbonate as prescribed for myoglobinuria, hemoglobinuria

III. Monitor for and treat clinical indications of intracranial hypertension

A. Administer glucose, thiamine, and naloxone (Narcan) as prescribed in unconscious patients in case hypoglycemia or narcotics are the cause of the unconsciousness

B. Monitor ICP and calculate CPP as indicated

C. Maintain SpO_2 more than or equal to 95%

D. Treat hyperglycemia with sliding-scale insulin: keep serum glucose less than 250 mg/dl

E. Elevate head of bed at 30 degrees

F. Utilize osmotic diuretics, barbiturate-induced coma, induced hypothermia as prescribed for intracranial hypertension

IV. Prevent infection

A. Monitor for persistent fever, leukocytosis, purulent sputum, positive blood cultures, or changing infiltrates on chest X-ray

B. Administer antibiotics as indicated and prescribed; prophylactic antibiotics are not indicated

C. Assist with bronchoscopy as necessary

V. Restore normal body temperature

A. Monitor core body temperature via pulmonary artery thermister or rectal probe

B. Monitor closely for dysrhythmias

C. Utilize central warming techniques (e.g., intravenous fluids warmed to 37° C (98.6° F), humidified oxygen warmed to 40° C (104° F), gastric lavage, peritoneal lavage, and/or enemas warmed to 37° C (98.6° F) initially

D. Utilize surface warming techniques (e.g., warm blankets, radiant heat lamps) after core body temperature is at least 32° C (90° F)

E. Monitor for afterdrop (hypotension due to rewarming causing peripheral vasodilation and the shifting of acidotic blood back into the central circulation)

F. Monitor skin perfusion

G. Continue cardiopulmonary resuscitation efforts if required until after body temperature is normal

VI. Monitor gastrointestinal and nutritional status

A. Insert nasogastric tube to decompress the stomach and to prevent vomiting and aspiration

B. Provide nutritional support as soon as possible

VII. Monitor for complications

A. Postimmersion syndrome: respiratory distress,

hypoxemia, pulmonary edema, fever, leukocytosis
B. ARDS
C. Dysrhythmias
D. Cerebral edema with or without residual neurologic deficits
E. Renal failure
F. DIC
G. Infection, sepsis

Drug Intoxication and Poisoning

Definition: Drug ingestion in amounts greater than recommended or the ingestion or absorption of a substance toxic to the human body

Etiology

I. Accidental or intentional overdosage of prescribed medication
   A. Intentional overdosage often involves more than one agent; often includes alcohol and/or illegal drugs
   B. Intentional overdosage may be a suicide attempt or an attention-seeking behavior
   C. Accidental overdosage is most often due to knowledge deficit regarding drug dosing or confusion
II. Accidental overdosage of illegal drugs
   A. Overdosage often caused by changes in drug purity
   B. Patient may be mentally ill and have tendency to be violent
III. Ingestion/absorption of poison or toxin

Pathophysiology: Dependent on the following:

I. Drug ingested
II. Amount of drug(s) or toxin ingested or absorbed
III. Time from ingestion to treatment
IV. Preexisting condition of patient

Clinical Presentation (Table 12-14)

I. Subjective: for drug-specific, see Table 12-14
   A. History of drug ingestion or exposure to toxin
      1. Patient may minimize or exaggerate the amount of the drug
      2. Identify the drug or toxin, the route, amount (number of pills, dose), and length of time elapsed since drug or toxin was taken
   B. May have history of depression or psychologic crisis
   C. May have history of previous toxic ingestion
   D. May have history of chemical dependency
   E. May have history of complicated drug regimen with or without confusion
   F. Note any history of renal or hepatic disease
II. Objective: for drug-specific signs, see Table 12-14
III. Diagnostic
   A. Serum
      1. Toxicology screen
      2. Alcohol level

B. Urine: toxicology screen
C. ECG: dysrhythmias often seen, depending on the drug or toxin
D. CT scan: may be done to rule out pathology
E. Lumbar puncture: may be done to rule out pathology

Nursing Diagnoses

I. Ineffective Airway Clearance related to drug effects on respiratory center, artificial airway
II. Ineffective Breathing Patterns related to drug effects on respiratory center
III. Decreased Cardiac Output related to dysrhythmias, diuresis, vasodilation, negative inotropic effects
IV. Altered Cerebral Tissue Perfusion related to hypoxia, cerebral hypoperfusion, intracranial hypertension
V. Risk for Injury related to seizures, intubation, aspiration, invasive procedures, hemorrhage
VI. Ineffective Individual and Family Coping related to sudden critical illness

Collaborative Management

I. Maintain airway, oxygenation, and ventilation
   A. Administer dextrose and thiamine and naloxone (Narcan) (sometimes referred to as a *coma cocktail*) as prescribed for loss of consciousness with no known cause
      1. Administer 50 to 100 ml of 50% dextrose; thiamine 50 to 100 mg IV or IM is also given to prevent Wernicke's encephalopathy, especially if a history of alcoholism or chronic drug abuse is present
      2. Administer naloxone (Narcan) 2 mg IV, IM, or transtracheally
   B. Maintain head-tilt, chin-lift position to maintain open airway; use jaw-thrust technique if cervical spine injury may exist
   C. Use an oropharyngeal or nasopharyngeal airway to keep the tongue away from the hypopharynx; oropharyngeal airways should not be used in conscious patients due to their propensity to cause vomiting by stimulating the gag reflex
   D. Assist with endotracheal intubation if gag and cough reflexes are depressed or if gastric lavage is to be initiated in lethargic patient
   E. Monitor breath sounds and chest X-ray for aspiration, pulmonary edema
   F. Administer oxygen therapy; adjust flow rate or oxygen concentration to keep SpO_2 approximately 95% unless contraindicated; in patients with chronic hypercapnia, adjust flow rate or oxygen concentration to keep SpO_2 approximately 90%
   G. Assist with initiation of mechanical ventilation for acute respiratory failure and respiratory acidosis
II. Maintain cardiovascular function
   A. Monitor ECG rhythm for conduction changes

Table 12-14 Drugs and Toxins

Drug or Toxin	Clinical Presentation of Intoxication	Specific Collaborative Management

Acetaminophen	**Mild/early stage**
	• May be asymptomatic
	• Anorexia, nausea, vomiting
	• Diaphoresis
	• Hypotension
	• Pallor
	12 hr to 4 days later
	• Signs of hepatotoxicity may occur: liver enzymes, bilirubin, PT increased; right upper quadrant pain
	• Gradual return to normal may occur
	Late: indications of hepatic failure
	• Anorexia, nausea, vomiting
	• Jaundice
	• Hepatosplenomegaly
	• Clinical indications of hepatic encephalopathy: confusion to coma
	• Bleeding
	• Hypoglycemia
	• Acute renal failure may develop
	• Dysrhythmias and shock may occur
		• Gastric lavage only if within 2 hr of ingestion
		• Activated charcoal if patient arrives within 4-6 hr after ingestion (although activated charcoal does adsorb N-acetylcysteine and reduces its peak serum levels, the loading dose of N-acetylcysteine does not need to be increased)
		• N-acetylcysteine (Mucomyst) 140 mg/kg initially, then 70 mg/kg every 4 hr × 17 doses to total of 1330 mg/kg
		  • If given PO, dilute in juice or carbonated beverage; if given via nasogastric or duodenal tube, dilute with water
		  • May cause anorexia, nausea, vomiting; repeat dose if vomiting occurs within 1 hr
		• Vitamin K may be prescribed, especially if hepatic failure occurs
		• Dextrose (e.g., $D_{50}W$) may be needed
		• Antidysrhythmics may be needed

Amphetamines	• Tachycardia
	• Hypertension
	• Tachypnea
	• Dysrhythmias
	• Hyperthermia, diaphoresis
	• Dilated but reactive pupils
	• Dry mouth
	• Urinary retention
	• Headache
	• Paranoid-type psychotic behavior
	• Hallucinations
	• Hyperactivity, anxiety
	• Hyperactive deep tendon reflexes, tremor, seizures
	• Confusion, stupor, coma
		• Calm, quiet environment
		  • Avoid overstimulation of patient
		  • Do not speak loudly or move quickly
		  • Do not approach from behind
		  • Avoid touching the patient unless you speak to the patient first or are sure it is safe
		• Gastric lavage, activated charcoal
		• Diazepam (Valium) for agitation
		• Phentolamine (Regitine) for hypertension
		• Anticonvulsants (e.g., diazepam, phenytoin, phenobarbital) for seizures
		• Antidysrhythmics (e.g., lidocaine) for ventricular dysrhythmias
		• Haloperidol (Haldol) for acute psychotic reactions
		• Hypothermia blanket, ice packs, ice-water sponge baths for hyperthermia
		  • Dantrolene (Dantrium) may be prescribed for malignant hyperthermia

Barbiturates, sedatives, hypnotics, tranquilizers	• Bradycardia, cardiac dysrhythmias • Hypotension • Hypothermia • Respiratory depression to respiratory arrest • Headache • Nystagmus, dysconjugate eye movements • Dysarthria • Ataxia • Depressed deep tendon reflexes • Confusion, stupor, coma • Hemorrhagic blisters • Gastric irritation (chloral hydrate) • Pulmonary edema (meprobamate) • Hypertonicity, hyperreflexia, myoclonus, seizures (methaqualone)	• Gastric lavage, multiple-dose activated charcoal, cathartics • Phenobarbital: sodium bicarbonate to alkalinize the urine and increase rate of barbiturate excretion; maintain urine pH >7.50 • Monitor potassium, calcium, and magnesium levels • Anticonvulsants (e.g., diazepam, phenytoin, phenobarbital) for seizures • Hemodialysis or hemoperfusion may be required

Continued

Table 12-14 Drugs and Toxins—cont'd

Drug or Toxin	Clinical Presentation of Intoxication	Specific Collaborative Management

Benzodiazepines	• Hypotension
	• Respiratory depression
	• Diminished or absent bowel sounds
	• Decreased deep tendon reflexes (DTR)
	• Confusion, drowsiness, stupor, coma
		• Gastric lavage, multiple-dose activated charcoal, cathartics
		• Flumazenil (Romazicon), a benzodiazepine receptor antagonist may be prescribed
		  • Contraindicated if patient has coingested tricyclic antidepressants; use cautiously if patient has history of long-term use of benzodiazepines
		  • Monitor for seizures, agitation, flushing, nausea and vomiting as side effects of flumazenil
		• Intubation and mechanical ventilation may be necessary

Beta-blockers	• Sinus bradycardia, arrest, block • Junctional escape rhythm • AV nodal block • Bundle branch block (usually right) • Hypotension • Heart failure • Cardiogenic shock • Cardiac arrest • Decreased LOC • Seizures • Respiratory depression, apnea • Bronchospasm • Hyperglycemia or hypoglycemia	• Gastric lavage, activated charcoal, cathartic • Bowel irrigation if sustained-release preparations ingested • Glucagon 3-5 mg IV, IM, or SC, followed by infusion of 1-5 mg/hr • Epinephrine, dopamine, isoproterenol, or atropine for bradycardia and hypotension; temporary pacing may be required • $D_{50}W$ for hypoglycemia • Anticonvulsants (e.g., diazepam, phenobarbital) for seizures; phenytoin is contraindicated
Calcium channel blockers	• Sinus bradycardia, arrest, block • SA blocks (diltiazem) • AV blocks (verapamil) • Hypotension • Heart failure • Confusion, agitation, dizziness, lethargy, slurred speech • Seizures • Nausea, vomiting • Paralytic ileus • Hyperglycemia	• Gastric lavage, activated charcoal, cathartic • Bowel irrigation if sustained-release preparations ingested • Calcium chloride 5 (500 mg)-10 (1 g) ml of 10% solution • Glucagon 3-5 mg IV, IM, or SC, followed by infusion of 1-5 mg/hr • Anticonvulsants (e.g., diazepam, phenytoin, phenobarbital) for seizures • Atropine, isoproterenol, temporary pacing for bradycardia

Carbon monoxide
Note: the affinity between carbon monoxide and hemoglobin is approximately 200 times the affinity between oxygen and hemoglobin
	• Dysrhythmias
	• Impaired hearing or vision
	• Pallor; cherry-red skin coloring may be seen
	• 10%-20%: mild headache, flushing, dyspnea or angina on vigorous exertion, nausea, dizziness
	• 20%-30%: throbbing headache, nausea, vomiting, weakness, dyspnea on moderate exertion, ST segment depression
	• 30%-40%: severe headache, visual disturbances, syncope, vomiting
	• 40%-50%: tachypnea, tachycardia, chest pain, worsening syncope
	• 50%-60%: chest pain, respiratory failure, shock, seizures, coma
	• 60%-70%: respiratory failure, shock, coma, death
		• Removal from contaminated area
		• Oxygenation
		  • 100% oxygen via mask initially; CPAP by mask may be utilized
		  • Intubation and mechanical ventilation until COHb level <5%; PEEP may be utilized
		  • Hyperbaric oxygen (at 2-3 atmospheres) as soon as available if:
		    • COHb >25%
		    • COHb >15% if history of cardiovascular disease, acute ECG changes, or CNS symptoms
		• Fluids, diuretics, urine alkalinization to treat myoglobinuria if present
		• Anticonvulsants (e.g., diazepam, phenytoin, phenobarbital) for seizures

Table 12-14 Drugs and Toxins—cont'd

Drug or Toxin	Clinical Presentation of Intoxication	Specific Collaborative Management
Caustic poisoning Acids (e.g., battery acid, drain cleaners, hydrochloric acid) Alkalis (e.g., drain cleaners, refrigerants, fertilizers, photographic developers)	• Burning sensation in the oral cavity, pharynx, esophageal area • Dysphagia • Respiratory distress: dyspnea, stridor, tachypnea, hoarseness • Soapy-white mucous membrane **Acid** • Oral ulcerations and/or blisters • May have signs of gastric perforation (e.g., abdominal pain, distention, absent bowel sounds, rebound tenderness) • May have signs of shock **Alkali** • May have signs of esophageal perforation (e.g., chest pain, subcutaneous emphysema)	• Diluent: flush mouth with copious volumes of water; drink water or milk (approximately 250 ml) • Do not induce vomiting or perform gastric lavage • Activated charcoal • Esophagogastroscopy to assess damage • Corticosteroids may be prescribed for alkali poisoning
Cocaine, including "crack" cocaine	• Tachycardia, dysrhythmias • Hypertension or hypotension • Tachypnea or hyperpnea • Cocaine-induced MI • Pallor or cyanosis • Hyperexcitability, anxiety • Headache • Hyperthermia, diaphoresis • Nausea, vomiting, abdominal pain • Dilated but reactive pupils • Confusion, delirium, hallucinations • Seizures • Coma • Respiratory arrest	• Swabbing of inside of nose to remove any residual drug if cocaine was snorted • Gastric lavage, multiple-dose activated charcoal if ingested • Bowel irrigation for "body packers" • Anticonvulsants (e.g., diazepam, phenytoin, phenobarbital) for seizures • Antidysrhythmics, usually lidocaine; calcium channel blockers may also be used (they may also help with coronary artery spasm) • Antihypertensives: alpha-blockers (e.g., phentolamine), alpha and beta-blockers (e.g., labetalol [Normodyne]), or vasodilators (e.g., nitroprusside [Nipride]) • Hypothermia blanket, ice packs, ice-water sponge baths for hyperthermia • Dantrolene (Dantrium) may be prescribed for malignant hyperthermia • Fluids, diuretics, urine alkalinization to treat myoglobinuria if present

Cyanide	• Anxiety, restlessness, hyperventilation initially
	• Bradycardia followed by tachycardia
	• Hypertension followed by hypotension
	• Dysrhythmias
	• Bitter almond odor to breath
	• Cherry red mucous membranes
	• Nausea
	• Dyspnea
	• Headache
	• Dizziness
	• Pupil dilation
	• Confusion
	• Stupor, seizures, coma, death
		• 100% oxygen initially by mask
		  • Hyperbaric oxygen may be needed
		  • Intubation and mechanical ventilation is frequently necessary
		• Supportive care if only anxiety, restlessness, hyperventilation
		• Discontinuance of causative agent (e.g., nitroprusside)
		• Antidotes for more serious symptoms
		  • Amyl nitrite by inhalation
		  • Sodium nitrite IV
		  • Sodium thiosulfate IV
		• Gastric lavage, activated charcoal if cyanide was ingested
		• Flushing of eyes and/or skin with water if dermal contamination; removal and isolation of clothing
		• Fluids, vasopressors for BP support
		• Anticonvulsants (e.g., diazepam, phenytoin, phenobarbital) for seizures
		• Antidysrhythmics (e.g., lidocaine) for ventricular dysrhythmia, atropine for bradydysrhythmias
		• Vitamin B_{12} may be prescribed

Continued

Table 12-14 **Drugs and Toxins—cont'd**

Drug or Toxin	Clinical Presentation of Intoxication	Specific Collaborative Management

Digitalis preparations	• Anorexia
	• Nausea
	• Vomiting
	• Headache
	• Restlessness
	• Visual changes
	• Sinus bradycardia, block, or arrest
	• PAT with AV block
	• Junctional tachycardia
	• AV blocks: 1st, 2nd Type I, 3rd
	• PVCs: bigeminy, trigeminy, quadrigeminy
	• Ventricular tachycardia: especially bidirectional
	• Ventricular fibrillation
		• Activated charcoal, cholestyramine
		• Correction of hypoxia, electrolyte imbalance (especially potassium)
		• Treatment of dysrhythmias
		  • For symptomatic bradydysrhythmias and blocks
		    • Atropine
		    • External pacemaker
		  • For symptomatic tachydysrhythmias
		    • Lidocaine
		    • Phenytoin
		    • Magnesium if hypomagnesemia or hyperkalemia present
		    • Cardioversion at lowest effective voltage and only if life-threatening dysrhythmias exist
		    • Defibrillation for ventricular fibrillation
		    • Verapamil if SVT
		• Digoxin immune FAB (Digibind) if >10 mg ingested (adult), serum digoxin >10 ng/ml, or serum potassium >5.0 mEq/L
		  • Monitor closely for exacerbation of condition digitalis was being used for (i.e., increase in heart rate, heart failure)

Ethanol	Ethanol concentration (mg/dl) • <25: sense of warmth and well-being, talkativeness, self-confidence, mild incoordination • 25-50: euphoria, decreased judgment and control • 50-100: decreased sensorium, worsened coordination, ataxia, decreased reflexes and reaction time • 100-250: nausea, vomiting, ataxia, diplopia, slurred speech, visual impairment, nystagmus, emotional lability, confusion, stupor • 250-400: stupor or coma, incontinence, respiratory depression • >400: respiratory paralysis, loss of protective reflexes, hypothermia, death **Note:** These signs/symptoms and blood ethanol levels vary widely; these signs/symptoms are for a non-alcohol-dependent person Also: • Alcohol odor to breath • Hypoglycemia • Seizures • Metabolic acidosis	• Gastric lavage if within 1 hour of ingestion • Fluid and electrolyte replacement (potassium, magnesium, calcium may be needed) • Anticonvulsants (e.g., diazepam, phenytoin, phenobarbital) for seizures • Glucose for hypoglycemia along with multivitamins including thiamine and folic acid • **Note:** Thiamine is necessary for the brain to utilize glucose; thiamine deficiency in alcoholic patients may cause Wernicke's encephalopathy • Hemodialysis may be necessary
Ethylene glycol	First 12 hours after ingestion • Appears "drunk" without the odor of ethanol on breath • Nausea, vomiting, hematemesis • Focal seizures, coma • Nystagmus, depressed reflexes, tetany • Metabolic acidosis with increased anion gap 12-24 hours after ingestion • Tachycardia • Mild hypertension • Pulmonary edema • Heart failure 24-72 hours after ingestion • Flank pain, costovertebral tenderness • Acute renal failure	• Gastric lavage (especially helpful if within 2 hours of ingestion) • 10% ethanol in D$_5$W IV to maintain serum ethanol level at 100-200 mg/dl • Fomepizole (Antizol) may be used instead of ethanol • Fluid and electrolyte replacement (particularly calcium but potassium and magnesium may also be needed) • Sodium bicarbonate for severe metabolic acidosis • Glucose for hypoglycemia and multivitamins, including thiamine, folic acid, and pyridoxine • **Note:** Thiamine is necessary for the brain to utilize glucose; thiamine deficiency in alcoholic patients may cause Wernicke's encephalopathy • Anticonvulsants (e.g., diazepam, phenytoin, phenobarbital) for seizures • Hemodialysis may be needed

Table 12-14   Drugs and Toxins—cont'd

Drug or Toxin	Clinical Presentation of Intoxication	Specific Collaborative Management
Hallucinogens (e.g., D-lysergic acid diethylamide [LSD])	• Tachycardia, hypertension • Hyperthermia • Anorexia, nausea • Headaches • Dizziness • Agitation, anxiety • Impaired judgment • Distortion and intensification of sensory perception • Toxic psychosis • Dilated pupils • Rambling speech • Polyuria	• Reassurance • Quiet environment with soft lighting • If ingested orally: activated charcoal may be used • Benzodiazepines (e.g., diazepam) for anxiety and agitation • Anticonvulsants (e.g., diazepam, phenytoin, phenobarbital) for seizures • Restraints only if necessary to protect patient
Isopropyl alcohol	• Gastrointestinal distress (e.g., nausea, vomiting, abdominal pain) • Headache • CNS depression, areflexia, ataxia • Respiratory depression • Hypothermia, hypotension	• Gastric lavage (especially helpful if within 2 hours of ingestion), activated charcoal • Fluids and vasopressors for hypoperfusion • Hemodialysis may be needed
Lithium	Mild • Vomiting, diarrhea • Lethargy, weakness • Polyuria, polydipsia • Nystagmus • Fine tremors Severe • Hypotension • Severe thirst • Tinnitus • Hyperreflexia • Coarse tremors • Ataxia • Seizures • Confusion • Coma • Dilute urine, renal failure • Heart failure	• Gastric lavage • Hydration • Anticonvulsants (e.g., diazepam, phenytoin, phenobarbital) for seizures • Hemodialysis may be necessary
Methanol	• Nausea and vomiting • Hyperpnea, dyspnea • Visual disturbances ranging from blurring to blindness • Speech difficulty • Headache • CNS depression • Motor dysfunction with rigidity, spasticity, and hypokinesis • Metabolic acidosis with anion gap	• Gastric lavage (especially helpful if within 2 hours of ingestion) • 10% ethanol in D_5W IV to maintain serum ethanol level at 100-200 mg/dl • Sodium bicarbonate for severe metabolic acidosis • Hemodialysis if visual impairment, base deficit >15, renal insufficiency, or blood methanol concentration >30 mmol/L

Methemoglobinemia caused by nitrites, nitrate, sulfa drugs, and others	• Tachycardia
	• Fatigue
	• Nausea
	• Dizziness
	• Cyanosis in the presence of a normal PaO_2; failure of cyanosis to resolve with oxygen therapy
	• Dark red or brown blood
	• Elevated methemoglobin levels
	• Headache, weakness, dyspnea (30%-40%)
	• Stupor, respiratory depression (60%)
		• Oxygen
		• Removal of cause
		  • Stop nitroglycerin, nitroprusside, sulfa drugs, anesthetic agents, or other causative agent
		  • Gastric lavage, activated charcoal, cathartic if agent ingested
		• Methylene blue
		  • If stupor, coma, angina, or respiratory depression or if level 30%-40% or more
		  • Administered at 2 mg/kg over 5 min; repeated at 1 mg/kg if patient still symptomatic after 30-60 min
		• Ascorbic acid may be administered in large doses

Continued

Table 12-14

Drugs and Toxins—cont'd

Drug or Toxin	Clinical Presentation of Intoxication	Specific Collaborative Management
Opioids and opiates	• Bradycardia • Hypotension • Decreased level of consciousness • Respiratory depression to respiratory arrest • Hypothermia • Miosis • Diminished bowel sounds • Needle tracks, abscesses • Seizures • Pulmonary edema (especially with heroin)	• Gastric lavage, activated charcoal, cathartics if ingested • Bowel irrigation for "body packers" • Naloxone (Narcan) 0.4-2 mg IV, IM, or transtracheally or nalmefene (Revex) 0.5 mg IV • Duration of action of naloxone is 1-2 hours, whereas nalmefene has a duration of action of 4-8 hours (heroin and morphine 4-6 hours, meperidine 2-4 hours) • Anticonvulsants (e.g., diazepam, phenytoin, phenobarbital) for seizures • Intubation and mechanical ventilation may be required; PEEP may be needed for pulmonary edema
Organophosphate and carbamate (cholinesterase inhibitors)	• Bradycardia • Nausea, vomiting, diarrhea • Abdominal pain and cramping • Increased oral secretions • Dyspnea • Slurred speech • Constricted pupils • Visual changes • Unsteady gait • Urinary incontinence • Poor motor control • Twitching • Change in level of consciousness • Seizures	• Gastric lavage, activated charcoal, cathartic if ingested • Removal and isolation of clothing • Washing of skin with ethyl alcohol and then soap and water if dermal contamination • Atropine 1-2 mg IV or IM; repeated as required • Pralidoxime chloride (Protopam) 1-2 grams IV over 15-30 min followed by infusion of 10-20 mg/kg may be used for organophosphates • Anticonvulsants (e.g., diazepam, phenytoin, phenobarbital) for seizures
Petroleum distillates	• Flushed skin • Hyperthermia • Vomiting • Diarrhea • Abdominal pain • Tachypnea • Dyspnea • Cyanosis • Coughing • Breath sound changes: crackles, rhonchi, diminished breath sounds • Staggering gait • Confusion • CNS depression or excitation	• Gastric lavage, activated charcoal, cathartic may be indicated; endotracheal tube should be inserted prior to gastric lavage if patient's LOC diminished • Washing of skin with soap and water if dermal contamination; removal and isolation of clothing • Oxygen, mechanical ventilation may be required
Phencyclidine (PCP)	• Tachycardia • Hypertensive crisis • Hyperthermia • Agitation, hyperactivity • Nystagmus • Blank stare • Hypoglycemia • Violent, psychotic behavior • Ataxia • Seizures • Myoglobinuria, renal failure • Lethargy, coma • Cardiac arrest	• Quiet environment • Gastric lavage if within 1 hour of ingestion, multiple dose activated charcoal, cathartic • Gastric suction • Benzodiazepines (e.g., diazepam) for anxiety and agitation • Haloperidol (Haldol) to improve schizophrenic symptoms • Fluids and diuretics for forced diuresis • Beta-blockers for dysrhythmias • Antihypertensives: vasodilators (e.g., nitroprusside [Nipride]) • Hypothermia blanket, ice packs, ice-water sponge baths for hyperthermia • Dantrolene (Dantrium) may be prescribed for malignant hyperthermia • Anticonvulsants (e.g., diazepam, phenytoin, phenobarbital) for seizures • Haloperidol (Haldol) for acute psychotic reactions • Fluids and diuretics for myoglobinuria; urinary alkalinization interferes with urinary elimination of PCP so sodium bicarbonate contraindicated

Table 12-14   Drugs and Toxins—cont'd

Drug or Toxin	Clinical Presentation of Intoxication	Specific Collaborative Management

Salicylates	**Initial**
	• Hyperthermia
	• Burning sensation in mouth or throat
	• Change in level of consciousness
	• Petechiae, rash, hives
	Later
	• Hyperventilation (respiratory alkalosis)
	• Nausea, vomiting
	• Thirst
	• Tinnitus
	• Diaphoresis
	Late
	• Hearing loss
	• Motor weakness
	• Vasodilation and hypotension
	• Respiratory depression to respiratory arrest
	• Metabolic acidosis
		• Gastric lavage, activated charcoal, cathartic
		• Bowel irrigation if enteric-coated salicylates ingested
		• Fluids with dextrose (e.g., $D_5\frac{1}{2}NS$)
		• Hypothermia blanket, ice packs, ice-water sponge baths for hyperthermia
		  • Dantrolene (Dantrium) may be prescribed for malignant hyperthermia
		• Sodium bicarbonate to alkalinize the urine and increase rate of salicylate excretion; maintain urine pH >7.50
		  • Monitor potassium, calcium, and magnesium levels
		• Vitamin K may be needed
		• Anticonvulsants (e.g., diazepam, phenytoin, phenobarbital) for seizures
		• Hemodialysis may be necessary

Tricyclic antidepressants (TCA)	**Anticholinergic** • Tachycardia, palpitations • Dysrhythmias • Hyperthermia • Headache • Restlessness • Mydriasis • Dry mouth • Nausea, vomiting • Dysphagia • Decreased bowel sounds • Urinary retention • Decreased deep tendon reflexes • Restlessness, euphoria • Hallucinations • Seizures • Coma **Anti-alpha adrenergic** • Hypotension • QT prolongation and quinidine-like dysrhythmias (including torsades de pointes) • AV and bundle branch blocks • Clinical indications of heart failure	• Gastric lavage, multiple-dose activated charcoal, cathartic • Sodium bicarbonate to alkalinize the urine and increase rate of TCA excretion; maintain urine pH >7.50 • Monitor potassium, calcium, magnesium levels • Hyperventilation may be used to produce alkalosis • Physostigmine (Antilirium) may be prescribed • Cardioversion, defibrillation, pacemaker as needed for dysrhythmias; avoid quinidine, lidocaine, digitalis; phenytoin or beta-blockers may be used to shorten QRS duration; overdrive pacing for torsades de pointes • Anticonvulsants (e.g., diazepam, phenytoin, phenobarbital) for seizures • Fluids and vasopressors for hypotension • Bethanechol (Urecholine) for urinary retention

or dysrhythmias, especially if tricyclic antidepressant (TCA) overdosage

  B. Insert intravenous catheter and treat hypovolemia as prescribed, usually initially with crystalloids

  C. Apply blankets and radiant heat lamps if needed for hypothermia

III. Identify causative agents: blood, urine, gastric contents for toxicology screen

IV. Prevent further absorption of drug

  A. Dilution: if drug or toxin cannot be removed by emesis or gastric lavage (e.g., caustic liquids), give water or milk (usually approximately 250 ml)

  B. Emesis: used only in alert patients with active gag reflex and rarely used in hospital setting

    1. Administer ipecac syrup 30 ml in 240 ml of water if prescribed

      a) Vomiting occurs within 15 to 30 minutes; repeat dosage if no vomiting after 30 to 40 minutes

      b) Contraindicated if the patient has seizures, decreased level of consciousness, or if corrosive, strong irritants or hydrocarbons have been ingested

      c) Monitor for complications of ipecac (e.g., protracted vomiting, abdominal cramping, diarrhea, mild CNS depression)

    2. Place patient in a left-side-lying position; have suction equipment available

  C. Gastric lavage: especially helpful if patient arrives within 30 minutes to 1 hour of ingestion of drug

    1. Assist with endotracheal intubation prior to gastric lavage in patients who have decreased level of consciousness and a diminished gag reflex

2. Contraindicated in patients who have ingested caustic agents or gastric irritants, are having seizures, or have a history of GI bleeding
3. Use large-bore (32-40 French) orogastric tube (Ewald)
   a) Viscous lidocaine on tube may decrease gag reflex
   b) Confirm placement by aspirating gastric contents
4. Place patient in a left-side-lying position; have suction equipment available
5. Use approximately 5 to 10 L of warm tap water; inject 150 to 200 ml at a time and aspirate completely before injecting any more lavage fluid
6. Monitor for potential complications (e.g., esophageal perforation, aspiration pneumonitis, laryngospasm, gastric erosion, epistaxis, mediastinitis)
7. Do not remove tube until after activated charcoal has been given

D. Adsorbent therapy
1. Administer activated charcoal as prescribed; usually 1 g/kg
2. Give multiple doses of activated charcoal as prescribed for theophylline, phenobarbital, carbamazepine (Tegretol), phenylbutazone, tricyclic antidepressants; usually administered as 25 g every 2 hours or 50 g every 4 to 6 hours after the initial dose until serum drug level is normal

E. Cathartics
1. Administer sorbitol with first dose of activated charcoal as prescribed
2. Administer magnesium sulfate or magnesium citrate as prescribed; magnesium-containing cathartics are contraindicated in renal insufficiency

F. Bowel irrigation
1. Administer nonabsorbable, osmotically active solution (e.g., polyethylene glycol lavage electrolyte solution [GoLYTELY, Colyte]) as prescribed orally or by nasogastric tube; usually at a rate of 1 to 2 L/hr for 4 to 6 hr or until the patient is having clear stools
   a) May be effective for overdosages of sustained-release drugs or drugs not adsorbed by activated charcoal
   b) May also be used by "body packers" and "body stuffers"; surgical intervention may also be required in these situations
      (1) "Body packers" swallow condoms or balloons filled with a drug to smuggle it
      (2) "Body stuffers" swallow drugs to prevent detection by police; these drugs are not specially prepared to prevent absorption in the GI tract so they present great risk of overdosage

c) Contraindicated if the patient has significant gastrointestinal pathology or dysfunction
2. Monitor for vomiting

G. Assist with gastroscopy if indicated: may be necessary to remove coalesced mass of pills

H. Assist with dermal decontamination for external toxins
1. Protect yourself with gloves, gown, goggles
2. Remove and discard clothing
3. Rinse skin with water until pH is normal if toxin is a strong acid or alkaline
4. Wash body with soap and water or wash body with alcohol, followed with soap and water

V. Facilitate removal of drug
A. Administer intravenous fluids and osmotic or loop diuretics as prescribed to cause a forced osmotic diuresis; most often used for ethanol, methanol, ethylene glycol
B. Administer appropriate agents to cause urinary alkalinization or acidification
1. Urinary alkalinization: administer sodium bicarbonate; used primarily for salicylates and tricyclic antidepressants
2. Urinary acidification: administer ammonium chloride or ascorbic acid
   a) May be used for PCP and amphetamines
   b) Usually currently avoided due to incidence of rhabdomyolysis and resultant myoglobinuria which may cause acute renal failure
C. Prepare patient for hemodialysis if appropriate; indications include the following:
1. Ethylene glycol or methanol serum level more than 50 mg/dl
2. Lithium intoxication
3. Heavy metal ingestion
4. Drug-induced renal or hepatic toxicity
5. Salicylate intoxication with severe acid-base imbalance or seizures unresponsive to treatment
6. Ingestion of an agent known to produce delayed toxicity
7. Severe poisoning of a dialyzable drug (Box 12-1)
D. Assist with hemoperfusion if prescribed; hemoperfusion is more effective for drugs

---

BOX 12-1   **Selected Dialyzable Drugs**

Acetaminophen
Alcohols: ethanol, ethylene glycol, methanol
Amphetamines
Antibiotics (most)
Barbiturates
Electrolytes: potassium, calcium, magnesium
Lithium
Phenobarbital
Salicylates
Theophylline

that are bound to plasma proteins, but it is not effective in correcting acid-base imbalances

    E. Administer appropriate antidote if available and prescribed (listed where applicable in Table 12-11)

VI. Maintain renal function

    A. Administer intravenous fluids to maintain urine output at 0.5 to 1.0 ml/kg/hr

    B. Monitor for myoglobinuria; administer fluids, diuretics, and sodium bicarbonate as prescribed

VII. Monitor hepatic function: liver function studies, coagulation studies

VIII. Monitor for complications

    A. Acute respiratory failure (type II) due to respiratory depression

    B. Aspiration pneumonitis

    C. Dysrhythmias

    D. Heart failure

    E. Nephrotoxicity, acute renal failure

    F. Hepatotoxicity, acute hepatic failure

    G. Seizures

    H. Coma, neurologic injury

    I. Repeat overdosage

IX. Ensure appropriate psychologic counseling

    A. Allow patient to express feelings in a noncondemning fashion

    B. Monitor environment for safety hazards; maintain suicide precautions if indicated

    C. Refer patient to a substance abuse program if appropriate

    D. Request psychiatric consultation for destructive behavior if appropriate

LEARNING ACTIVITIES

1. **DIRECTIONS:** Complete the following crossword puzzle related to shock, SIRS, and MODS.

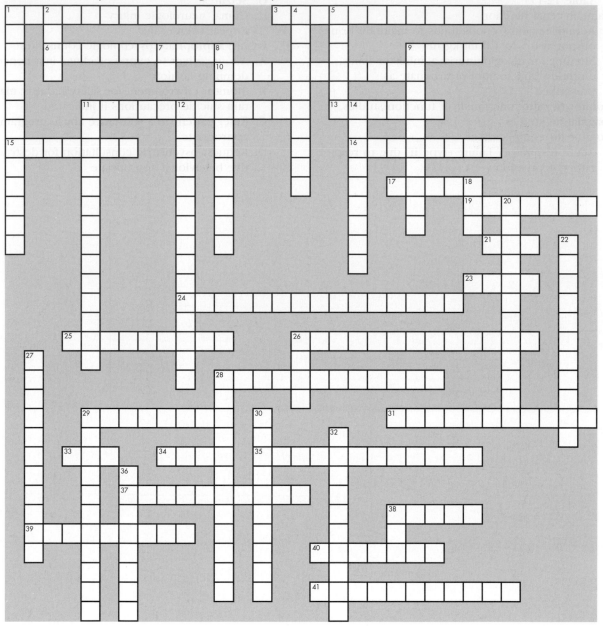

Across

1. Type of shock caused by antigen-antibody response, IgE, and the release of histamine and other mediators
3. Type of fluids that contain solutes to affect osmotic pressure (plural)
6. Inotropic agent used most often in cardiogenic shock
9. Hemodynamic parameter that differentiates hypovolemic shock from cardiogenic shock and cardiac pulmonary edema from noncardiac pulmonary edema (abbrev.)
10. Stage of shock when compensatory mechanisms are no longer effective in maintaining tissue perfusion
11. Stage of septic shock with fever, increased CO/CI, decreased SVR
13. Type of shock associated with the physiologic response to endotoxin
15. Protein component of blood used in fluid resuscitation to increase intravascular colloidal oncotic pressure
16. DO_2 is oxygen ____
17. Type of fluid required for hemorrhage to the point of hypoperfusion
19. Stage of shock associated with a decrease in tissue oxygenation but no clinical indications of hypoperfusion
21. Type of acute renal failure seen in MODS (abbrev.)
23. Systemic response of the immune system to microorganisms, tissue trauma, toxins, burns, etc. (abbrev.)
24. Method of returning the patient's own hemorrhaged blood to his or her intravascular space
25. Mediator seen in anaphylactic shock, which causes vasodilation and increased capillary permeability
26. Consequence of muscle destruction; may cause renal failure
28. Drugs that may be used to decrease preload or afterload in cardiogenic shock
29. Type of fluids that increase intravascular colloidal oncotic pressure; contraindicated in situations associated with increased capillary permeability (plural)
31. Type of shock caused by loss of intravascular blood volume
33. Branch of the autonomic nervous system of primary importance in the compensatory response to hypoperfusion in shock (abbrev.)
34. Mechanical therapy used in cardiogenic shock to increase coronary artery perfusion and decrease afterload (abbrev.)
35. Stage of shock dominated by neuroendocrine responses to hypoperfusion
37. Edema of mucous membranes, seen in anaphylactic shock
38. Condition of insufficient perfusion of cells and vital organs, causes tissue hypoxia
39. Antiprostaglandin (generic)
40. Colloid that contains large starch molecules; affects platelet aggregation
41. Alkaline buffer used for severe metabolic acidosis (pH 7.0 or less)

Down

1. Anaphylactic-like reaction when previous exposure is not required, not mediated by IgE, probably triggered by complement system
2. Type of acute respiratory failure seen in MODS (abbrev.)
4. Stage of shock associated with irreversible organ damage
5. Systemic state characterized by the presence of invading microorganisms and their toxins in the blood
7. Most common cause of cardiogenic shock (abbrev.)
8. First-line drug in anaphylactic shock (generic)
9. Drug most commonly associated with anaphylactic shock
11. Consequence of hemolytic blood transfusion reaction; may cause renal failure
12. H_1 antihistamine (generic)
14. Substance contained in the cell wall of some microorganisms that is released when the organism dies; the body responds to this substance with the release of mediators, which causes septic shock
18. Type of coagulopathy seen in MODS (abbrev.)
20. Third-spacing is the shift of fluid from intravascular space to ____ space, pleural space, pericardial space, or peritoneal space
22. Type of shock caused by inability of the heart to effectively pump blood
26. Often fatal result of SIRS; previously referred to as multisystem organ failure (MSOF) (abbrev.)
27. Complication of administering large volumes of IV fluid and blood that may shift the oxyhemoglobin dissociation curve to the left and impair oxygen delivery to the tissues
28. Drugs that may be used to increase BP in the refractory stage of shock
29. VO_2 is oxygen ____
30. Presence of viable bacteria in the blood
32. Type of shock caused by suppression of sympathetic nervous system
36. Narcotic antagonist (generic); may be useful in blocking the effects of endorphin in septic shock
38. Hemodynamic parameter that is increased in hypovolemic and cardiogenic shock but decreased in early septic, anaphylactic, and neurogenic shock

2. **DIRECTIONS:** Identify which type of shock the following pathologic conditions or procedures may cause (more than one may be checked).

Condition	Hypovolemic	Cardiogenic	Septic	Anaphylactic	Neurogenic
Myocardial infarction					
Bee sting					
Head injury					
Diarrhea					
Pulmonary embolism					
Ruptured gallbladder					
Esophageal varices					
Ruptured papillary muscle					
Insulin shock					
Ascites					
IVP dye					
Spinal cord injury					
Invasive procedures					
Burns					
Blood transfusion reaction					
Spinal anesthesia					
Trauma					
Malnutrition					
Chemotherapy					

3. **DIRECTIONS:** Match the pathophysiology with the type of shock.

_____a. Vasodilation resulting from stimulation of the inflammatory and immune systems by endotoxins

_____b. Inability of the heart to effectively pump

_____c. Inadequate amount of circulating volume

_____d. Vasodilation resulting from the release of histamine from mast cells caused by major allergic reaction

_____e. Vasodilation resulting from suppression or loss of the sympathetic nervous system

1. cardiogenic
2. septic
3. anaphylactic
4. neurogenic
5. hypovolemic

4. DIRECTIONS: Identify the following clinical indications of shock as occurring during the compensatory, progressive, and/or refractory stages of shock.

Clinical Finding	Compensatory	Progressive	Refractory
Tachycardia			
Dysrhythmias			
Cool, pale skin			
Uncontrollable bleeding (DIC)			
Mottling of extremities			
Neurologic changes: lethargy, coma			
Oliguria			
Anuria			
Profound hypoxemia, increased PVR, decreased lung compliance (ARDS)			
Narrow pulse pressure			
Profound hypotension despite vasopressors			
Hypotension			
Decreased bowel sounds			
Thirst			
Neurologic changes: irritability, confusion			
Nausea			
Neurologic changes: coma, focal signs			
Absent bowel sounds			

5. DIRECTIONS: Complete this table by putting ↑, ↓, or normal in the empty cells.

Type of Shock	CO/CI	RAP/PAP/PAOP	SVR	SvO$_2$
Hypovolemic				
Cardiogenic				
Early Septic				
Late Septic				
Anaphylactic				
Neurologic				

Key: *CO*, cardiac output; *CI*, cardiac index; *RAP*, right atrial pressure; *PAP*, pulmonary artery pressure; *PAOP*, pulmonary artery occlusive pressure; *SVR*, systemic vascular resistance; *SvO$_2$*, oxygen saturation of venous blood

6. DIRECTIONS: List two fluids in each category.

Crystalloids		
Isotonic		
Hypotonic		
Hypertonic		
Colloids		
Blood or blood products		

7. DIRECTIONS: Identify the three factors that affect oxygen delivery.

1. _____
2. _____
3. _____

8. **DIRECTIONS:** Calculate the following according to this brief case study.
   A patient is admitted after an explosion. His anterior chest, abdomen, and upper arms have a dark brown to black appearance. His hands also have a dark brown appearance. His face is red with blisters, and the skin is weeping. His weight is 75 kg.

   a. What percentage of the body has partial thickness burns?_____

   b. What percentage of the body has full thickness burns?_____

   c. Would this patient be categorized as having a minor, moderate, or major burn?_____

   d. In what type of facility should this patient receive definitive care?_____

   e. Calculate his fluid requirements for the first 24 hours._____

   f. How much should be given during the first 8 hours _____ , second 8 hours _____, third 8 hours _____ ?

9. **DIRECTIONS:** Identify the following as occurring with salt water near-drowning and/or fresh water near-drowning (assuming that significant aspiration into the lungs occurred).

	Salt Water Near-drowning	Fresh Water Near-drowning
Hypernatremia		
Hyponatremia		
ARDS		
Hemoconcentration		
Hemodilution		

10. **DIRECTIONS:** Identify the three actions used for most (but not all) drug intoxication to decrease absorption of the drug.

    1. _____

    2. _____

    3. _____

11. **DIRECTIONS:** Match the following antidotes to the appropriate drug or toxin.

    _____a. Methemoglobinemia

    _____b. Cyanide

    _____c. Methanol

    _____d. Organophosphates

    _____e. Carbon monoxide

    _____f. Acetaminophen

    _____g. Benzodiazepines (e.g., diazepam)

    _____h. Opiates (e.g., morphine sulfate)

    _____i. Ethylene glycol

    _____j. Beta-blocker

    _____k. Digoxin

    _____l. Calcium channel blockers

    1. Glucagon
    2. 100% oxygen, hyperbaric oxygenation if possible
    3. Digibind
    4. Fomepizole (Antizol)
    5. Ethanol
    6. Methylene blue
    7. Calcium
    8. Amyl nitrate
    9. Atropine
    10. Acetylcysteine (Mucomyst)
    11. Flumazenil (Romazicon)
    12. Naloxone (Narcan)

12. **Directions:** Complete the following crossword puzzle related to burns, near-drowning, and drug overdosage.

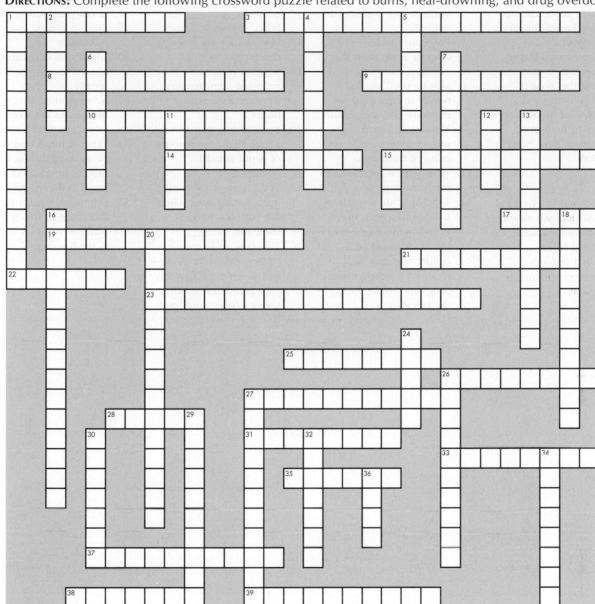

Across

1. Type of burn that often initially causes gastrointestinal symptoms
3. Condition caused by nitrates and nitrites, which causes a change in hemoglobin so that it cannot effectively carry oxygen
8. Fluid shift in burns is from intravascular to _____ space
9. Zone in the center of the burn that has the most contact with the heat source
10. Drug often used by adolescents in suicide gesture that can cause fatal hepatic damage (generic)
14. Suspect this type of injury if the patient has facial burns or if the fire was in an enclosed area
15. Procedure that involves removal of necrotic tissue
17. Technique of estimating burn surface area where percentages are assigned to body parts; rule of _____
19. Phase of burn care when the major complications are acute respiratory failure and shock
21. Type of antidepressant that may cause torsades de pointes, especially at toxic levels
22. Zone of burn injury that surrounds the center
23. Hemoglobin saturated with carbon monoxide rather than oxygen
25. Adsorbent agent used in drug overdosage
26. Osmotic laxative that is added to the first dose of charcoal
27. Complication of near-drowning that makes initial resuscitation efforts unsuccessful
28. Drowning in this type of water may cause hyponatremia and seizures
31. This vitamin must be given with dextrose to malnourished patients to prevent Wernicke's encephalopathy
33. Type of burn caused by caustic agents
35. Curling's ulcer seen in patients with burns is this type of ulcer

37. Type of burn that causes extensive tissue damage but may look minimal on the body surface
38. Dilution is used rather than emesis or gastric lavage if this type of chemical is ingested
39. This type of blood screen is done to determine what drugs have been ingested

Down

1. Complication of electrical burns, which may result in myoglobinuria and acute renal failure
2. Reflex that reduces oxygen requirements in submersion

4. Outermost zone of the burn, which is minimally injured
5. Procedure to flush the drug or toxin from the stomach
6. May be used intravenously in methanol or ethylene glycol ingestion
7. Type of skin graft that provides permanent covering of burn areas
11. This "gap" is increased in methanol ingestion
12. Type of acute respiratory failure often seen in near-drowning (abbrev.)
13. Blood cleansing procedure that may be required to remove some drugs and toxins from the blood

15. Type of drowning where no water gets into the lungs; asphyxia occurs
16. Insecticides are often this type
18. Surgical procedure for relieving compression from circumferential burns
20. Burn all the way around a limb that causes risk of acute arterial occlusion
24. Technique of estimating burn surface area when the patient's hand is used; rule of _____
26. This type of overdose causes metabolic acidosis and respiratory alkalosis
27. Skin graft from another species (e.g., cow, pig)

29. High pressure; this type of oxygen therapy is used in carbon monoxide poisoning
30. Toxin that may cause a bitter almond odor to the breath
32. New antidote that may be used in antifreeze ingestion (brand name)
34. Type of fluids that should be avoided during the first 24 hours after a major burn (plural)
36. Submersion and near-drowning in this type of water is twice as lethal as in fresh water

LEARNING ACTIVITIES ANSWERS

1.

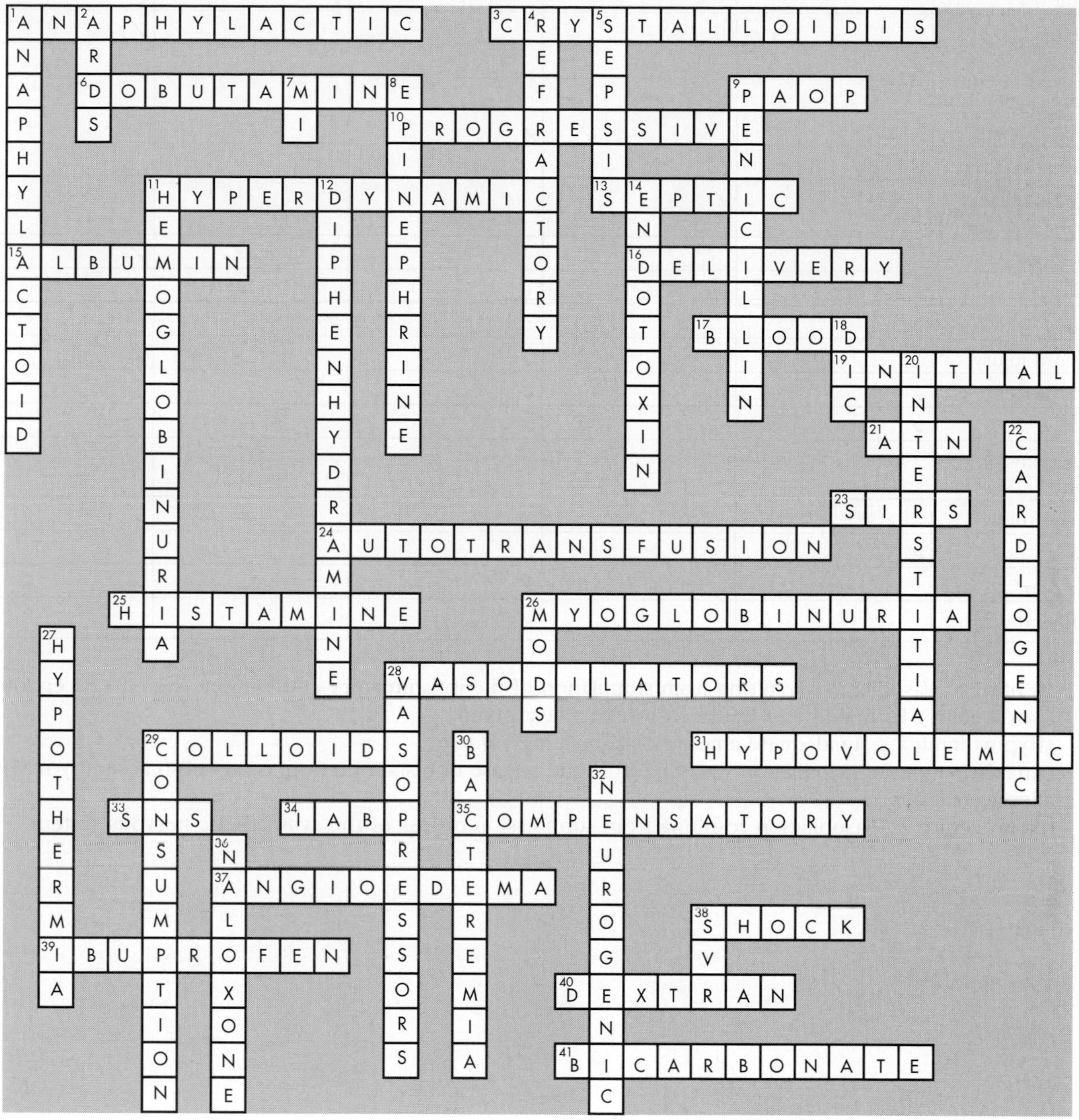

1 ANAPHYLACTIC
2 ARDS
3 CRYSTALLOIDIS
4 REFRACTORY
5 SEPSIS
6 DOBUTAMINE
7 MI
8 EPINEPHRINE
9 PAOP
9 PENICILLIN
10 PROGRESSIVE
11 HYPERDYNAMIC
11 HEMOGLOBINURIA
12 DIPHENHYDRAMINE
13 SEPTIC
14 ENDOTOXIN
15 ALBUMIN
1 ANAPHYLACTOID
16 DELIVERY
17 BLOOD
18 DIC
19 INITIAL
20 INTERSTITIA
21 ATN
22 CARDIOGENIC
23 SIRS
24 AUTOTRANSFUSION
25 HISTAMINE
26 MYOGLOBINURIA
26 MODS
27 HYPOTHERMIA
28 VASODILATORS
28 VASOPRESSORS
29 COLLOIDS
29 CONSUMPTION
30 BACTEREMIA
31 HYPOVOLEMIC
32 NEUROGENIC
33 SNS
34 IABP
35 COMPENSATORY
36 NALOXONE
37 ANGIOEDEMA
38 SHOCK
38 SVR
39 IBUPROFEN
40 DEXTRAN
41 BICARBONATE

2.

Condition	Hypovolemic	Cardiogenic	Septic	Anaphylactic	Neurogenic
Myocardial infarction		✓			
Bee sting				✓	
Head injury					✓
Diarrhea	✓				
Pulmonary embolism		✓			
Ruptured gallbladder			✓		
Esophageal varices	✓				
Ruptured papillary muscle		✓			
Insulin shock					✓
Ascites	✓				
IVP dye	✓			✓	
Spinal cord injury					✓
Invasive procedures	✓		✓		
Burns	✓		✓		
Blood transfusion reaction				✓	
Spinal anesthesia					✓
Trauma	✓		✓		
Malnutrition			✓		
Chemotherapy			✓		

3.   __2__ (septic): a. Vasodilation resulting from stimulation of the inflammatory and immune systems by endotoxins
   __1__ (cardiogenic): b. Inability of the heart to effectively pump
   __5__ (Hypovolemic): c. Inadequate amount of circulating volume
   __3__ (Anaphylactic): d. Vasodilation resulting from the release of histamine from mast cells caused by major allergic reaction
   __4__ (Neurogenic): e. Vasodilation resulting from suppression or loss of the sympathetic nervous system

4.

Clinical Finding	Compensatory	Progressive	Refractory
Tachycardia	✓	✓	
Dysrhythmias		✓	✓
Cool, pale skin	✓		
Uncontrollable bleeding (DIC)			✓
Mottling of extremities		✓	✓
Neurologic changes: lethargy, coma		✓	✓
Oliguria	✓		
Anuria		✓	✓
Profound hypoxemia, increased PVR, decreased lung compliance (ARDS)			✓
Narrow pulse pressure	✓		
Profound hypotension despite vasopressors			✓
Hypotension		✓	✓
Decreased bowel sounds	✓	✓	
Thirst	✓		
Neurologic changes: irritability confusion	✓		
Nausea		✓	
Neurologic changes: coma, focal signs			✓
Absent bowel sounds			✓

5.

Type of Shock	CO/CI	RAP/PAP/PAOP	SVR	Svo2
Hypovolemic	↓	↓	↑	↓
Cardiogenic	↓	↑	↑	↓
Early Septic	↑	↓	↓	↑
Late Septic	↓	↑↓ or normal	↑	↓
Anaphylactic	↓	↓	↓	↓
Neurologic	↓	↓	↓	↓

Key: *CO*, cardiac output; *CI*, cardiac index; *RAP*, right atrial pressure; *PAP*, pulmonary artery pressure; *PAOP*, pulmonary artery occlusive pressure; *SVR*, systemic vascular resistance; *Svo$_2$*, oxygen saturation of venous blood

6.

Crystalloids		
Isotonic	Normal (0.9%) saline	Lactated Ringer's
Hypotonic	Half-normal (0.45%) saline	5% dextrose in water
Hypertonic	3% saline	Hypertonic dextrose (e.g., 10%, TPN)
Colloids	Albumin	Dextran 70 or Hespan
Blood or blood products	Whole blood	Red blood cells

7.   1. Sao$_2$; 2. Hemoglobin; 3. Cardiac output

8. a. What percentage of the body has partial thickness burns? approximately 4.5%

  b. What percentage of the body has full thickness burns? approximately 27%

  c. Would this patient be categorized as having a minor, moderate, or major burn? major: full thickness more than 10% plus involvement of hands and face plus high likelihood of inhalation injury (facial burns)

  d. In what type of facility should this patient receive definitive care? tertiary (e.g., burn unit or burn center)

  e. Calculate his fluid requirements for the first 24 hours. Approximately 9,450 ml (using 4 ml/kg/%BSA)

  f. How much should be given during the first 8 hours (4,725 ml), second 8 hours (2,365 ml), third 8 hours (2,365 ml)?

9.

	Salt Water Near-drowning	Fresh Water Near-drowning
Hypernatremia	✔	
Hyponatremia		✔
ARDS	✔	✔
Hemoconcentration	✔	
Hemodilution		✔

10. 1. gastric lavage; 2. activated charcoal; 3. cathartic

11. _6_ (Methylene blue): a. Methemoglobinemia

  _8_ (Amyl nitrate): b. Cyanide

  _5_ (Ethanol): c. Methanol

  _9_ (Atropine): d. Organophosphates

  _2_ (Oxygen): e. Carbon monoxide

  _10_ (Acetylcysteine [Mucomyst]): f. Acetaminophen

  _11_ (Flumazenil [Romazicon]): g. Benzodiazepines (e.g., diazepam)

  _12_ (Naloxone [Narcan]): h. Opiates (e.g., morphine sulfate)

  _4_ (Fomepizole [Antizol]): i. Ethylene glycol

  _1_ (Glucagon): j. Beta-blocker

  _3_ (Digibind): k. Digoxin

  _7_ (Calcium): l. Calcium channel blockers

12.

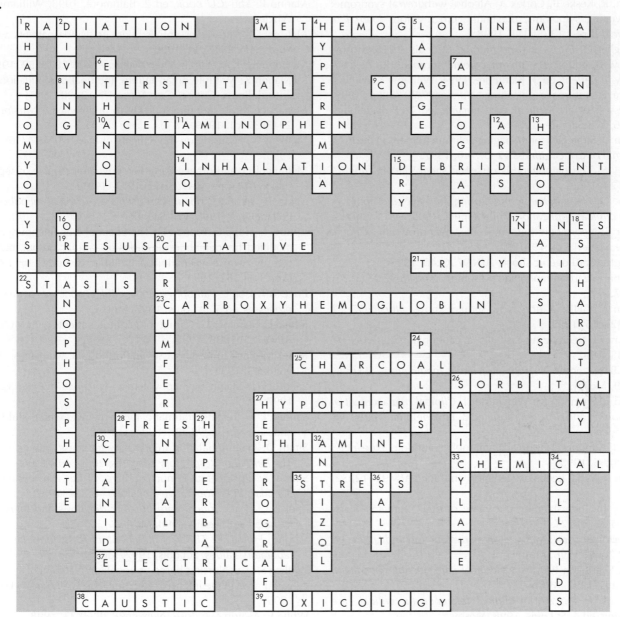

Bibliography and Selected References

Alspach J, editor: *Core curriculum for critical care nursing,* ed 5, Philadelphia, 1998, WB Saunders.

Barbarito C: Anaphylaxis, *AJN* 99 (1):33, 1999.

Barkauskas V, et al: *Health and physical assessment,* St Louis, 1994, Mosby.

Beare P, Myers J: *Adult health nursing,* ed 3, St Louis, 1998, Mosby.

Benner P: From novice to expert, *AJN* 82(3):402, 1982.

Benner P, Tanner C: How expert nurses use intuition, *AJN* 87 (1):23, 1987.

Boggs R, Wooldridge-King M: *AACN procedure manual for critical care,* ed 3, Philadelphia, 1993, WB Saunders.

Boghdadi M, Henning R: Cocaine: pathophysiology and clinical toxicology, *Heart and Lung* 26 (6):466, 1997.

Bone R: Managing sepsis: what treatments can we use today? *Journal of Critical Illness* 12 (1):15, 1997.

Brar R, Hollenberg S: Administering fluid resuscitation effectively for traumatic shock, *Journal of Critical Illness* 11 (10):672, 1996.

Brar R, Hollenberg S: The technique of fluid resuscitation, *Journal of Critical Illness* 11 (8):550, 1996.

Byers J, Flynn M: Acute burn injury: a trauma case report, *Critical Care Nurse* 16 (4):55, 1996.

Cancio L, Mozingo D, Pruitt B: Administering effective emergency care for severe thermal injuries, *Journal of Critical Illness* 12 (2):85, 1997.

Cancio L, Mozingo D, Pruitt B: Strategies for diagnosing and treating asphyxiation and inhalation injuries, *Journal of Critical Illness* 12 (4):217, 1997.

Cancio L, Mozingo D, Pruitt B: The technique of fluid resuscitation for patients with severe thermal injuries, *Journal of Critical Illness* 12 (3):183, 1997.

Cardona VD: *Trauma nursing from resuscitation through rehabilitation,* Philadelphia, 1995, WB Saunders.

Carlson, R, Keske B, Cortex A: Alcohol withdrawal syndrome: alleviating symptoms, preventing progresssion, *Journal of Critical Illness* 13 (5):311, 1998.

Carrougher G: *Burn care and therapy,* St Louis, 1998, Mosby.

Chernow B, editor: *The pharmacologic approach to the critically ill patient,* ed 3, Baltimore, 1994, Williams & Wilkins.

Chiocca E: Antifreeze poisoning, *Nursing99* 29 (5):64, 1999.

Clochesy J, et al.: *Critical care nursing,* ed 2, Philadelphia, 1996, WB Saunders.

Crippen D: Strategies for managing delirium tremens in the ICU, *Journal of Critical Illness* 12 (3):140, 1997.

Crowley S: The pathogenesis of septic shock, *Heart Lung* 25 (2):124, 1996.

Darovic G: *Hemodynamic monitoring: invasive and noninvasive clinical application,* Philadelphia, 1995, WB Saunders.

DeBoer S: Neurologic outcomes after near-drowning, *Critical Care Nurse* 17 (4):19, 1997.

DeJong M: Cardiogenic shock, *AJN* 97 (6):40, 1997.

DiDonna T: Carbon monoxide poisoning, *Nursing97* 27 (1):33, 1997.

Dillman J: GHB: a drug you should know, *Nursing97* 27 (9):32cc15, 1997.

Freeman Z: Necrotizing fasciitis: a cautionary tale, *AJN* 97 (3):35, 1997.

Gahart B, Nazareno A: *1999 intravenous medications,* St Louis, 1999, Mosby.

Haddad L, Shannon M, Winchester J: *Clinical management of poisoning and drug overdose,* ed 3, Philadelphia, 1998, WB Saunders.

Hanks B: Administering an acetaminophen antidote, *Nursing95* 25 (8):66, 1995.

Hayden R: What keeps oxygenation on track? *AJN* 92 (12):32, 1992.

Headley J: Understanding the value of dual oximetry, *Nursing95* 25 (6):32T, 1995.

Huddleston Secor V: *Multiple organ dysfunction and failure,* ed 2, St Louis, 1996, Mosby.

Keen J, Searingen P: *Mosby's critical care nursing consultant,* St Louis, 1997, Mosby.

Kinney M, et al.: *AACN clinical reference for critical care nursing,* ed 4, St Louis, 1998, Mosby.

Laskowski-Jones L: Managing hemorrhage—taking the right steps to protect your patient, *Nursing97* 27 (9):36, 1997.

Lieberman P: Anaphylaxis: how to quickly narrow the differential diagnosis, *The Journal of Respiratory Diseases* 20 (3):221, 1999.

Marino P: *The ICU book,* ed 2, Baltimore, 1998, Williams & Wilkins.

McCain D: Nursing essentials: skin grafts for patients with burns, *AJN* 98 (7):34, 1998.

McDonough J: Acetaminophen overdose, *AJN* 98 (3):52, 1998.

McMahon K: Multiple organ failure: the final complication of critical illness, *Critical Care Nurse* 15 (12):20, 1995.

Menapace M: Responding quickly to anaphylaxis, *Nursing99* 29 (3):32cc1, 1999.

Metheny N: Focusing on the dangers of D_5W, *AJN* 97 (10):55, 1997.

Metrangolo L and others: Early hemodynamic course of septic shock, *Crit Care Med* 23 (12):1971, 1995.

Mims B, et al.: *Critical care skills: a clinical handbook,* Philadelphia, 1996, WB Saunders.

Ostrow L, Hupp E, Topjian D: The effect of Trendelenburg and modified Trendelenburg positions on cardiac output, blood pressure, and oxygenation: a preliminary study, *Am J Crit Care* 3 (5):382, 1994.

Price S, Wilson L: *Pathophysiology: clinical concepts of disease processes,* ed 5, St Louis, 1997, Mosby.

Rauen C, Stamatos C: Caring for geriatric patients with MODS, *AJN* 97 (5):16BB, 1997.

Roper M: Back to basics: assessing orthostatic vital signs, *AJN* 96 (8):43, 1996.

Sandrock J: Managing hypovolemia, *Nursing97* 27 (2):32aa, 1997.

Sandrock J: Treating traumatic hypovolemia: which fluid to choose?, *Nursing98* 28 (1):32cc1, 1998.

Smith D: Acute inhalation injury: how to assess, how to treat, *The Journal of Respiratory Diseases,* 20 (6):405, 1999.

Sulton L: Postoperative nursing care of the burn patient, *Seminars in Perioperative Nursing* 6 (4):236, 1997.

Thelan L, et al: *Critical care nursing: diagnosis and management,* ed 3, St Louis, 1998, Mosby.

Varon J, Fromm R: *The ICU handbook of facts, formulas, and laboratory values,* St Louis, 1997, Mosby.

Watling S, et al: Nursing-based protocol for treatment of alcohol withdrawal in the intensive care unit, *Am J Crit Care* 4 (1):66, 1995.

White V: Aspirin overdose, *Nursing98* 28 (4):33, 1998.

Young J: A closer look at IV fluids, *Nursing98* 28 (10):52, 1998.

Zimmerman J: Managing acute poisonings and drug overdoses in the ICU, *Journal of Critical Illness* 12 (6):368, 1997.

Zimmermann P: Tricyclic antidepressant overdose, *AJN* 97 (10):39, 1997.

Professional Caring and Ethical Practice

Clinical Judgment

I. Description: clinical reasoning, which includes clinical decision making, critical thinking, and a global grasp of the situation, coupled with the skills required

II. Decision making
   A. Involves several steps by which information is assimilated, integrated, weighed, and valued to arrive at the selection of a course of action from among several possible alternatives
   B. Consists of the following six steps:
      1. Information collection and problem identification
      2. Identification of possible solutions or actions
      3. Analysis of the possible consequences of each solution or action
      4. Selection of the best possible solution or action for implementation
      5. Implementation of the solution or action
      6. Evaluation of the results

III. Critical thinking
   A. Definition: controlled, purposeful, goal-directed reasoning; thinking based on evidence rather than conjecture
   B. Eight key questions in critical thinking (Alfaro-LeFevre, 1995)
      1. What is the goal of my thinking?
      2. What are the circumstances?
      3. What knowledge is required?
      4. How much room is there for error?
      5. How much time do I have?
      6. What resources can help me?
      7. Whose perspectives must be considered?
      8. What factors are influencing my thinking?
   C. Strategies enhancing critical thinking (Alfaro-LeFevre, 1995)
      1. Anticipate the questions others might ask
      2. Ask "why?"
      3. Ask "what else?"
      4. Ask "what if?"
      5. Paraphrase in your own words
      6. Compare and contrast
      7. Organize and reorganize information
      8. Look for flaws in your thinking
      9. Ask someone else to look for flaws in your thinking
      10. Develop good habits of inquiry
      11. Revisit information
      12. Replace the phrases "I don't know" or "I'm not sure" with "I need to find out"
      13. Turn errors into learning opportunities
      14. Share your mistakes—they're valuable

IV. Clinical knowledge and skills (refer to Chapters 2-12)

Advocacy/Moral Agency

I. Description: working on another's behalf and representing the concerns of the patient, family, and community; serving as a moral agent in identifying and helping to resolve ethical and clinical concerns within the clinical setting

II. Advocacy
   A. Advocacy refers to respecting and supporting the basic values, rights, and beliefs of the critically ill patient (AACN: Position statement: role of the critical care nurse as patient advocate, 1989)
   B. The nurse should do the following (AACN: Position statement: role of the critical care nurse as patient advocate, 1989):
      1. Respect and support the right of the patient or the patient's designated surrogate to autonomous, informed decision making
      2. Intervene when the best interest of the patient is in question
      3. Help the patient obtain necessary care
      4. Respect the values, beliefs, and rights of the patient
      5. Provide education and support to help the patient or the patient's designated surrogate make decisions

6. Represent the patient in accordance with the patient's choices
7. Support the decisions of the patient or the patient's designated surrogate or transfer care to an equally qualified critical care nurse
8. Intercede for patients who cannot speak for themselves in situations that require immediate action
9. Monitor and safeguard the quality of care the patient receives
10. Act as liaison between the patient, the patient's family, and healthcare professionals

III. Definitions and concepts related to ethical decision making
A. Ethics: systems of valued behaviors and beliefs that govern proper conduct to ensure the protection of an individual's rights; involves judgments that help to differentiate right from wrong or indicate how things ought to be
B. Accountability: answerability or responsibility
1. Personal accountability: to oneself and to the patient
2. Public accountability: to employer and to society
C. Ethical concepts: the four main concepts include autonomy, justice, fidelity, and beneficence; nonmaleficence, veracity, and confidentiality are also considered important ethical concepts
1. Autonomy
a) Autonomy refers to the right of self-determination, independence, and freedom; actions are based on the patient's values and beliefs
b) The nurse must be willing to respect the patient's right to make decisions about his or her own care, even if the nurse does not agree with those decisions
c) Limitations to autonomy include the following:
(1) When the rights of one person interfere with another individual's rights, health, or well being
(2) When a person is likely to injure himself or herself or others
2. Justice
a) Justice refers to the obligation to be fair to all people
b) Individuals have the right to be treated fairly and equally regardless of race, sex, marital status, medical diagnosis, social standing, economic level, or religious belief; also includes equal access to health care for all
3. Fidelity
a) Fidelity refers to an individual's faithfulness or loyalty to agreements and responsibilities that the individual has accepted
b) It is one of the key elements of accountability

c) A conflict may occur between fidelity to patients and fidelity to employer, government, and society
4. Beneficence
a) Beneficence refers to an individual's obligation to do good and not harm
b) Conflicts that may occur include the following decisions:
(1) What is best for another person
(2) Who should make the decision
(3) Long-term or short-term benefit (a temporary harm may eventually produce a greater good)
5. Nonmaleficence
a) Nonmaleficence refers to an individual's requirement to do no harm, intentionally or nonintentionally
b) It includes protecting mentally incompetent persons, nonresponsive persons, children, and any other person who cannot protect himself or herself
c) This principle is not absolute; an example of a conflict related to nonmaleficence is when surgical trauma causes an ultimate cure or improvement in the patient's condition
6. Veracity
a) Veracity refers to an individual's obligation to tell the truth and to not intentionally deceive or mislead the patient
b) This principle is not absolute; an example of a conflict related to veracity is when telling the patient the truth may cause harm
7. Confidentiality: refers to respecting privileged information

IV. Ethical approaches: vary in the basis for ethical decisions
A. Deontology: actions are right or wrong based on a set of morals or rules
1. Emphasizes duty or obligation to another person
2. Only acceptable ethical theory for decision making in health care
B. Teleology: actions are right or wrong based on the action's consequences and usefulness; looks at outcome; the end justifies the means
C. Utilitarianism: the morally right thing to do is whatever produces the greatest good for the greatest number; it is derived from teleology
D. Egoism: actions are right or wrong based on self-interest and self-preservation
E. Paternalism: beneficence should take precedence over autonomy
F. Obligationism: actions are right or wrong based on balancing distributive justice with beneficence
G. Social contract theory: actions are considered with distributive justice, with each person having equal right to the greatest degree of liberty possible

H. Natural law: actions are morally or ethically right when they are in accord with human nature

V. Ethical dilemmas: situation that requires a choice between two equally unfavorable alternatives
   A. Conflicts related to rights of the individual: autonomy versus paternalism
      1. Informed consent
      2. Technology versus quality of life
      3. Resuscitate versus do-not-resuscitate (DNR)
      4. Behavior control
         a) Behavior control may be misused to suppress personal freedom (e.g., use of restraints or sedating drugs)
         b) Individual's right to freedom may conflict with society's obligation to maintain social order
   B. Conflicts related to resource allocations: justice versus utilitarianism
      1. Triage decisions
      2. Quality-of-life decisions
      3. Inability to pay and/or lack of health insurance
      4. Organ transplantation decisions
         a) Living donors: rights of donor, recipient, families, society
         b) Choice of one recipient over another: potential for elitism
         c) Utilization of healthcare resources: tremendous cost of organ transplantation
         d) Designation of death: when an organ or organs can be removed
   C. Conflicts related to the role of the nurse: veracity versus fidelity
      1. Withholding therapy
      2. Right to die
         a) Positive euthanasia (also referred to as *active euthanasia* or *mercy killing*): life support systems are withdrawn or a medication, treatment, or procedure is used to cause death (e.g., assisted suicide)
         b) Negative euthanasia (also referred to as *passive euthanasia*): no extraordinary or heroic life-support measures are used to save a person's life (e.g., DNR orders)
   D. Conflicts related to personal values: professional integrity versus personal ethical and moral beliefs
      1. Nurse participation in treatments or therapies against their ethical or moral beliefs (e.g., abortion)
      2. Nurse providing care for patients whose practices are against their ethical or moral beliefs (e.g., domestic violence)

VI. Factors affecting ethical issues and ethical decision making (Fig. 13-1)

VII. Ethical decision-making process
   A. Collect, analyze, and interpret the data
   B. State the dilemma as clearly as possible

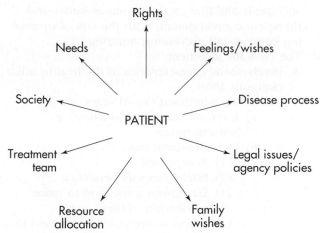

Figure 13-1 Factors affecting ethical issues and ethical decision making in nursing. (From Kinney M, et al: *AACN clinical reference for critical care nursing,* ed 4, St Louis, 1998, Mosby.)

   C. Identify the ethical principles involved in the dilemma
   D. Consider whether this dilemma could be resolved or influenced by the nurse
   E. Examine all possible solutions to the dilemma
   F. Evaluate the likely outcome of each solution and the advantages and consequences of each solution
   G. Choose the solution with the outcome most consistent with personal values and ethical principles
   H. Carry out the decision
   I. Evaluate the impact of the action

VIII. Ethical codes: guidelines that outline the nurse's responsibility to the patient, to the employer, and to society
   A. American Nurses Association (ANA) Ethical Code for Nurses (Box 13-1)

IX. Rights
   A. Legal rights: life, liberty, property, individual freedoms, due process
      1. Based on a legal entitlement to some good or benefit
      2. Guaranteed by laws, and if violated, can be upheld in the legal system
   B. Ethical rights (moral rights)
      1. Based on moral or ethical principles
      2. Backed by general opinion of society or culture
      3. Privileges often allotted to certain individuals or groups of individuals
   C. Entitlements: statutory rights for a defined group (e.g., Medicare)
   D. American Hospital Association (AHA) Patient's Bill of Rights (Box 13-2)

Caring Practices

I. Description: the constellation of nursing activities that are responsive to the uniqueness of the patient and family and that create a compassionate and therapeutic environment, with the aim of promoting comfort and preventing suffering

II. The critically ill patient
- A. Psychosocial characteristics of the healthy adult (Ericson, 1969)
  1. Young adulthood (18-40 years of age)
     - a) Intimacy versus self-isolation or self-absorption
     - b) Developmental tasks
       (1) Accepts self
       (2) Establishes independence
       (3) Establishes a vocation to make worthwhile contributions
       (4) Learns to appraise and express love responsibly
       (5) Establishes intimate bond with another
       (6) Establishes and manages residence
       (7) Finds congenial social group
       (8) Decides on option of a family
       (9) Formulates philosophy of life
       (10) Establishes role in community
  2. Middle adulthood (40-60 years of age)
     - a) Generativity versus self-absorption and stagnation
       - b) Developmental tasks
         (1) Develops new satisfaction as a mate
         (2) Supportive to mate
         (3) Develops sense of unity with mate
         (4) Assists offspring to become happy, responsible adults
         (5) Takes pride in accomplishments of self and mate
         (6) Balances work with other roles; assists aging parents
         (7) Achieves social and civic responsibility
         (8) Maintains active organizational membership
         (9) Accepts physical changes of middle age
         (10) Makes an art of friendship
         (11) Balances leisure with service pursuits
         (12) Develops more depth of personal philosophy by reevaluating values and examining assets
  3. Older adulthood (60 years of age to death)
     - a) Integrity versus despair
     - b) Developmental tasks
       (1) Continued self-development
       (2) Adapting to family responsibilities
       (3) Maintaining self-worth, pride, and usefulness
       (4) Dealing with loss of spouse, friends, upcoming end to life
- B. Basic human needs
  1. Basic needs may be the same, but the manner in which they are fulfilled depends on personal abilities, environment, and life experience
  2. Maslow's hierarchy of needs (Maslow, 1968) is progressive; primary needs must be met

---

BOX 13-1 **American Nurses Association (ANA) Ethical Code for Nurses**

The nurse provides services with respect for human dignity and the uniqueness of the client, unrestricted by considerations of social or economic status, personal attributes, or the nature of health problems.

The nurse safeguards the client's right to privacy by judiciously protecting information of a confidential nature.

The nurse acts to safeguard the client and the public when health care and safety are affected by incompetent, unethical, or illegal practice by any person.

The nurse assumes responsibility and accountability for individual nursing judgments and actions.

The nurse maintains competence in nursing.

The nurse exercises informed judgment and uses individual competency and qualifications as criteria in seeking consultation, accepting responsibilities, and delegating nursing activities to others.

The nurse participates in activities that contribute to the ongoing development of the profession's body of knowledge.

The nurse participates in the profession's efforts to implement and improve standards of nursing.

The nurse participates in the profession's efforts to establish and maintain conditions of employment conducive to high-quality nursing.

The nurse participates in the profession's efforts to protect the public from misinformation and misrepresentation and to maintain the integrity of nursing.

The nurse collaborates with members of the health professions and other citizens in promoting community and national efforts to meet the health needs of the public.

BOX 13-2 **American Hospital Association (AHA) Patient's Bill of Rights**

The Patient has the Right to:

Considerate and respectful care

Obtain from the physician information regarding diagnosis, treatment, and prognosis

Give informed consent before the start of any procedure or treatment

Refuse treatment to the extent permitted by law

Privacy concerning own medical care program

Confidential communication and records

Expect that the hospital will make a reasonable response to a patient's request for service

Information regarding the relationship of his or her hospital to other health and educational institutions as far as care is concerned

Refuse to participate in research projects

Expect reasonable continuity of care

Examine and question the bill

Know the hospital rules and regulations that apply to patients' conduct

prior to dealing with higher level needs
(Table 13-1)
C. Human needs of the critically ill patient
(Fig. 13-2)
D. Psychosocial responses to the critical illness and
critical care environment
1. Stress
a) Definition: mental, emotional, or physical tension or strain
b) Two types: distress (to noxious stimuli)
and eustress (to nonthreatening stimuli)
c) Admission to a critical care unit is fright-
ening and anxiety-producing
d) Sensory deprivation and sensory overload are stress factors within a critical
care unit
e) Interventions to decrease or eliminate
stress
(1) Maintain a calm, restful environment
(2) Provide for as much independence
of the patient as possible
(3) Provide contact with reality and
outside world
(4) Encourage use of coping mechanisms (Table 13-2)

Table 13-1	**Maslow's Hierarchy of Needs**
Physiologic	Oxygen, food, water, sleep
Safety and security	Protection, freedom from anxiety
Love and belonging	Freedom from loneliness, alienation
Esteem and recognition	Freedom from sense of worthlessness, inferiority, and helplessness
Self-actualization	Aesthetic needs, self-fulfillment, creativity, spirituality

2. Crisis
a) Definition: an acute state of stress in
which the person feels overwhelmed by
stressors
(1) Involves an attempt to regain
equilibrium
(2) Self-limited and allows for growth
b) May be maturational, adventitious, or situational in focus
(1) Maturational: arise as a result of
growth and development and involve
changes in self-concept and roles
(2) Adventitious: follow accidental and
uncommon events leading to major
environmental changes (e.g.,
natural disasters)
(3) Situational: follow an external event
or experience and its associated
losses and changes
c) Stages
(1) Shock and disbelief
(2) Disorganization: may be demanding,
irrational, angry
(3) Reorganization: difficulty making
decisions, forced to confront critical
questions
(4) Resolution
d) Interventions to assist the patient in
crisis
(1) Listen to the patient's perception of
the situation
(2) Encourage the patient to express his
or her feelings about the situation
(3) Assist the patient to gain an understanding of the situation by discussing losses and positive outcomes
(4) Assist the patient in developing a
viable solution
3. Fear/anxiety
a) Definition: fear is an unpleasant feeling specific to a known threat; anxiety is

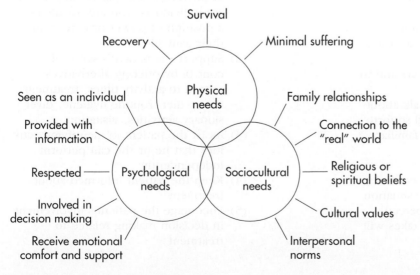

Figure 13-2 Human needs of the critically ill
patient. (From Kinney M, et al.: *AACN clinical reference for critical care nursing,* ed 4,
St Louis, 1998, Mosby.)

Table 13-2 Coping Mechanisms to Stress

Type	Example
Action	Taking walks, cleaning house, gardening, singing
Cognitive	Problem solving, reading about issue
Spiritual	Prayer
Interpersonal	Talking with support person
Emotional	Use of psychologic defense mechanisms (Table 13-3)

Table 13-3 Psychologic Defense Mechanisms

Defense Mechanism	Description
Suppression	Conscious, deliberate forgetting of unacceptable or painful thoughts, impulses, feelings, or acts
Repression	Unconscious, involuntary forgetting of unacceptable or painful thoughts, impulses, feelings, or acts
Denial	Treating obvious reality factors as though they do not exist because they are consciously intolerable
Rationalization	Attempting to justify feelings, behavior, and motives that would otherwise be intolerable, by offering a socially acceptable, intellectual, and apparently logical explanation for an act or decision
Compensation	Making extra effort to achieve in one area to offset real or imagined deficiencies in another area
Sublimation	Directing energy from unacceptable drives into socially acceptable behavior
Projection	Unconsciously attributing one's own unacceptable qualities and emotions to others
Regression	Going back to an earlier level of emotional development and organization
Withdrawal	Separating oneself from interpersonal relationships in order to avoid emotional expression or responsiveness

an unpleasant feeling to an unknown threat

  b) Anxiety can produce both psychologic and physiologic symptoms; manifestations may include restlessness, irritability, increase in questions, insomnia, tachycardia, tremors

  c) Interventions to decrease feelings of fear and anxiety

    (1) Communicate honestly and empathetically

    (2) Consult psychologist, psychiatric liaison nurse, chaplain if appropriate

    (3) Identify defense mechanisms being used (Table 13-3)

    (4) Encourage expression of fears and concerns

    (5) Reduce sensory overload

    (6) Teach relaxation and imagery techniques

    (7) Encourage the patient to ask questions

    (8) Encourage the patient to participate in care

    (9) Explore the patient's desire for spiritual or psychological counseling

4. Loneliness

  a) Definition: discomfort caused by separation from significant relationships, places, events, and objects

  b) Manifestations may include crying, withdrawal

  c) Interventions to decrease loneliness

    (1) Encourage participation in decision making and self-care

    (2) Encourage discussion of fears and to ask questions

    (3) Encourage the patient to talk about life, family, work, pet, and so forth

    (4) Ask the family to bring in familiar and loved objects

5. Powerlessness

  a) Definition: a perceived lack of control over the outcome of a specific situation or problem and the patient's perception that any action he or she takes will not affect the outcome

  b) May be manifested by apathy, withdrawal, resignation, fatalism, lack of decision making, aggression, anger

  c) Interventions to decrease feelings of powerlessness

    (1) Recognize the potential for feelings of powerlessness; particularly at risk are individuals who are usually in a position of power or control in their daily life

    (2) Support the patient's sense of control by offering alternatives related to activity times, treatment times, diet, routine hygiene, diversionary activities, visitation

    (3) Assist the patient in identifying activities that he or she can perform independently

    (4) Keep the patient informed about treatment

    (5) Encourage the patient's involvement in decision making related to treatment

(6) Increase the patient's control as his or her condition improves

6. Sensory overload
   a) Definition: increased frequency and intensity of stimulation of the senses with nonmeaningful stimuli
   b) Contributing factors: constant noise and lights, alarms, chatter of unfamiliar voices, offensive orders
   c) Intervention: eliminate or limit nonmeaningful sensory stimulation

7. Sensory deprivation
   a) Definition: decreased frequency, intensity, or variety of stimulation of the senses with meaningful stimuli
   b) Contributing factors: absence of windows, clocks, calendars; loss of normal light/dark patterns lack of familiar faces; deprivation of familiar touches, sounds, smells, and tastes of usual environment
   c) Interventions
      (1) Encourage family visitation
      (2) Encourage the family to bring familiar objects to the hospital
      (3) Place calendar and clock where the patient can see them; darken room at night

8. Anger
   a) Definition: feeling of great displeasure, hostility, exasperation
   b) May be manifested by clenching of teeth or muscles, avoidance of eye contact, sarcasm, insulting comments, screaming, argumentativeness, demanding behavior
   c) Interventions to decrease feelings of anger
      (1) Assist in identifying the cause of anger
      (2) Give the patient permission to be angry
      (3) Assist the patient in identifying appropriate ways to express the anger

9. Depression
   a) Definition: feeling of sadness, hopelessness
   b) May be manifested by loss of interest in people, dissatisfaction, difficulty making decisions, crying; patient may say that he or she is a failure, that he or she is being punished, or that he or she is considering hurting himself or herself
   c) Interventions to decrease feelings of depression
      (1) Provide information necessary to assist the patient to realistically visualize the future
      (2) Inspire hope and facilitate coping

10. Denial
    a) Definition: refusal to acknowledge the truth; allows the patient to come to grips with reality a little at a time
    b) Denial may be manifested by shrugging off symptoms, refusing to discuss the illness, appearing cheerful, and verbalizing the illness while ignoring restrictions
    c) Interventions
       (1) Allow the patient to express feelings
       (2) Do not confront the patient with the truth

11. ICU syndrome
    a) Definition: confusion or psychosis associated with the critical care environment
    b) Also called ICU psychosis, postcardiotomy delirium, postoperative psychosis, intensive care delirium, acute confusion, impaired psychologic response
    c) Usually occurs after 48 hours in the critical care unit; usually clears within 48 hours after transfer from the critical care unit
    d) Contributing factors include sleep deprivation, sensory deprivation, sensory overload, age, severe illness, history of mental illness or psychologic problems, cardiopulmonary bypass, prolonged surgery, electrolyte imbalance, hypothermia, endocrine disorders, medication
    e) May be manifested by altered consciousness, decreased attention span, disorientation, memory loss, labile emotions, perceptual distortions, hallucinations, paranoia, combativeness
    f) Interventions to decrease incidence or severity of ICU syndrome
       (1) Reduce the sleep deprivation, sensory deprivation, and sensory overload
       (2) Provide continuity of nursing staff to lessen the number of adjustments required by the patient
       (3) Reorient the patient often
       (4) Plan uninterrupted sleep time
       (5) Decrease noise level on alarms and decrease extraneous conversation and other noise
       (6) Adjust lighting to simulate night and day
       (7) Place a clock and calendar in the room
       (8) Encourage the family to visit and reorient the patient
       (9) Encourage placement of personal belongings at bedside

12. Near-death experience (NDE)
    a) Definition: a vivid series of events reported by some individuals after periods of clinical death

b) Manifestations include the following events (Sommers, 1994):
   (1) Time interval without feeling
   (2) Separation of mind and body
   (3) Propulsion through space or a long, dark tunnel
   (4) Interaction with a bright light
   (5) Meeting an escort (often a deceased family member or friend) who accompanies them to a warm, peaceful, bright area
   (6) Experiencing a life review
   (7) The choice of whether to go back or being told to go back
   (8) Return to the body
c) Interventions
   (1) Be alert for indications that the patient has experienced an NDE, especially in patients who have experienced cardiac arrest, electro-physiologic studies, any life-threatening crisis; the patient may do any of the following:
      (a) Say "I had the strangest dream" or something similar
      (b) Be angry, withdrawn, or unusually calm
   (2) Provide the patient with an opportunity to discuss the experience, such as "Did anything happen when you were very sick yesterday that you want to talk about?"
   (3) Explore your own feelings about NDE
   (4) Listen to the patient and avoid judgment
   (5) Reassure the patient who experiences an NDE that he or she is not "crazy" and that many people have had this experience
   (6) Refer the patient to books to read or a support group if available
13. Death and dying
   a) Definition: dying is a psychophysiologic process that ultimately terminates in death for the individual and grieving for significant others
   b) Stages of death and dying (Kubler-Ross, 1969) (Table 13-4)
   c) Interventions to assist the patient in dealing with death and dying
      (1) Develop a personal philosophy of death in order to deal effectively with dying patients and living families
      (2) Do not eliminate hope
         (a) Hope is the expectation that a desire will be fulfilled
         (b) Hope aids in the tolerance of pain and suffering throughout the dying process

Table 13-4	**Stages of Death and Dying (Kubler-Ross, 1969)**
Stage	**The patient may say:**
Shock and disbelief	"I can't be dying; you're wrong" "No, not me"
Denial	"Most people with this disease die but not me"
Anger	"Why me? What have I done to deserve this?"
Bargaining	"If I do this. . ., let me live until. . ."
Depression	"What's the use?"
Acceptance	"I'm ready to die"

   (3) Encourage the patient and family to discuss their fears and concerns; listen attentively
   (4) Provide your presence and your compassion
   (5) Provide comfort measures and analgesia
   d) Interventions to assist the family
      (1) Allow the family to be with the patient
      (2) Encourage the family to participate in the patient's care
      (3) Reassure the family of the patient's analgesia and comfort
      (4) Provide information about the patient's status often, especially the patient's imminent death
      (5) Encourage ventilation of anxiety, fears, concerns
      (6) Ensure a private, comfortable area for the family
      (7) Refer the family to other sources of support, such as the chaplain, social worker, support group
14. Transfer anxiety
   a) Definition: anxiety caused by anticipation of transfer from one nursing unit to another; often most significant when moving from a more closely monitored unit such as a critical care unit to a unit with lower nurse-to-patient ratios
   b) Represents the need to start over in developing trust and security with a new environment and staff
   c) Interventions to decrease transfer anxiety
      (1) Provide opportunities for the patient and family to voice their concerns and fears
      (2) Demonstrate trust in the competence of the receiving nurse and unit
      (3) Emphasize that the transfer is an indication of patient progress

Table 13-5	The Seven Dimensions of Patient-Centered Care	
Dimension	**Key Aspects and Activities Associated with the Dimension**
Respect for patient values, preferences, and expressed needs	• Recognition of patient needs and his or her autonomy • Preservation of patient dignity • Involvement of patient in decision making • Active attention to quality-of-life issues
Coordination and integration of care	• Direct clinical care • Includes support and ancillary services
Information, communication, and education	• Information on clinical status, progress, and prognosis • Information regarding the process of care delivery • Education to enable autonomy, self-care, and health promotion
Physical comfort	• Pain management • Help with activities of daily living • Modification of the hospital environment
Emotional support and alleviation of fear and anxiety	• Placing anxiety as the major priority • Attention to emotional impact of the clinical condition, treatment, and prognosis • Attention to emotional impact on both patient and family • Attention to reality of financial concerns regarding the illness
Involvement of family and friends	• Recognition of need for family and friends, as well as their needs • Accommodation of visiting • Involvement in decision making • Provision of support to family and friends
Transition and continuity	• Sensitive to patient concerns about medications, treatment, follow-up, danger signals to watch for, health promotion, and prevention of reoccurence • Coordination and planning for continued care needs • Access to ongoing care and assistance as needed

From Kinney M, et al.: *AACN clinical reference for critical care nursing,* ed 4, St Louis, 1998, Mosby.

E. Dimensions of patient-centered care (Kinney, 1998) (Table 13-5)

F. Complementary therapies: therapies used in conjunction with conventional therapies; most are intended to cause relaxation, decrease anxiety, and augment pain management
  1. Progressive muscle relaxation (PMR)
     a) Involves progressive tensing and relaxing of successive muscle groups
     b) Helps the patient to eventually sense muscle tension without having to progress through the tensing and relaxing of successive muscle groups
     c) Decreases stress and anxiety
     d) Often accompanied by diaphragmatic breathing
  2. Breathing
     a) Involves instruction, practice, and encouragement in the use of breathing techniques, such as diaphragmatic breathing or pursed-lip breathing
     b) Decreases stress and anxiety, may improve effectiveness of ventilation, especially in dyspneic patients
  3. Meditation
     a) Involves intentional concentration and repetition of a word, phrase, or muscular activity
     b) Encourage use of a word or phrase that holds a special meaning for the patient
     c) Decreases stress and anxiety
  4. Co-meditation
     a) Involves concentrating on certain sounds, images, or words
        (1) An assistant utters the words, which is often a script written by the patient
        (2) Efforts are made to synchronize the word with the rhythm of the patient's exhalations
     b) Decreases stress and anxiety
  5. Guided imagery
     a) Involves focusing and directing the imagination through the use of specific words and suggestions
     b) Identify the patient's concept of a relaxing location or situation and verbally guide thoughts there
     c) Decreases stress and anxiety, decreases fear, enhances the immune system
  6. Massage
     a) Involves a technique of controlled touch to manipulate soft tissue
     b) Effects depend on type and speed of movements, pressure exerted by the

hands, fingers, or thumbs, and the area of the body being massaged
c) Decreases stress and anxiety, reduces muscle tension and spasm, reduces edema, causes release of endorphin to augment pain relief
d) Aromatherapy and music may enhance the effectiveness
7. Hypnosis
a) Involves suggestion to enable a person to experience the imaginary as real, allowing deep relaxation
b) Decreases stress and anxiety
8. Biofeedback
a) Involves use of conscious mental effort to control involuntary body function, such as BP, heart rate, and respiratory rate
(1) A biofeedback instrument is used initially to alert the patient to the cues that signal a developing symptom (e.g., tension in neck and shoulders); audible tones are given
(2) Relaxation techniques are taught to decrease muscle tension
b) Decreases stress and anxiety, causes muscle relaxation
9. Therapeutic (or healing) touch
a) Involves the transfer of energy from the practitioner's hands to the patient, without actually touching, to potentiate the healing process of one who is ill or injured
b) Consists of the following steps: centering, assessment, unruffling, modulating, and evaluation
c) Used to help restore the balance of the energy field and to provide additional energy to be used for healing
10. Purposeful touch
a) Involves handholding, stroking or patting a patient's arm, hand, or face, placing one's hand on the patient's shoulder, placing one's arm around the patient's shoulder, or hugging
b) May also be referred to as affective touch, comforting touch, or empathetic touch
c) Reduces stress and communicates encouragement, support, or affection
11. Music therapy
a) Involves use of music to soothe and relax
b) Identify the patient's music preferences; any simple, repetitive, low-pitched music is appropriate for relaxation
c) The most soothing music has a ¾ beat; chants, folk songs, lullabies are very relaxing
d) Causes endorphin release, distraction

from pain or anxiety, and relaxation, improves quantity and quality of sleep
12. Aromatherapy
a) Involves the use of essential oils extracted from flowers, leaves, stalks, fruits, and roots for therapeutic purposes
b) May be used in massage, baths, compresses, or inhalation
c) Effects vary depending on the essential oil used; may alter mood, reduce anxiety, cause relaxation, cause decongestion, reduce inflammation, increase circulation, relieve pain (Table 13-6)
13. Pet therapy
a) Involves visitation by the patient's own pet or one from a list of pet visitation animals (usually a dog but may be a cat or rabbit)
b) Decreases stress and anxiety, may decrease heart rate and blood pressure
c) Adhere to specific guidelines to ensure the safety and security of the patient, families, and staff
14. Humor
a) Involves using words and images to elicit laughter
b) Decreases stress and anxiety, enhances the patient's ability to cope and feelings

Table **13-6**	**Effects of Commonly Used Essential Oils and Fragrances**
Basil	• Increases sense of well-being
Chamomile	• Promotes relaxation and sleep • May relieve allergy symptoms • Should not be used in patients with inhalation allergy to ragweed
Eucalyptus	• Stimulates • May act as a decongestant
Frankincense	• Reduces stress and promotes calm
Geranium	• Promotes balance
Ginger	• Relieves nausea and pain
Lavender	• Promotes relaxation, comfort, and coping • May have antidepressant qualities
Lemon	• Increases sense of well-being
Marjoram	• Reduces stress and muscle spasms
Peppermint	• Stimulates • Relieves nausea and pain • May act as a decongestant
Rosemary	• Increases sense of well-being
Sandalwood	• Promotes relaxation
Tea tree	• Acts as a topical antiseptic (especially antifungal)
Ylang-ylang	• Promotes relaxation and sleep

of well-being, decreases tension in a difficult situation, causes endorphin release, augments the immune system, causes muscle relaxation

   c) Conduct a humor assessment to determine the patient's receptiveness to humor and which type of humor is appropriate or inappropriate

   d) Timing of humor is crucial; humor is inappropriate during a crisis or when laughing will cause pain

   e) Some forms of humor are inappropriate, such as humor that demeans (e.g., racial or ethnic jokes) or sexually oriented humor (e.g., "dirty" jokes)

15. Acupuncture

   a) Involves the insertion of needles into specific points in the body for therapeutic purposes; may also involve use of heat (moxibustion), pressure (acupressure), or electromagnetic energy to stimulate acupuncture points

   b) Causes endorphin release and decrease in pain

III. The family of the critically ill adult

A. Assessment

1. Availability of family

2. Structure and communication patterns within the family
   a) Role of patient within family
   b) Primary decision maker
   c) Family spokesperson
   d) Conflicts within the family

3. Perceptions and understanding
   a) Knowledge of patient condition
   b) Past experience with critical care
   c) Past experience with similar health situations (e.g., MI, cancer)
   d) Need for information about the patient
   e) Expectations of outcome

4. Coping patterns
   a) Previous responses to crises
   b) Usual coping mechanism

5. Family resources and needs related to resources
   a) Transportation
   b) Lodging
   c) Finances
   d) Spiritual support

6. Family health maintenance needs
   a) Dietary
   b) Hygiene
   c) Rest/sleep
   d) Medications

B. Stressors

1. Observation of a loved one in a life-threatening situation

2. Overwhelming technology in the critical care environment

3. Separation from the family member

4. Effect of illness on family's financial stability

C. Most important needs of families (Leske, 1991)

1. To have questions answered honestly

2. To be assured the best care possible is being given to the patient

3. To know the prognosis

4. To feel hopeful

5. To know specific facts about the patient's progress

6. To be called at home about changes in the patient's condition

7. To know how the patient is being treated medically

8. To feel that hospital personnel care about the patient

9. To receive information about the patient daily

10. To have understandable explanations

11. To know exactly what is being done for the patient

12. To know why things were done for the patient

13. To see the patient often

14. To talk to the doctor every day

15. To be told about transfer plans

D. Responses

1. Anxiety

2. Fear of death, pain, discomfort of their loved one

3. Financial concerns

4. Fear of temporary or permanent changes in the roles of the patient and other family members

5. Severe dysfunction: argumentativeness, aggression, intoxication, guilt, blame, verbal or physical abuse toward healthcare workers

E. Interventions

1. Provide information about the status of the patient; on request, at designated times, including during visiting hours, at the time of any significant change in condition

2. Be available during family visitation to answer questions and provide explanations

3. Encourage family members to make notes regarding information that the physician or nurse have given or questions that they would like to ask during the next interaction with the nurse or physician

4. Encourage the designation of one family member to phone or be phoned who will then communicate to the other family members

5. Provide a brochure describing the unit, usual activities, visitation policies, and other useful information

6. Introduce yourself and ask names and relationships of family members

7. Identify family members by name if possible

8. Use touch therapeutically as allowed by the family members

9. Individualize visiting times based on the

needs and response of the patient and the family

10. Explain to the family if visitation must be interrupted or postponed by a procedure or crisis

11. Warn the family and explain the reason for a patient's unusual behavior (e.g., confusion)

12. Encourage the family to touch the patient, hold hands, express their feelings

13. Involve the family in decision making

14. Encourage family participation in care if they desire

15. Respect the cultural beliefs and rituals of the family; accommodate these beliefs and rituals if at all possible

16. Encourage the family members to take care of their own basic needs (eat, sleep, bathe)

17. Provide a comfortable area for visitors close to the unit with bathroom facilities and a telephone; have a private area available for family meetings and family-physician discussion

18. Encourage participation in a support group if available

19. Be empathetic

Collaboration

I. Description: working with others in a way that promotes and encourages each person's contributions toward achieving optimal and realistic patient goals; collaboration involves intra- and interdisciplinary work with all colleagues

II. Definitions
   A. Collaboration: working together
   B. Collaborative practice: when members of the medical and nursing professions, together with members of other related healthcare disciplines, work together to ensure quality patient and family care; includes the following critical aspects:
      1. Sharing in planning, decision making, problem solving, goal setting, and responsibility
      2. Communicating openly and respectfully
      3. Coordinating
      4. Cooperating
      5. Recognizing and accepting separate and interrelated spheres of practice
   C. Consultation: process of seeking, giving, and receiving help; may be formal (written) or informal (verbal)

III. Essential elements of collaboration
   A. Communication
   B. Trust
   C. Respect
   D. Understanding and acceptance of team members' roles
   E. Competence
   F. Shared responsibility and accountability
   G. Shared goal setting

H. Flexibility
I. Administrative support

IV. Components of collaborative practice
   A. Unit co-directors: a physician and a nurse
   B. Collaborative practice committee
   C. Primary nurse and primary physician
   D. Autonomy for clinical decision making
   E. Integrated patient records
   F. Multidisciplinary review of care

V. Blocks to collaboration
   A. Nurses and physicians
      1. Authoritative (sometimes aggressive) physicians
      2. Nonassertive (sometimes submissive) nurses
      3. Team members satisfied with traditional hierarchy
   B. Misunderstanding or lack of understanding regarding the role and practice of professional nursing
      1. Nurses have their own license; they do not practice under the license of the physician
      2. Physicians cannot discipline or fire nurses employed by the hospital
      3. Nursing is not medicine; these professions are separate yet interrelated; if an umbrella term is needed, let it be "healthcare," not "medicine"
      4. Nurses are nurses because they chose to be; it wasn't because they weren't or aren't intelligent enough to be physicians
      5. Nurses have independent functions as well as dependent functions; they can perform these independent functions without a physician's order (prescription is a much better word than order)
      6. Nursing research has established a limited body of scientific knowledge
      7. Nurses control nursing practice
   C. Ineffective or lack of communication between the professions
   D. Lack of administrative support
   E. Systems issues

VI. Strategies for improving collaboration
   A. Evaluate current interdisciplinary relationships in your institution and on your unit
      1. Are team members sought out for communication about the patient?
      2. Is communication peer-to-peer?
      3. Is recognition of each team member's role in enhancing patient outcomes given?
      4. Are team members willing to accept responsibility and accountability for patient outcomes?
      5. What are the steps taken when conflicts arise between team members?
   B. Establish a multidisciplinary critical care committee co-chaired by a nurse and a physician
      1. Disciplines have equal representation and decision making
      2. The committee should deal with issues

related to practice, communication, and improving effectiveness or efficiency

C. Establish multidisciplinary professional activities such as the following:
1. Rounds
2. Patient records
3. Orientation
4. Education programs
5. Task forces for problem resolution
6. Research

D. Establish a professional nursing environment
1. Assurance of competency
2. Knowledge of and ability to articulate the unique role of nursing
3. Encouragement of professional development of nursing staff

Systems Thinking

I. Description: the body of knowledge and tools that allow the nurse to appreciate the care environment from a perspective that recognizes the holistic interrelationship that exists within and across healthcare systems

II. Nursing is one aspect of patient care; nurses must work together with other members of the healthcare team and understand the organizational structure of the institution

III. Patient care delivery systems (Table 13-7)

IV. Delivery-of-care models
A. Patient-focused care
1. Goal: provide patients with a "seamless" healthcare experience and decrease fragmentation of care; focus is on meeting the patient's needs
2. Key components
a) Care for each patient coordinated by an RN or case manager
b) Cross-training of staff to provide up to 90% of patient services
c) Assignment of ancillary personnel to patient care units
d) Team approach among licensed and unlicensed members
e) Location of services closer to the patient

3. Benefits
a) To hospital
(1) Reduction in management layers
(2) Emphasis on shared governance and self-directed work teams
b) To patient
(1) Interaction with a decreased number of healthcare providers
(2) Improved coordination of care to enhance quality of care and increase patient satisfaction
c) To society: reduction of healthcare costs

B. Family-centered care
1. Seen most often in maternity and pediatric populations
2. Goal: allow the patient and family members to maintain their normal roles as much as possible, including communication between the interdisciplinary team and patient and family members
3. Considers the nurse, patient, and family as partners in the patient's care and the impact of the patient's illness on the family unit

C. Cooperative care
1. Similar to that of home health care: the patient and the family are in charge
2. Goal: early self-management by providing patients with a wellness-oriented hospital environment
3. Hospital environment viewed as an extension of the home rather than as an interruption
4. An integrated, multidisciplinary healthcare team focusing on therapeutic care and education allows response to patient's need in a timely manner
5. Patients have the right and responsibility to participate in their own health care as full partners to maximize their ability for self-management on discharge
6. Inclusion of the patient's family and support system as care partners during the hospital stay leads to more humanistic hospital

Table 13-7 | Patient Care Delivery Systems

	Functional Nursing	Team Nursing	Primary Nursing
Description	Task oriented; nurses perform tasks (e.g., charge, medicine, treatments) as assigned	Group oriented; team leader (RN) with team members deliver care to a group of patients	Patient oriented; nurse is responsible for all aspects of care for assigned patients; accountable for care delivered during entire hospitalization
Advantages	Cost effective	Cost effective Increased staff satisfaction	Increased staff satisfaction Improved continuity of care Improved quality of care May be more cost effective
Disadvantages	Fragmented nursing care Diminished continuity of care Diminished staff satisfaction	Diminished continuity of care	Restricted opportunity for evening and night shift nurses to be assigned as "primary nurse"

care and enhances the potential for improved treatment compliance and self-management after discharge

D. Holistic care
  1. Designed for the chronically ill patient with complex medical conditions that require frequent acute care admissions; addresses the physical, mental, emotional, and spiritual health of the patient and family—mind, body, and spirit
  2. Goal: maximize wellness, minimize complications, and provide an inner peace
  3. Includes common holistic therapies such as relaxation therapy, humor, massage, music, art, recreation, imagery, and pet therapy to reduce physiologic and psychologic stress
  4. Characteristics of the holistic team include the following:
     a) Excellent psychosocial and physical assessment skills
     b) Flexibility
     c) Ability to manage without the security of routines
     d) Mature and refined interpersonal skills and self-awareness
     e) Knowledge of family theory and the impact of illness on family functioning

E. Transitional care (also known as *sub-acute care*)
  1. Developed to provide the need for a more cost-effective approach to the treatment of patients with complex medical conditions and rehabilitation needs
  2. Goal: to achieve desired outcomes in a low-cost, humane setting
  3. Severity of the patient's condition requires:
     a) Frequent on-site visits from the physician
     b) Professional nursing care
     c) Significant ancillary services
     d) Outcome-focused, interdisciplinary approach using a professional team
     e) Complex medical and/or rehabilitation care

V. Outcomes management
  A. Definition
    1. Outcomes: the end results of care; what happens as a result of our care delivery structure and process
    2. Outcomes management: management with outcomes used to evaluate efficiency, improve patient care, reduce unintended variation, and compare facilities
  B. Goal: to improve efficiency in healthcare delivery by reducing unintended variation
  C. Focus
    1. Profession-independent and patient-focused outcomes
       a) Internal evaluation is to improve the results of patient care

       b) External evaluation is used to compare care delivery among facilities to assist the public in evaluating health care, reduce cost, and maintain quality
    2. Patient care improvement
  D. Variables
    1. Diagnosis
       a) Not sufficient as only variable
       b) Co-morbidities, severity of illness, and age contribute to outcomes
    2. Interventions
       a) Must mirror the complex realities of care delivery
       b) Monitoring one intervention and demonstrating its impact on patient outcomes is difficult
    3. Outcome indicators
       a) Early indicators of outcomes were the "five Ds": death, disease, disability, discomfort, and dissatisfaction
       b) Second generation indicators are more positive and broader in scope (e.g., functional status, quality of life)
       c) Clinical indicators should reflect desired outcomes and represent high-quality care delivery
  E. Care continuum
    1. Healthcare delivery traditionally has been fragmented
    2. The care continuum must provide a seamless integration of services across an entire illness, not emergent care, critical care, stepdown care, then rehabilitation
  F. Care environment
    1. Environments where nursing leaders have patient-centered expectations and nurses feel valued, trusted, and respected are associated with higher quality of patient care
    2. Mutual respect, interaction, coordination, and communication among medical and nursing staff members have a greater influence on patient outcomes than do specific therapies

VI. Change process
  A. Change is one constant in healthcare organizations
  B. Types of change
    1. Planned: active process with predetermined goals
       a) Three-step process
          (1) Unfreezing: restraining forces emerge that threaten the change, causing resistance to change
          (2) Moving: driving forces overcome restraining forces; movement toward acceptance
          (3) Refreezing: acceptance and incorporation of the change
    2. Unplanned: reactive process to change that was not planned

VII. Conflict resolution
  A. Communicate with the angry person
  B. Identify common goals (e.g., quality patient care)
  C. Discuss only one issue at a time; don't bring up old issues and anger
  D. Discuss facts, not opinions, judgments, or what others are saying; do not make personal attacks
  E. Communicate with the person involved; do not jump to a higher organizational level
VIII. Strategies for keeping patients satisfied (Long and Greeneich, 1994)
  A. Recognize that you own the problem, even if it is not your fault
  B. Do not just assess your patient's needs—reassess them
  C. Try to exceed your patient's expectations
IX. Remember that patients are healthcare consumers who want good service

Response to Diversity

I. Description: the sensitivity to recognize, appreciate, and incorporate differences into the provision of care
II. Cultural diversity
  A. Definitions
    1. Diversity: those differences that make each person unique; includes, but is not limited to, national origin, religion, age, gender, sexual orientation, race, ethnicity, education, socioeconomic status, abilities/disabilities
    2. Culture: the learned, shared, and transmitted values, beliefs, and practices of a particular group that guide thinking, actions, behaviors, interactions with others, emotional reactions to daily living, and one's world view; subculture: a recognizable segment of a larger cultural group that shares some characteristics of the larger group but with unique features of its own
    3. Cultural sensitivity: a learned skill in which a person has an awareness of and appreciation for another's cultural uniqueness; also referred to as *ethnosensitivity*
    4. Culturally congruent nursing care: use of cognitively based nursing techniques that incorporate an individual's cultural values, beliefs, and lifeways; these techniques facilitate, assist, support, and/or enable an individual toward health and well being, to face illness or death in culturally meaningful ways
    5. Race: a group of people related by common descent of heredity who have similar physical characteristics, such as skin color, facial form, eye shape, and so on
    6. Ethnic group: subset of culture; a smaller group that identifies itself as distinct because of shared characteristics, such as culture, language, traditions, appearance, and social heritage
    7. Nationality: a people from a place with specified political and geographic boundaries
    8. Customs: patterns and practices within a cultural group that encompass collective learned behaviors (includes diet and health behaviors)
    9. Rituals: culturally prescribed codes of behavior (may guide practices and decisions, including health and wellness)
    10. Values: personal standards of what is good or useful in relationship to oneself and to others
    11. Norms: commonly shared customs and standards of behavior that are acceptable within a given group of people
    12. Cultural paradigms: abstract explanation used by a cultural group to account for major life events
    13. Enculturation: the process by which culture is transmitted from one generation to the next by means of social learning
    14. Acculturation: the process by which an individual or group takes on the behaviors and practices of the dominant culture; factors that influence the degree and pace of an individual's acculturation include length of time in the new culture, age, economic/educational status, discriminatory practices of the dominant culture, and so on
    15. Ethnocentrism: the belief that one's own ethnic group, way of life, beliefs, values are superior to others
    16. Cultural imposition: the practice of imposing one's cultural beliefs on others with the belief that they are superior
    17. Cultural relativism: the attitude that the differences in ways of doing things hold equal validity
    18. Cultural pain: the discomfort or suffering experienced by an individual or group resulting from the insensitivity of others who have different beliefs and/or cultural norms
  B. Significance
    1. Of the developed countries in the world, the United States will experience the greatest increase in population and diversity of inhabitants; immigration will account for at least one third of the increase
      a) The percentage of whites of European origin (the dominant culture in the United States) will continue to decline, creating a more multicultural power base
    2. Nurses must be aware that issues of culture, race, gender, race and socioeconomics strongly influence health status and utilization of the healthcare system
      a) Culturally inappropriate care and inatten-

tion to cultural differences in care may negatively affect health outcomes

   b) Individuals from different cultures and illegal immigrants often delay seeking medical attention because of language, cost, and cultural barriers; these delays often result in more serious conditions

3. Healthcare reform is resulting in cultural competence guidelines and enforcement by state agencies

C. Aspects of cultural sensitivity

   1. Acknowledgment that cultural diversity exist

   2. Appreciation of the uniqueness of all patients, with culture as one aspect that enhances their uniqueness

   3. Respect of the unfamiliar

   4. Appreciation that cultural values are ingrained and difficult to change

   5. Modification of care to include consistency with the patient's culture

   6. Examination of personal cultural beliefs and values

   7. Realization that the patient's health practices may be very different from yours but that each cultural group has health practices that attempt to improve health and temper illness

   8. Recognition that all people within a cultural group do not respond to illness the same; diversity exists within cultures

D. Cultural assessment

   1. Assess degree of acculturation (how well language of the dominant culture is spoken, language spoken in the home, length of time in country, food preferences, etc.)

   2. Encourage the patient to discuss cultural beliefs and practices; definitions of health/ illness, origin of illnesses may differ within cultures

3. Make efforts to respect and understand different communication styles

4. Honor time and value orientation

5. Provide privacy according to individual's needs; be aware that in many cultures, it is extremely important for family members to be present during assessments

6. Identify the decision-maker within families; it may be someone other than the patient

7. Recognize that patients' reactions to pain are culturally driven

8. Be aware of biologic variations among cultures, such as body structure, skin/hair color, population-specific diseases, psychologic coping characteristics

9. Recognize that dietary/religious practices and cultural taboos have important implications related to nursing care

10. Identify hobbies

11. Note cultural practices and modify care as necessary

E. Cultural phenomena impacting nursing care (Fig. 13-3 and Table 13-8)

F. Cultural aspects of pain

   1. Pain is not purely a neurophysiologic response; cultural, social, and psychologic denominators influence pain

   2. Pain intensity, expression, tolerance, and expected responses from caretakers are influenced by culture

   3. A patient's attitude and beliefs about pain are determined by culture

   4. Each culture has its own language of distress

     a) Facial expressions

     b) Sounds

     c) Changes in activity

     d) Words to describe feelings

   5. Nurses must always remember that regardless

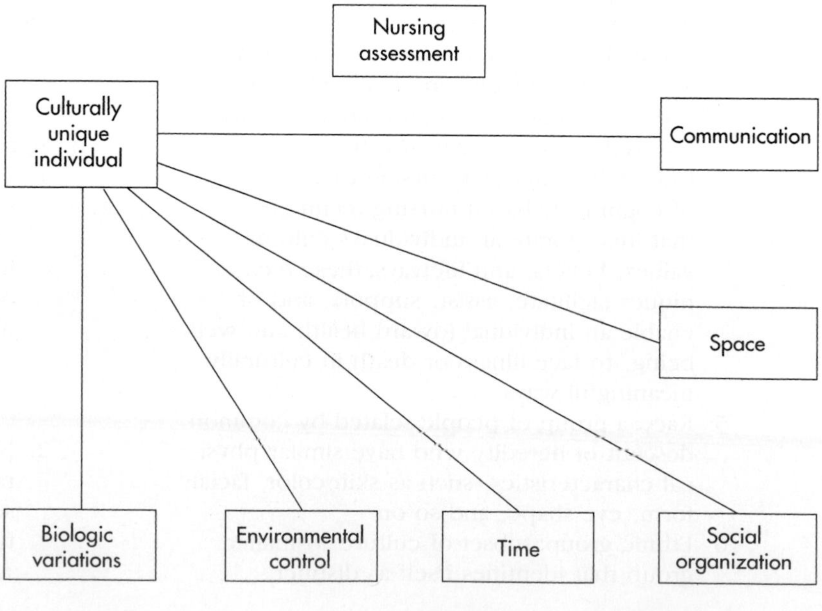

Figure 13-3 Application of cultural phenomena to nursing care and nursing practice. (From Davidhizer R, Giger J: *Transcultural nursing assessment and intervention*, ed 3, St Louis, 1999, Mosby.)

Table 13-8 **Cross-cultural Examples of Cultural Phenomena That Have an Impact on Nursing Care**

Nations of Origin	Communication	Space	Time Orientation	Social Organization	Environmental Control	Biological Variations
Asian China Hawaii Philippines Korea Japan Southeast Asia (Laos, Cambodia, Vietnam)	National language preference Dialects, written characters Use of silence Nonverbal and contextual cuing	Noncontact people	Present	Family: hierarchical structure, loyalty Devotion to tradition Many religions, including Taoism, Buddhism, Islam, and Christianity Community social organizations	Traditional health and illness beliefs Use of traditional medicines Traditional practitioners: Chinese doctors and herbalists	Liver cancer Stomach cancer Coccidioidomycosis Hypertension Lactose intolerance
African West Coast (as slaves) Many African countries West Indian Islands Dominican Republic Haiti Jamaica	National languages Dialect: pidgin, creole, Spanish, and French	Close personal space	Present over future	Family: many female, single parent Large, extended family networks Strong church affiliation within community Community social organizations	Traditional health and illness beliefs Folk medicine tradition Traditional healer: root-worker	Sickle cell anemia Hypertension Cancer of the esophagus Stomach cancer Coccidioidomycosis Lactose intolerance
Europe Germany England Italy Ireland Other European countries	National languages Many learn English immediately	Noncontact people Aloof Distant Southern countries: closer contact and touch	Future over present	Nuclear families Extended families Judeo-Christian religions Community social organizations	Primary reliance on modern health care system Traditional health and illness beliefs Some remaining folk medicine traditions	Breast cancer Heart disease Diabetes mellitus Thalassemia
Native American 500 Native American tribes Aleuts Eskimos	Tribal languages Use of silence and body language	Space very important and has no boundaries	Present	Extremely family oriented Biological and extended families Children taught to respect traditions Community social organizations	Traditional health and illness beliefs Folk medicine tradition Traditional healer: medicine man	Accidents Heart disease Cirrhosis of the liver Diabetes mellitus
Hispanic countries Spain Cuba Mexico Central and South America	Spanish or Portuguese primary language	Tactile relationships Touch Handshakes Embracing Value physical presence	Present	Nuclear family Extended families *Compadrazza:* godparents Community social organizations	Traditional health and illness beliefs Folk medicine tradition Traditional healers: *curandero, espiritisco, portera, señoro*	Diabetes mellitus Parasites Coccidioidomycosis Lactose intolerance

Compiled by Rachel Spector, RN, PhD, from Davidhizer R, Giger J: *Transcultural nursing assessment and intervention,* ed 3, St Louis, 1999, Mosby.

of the patient's cultural background, pain is what the patient says it is and it occurs when he or she says it does

   a) All pain should be considered "real" and treated compassionately

   b) Be aware that patients who do not verbally express the presence of pain may not be pain-free

G. Drug polymorphism

  1. Age, drug, gender, body size, and body composition affect individual response to drugs

  2. Factors that influence drug polymorphism vary among ethnic groups and can be categorized as environmental, genetic, and cultural; these do not include all the aspects that affect patient's response to drugs but raise awareness regarding possible differences in response

  3. Drug metabolism is genetically determined

  4. Race may affect response; also called *genetic polymorphism*

  5. Environmental factors include diet, alcohol, smoking, malnutrition, vitamin deficiencies, stress, fever, and physiologic rhythms; each of these factors can affect drug absorption

  6. Cultural factors include values, beliefs, compliance, family influence, and prior drug experience; patients may be taking herbal or homeopathic remedies that can alter response to drug absorption

  7. Nurses must become familiar with drugs that affect patients of different ethnicities; one example of this difference is that ACE inhibitors (e.g., captopril) are ineffective or minimally effective in African Americans (the angiotensin II blocker valsartan [Diovan] or a calcium channel blocker or beta-blocker are more likely to be used for hypertension in African Americans)

H. Cultural behaviors relevant to nursing care (Table 13-9)

I. Problems in providing culturally congruent health care; all of the following issues can lead to poor health outcomes:

  1. Stereotyping, prejudice, ignoring blind spots, and labeling

  2. Personal biases and bigotry

  3. Cultural differences, patients being labeled by nurses as "the difficult patient and/or family"

  4. Lack of interpreters and educational materials in patient's language

  5. Lack of diversity among nursing staff

  6. Lack of time (with culturally congruent care, listening to stories is important)

  7. Lack of flexibility with teaching methods

III. Religious diversity

A. Definitions

  1. Spirituality: a basic human phenomenon that helps create meaning in the world

    a) Encompasses a person's ideology, view of the world, and meaning of life

    b) It gives an individual a sense of inner peace and harmony

  2. Spiritual distress: disruption in the life principle that pervades a person's entire being and that integrates and transcends one's biologic and psychosocial nature

  3. Religion: a specific unified system of an expression of the belief in and reverence for a supernatural power accepted as the creator and governor of the universe

  4. Religious symbols: symbols used in the expression of faith (e.g., rosary, prayer cloth, prayer rug, medicine bundles, red ribbon, charms, "the garment")

  5. Meditation: a devotional exercise of contemplation

  6. Prayer: an intimate conversation between an individual and God or other Higher Being

  7. Hope: to wish for something with expectation of its fulfillment

  8. Faith: confident belief in the truth of a person, idea, or thing (e.g., God); belief not based on logical proof or material evidence

B. Significance

  1. Exclusion of the important role of spirituality for patients and families can have an impact on recovery and health

  2. Care of the whole person enhances healing and health

  3. Spiritual beliefs of providers may be an important consideration for many patients when selecting a healthcare provider

C. Causes of spiritual distress

  1. Separation from religious and cultural ties

  2. Challenged belief and value systems

  3. Sense of meaninglessness or purposelessness

  4. Remoteness from God

  5. Disrupted spiritual trust

  6. Moral or ethical nature of therapy

  7. Sense of guilt and shame

  8. Intense suffering

  9. Unresolved feelings about death

  10. Anger toward God

D. Aspects of spiritual sensitivity include the following:

  1. Perform self-exploration of your own values and beliefs

  2. Acknowledge that you may not agree with every aspect of the patient's spiritual beliefs and practices; be nonjudgmental and respect the patient's right to worship the Supreme Being of his or her choice

  3. Develop good listening skills; encourage patient to discuss spiritual concerns

  4. Know your limits; if you are uncomfortable discussing spiritual needs with the patient or praying with the patient, contact the patient's personal spiritual advisor or consult hospital chaplain service as requested by the patient and/or family

Table 13-9   Cultural Behaviors Relevant to Health Assessment

Cultural Group	Cultural Variations (Common Belief/Practice)	Nursing Implications
African Americans	Dialect and slang terms require careful communication to prevent error (e.g., "bad" may mean "good").	Question the client's meaning or intent.
Mexican Americans	Eye behavior is important. An individual who looks at and admires a child without touching the child has given the child the "evil eye."	Always touch the child you are examining or admiring.
Native Americans	Eye contact is considered a sign of disrespect and is thus avoided.	Recognize that the client may be attentive and interested even though eye contact is avoided.
Appalachians	Eye contact is considered impolite or a sign of hostility. Verbal patter may be confusing.	Avoid excessive eye contact. Clarify statements.
American Eskimos	Body language is very important. The individual seldom disagrees publicly with others. Client may nod yes to be polite, even if not in agreement.	Monitor own body language closely as well as client's to detect meaning.
Jewish Americans	Orthodox Jews consider excess touching, particularly from members of the opposite sex, offensive.	Establish whether client is an Orthodox Jew and avoid excessive touch.
Chinese Americans	Individual may nod head to indicate yes or shake head to indicate no. Excessive eye contact indicates rudeness. Excessive touch is offensive.	Ask questions carefully and clarify responses. Avoid excessive eye contact and touch.
Filipino Americans	Offending people is to be avoided at all cost. Nonverbal behavior is very important.	Monitor nonverbal behaviors of self and client, being sensitive to physical and emotional discomfort or concerns of the client.
Haitian Americans	Touch is used in conversation. Direct eye contact is used to gain attention and respect during communication.	Use direct eye contact when communicating.
East Indian Hindu Americans	Women avoid eye contact as a sign of respect.	Be aware that men may view eye contact by women as offensive. Avoid eye contact.
Vietnamese Americans	Avoidance of eye contact is a sign of respect. The head is considered sacred; it is not polite to pat the head. An upturned palm is offensive in communication.	Limit eye contact. Touch the head only when mandated and explain clearly before proceeding to do so. Avoid hand gesturing.

From Davidhizer R, Giger J: *Transcultural nursing assessment and intervention*, ed 3. St Louis, 1999, Mosby.

5. Schedule physical care to allow religious rituals and practices
6. Respect the patient's rights and privacy
7. Increase your knowledge regarding different faiths (Table 13-10 identifies selected faiths and nursing implications)
E. Perform spiritual needs assessment
1. Assess the patient's spiritual or religious beliefs, values, and practices
2. Listen for verbal cues regarding spirituality (e.g., referring to God/spiritualist, talking about church, prayer, synagogue, etc.)
3. Note the presence of religious symbols (e.g., crucifix, star of David, Bible, Torah, Qur'an, or other spiritual books, prayer cloth) in room during interview
4. Listen for expressions of spiritual distress (expressed hopelessness or guilt, crying,

sleep disturbances, disrupted spiritual trust, loss of meaning and purpose in life)
5. Be alert to comments related to spiritual concerns or conflicts (e.g., "Why me, God?" "I'm being punished for my sins")
6. Determine if the patient wishes to participate in religious or spiritual practices (such as communion) during hospitalization
7. Identify specific religious concerns such as dietary needs, refusal to accept blood
F. Provide care sensitive to the patient's spiritual/ religious needs
1. Convey a caring, nonjudgmental attitude
2. Inform the patient and family of the availability of spiritual/religious services (e.g., pastoral care, chapel, religious services, religious books, communion, baptism, last rites)

Table 13-10	Religious Beliefs of Selected Religions and Appropriate Nursing Interventions	
Religion	**Belief**	**Interventions**
Catholicism	• God does not cause suffering but allows it for furthering human growth • Baptism is necessary for salvation	• Inform patient that Holy Communion is available • Have Catholic priest available to perform Anointing of the Sick • If patient is close to death and a Catholic religious representative is not available, any Christian may perform the baptism and then notify the priest immediately • Make all efforts to leave religious symbols (e.g., rosary) in place
Christian Scientist	• Sin, sickness, and death can be overcome by a full understanding of the divine principle of Jesus' teaching and healing • Disease and illness is a delusion of the nonspiritual mind and can be overcome by prayer	• Be aware that medical care may be refused • May utilize the services of physicians for the purpose of setting bones, treatment of malignancies, and delivering babies • Pain medications may be accepted for severe pain only • There is no clergy or priesthood but there are "readers"
Hinduism	• Illness may result from misuse of the body or sins from a previous lifetime • Meditation and prayer must be done at specific times throughout the day • Females cannot be left in the presence of an unfamiliar male	• Plan care around religious practices • Provide same-sex caregivers • Provide vegetarian meals as requested • May refuse medication by capsule since many capsules are made from meat • Allow the family to wash the family member's body following death if desired; do not remove any sacred threads that are placed on the body
Islam (Muslim)	• Submit to Allah's will in matters of health • Prayer and washing required five times a day • The left hand is considered unclean; food will not be handled with the left hand	• Provide privacy and plan care to accommodate prayer times • Educate regarding pain-reducing techniques • Provide diet with dietary restrictions as requested • Pork and some other foods prohibited • May refuse to take capsules since many are made from pork • Follow patient and family wishes regarding therapies; prolonging life by life support machinery is often seen as unacceptable • Allow family to stay with relative during process of dying • Allow family to wash body after death • Turn deceased person's face toward the right
Jehovah's Witnesses	• Opposed to transfusions of blood obtained from a blood bank and some blood products (the source of the soul is believed to be in the blood) • Opposed to eating foods to which blood has been added • Do not celebrate national holidays (including Christmas), birthdays, or salute flags; it is believed that violators will spend an eternity in nothingness	• Assess the patient's religious beliefs and practices before administering blood or blood products • Most Witnesses carry cards indicating types of acceptable transfusions • "Mature minors," according to Jehovah's Witness standards, may refuse blood transfusions • Be aware that the patient may refuse surgical or medical interventions that will require blood transfusion • Consider the use of volume expanders such as saline, lactated Ringer's solution, hetastarch (Hespan) • Implement blood-conservation strategies, especially in children • Consult hematologist and/or medical centers familiar with bloodless medicine and surgery management, if needed • Respect patient and family decisions to refuse blood products • Avoid foods to which blood has been added (e.g., certain sausages, lunch meats) • Avoid attempts to involve the patient in preparations for celebrations of national holidays

Table 13-10 Religious Beliefs of Selected Religions and Appropriate Nursing Interventions—cont'd

Religion	Belief	Interventions
Judaism	• Sabbath begins at sundown on Friday and ends at sundown on Saturday • There is hope for recovery until death is imminent • May not eat non-Kosher foods • Orthodox Jews: work of any kind is prohibited on the Sabbath, including driving or using the telephone • Orthodox Jews: prayer required three times a day • A person must stay with a critically ill or dying family member until death so that the soul will not feel alone	• Provide Kosher diet as requested • Provide privacy and plan care considering prayer times • Allow a relative to stay with the dying patient • Notify Rabbi/Rebbe according to family's wishes • Caregivers should leave the body untouched for approximately one half hour after death to allow the soul to depart • After death, by Judaic law, the body cannot be left alone • Autopsies generally not allowed unless required by law • Assist and respect practices of the Sabbath • Do not shave body hair of Hasidic Jews • Hasidic/Orthodox: provide same-sex caregivers
Seventh-Day Adventist	• Sabbath is recognized as dusk on Friday to dusk on Saturday • The body is a temple of God and should be kept healthy	• Provide diet with dietary restrictions as requested • The Church encourages a vegetarian diet • Be aware that patient may avoid seafood, meat, caffeine, alcohol, drugs, and tobacco • Protein and iodine deficiency may occur • Be aware that the patient may refuse procedures (medical or surgical) that occur on the Sabbath

3. Inform the patient and family of policies related to clergy visitation
4. Provide privacy and opportunities for religious practices, such as prayer and meditation
5. Prepare the patient for desired religious rituals
6. Join in prayer or reading of scripture if comfortable
    a) If you are comfortable praying with the patient and family, the following suggestions may be helpful:
        (1) Trust God or other Higher Power to enable you to know what to do and what to say
        (2) Really listen to the patient so that you know what the patient's and family's greatest concerns are
        (3) Explore the spiritual needs of the patient; ask the patient what he or she would like for God or other Higher Power to do
        (4) Be sensitive and respectful
        (5) Hold the patient's hand or stroke his or her arm, if culturally appropriate
    b) If you are not comfortable praying with or providing other spiritual support for the patient and family, call patient's own spiritual advisor or a representative of pastoral care to pray with or comfort the patient and family
7. Notify chaplain or patient's own spiritual advisor of the patient's spiritual distress (with the patient's permission)

8. Provide honest information to aid in informed decision making when spiritual beliefs and therapeutic regimens are in conflict
G. Problems in providing spirituality-sensitive health care
    1. Avoiding or minimizing the role of spirituality in patient healing
    2. Treating religious beliefs as mental illness
    3. Failure to involve patient and family in decision making
    4. Giving information that can lead to false hope
    5. Not allowing the patient an opportunity to work through grief

Clinical Inquiry or Innovator/Evaluator

I. Description: the ongoing process of questioning and evaluating practice, providing informed practice, and innovating through research and experimental learning
II. Nursing research
    A. Primary goal of nursing research: develop a specialized, scientifically based body of nursing knowledge to facilitate improvement in patient care
    B. Definitions
        1. Scientific method: systematic approach to solving problems that controls variables and biases
        2. Basic research: research to advance knowledge; helps in understanding relationships among phenomena
        3. Applied research: research to solve a particu-

lar problem; helps in making decisions or evaluating techniques

4. Variable: concept examined in a research study
   a) Independent variable: the presumed cause manipulated by the researcher to observe the effect in a cause-and-effect relationship
   b) Dependent variable: the response or outcome the researcher would like to explain or predict
   c) Extraneous variable: a factor that can affect the dependent variable and interfere with research results

5. Hypothesis: statement that predicts a relationship among two or more variables; may be simple, complex, directional, nondirectional, or null

C. Research types
   1. Quantitative research: deductive process that tests hypotheses and examines cause-and-effect relationships to explore specific phenomena; emphasizes facts and data to validate or extend existing knowledge
      a) Experimental: uses randomization and a control group to test the effects of an intervention
      b) Quasi-experimental: involves manipulation of variables but lacks a comparison group or randomization
      c) Nonexperimental
         (1) Descriptive: describes situations, experiences, and phenomena as they exist
         (2) Ex post facto (correlational): describes relationships among variables
   2. Qualitative: inductive process used to understand phenomena in a defined context; emphasizes development of new insights, theory, and knowledge
      a) Relies less on numbers and measurements and more on nursing strategies, interpersonal communication techniques, intuition, and collaboration between nurse and patient to discover underlying relationships
      b) Includes case studies, open–ended questions, field studies, and participant observation

D. Steps in the research process:
   1. Formulate the research problem
   2. Review related literature
   3. Formulate the hypothesis
   4. Select the research design
   5. Identify the population to be studied
   6. Specify methods of data collection
   7. Design the study
   8. Conduct the study
   9. Analyze the data
   10. Interpret the results
   11. Communicate the findings
   12. Utilize the findings to improve patient care

E. Ethical responsibilities related to nursing research studies
   1. Protect the rights of research subjects
   2. Ensure that the potential benefits of the study outweigh any potential risk to the subjects
   3. Submit the proposed study for review by the investigational review committee
   4. Obtain informed consent from each subject

F. Nursing responsibilities related to research
   1. Identifying problem areas and research questions for investigation
   2. Assist in collection of data as requested
   3. Read and interpret reports of nursing research
   4. Assess the quality of nursing research studies and applicability to practice
   5. Apply research findings to change clinical practice and improve patient care
   6. Share research findings with peers
   7. Design and conduct nursing research

G. Use of nursing research in clinical practice
   1. Transferring research-based findings to the clinical setting
      a) Identify the clinical problem
      b) Conduct a literature review for pertinent research studies
      c) Evaluate and critique the research studies
      d) Determine the relevance of the research findings to clinical practice
      e) Identify the desired outcome(s)
      f) Use research findings to modify current clinical practice
      g) Teach clinicians about change in clinical practice
      h) Evaluate the outcomes and compare with desired outcomes
      i) Revise as necessary
   2. Keep clinical practice current and optimal
      a) Share current research findings with other nurses
         (1) Bulletin boards for current articles
         (2) Journal clubs
         (3) Patient care conferences
         (4) Protocol and procedure development
         (5) Care paths
      b) Keep procedure descriptions current
         (1) Procedures should be written by staff nurses who actually perform the procedure
         (2) Nurses assigned to rewrite a procedure should thoroughly research current practice recommendations related to the procedure rather than just confirming how it is currently being performed at the institution

III. Quality assurance and improvement
   A. Goal: ensure a specified degree of quality in patient care through continuous measurement and evaluation; the focus is on change and improvement

B. Stages of quality assurance
   1. Measurement of observed nursing practice
      a) Structure evaluation: examines the components of services, such as the setting and environment, that affect quality of care
      b) Process evaluation: examines activities and behaviors of the healthcare provider (e.g., nurse)
      c) Outcome evaluation: measures changes in behaviors and attitudes of patients
   2. Comparison of observed practice with expectations
      a) Retrospective review: examination of completed healthcare delivery by reviewing charts, conducting conferences or interviews, reviewing questionnaires
      b) Concurrent review: evaluation of a patient's health status (outcome audit) or management (process) while ongoing by chart reviews, interviews, and observation of the patient
   3. Implementation of change to reconcile discrepancies between observations and expectations
C. Total quality management (TQM) and Continuous Quality Improvement (CQI)
   1. Healthcare team members monitor quality, identify problems, and devise solutions; more decentralized
   2. The philosophy of these techniques is more consumer-based; change is based on the patient's needs, not the values of the healthcare providers
   3. Goals may include improved patient care, patient satisfaction, or improved employee morale, decreased cost, elimination of duplication of services; the focus is on results rather than on daily activities

Facilitator of Learning of Patient/Family Educator

I. Description: the ability to facilitate patient and family learning
II. Definitions
   A. Teaching: the process of facilitating learning; an interaction designed to help a person learn to do something that he or she is currently unable to do; a two-way interaction
   B. Learning: the process by which a person becomes capable of doing something he or she could not do before, including a wide range of behavior, from motor skills to intellectual skills; an emotional experience that can be negative or positive, traumatic, or pleasant
   C. Patient education: the process of teaching patients and their families about the illness, treatment, and other health-related matters, including how to adhere to the regimen and helping them change their behavior
III. Reasons for patient education
   A. Because the patient has a need and a right to know those things that are relevant to his or her condition, disease, or situation
   B. To produce changes in knowledge, skills, attitudes, appreciation, and understanding
   C. To promote and improve health
   D. To encourage the patient to assume responsibility for disease management
   E. To prevent illness and complications
   F. To aid in coping with illness and adaptation to change
   G. To promote compliance with the therapeutic regimen
   H. To reduce anxiety (including family stress and anxiety)
   I. To reduce number of physician's office and/or emergency department visits and number and length of hospitalizations
IV. Principles of adult education
   A. Qualities of the adult learner: a self-directed independent person who becomes ready to learn when the need to know or to perform is experienced; characteristics of the adult learner include the following:
      1. Goal-oriented
      2. Less flexible
      3. Requires longer time in the performance of learning tasks
      4. Impatient in the pursuit of objectives
      5. Finds little use for isolated facts
      6. Strives for recognition and success
      7. Has multiple responsibilities, all of which draw on his or her time
      8. Experienced in the "school of life"
      9. Requires a more constant and ideal learning environment
      10. Usually comes to the teaching program on a voluntary basis
      11. Wishes to be involved in mutual planning of learning experiences
      12. Likes to participate in diagnosing needs for learning, formulating learning objectives, and evaluating learning
      13. Expects a climate of mutual respect, trust, and collaboration that supports learning
   B. Educational concepts useful with adults
      1. Pacing
         a) Allow adults to set their own pace, if possible
         b) Tasks or methods involving significant time pressure are likely to be difficult for adults
      2. Arousal anxiety
         a) Some degree of arousal is necessary for learning; however, older adults may become anxious in a learning situation
         b) Allow individuals an opportunity to become familiar with the situation
         c) Minimize the role of competition and evaluation
      3. Fatigue
         a) Some tasks may produce considerable mental or physical fatigue, a problem

that is likely to particularly affect older adults

b) Shorten the instruction sessions or provide frequent rest breaks

4. Difficulty: arrange materials from the simple to the complex in order to build individual's confidence and skills

5. Errors: structure the tasks so errors are avoided and do not have to be unlearned

6. Practice: provide an opportunity for practice on similar but different tasks; such practice helps to develop generalizable skills

7. Feedback: provide information on the adequacy of previous responses

8. Cues
   a) Materials should be presented to compensate for the potential sensory problems of older adults
   b) Direct attention toward the relevant aspects of the task
   c) Reduce the level of irrelevant information to a minimum

9. Organization
   a) Learning and remembering often require that information be grouped or related in some way
   b) Instruct individuals in the use of various mnemonic techniques (mental images, verbal associations, etc.), which may be used to elaborate or organize the material

10. Relevance/experience
    a) People learn and remember what is important to them
    b) Attempt to make the task relevant to individual's concerns
    c) Performance is likely to be facilitated to the extent that the individuals are able to integrate the new information with known information

V. Barriers to teaching/learning
   A. Nurse factors: lack of time, lack of knowledge, consideration of teaching as a lower priority than physical care
   B. Physician interference
   C. Patient factors
      1. Physiologic instability
      2. Psychologic factors (e.g., anxiety, pain)
      3. Poor language or reading skills
      4. Sensory deficits: vision, hearing
      5. Poor manual dexterity for psychomotor skills
      6. Attitudes and beliefs that conflict with teaching

VI. Teaching/learning process
   A. Assessment
      1. Readiness to learn
         a) Desire to know (e.g., asking questions)
         b) Absence of acute distress (e.g., pain, dyspnea)
         c) Adequate energy

2. Sensory deficits (e.g., use of eyeglasses, hearing aid)
3. Educational level and reading ability
4. Learning style
   a) Environment
      (1) Formal or informal
      (2) Tolerance to distraction
   b) Alone or in a group
   c) Preferred learning mode
      (1) Reading: print materials
      (2) Seeing: pictorial materials
      (3) Listening: auditory
      (4) Manipulating: tactile, kinesthetic

B. Plan
   1. Identify objectives; parts of the objective should include the following:
      a) What should the learner be able to do? (behavior)
         (1) Cognitive
         (2) Affective
         (3) Psychomotor
      b) How well should he or she be able to do it? (the criteria)
      c) Under what conditions should he or she be able to do it? (the condition)
   2. Identify content to teach
      a) Language and terminology
      b) Healthcare system: personnel, organization and structure, routines and procedures, norms and expectations, immediate environment
      c) Basic anatomy and physiology of affected body system
      d) Diagnosis, disease process
      e) Therapy: treatments, medications, diet, activity, personal health habits
      f) Prevention of complications
      g) Skills (e.g., insulin administration, pulse taking)
      h) Community resources
   3. Determine methods
      a) Individual or group
         (1) Use individual method when you are assessing patient's knowledge, when family members or friends try to dominate teaching sessions, when the information you'll teach provokes anxiety or is considered a topic not generally discussed in public
         (2) Individual methods include programmed instruction, reading materials, audiovisual aids, one-to-one instruction
         (3) Group sessions lessen feelings of alienation and being "different"; learners learn from other learners
         (4) Patient-operated groups and self-help groups offer the benefit of encouraging patients to share coping techniques and useful hints

(5) Group teaching saves time and money

(6) Family members gain support from health professionals as well as other patients and their families

(7) Combinations may be helpful to meet the patient's individual needs

b) Teaching methods: the teacher of adults is a facilitator more than a teacher; use various methods

  (1) Lecture

    (a) May be in group session, on videotape, or on closed-circuit television

    (b) Is usually no longer than 20 minutes

    (c) Includes introduction to establish the need to know, body to deliver content that needs to be known, and summary to review what was covered

  (2) Discussion

    (a) Helps the patient to ask any questions about information that is in doubt

    (b) Guides the nurse to assess what the patient needs to know more about

  (3) Audiovisuals

    (a) Includes visual and auditory stimulation to teach content

  (4) Printed materials

    (a) May be used in place of other techniques but should include a discussion with the nurses after reading for clarification of content

    (b) May be used as a supplement to other methods

    (c) Useful as an aid to review at a later date

    (d) Should be written at approximately fourth-grade level; picture books may be especially helpful in multilanguage areas

  (5) Explanations

    (a) Give only as much information as requested

    (b) Ask for feedback

  (6) Exploration: encourage patient to answer own questions

  (7) Demonstration and return demonstration

    (a) Used when the patient must learn a new skill

    (b) Describe what you are going to do, then do it while the patient observes; then talk to the patient through the process while he or she does it; finally, have the patient perform the skill while he or she tells you what he or she is doing

  (8) Role playing

    (a) Provides practice in a safe setting

    (b) Useful to see how others might respond

C. Implement

1. Assign one person to teach the patient to minimize confusion, contradiction, and incompleteness

2. Schedule teaching sessions according to the patient's receptiveness; let the patient set the pace and choose topics of most interest first

3. Provide ideal setting: control the environment

4. Know your subject area: be competent and confident

5. Speak the patient's language: minimize use of medical terminology

6. Consider your presentation style

  a) Keep the presentations of material short

  b) Place key points up front

  c) Use verbal headings

  d) Summarize at the end

  e) Obtain feedback and request questions

7. Include "why" where appropriate

8. Use visual aids

9. Remember that successful learning takes time and reinforcement

10. Provide a means for the patient to learn more, such as written information for reading and review, resource groups

11. Coordinate education through written teaching plans, patient care conferences, and documentation

  a) Written teaching plans should include the following:

    (1) Objectives

    (2) Content

    (3) Teaching methods

    (4) Methods of evaluation

  b) Documentation should include the following:

    (1) Objectives

    (2) Content outline

    (3) Method used

    (4) Evaluation of learning

      (a) How was learning evaluated?

      (b) Evaluation of learning

        (i) Objective met

        (ii) Objective partially met—needs reinforcement

        (iii) Objective not met—needs repetition

    (5) Comments

    (6) Signature

D. Evaluate learning using any of the following methods:

1. Written tests

2. Oral evaluation

3. Return demonstration
4. Analysis of physical findings (e.g., serum glucose, weight)
5. Follow-up questionnaire

VII. Education for low-literacy individuals
   A. Definition: adults with poorly developed skills in reading, writing, listening and speaking
   B. Assessing literacy level
      1. Individuals reading at a fifth-grade or higher level are considered literate; hand printing instructions and asking the patient to read them back to you is a nonthreatening way to assess reading ability
      2. Incongruent behavior may signal a literacy problem; be alert for behavior that does not match the reported level of understanding
      3. Low-literacy materials are preferred for low-literacy individuals
   C. Teaching strategies for low-literacy patients
      1. Identify and eliminate or minimize stress, anxiety, or other distractions before teaching
      2. Correct misconceptions that affect learning
      3. Personalize the health message and explain the need for the information

4. Relate information to patient's past experiences and actively involve the patient and family in discussions
5. Consider qualities of poor readers and utilize teaching strategies that are helpful (Table 13-11)

Table 13-11	Qualities of Poor Readers and Appropriate Teaching Strategies	
Qualities of Poor Readers	**Teaching Strategies**
Take words literally	Explain the meaning of all words
Read slowly; miss meaning	Use common words and examples
Skip over uncommon words	Use examples, review content often
Miss content	Describe content first, use verbal heading and visuals
Tire quickly	Use short segments

LEARNING ACTIVITIES

1. **DIRECTIONS:** Complete the following crossword puzzle.

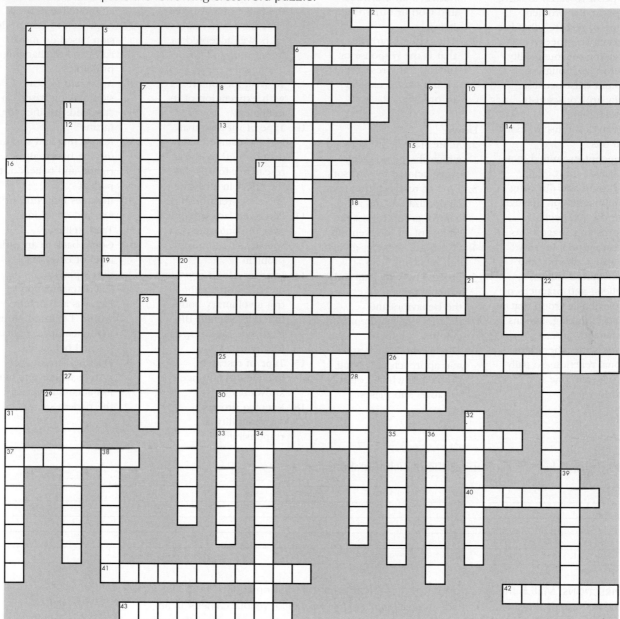

Across

1. Involves the insertion of needles into specific points in the body for therapeutic purposes
4. Working together
6. Basic human phenomenon that helps create meaning in the world

7. Approach to ethical decision making where beneficence should take precedence over autonomy
10. Type of consent that must be obtained prior to procedures and inclusion in study groups

12. Type of evaluation or review that might look at physiologic parameter
13. Process by which a person becomes capable of doing something he or she could not previously do
15. Doing good

16. Group of people related by common descent of heredity who have similar physical characteristics, such as skin color, facial form, eye shape, etc.
17. Belief not based on logical proof or material evidence

19. Avoiding harm
21. Process of facilitating learning
24. Respecting privileged information
25. Type of research to solve a particular problem
26. Type of research that is a deductive process
29. Treating obvious reality factors as though they do not exist because they are consciously intolerable
30. Involves the use of essential oils
33. Concept examined in a research study
35. Focusing and directing the imagination through the use of specific words and suggestions
37. Treating people fairly
40. Learned, shared, and transmitted values, beliefs, and practices of a particular group that guide thinking, actions, behaviors, interactions with others, emotional reactions to daily living, and one's world view

41. Directing energy from unacceptable drives into socially acceptable behavior
42. Intimate conversation between an individual and God or other Higher Being
43. The type of variable that is the response or outcome the researcher would like to explain or predict

Down
2. Acute state of stress in which the person feels overwhelmed by stressors
3. Type of research that uses randomization and a control group to test the effects of an intervention
4. Process of seeking, giving, and receiving help
5. Process by which an individual or group takes on the behaviors and practices of the dominant culture
6. This method is a systematic approach to solving problems, which controls variables and biases

7. Unconsciously attributing one's own unacceptable qualities and emotions to others
8. Specific unified system of an expression of the belief in and reverence for a supernatural power accepted as the creator and governor of the universe
9. To wish for something with expectation of its fulfillment
10. Type of variable that is the presumed cause manipulated by the researcher to observe the effect in a cause-and-effect relationship
11. Perceived lack of control over the outcome of a specific situation or problem
14. Involves use of conscious mental effort to control involuntary body function, such as BP, heart rate, and respiratory rate
15. Type of research intended to advance knowledge
18. Keeping promises
20. Answerability or responsibility

22. Statement that predicts a relationship among two or more variables
23. Culturally prescribed codes of behavior
26. Type of research that is an inductive process
27. Approach to ethical decision based on moral rules and unchanging principles
28. Approach to ethical decision making based on "the ends justifies the means"
30. Respecting and supporting the basic values, rights, and beliefs of the patient
31. Includes behavior, criteria, and condition
32. Truth telling
34. Going back to an earlier level of emotional development
36. Self-determination
38. Patterns and practices within a cultural group that encompass collective learned behaviors
39. Nursing care delivery system where one nurse has accountability for the patient's care

2. **Directions:** List the six steps of the decision-making process.
1. _____
2. _____
3. _____
4. _____
5. _____
6. _____

3. **Directions:** Match the situation with the ethical principle demonstrated.

____ The new surgical resident has made three attempts to place a central venous catheter in an elderly patient. The nurse insists that no more attempts be made until the attending physician is present.

____ There is a code on the patient in the bed next to your patient. Your patient asks you if the patient died. You reply that despite exhaustive efforts, the patient did die.

____ The patient has decided that he or she does not want to be intubated again.

____ The nurse explains to the patient that care will still be provided despite the fact that he or she has no health insurance.

____ The nurse's next-door neighbor is in the hospital. She visits him, but she does not read his chart.

____ The nurse begins on time, takes only the allotted time for lunch, and leaves after completion of work and report.

____ The confused patient keeps reaching for his or her endotracheal tube. The nurse applies soft restraints to prevent self-extubation.

a. Veracity
b. Confidentiality
c. Autonomy
d. Nonmaleficence
e. Fidelity
f. Justice
g. Advocacy

4. **DIRECTIONS:** Match the level of Maslow's Hierarchy of Needs to the example.

____Physiologic   a. Art and music
____Safety and security   b. Water
____Love and belonging   c. Promotion at work
____Esteem and recognition   d. Marriage
____Self-actualization   e. Home security

5. **DIRECTIONS:** List eight complementary therapies that are helpful with patients with stress, anxiety, or pain.

1. _____
2. _____
3. _____
4. _____
5. _____
6. _____
7. _____
8. _____

6. **DIRECTIONS:** List five of the most important needs of families as identified by Leske.

1. _____
2. _____
3. _____
4. _____
5. _____

7. **DIRECTIONS:** List five of the essential elements of collaboration.

1. _____
2. _____
3. _____
4. _____
5. _____

8. **DIRECTIONS:** List and describe the three steps in the change process.

1. _____
2. _____
3. _____

9. **DIRECTIONS:** Identify the following as T (true) or F (false).

a. The nurse's own values and beliefs will not affect his or her sensitivities with patients.   True   False
b. Pain is influenced by culture.   True   False
c. Race is not a factor in drug absorption and action.   True   False
d. It is never appropriate for a nurse to pray with a patient; he or she should call the chaplain.   True   False
e. Decisions concerning medical care should be made by the physician alone.   True   False
f. Physical care should always take precedence over psychosocial and spiritual care.   True   False
g. Inability to speak English is an indication of ignorance.   True   False

10. **DIRECTIONS:** Match the religion with the implication.

____Islam (Muslim)   a. Provide Kosher diet as requested
____Catholicism   b. Opposed to blood transfusions
____Judaism   c. Provide same-sex caregivers
____Hinduism   d. Medical care may be refused; prayer is used as the primary treatment of illness
____Christian Scientist   e. The patient must be baptized before death
____Seventh-Day Adventist   f. Procedures may be refused between dusk on Friday to dusk on Saturday
____Jehovah's Witnesses   g. The patient's head is turned to the right after death

11. **DIRECTIONS:** List five ways to share research findings with colleagues.

1. _____
2. _____
3. _____
4. _____
5. _____

12. **DIRECTIONS:** List five qualities of an adult learner.

1. _____
2. _____
3. _____
4. _____
5. _____

LEARNING ACTIVITIES ANSWERS

1.

2. 1. Information collection and problem identification
2. Identification of possible solutions or actions
3. Analysis of the possible consequences of each solution or action
4. Selection of the best possible solution or action for implementation
5. Implementation of the solution or action
6. Evaluation of the results

3. g. (Advocacy) The new resident has made three attempts to place a central venous catheter in an elderly patient. The nurse insists that no more attempts are made until the attending physician is present.

a. (Veracity) There is a code in the bed next to your patient. Your patient asks you if the patient died. You reply that despite exhaustive efforts, the patient did die.

c. (Autonomy) The patient has decided that he or she does not want to be intubated again.

f. (Justice) The nurse explains to the patient that care will still be provided despite the fact that he or she has no health insurance.

b. (Confidentiality) The nurse's next-door neighbor is in the hospital. She visits him, but she does not read his chart.

e. (Fidelity) The nurse begins on time, takes only the allotted time for lunch, and leaves after completion of work and report.

d. (Nonmaleficence) The confused patient keeps reaching for his or her endotracheal tube. The nurse applies soft restraints to prevent self-extubation.

4. _b_ Physiologic
    _e_ Safety and security
    _d_ Love and belonging
    _c_ Esteem and recognition
    _a_ Self-actualization

5. Any eight of the following:
    - Progressive muscle relaxation (PMR)
    - Breathing
    - Meditation
    - Co-meditation
    - Guided imagery
    - Massage
    - Hypnosis
    - Biofeedback
    - Therapeutic (or healing) touch
    - Purposeful touch
    - Music therapy
    - Aromatherapy
    - Pet therapy
    - Humor
    - Acupuncture

6. Any five of the following:
    - To have questions answered honestly
    - To be assured the best care possible is being given to the patient
    - To know the prognosis
    - To feel hopeful
    - To know specific facts about the patient's progress
    - To be called at home about changes in the patient's condition
    - To know how the patient is being treated medically
    - To feel that hospital personnel care about the patient
    - To receive information about the patient daily
    - To have understandable explanations
    - To know exactly what is being done for the patient
    - To know why things were done for the patient
    - To see the patient often
    - To talk to the doctor every day
    - To be told about transfer plans

7. Any five of the following:
    - Communication

- Trust
- Respect
- Understanding and acceptance of team members' roles
- Competence
- Shared responsibility and accountability
- Shared goal-setting
- Flexibility
- Administrative support

8. 1. Unfreezing: resistance
    2. Moving: movement toward acceptance
    3. Refreezing: acceptance and incorporation of the change

9. a. False
    b. True
    c. False
    d. False
    e. False
    f. False
    g. False

10. _g_ Islam (Muslim)
    _e_ Catholicism
    _a_ Judaism
    _c_ Hinduism
    _d_ Christian Scientist
    _f_ Seventh-Day Adventist
    _b_ Jehovah's Witnesses

11. - Bulletin boards for current articles
    - Journal clubs
    - Patient care conferences
    - Protocol and procedure development
    - Care paths

12. Any five of the following:
    - Goal-oriented
    - Less flexible
    - Requires longer time in the performance of learning tasks
    - Impatient in the pursuit of objectives
    - Finds little use for isolated facts
    - Strives for recognition and success
    - Has multiple responsibilities, all of which draw on his or her time
    - Experienced in the "school of life"
    - Requires a more constant and ideal learning environment
    - Usually comes to the teaching program on a voluntary basis
    - Wishes to be involved in mutual planning of learning experiences
    - Likes to participate in diagnosing needs for learning, formulating learning objectives, and evaluating learning
    - Expects a climate of mutual respect, trust, and collaboration that supports learning

Bibliography and Selected References

Alexander R, Steefel L: Biofeedback: listen to the body, *RN* 58 (8):51, 1995.

Alfaro-LeFevre R: *Critical thinking in nursing: a practical approach*, Philadelphia, 1995, WB Saunders.

Allen L: Treating agitation without drugs, *AJN* 99 (4):36, 1999.

Alspach G: Alternative and complementary therapies: treading tentatively out of the mainstream, *Critical Care Nursing* 18 (5):13, 1998.

Andrews J: *Cultural, ethnic, and religious reference manual for healthcare providers*, ed 2, Winston-Salem, 1999, JAMARDA Resources.

Andrews M, Boyle J: *Transcultural concepts in nursing care*, ed 3, Philadelphia, 1999, Lippincott.

Angelucci P: Spirituality and the use of an intensive care unit on-staff/on-site chaplain, *Critical Care Nurse* 19 (4):62, 1999.

Antai-Otong D: Active listening at work, *AJN* 99 (2):24L, 1999.

Atsberger D: Relaxation therapy: its potential as an intervention for acute postoperative pain, *Journal of Post Anesthesia Nursing* 10 (1):2, 1995.

Barkauskas V, et al.: *Health assessment*, ed 2, St Louis, 1998, Mosby.

Barter M: Delegation and supervision outside the hospital, *AJN* 99 (7):24A, 1999.

Benson H: Commentary: self-care, the three-legged stool, and remembered wellness, *Journal of Cardiovascular Nursing* 10 (3):1, 1996.

Berrio M, Levesque M: Advance directives: most patients don't have one. Do yours? *AJN* 96 (8):25, 1996.

Bryan-Brown C, Dracup K: Alternative therapies, *American Journal of Critical Care* 4 (6): 416, 1995.

Buckle J: Clinical aromatherapy and touch: complementary therapies for nursing practice, *Critical Care Nurse* 18 (5):54, 1998.

Byers J, Smyth K: Effect of a music intervention on noise annoyance, heart rate, and blood pressure in cardiac surgery patients, *American Journal of Critical Care* 6 (3):183, 1997.

Camp P: Having faith: experiencing coronary artery bypass grafting, *Journal of Cardiovascular Nursing* 10 (3):55, 1996.

Casey A: Complementary therapies resource list, *Journal of Cardiovascular Nursing* 10 (3):87, 1996.

Cassidy C: Want to know how you're doing, *AJN* 99 (9):51, 1999.

Catalano J: *Ethical and legal aspects of nursing*, ed 2, Springhouse, PA, 1995, Springhouse Corporation.

Cerrato P, Amara A: Use research to weigh the alternatives, *RN* 60 (2):53, 1997.

Cerrato P: Aromatherapy: is it for real? *RN* 60 (6):51, 1998.

Chally P, Loriz L: Ethics in the trenches—decision making in practice *AJN* 98 (6):17, 1998.

Champagne M, Tornquist E, Funk S: Achieving research-based practice, *AJN* 97 (5): 16AAA, 1997.

Chapple H: Changing the game in the intensive care unit: letting nature take its course, *Critical Care Nurse* 19(3):25, 1999.

Chlan L, Tracy M: Music therapy in critical care: indications and guidelines for intervention, *Critical Care Nurse* 19 (3):35, 1999.

Clark C: Spiritual care for the critically ill, *American Journal of Critical Care* 4 (1):77, 1995.

Colbath JD: Holistic health options for women, *Critical Care Nursing Clinics of North America* 9 (4):589, 1997.

Collopy K: Advanced practice nurses guiding families through systems, *Critical Care Nurse* 19(5):80, 1999.

Corley M: Moral distress of critical care nurses, *American Journal of Critical Care* 4 (4):280, 1995.

Cullen L, Titler M, Drahozal R: Family and pet visitation in the critical care unit, *Critical Care Nurse* 19 (3):84, 1999.

Cummins K, Hill M: Charting by exception, *AJN* 99 (3):24G, 1999.

Cyrus V: *Experiencing race, class, and gender in the United States*, Mountain View, CA, 1993, Mayfield Publishing.

Czerwinski S, Blastic L, Rice B: The synergy mode: building a clinical advancement program, *Critical Care Nurse* 19 (4):72, 1999.

Daly B: Why a new code? *AJN* 99 (6):64, 1999.

Davidhizer R, Giger J: *Transcultural nursing assessment and intervention*, ed 3, St Louis, 1999, Mosby.

Davidson S, Scott R: Thinking critically about delegation, *AJN* 99 (6):61, 1999.

Day L, Stannard D: Developing trust and connection with patients and their families, *Critical Care Nurse* 19(3):66, 1999.

Deering C: To speak or not to speak? *AJN* 99 (1):34, 1999.

DePalma J, Townsend R: Ethical issues in organ donation and transplantation: are we helping a few at the expense of many? *Critical Care Nursing Quarterly* 19 (1):1, 1996.

Dossey B, Dossey L: Body mind-spirit—attending to holistic care, *AJN* 98 (8):35, 1998.

Dossey B, Guzzetta C: Implications for bio-psycho-social-spiritual concerns in cardiovascular nursing, *Journal of Cardiovascular Nursing* 10 (3):72, 1996.

Dossey B: Help your patient break free from anxiety, *Nursing96* 26 (10):52, 1996.

Dossey B: Holistic modalities and healing moments, *AJN* 98 (6):44, 1998.

Dossey B: Using imagery to help your patient heal, *AJN* 95 (6):41. 1995.

Dossey B: Attending to holistic care, *AJN* 98 (99):8, 1998.

Dossey L: *Prayer is good medicine*, San Francisco, 1996, Harper Collins.

Dossey L: *Healing words: the power of prayer and the practice of medicine*, San Francisco, 1993, Harper Collins.

Dunn D: Exploring the gray areas of informed consent, *Nursing 99* 29 (7):41, 1999.

Egan P, Nemcek M, Egan P: Forward vision: navigating health care changes, *AJN* 99 (2):24Q, 1999.

Erikson E: *Identity, youth and crisis*, New York, 1968, WW Norton.

Eskreis T: Seven common legal pitfalls in nursing, *AJN* 98 (4):34, 1998.

Esposito J: *Islam: the straight path*, ed 3, New York, 1998, Oxford University Press.

Evers K, Lewis D, Schaeffer M: Sociological and cultural factors affecting consent for organ donation, *Critical Care Nurse* 19 (4):57, 1999.

Floriani C: The spiritual side of pain, *AJN* 99 (3):24PP, 1999.

Forward D: Managing malpractice insurance, *AJN* 98 (3):16BB, 1998.

French M: The mind-body-spirit connection: an introduction to alternative therapies, *ADVANCE for Nurse Practitioners*, November 1996.

Furukawa M: Meeting the needs of the dying patient's family, *Critical Care Nurse* 16 (1):51, 1996.

Galanti G: *Caring for patients from different cultures*, Philadelphia, 1991, University of Pennsylvania.

Geissler E: *Mosby's pocket guide series: cultural assessment*, St Louis, 1998, Mosby.

Gigar J, Davidhizar R: Transcultural nursing, ed 3, St Louis, 1999, Mosby.

Gillman J, et al: Pastoral care in a critical care setting, *Critical Care Nursing Quarterly* 19 (1):10, 1996.

Giuliano K, Bloniasz E, Bell J: Implementation of a pet visitation program in critical care, *Critical Care Nurse* 19 (3):43, 1999.

Giuliano K: Organ transplants—tackling the tough ethical questions, *Nursing97* 27 (5):35, 1997.

Good M: Relaxation techniques for surgical patients, *AJN* 95 (5):39, 1995.

Goode M, Witmer S: The 'Least Worst Death': who makes the call? *AJN* 99 (5):41, 1999.

Grossman D: Cultural dimension in home health nursing, *AJN* 96 (7):33, 1996.

Grotbo A: Giving your patients some time out, *AJN* 99 (7):24HH, 1999.

Guzzetta C: Weaving a tapestry of holism, *Journal of Cardiovascular Nursing* 12 (2):18, 1998.

Hall P: Providing psychosocial support, *AJN* 96 (10):16N, 1996.

Hansten R, Washburn M: Knowing how to delegate, *AJN* 95 (7):16H, 1995.

Hayden L: Helping patients with end-of-life decisions, *AJN* 99 (4):24BB, 1999.

Haynor P: Meeting the challenge of advance directives, *AJN* 98 (3):26, 1998.

Heitman L, Robinson B: Developing a nursing ethics roundtable, *AJN* 97 (1):36, 1997.

Helmlinger C, Whittaker S: Safeguarding nurses and patients, *AJN* 99 (8):55, 1999.

Hester L: Coordinating a successful discharge plan, *AJN* 96 (6):35, 1996.

Hoppe B: Cost containment in critical care, *American Journal of Critical Care* 5 (1):4, 1996.

Huber D: Understanding the sources of stress for nurses, *AJN* 95 (12):16J, 1995.

Hughes K, Dvorak E: The use of decision analysis to examine ethical decision making by critical care nurses, *Heart and Lung* 26 (3):238, 1997.

Hutchison C: Healing touch—an energetic approach, *AJN* 99 (4):43, 1999.

Kallenbach A, Meyer D: Patient care conference: a coordinated, collaborative effort, *Critical Care Nurse* 16 (5):77, 1996.

Karlawish J: Shared decision making in critical care: a clinical reality and an ethical necessity, *American Journal of Critical Care* 5 (6):391, 1996.

Keegan L: Alternative and complementary therapies, *Nursing98*, 28 (4):51, 1998.

Kelly D: Three tips for closer caring, *Nursing95*, 25 (5):72, 1995.

Kinney M, et al.: AACN clinical reference for critical care nursing, ed 4, St Louis, 1998, Mosby.

Kolcaba K: The art of comfort care, *IMAGE* 27 (4):287, 1995.

Kornfeld H: Co-meditation: guiding patients through the relaxation process, *RN* 58 (11):57, 1995.

Kowalski S: Assisted suicide: is there a future? ethical and nursing considerations, *Critical Care Nursing Quarterly* 19 (1):45, 1996.

Kubler-Ross E: *On death and dying*, New York, 1969, Macmillan.

Kudzma E: Culturally competent drug administration, *AJN* 99 (8):46, 1999.

Lake D: No code, *AJN* 96 (2):38, 1996.

Lamm M: *The Jewish way in death and mourning*, New York, 1996, Jonathan David.

Leash R: Death notification: practical guidelines for health care professionals, *Critical Care Nursing Quarterly* 19 (1):21, 1996.

Leininger M: *Transcultural nursing: concepts, theories, research, and practices*, ed 2, New York, 1995, McGraw-Hill.

Leith B: Patients' and family members' perceptions of transfer from intensive care, *Heart and Lung* 28 (3):210, 1999.

Leske J: Overview of family needs after critical illness: from assessment to intervention, *AACN Clinical Issues in Critical Care Nursing* 2:220, 1991.

Leske J: Interventions to decrease family anxiety, *Critical Care Nurse* 18 (4):92, 1998.

London F: Return demonstrations: how to validate patient education, *Nursing97* 27 (2):32j, 1997.

Long C, Greeneich D: Four strategies for keeping patients satisfied, *AJN* 94 (6):26, 1994.

Mackey R: Discover the healing power of therapeutic touch, *AJN* 95 (4):27, 1995.

Mandle C, et al: The efficacy of relaxation response interventions with adult patients: a review of the literature, *Journal of Cardiovascular Nursing* 10 (3):4, 1996.

Manion J: Understanding the seven stages of change, *AJN* 95 (4):41, 1995.

Martin K, Cepero K: You're being deposed? remain calm, *Nursing99* 29 (3):61, 1999.

Maslow A: *Toward a psychology of being*, ed 2, Princeton, MA, 1968, Van Nostrand.

Massey V: *Nursing research*, ed 2, Springhouse, PA, 1995, Springhouse Corporation.

McCullough M, et al: *Hope, faith, and healing*, Lincolnwood, Illinois, 1997, Publications International.

McGhee P: Rx: Laughter, *RN* 60 (7):50, 1998.

McKee R: Clarifying advance directives, *Nursing99* 29 (5):52, 1999.

McLaughlin K, Miller J, Wooten C: Ethical dilemmas in critical care: nurse case managers' perspective, *Critical Care Nursing Quarterly* 22 (3):51, 1999.

Meintz S: Whatever became of the back rub? *RN* 58 (4):49, 1995.

Miles A: Anger at God after a loved one dies, *AJN* 98 (3):64, 1998.

Mitchell P, et al: Critical care outcomes: linking structures, processes, and organizational and clinical outcomes, *American Journal of Critical Care* 5 (5):353, 1996.

Moch S, et al: Linking research and practice through discussion, *IMAGE* 29 (2):189, 1997.

Moyers, B: *Healing and the mind*, New York, 1993, Doubleday.

Mulloney S, Wells-Federman C: Therapeutic touch: a healing modality, *Journal of Cardiovascular Nursing* 10 (3):4, 1996.

Murray C: Addressing your patient's spiritual needs, *AJN* 95 (11):16N, 1995.

Murray C: Getting in touch with massage, *Nursing96*, 26 (10):32f, 1996.

Murray C: Helping your patient relax, *Nursing96*, 26 (2):32h, 1996.

Murray C: Addressing your patient's spiritual needs, *AJN* 95 (95): 11,1995.

O'Brien M: *Spirituality in nursing: standing on holy ground*, Boston, 1999, Jones and Bartlett.

Oermann M, Huber D: Patient outcomes: a measure of nursing's value, *AJN* 99 (9):40, 1999.

Osguthorpe S: Managing a shift effectively: the role of the charge nurse, *Critical Care Nurse* 17 (2):64, 1997.

Parkman C: Bringing advance directives into focus, *Nursing98* 28 (10):32hn6, 1998.

Petterson M: Integrated patient records benefit both patients and healthcare team. *Critical Care Nurse* 19 (2):120, 1999.

Polston M: Whistleblowing: does the law protect you? *AJN* 99 (1):26, 1999.

Pope D: Music, noise, and the human voice in the nurse-patient environment, *IMAGE* 27 (4):291, 1995.

Porter B: Learning how to cope with tragedy, *Nursing96* 26 (1):32f, 1996.

Proulx D: Animal-assisted therapy, *Critical Care Nurse* 18 (2):80, 1998.

Puopolo A: Gaining confidence to talk about end-of-life care, *Nursing99* 29 (7):49, 1999.

Rankin M, Esteves M: How to assess a research study, *AJN* 96 (12):33, 1996.

Richards K: Effect of a back massage and relaxation intervention on sleep in critically ill patients, *American Journal of Critical Care* 7 (4):288, 1998.

Sachs P, Deflecting harsh words when tempers flare, *Nursing99* 29 (3):63, 1999.

Schweitzer A: Contemplating a death, *AJN* 99 (5):24LL, 1999.

Sell S: Reiki: an ancient touch therapy, *RN* 58 (2):57, 1996.

Shermont H, Russell G: Making work assignments that really work, *AJN* 96 (1):16M, 1996.

Shinkarovsky L: Hypnotherapy, not just hocus-pocus, *RN* 59 (6):55, 1996.

Shipler D: *A country of strangers—blacks and whites in America*, New York, 1997, Knopf.

Simon S, et al: Current practices regarding visitation policies in critical care units, *American Journal of Critical Care* 6 (3):210, 1997.

Simpson T, et al: Implementation and evaluation of a liberalized visiting policy, *American Journal of Critical Care* 5 (6):420, 1996.

Skinner S: The world according to homeopathy, *Journal of Cardiovascular Nursing* 10 (3):65, 1996.

Smith-Stoner M, Frost A: How to build your "hope skills," *Nursing99* 29 (9):1999.

Snyder M, Lindquist R: *Complementary/alternative therapies in nursing*, New York, 1998, Springer.

Sommers MS: The near-death experience following multiple trauma, *Critical Care Nurse* 14 (4):62, 1994.

Spital J: What you should expect from your attorney. . . and what your attorney expects from you, *Nursing99* 29 (6):62, 1999.

Stewart K: Written patient education materials—are they on the level? *Nursing96* 26 (1):32j, 1996.

Strevy S: Listen to the music, *Nursing99* 29 (4):32hn6, 1999.

Sullivan M: Nursing leadership and management, ed 2, Springhouse, PA, 1995, Springhouse Corporation.

Sumner C: Recognizing and responding to spiritual distress, *AJN* 98 (1):26, 1998.

Sumner C: Recognizing and responding, *AJN* 98 (98): 1, 1998.

Trevelyan J: A true complement?. . . nurses' view of complementary therapies, *Nursing Times* 92 (5):42, 1996.

Trossman S: Nurse researchers open doors, *AJN* 99 (9):68 1999.

Ufema J: Reflections on death and dying, *Nursing99* 29 (6):57, 1999.

Wesley R: *Nursing theories and models,* ed 2, Springhouse, PA, 1995, Springhouse Corporation.

Wheeler S: Helping families cope with death and dying, *Nursing96* 26 (7):25, 1996.

Wilkinson A: Nursing malpractice, *Nursing98* 28 (6):34, 1998.

Wright K: Professional, ethical, and legal implications for spiritual care in nursing, *Image* 30 (1):81, 1998.

Youngkin EQ, Israel D: A review and critique of common herbal alternative therapies, *Nurse Practitioner* 21 (10):39, 1996.

Ziment I: Eastern "alternative" medicine: what you need to know, *The Journal of Respiratory Diseases* 19 (8):630, 1998.

Ziment I: Western "alternative" medicine: what you need to know, *The Journal of Respiratory Diseases* 19 (9):747, 1998.

Selected Nursing Diagnoses Commonly Seen in Critically Ill Patients

Nursing Diagnosis	Defining Characteristics	Nursing Interventions	Expected Outcomes

Activity Intolerance related to:
• Changes in heart rate, rhythm, or conduction
• Inability to increase heart rate in response to exercise
• Effects of drugs (e.g., beta-blockers)
• Imbalance between oxygen supply and demand
• Hypoxemia
• Dyspnea
• Anemia
• Weakness, fatigue
• Uremia
• Osteomalacia, osteoporosis
• Pain
• Fluid and electrolyte imbalance
• Immobility
• Malnutrition
• Obesity
	• Verbal report of dyspnea, pain, weakness, fatigue, or syncope
	• Abnormal physiologic response to exercise
	  • Tachycardia or dysrhythmia
	  • Hypotension
	  • Tachypnea or dyspnea
	  • Arterial blood gas changes: hypoxemia and/or hypercapnia during exercise
	  • Heart sound changes with exercise: S_4, S_3
	  • Breath sound changes with exercise: crackles, rhonchi, wheezes
	• Clinical indications of anemia: chest pain, syncope, hypotension, dyspnea
	• Lack of desire to engage in physical activity
	• Radiologic evidence of demineralization
	• Bone pain, pathologic fractures
		• Monitor for changes in defining characteristics
		  • Monitor ECG during exercise if indicated
		  • Monitor SpO_2 during physical activity if indicated
		• Explain all procedures thoroughly to decrease anxiety
		• Assess need for ambulation aids (e.g., cane, walker)
		• Assess muscle tone and strength daily
		• Teach relaxation techniques
		• Teach patient to monitor physiologic response (e.g., pulse rate, shortness of breath) to activity
		• Monitor the patient's participation in activities of daily living (e.g., bathing, eating); assist with activities of daily living if appropriate
		• Perform passive range-of-motion (ROM) exercises during bed rest
		• Encourage active range-of-motion exercises when tolerated; instruct patient how to avoid Valsalva maneuver
		• Assist with postural changes gradually; monitor HR and BP response to postural changes as indicated
		• Collaborate with physical, occupational, and/or recreational therapy to plan and monitor an activity program
		  • Focus on what the patient can do rather than on deficits
		  • Encourage participation in graded exercise program
		  • Schedule activities (e.g., active ROM, ambulation) when energy levels are highest
		  • Avoid activity after meals
		  • Group activities to provide rest periods
			• Patient reports increased ability to perform daily activities without pain, dyspnea, weakness, fatigue, or syncope
			• Absence of abnormal responses to exercise
			• HR within 20 bpm of patient's normal
			• ECG rhythm: normal sinus rhythm or patient's usual rhythm (e.g., chronic atrial fibrillation) without ventricular ectopy
			• BP within 20 mm Hg of patient's normal
			• RR <24/min
			• SaO_2, SpO_2 >90%
			• $PaCO_2$ 35-45 mm Hg or within 5 mm Hg of patient's normal
			• Participation in activities (e.g., active ROM, ambulation, resistive exercises)

Nursing Diagnosis	Defining Characteristics	Nursing Interventions	Expected Outcomes
		• Plan rest periods before and after activity	
		• Plan rest periods after meals	
		• Provide positive reinforcement for participation in graded activity	
		• Administer analgesics prior to activity as indicated	
		• Administer oxygen during activity as indicated	
		Coronary artery disease or heart failure	
		• Assist the patient to identify activities that cause chest pain or dyspnea; encourage avoidance of these activities or slowing the pace of these activities	
		• Teach the patient how to use NTG prophylactically before activities likely to cause chest pain	
		Pulmonary disease	
		• Assist the patient to identify activities that cause dyspnea; encourage avoidance of these activities or slowing the pace of these activities	
		• Encourage the use of relaxation techniques prior to exercise	
		• Teach the patient how to cough effectively; encourage airway clearance techniques prior to exercise	
		• Administer oxygen before and during exercise if SpO_2 is <90% or patient is dyspneic during activity	
		Anemia	
		• Administer erythropoietin and/or blood and blood products as prescribed	
		Renal failure	
		• Restrict dietary phosphorus; administer phosphate-binding gels as prescribed	
		• Administer large doses of vitamin D, dihydrotachysterol, or 1,25-vitamin D as prescribed	
		• Dihydrotachysterol does not require 1-hydroxylation by the kidney	
		• 1,25-vitamin D is a completely activated form of vitamin D	
		• Administer calcium supplements with vitamin D preparations	
		• Evaluate and encourage compliance to prevent secondary hyperparathyroidism	

Continued

Nursing Diagnosis	Defining Characteristics	Nursing Interventions	Expected Outcomes

Altered Nutrition: Less Than Body Requirements related to:
• Inability to obtain or prepare adequate amount or quality of food
  • Poverty
  • Disability or chronic illness
• Inability to ingest food
  • Food restriction (e.g., NPO)
  • Anorexia
  • Altered sense of taste
  • Nausea, vomiting
  • Abdominal pain
  • Alcoholism
  • Gingivitis
  • Stomatitis
  • Esophagitis
  • Dysphagia
• Unwillingness to ingest food
  • Eating disorders
  • Dislike for dietary restrictions
  • Depression
• Inability to digest food
  • Altered digestive enzymes
• Inability to absorb or metabolize food
  • Insulin deficiency: absolute or relative
  • Increase in gastric or intestinal mobility
• Increase in metabolic requirements causing a relative deficiency of nutrients
  • Burns
  • Sepsis
  • Hyperthyroidism
• Adverse drug effects
	• Patient verbalizes complaints of anorexia, nausea, vomiting, diarrhea, dysphagia, sore mouth
	• Apathy
	• Fatigue, weakness
	• Headache
	• Poor muscle tone
	• Evidence of delayed wound healing
	• Unplanned weight loss of 20% within 6 months
	• Daily caloric intake less than estimated nutritional requirements
	• Decreased serum total protein, albumin, transferrin, folic acid, total lymphocytes
	• Diminished skinfold and arm circumference measurement
	• Elevated serum ketones and urine ketones
	• Absence of response to skin antigen testing (anergy)
		• Monitor for changes in defining characteristics
		  • Weigh daily at same time on same scale
		  • Record daily food intake and calorie count
		• Evaluate bowel sounds and appropriateness to feed
		• Assess adequate dentition; assess fit of dentures; request dental consultation if necessary
		• Administer antiemetics as prescribed for nausea, especially prior to meals
		• Utilize prescribed drugs for oral infections
		  • Nystatin or clotrimazole (Mycelex) are often used for oral candida (thrush)
		  • Acyclovir (Zovirax) is often used for oral herpes infections
		  • Viscous lidocaine may be utilized prior to meals with patients with stomatitis
		• Utilize appetite-enhancing methods
		  • Removal of any noxious stimuli (e.g., emesis pan, bedpan)
		  • Oral hygiene prior to meals
		  • Small servings
		  • Attractive presentation
		  • Comfortable environment: lighting, temperature, family present if possible
		• Collaborate with physician, dietician, and pharmacist to estimate patient's metabolic needs and establish a plan for meeting these needs
		  • Provide sufficient calories and nutrients
		    • Oral feedings
		      • Provide small, frequent feedings and dietary supplements as indicated
		      • Identify and provide patient's food preferences unless contraindicated by dietary restrictions
		    • Enteral feedings
		    • Parenteral feedings if GI tract cannot be utilized
		  • Maintain protein intake of approximately 1g/kg of ideal body weight/24 hr; more will be needed in patients with protein malnutrition for repletion
			• Caloric intake equals estimated nutritional requirements
			• Cessation of weight loss and gradual weight gain
			• Normal muscle tone and strength
			• Evidence of wound healing
			• Serum albumin >3.5 g/dl
			• Total lymphocytes >1500/mm^3
			• Negative serum ketones and urine ketones
			• Normal serum total protein and albumin
			• Patient verbalizes understanding of dietary guidelines and intention to follow guidelines

Nursing Diagnosis	Defining Characteristics	Nursing Interventions	Expected Outcomes

		• If protein is restricted, ensure that protein is of high biologic value (i.e., contains essential amino acids); egg white has all essential amino acids
		• Provide carbohydrates and calories in sufficient amounts so that protein is not utilized for energy needs
		• Maintain caloric intake of approximately 50 kcal/kg of ideal body weight/24 hr; more will be needed for repletion or if patient is hypermetabolic (e.g., sepsis)
		  • Provide carbohydrates and calories in sufficient amounts so that protein is not utilized for energy needs; 30% of nonprotein calories are usually in the form of fat (e.g., intralipid)
		    • Acute respiratory failure: carbohydrates may be decreased and fats increased, especially during weaning from mechanical ventilator because carbohydrate metabolism produces more CO_2 than fat metabolism
		    • Diabetes mellitus: 50% to 60% of calories are usually provided in the form of carbohydrates, with the remainder provided as 12% to 20% protein and less than 30% fat
		• Administer vitamin, iron, and trace elements as prescribed
		• Maintain nutrient and/or electrolyte restrictions as indicated
		• Administer insulin as prescribed
		• Provide rest periods before and after meals
		• Consult psychologic or social services if needed
		  • Meals-on-wheels referral may be needed at time of discharge due to fatigue and decreased energy	

Continued

Nursing Diagnosis	Defining Characteristics	Nursing Interventions	Expected Outcomes

Altered Protection related to electrolyte imbalance caused by:
• Acid-base imbalance
• Acute pancreatitis
• ADH deficiency or excess
• Decreased electrolyte excretion
• Dietary restrictions
• Diuretic therapy
• Excessive intake
• Gastric or intestinal suction
• Hemorrhage
• Increased insensible losses due to increased ventilatory rate, fever
• Increased secretion of ADH
• Insulin deficiency
• Therapeutic dietary restrictions
• Vomiting
	• Clinical manifestations of hyponatremia
	  • Anorexia
	  • Nausea/vomiting
	  • Muscle cramps and twitching
	  • Hypotension
	  • Seizures
	  • Coma
	• Clinical manifestations of hypernatremia
	  • Low-grade fever
	  • Dry, sticky mucous membranes
	  • CNS irritability: restlessness, agitation
	  • Muscle cramps, increased deep tendon reflexes
	  • Seizures
	• Clinical manifestations of hyperkalemia
	  • Nausea, vomiting, intestinal colic, diarrhea
	  • Muscle weakness progressing to flaccid paralysis
	  • Increased deep tendon reflexes
	  • Lethargy, mental confusion
	  • ECG changes: tall, peaked T-waves
	  • Respiratory muscle weakness, respiratory distress or arrest
	• Clinical manifestations of hypokalemia
	  • Anorexia, nausea, vomiting
	  • Decreased bowel motility
	  • Muscle cramps, muscle weakness progressing to flaccid paralysis
	  • Mental apathy, confusion, drowsiness
	  • Dysrhythmias
	• Clinical manifestations of hypomagnesemia
	  • Hyperactive deep tendon reflexes
	  • Circumoral paresthesia
	  • Carpopedal spasm
	  • Seizures
	  • Dysrhythmias
	• Clinical manifestations of hypocalcemia
	  • Hyperactive deep tendon reflexes
	  • Circumoral paresthesia
	  • Carpopedal spasm
	  • Laryngospasm
		• Monitor for changes in defining characteristics
		• Identify cause or causes of electrolyte balance
		• Monitor serum electrolyte values
		• Monitor ECG for indications of electrolyte imbalance
		• Initiate IV infusion and administer solution as prescribed
		• Initiate electrolyte replacement as indicated and prescribed
		  • Intravenous replacement
		  • Dietary replacement
		• Restrict dietary and drug intake of elevated electrolytes as indicated
		• Administer other drug therapies as prescribed (e.g., glucose and insulin for critical hyperkalemia)
			• Absence of clinical manifestations of electrolyte imbalance
			• Absence of laboratory indicators of electrolyte imbalance

Nursing Diagnosis	Defining Characteristics	Nursing Interventions	Expected Outcomes

	• Dysrhythmias
	 • Seizures
	 • Clinical manifestations of hypophosphatemia
	   • Anorexia, nausea, vomiting
	   • Malaise, fatigue
	   • Muscle weakness, especially respiratory muscles
	   • Dysrhythmias
	 • Laboratory indicators of electrolyte imbalance (e.g., serum electrolyte below or above laboratory-defined normal values)		

Altered Protection related to:
 • Congenital clotting abnormality (e.g., hemophilia)
 • Thrombolytic, anticoagulant, platelet aggregation inhibitor therapy
 • Inadequate intake or absorption of vitamin K
 • Decreased fibrinogen production (e.g., liver disease)
 • Decreased production of clotting factors
	• Increased PT, aPTT, bleeding times; decreased platelet count
	 • Petechiae, bruising
	 • Evidence of bleeding
	   • Bleeding from wounds, punctures
	   • Bleeding from gums, mouth, nose
	   • Blood in emesis
	   • Blood in sputum
	   • Blood in urine
	   • Blood in stool
	   • Vaginal bleeding
		• Monitor clotting parameters and bleeding times
		 • Detect bleeding
		   • Monitor for oral, nasal, scleral, rectal, or vaginal bleeding
		   • Monitor for petechiae, ecchymosis, hematoma, bleeding from puncture points, catheter insertion sites, wounds
		   • Monitor gastric aspirate and/or stools for occult blood
		   • Monitor bowel habits; observe for tarry or bloody stools
		   • Monitor for joint or bone pain
		   • Monitor for changes in neurologic status
		 • Prevent bleeding
		   • Keep nails cut short to prevent scratches that may bleed
		   • Administer antipruritics as prescribed
		   • Encourage use of soft toothbrush
		   • Encourage avoidance of blade razor
		   • Avoid unnecessary injections and blood sampling
		     • If arterial puncture is necessary: hold pressure for 10-15 minutes
		     • If venous puncture is necessary: hold pressure for 5 minutes
		   • Suction only if necessary
		   • Avoid use of noninvasive blood pressure (NIBP) cuffs
		   • Avoid aspirin and aspirin-containing drugs unless specifically prescribed
		   • Assess gastric pH; antacids, histamine$_2$ receptor antagonists, or mucosal barriers may be prescribed to decrease the acidity of gastric contents
		   • Have vitamin K and/or protamine available for reversal of anticoagulants
			• Absence of bleeding from surface wounds, body systems
			 • PT, aPTT, bleeding time within normal limits or within therapeutic range if drugs are being given to affect these parameters

Continued

Nursing Diagnosis	Defining Characteristics	Nursing Interventions	Expected Outcomes
Altered Thermoregulation related to: • Brain or spinal cord injury • Aging • Thyroid disorder	• Fluctuations in body temperature above or below the normal range • Warm or cool skin • Flushed or pale skin • Piloerection • Shivering • Decreased capillary refill (>3 seconds)	• Monitor for changes in defining characteristics • Monitor body temperature at least every 4 hours; more often if abnormalities noted • Monitor for clinical indications of infection as a possible cause of hyperthermia • Regulate room temperature *For hypothermia* • Provide warm fluids and food • Apply warmed blankets • Use radiant heat lamps (especially helpful in patients with burns) • Place warming blanket on bed; place sheet between patient and blanket • Infuse warm IV fluids, assist with peritoneal lavage with warm fluid, irrigate bladder with warm fluid, and warm inhaled air for severe hypothermia *For hyperthermia* • Remove excess bedding • Place cooling blanket on bed; place sheet between patient and blanket • Use fans to circulate air • Sponge patient with tepid water if necessary • Place ice bags to axilla and groin • Administer antipyretics as prescribed; may be helpful depending on cause of hyperthermia • Administer chlorpromazine (Thorazine) or meperidine (Demerol) as prescribed for shivering	• Normal body temperature • Patient verbalizes comfort with temperature • Normal skin color and temperature • No piloerection or shivering • Normal capillary refill (<3 seconds)
Altered Thought Processes related to: • Sensory overload (of nonmeaningful stimuli) • Sensory deprivation (of meaningful stimuli) • Sleep deprivation • "ICU psychosis" • CNS injury • Organic mental disorder • Drug ingestion • Uremia • GI hemorrhage • Hepatic encephalopathy	• Disorientation to person, place, time, and/or situation • Confusion regarding purpose of hospitalization, confinement • Sleep disturbances • Agitation, anxiety, irritability • Hallucinations	• Monitor for changes in defining characteristics • Use the patient's name when speaking to him or her • Speak slowly and clearly • Reorient patient to person, place, time, and situation verbally often; have clock, calendar in room • Be respectful when correcting the patient's misperceptions • Maintain light-dark patterns using windows and lighting • Eliminate as much nonmeaningful visual, auditory, and tactile stimulation as possible • Allow family visitation as indicated; encourage the family to bring in familiar objects (e.g., photos) • Eliminate invasive and intrusive procedures if possible • Protect from self-injury through use of siderails; use restraints only as needed for self-protection	• Patient alert and oriented • Absence of agitation, irritability • Patient verbalizes absence of anxiety; absence of nonverbal indicators of anxiety • Absence of injury

Nursing Diagnosis	Defining Characteristics	Nursing Interventions	Expected Outcomes
		Renal failure • Restrict protein intake but provide adequate calories so that protein is not utilized for energy (catabolism increases BUN) • Institute dialysis as prescribed to keep BUN <100 mg/dl *GI hemorrhage* • Check stools and NG aspirate for occult blood; blood (being primarily protein) metabolism increases BUN and ammonia • Treat GI bleeding by irrigating nasogastric tube with room temperature saline until clear • Administer antacids and histamine$_2$-receptor antagonists as prescribed • Administer osmotic laxative (e.g., sorbitol) as prescribed • Prevent constipation *Hepatic encephalopathy* • Restrict protein intake but provide adequate calories so that protein is not utilized for energy • Administer neomycin as prescribed to decrease bacterial action in intestine • Administer osmotic laxative (e.g., sorbitol) as prescribed • Prevent constipation	

Altered Tissue Perfusion related to:
• Arterial thrombus, embolus, spasm, hemorrhage
• Decreased cardiac output
• Inadequate hemoglobin
• Vasopressor therapy
• Intraarterial catheter or sheath
• Fracture or circumferential burn
• Poor positioning and arterial compression
	• Myocardial
	  • Chest pain
	  • Tachycardia, hypotension
	  • ST-T-wave changes on ECG
	  • Decreased cardiac output/cardiac index
	• Cerebral
	  • Change in level of consciousness: restlessness to confusion to lethargy to coma
	  • Syncope
	  • Pupillary changes
	  • Motor or sensory changes
	  • Aphasia
	  • Altered thought processes
	• Pulmonary
	  • Dyspnea
	  • Hemoptysis
	  • Pleuritic pain
	  • Pleural friction rub
	  • Decreased Sao$_2$, Spo$_2$, Pao$_2$
	• Renal
	  • Decrease in urine output
	  • Hematuria
	  • Pyuria
		• Monitor for changes in defining characteristics
		• Affirm or establish airway; intubation may be necessary
		• Administer oxygen therapy as indicated and prescribed; mechanical ventilation and PEEP may be necessary
		• Decrease oxygen requirements by limiting activity, anxiety, pain
		  • Administer analgesics as indicated and prescribed
		  • Identify and treat anxiety
		• Initiate IV infusion in a nonischemic limb and administer solution as prescribed
		  • Crystalloids (e.g., normal saline, lactated Ringer's)
		  • Colloids (e.g., albumin, dextran 70, hetastarch)
		  • Blood and blood products (e.g., packed red blood cells)
		    • Blood and/or blood products are indicated for signs/symptoms such as hypotension, chest pain, syncope, dyspnea not simply by a certain hematocrit level
		• Assess cause of anemia if present (e.g., actual blood loss versus suppression of erythropoietin as in renal failure)
			Cardiac
			• Absence of chest pain, tachycardia, hypotension, ST-T-wave changes
			Cerebral
			• Patient alert and oriented
			• Absence of pupil changes, motor or sensory changes, speech changes
			Pulmonary
			• Absence of dyspnea, hemoptysis, pleuritic pain, pleural friction rub
			Renal
			• Urine output >0.5 ml/kg/hr
			• Normal BUN and creatinine
			• Absence of hematuria, pyuria, flank pain
			Splenic
			• Absence of LUQ pain, abdominal rigidity

Nursing Diagnosis	Defining Characteristics	Nursing Interventions	Expected Outcomes

	• Flank pain
	• Changes in BUN, creatinine
	• *Splenic*
	• LUQ pain radiating to left shoulder
	• Abdominal rigidity
	• *Mesenteric*
	• Abdominal pain
	• Watery, bloody diarrhea
	• *Peripheral*
	• Pain and/or intermittent claudication
	• Pale and/or cyanotic extremities
	• Diminished or absent peripheral pulses
	• Motor or sensory changes
	• Cool or cold extremities
	• Decreased capillary refill (>3 seconds)
	• Dry, thick, brittle nails
	• Hair loss
	• Bruits
	• Ulcerations
	• Poor healing of wounds
		• Administer recombinant erythropoietin (Epogen) as prescribed for the anemia caused by erythropoietin deficiency in chronic renal failure; iron, folic acid, pyridoxine, and vitamin B_{12} may be indicated in anemia seen in chronic renal failure
		• Insert a urinary catheter if indicated and prescribed and monitor urine output hourly
		Myocardial
		• Assist with insertion of pulmonary artery catheter and measure hemodynamic parameter if indicated
		• Administer thrombolytics, anticoagulants, and/or platelet aggregation inhibitors as prescribed
		• Prepare patient for percutaneous coronary intervention (PCI) or coronary artery bypass grafting (CABG) as requested
		• Administer inotropes (e.g., dobutamine) and/or vasodilators (e.g., nitrates) as prescribed
		• Assist with insertion of IABP, LVAD, RVAD, or bi-VAD as requested
		Cerebral
		• Assist with insertion of ICP monitoring device and measure ICP and calculate CPP if indicated
		• Prepare patient for surgery if indicated
		• Maintain patent airway and ventilation
		• Elevate head of bed 30 degrees; keep head aligned with body; prevent compression of the jugular veins by head position, cervical collar, tracheostomy ties, etc.
		• Teach patient how to avoid Valsalva maneuver
		• Avoid activities that increase ICP if possible; if activity is necessary, allow time between multiple activities that increase ICP
		Pulmonary
		• Prevention
		  • Establish and maintain position of comfort
		  • Encourage patient to turn and breathe deeply
		  • Perform passive ROM or encourage active ROM
		  • Encourage patient to move toes, dorsiflex and hyperextend feet, bend legs at knees
		  • Apply antiembolic stockings or sequential compression devices
		  • Administer mini-heparin as prescribed
			Mesenteric
			• Absence of abdominal pain
			• Absence of bloody diarrhea
			Peripheral
			• Absence of limb pain, diminished pulses, pallor, motor or sensory changes, coolness or coldness

Nursing Diagnosis	Defining Characteristics	Nursing Interventions	Expected Outcomes

		• *Treatment*
		  • Administer oxygen to maintain SpO_2 at 95% or greater unless contraindicated
		  • Administer heparin by IV infusion as prescribed
		  • Administer thrombolytics as prescribed
		  • Prepare patient for embolectomy if requested
		Renal, mesenteric, splenic
		• Ensure adequate hydration; low dose (1-2 µg/kg/min) dopamine may be prescribed
		• Monitor for clinical indications of bowel perforation
		• Prepare patient for angioplasty or surgical procedure as requested
		Peripheral
		• Eliminate/minimize vasoconstrictive activities and agents
		  • Smoking
		  • Stress
		  • Vasoconstrictive agents (e.g., phenylephrine, norepinephrine, dopamine)
		• Decrease oxygen requirements by limiting activity, anxiety, pain
		• Keep patient warm with extremities flat; avoid bending of limb at a cannulation, injury, or surgical site
		• Assist with removal of IABP or sheath as requested
		• Assist with intraarterial thrombolytic or prepare patient for embolectomy or surgical procedure as requested
		• Assist with escharotomy (circumferential burn) or fasciotomy (compartment syndrome)	

Anxiety related to: • Acute change in health status • Unfamiliar environment • Recommended lifestyle changes • Altered body image • Change in self-concept • Change in role in family • Threat of death • Social isolation • Hemorrhage • Pain • Fear of unknown • Financial concerns	• Patient verbalizes anxiety, apprehension, nervousness, uncertainty, fear, worry, inability to cope, feeling of impending doom • Tachycardia, palpitations • Mild hypertension • Tachypnea • Restlessness, fidgeting • Diaphoresis • Anorexia, nausea, vomiting, and/or diarrhea • Dry mouth • Increased muscle tension • Poor eye contact • Inability to concentrate • Concentration on self; narrow focus of attention • Wrinkled brow, worried facial expression • Crying	• Monitor for changes in defining characteristics • Establish rapport; give patient undivided attention; listen to patient • Consider individuality of this patient; treat the patient as a unique person • Identify prior coping strategies; assist the patient to utilize coping mechanisms that have been helpful (e.g., prayer, family, relaxation techniques, breathing techniques) • Explain all procedures, the reasons for them, and their importance in a simple, concise, reassuring manner • Explain critical care unit environment including noises, visiting policy, meal times, what is scheduled today	• Patient verbalizes absence of anxiety • Absence of nonverbal indicators of anxiety • Patient able to verbalize fears and concerns

Continued

Nursing Diagnosis	Defining Characteristics	Nursing Interventions	Expected Outcomes

	• Tremor, trembling, shakiness
	• Expresses feelings of helplessness, inadequacy, regret, concern
	• Withdrawal
	• Verbalization of inability to cope
	• Inability to solve problem effectively
	• Inability to meet role expectations
	• Inappropriate or ineffective use of defense mechanisms
	• Verbal manipulation
	• Excessive food intake, alcohol consumption, smoking
	• Digestive, bowel disturbance
	• Chronic fatigue or sleep pattern disturbance
		• Provide opportunity for patient to verbalize feelings, concerns, fears, anxieties
		• Talk to patient and reassure him or her in a calm, firm voice; be unhurried; maintain calm, confident attitude
		• Provide for comfort: decrease stimuli, adjust room temperature, allow for rest periods
		• Allow patient to make decisions regarding environment and self-care activities
		• Assist the patient to develop anxiety-reducing skills (e.g., relaxation, deep breathing, imagery, positive self-statements)
		• Administer minor tranquilizers as prescribed and indicated
		• Provide diversionary activities (e.g., music, television, books)
		• Allow visitation by family/significant other and encourage their participation in care
		  • Evaluate patient's physiologic and psychologic response to visitation; utilize this assessment in decision making regarding frequency and duration of visits
		  • Allow private family time daily
		• Answer questions simply and concisely; begin teaching about disease process, treatments, recommended lifestyle changes when the patient indicates readiness to learn
		• Assess usual roles and discuss feelings about changes in role performance
		• Refer for rehabilitation as appropriate	

Body Image Disturbance related to: • Change in body function and/or appearance	• Missing body part • Not touching or looking at body part • Hiding or overexposing body part • Refusal to verify actual change • Preoccupation with change or loss • Personalization of part or loss by name • Depersonalization of part or loss by impersonal pronouns	• Monitor for changes in defining characteristics • Assess patient's prehospital perception of body image • Listen to patient's verbalization of alterations in body image • Assess perceived impact of change on ADLs, social behavior, personal relationships, occupation, and recreation • Use simple explanations when describing patient's illness, surgery, treatments, progress, status	• Patient looks at and touches affected body part or area • Patient participates in care of affected body part or area • Patient sets realistic goals regarding changes in lifestyle, return to work, etc. • Patient participates in self-care and physical activity

Nursing Diagnosis	Defining Characteristics	Nursing Interventions	Expected Outcomes
	• Verbalization of negative feelings about body • Verbalization about change in lifestyle • Focus on past strength, function, or appearance	• Provide information regarding healing status of body part • Assist the patient to identify actual changes and establish realistic goals • Encourage physical mobility and activity • Encourage the patient to participate in his or her own care and ADLs • Refer patient to appropriate support groups	
Constipation related to: • Inactivity, immobility • Emotional stress • Drug effect (e.g., opiates) • Electrolyte imbalance • Inadequate dentition • Inadequate fiber intake • Decreased GI motility • Inadequate fluid intake • Hemorrhoids • Chronic enema or laxative use • Lack of privacy	• Change in bowel pattern • Decreased frequency or amount of stool • Dry, hard, formed stool and/or oozing liquid stool • Pain with defecation • Straining at stool • Anorexia, nausea, vomiting, abdominal distention, abdominal pain • Change in bowel sounds • Palpable mass in left lower quadrant • Blood on stool or toilet tissue • Feeling of pressure in rectum or abdominal fullness	• Monitor for changes in defining characteristics • Discuss usual pattern of bowel elimination • Evaluate usual dietary habits, eating habits, eating schedule, liquid intake, activity, medications • Inspect the color, consistency, amount of stool • Auscultate bowel sounds • Examine abdomen for distention, palpable masses • Encourage fluids unless contraindicated; fruit juices and warm fluids are especially helpful • Collaborate with physician and dietician regarding patient's diet • Encourage dietary fiber unless contraindicated • Teach patient about foods high in fiber • Encourage physical activity as tolerated • Provide privacy for the patient at the time of day that bowel elimination usually occurs • Digitally remove fecal impaction if necessary • Administer pharmacologic agents as prescribed • Stool softeners • Chemical irritants • Bulk fiber • Suppositories • Oil retention enema	• Normal amount and frequency of stool • Absence of abdominal pain or pain with stool • Absence of blood with stool • Absence of abdominal mass

Continued

Nursing Diagnosis	Defining Characteristics	Nursing Interventions	Expected Outcomes

Decreased Adaptive Capacity: Intracranial related to:
• Cerebral edema
• Cerebral hemorrhage
• Intracranial hematoma
• Cerebral vasodilation caused by hypercapnia, hypoxemia, vasodilators
• Hydrocephalus
• Intracranial mass (e.g., tumor, abscess, or other space-occupying lesions)
	• Change in level of consciousness
	• Pupillary change
	  • Oval pupil
	  • Unequal pupil
	  • Nonreactive pupil(s)
	• Papilledema
	• Respiratory pattern change
	• Motor changes
	• Sensory changes
	• Vital sign changes
	  • Increased systolic BP
	  • Decreased diastolic BP
	  • Bradycardia
	• Headache
	• Visual changes
	• Seizures
	• Vomiting
	• Pathologic reflexes (e.g., Babinski reflex, grasp reflex)
	• GCS <13
	• ICP >15 mm Hg
	• CPP <60 mm Hg
	• Decreased brain compliance as evidenced during volume pressure response testing
		• Monitor for changes in defining characteristics
		• Assist with insertion of ICP monitoring device and measure ICP and calculate CPP if indicated
		• Maintain patent airway and ventilation
		• Elevate head of bed 30 degrees
		• Keep head in neutral alignment; avoid pillow or allow only small pillow
		• Prevent compression of the jugular veins by head position, cervical collar, tracheostomy ties, etc.
		• Avoid hip flexion
		• Teach patient how to avoid Valvalsa maneuver
		  • Teach patient to cough with mouth open if coughing is necessary
		  • Teach patient to avoid straining, bending, sneezing
		  • Administer stool softeners and antiemetics as prescribed
		• Avoid activities that increase ICP if possible; if activity is necessary, allow time between multiple activities that increase ICP
		• Reorient patient often to person, place, date, time, and situation
		• Explain procedures thoroughly
		• Monitor for clinical indications of infection; administer antibiotics as prescribed
		• Maintain normothermia with antipyretics, cooling blanket
		• Administer prescribed pharmacologic agents (e.g., mannitol [Osmitrol], barbiturates) to decrease ICP
		• Drain CSF via ventriculostomy if indicated and intraventricular catheter in place
		• Prepare patient for surgery for evacuation of clot, drainage of abscess, etc., as requested
			• Alert and oriented to person, place, and date
			• Pupils round, equal, and reactive to light
			• Eupnea
			• Able to move all extremities spontaneously and/or on verbal request
			• Absence of sensory deficits
			• Vital signs within normal range or within 10% of patient's normal
			• GSC of 15
			• ICP 15 mm Hg or less
			• CPP >60-70 mm Hg

Decreased Cardiac Output related to:
• Increased or decreased heart rate; dysrhythmias
• Decreased or increased preload
• Decreased contractility
	• Clinical indications of sympathetic nervous system innervation initially
	  • Tachycardia
	  • Tachypnea
	  • BP changes: narrowed pulse pressure
	  • Increased SVR, SVRI
		• Monitor for changes in defining characteristics
		• Obtain baseline vital signs and monitor as indicated
		• Monitor ECG for dysrhythmias
		• Assess for chest pain
		• Auscultate heart and lung sounds
		• Monitor intake and output and daily weights
			• Alert and oriented
			• HR 60-100 bpm
			• MAP >70 mm Hg
			• CI 2.5-4.0 L/min/m^2
			• PAOP 18 mm Hg or less
			• Urine output >0.5 ml/kg/hr

Nursing Diagnosis	Defining Characteristics	Nursing Interventions	Expected Outcomes

• Increased afterload
• Drug effects
• Vasodilation causing a relative hypovolemia
• Structural or valvular defects
	• Clinical indications of hypoperfusion eventually
	  • Chest pain
	  • Dysrhythmias
	  • Hypotension
	  • Cool or cold, clammy skin
	  • Decreased bowel sounds
	  • Decreased urine output
	  • Elevation in BUN, creatinine
	  • Syncope, vertigo
	  • Changes in level of consciousness: restlessness to confusion to lethargy to coma
	• Clinical indications of LVF
	  • Dyspnea, orthopnea
	  • S_3
	  • Crackles
	  • Increased PAP, PAOP
	• Clinical indications of RVF
	  • Jugular venous distention (JVD)
	  • Peripheral edema
	  • Hepatomegaly
	  • Fatigue, weakness
	  • Weight gain
	  • Increased RAP
	• Changes in hemodynamic parameters
	  • Decreased cardiac output and index
	  • Decreased or increased PAOP: decreased if hypovolemia or vasodilation; increased if heart failure
	  • Decreased Svo_2
	• Metabolic acidosis; elevated serum lactate levels
		• Assess arterial blood gases as indicated
		• Initiate IV with prescribed fluid at prescribed rate
		• Assist with insertion of hemodynamic monitoring catheters
		  • Provide standardized care for monitoring and maintaining invasive catheters
		• Evaluate adequacy of airway and ventilation ($Paco_2$); intubation and mechanical ventilation may be necessary
		• Evaluate adequacy of oxygenation (Sao_2, Spo_2, Pao_2); administer oxygen therapy as prescribed and indicated to maintain Spo_2 >95% unless contraindicated
		• Insert a urinary catheter as prescribed; monitor hourly urine output
		• Administer fluids, inotropes, and/or vasodilators as indicated and prescribed; monitor for effectiveness and adverse effects; diuretics may also be indicated if preload (PAOP) increased
		• Assist with insertion of intraaortic balloon pump if indicated
		  • Provide standardized care for monitoring, maintaining, and timing of the intraaortic balloon pump
		• Establish and maintain position of comfort
		• Maintain environment conducive to rest and sleep
		• Allow patient to rest between nursing activities
		• Assess for and treat anxiety
		• Minimize excessive nonmeaningful stimuli
		• Administer stool softeners as prescribed
		• Encourage patient to turn and breathe deeply
		• Keep patient warm to prevent vasoconstriction and shivering
		• Assist with activities of daily living (ADL)
		• Provide nutrition appropriate to needs and digestive capabilities
		  • Low sodium
		  • Low cholesterol and saturated fat
		  • High fiber
		  • High potassium if patient receiving potassium-wasting diuretics	

Continued

Nursing Diagnosis	Defining Characteristics	Nursing Interventions	Expected Outcomes

Diarrhea related to:
• Anxiety
• Viral, bacterial, parasitic infection
• Antibiotics causing change in normal intestinal flora and proliferation of *Clostridium difficile*
• Adverse drug effects
• Enteral feedings
  • Hyperosmolality
  • Bolus feeding
  • Bacterial contamination
  • Lactose intolerance
  • Low-fiber enteral formula
• Increased GI motility
  • Inflammatory bowel disease
  • Irritable bowel syndrome
  • GI bleeding
• Lactose intolerance
• Excessive intake of fruit, fruit juice, vegetables, whole grains
	• Change in bowel pattern
	• Increased frequency or amount of stool
	• Liquid or semi-liquid stool
	• Abdominal pain or cramping
	• Change in bowel sounds
	• Urgency to have bowel movement
	• Weight loss
	• Dehydration
		• Monitor for changes in defining characteristics
		• Inspect the color, consistency, amount of stool
		• Examine abdomen for distention
		• Auscultate bowel sounds
		• Encourage fluids; avoid fruit juices
		• Provide perianal care with each diarrheal stool
		• Collaborate with physician and dietician regarding patient's diet
		  • Small, soft feedings
		  • Avoidance of raw fruit and vegetables
		  • Whole-grain fiber may be helpful
		• Collaborate with physician and dietician regarding patient's enteral feedings
		  • Provide isotonic feeding
		  • Deliver feedings slowly or continuously with an infusion pump
		  • Deliver feeding at room temperature
		  • Prevent bacterial contamination by allowing feeding to hang at room temperature no longer than 4 hours
		  • Use fiber additives or high-fiber formula
		  • Use lactose-free formula if indicated
		• Provide rest to decrease bowel motility
		• Provide privacy for the patient during bowel movements
		• Administer pharmacologic agents as prescribed
		  • Antidiarrheals
		  • Antispasmodics
		  • Fluid and electrolyte replacement
		• Collect stool specimen for *C. difficile* toxin; if positive, administer antibiotic as prescribed (usually metronidazole [Flagyl])
			• Normal amount and frequency of stool
			• Absence of abdominal pain or cramping
			• No clinical indications of dehydration

Nursing Diagnosis	Defining Characteristics	Nursing Interventions	Expected Outcomes

Dysfunctional Ventilatory Weaning Response related to:
• History of mechanical ventilation of more than 1 week
• Pain or discomfort
• Muscle weakness
• Malnutrition
• Anemia
• Ineffective airway clearance
• Inappropriate pacing of diminished ventilator support
• Adverse environment
• Decreased motivation
• Fear, anxiety
• Hopelessness, powerlessness
• Sleep pattern disturbance
• Knowledge deficit of weaning process
• History of multiple unsuccessful weaning attempts
• Patient-perceived inability to wean
	Responds to weaning attempts with:
	• Tachycardia
	• Tachypnea
	• Hypertension
	• Restlessness
	• Anxiety
	• Agitation
	• Dyspnea
	• Increased concentration on breathing
	• Inability to cooperate
	• Diaphoresis
	• Accessory muscle use
	• Paradoxical abdominal breathing
	• Inability to breathe in "synch" with ventilator
	• Decreased level of consciousness
	• Abnormal breath sounds
	• Decreased SpO_2
	• Arterial blood gas changes
	  • Decreased SaO_2, PaO_2
	  • Increased $PaCO_2$
	  • Respiratory acidosis
		• Monitor for changes in defining characteristics
		• Ensure adequate nutritional status, hemodynamics, and psychologic readiness
		• Carbohydrates may need to be decreased with equivalent calories supplies in the form of fats since the metabolism of CHO increases CO_2 production
		  • Enterally: Pulmocare or similar formula
		  • Parenterally: substitute increased lipids for decrease in CHO
		• Establish a plan for weaning with other members of the healthcare team; involve the patient in planning
		• Convey confidence regarding patient's ability to succeed
		• Time weaning efforts when the patient is rested and support staff is available (e.g., anesthesia, respiratory therapy)
		• Administer oxygen as prescribed
		• Suction airway as indicated
		• Administer analgesics as prescribed and indicated
		• Control the environment: quiet, cool room
		• Provide positive reinforcement and reassurance
		• Stay with patient during weaning attempts or as ventilator settings are changed; touch the patient, hold his or her hand
		• Maintain a calm, confident attitude
		• Increase or decrease family visitation depending on their effect on the weaning process
			• Successful weaning from mechanical ventilation with:
			• HR, BP, RR within normal range
			• ABGs within normal limits or patient's normal

Continued

Nursing Diagnosis	Defining Characteristics	Nursing Interventions	Expected Outcomes

Fluid Volume Deficit related to:
• Inadequate fluid intake or fluid restriction
• Inadequate fluid replacement
• Fluid loss (e.g., diaphoresis, vomiting, gastric suction, diarrhea, diuresis, draining wounds)
• Increased insensible loss caused by hyperventilation, fever
• Fluid sequestration (e.g., ascites, pleural effusion, pericardial effusion)
• Blood loss (e.g., trauma, coagulopathy)
• Blood sequestration (e.g., hemothorax, intraabdominal, retroperitoneal)
• Decreased ADH or aldosterone synthesis, secretion, or effect
	• Orthostatic changes in HR and BP
	• Tachycardia
	• Hypotension
	• Increased body temperature
	• Decreased RAP, PAOP
	• Decreased CO and CI
	• Decrease in urine output (oliguria)
	• Increase in urine concentration
	• Weight loss
	• Peripheral pulses 1+/3+ in quality
	• Decreased skin turgor
	• Dry skin; dry, sticky mucous membranes and tongue; and longitudinal furrowing of the tongue
	• Weakness and/or fatigue
	• Change in level of consciousness
	• Hemoconcentration: increased serum sodium; increased hematocrit; increased serum osmolality; hematocrit will be decreased if blood is lost
	• Increased blood urea nitrogen (BUN)
	• Thirst (polydipsia)
		• Monitor for changes in defining characteristics
		• Weigh daily with same scale and at same time of day (1 kg = 1 L)
		• Record accurate intake and output hourly
		• Assist with insertion of CVP, PAP, or arterial catheter as indicated
		  • Provide standardized care for monitoring and maintaining invasive catheters
		• Assess renal function: urine volume, urine creatinine clearance, serum creatinine, blood urea nitrogen
		  • Insert urinary catheter and monitor urine output hourly
		• Administer oral fluids as tolerated
		  • Keep water pitcher within reach; keep fluids of choice available
		• Assist patient with diet and fluids
		• Administer parenteral fluids as prescribed
		  • Volume: based on patient losses, including insensible losses in the calculation; often administered on a milliliter for milliliter loss basis
		    • Monitor closely for clinical indications of fluid overload (e.g., tachycardia, tachypnea, dyspnea, S_3, crackles)
		  • Solution: based on patient losses and serum osmolality and serum sodium
		    • Type and crossmatch for multiple units of blood for patients who are actively bleeding
		  • Monitor response to fluid and/or blood replacement
		  • Administer appropriate electrolyte replacement as prescribed
		• Administer antiemetics or antidiarrheals as indicated and prescribed
		• Administer prescribed pharmacologic agents for endocrine dysfunction (e.g., DI, DKA)
		  • Hormone replacement
		  • Agents that stimulate secretion of a hormone
		  • Agents that increase the effect of a hormone at its target organ
		• Maintain skin and mucous membrane integrity
		  • Careful assessment of skin and mucous membranes
		  • Turn at least every 2 hours
		  • Provide mouth care every 4 hours
			• HR and BP within 10% of patient baseline
			• Normothermia
			• RAP: 2-6 mm Hg
			• PAOP: 6-12 mm Hg
			• CI 2.5-4.0 L/min/m²
			• Normalization of urine output (usually 0.5 ml/kg/hour)
			• Normalization in urine concentration: specific gravity 1.005-1.030; urine osmolality 50-1,200 mOsm/L as appropriate for serum osmolality
			• Weight normalization in relation to patient's usual body weight
			• Peripheral pulses 2+/3+ in quality
			• Normal skin turgor, moist skin, mucous membranes, intact skin and mucous membranes
			• Alert and oriented to person, place, and date
			• Normal serum sodium: 136-145 mEq/L
			• Normal hematocrit: 40%-52% for males; 35%-47% for females
			• Serum osmolality: 280-295 mOsm/L

Nursing Diagnosis	Defining Characteristics	Nursing Interventions	Expected Outcomes

Fluid Volume Excess related to:
• Excessive fluid intake or replacement
• Excessive sodium intake or replacement
• Inadequate renal perfusion or function
• Sodium and/or water retention
• Increased ADH or aldosterone synthesis, secretion, or effect
• Stress
• Decreased CO
	• Tachycardia
	• Hypertension or hypotension
	• Increased RAP, PAOP
	• Abnormal CO and CI
	• Change in urine output
	• Change in urine concentration
	• Weight gain
	• Edema, ascites, pericardial or pleural effusion, and/or anasarca
	• Jugular venous distention, positive hepatojugular reflux
	• Peripheral pulses 3+/3+ in quality
	• S_3
	• Dyspnea, orthopnea, tachypnea
	• Breath sound changes: crackles
	• Anorexia, nausea, vomiting, abdominal pain
	• Weakness, fatigue
	• Restlessness, anxiety
	• Change in level of consciousness
	• Seizures
	• Hemodilution: decreased serum sodium, decreased hematocrit, decreased serum osmolality
		• Monitor for changes in defining characteristics
		• Record accurate intake and output hourly and weights daily
		• Assess renal function: urine volume, urine creatinine clearance, serum creatinine, BUN
		• Monitor closely for clinical indications of pulmonary edema and/or cerebral edema
		• Administer dopamine (Intropin) at 1-2 µg/kg/min as prescribed to improve renal blood flow and glomerular filtration rate (effectiveness controversial)
		• Restrict fluids and/or sodium depending on serum sodium and serum osmolality; include oral fluids, parenteral fluids, irrigation fluids, ice chips, cardiac output injectates, medication volumes
		  • For accuracy in intravenous infusion volumes
		    • Use volumetric infusion pump
		    • Use decanting method in which volume equal to the volume of medication to be added if removed prior to addition of medication
		• Administer diuretics as prescribed and monitor urinary output response; do not administer diuretics to anuric patients
		• Administer parenteral fluids carefully as prescribed: use minidrip and/or volumetric pump
		  • Volume: based on patient losses, including insensible losses in the calculation; often administered on a milliliter for milliliter loss basis
		  • Solution: based on patient losses, and serum osmolality and serum sodium
		• Monitor serum electrolytes and administer appropriate electrolyte replacement as prescribed
		  • Severe hyponatremia may be treated with hypertonic (3%) saline
		    • Institute seizure precautions for serum sodium level 125 mEq/L or less
		  • Potassium replacement may be required
		• Prepare patient for hemodialysis if necessary (pulmonary edema is an indication for emergency dialysis in a patient with renal failure)
			• Normalization of urine output (usually 0.5 ml/kg/hr)
			• Normalization in urine concentration: specific gravity 1.005-1.030; urine osmolality 50-1,200 mOsm/L as appropriate for serum osmolality
			• Weight normalization
			• Absence of edema, ascites, pericardial or pleural effusion, and/or anasarca
			• Absence of jugular venous distention, positive hepatojugular reflux
			• Peripheral pulses 2+/3+ in quality
			• Absence of S_3
			• Absence of dyspnea, orthopnea, tachypnea
			• Absence of crackles
			• Absence of anorexia, nausea, vomiting, abdominal pain
			• Alert and oriented to person, place, and date
			• Absence of seizures
			• Normal serum sodium: 136-145 mEq/L
			• Normal hematocrit: 40%-52% for males; 35%-47% for females
			• BP within 10% of patient baseline
			• RAP: 2-6 mm Hg
			• PAOP: 6-12 mm Hg
			• CI 2.5-4.0 L/min/m^2

Continued

Nursing Diagnosis	Defining Characteristics	Nursing Interventions	Expected Outcomes

		• Administer prescribed pharmacologic agents for endocrine dysfunction (e.g., SIADH)
		   • Agents that inhibit secretion of a hormone
		   • Agents that decrease the effect of a hormone at its target organ
		 • Maintain skin and mucous membrane integrity
		   • Careful assessment of skin and mucous membranes
		   • Turn at least every 2 hours
		   • Provide mouth care every 4 hours	

Impaired Gas Exchange related to:
 • Decreased driving pressure of oxygen
   • Decreased inspired oxygen content (e.g., smoke)
   • Decreased barometric pressure (high altitude)
 • Alveolar hypoventilation
 • Increased alveolar deadspace
 • Shunt
 • Ventilation-perfusion mismatch
 • Alveolar-capillary membrane changes
 • Decreased hemoglobin and/or abnormal hemoglobin
 • Decreased 2,3-DPG levels
	• Tachycardia
	 • Dysrhythmias
	 • Mild hypertension
	 • Tachypnea
	 • Dyspnea, orthopnea
	 • Use of accessory muscles
	 • Cyanosis (depending on hemoglobin level)
	 • Cough: sputum may be pink-tinged and frothy in pulmonary edema
	 • Breath sound changes: diminished intensity of breath sounds; presence of adventitious sound (e.g., crackles)
	 • Decreased exercise capacity, fatigue
	 • Neurologic changes: restlessness to confusion to lethargy
	 • Pulmonary hypertension
	   • PAm >20 mm Hg
	   • PAd more than 5 mm Hg greater than PAOP
	   • PVR >250 dynes/sec/cm^{-5}
	 • Decreased SpO_2
	 • Arterial blood gas changes
	   • Decreased SaO_2, PaO_2
	   • $PaCO_2$ may be decreased or increased depending on ventilation status
	 • Elevated serum arterial lactate levels
	 • May have abnormal chest X-ray
		• Monitor for changes in defining characteristics
		 • Assess respiratory effort, rate, depth, rhythm, and use of accessory muscles
		 • Assess breath sounds as indicated
		 • Assess pulse oximetry and arterial blood gases as indicated
		 • Monitor pH and serum arterial lactate levels
		 • Assess patient for chest pain; administer analgesics as indicated and prescribed
		 • Monitor hemoglobin and CO
		   • Administer blood as prescribed for anemia
		   • Administer fluids replacement as prescribed for hypovolemia
		   • Administer inotropes, venous vasodilators, diuretics as prescribed for heart failure
		   • Monitor for effectiveness and adverse effects
		 • Position for optimal ventilation and optimal ventilation-perfusion matching
		   • Elevate head of bed 30-45 degrees for optimal chest excursion
		   • Prone and semiprone positions may also be used to improve ventilation
		   • Turn from good lung down to back every 2 hours
		 • Administer oxygen at 2-6 L/min to maintain SpO_2 of 95% or greater if patient is hypoxemic; if patient has chronic hypercapnia, administer oxygen to maintain SpO_2 at 90%-92%
		 • Keep artificial airways and manual resuscitation bag readily available; intubation and mechanical ventilation may be necessary
		 • Encourage the patient to turn and breathe deeply; encourage the patient to cough if rhonchi are audible
			• Alert and oriented
			 • Absence of dyspnea, orthopnea, use of accessory muscles, cough
			 • RR <24/min
			 • Clear and equal breath sounds
			 • Absence of crackles, rhonchi
			 • Skin color normal for race; absence of cyanosis
			 • Absence of dysrhythmias
			 • BP and HR within 10% of patient's normals
			 • PaO_2 >60 mm Hg; SaO_2 >90%
			 • $PaCO_2$ 35-45 mm Hg or at patient's normal level

Nursing Diagnosis	Defining Characteristics	Nursing Interventions	Expected Outcomes
		• Suction only if coughing is ineffective in clearing secretions or patient is too fatigued to cough (intubated patients cannot cough effectively and must be suctioned when secretions are present)	
		• Instruct and assist in splinting for deep breathing and coughing	
		• Encourage rest periods between coughing sessions and chest physiotherapy	
		• Utilize techniques to prevent complications of suctioning (e.g., hyperoxygenation)	
		• Encourage noncaffeinated oral fluids to thin secretions	
		• Two to three L of fluid/24 hr unless contraindicated by cardiac or renal disease	
		• Provide humidification of inspired air and therapeutic oxygen	
		• Keep room cool and comfortable	
		• Provide calm and quiet environment	
		• Identify and treat anxiety	
		• Assist in insertion of chest tube and institution of water-seal drainage system if necessary for pneumothorax or hemothorax	

Impaired Verbal Communication related to
• Artificial airway
• Aphasia
• Laryngectomy
	• Inability to speak
	• Difficulty expressing thoughts, needs, desires
		• Monitor for changes in defining characteristics
		• Emphasize temporary nature of loss of ability to speak if inability to communicate caused by artificial airway
		• Establish acceptable method of communication
		  • Picture communication board
		  • Alphabet board
		  • Felt-tip pen or marker and paper
		    • Pencils and ballpoint pens require more pressure
		  • "Magic" slate
		  • Lip reading is usually not an acceptable method, especially if oral tube is in place
		• Use short, simple questions that elicit "yes" or "no" answers
		• Use nonverbal communication (e.g., facial expressions, gestures, pointing)
		• Be calm and unhurried
		• Allow time for communication; be patient
		• Minimize distractions
		• Utilize family and significant others to assist with communication
			• Patient, nurse, and significant others are satisfied with ability to communicate
			• Patient able to communicate needs and desires

Continued

Nursing Diagnosis	Defining Characteristics	Nursing Interventions	Expected Outcomes

Ineffective Airway Clearance related to:
• Altered level of consciousness
• Airway obstruction
• Artificial airway
• Decreased energy/fatigue
• Increased amount or viscosity of mucus
• Ineffective cough
• Tracheobronchial infection
• Tracheobronchial trauma
• Mucosal swelling and/or bronchospasm
• Neuromuscular or impairment
• Perceptual/cognitive impairment
• Smoking: ineffective cilia
• Thoracic, abdominal, or flank pain
	• Tachycardia
	• Tachypnea
	• Dyspnea
	• Cough
	• Cyanosis (depending on hemoglobin level)
	• Clinical indicators of respiratory distress (see Table 4-2)
	• Clinical indicators of hypoxemia/hypoxia (see Table 4-3)
	• Clinical indicators of hypercapnia (see Table 4-4)
	• Fever
	• Adventitious breath sounds (e.g., crackles, rhonchi, wheezes)
	• Arterial blood gas changes
	  • Decreased SaO_2, PaO_2
	  • $PaCO_2$ may be decreased or increased depending on ventilation status
	• May have abnormal chest X-ray
		• Monitor for changes in defining characteristics
		• Monitor oxygenation and ventilation
		  • Bedside ventilatory parameters: tidal volume, vital capacity, maximal inspiratory pressure
		  • Arterial blood gases
		  • Pulse oximetry
		  • Capnography
		• Assess ability to clear secretions
		• Maintain a patent airway
		  • Ensure proper positioning of head and neck (e.g., sniffing position)
		  • Encourage deep breathing and sustained inspiratory maneuvers
		  • Utilize chest physiotherapy to mobilize secretions if indicated and not contraindicated
		    • Postural drainage
		    • Percussion
		    • Vibration
		  • Encourage coughing if rhonchi are audible
		    • Instruct and supervise controlled coughing
		  • Suction only if coughing is ineffective in clearing secretions or patient is too fatigued to cough
		    • Endotracheal tubes hold the epiglottis open and prevent effective coughing
		    • Utilize techniques to prevent complications of suctioning (e.g., hyperoxygenation)
		  • Encourage rest periods between coughing sessions and chest physiotherapy
		  • Utilize artificial airways if necessary
		    • Secure tube with tape, ties, or stabilization devices designed for ET tubes
		    • Restrain patient's wrists if necessary to prevent self-extubation
		    • Maintain cuff inflation to provide a relative seal if endotracheal tube or tracheostomy tube utilized
		• Assess color, consistency, amount, and odor of mucus
		  • Obtain sputum for culture and sensitivity if indicated
		• Assess for indications of pulmonary infection: fever, tachycardia, tachypnea, yellow, green, or brown sputum, rhonchi on auscultation, abnormal chest X-ray
			• Patient able to cough effectively to clear airways
			• Sputum: thin, clear
			• Vital capacity of at least 10 ml/kg and maximal inspiratory pressure of at least −20 cm H_2O
			• Breath sounds clear and equal bilaterally
			• PaO_2 of at least 60 mm Hg; SaO_2 of at least 90%; SvO_2 >60%
			• $PaCO_2$ 35-45 mm Hg or within 5 mm Hg of the patient's normal

Nursing Diagnosis	Defining Characteristics	Nursing Interventions	Expected Outcomes
		• Encourage noncaffeinated oral fluids to thin secretions • Two to three L fluid/24 hr unless contraindicated by cardiac or renal disease • Adequate humidification provided via mask, humidifier, nebulizer in patients with artificial airways • Administer oxygen if patient is hypoxemic; oxygen must be humidified • Position the patient for optimal chest excursion and optimal coughing: high-Fowler's position with knees drawn up; reposition at least every 2 hours • Administer pharmacologic therapies as prescribed: expectorants, mucolytics, antibiotics • Teach patient abdominal muscle-tightening exercises and diaphragmatic breathing if muscle weakness is a factor • Teach family assisted coughing techniques if indicated (e.g., cervical or high thoracic level spinal cord injury) • Teach and provide incisional splinting if thoracic pain is a factor	

Ineffective Breathing Pattern related to:
• Anxiety
• Airway or tracheobronchial obstruction
• Abdominal distention
• Barotrauma
• CNS depression (e.g., opiates, head injury)
• Increased work of breathing
  • Decreased compliance
  • Increased airway resistance
• Decreased energy/fatigue
• Immobility
• Morbid obesity
• Muscle deconditioning
• Neuromuscular or musculoskeletal impairment
• Thoracic or abdominal pain
• Ventilator malfunction
	• Tachycardia
	• Tachypnea
	• Dyspnea
	• Cough
	• Prolonged expiratory time
	• Diminished chest excursion
	• Asymmetric chest excursion
	• Clinical indicators of respiratory distress (see Table 4-2)
	• Clinical indicators of hypoxemia/hypoxia (see Table 4-3)
	• Clinical indicators of hypercapnia (see Table 4-4)
	• Breath sound changes: diminished and/or unequal breath sounds, crackles, wheezes
	• Decreased tidal volume and vital capacity
	• Arterial blood gas changes
	  • Decreased SaO_2, PaO_2
	  • $PaCO_2$ may be decreased or increased depending on ventilation status
	• May have abnormal chest X-ray
		• Monitor for changes in defining characteristics
		• Monitor oxygenation and ventilation
		  • Bedside ventilatory parameters: tidal volume, vital capacity, maximal inspiratory pressure
		  • Arterial blood gases
		  • Pulse oximetry
		  • Capnography
		• Position for optimal ventilation and optimal ventilation-perfusion matching
		  • Elevate head of bed 30-45 degrees for optimal chest excursion
		  • Prone and semiprone positions may also be used to improve ventilation
		  • Turn from good lung down to back every 2 hours
		• Encourage deep breathing every 2 hours; incentive spirometry may also be helpful
		• Utilize chest physiotherapy as indicated
		• Administer oxygen if patient is hypoxemic to maintain SaO_2 95% or greater unless contraindication; if patient has chronic hypercapnia, maintain SaO_2 90%-92%
		• Encourage coughing if rhonchi are audible
		• Suction patient if coughing is inadequate
			• HR <120/min or within 20 bpm of patient's normal
			• RR < 24/min
			• Absence of subjective reports of dyspnea
			• Absence of intercostal retractions or use of accessory muscles
			• Chest excursion of at least 3 cm
			• Clear and equal breath sounds
			• Symmetrical breath sounds
			• Tidal volume at least 5 ml/kg; vital capacity at least 10 ml/kg
			• PaO_2 of at least 60 mm Hg; SaO_2 or SpO_2 of at least 90%
			• $PaCO_2$ 35-45 mm Hg with pH between 7.35 and 7.45

Continued

Nursing Diagnosis	Defining Characteristics	Nursing Interventions	Expected Outcomes

		• Encourage rest periods between coughing sessions and chest physiotherapy
		• Administer pharmacologic therapies as prescribed
		  • Beta$_2$-stimulants and xanthines for bronchospasm
		  • Expectorants and mucolytics for excess mucus
		  • Antibiotics for infection
		  • Analgesics for pain
		  • Sedatives should be avoided if possible
		• Keep artificial airways and manual resuscitation bag readily available
		• Institute mechanical ventilation as indicated by inadequate ventilation (elevated PaCO_2 with respiratory acidosis)
		  • Assess ability to breathe in "synch" with ventilator
		  • Sedate as necessary
		• Maintain nutritional status and prevent muscle wasting by providing appropriate meals and/or supplements
		  • Provide high-protein, high-calorie meals and supplements; increased calories are provided by increasing fat as carbohydrate metabolism increases CO_2 production
		• Assess and maintain functioning of chest tubes if appropriate
		If esophageal-gastric balloon tamponade
		• Keep scissors at the bedside in patients with balloon tamponade tube in place; if tube accidentally becomes displaced upward blocking the airway, cut across all lumens and remove tube
		• Keep an extra tube in the room for immediate replacement if needed to control bleeding
		• Always electively deflate the esophageal balloon before the gastric balloon	

Ineffective Individual and Family Coping related to:
• Overwhelming disease process
• Dependence on technology
• Situational crisis
	• Patient and/or significant others verbalize anxiety, apprehension, nervousness, uncertainty, fear, worry, grief, hopelessness, powerlessness, isolation
	• Patient and/or significant others express inability to cope
		• Monitor for changes in defining characteristics
		• Recognize common causes of stress in patient
		  • Sudden, unexpected change in health status
		  • Body image changes (e.g., incision, wounds, loss of limb, skin color, vascular access)
			• Patient and/or significant others express fears and concerns
			• Patient and/or significant others able to participate in decision making and care

Nursing Diagnosis	Defining Characteristics	Nursing Interventions	Expected Outcomes
• Disruption of usual family functions and roles	• Patient and/or significant others demonstrate nonverbal indicators of anxiety • Hesitancy of significant others to spend time with critically ill patient or inappropriate behavior when visiting • Misinterpretation of information • Inability to make decisions • Lack of cooperation among family members • Inappropriate emotional outbursts • Arguments among family members; arguments with patient • Inability to respond to each other's feelings and support each other	• Fear of unknown • Long-term hospitalization • Role changes • Sexuality changes • Fear of death • Establish rapport; give patient undivided attention; *listen* to patient • Consider individuality of this patient; treat the patient as a unique person • Identify patient's perception of the situation; identify significant other's assessment of the situation • Assess past and current coping mechanisms; support effective copying mechanisms • Explain all procedures, the reasons for them, and their importance in a simple, concise, reassuring manner • Provide honest and accurate information • Provide opportunity for patient to verbalize feelings, concerns, fears, anxieties • Talk to and reassure patient in a calm, firm voice; be unhurried; maintain calm, confident attitude • Provide for comfort: decrease stimuli, adjust room temperature, allow for rest periods • Teach and encourage utilization of relaxation techniques • Allow patient to make decisions regarding environment and self-care activities • Encourage the patient to participate in self-care activity if he or she is able; praise efforts • Allow visitation by family/significant others and encourage their participation in care • Encourage family and significant others participation in care • Observe family and significant others for signs of fatigue and need for emotional or spiritual support; utilize psychiatric liaison nurse, psychologists, social workers, and chaplain • Assess usual roles and discuss feelings about changes in role performance • Promote hope and positive attitude • Identify and encourage utilization of community resources and support groups	• Patient and/or significant others able to utilize psychosocial support

Continued

Nursing Diagnosis	Defining Characteristics	Nursing Interventions	Expected Outcomes

Pain related to:
• Biologic injury
• Chemical injury
• Physical injury
• Psychologic factors
	• Verbal complaints of pain
	• Tense, guarded posture
	• Sympathetic responses: tachycardia, mild hypertension, tachypnea, pupillary dilation, diaphoresis
	• Grimacing, moaning, crying, restlessness, withdrawal
	• Impaired concentration, irritability
	• Knees flexed to relieve pain in peritoneal irritation
	• Tense, guarded posture
	• Rebound tenderness may be present
		• Monitor for changes in defining characteristics
		• Observe patient for verbal and nonverbal expression of pain or discomfort
		• Assess pain: PQRST
		  • P: provocation, palliation
		  • Q: quality
		  • R: region, radiation
		  • S: severity
		  • T: timing
		• Utilize nonpharmacologic approaches
		  • Place patient in position of comfort
		  • Encourage relaxation techniques including imagery
		  • Provide distraction
		• Administer analgesics as prescribed
		  • Narcotics (e.g., morphine)
		    • Intravenous: intermittent bolus, basal continuous dose
		    • Epidural: basal continuous dose, intermittent bolus
		    • Oral: absorption is affected by GI perfusion; seldom used in critical care situations
		  • Nonnarcotics: NSAIDs are particularly helpful for surgical and inflammatory pain
		  • Local anesthetics (e.g., bupivacaine [Marcaine])
		    • Interpleural
		    • Intercostal
		• Provide environment conducive to rest whenever possible
		  • Comfortable temperature
		  • Dim lighting
		  • Quiet or relaxing music
		• Prepare patient for procedures to be performed and any anticipated pain
		• Instruct patient to inform nurse of any new pain
		Chest pain
		• Obtain baseline vital signs and monitor as indicated
		• Obtain multiple-lead ECG with each episode of chest pain
		  • Assess ECG for:
		    • ST-T-wave changes
		    • Conduction defects
		  • Monitor continuous ECG for rate, rhythm, and dysrhythmias
		• Monitor for accompanying signs/symptoms
		• Obtain cardiac enzymes and isoenzymes as indicated
		• Initiate IV infusion and administer solution at prescribed rate or to keep vein open (KVO)
			• Patient verbalizes relief of pain
			• Absence of nonverbal indicators of pain
			• BP and HR within 10% of patient's normals
			If chest pain
			• Absence of ST-T-wave changes
			• Absence of dysrhythmias

Nursing Diagnosis	Defining Characteristics	Nursing Interventions	Expected Outcomes
		• Administer oxygen at 5 L/min via nasal cannula unless contraindicated	
		• Administer antianginal agents (e.g., nitroglycerin) or analgesics (e.g., morphine) as prescribed	
		• Remain with patient during chest pain	
		• Report persistent chest pain, significant changes in blood pressure, heart rate, or rhythm, respiratory rate and rhythm to physician	
		Abdominal pain	
		• Assess for changes in bowel sounds, abdominal distention, rebound tenderness	
		• Maintain gastric suction and NPO status as indicated	
		• Prepare patient for procedures to be performed and any anticipated pain	
		Headache	
		• Do not give narcotics if clinical indications of intracranial hypertension are present; nonnarcotic analgesics are usually used	
Risk for Aspiration related to:	• Tachycardia	• Monitor for changes in defining characteristics	• Absence of dyspnea, cough, tachypnea, tachycardia, or fever
• Decreased level of consciousness	• Tachypnea	• Assess gag and cough reflex; assess ability to swallow	
• Oropharyngeal airway in conscious patient	• Dyspnea	• Keep suction equipment available	• Breath sounds clear and equal
	• Cough	• Position unconscious patients on their side	
• Presence of endotracheal tube (splints epiglottis open)	• Fever	• Offer foods with consistency that patient can swallow; cut food into small pieces; soft and semi-liquid foods may be easier for the patient to swallow than liquids	• Normal arterial blood gases and chest X-ray
	• Breath sound changes: diminished breath sounds; presence of adventitious sounds (e.g., crackles, rhonchi, wheezes)		
• Facial/oral/neck surgery or trauma	• Arterial blood gas changes: hypoxemia with hypocapnia	• Encourage the patient to chew thoroughly and eat slowly; discourage talking while eating	
• Wired jaws	• Abnormal chest X-ray	• Maintain upright position for 30-45 minutes after feeding	
• Impaired gag and/or cough reflex		• Administer antacids and/or histamine$_2$-receptor antagonists as prescribed to decrease the acidity of gastric contents in patients at high risk of aspiration	
• Impaired swallowing			
• Increased gastric volume or retention			
• Increased intraabdominal pressure		*Nasogastric suction*	
• Gastrointestinal tubes, especially large-bore nasogastric tubes		• Maintain nasogastric suction as prescribed	
		• Use appropriate suction	
		• Nonvented tubes should be on intermittent low suction	
• Decreased gastric motility		• Vented nasogastric tubes should be on continuous low suction	
• Enteral feedings		• Reposition tube as needed to maintain drainage	

Nursing Diagnosis	Defining Characteristics	Nursing Interventions	Expected Outcomes
		Enteral nutrition • Check placement of tube prior to use; chest X-ray is required for small-lumen feeding tube • Elevate head of bed 30 degrees during and after intermittent enteral feedings; keep head of bed elevated at all times if continuous enteral feedings are used • Utilize small-lumen feeding tubes, which cause less gastroesophageal incompetence than do larger lumen nasogastric tubes; percutaneous gastroscopy or jejunostomy tubes also help to prevent aspiration • Check for gastric retention prior to intermittent enteral feedings and at least every four hours if receiving continuous enteral feedings; hold feeding for 1 hour if greater than 100 ml is aspirated • Administer metoclopramide HCl (Reglan) as prescribed to promote gastric motility *Endotracheal tube* • Keep endotracheal or tracheostomy tube cuff inflated utilizing minimal occlusive volume or minimal leak technique; tracheal pressure should be less than 20 mm Hg (25 cm H_2O) to prevent tracheal ischemia • Do not routinely deflate cuff because upper airway secretions are allowed to fall down into airway	
Risk for Impaired Skin Integrity related to: • Dry skin • Edema • Diaphoresis • Dermatitis • Skin lesions • Pruritus	• Breaks in skin or mucous membranes • Reddened excoriated skin • Edematous skin • Incisions or other wounds	• Monitor for changes in defining characteristics • Turn patient or assist patient in turning at least every 2 hours • Inspect skin for erythema or prolonged blanching with each position change • Use turning sheets to turn patients rather than letting them scoot	• Skin is clean, dry, intact • Absence of reddened areas or breaks in skin or mucous membranes • Absence of redness, induration at intravenous or intraarterial catheter sites

Nursing Diagnosis	Defining Characteristics	Nursing Interventions	Expected Outcomes

• Prolonged skin contact with body secretions
  • Incontinence
  • Diarrhea
  • Fistula
  • Stoma
• Adhesives
• Surgical procedures
• Invasive procedures and catheters
• Bacterial or fungal infections
• Immobility
• Malnutrition
• Age
• Pronounced body prominences
• Radiation therapy
• Hypothermia or hyperthermia
	• Breaks in skin or mucous membranes
	• Reddened excoriated skin
	• Edematous skin
	• Incisions or other wounds
		• Position with pillows to relieve pressure
		• Keep head of bed elevated no more than 30 degrees to prevent shearing forces
		• Keep linens dry and wrinkle-free
		• Special beds may be necessary for patients with increased risk of skin breakdown (e.g., malnutrition, incontinence)
		• Limit time sitting in chair to 2 hours at a time
		• Keep skin clean and dry
		• Apply water-soluble lubricant to each nostril every 8 hours for patients with nasogastric tube
		• Clean rectal area after each episode of diarrhea using a mild soap
		• Avoid tape and adhesives if possible
		• Keep edematous limbs elevated
		• Administer medications for itching (e.g., antihistamines) as prescribed
		• Administer topical antibiotics as prescribed
		• Provide active and/or passive ROM exercises
		• Collaborate with physician and dietician to provide adequate nutritional support
		  • High-protein diet unless contraindicated
		  • Enough carbohydrates that the protein will not be used for energy
		  • Monitor serum total protein, serum albumin, and serum transferrin levels for improvement in nutritional status
		• Provide standardized care for monitoring and maintaining intravenous and arterial catheters
		• Apply gentle consistent pressure to bleeding sites
		• Limit injections, invasive procedures if possible
		• Avoid rectal temperatures, tubes
		• Provide oral hygiene every 4 hours
		• Avoid drying solutions (e.g., alcohol-containing mouthwashes, lemon and glycerin swabs)
		• Moisturize lips with lubricant
			• Indicators of adequate healing of surgical incisions or wounds
			• Decrease in clinical indications of inflammation (redness, swelling, warmth, pain)

Continued

Nursing Diagnosis	Defining Characteristics	Nursing Interventions	Expected Outcomes

Risk for Infection related to:
• Artificial airway
• Decreased activity of the Kupffer cells
• Decreased function of immune system
• Decreased number or function of leukocytes
• Exposure to unusually virulent (e.g., hospital-acquired) organism
• Humidifiers and nebulizers
• Hyperglycemia
• Immunodeficiency
• Impaired or absent protective reflexes
• Inadequate primary defenses
• Increased amounts of circulating corticosteroids
• Intestinal perforation
• Invasive procedures and/or catheters
• Loss of normal flora
• Malnutrition
• Side effects of drugs
• Surgical procedures
• Translocation of GI bacteria to blood or lymph
• Uremic toxins
	• Tachycardia
	• Fever
	• Leukocytosis (especially with increased neutrophils with increased bands)
	• Redness, warmth, induration, purulent drainage at catheter insertion site or surgical wound
	• Positive blood, sputum, urine, or wound cultures
	• Cloudy, foul-smelling urine
	• Crackles, abnormal chest X-ray
	• Yellow, brown, or green sputum; may be foul-smelling
		• Monitor for changes in defining characteristics
		• Practice handwashing for at least 10 seconds using mechanical friction and soap and water before catheter insertion, catheter manipulation, blood sampling, dressing changes
		• Utilize universal blood and body fluid precautions
		  • Wear gloves for suctioning, oral care, repositioning of ET, IV care, indwelling urinary bladder catheter care, wound care, and for any other procedure that involves contact with body fluids, secretions, or blood
		  • Utilize disposable gowns in situations when clothing may be contaminated by body fluids
		  • Utilize eye protection during tracheobronchial suctioning or any other time when spraying of secretions may occur
		• Avoid invasive procedures if possible; discontinue invasive catheters as soon as possible
		• Utilize aseptic techniques to protect from cross-contamination and nosocomial infection
		• Monitor environment, visitors, personnel caring for patient for possible contamination sources
		• Change catheters, tubings, dressings at regular intervals; meticulous aseptic technique when caring for invasive lines
		  • Handle all IVs aseptically
		  • Secure catheters to prevent catheter movement and vein irritation
		  • Maintain an occlusive, sterile dressing on invasive lines; change at least every 48-72 hours and more often if soiled
		  • Change IV tubing every 48-72 hours or per hospital policy
		  • Eliminate all nonessential stopcocks; cover stopcock ports with occlusive covers
		  • Remove and replace catheters inserted in an emergency, without proper asepsis as soon as possible under aseptic conditions
		  • Inspect skin for redness, localized warmth, or drainage from incisions, venous catheter sites, arterial catheter sites
		  • Remove and culture catheters at any sign of infection
			• Normothermia
			• WBC: less than 11,000 mm^3
			• Absence of clinical indications of local infection: redness, swelling, purulent drainage from IV sites, wounds, incision lines
			• Urine: clear and faintly ammonia scented
			• Breath sounds: clear and equal
			• Chest X-ray: absence of changes indicative of pneumonia, atelectasis
			• Negative culture if obtained

Nursing Diagnosis	Defining Characteristics	Nursing Interventions	Expected Outcomes

		• Avoid indwelling urinary catheter if possible; straight catheterization intermittently is usually preferable unless hourly urine output monitoring is necessary
		• Ensure maintenance of a closed drainage system if indwelling urinary catheter is used; empty collection bag at least every 8 hours and measure carefully; observe urinary drainage for color, odor, and sediment
		• Provide meticulous skin care to avoid breaks in skin integrity; apply lotion to dry skin
		• Provide aseptic vascular access care; monitor for redness, induration, purulent drainage
		• Keep nails clipped short to decrease scratching trauma; pruritus is a serious problem in renal failure
		• Provide meticulous pulmonary care: encourage deep breathing, incentive spirometry, coughing or suctioning if needed, monitor sputum production and appearance
		  • Encourage patient to cough if rhonchi are audible
		  • Observe and record amount and character of sputum; culture as indicated
		  • Provide oral hygiene every 4-8 hours
		  • Provide stoma care every 8 hours; change gauze dressing more often if copious secretions are present
		  • Maintain sterile technique in suctioning endotracheal tubes or tracheostomy tubes; aseptic technique for oropharyngeal or nasopharyngeal airways
		  • Empty humidifier condensation into water trap; not back into humidifier reservoir
		  • Change ventilator tubing circuit every 48 hours or per hospital policy
		• Utilize appropriate isolation techniques for patients with positive hepatitis antigen: private room, separate hemodialysis machine if on dialysis, caution with all body secretions
		• Obtain culture and sensitivity studies of purulent drainage, malodorous and/or cloudy urine, malodorous or discolored sputum as indicated; blood cultures are indicated for temperatures above 101° F or 38.3° C	

Continued

Nursing Diagnosis	Defining Characteristics	Nursing Interventions	Expected Outcomes

		• Evaluate nutritional status and provide appropriate nutritional support and vitamin supplementation
		• Assess for early clinical indications of sepsis (e.g., cognitive changes, tachycardia, tachypnea, fever)
		• Assess for hemodynamic monitoring for changes of septic shock (e.g., decreased SVR, increased CO/CI, increased SvO_2)
		• Administer antibiotics as prescribed
		  • Administer antibiotics on time to ensure maintenance of therapeutic blood levels
		  • Monitor peak and trough levels and for clinical indications of toxicity
		  • Monitor creatinine clearance as indicated, especially when giving aminoglycoside antibiotics	

Risk for Injury related to:
• Altered cerebral function
  • CNS infection or malignancy
  • Inadequate cerebral perfusion or oxygenation
  • Increased ammonia levels
  • HIV encephalopathy
  • Hypoglycemia
• Seizures
• Endotracheal intubation
• Intravenous and/or arterial catheters
• Microshock
• Stress ulcer
• Vascular access
• Increased intrathoracic pressure
• Inadequate blink reflex
	• Disorientation
	• Impaired judgment
	• Sensory-perceptual deterioration
	• Patient reaching for endotracheal tube
	• Clinical manifestations of air embolism
	  • Respiratory distress
	  • Hypotension
	  • Change in level of consciousness
	• Clinical manifestations of venous thrombosis
	  • Edema
	  • Erythema
	  • Ipsilateral swelling of arm, neck, face
	  • Pain at site
	• Clinical manifestations of arterial thrombosis
	  • Pain of limb distal to puncture and occlusion
	  • Pallor
	  • Pulselessness and decreased capillary refill rate
	  • Motor and/or sensory changes
	  • Coolness or coldness
	• Dysrhythmias caused by microshock
	• Stress caused by critical care environment and critical illness and/or administration of corticosteroids
	• Presence of vascular access
	• History of emphysema, congenital blebs, or use of large tidal volumes or levels of PEEP
		• Monitor for changes in defining characteristics
		Altered cerebral function
		• Maintain a quiet environment to reduce environmental stimuli
		  • Dim lights
		  • Minimize noise
		• Reorient patient often: have clock, calendar, family pictures in room
		• Keep needed items (e.g., call light) placed within easy reach
		• Provide simple, brief explanations
		• Provide consistency in caregiver assignment
		• Caution visitors to avoid stress-provoking discussions
		• Maintain siderails up and bed in low position
		• Monitor closely for clinical indications of hypoglycemia, especially during peak times of insulin effect, if meals are missed, or if exertion is increased
		• Reduce and maintain BUN < 100 mg/dl by dialysis, prevention of constipation, dehydration, and GI bleed
		Seizures
		• Initiate seizure precautions if indicated
		  • Instituted if serum sodium <125 mEq/L or if patient has a history of or predisposition to seizures
		  • Includes close observation, padded siderails, supplemental oxygen, oral airway at bedside
		Intubation
		• Restrain only as necessary for patient protection
		• Reorient patient often and inform of purpose of tube, why he or she cannot speak, etc.
			• Absence of injury
			• Patient does not self-extubate
			• Absence of clinical manifestations of air embolism
			• Absence of clinical manifestations of venous thrombosis
			• Absence of clinical manifestations of arterial thrombosis
			• Absence of dysrhythmias caused by microshock
			• Negative guaiac stools and vomitus
			• Patient does not develop pneumothorax, pneumomediastinum, or subcutaneous emphysema
			• Absence of bleeding from vascular access
			• Absence of corneal abrasion

Nursing Diagnosis	Defining Characteristics	Nursing Interventions	Expected Outcomes
	• Use of muscle paralytic agents • Absence of blink reflex	*Intravenous and/or arterial catheters* • Use Luer-Lok connections on all intravenous and intraarterial catheters • Instruct patient to hold breath during tubing changes on central venous catheter • Monitor for clinical manifestations of venous thrombosis; catheter should be removed as soon as possible • Monitor for clinical manifestations of arterial thrombosis; catheter should be removed immediately *Microshock* • Recognize patients at risk of microshock (e.g., patients with intracardiac catheter, pacemaker leads) • Do not touch a piece of electrical equipment at the same time as you touch the patient • Touch the siderail before you touch the patient to discharge static electricity • Report 60-cycle interference or any piece of malfunctioning equipment to the biomedical department immediately • Ensure proper grounding of all electrical equipment *Stress ulcer* • Assess gastric pH; monitor gastric aspirate and/or stools for occult blood • Monitor bowel habits; observe for tarry or bloody stools • Provide oral or enteral feedings to decrease gastric acidity and protect the gastric mucosa; antacids and/or histamine$_2$-receptor antagonists may be prescribed to decrease the acidity of gastric contents (maintain pH 3.5 to 5.0); sucralfate (Carafate) may be used as a mucosal barrier *Potential for barotrauma* • Monitor peak inflation pressure and compliance • Monitor for clinical indications of pneumothorax: sudden increase in peak inflation pressure, diminished breath sounds on affected side, hypoxemia • Assist with emergency decompression with needle tap and/or insertion of chest tube as requested *Vascular access* • Assess external vascular access connections to ensure that they are tightly connected • Perform frequent neurovascular assessments of limb with vascular access	

Nursing Diagnosis	Defining Characteristics	Nursing Interventions	Expected Outcomes

Sleep-Pattern Disturbance related to:
• Noise
• Unfamiliar surrounding
• Discomfort with room temperature, humidity, lighting, odor
• Frequent awakenings by healthcare professionals
• Physical restraint
• Immobility
• Lack of privacy
• Absence of sleep partner
• Nocturia
• Pain
• Dyspnea
• Nausea, vomiting, dyspepsia
• Disturbance of circadian rhythm
• Daylight/darkness exposure
• Anxiety, fear
• Worry about home, health, problems
• Depression
• Loneliness
• Drug effect
	• Inability to go to sleep
	• Frequent awakenings
	• Early awakening
	• Verbalization of difficulty falling asleep
	• Verbalization of not feeling rested
	• Decreased proportion of REM sleep
		Inadequate blink reflex
		• Instill artificial tears or Lacrilube as indicated
		• Monitor for changes in defining characteristics
		• Provide daytime activities (e.g., ROM, ambulation) as tolerated
		• Encourage the patient to discuss fears and concerns
		• Maintain light-dark patterns and wake-sleep patterns; discourage excessive sleep during the day
		• Assess the patient's usual presleep nighttime rituals; assist the patient to perform these rituals (e.g., assist with mouth care, washing of face and hands, beverage at bedside, etc.)
		• Avoid stimulants close to bedtime (e.g., caffeine-containing beverages, chocolate)
		• Avoid heavy meal prior to sleep; a small snack may be helpful
		• Provide backrub at bedtime if desired
		• Provide relaxing music if desired
		• Assist the patient to a position of comfort
		• Allow the patient's significant other to sleep in the patient's room if possible
		• Ensure comfort
		  • Room temperature and bed coverings
		  • Lighting
		  • Elimination of offensive odors
		  • Elimination of unnecessary noise (e.g., decrease volume of alarms, close door, ask staff to lower voices)
		• Administer pharmacologic agents as prescribed
		  • Anxiolytics
		  • Sedatives
		  • Hypnotics
		  • Analgesics
		• Avoid interrupting the patient's sleep unless absolutely necessary (e.g., omit vital sign measurement during sleep if possible, schedule medications before sleep)
			• Patient verbalizes satisfaction with amount and quality of sleep

Common Abbreviations Used in Critical Care

2,3-DPG	2,3-diphosphoglyceric acid
A	Alveolar
a	Arterial
A_2	Aortic (first) component of S_2
AAA	Abdominal aortic aneurysm
AACN	American Association of Critical-Care Nurses
AAL	Anterior axillary line
ABG	Arterial blood gas
ABI	Anklc-brachial index
AC	Assist-control
ACE	Angiotensin-converting enzyme
ACLS	Advanced cardiac life support
ACT	Activated clotting time
ACTH	Adrenocorticotropic hormone
ADH	Antidiuretic hormone
ADL	Activities of daily living
ADP	Adenosine diphosphate
AF	Atrial fibrillation
AHA	American Hospital Association
AICD	Automatic implantable cardioverter defibrillator
AIDS	Acquired immune deficiency syndrome
AIVR	Accelerated idioventricular rhythm
ALS	Amyotrophic lateralizing sclerosis
ALT	Alanine aminotransferase
ANA	Antinuclear antibody
ANA	American Nurses' Association
ANF	Atrial natriuretic factor
aPTT	Activated partial thromboplastin time
AR	Aortic regurgitation
ARDS	Acute respiratory distress syndrome
ARF	Acute respiratory failure
AS	Aortic stenosis
ASA	Acetylsalicylic acid (aspirin)
AST	Aspartate aminotransferase

ATN	Acute tubular necrosis
ATP	Adenosine triphosphate
AV	Atrioventricular
AVM	Arteriovenous malformation
BBB	Bundle branch block
BCLS	Basic cardiac life support
Bi-PAP	Positive airway pressure on both inspiration and expiration
Bi-VAD	Biventricular assist device
BP	Blood pressure
BSA	Body surface area
BUN	Blood urea nitrogen
C	Celsius (also referred to as *centigrade*)
CABG	Coronary artery bypass graft
CAD	Coronary artery disease
Cao_2	Oxygen content in arterial blood
CAPP	Coronary artery perfusion pressure
CAVH	Continuous arteriovenous hemofiltration
CAVHD	Continuous arteriovenous hemodialysis
CBC	Complete blood count
CBF	Cerebral blood flow
CCO	Continuous cardiac output
CCU	Critical care unit
CDC	Centers for Disease Control and Prevention
CHB	Complete heart block
CHO	Carbohydrate
CHP	Capillary hydrostatic pressure
CI	Cardiac index
CK	Creatine kinase
CK-MB	Creatine kinase-myocardial band
cm	Centimeter
CMV	Cytomegalovirus
CNS	Central nervous system
CO	Cardiac output
CO_2	Carbon dioxide
COP	Colloidal oncotic pressure
COPD	Chronic obstructive pulmonary disease
CPAP	Continuous positive airway pressure
CPD	Citrate phosphate dextrose
CPP	Cerebral perfusion pressure
CPR	Cardiopulmonary resuscitation
CQI	Continuous quality improvement
CRRT	Continuous renal replacement therapy
CSF	Cerebrospinal fluid
CT	Computed atrial tomography
CVA	Costovertebral angle
CVA	Cerebrovascular accident
CvO_2	Oxygen content in venous blood
CVP	Apcentral venous pressure
CVVHD	Continuous venovenous hemodialysis
D_5LR	5% dextrose in lactated Ringer's

D_5NS	5% dextrose in normal saline
D_5W	5% dextrose in water
DAI	Diffuse axonal injury
DBP	Diastolic blood pressure
DI	Diabetes insipidus
DIC	Disseminated intravascular coagulation
DKA	Diabetes ketoacidosis
dl	Deciliter
DM	Diabetes mellitus
DNA	Deoxyribonucleic acid
DNR	Do not resuscitate
DO_2	Oxygen delivery to the tissues
DO_2I	Delivery of oxygen to the tissue index
DTR	Deep tendon reflexes
DVT	Deep vein thrombosis
ECF	Extracellular fluid
ECG	Electrocardiogram (may also be abbreviated EKG)
ECMO	Extracorporeal membrane oxygenator
EDH	Epidural hematoma
EEG	Electroencephalogram
ELCA	Excimer laser coronary arthrectomy
EMG	Electromylogram
EMI	Electromagnetic interference
EPS	Electrophysiology studies
ERCP	Endoscopic retrograde cholangiopancreatography
ERV	Expiratory reserve volume
ESR	Eosinophil sedimentation rate
ET	Endotracheal
F	Fahrenheit
f	Frequency of ventilation
FDA	Food and Drug Administration
FEV	Forced expiratory capacity
FFP	Fresh frozen plasma
FIo_2	Fraction of inspired oxygen
FRC	Functional residual capacity
FSP	Fibrin split products (also referred to as *fibrin degradation products*)
FVC	Forced vital capacity
g	Gram
GCS	Glasgow Coma Scale
GFR	Glomerular filtration rate
GI	Gastrointestinal
GP	Glycoprotein
GU	Genitourinary
H^+	Hydrogen ion
H_2O	Water
HBV	Hepatitis B virus
HCO_3	Bicarbonate
Hct	Hematocrit
HDL	High-density lipoproteins
HF	Heart failure

HFV	High-frequency ventilation
Hg	Mercury
Hgb	Hemoglobin
HHNK	Hyperglycemic hyperosmolar nonketotic (condition or coma)
HIV	Human immunodeficiency virus
HLA	Human leukocyte antigen
HOB	Head of bed
HR	Heart rate
HRT	Hormone replacement therapy
I:E	Inspiration:expiration
IABP	Intraaortic balloon pump
IAP	Intraabdominal pressure
IC	Inspiratory capacity
ICH	Intracranial hematoma
ICOP	Interstitial colloidal oncotic pressure
ICP	Intracranial pressure
ICS	Intercostal space
ICU	Intensive care unit
IFD	Intermittent flush device
Ig	Immunoglobulin
IHD	Inflammatory heart disease
IHP	Interstitial hydrostatic pressure
IHSS	Idiopathic hypertrophic subaortic stenosis (now referred to as *hypertrophic cardiomyopathy*)
IL	Interleukin
ILV	Independent lung ventilation
IM	Intramuscular
IMV	Intermittent mandatory ventilation
INR	International normalized ratio
IPPB	Intermittent positive-pressure breathing
IRA	Infarct-related artery
IRV	Inspiratory reserve volume
IRV	Inverse ratio ventilation
IU	International units
IV	Intravenous
IVP	Intravenous pyelogram
JVD	Jugular venous distention
kg	Kilogram
KS	Kaposi's sarcoma
KUB	Kidneys, ureters, bladder (same as flat plate of abdomen)
L	Liter
LA	Left atria
LAAL	Left anterior axillary line
LAD	Left anterior descending (artery)
LAD	Left axis deviation
LAH	Left anterior hemibundle
LAP	Left atrial pressure
LBB	Left bundle branch
LBBB	Left bundle branch block
LCA	Left circumflex artery
LDH	Lactic dehydrogenase

LDL	Low-density lipoproteins
LES	Lower esophageal sphincter
LICS	Left intercostal space
LLQ	Left lower quadrant
LMAL	Left midaxillary line
LMN	Lower motor neuron
LOC	Level of consciousness
LP	Lumbar puncture
LPAL	Left posterior axillary line
LPH	Left posterior hemibundle
LR	Lactated Ringer's
LSB	Left sternal border
LUQ	Left upper quadrant
LV	Left ventricle
LVAD	Left ventricular assist device
LVEDP	Left ventricular end-diastolic pressure
LVEDV	Left ventricular end-diastolic volume
LVF	Left ventricular failure
LVH	Left ventricular hypertrophy
LVSWI	Left ventricular stroke work index
M_1	Mitral (first) component of S_1
mA	Milliampere (unit of measurement for electrical current)
MAL	Midaxillary line
MAO	Monoamine oxidase (as in MAO inhibitors)
MAP	Mean arterial pressure
MCL	Midclavicular line
mEq	Milliequivalent (unit of measurement for solutes in solution)
mg	Milligram (unit of measurement for weight)
MI	Myocardial infarction
MIDCABG	Minimally invasive coronary artery bypass graft
MIP	Maximal inspiratory pressure (or force) (also referred to as negative inspiratory pressure [or force])
ml	Milliliter (unit of measurement for volume)
mm	Millimeter (unit of measurement for length)
mm Hg	Millimeters of mercury
MODS	Multiple organ dysfunction syndrome
mOsm/kg	Milliosmols per kilogram (unit of measure for osmolality)
MR	Mitral regurgitation
MRI	Magnetic resonance imaging
MS	Mitral stenosis
MSL	Midsternal line
MUGA	Multiple-gated acquisition scan
MVO_2	Myocardial oxygen consumption
MVP	Mitral valve prolapse
μg	Microgram (unit of measurement for weight)
NBHD	Nonbeating heart donor
NDE	Near death experience
NG	Nasogastric
NIF	Negative inspiratory force
NK	Natural killer
NNRTI	Nonnucleoside reverse transcriptase inhibitor

NPO	Nothing by mouth
NS	Normal saline
NSAID	Nonsteroidal antiinflammatory drug
NSR	Normal sinus rhythm
NTG	Nitroglycerin
NTP	Nitroprusside
NYHA	New York Heart Association
O_2	Oxygen
O_2EI	Oxygen extraction index
O_2ER	Oxygen extraction ratio
P_2	Pulmonic (second) component of S_2
PA	Pulmonary artery
PAC	Premature atrial contraction
$Paco_2$	Partial pressure of carbon dioxide in arterial blood
PAd	Pulmonary artery diastolic pressure
PAL	Posterior axillary line
PAm	Pulmonary artery pressure mean
Pao_2	Pressure of oxygen in arterial blood
PAO_2	Pressure of oxygen in alveolar blood
PAOP	Pulmonary artery occlusive pressure (previously referred to as *pulmonary capillary wedge pressure* or *pulmonary artery wedge pressure*)
PAP	Pulmonary artery pressure
PAs	Pulmonary artery systolic pressure
PAT	Paroxysmal atrial tachycardia
PC/IRV	Pressure-controlled/inverse ratio ventilation
PCA	Patient-controlled analgesia
PCI	Percutaneous coronary intervention
PCP	*Pneumocystis carinii* pneumonia
PD	Postural drainage
PDE	Phosphodiesterase
PE	Pulmonary embolism
PEA	Pulseless electrical activity
P_Eco_2	Partial pressure of carbon dioxide in exhaled air
PEEP	Positive end-expiratory pressure
PEG	Percutaneous endoscopic gastrostomy
PET	Positron emission tomography
$P_{et}co_2$	Partial pressure of carbon dioxide in end-tidal air
pH	Hydrogen ion concentration
pHi	Intramucosal pH
PICC	Peripherally inserted central catheter
PIP	Peak inspiratory pressure
PJC	Premature junctional contraction
PMI	Point of maximal impulse
PML	Progressive multifocal leukoencephalopathy
PMN	Polymorphonuclear leukocytes
PMR	Papillary muscle rupture
PMR	Progressive muscle relaxation
PND	Paroxysmal nocturnal dyspnea
PNS	Parasympathetic nervous system
PO	Oral

PPF	Plasma protein fraction
PSV	Pressure support ventilation
PT	Prothrombin time
PT	Physical therapy
PTCA	Percutaneous transluminal coronary angioplasty
PTT	Partial prothrombin time
Ptco$_2$	Transcutaneous Pao$_2$
PVC	Premature ventricular contraction
PVR	Pulmonary vascular resistance
PVRI	Pulmonary vascular resistance index
Q	Perfusion
QA	Quality Assurance
RA	Right atrium
RAA	Renin-angiotensin-aldosterone
RAD	Right axis deviation
RAP	Right atrial pressure
RAS	Reticular activating system
RBB	Right bundle branch
RBBB	Right bundle branch block
RBC	Red blood cell
RCA	Right coronary artery
REF	Right (ventricular) ejection fraction
REM	Rapid eye movement
RHD	Rheumatic heart disease
RICS	Right intercostal space
RIND	Reversible ischemic neurologic deficit
RLQ	Right lower quadrant
RNA	Ribonucleic acid
ROM	Range of motion
rPA	Recombinant plasminogen activator
RQ	Respiratory quotient
RR	Respiratory rate
RSB	Right sternal border
rtPA	Recombinant tissue plasminogen activator
RUQ	Right upper quadrant
RV	Right ventricle
RV	Residual volume
RVAD	Right ventricular assist device
RVEDP	Right ventricular end-diastolic pressure
RVEDV	Right ventricular end-diastolic volume
RVF	Right ventricular failure
RVH	Right ventricular hypertrophy
RVSWI	Right ventricular stroke work index
SA	Sinoatrial
SAH	Subarachnoid hemorrhage
Sao$_2$	Oxygen saturation of arterial blood
SC	Subcutaneous
SCI	Spinal cord injury
SCUF	Slow continuous ultrafiltration
SDH	Subdural hematoma

SIADH	Syndrome of inappropriate antidiuretic hormone
SIMV	Synchronized intermittent mandatory ventilation
SIRS	Systemic inflammatory response syndrome
Sjo_2	Oxygen saturation of jugular venous blood
SK	Streptokinase
SNS	Sympathetic nervous system
Spo_2	Oxygen saturation in plasma (e.g., pulse oximetry)
SRS-A	Slow-reacting substance of anaphylaxis
SV	Stroke volume
SVI	Stroke volume index
Svo_2	Oxygen saturation of mixed venous blood
SVR	Systemic vascular resistance
SVRI	Systemic vascular resistance index
SVT	Supraventricular tachycardia
T_1	Tricuspid (second) component of S_1
TAA	Thoracic aortic aneurysm
TB	Tuberculosis
TCA	Tricyclic antidepressants
TEC	Transluminal extraction catheter
TENS	Transcutaneous electrical nerve stimulation
TIA	Transient ischemic attack
TIPS	Transjugular intrahepatic portosystemic shunt
TLC	Total lung capacity
TNF	Tumor necrosis factor
TPN	Total parenteral nutrition
TQM	Total quality management
TT	Thrombin time
UES	Upper esophageal sphincter
UMN	Upper motor neuron
UTI	Urinary tract infection
V	Ventilation
V/Q	Ventilation/perfusion ratio
V_A	Alveolar minute ventilation
VAD	Ventricular assist device
VAPSV	Volume-assured pressure support ventilation
VC	Vital capacity
V_D	Anatomical deadspace
V_E	Minute ventilation
VF	Ventricular fibrillation
VO_2	Oxygen consumption by the tissues
VO_2I	Consumption of oxygen by the tissue index
VPR	Volume pressure response
V/Q	Ventilation/perfusion
VSD	Ventricular septal defect
VT	Ventricular tachycardia
V_T	Tidal volume
WBC	White blood cell
WPW	Wolff-Parkinson-White syndrome

Normal Laboratory Values

Blood

Chemistries

I. Sodium: 136 to 145 mEq/L
II. Potassium: 3.5 to 5.0 mEq/L
III. Chloride: 96 to 106 mEq/L
IV. Calcium: 8.5 to 10.5 mg/dl
V. Phosphorus: 3.0 to 4.5 mg/dl
VI. Magnesium: 1.5 to 2.5 mEq/L or 1.8 to 2.4 mg/dl
VII. CO_2: 23 to 30 mEq/L
VIII. Glucose: 70 to 110 mg/dl
IX. BUN: 5 to 20 mg/dl
X. Creatinine: 0.7 to 1.5 mg/dl
XI. Uric acid: 3 to 7 mg/dl
XII. Osmolality: 280 to 295 mOsm/L
XIII. Lactate: 1 to 2 mmol/L
XIV. Ammonia: 15 to 110 mg/dl
XV. Iron: 50 to 150 µg/dl
XVI. Iron-binding capacity: 250 to 410 µg/dl
XVII. Carcinoembryonic antigen (CEA): less than 2 ng/ml
XVIII. Bilirubin
    A. Total: 0.3 to 1.3 mg/dl
    B. Direct: 0.1 to 0.3 mg/dl
    C. Indirect: 0.1 to 1.0 mg/dl
XIX. Proteins
    A. Total protein: 6 to 8 g/dl
    B. C-reactive protein: less than 0.8 mg/dl
    C. Albumin: 3.5 to 4.5 g/dl
    D. Prealbumin: 15 to 32 mg/dl
    E. Transferrin: 250 to 300 mg/dl
    F. Globulin: 2.3 to 3.5 g/dl
    G. Albumin/globulin ratio (A/G): 1.5:1 to 2.5:1
    H. Fibrinogen: 200 to 400 mg/dl or 2 to 4 g/L
XX. Lipids
    A. Cholesterol: 150 to 200 mg/dl
    B. Triglycerides: 40 to 150 mg/dl
    C. Lipoprotein-cholesterol fractionation
        1. HDL: 29 to 77 mg/dl
        2. LDL: 62 to 185 mg/dl

XXI. Enzymes
    A. Total CK: normal 55 to 170 U/L for males; 30 to 135 U/L for females
    B. CK to MB: 0 to 4% of total CK
    C. LDH: 90 to 200 IU/L
    D. LDH-1: 17 to 25% of total LDH
    E. Alanine aminotransferase (ALT): 5 to 36 units/ml (formerly called *SGPT*)
    F. Aspartate aminotransferase (AST): 15 to 45 units/ml (formerly called *SGOT*)
    G. Gammaglutamyl transferase (GGT): 5 to 38 IU/L
    H. Alkaline phosphatase: 30 to 85 IU/L
    I. Amylase: 56 to 190 IU/L
    J. Lipase: 0 to 1.5 U/ml
XXII. Muscle proteins
    A. Myoglobin: normal less than 110 ng/ml
    B. Troponin I: normal less than 1.5 ng/ml
    C. Troponin T: normal less than 0.1 ng/ml

Arterial Blood Gases

I. pH: normal 7.35 to 7.45
II. $Paco_2$: normal 35 to 45 mm Hg
III. HCO_3: normal 22 to 26 mEq/L
IV. Base excess: −2 to +2
V. Pao_2: normal 80 to 100 mm Hg
VI. Sao_2: more than 95%

Hematology

I. Red blood cells (RBC): 4.4 to 5.9×10^6/ml for males; 3.8 to 5.2×10^6/ml for females; red cell indices include the following:
    A. Mean corpuscular volume (MCV): 80 to 100 μm^3
    B. Mean corpuscular hemoglobin (MCH): 27 to 31 pg
    C. Mean corpuscular hemoglobin concentration (MCHC): 32 to 36 g/dl
II. Reticulocyte count: 0.5 to 1.5% of RBC

III. Erythrocyte sedimentation rate (ESR or sed rate): 1 to 13 mm/hr for males, 1 to 20 mm/hr for females

IV. Hematocrit: 40% to 52% for males; 35% to 47% for females

V. Hemoglobin: 13 to 18 g/dl for males; 12 to 16 g/dl for females

VI. Platelets: 150,000 to 400,000/mm^3

VII. White blood cells (WBC): 3,500 to 11,000 mm^3
  A. Differential
    1. Neutrophils: 40% to 80%
    2. Eosinophils: 0% to 5%
    3. Basophils: 0% to 2%
    4. Monocytes: 3% to 8%
    5. Lymphocytes: 10% to 40%

VIII. Immune profile
  A. CD4 cell count: 800 cells/mm^3; varies with age
  B. CD4/CD8 ratio: helper cells:suppressor/cytotoxic cells ratio: >1

IX. HIV antibody screening: negative

Clotting Profile

I. Prothrombin time (PT): 12 to 15 seconds

II. Activated partial thromboplastin time (aPTT): 25 to 38 seconds

III. Activated clotting time (ACT): 70 to 120 seconds

IV. Thrombin time: 10 to 15 seconds

V. Bleeding time: 1 to 9.5 minutes

VI. Lee White clotting time: 6 to 12 minutes

VII. Platelets: 150,000 to 400,000/mm^3

VIII. Fibrinogen: 200 to 400 mg/dl or 2 to 4 g/L

IX. Fibrin split products (FSPs) (also referred to as *fibrin degradation products* [FDPs]): 0 to 10 µg/dl

X. D-dimer: normal less than 250 ng/ml

Hormones

I. Thyroid-stimulating hormone (TSH): normal 2 to 10 mU/L

II. Triiodothyronine (T3): 0.2 to 0.3 µg/dl

III. Thyroxine (T4): 6 to 12 µg/dl

IV. ACTH: 15 to 100 pg/ml in a.m., 10 to 50 pg/ml in p.m.

V. Cortisol: 6 to 28 µg/dl at 8 a.m., 4 to 12 µg/dl at 4 p.m.; 2 to 12 µg/dl at 8 p.m.

VI. ADH: 1 to 5 pg/ml

Toxicology

I. Alcohol: 0 mg/dl

II. Dilantin: therapeutic 10 to 20 µg/ml

III. Digoxin: therapeutic 0.5 to 2.0 ng/ml

IV. Lidocaine: therapeutic 1.5 to 5.0 µg/ml

V. Phenobarbital: therapeutic 10 to 40 µg/ml

VI. Theophylline: therapeutic 10 to 20 ng/dl

Urine

I. Glucose: negative

II. Ketones: negative

III. Protein: 0 to 8 mg/dl; less than 150 mg/24 hr urine output

IV. Amylase: 3 to 21 IU/hr

V. Bilirubin: negative

VI. Bilinogen: 0.3 to 3.5 mg/dl

VII. RBCs: 0 to 2/low power field

VIII. WBCs: 0 to 4/low power field

IX. Hemoglobin/myoglobin: negative

X. Bilirubin: none

XI. Specific gravity: 1.005 to 1.030

XII. Osmolality: 50 to 1,200 mOsm/L

XIII. Creatinine clearance: 85 to 135 ml/min

XIV. Culture and sensitivity: no bacteria present; if bacteria are present, appropriate antibiotic therapy is identified

XV. pH: 4.0 to 8.0 with average of 6.0

XVI. Spot urine electrolytes
  A. Sodium: 40 to 220 mEq/L/day
  B. Potassium: 25 to 120 mEq/L/day
  C. Chloride: 110 to 250 mEq/day

XVII. Hormone metabolites
  A. 17-Hydroxycorticosteroids: 4.5 to 10 mg/24 hr for males, 2.5 to 10 mg/24 hr for females
  B. 17-Ketosteroids: 8 to 15 mg/24 hr for males, 6 to 12 mg/24 hr for females

Stool

I. Fecal occult blood test: negative

II. Ova, parasites, blood (OPB): negative

III. Fecal fat: 5 g/24 hr

IV. Urobilinogen: 0 to 4 mg/day

V. Culture: intestinal flora

VI. Assay for *Clostridium difficile* toxin A or B: normal negative; positive if diarrhea is caused by *C. difficile*

Note: Values may vary depending on laboratory.

Formulae Significant to Critical Care Nursing

General

Conversion	
To convert pounds to kilograms	1 lb = 0.45 kg
To convert inches to cm	1 in = 2.54 cm
To convert mm Hg to cm of H_2O	1 mm Hg = 1.36 cm H_2O
To convert Fahrenheit to Celsius	$(°F - 32) ÷ 1.8$

Drug Administration	
To calculate μg/kg/min if you know the rate of the infusion	$\dfrac{(μg/ml) \times (ml/hr)}{(60\ min/hr) \times (kg\ of\ body\ weight)}$
To calculate rate in ml/hr if you know the dose in μg/kg/min	$\dfrac{(dose\ in\ μg/kg/min) \times (60\ min/hr) \times (wt\ in\ kg)}{μg/ml\ of\ the\ solution}$
To calculate mg/min if you know the rate of the infusion	$\dfrac{(mg/ml) \times (ml/hr)}{(60\ min/hr)}$
To calculate rate in ml/hr if you know the dose in mg/min	$\dfrac{(dose\ in\ mg/min) \times (60\ min/hr)}{mg/ml\ of\ the\ solution}$
To calculate μg/min if you know the rate of the infusion	$\dfrac{(μg/ml) \times (ml/hr)}{(60\ min/hr)}$
To calculate rate in ml/hr if you know the dose in μg/min	$\dfrac{(dose\ in\ μg/min) \times (60\ min/hr)}{μg/ml\ of\ the\ solution}$

Cardiovascular

Parameter	Method of Calculation	Normal
Mean arterial pressure (MAP)	[BP systolic + (BP diastolic × 2)] ÷ 3	70-105 mm Hg (Normal systolic BP 90-140 mm Hg; normal diastolic BP 60-90 mm Hg)
Cardiac index (CI)	CO ÷ BSA	2.5-4.0 L/min/m^2
Stroke volume (SV)	CO ÷ HR	60-120 ml/beat
Stroke index (SI)	SV/BSA	30-65 ml/m^2/beat
Systemic vascular resistance (SVR)	[(MAP − RAP) × 80] ÷ CO	900-1,400 dynes/sec/cm^{-5}
Systemic vascular resistance index (SVRI)	[(MAP − RAP) × 80] ÷ CI	1,700-2,600 dynes/sec/cm^{-5}/m^2
Pulmonary vascular resistance (PVR)	[(PAm − PAOP) × 80] ÷ CO	100-250 dynes/sec/cm^{-5}
Pulmonary vascular resistance index (PVRI)	[(PAm − PAOP) × 80] ÷ CI	225-315 dynes/sec/cm^{-5}/m^2
Left ventricular stroke work index (LVSWI)	[SI × (MAP − PAOP)] × 0.0136	45-65 g•m/m^2

Parameter	Method of Calculation	Normal
Right ventricular stroke work index (RVSWI)	$[SI \times (PAm - RAP)] \times 0.0136$	5-12 g•m/m^2
Coronary artery perfusion pressure (CAPP)	Diastolic BP – PAOP	60-80 mm Hg
Right ventricular end-diastolic volume index (RVEDVI)	RVEDV ÷ BSA	60-100 ml/m^2
Right ventricular end-systolic volume index (RVESVI)	RVESV ÷ BSA	30-60 ml/m^2
Arterial oxygen content (Cao$_2$)	$1.34 \times Hgb \times Sao_2$	18-20 ml/dl
Venous oxygen content (Cvo$_2$)	$1.34 \times Hgb \times Svo_2$	12-16 ml/dl
Oxygen delivery (DO$_2$)	$CO \times Cao_2 \times 10$	900-1,100 ml/min
Oxygen delivery index (DO$_2$I)	$CI \times Cao_2 \times 10$	550-650 ml/min/m^2
Oxygen consumption (VO$_2$)	$CO \times Hgb \times 13.4 \times (Sao_2 - Svo_2)$	200-300 ml/min
Oxygen consumption index (VO$_2$I)	$CI \times Hgb \times 13.4 \times (Sao_2 - Svo_2)$	110-160 ml/min/m^2
Oxygen extraction ratio (O$_2$ER)	Cao$_2$ – Cvo$_2$ ÷ Cao$_2$	22%-30%
Oxygen extraction index (O$_2$EI)	Sao$_2$ – Svo$_2$ ÷ Sao$_2$	20%-27%
Coronary artery perfusion pressure (CAPP)	Diastolic BP – PAOP	60-80 mm Hg
Corrected QT	$QT \div \sqrt{RR}$	0.35-0.43 seconds

Pulmonary

Parameter	Method of Calculation	Normal
Static compliance	(Tidal volume/Plateau pressure) – PEEP	50-100 ml/cm H$_2$O
Dynamic compliance	(Tidal volume/Peak pressure) – PEEP	35-55 ml/cm H$_2$O
a/A ratio	(Pao$_2$/Pao$_2$) Note: Pao$_2$ is calculated as: Fio$_2$ (760 – 47) – (Paco$_2$ ÷ 0.8) **Note:** Fio$_2$: fraction of inspired oxygen (written as a decimal) Pb: barometric pressure (760 mm Hg at sea level, adjust for higher altitudes) (47 is the pressure of water vapor at sea level and is subtracted from barometric pressure); Paco$_2$: arterial carbon dioxide tension 0.8 is the usual respiratory quotient	normal >0.8 moderately abnormal 0.5-0.8 significantly abnormal 0.25-0.5 critically abnormal <0.25
A:a gradient	Pao$_2$ – Pao$_2$	<10 mm Hg **Note:** A:a gradient × 0.05 = approximate % shunt
Pao$_2$/Fio$_2$ ratio	Pao$_2$/Fio$_2$ (decimal)	>300 300 = ~15% shunt 200 = ~20% shunt
Respiratory index	(Pao$_2$ – Pao$_2$)/Pao$_2$	<1.0

Neurologic

Parameter	Method of Calculation	Normal
Cerebral perfusion pressure (CPP)	MAP – ICP	60-100 mm Hg

Nutrition

Parameter	Method of Calculation	Normal
Body mass index (BMI)	Weight (kg)/Ht (m) × Ht (m)	Optimal: 20-25 Obesity: >25 Underweight: <20

Fluid, Electrolyte, Acid-Base

Parameter	Method of Calculation	Normal
Serum osmolality	$(2 \times Na) + \dfrac{BUN}{2.6} + \dfrac{glucose}{18}$	280-295 mOsm/L
Anion gap	$(Na + K) - (Cl + HCO_3)$	5-15

Critical Care Pharmacology: Selected Drugs Often Used in Critical Care

Drug	Classification/ Actions	Indications	Administration	Adverse Effects	Nursing Implications
Abciximab (ReoPro)	**Platelet aggregation inhibitor** (GP IIb/IIIa platelet receptor blocker) • Inhibits platelet aggregation and platelet-mediated thrombosis	• Acute coronary syndrome with or without percutaneous coronary intervention (PCI) • PCI when risk for thrombosis is high	• IV injection: 0.25 mg/kg administered between 10 minutes and 1 hour before the start of the PTCA or atherectomy followed by infusion • IV infusion: 0.125 μg/kg/min (10 μg/min maximum) for 12 hours	• Bleeding • Intracranial hemorrhage • Hematuria • Hematemesis • Bleeding at sheath site or other puncture point • Thrombocytopenia • Hypotension • Bradycardia • Nausea, vomiting, abdominal pain • Chest pain • Back pain • Headache • Pain at injection site • Allergic reaction, anaphylaxis (especially with repeat administration)	• Monitor PT, aPTT, or ACT, platelet count • Administer with aspirin and heparin therapy as prescribed • Note contraindications: patients with active internal bleeding, clinically significant bleeding in the GI or GU tract within the last 6 weeks, bleeding diathesis, history of CVA within the last two years or CVA with significant residual neurologic deficit, intracranial neoplasm, aneurysm, or AV malformation, severe uncontrolled hypertension, oral anticoagulants within 7 days unless prothrombin time is less than 1.2 × control, thrombocytopenia, presumed or documented history of vasculitis, major surgery or trauma within the last 6 weeks, pericarditis, known hypersensitivity to abciximab or murine proteins • Use cautiously in patients who weigh less than 75 kg, patients older than 65 years of age, patients with a history of GI disease, patients receiving thrombolytics • Do not administer with dextran • Monitor oral secretions, sputum, vomitus, NG aspirate, stool, urine for blood • Limit venipuncture and urinary catheterization as possible; use IV catheter with saline lock for blood sampling; avoid noncompressible IV sites • Avoid nasotracheal and nasogastric tubes if possible • Avoid automatic BP cuffs • Administer platelets as prescribed for thrombocytopenia • Store refrigerated, do not shake (should be clear), administer through filter

Continued

Drug	Classification/ Actions	Indications	Administration	Adverse Effects	Nursing Implications
Adenosine (Adenocard)	**Endogenous Nucleoside** **Unclassified Antidysrhythmic** • Slows conduction through the AV node • Interrupts the reentry pathways through the AV node to restore normal sinus rhythm	• Supraventricular tachycardias, including those associated with WPW • Not effective in atrial fibrillation or atrial flutter but may slow rate so that fibrillatory or flutter waves can be identified	• IV injection: 6 mg IV; must be given within 6 seconds; repeat at 12 mg IV if conversion is not achieved within 1-2 minutes; 12-mg dose may be repeated once • Must be administered as quickly as possible (referred to as IV "slam") due to very short half-life (10 seconds); administer as quickly as possible into NS flush or insert Y connector into line to push NS flush as quickly as possible after pushing adenosine as quickly as possible	• Transient dysrhythmias at the time of conversion (including short asystolic pause) • Pause may be prolonged, especially in patients with sick sinus syndrome • Hypotension if large doses are used • Nausea • Facial flushing • Headache • Dyspnea • Bronchospasm • Chest pressure • Recurrence of dysrhythmias	• Monitor HR, BP, ECG, RR and depth, breath sounds • Note contraindications: known hypersensitivity, second- or third-degree AV block, sick sinus syndrome, ventricular dysrhythmias • Use cautiously in patients with asthma or older adults • Decrease initial dosage as prescribed in patients receiving dipyridamole (Persantine), diazepam (Valium), phenobarbital, or carbamazepine (Tegretol); initial dose may be prescribed as 3 mg • Increase initial dosage as prescribed if patient receiving aminophylline or another xanthine; initial dose may be prescribed as 12 mg • Store at room temperature; solution must be clear at time of use
Albuterol (Proventil, Ventolin)	**Sympathomimetic Bronchodilator (beta₂-specific)** • Relaxes smooth muscle of bronchi	• Bronchospasm, asthma	• PO: 2-4 mg every 6-8 hours • Hand-held inhaler: 1-2 inhalations every 4-6 hours • Nebulizer: 0.5 ml (2.5 mg) in 3-5 ml of normal saline over 10-15 minutes every 6 hours	• Tachycardia • Palpitations • Nausea, vomiting • Anxiety • Tremor • Headache	• Monitor HR, BP, breath sounds • Note contraindications: known hypersensitivity, glaucoma, tachydysrhythmias; do not give with MAO inhibitors • Use cautiously in older adults and patients with diabetes mellitus, hypertension, hyperthyroidism, cardiac disease, seizure disorder, prostatic hypertrophy • Do not administer with beta-blockers (they block effect)
Aminophylline (Theophylline, Elixophyllin, Tedral, Quibron, Choledyl)	**Xanthine Bronchodilator** • Relaxes smooth muscle of bronchi and pulmonary vessels • Decreases PVR	• Bronchospasm, asthma • Pulmonary edema • Pulmonary hypertension	• PO: 250-500 mg every 6-8 hours • IV: loading dose of 5-6 mg/kg (250-500 mg) over 20 minutes followed by infusion	• Tachycardia • Hypotension • Palpitations • Anxiety • Restlessness • Insomnia • Dizziness	• Monitor HR, BP, ECG, RR and rhythm, breath sounds, urine output, and fluid status • Note contraindications: known sensitivity, cardiac dysrhythmias

	• Increases cardiac contractility causing increased CO and GFR • Inhibits histamine and slow-reacting substance of anaphylaxis (SRA)	• IV infusion: mix 500 mg in 250 ml (2 mg/ml) and infuse at 0.5-0.7 mg/kg/hr 　• HF, liver disease: ~0.1-0.2 mg/kg/hr 　• COPD: ~0.3 mg/kg/hr 　• Smokers: ~0.8 mg/kg/hr • Therapeutic blood level 10-20 µg/ml	• Tremors • Headache *Signs of toxicity:* • Anorexia, nausea, vomiting • Ventricular dysrhythmias • Agitation, seizures	• Use cautiously in older adult and patients with acute MI, HF, hypertension, hepatic disease, acute peptic ulcer, hyperthyroidism, diabetes mellitus • Administer PO drug with meals to decrease GI adverse effects
Amiodarone hydrochloride (Cordarone)	**Class III Antidysrhythmic** • Prolongs the action potential and effective refractory period • Life-threatening or refractory ventricular dysrhythmias • Refractory supraventricular dysrhythmias, especially those caused by WPW	• PO: loading dose of 800-1,600 mg/day for 1-3 weeks; then 600-800 mg/day for 1 month; then 200-800 mg/day • IV injection (loading dose): 150 mg over 10 minutes followed by: • IV infusion: mix 900 mg in 500 ml (1.8 mg/ml); usual dose is 1 mg/min for the next 6 hours followed by 0.5 mg/min 　• Use central venous catheter if more concentrated solution is used 　• Use solutions diluted in PVC containers within 2 hours; solutions diluted in glass or polyolefin containers within 24 hours 　• Administer through PVC tubing since dosing has taken into account adsorption to tubing • Therapeutic blood level 1.5-2.5 µg/ml	• Hypotension • Proarrhythmia including PVCs, ventricular tachycardia, torsades de pointes, PACs, supraventricular tachycardia, bradycardia, SA block or arrest, AV block, bundle branch block • HF • Nausea, vomiting • Dizziness • Headache • Fatigue, malaise, muscle weakness • Corneal microdeposits • Rash, photosensitivity • Altered liver enzymes, hepatotoxicity • Hyperthyroidism, hypothyroidism • Blue-gray skin discoloration • Tremors, peripheral neuropathies, extrapyramidal symptoms • Cough, progressive dyspnea, pulmonary fibrosis	• Monitor HR, BP, ECG, RR and depth, breath sounds, electrolytes, liver function studies, thyroid function studies, pulmonary function studies, chest X-ray, neurologic symptoms • Monitor for clinical indications of heart failure, pulmonary fibrosis • Note contraindications: known hypersensitivity, marked sinus bradycardia, second- or third-degree AV block unless functioning pacemaker, cardiogenic shock • Use cautiously in patients with sinus node disease, conduction disturbances, severely depressed ventricular function, and marked cardiomegaly • Do not confuse amiodarone (an antidysrhythmic agent) with amrinone (an inotropic agent) • Advise methylcellulose ophthalmic solution and annual eye examinations for patients on long-term therapy • Advise use of SPF 15 sunscreen and sunglasses for patients on long-term therapy • Monitor for drug interactions: interacts with digitalis, anticoagulants, beta-blockers, calcium channel blockers, phenytoin, and class I antidysrhythmics • If used concurrently with digitalis, monitor closely for indications of digitalis toxicity • Administer PO drug with food to decrease GI adverse effects

Continued

Drug	Classification/Actions	Indications	Administration	Adverse Effects	Nursing Implications
Amrinone (Inocor)	**PDE Inhibitor Inotrope** • Increases cardiac contractility • Relaxes vascular smooth muscle to cause vasodilation of arteries and veins and decrease afterload and preload	• Short-term management of patients with HF who have not responded to traditional therapy of digitalis, diuretics, and/or vasodilators	• IV injection: 0.75 mg/kg over 2-3 minutes; may repeat in 30 minutes • IV infusion: mix 500 mg in 500 ml (1000 μg/ml) and infuse at 5-15 μg/kg/min • Maximum: 10 mg/kg/day • Do not reconstitute with dextrose	• Hypotension • Dysrhythmias • Anorexia, nausea, vomiting, abdominal pain, diarrhea • Increased liver enzymes, hepatotoxicity • Thrombocytopenia • Chest pain • Hypersensitivity reactions • Burning at injection site	• Monitor HR, BP, ECG, PA, PAOP, CI, SVR, platelet counts, liver function studies, electrolytes (especially potassium), BUN, creatinine • Platelet count below 150,000/mm³ usually requires dosage reduction • Platelet count below 100,000/mm³ usually requires discontinuance • Note contraindications: known hypersensitivity to this drug or bisulfites (preservative), severe aortic or pulmonic valvular disease, hypertrophic cardiomyopathy, ventricular dysrhythmias • Use cautiously in renal disease, liver disease, atrial dysrhythmias, older adult • Use cautiously in acute MI since myocardial oxygen consumption is increased • Correct hypokalemia and hypovolemia before or during amrinone use • Note that milrinone is prescribed more often than amrinone because of the greater incidence of thrombocytopenia with amrinone • Do not confuse amiodarone (an antidysrhythmic agent) with amrinone (an inotropic agent)
Atropine sulfate Ipratropium (Atrovent)	**Anticholinergic (also called parasympatholytic)** • Decreases vagal tone • Increases sinus rate • Slightly increases conduction through the AV node • Relaxes smooth muscle; prevents bronchospasm • Decreases GI, tracheobronchial secretions	• Symptomatic sinus bradycardia • Asystole • Preoperative preparation for surgery • Anticholinesterase insecticide (organophosphate) poisoning • Bronchospasm; asthma	• IV injection: 0.5-2 mg (0.5 mg given as initial dose in sinus bradycardia, 1 mg given as initial dose in asystole, 2 mg given as initial dose in organophosphate poisoning); repeated as needed at 3- to 5-minute intervals • Maximum: 0.04 mg/kg (usually approximately 3.0 mg) • Nebulizer: 0.025 mg/kg diluted with 3-5 ml of normal saline every 6-8 hours • Hand-held inhaler: 2 puffs every 6-8 hours	• Tachycardia, palpitations • Bradycardia if given slowly or in dose of <0.5 mg • Hypotension • Dry mouth • Blurred vision, dilated pupils • Urinary retention • Constipation, paralytic ileus • Headache • Dizziness • Restlessness • Increased myocardial oxygen consumption and chest pain in patients with CAD Note: ipratropium (by inhalation) causes virtually no systemic adverse effects	• Monitor HR, BP, ECG, urine output, bowel sounds • Note contraindications: known hypersensitivity to belladonna, glaucoma, GI obstruction, myasthenia gravis, thyrotoxicosis, ulcerative colitis, prostatic hypertrophy, tachydysrhythmias • Use cautiously in renal disease, HF, hyperthyroidism, hepatic disease, hypertension • Use cautiously in acute MI: do not administer atropine for bradycardia unless the patient is symptomatic; increasing heart rate increases myocardial oxygen consumption and can increase infarction size • Do not use pupils as a reflection of brain status after atropine: pupils will be dilated and nonreactive • Use hard candy to help alleviate side effect of dry mouth unless contraindicated

Drug	Action	Indications	Dosage	Adverse Effects	Nursing Considerations
Bretylium (Bretylol)	**Class III Antidysrhythmic** • Initially exerts short-lived adrenergic stimulatory effects: increased contractility and automaticity • Later adrenergic blocking effects dominate: decreased contractility and automaticity • Increased ventricular fibrillation threshold	• Ventricular dysrhythmias	• IV injection: • VT: 5-10 mg/kg slowly (over 8 minutes) • VF: 5 mg/kg; may be repeated at 10 mg/kg every 5 minutes • Maximum: 30 mg/kg • IV infusion: mix 2 g in 500 ml (4 mg/ml) and infuse at 1-2 mg/min • Therapeutic blood level 0.5-1.5 µg/ml	• Transient tachycardia, hypertension • Bradycardia • AV block • Hypotension • Nausea, vomiting • Vertigo • Nasal congestion • Dizziness, lightheadedness, syncope • Chest pain • HF	• Monitor HR, BP, ECG • Note contraindications: known hypersensitivity, digitalis toxicity, aortic stenosis, pulmonary hypertension • This drug may aggravate digitalis toxicity and is contraindicated in ventricular dysrhythmias caused by digitalis toxicity • Use cautiously in renal disease • Monitor for potentiation of the effects of catecholamines • Monitor for vomiting, a common adverse effect; be prepared to suction the patient's airway
Calcium chloride	**Electrolyte** • Increases vascular tone and cardiac contractility in hypocalcemia • Reverses calcium channel blocker toxicity • Decreases cardiac effects of hyperkalemia • Decreases neuromuscular effects of hypermagnesemia	• Hypocalcemia • Calcium channel blocker toxicity • Hyperkalemia • Hypermagnesemia	• IV injection: 500 mg-1 g (7-14 mEq) at rate <50 mg/min; may repeat at 10-minute intervals • Administer into central venous catheter or large peripheral vein	• Bradycardia (especially if injected rapidly) • Hypotension • Shortened QT • Ventricular dysrhythmias • Cardiac arrest • Hypercalcemia • Pain or burning at injection site, phlebitis	• Monitor HR, BP, ECG, serum calcium • Note contraindications: hypercalcemia, digitalis toxicity, ventricular fibrillation, renal calculi • Use cautiously in renal disease, pulmonary disease, cor pulmonale, digitalized patients, sarcoidosis • Monitor for clinical indications of hypercalcemia: lethargy, confusion, muscle weakness, dysrhythmias • Maintain patient in supine position for 30 minutes after IV dose • Do not give with sodium bicarbonate • Prevent extravasation: necrosis may result

Continued

Drug	Classification/ Actions	Indications	Administration	Adverse Effects	Nursing Implications

Captopril (Capoten)	**ACE (Angiotensin-Converting Enzyme) Inhibitor**
	• Inhibits conversion of angiotensin I to angiotensin II
	• Prevents vasoconstriction and aldosterone secretion to decrease preload and afterload
		• HF
		• Hypertension
			• PO: 6.25-150 mg every 8-12 hours
			  • Administer 1 hour before meals
			  • Maximum: 450 mg/day
			Other ACE inhibitors:
			• Enalapril (Vasotec)
			  • PO: 5-40 mg/day
			  • IV injection: 1.25-5 mg every 6 hours
			• Lisinopril (Zestril): PO: 10-80 mg/day
			• Ramipril (Altace): PO: 1.25-20 mg/day
			• Benazepril (Lotensin): PO: 10-40 mg/day in one or two equally divided doses
			• Quinapril (Accupril): PO: 5-80 mg/day
			• Fosinopril (Monopril): PO: 10-80 mg/day
				• Tachycardia
				• Hypotension, especially after first dose
				• Anorexia
				• Loss of taste
				• Rash, angioedema
				• Dizziness
				• Photosensitivity
				• Proteinuria, nephrotic syndrome, renal failure
				• Leukopenia
				• Hyperkalemia
				• Bronchospasm
				• Cough
					• Monitor HR, BP, urine output, protein in urine, serum potassium, WBC
					  • Check periodically for proteinuria
					  • Monitor WBC and differential before treatment and periodically during treatment
					• Note contraindications: known hypersensitivity, AV block, hypotension
					• Use cautiously in renal disease, lupus, scleroderma, hypovolemia, leukemia, diabetes mellitus, thyroid disease, COPD, asthma, hyperkalemia and in patients on drugs that may affect WBC counts or immune response
					• Monitor for allergic reaction: rash, fever, pruritus, urticaria; antihistamines may be used; discontinuance may be necessary
					• Administer thiazide diuretics as prescribed; often given together
					• Angiotensin II blocker (e.g., losartan [Cozaar], valsartan [Diovan] may be prescribed if cough develops

Carvedilol (Coreg)	**Alpha and Beta Adrenergic Blocker** • Blocks response to alpha and beta stimulation • Causes decrease in SVR and BP without reflex tachycardia • Causes decrease in heart rate	• NYHD class II or III heart failure • Hypertension • Angina	• PO: 6.25 mg bid initially; after 7-14 days, if tolerated well, may be increased to 12.5 bid; after 7-14 days, if tolerated well, may be increased to 25 mg bid • Maximum: 50 mg/day	• Bradycardia • Orthostatic hypotension • Ventricular dysrhythmias • AV blocks • HF • Nausea, vomiting, diarrhea • Dizziness • Lethargy • Hyperglycemia in type 2 DM • Hypoglycemia without symptoms in type 1 DM • Agranulocytosis, thrombocytopenia • Bronchospasm in patients with asthma, COPD	• Monitor HR, BP, ECG, breath sounds, daily weight • Note contraindications: known hypersensitivity, shock, second- or third-degree AV block, sinus bradycardia, sick sinus syndrome, NYHD class IV HF, asthma • Use cautiously in diabetes mellitus, renal disease, hepatic disease, thyroid disease, COPD, CAD, bronchospasm, peripheral vascular disease • Do not discontinue suddenly

Drug	Action/Uses	Dosages	Adverse Effects	Nursing Considerations
Cimetidine (Tagamet)	**Histamine₂-Receptor Antagonist** • Inhibits histamine at H₂-receptor site in parietal cells, which inhibits gastric acid secretion • Peptic ulcer disease • Prophylaxis for patients with high potential for stress ulcer • Hyperacidity	• PO: 300 mg every 6 hours with meals • IV injection: 300 mg in 20 ml over 5 minutes every 6-8 hours or 300 mg in 50 ml over 15-20 minutes • IV infusion: mix 1,200 mg in 250 ml (4.8 mg/ml); usual dose 35-50 mg/hr	• Bradycardia • Headache • Jaundice • Diarrhea • Gynecomastia • Slurred speech • Elevated BUN, creatinine • Agranulocytosis, thrombocytopenia, aplastic anemia • Prolonged prothrombin time • Confusion, especially in the older patient • Seizures	• Monitor HR, BP, BUN, creatinine, platelet count, neurologic status, gastric pH • pH is maintained 3.5 or greater • Note contraindications: known hypersensitivity • Use cautiously in liver disease, renal disease, older adults • Encourage increase in fluids to ~3 L/day unless contraindicated • Note that cimetidine inhibits oxidative metabolism of many drugs; ranitidine is preferred since it does not interfere with metabolism of other drugs
Dexamethasone (Decadron) Hydrocortisone sodium succinate (Solu-Cortef) Methylprednisolone sodium succinate (Solu-Medrol) Beclomethasone (Vanceril) Prednisone Cortisone	**Glucocorticoid Hormones** • Suppress immune response • Decrease inflammation • Methylprednisolone sodium succinate exerts a weak mineralocorticoid effect • Cortisone exerts a potent mineralocorticoid effect • Anaphylaxis • Asthma • Aspiration pneumonitis • Cerebral edema • Need for immunosuppression (e.g., posttransplant, autoimmune diseases) • Adrenal insufficiency	PO, inhalation, IM, IV • Dexamethasone 10-40 mg IV initially and then decreasing dosages • Hydrocortisone sodium succinate 100 mg-2.0 g IV every 2-6 hours • Methylprednisolone sodium succinate 100-250 mg IV every 2-6 hours • Cortisone 25-300 mg PO or IM daily or on alternate days • Prednisone 1.5-15 mg PO bid, tid, or qid • Beclomethasone 2-4 metered-dose inhalations tid or qid	• Hypertension • Sodium and water retention • Potassium loss • Muscle weakness • Peptic ulcer, GI hemorrhage • Hyperglycemia • Leukocytosis • Thrombocytopenia • Increased susceptibility to infection • Delayed wound healing • Hirsutism • Apnea with rapid IV administration • Oral fungal (*Candida*) infection with inhaled steroids	• Monitor HR, BP, serum glucose, serum electrolytes, daily weight • Note contraindications: known hypersensitivity, psychosis, idiopathic thrombocytopenia, acute glomerulonephritis, fungal infection, AIDS, tuberculosis • Use cautiously in diabetes mellitus, glaucoma, osteoporosis, seizure disorders, ulcerative colitis, HF, myasthenia gravis, renal disease, peptic ulcer disease, esophagitis • Note that steroids may worsen latent diabetes and cause hyperglycemic hyperosmolar nonketotic syndrome; also note that steroids may mask signs of infection • Administer daily PO steroids on awakening • Administer IV steroid slowly to reduce the risk of steroid apnea • Instruct patient to rinse mouth after inhaled steroids

Continued

Drug	Classification/ Actions	Indications	Administration	Adverse Effects	Nursing Implications
Diazepam (Valium) and other benzodiazepines	**Benzodiazepine Tranquilizer** • Reduces skeletal muscle tension • Causes mild sedation	• Anxiety • Sedation for minor surgical or nonsurgical procedures • Acute alcohol withdrawal • Seizures	• PO: 2-10 mg every 6-8 hours • IV injection: 2-20 mg at rate no faster than 2 mg/min; may repeat every 5-10 minutes • Maximum: 100 mg/24 hr • Do not mix with any other drugs or dextrose solution Other benzodiazepines • Lorazepam (Ativan): PO: 2-6 mg/day in divided doses • Alprazolam (Xanax): PO: 0.25-0.5 mg tid	• Tachycardia • Hypotension (IV) • Nausea, vomiting • Urinary retention • Drowsiness • Dizziness, ataxia • Blurred vision • Slurred speech • Confusion • Respiratory depression (IV) • Drug dependence may occur	• Monitor HR, BP, ECG, RR and depth • Note contraindications: known hypersensitivity, glaucoma, psychosis • Use cautiously in liver disease, renal disease, older adult • Use large veins for IV injection • Administer flumazenil (Romazicon), a benzodiazepine antagonist, if necessary and prescribed
Digitalis (Digoxin, Lanoxin, Digitoxin, lanatoside C)	**Cardiac Glycoside** • Increases cardiac contractility to increase CO • Increases the refractory period of the AV node • Decreases sinus node firing rate • Decreases atrial automaticity • Increases ventricular automaticity • Increases GFR and urine output	• HF • Supraventricular tachycardias, especially in patients with HF	IV, PO • Digitalizing dose: 0.75-1.5 mg dose over 24 hours, usually in 4 doses of 0.25 mg • Administer IV dose over 5 minutes • Maintenance dose: 0.125-0.5 mg daily • Therapeutic blood level 0.5-2.0 ng/ml	*Toxic effects* • Anorexia, nausea, vomiting, diarrhea • Fatigue, muscle weakness • Agitation • Hallucinations • Visual disturbances • SA and AV blocks • Junctional and ventricular dysrhythmias *Treatment of toxicity* • Discontinue drug • Correct hypoxemia, ischemia, acid-base or electrolyte imbalance • Treat tachydysrhythmias as prescribed: usually lidocaine • Treat bradydysrhythmias as prescribed: usually atropine or pacemaker • Administer Digibind as prescribed for life-threatening dysrhythmias or blocks • Correction of hypokalemia is recommended before Digibind	• Monitor apical HR, ECG, serum electrolytes, especially potassium, calcium, magnesium • Note contraindications: known hypersensitivity, sick sinus syndrome, SA or AV block, ventricular tachycardia, hypertrophic cardiomyopathy, WPW • Use cautiously in patients with acute MI, hypothyroidism, liver disease, renal disease, hypothyroidism, older adult • Assess patient for clinical indications of digitalis toxicity • Withhold for 1-2 days before elective electrical cardioversion

			• Average dose is 400-800 mg over 30 min or IV bolus if cardiac arrest • Administered through inline filter • Reversal of digitalis toxicity occurs within 30-60 min but digoxin levels remain elevated		
Diltiazem (Cardizem)	**Calcium Channel Blocker** • Relaxes vascular smooth muscle decreasing preload and afterload • Relieves coronary artery spasm • Slows SA and AV nodal conduction times	• Angina • Coronary artery spasm • Mild HF • Hypertension • Hypertrophic cardiomyopathy • Supraventricular tachycardia	• PO: 30-60 mg every 6 hours • IV injection: 0.15-0.25 mg/kg (20 mg average) over 2 minutes, may be repeated in 15 minutes at 0.35 mg/kg (25 mg average) over 2 minutes • IV infusion: mix 125 mg in 100 ml for a total volume of 125 ml (1 mg/ml) and infuse at 5-15 mg/hr	• Bradycardia • Dysrhythmias • AV block • Hypotension • Nausea • Headache • Flushing • Fatigue • Drowsiness • Edema • Rash • Renal failure • Transient elevation in liver enzymes	• Monitor HR, BP, ECG • Note contraindications: known hypersensitivity, severe hypotension, second- or third-degree AV block, SSS, WPW, acute MI, pulmonary edema • Use cautiously in HF, hypotension, liver disease, renal disease, older adult
Dobutamine hydrochloride (Dobutrex)	**Sympathomimetic** • Increases cardiac contractility and cardiac output • Decreases preload and possibly afterload	• Cardiogenic shock • Low cardiac output states	• IV infusion; mix 250 mg in 250 ml (1000 µg/ml) and infuse at 2-40 µg/kg/min • Maximum: 40 µg/kg/min • Administer through central venous catheter if possible; if administered peripherally, use a large vein • Do not administer with alkaline solutions	• Tachycardia • Ventricular ectopy • Hypertension or hypotension • Nausea, vomiting • Dyspnea • Headache • Anxiety • Paresthesia • Palpitations • Chest pain	• Monitor BP, HR, ECG, PA, PAOP, SVR, CI • Note contraindications: known hypersensitivity, hypertrophic cardiomyopathy • Use cautiously in patients with hypertension or ventricular dysrhythmias • Note that the increase in heart rate is less than with dopamine • Use with nitroprusside as prescribed in cardiogenic shock; dobutamine increases contractility and decreases preload (and to a lesser degree afterload) and nitroprusside decreases afterload and preload

Continued

Drug	Classification/Actions	Indications	Administration	Adverse Effects	Nursing Implications
Dopamine hydrochloride (Intropin)	**Sympathomimetic** Dosage determines action • 0.5-2 μg/kg/min causes dopaminergic stimulation (dilates the renal and mesenteric circulation) • 2-5 μg/kg/min causes beta stimulation (increases contractility) • 5-10 μg/kg/min causes alpha and beta stimulation (increases contractility and causes vasoconstriction) • Dosages > 10 μg/kg/min cause predominant alpha stimulation (vasoconstriction)	• Poor renal or mesenteric perfusion (0.5-2 μg/kg/min) • Low cardiac output states (2-10 μg/kg/min) • Vasogenic forms of shock (10 or > μg/kg/min)	• IV infusion: mix 400 mg in 250 ml (1600 μg/ml) and infuse at 0.5-20 μg/kg/min depending on desired effect • Maximum: 20 μg/kg/min • Administer through central venous catheter if possible; if administered peripherally, use a large vein • Do not administer with alkaline solutions	• Tachycardia • Ventricular ectopy • Hypertension or hypotension • Nausea, vomiting • Dyspnea • Headache • Palpitations • Chest pain in patients with CAD • Tissue necrosis with high dosages or extravasation	• Monitor HR, BP, ECG, PA, PAOP, SVR, CI, urine output • Note contraindications: known hypersensitivity, uncorrected tachydysrhythmias, ventricular fibrillation, pheochromocytoma, hypertrophic cardiomyopathy, and in patients receiving MAO inhibitors • Use cautiously in peripheral vascular disease • Consider the cause of hypotension instead of automatically initiating dopamine to increase the blood pressure; *improve perfusion* by treating the cause of hypotension (e.g., volume replacement, inotropes, preload or afterload reduction) • Provide volume expansion during weaning; taper gradually to wean • Do not administer if discolored • Prevent extravasation because necrosis may occur; treat extravasation with phentolamine (Regitine)
Epinephrine hydrochloride (Adrenalin)	**Sympathomimetic** • Increases heart rate, cardiac contractility, myocardial oxygen consumption, ectopic activity • Causes vasoconstriction	• Asystole • Ventricular fibrillation • Pulseless electrical activity (PEA) • Asthma • Anaphylaxis	Cardiac arrest • IV injection: 1 mg; may repeat at 3-5 minute intervals • IV infusion: mix 1 mg in 250 ml (4 μg/ml) and infuse at 2-10 μg/min; titrate to desired effect	• Tachycardia • Dysrhythmias • Palpitations • Anxiety • Restlessness • Headache • Dizziness • Tremor • Cerebral hemorrhage	• Monitor HR, BP, ECG, RR, breath sounds • Note contraindications: glaucoma, organic brain damage, cardiomegaly • Use cautiously in older adults and those with hyperthyroidism, chest pain, hypertension, psychoneurosis, diabetes mellitus • Prevent extravasation as necrosis may occur; treat with phentolamine (Regitine)

Drug	Action/Classification	Indications	Dosage	Adverse Effects	Nursing Considerations
	• Acts as a histamine antagonist		Asthma or anaphylaxis • Subcutaneous 0.1-0.5 mg or 0.1-0.25 mg IV	• Chest pain • Hyperglycemia	• Administer through central venous catheter if possible; if administered peripherally, use a large vein • Do not administer with alkaline solutions • Discard if discolored or precipitate present
Eptifibatide (Integrilin)	**Platelet aggregation inhibitor** (GP IIb/IIIa platelet receptor blocker) • Inhibits platelet aggregation and platelet-mediated thrombosis	• Acute coronary syndrome with or without percutaneous coronary intervention (PCI) • PCI when risk for thrombosis is high	For acute coronary syndrome • IV injection: 180 µg/kg over 1-2 minutes followed by: • IV infusion: 2 µg/kg/min for up to 72 hours; decreased to 0.5 µg/kg/min during PCI and continued for 24 hours after PCI For PCI without acute coronary syndrome • IV injection: 135 µg/kg over 1-2 minutes before procedure followed by: • IV infusion: 0.5 µg/kg/min for 24 hours	• Bleeding • Intracranial hemorrhage • Hematuria • Hematemesis • Bleeding at sheath site • Hypotension	• Monitor PT, aPTT, or ACT, platelet count • Keep ACT between 300-350 seconds • Note contraindications: active internal bleeding, clinically significant bleeding in the GI or GU tract within the last 6 weeks, bleeding diathesis, history of CVA within the last two years or CVA with significant residual neurologic deficit, intracranial neoplasm, aneurysm, or AV malformation, severe uncontrolled hypertension, oral anticoagulants within 7 days unless prothrombin time is less than 1.2 × control, thrombocytopenia, presumed or documented history of vasculitis, major surgery or trauma within the last 6 weeks, pericarditis, known hypersensitivity to eptifibatide, renal failure, thrombocytopenia • Administer with aspirin and heparin therapy as prescribed • Monitor oral secretions, sputum, vomitus, NG aspirate, stool, urine for blood • Limit venipuncture and urinary catheterization as possible; use IV catheter with saline lock for blood sampling; avoid noncompressible IV sites • Avoid nasotracheal and nasogastric tubes if possible • Avoid automatic BP cuffs • Administer platelets as prescribed for thrombocytopenia • Store refrigerated

Continued

Drug	Classification/ Actions	Indications	Administration	Adverse Effects	Nursing Implications
Esmolol (Brevibloc)	**Cardioselective Beta-Blocker Class II Antidysrhythmic** • Decreases heart rate, contractility, automaticity, excitability, conductivity • Depresses sinus node automaticity • Increases AV nodal refractoriness and decreases conduction velocity • Decreases myocardial oxygen consumption	• Supraventricular tachycardia • Intraoperative or postoperative tachycardia and/ or hypotension	• IV injection: loading dose of 500 µg/kg over 1 minute followed by maintenance dose of 50 µg/kg/min for 4 minutes • If desired effect does not occur, repeat the loading dose of 500 µg/kg over 1 minute and follow with a dose increased by 50 µg/kg/min for 4 minutes (e.g., 500 + 100, 500 + 150, 500 + 200) • IV infusion: when desired effect is achieved, no additional loading doses are needed, and the maintenance dose is increased by 50 µg/kg/min and maintained	• Bradycardia • Hypotension • AV block • Nausea, vomiting • Fatigue, lethargy • HF • Bronchospasm, especially in patients with asthma • Urinary retention • Inflammation and induration at injection site	• Monitor HR, BP, ECG • Monitor for clinical indications of heart failure • Note contraindications: known hypersensitivity, bradycardia, AV block greater than first degree, HF, shock, asthma • Use cautiously in diabetes mellitus, renal disease, hyperthyroidism, COPD, liver disease, myasthenia gravis, peripheral vascular disease, hypotension • May potentiate the hypoglycemic effects of insulin and prevents sympathetic symptoms of hypoglycemia; masks sympathetic clinical indications of shock since receptors are blocked
Fenoldopam mesylate (Corlopam)	**Vasodilator Antihypertensive** • Relaxes vascular smooth muscle decreasing preload (PAOP) and afterload (SVR) • Stimulates dopaminergic receptors causing diuresis	• Severe hypertension (short-term treatment)	• IV infusion: mix 10 mg in 250 ml (40 µg/ml); usual dose is 0.03-0.3 µg/kg/min • Maximum: 1.7 µg/kg/min	• Tachycardia, hypotension • Headache • Flushing • Nausea • Hypokalemia • Increased intraocular pressure • Increased intracranial pressure	• Monitor HR, BP, urine output, neurologic status • Note contraindications: known hypersensitivity to fenoldopam or sulfite, intracranial hypertension • Use caution in patients with glaucoma or ocular hypertension • Do not administer with beta-blockers

| Flecainide (Tambocor) | **Class IC Antidysrhythmic** • Blocks sodium influx during phase 0, which depresses the rate of depolarization • Does not change repolarization and action potential duration | • Life-threatening or refractory ventricular dysrhythmias • Atrial or ventricular dysrhythmias that do not respond to other drugs | • PO: 50-200 mg twice daily; maximum dose 400 mg/day | • Proarrhythmia including PVGs, ventricular tachycardia, torsades de pointes, PACs, supraventricular tachycardia, bradycardia, SA block or arrest, AV block, bundle branch block • Nausea, vomiting, abdominal pain, constipation • Dyspnea • Chest pain • Headache • Drowsiness • Dizziness • Blurred vision • Tremor • Dry mouth | • Monitor HR, BP, ECG • Report widening of QRS of greater than 25% • Monitor closely for heart failure • Note contraindications: known hypersensitivity, second- or third-degree AV block, cardiogenic shock • Use cautiously in heart failure, SA or bi-fascicular blocks or sick sinus syndrome without a pacemaker, renal disease, liver disease, myasthenia gravis • Use cautiously in patient also receiving another negative inotropic agent (e.g., verapamil, procainamide, beta-blocker) • Correct electrolyte imbalance prior to therapy if possible |
| Fosphenytoin sodium (Cerebyx) | **Anticonvulsant** • Thought to stabilize neurons | • Seizures • Seizure prophylaxis | • IV loading dose: 10-20 mg phenytoin sodium equivalent (PE)/kg at rate of 100-150 PE/min • IV or IM maintenance dose: 4-6 mg PE/kg/day | • Nystagmus, diplopia • Dizziness, ataxia • Pruritus • Paresthesia • Headache • Somnolence • CNS depression • Hypotension is given too rapidly IV | • Monitor HR, BP, RR and depth, ECG, and response to therapy • Note that fosphenytoin causes less pain, burning, tenderness, and erythema at injection site than phenytoin • Note contraindications: known hypersensitivity to fosphenytoin, phenytoin, sinus bradycardia, SA or AV block, sick sinus syndrome • Use cautiously in patients with renal or hepatic impairment, older adults, and patients with hypoalbuminemia; dosage adjustment may be required • Store in refrigerator • Concomitant administration of a benzodiazepine (e.g., diazepam [Valium]) is usually necessary to control seizures in status epilepticus |

Continued

Drug	Classification/ Actions	Indications	Administration	Adverse Effects	Nursing Implications
Furosemide (Lasix)	**Loop Diuretic** • Inhibits sodium reabsorption in the ascending loop of Henle • Promotes sodium, potassium, chloride, water excretion • Causes smooth muscle relaxation and vasodilation • Increases glomerular filtration rate (GFR)	• Hypertension • Fluid overload • HF/pulmonary edema • Hypercalcemia • Cerebral edema • Conditions refractory to thiazide diuretics	• PO: 20-80 mg daily • IV injection: 20-120 mg; administer at rate not to exceed 10 mg/min; if initial dose is ineffective, the next dose is usually double the original dose • IV infusion: mix 250 mg in 250 ml (1 mg/mL); usual dose is 0.1-0.75 mg/kg/hr; not to exceed 4 mg/min • Maximum: 1 g/day • Do not mix with acidic solutions Other loop diuretics • Torsemide (Demadex): 5-20 mg/day PO or IV (over 2 minutes); may be titrated to desired effect but single dose should not exceed 200 mg • Bumetanide (Bumex): 0.5-1.0 mg IV over 1-2 minutes; may be repeated at 2-3 hour intervals • Maximum 10 mg/day	• Hypotension • Hypovolemia • Nausea, vomiting, abdominal pain • Rash • Electrolyte imbalance: hypocalcemia, hypokalemia, hypomagnesemia, hyponatremia • Acid-base imbalance: hypochloremic alkalosis • Increased uric acid and BUN • Renal failure • Hyperglycemia • Photosensitivity • Thrombocytopenia, agranulocytosis, leukopenia, neutropenia, anemia • Transient deafness (with rapid IV injection)	• Monitor HR, BP, urine output, serum electrolytes, BUN, creatinine, uric acid, CBC, daily weights • Monitor patients also on digitalis for clinical indications of digitalis toxicity • Monitor serum glucose in patients with diabetes mellitus • Monitor for clinical indications of gout • Note contraindications: known hypersensitivity to sulfonamides, anuria, hypovolemia, electrolyte depletion • Sulfonamide-sensitive patients may have allergic reaction to these drugs (furosemide, bumetanide, torsemide) as they are all sulfa-derivatives • Use cautiously in diabetes mellitus, dehydration, severe renal disease, gout, hepatic disease • Do not administer if yellow or if precipitate is present • Teach patient about potassium-rich foods

| Heparin sodium | **Anticoagulant**
• Prevents conversion of prothrombin to thrombin
• Prevents conversion of fibrinogen to fibrin
• Prevents extension of existing clots
• Decreases platelet aggregation | • Unstable angina or myocardial infarction
• Maintenance of arterial patency after PCI or thrombolytic therapy
• Prevention of thrombus formation during periods of inactivity
• Deep vein thrombosis
• Pulmonary emboli
• Peripheral arterial emboli
• Transient ischemic attacks or reversible ischemic neurologic deficit
• Disseminated intravascular coagulation (controversial)
• Maintenance of arterial line patency | • Subcutaneous: usually prophylactic, dose is 5,000 U every 12 hours (also called mini-heparin)
• IV injection: 50-150 U/kg (usually 5000-10,000 U) followed by infusion
• IV infusion: mix 25,000 U in 500 ml (50 U/ml) and infuse at 10-20 U/kg/hour (usually 700-1,500 U/hr) or whatever dose is needed to achieve aPTT of 1½-2½ times the laboratory control
Note: The trend in IV weight-dosed heparin is to decrease the amount of heparin (60 U/kg for injection followed by 12 U/kg for injection) and the desirable aPTT (45-60 seconds)
• Maximum: 40,000 U/day | • Hemorrhage with excessive aPTT
• Hypertension or hypotension
• Hypersensitivity reaction including bronchospasm
• Fever
• Hepatitis
• Thrombocytopenia (caused by white clot syndrome; also called heparin-associated thrombocytopenia and thrombosis [HATT] or heparin-induced thrombocytopenia and thrombosis [HITT]) | • Monitor aPTT and platelet count and for signs of hemorrhage
• Note petechiae and request platelet count if petechiae noted; heparin usually discontinued if platelet count is <100,000/mm³
  • Administer lepirudin (Refludan) as prescribed for white clot syndrome; this recombinant DNA technology drug is indicated for anticoagulation in patients with white clot syndrome
• Note contraindications: known hypersensitivity, active bleeding, blood dyscrasias (except DIC), suspected intracranial hemorrhage, severe hypertension, peptic ulcer disease, open wounds, recent surgery, endocarditis, shock, threatened abortion
• Use cautiously in alcoholism, liver disease, renal disease, older adults
• Monitor oral secretions, sputum, vomitus, NG aspirate, stool, urine for blood
• Ensure that protamine sulfate (antidote) is available
• Avoid IM, arterial, or venous punctures if at all possible
• Hold pressure for longer than usual if punctures necessary
• Do not discontinue suddenly: warfarin will usually have already been started and the PT within therapeutic range before heparin is discontinued
• Do not aspirate before subcutaneous administration and do not massage after administration
• Note that NTG interacts with heparin, causing more heparin to be required to achieve therapeutic aPTT; monitor aPTT closely with significant NTG dosage changes or discontinuance |

Continued

Drug	Classification/ Actions	Indications	Administration	Adverse Effects	Nursing Implications
Heparin: low-molecular-weight enoxaparin (Lovenox) dalteparin sodium (Fragmin)	**Anticoagulant** • Inhibits anti-thrombin activity • Prevents DVT • Does not prevent platelet aggregation	• High risk for DVT • Acute coronary syndrome	• Enoxaparin (Lovenox) • SC: 30-40 mg bid dalte-parin sodium (Fragmin) • SC: 2,500 IU daily start-ing 1-2 hours before surgery and repeated daily for 5-10 days postoperatively	• Bleeding • Epidural or spinal hematoma (especially when used with patients with epidural or spinal anesthesia) • Fever • Elevation of liver enzymes • Thrombocytopenia	• Note that LMW heparin does not require routine laboratory monitoring because it does not usually alter PT or aPTT • Note contraindications and cautions as for heparin • Obtain baseline platelet count; monitor for petechiae • Monitor oral secretions, sputum, vomitus, NG aspirate, stool, urine for blood • Ensure that protamine sulfate (antidote) is available • Avoid IM, arterial, or venous punctures if at all possible • Hold pressure for longer than usual if punctures necessary • Administer deep subcutaneously but avoid IM injection
Hydralazine (Apresoline)	**Vasodilator Antihypertensive** • Relaxes arteriolar smooth muscle decreasing SVR, afterload, and BP	• Hypertension • Afterload reduction	• PO: 10-50 mg every 6-8 hours • IV injection: 5-40 mg over 3-5 minutes • Maximum: 400 mg/day	• Tachycardia • Orthostatic hypotension • Anorexia, nausea, vomiting, diarrhea • Sodium retention • Weight gain • Palpitations • Flushing • Headache • Tremors • Dizziness • Lupuslike syndrome • Exacerbation of HF or chest pain • Leukopenia, agranulocytosis	• Monitor HR, BP, ECG • Note contraindications: known hypersen-sitivity to hydralazine, coronary artery disease, mitral valve disease, severe aortic stenosis • Use cautiously in renal disease, cerebro-vascular disease • Administer beta-blockers as prescribed for reflex tachycardia because it may cause myocardial ischemia

Drug	Action	Indications	Dosage	Side Effects	Nursing Considerations
Ibutilide (Corvert)	**Class III Antidysrhythmic** • Blocks potassium movement during phase III • Increases action potential duration • Prolongs effective refractory period	• Recent onset atrial fibrillation or atrial flutter	• IV infusion: mix 1 mg in 50 ml and infuse over 10 minutes for patients weighing more than 60 kg (0.01 mg/kg in patients weighing less than 60 kg); may be repeated after 10 minutes if needed • Discontinue if atrial fibrillation or flutter terminates, a new dysrhythmia occurs, or if prolongation of the QT occurs	• Proarrhythmia including PVCs, ventricular tachycardia, torsades de pointes, PACs, supraventricular tachycardia, bradycardia, AV block, bundle branch block • Nausea • Heart failure • Syncope • Headache • Renal failure	• Monitor HR, BP, ECG • Report widening of QRS by greater than 25% or prolongation of QT interval to more than half of RR interval or hypotension • Correct electrolyte imbalances (especially hypokalemia) before initiating ibutilide • Administer anticoagulants for 2-3 weeks as prescribed for patients with atrial fibrillation of more than 2 to 3 days duration • Note contraindications: patients with second- or third-degree AV block, SA block without pacemaker • Use cautiously in patients receiving digitalis because this drug may mask the cardiotoxicity associated with excessive digoxin levels • Do not administer concurrently or within 4 hours of class IA antiarrhythmics or other class III antiarrhythmics; do not administer with other drugs that prolong the QT interval, such as phenothiazines, tricyclic antidepressants
Insulin	**Pancreatic Hormone** • Allows glucose to move into the cell • Lowers serum glucose	• Hyperglycemia • Diabetes mellitus • Hyperkalemia (insulin would be given with dextrose unless patient is hyperglycemic)	Subcutaneous, IM, IV • IV infusion: mix 100 u in 250 ml (0.4 U/ml); usual dose is 0.1 U/kg/hour or 5-10 U/hr; adjusted according to serum glucose levels: goal is to reduce serum glucose by 75-100 mg/dl/hr • Only regular insulin may be given IV	• Tachycardia, palpitations • Hypoglycemia • Hypokalemia, hypophosphatemia • Allergic reactions including anaphylaxis with pork or beef insulin not seen with humulin	• Monitor HR, serum glucose, serum electrolytes • Note contraindications: known hypersensitivity, hypoglycemia • Administer at room temperature

Continued

Drug	Classification/Actions	Indications	Administration	Adverse Effects	Nursing Implications
Isoproterenol (Isuprel)	**Sympathomimetic** • Increases HR and cardiac contractility • Relaxes smooth muscle, which causes vasodilation and bronchodilation	• Asystole • AV block • Bradycardia unresponsive to atropine when pacemaker is not available • Torsades de pointes	• IV infusion: mix 1 mg in 250 ml (4 µg/ml) and infuse at 2-10 µg/min; titrated to heart rate response • Maximum: 30 µg/min	• Tachycardia, palpitations • Dysrhythmias • Chest pain; increase in infarct size because of increase in myocardial oxygen consumption • Nausea, vomiting • Anxiety • Tremors • Insomnia • Dizziness • Headache • Hyperglycemia	• Monitor HR, BP, ECG • Note contraindications: known hypersensitivity, glaucoma • Use cautiously in acute MI, digitalis toxicity, hypertension, hypovolemia, hyperthyroidism, diabetes mellitus, prostatic hypertrophy • Avoid concurrent use of epinephrine • Discontinue infusion if chest pain or ventricular dysrhythmias occur • Decrease rate if heart rate is greater than 110 bpm • Do not administer with beta-blockers (they block effect)
Labetalol hydrochloride (Normodyne, Trandate)	**Alpha and Beta Adrenergic Blocker** • Blocks response to alpha and beta stimulation • Causes decrease in blood pressure without reflex tachycardia • Causes decrease in HR	• Hypertension • Hypertensive crisis	• PO: 100-400 mg every 12 hours • IV injection: 20 mg over 2 minutes, may repeat 40 mg every 10 minutes • IV infusion: mix 300 mg in 250 ml for a total volume of 300 mg in 300 ml (1 mg/ml); usual dose if 2 mg/min until satisfactory response is achieved • Maximum: 300 mg	• Bradycardia • Orthostatic hypotension • Ventricular dysrhythmias • AV blocks • HF • Nausea, vomiting, diarrhea • Dizziness • Lethargy • Hypoglycemia without symptoms in insulin-dependent diabetics • Agranulocytosis, thrombocytopenia • Bronchospasm in patients with COPD, asthma	• Monitor HR, BP, ECG, breath sounds, daily weight • Note contraindications: known hypersensitivity, shock, second- or third-degree AV block, sinus bradycardia, HF, asthma • Use cautiously in diabetes mellitus, renal disease, hepatic disease, thyroid disease, COPD, CAD, bronchospasm, peripheral vascular disease • Keep patient supine for 3 hours after IV administration • Do not discontinue suddenly

Drug	Classification/Action	Indications	Dosage	Side effects	Nursing considerations

Lidocaine hydrochloride (Xylocaine)	**Class IB Antidysrhythmic**
	• Decreases ventricular automaticity and excitability
	• Increases ventricular fibrillation threshold
		• Ventricular dysrhythmias	• IV injection:
			  • VF: 1.5 mg/kg repeated every 3-5 minutes
			  • VT: 1 mg/kg repeated every 5-10 minutes
			  • Maximum: 3 mg/kg
			• IV infusion: mix 2 g in 500 ml (4 mg/ml) and infuse at 1-4 mg/min
			• Therapeutic blood level: 2-5 µg/ml
				• Hypotension
				• SA arrest
				• AV block
				• Nausea, vomiting
				• Tremors
				• Restlessness
				• Lightheadedness
				• Anaphylaxis
				Clinical indications of toxicity (in relative order of occurrence)
				• Perioral paresthesias
				• Feelings of dissociation
				• Dizziness
				• Drowsiness
				• Euphoria
				• Mild agitation
				• Dysarthria
				• Hearing impairment
				• Disorientation
				• Confusion
				• Muscle twitching
				• Seizures
				• Respiratory arrest
					• Monitor HR, BP, ECG
					• Note contraindications: known hypersensitivity, AV block, supraventricular dysrhythmias, sick sinus syndrome
					• Use cautiously in liver disease, HF, respiratory depression, malignant hyperthermia, and in older adults
					• Note that toxicity incidence is increased if patient has HF or liver disease, has low lean body mass or is elderly, or is concurrently taking cimetidine (Tagamet) or beta-blocker
					• Note that the administration of prophylactic lidocaine after MI is no longer recommended; while the incidence of ventricular fibrillation is decreased, the incidence of asystole is increased

Magnesium sulfate	**Electrolyte** • Slows heart rate at SA node • Prolongs conduction time • Causes smooth muscle relaxation and vasodilation • Acts as a CNS depressant and has anticonvulsant effect	• Hypomagnesemia • Ventricular tachydysrhythmias, especially torsades de pointes • Prophylactically in acute MI • Eclampsia of pregnancy • Seizures • Asthma	Cardiac arrest • IV injection: 1-2 g over 1-2 minutes Other indications • IV infusion: mix 1-2 g in 100 ml and infuse over 1-4 hours	• Bradycardia • Hypotension • Diaphoresis • Flushing • Hypermagnesemia resulting in respiratory muscle weakness and arrest	• Monitor HR, BP, RR, ECG, urine output, deep tendon reflexes, mental status • Note contraindications: renal disease • Use cautiously in renal insufficiency, patients on digitalis • Monitor closely for clinical indications of hypermagnesemia: hypotension, AV block, CNS depression, depressed or absent DTR, muscle weakness or paralysis, respiratory arrest • Administer calcium IV as prescribed for hypermagnesemic effects • Have intubation equipment and mechanical ventilator available

Continued

Drug	Classification/ Actions	Indications	Administration	Adverse Effects	Nursing Implications
Mannitol (Osmitrol)	**Osmotic Diuretic** • Increases osmolality of the glomerular filtrate • Causes decreased reabsorption of water and electrolytes and increased excretion of sodium and chloride • Increases urine output	• Acute renal failure • Cerebral edema (patient must have intact blood–brain barrier) • Glaucoma • Drug toxicity (forced diuresis) • Renal pigments (e.g., hemoglobinuria, myoglobinuria)	• IV infusion: 1-2 g/kg over 30-60 minutes; average dose 50-100 g • Use inline filter when administering mannitol	• Tachycardia • Nausea, vomiting • Fluid and electrolyte imbalance • Pulmonary edema • Thirst • Phlebitis • Seizures • Rebound cerebral edema 8-12 hours after diuresis	• Monitor HR, BP, urine output, serum osmolality, serum electrolytes, BUN, uric acid, daily weights • Note contraindications: known hypersensitivity, active intracranial bleeding, anuria, severe dehydration • Use cautiously in severe renal failure, HF, dehydration • Check bottle or ampule for crystallization: discard and replace • Monitor closely for rebound effect: return of clinical indications of intracranial hypertension 8-12 hours after mannitol
Metaproterenol (Alupent, Metaprel)	**Sympathomimetic Bronchodilator (Beta₂ specific)** • Relaxes smooth muscle of bronchi	• Bronchospasm, asthma	• PO: 20 mg every 6-8 hours • Hand-held inhaler: 2-3 inhalations every 3-4 hours • Nebulizer: 0.2-0.3 ml of undiluted 5% solution or 2.5 ml of a 6% solution every 6-8 hours	• Tachycardia • Palpitations • Nausea, vomiting • Anxiety • Tremor • Headache	• Monitor HR, BP, RR, breath sounds • Note contraindications: known hypersensitivity, glaucoma, tachydysrhythmias; do not give with MAO inhibitors • Use cautiously in older adults and patients with diabetes mellitus, hypertension, hyperthyroidism, cardiac disease, seizure disorder, prostatic hypertrophy • Do not administer with beta-blockers (they block effect)
Metoprolol (Lopressor)	**Cardioselective Beta-Blocker** **Class II Antidysrhythmic** • Decreases heart rate, contractility, automaticity, excitability, conductivity • Depresses sinus node automaticity • Increases AV nodal refractoriness and decreases conduction velocity • Decreases myocardial oxygen consumption	• Hypertension • Angina • Myocardial infarction (primary prevention and secondary prevention of extension and reinfarction)	• PO: 100-450 mg daily in one or two doses • IV injection: 5 mg IV slowly at 5 minute intervals to a total of 15 mg	• Bradycardia • AV block • Hypotension • Nausea, vomiting, diarrhea, constipation • Fatigue, lethargy • Rash • Syncope • HF • Dyspnea, wheezing • Mental depression • Hyperglycemia in type 2 DM • Asymptomatic hypoglycemia in type 1 DM • Impotence • Emotional lability • Agranulocytosis, thrombocytopenia	• Monitor HR, BP, ECG • Monitor for clinical indications of heart failure • Note contraindications: known hypersensitivity, sinus bradycardia, AV block greater than first degree, HF, shock, asthma, Raynaud's syndrome • Use cautiously in diabetes mellitus, renal disease, hyperthyroidism, COPD, liver disease, myasthenia gravis, peripheral vascular disease, hypotension • May potentiate the hypoglycemic effects of insulin and prevents sympathetic symptoms of hypoglycemia • Note that this drug limits cardiac reserve and exercise capacity since heart rate cannot increase • Note that this drug masks sympathetic clinical indications of shock since receptors are blocked

Drug	Action	Use	Dosage	Side Effects	Nursing Considerations
Mexiletine (Mexitil)	**Class IB Antidysrhythmic** • Blocks sodium influx during phase 0, which depresses the rate of depolarization • Shortens repolarization and action potential duration • Suppresses ventricular automaticity in ischemic tissue	• Life-threatening or refractory ventricular dysrhythmias	• PO: initial dose of 200-400 mg followed by 200-400 bid, tid, or qid; maximum 1200 mg/day	• Proarrhythmia including PVCs, ventricular tachycardia, torsades de pointes, PACs, supraventricular tachycardia, bradycardia, AV block, bundle branch block • Hypotension • Nausea, vomiting • Diarrhea or constipation • Elevated liver enzymes • Palpitations • Chest pain • Dyspnea • Headache • Paresthesia, tremors, nystagmus, ataxia, dysarthria • Tinnitus • Blurred vision • Dizziness • Drowsiness, insomnia • Confusion • Seizures	• Monitor HR, BP, ECG • Note contraindications: second- or third-degree block or sick sinus syndrome without pacemaker, cardiogenic shock • Administer with meals to decrease GI adverse effects • Note that risk of toxicity is greater if patient is concurrently receiving cimetidine (Tagamet) or beta-blocker; dosage is adjusted in HF and liver disease • Monitor closely for clinical indications of toxicity: tremor, dizziness, ataxia, nystagmus
Midazolam hydrochloride (Versed)	**Benzodiazepine Tranquilizer; Anesthetic** • Depresses the CNS at the limbic and subcortical level • Allows conscious sedation and amnesia	• Preoperative sedation • Conscious sedation for short procedures (e.g., cardioversion, intubation) • Induction of general anesthesia	• IM injection: 0.07-0.35 mg/kg • IV injection: 0.15-0.35 mg/kg • IV infusion: mix 150 mg in 250 ml (0.6 mg/ml); usual dose is 0.05-0.10 mg/kg/hr	• Bradycardia • Dysrhythmias • Hypotension • Nausea, vomiting, hiccoughs • Headache • Agitation • Bronchospasm • Respiratory depression, apnea • Pain and tenderness at injection site	• Monitor HR, BP, RR and depth • Note contraindications: known hypersensitivity, shock, coma, acute alcohol intoxication, glaucoma • Use cautiously in COPD, HF, renal failure, older adult, debilitated person • Use large muscle mass if given IM; use large vein if given IV, avoid infiltration • Administer flumazenil (Romazicon), a benzodiazepine antagonist, if necessary and prescribed

Continued

Drug	Classification/Actions	Indications	Administration	Adverse Effects	Nursing Implications
Milrinone (Primacor)	**PDE Inhibitor; Inotrope** • Increases cardiac contractility • Relaxes vascular smooth muscle to cause vasodilation of arteries and veins and to decrease afterload and preload	• HF: short-term (<5 days) management of patients with HF who have not responded to traditional therapy of digitalis, diuretics, and/or vasodilators	• IV injection: 50 μg/kg over 10 minutes • IV infusion: mix 30 mg in 250 ml (120 μg/ml); usual dose 0.25-1 μg/kg/min (less if renal insufficiency)	• Dysrhythmias • Hypotension • Anorexia, nausea, vomiting, abdominal pain • Increased liver enzymes, hepatotoxicity • Hypokalemia • Tremor • Thrombocytopenia • Chest pain • Hypersensitivity reactions • Headache	• Monitor HR, BP, ECG, PA, PAOP, CI, SVR, platelet counts, liver function studies, electrolytes (especially potassium), BUN, creatinine • Platelet count below 150,000/mm³ usually requires dosage reduction • Platelet count below 100,000/mm³ usually requires discontinuance • Note contraindications: known hypersensitivity, severe aortic or pulmonic valvular disease, hypertrophic cardiomyopathy, ventricular dysrhythmias • Use cautiously in renal disease, liver disease, atrial dysrhythmias, older adult • Use cautiously in acute MI because myocardial oxygen consumption is increased • Correct hypokalemia and hypovolemia before or during amrinone use • Note that milrinone is more often prescribed than amrinone because of the greater incidence of thrombocytopenia with amrinone
Moricizine (Ethmozine)	**Class I Antidysrhythmic** • Blocks sodium influx during phase 0, which depresses the rate of depolarization • Shortens the action potential and increases the refractory period	• Life-threatening or refractory ventricular dysrhythmias	• PO: 200-300 mg tid	• Proarrhythmia including PVCs, ventricular tachycardia, torsades de pointes, PACs, supraventricular tachycardia, bradycardia, AV block, bundle branch block • Hypotension or hypertension • Nausea, vomiting, abdominal pain, constipation • Palpitations • Chest pain • HF • Dyspnea or apnea • Fatigue • Headache • Dizziness • Fever	• Monitor HR, BP, ECG • Note contraindications: second- or third-degree AV block or bifascicular intraventricular block without a pacemaker, contraindicated in cardiogenic shock • Use cautiously with sick sinus syndrome, HF, liver disease, renal disease • Administer with meals to decrease adverse GI effects • Monitor closely for proarrhythmias, especially in the first week of therapy • Correct electrolyte imbalance prior to therapy • Monitor patients with heart failure closely for worsening of condition

Drug	Action	Uses	Dosage	Side Effects/Adverse Reactions	Nursing Considerations
Morphine sulfate	**Opiate Narcotic** • Modifies pain perception and reaction • Dilates veins and decreases preload	• Severe pain • Left ventricular failure (preload reduction)	• PO: 10-30 mg every 4 hours • IM injection: 4-15 mg every 4 hours • IV injection: 10 mg in 9 ml of saline for total volume of 10 ml and concentration of 1 mg/ml; titration for pain • IV infusion: mix 200 mg in 250 ml (0.8 mg/ml) and titrate for pain management; usual dose 0.05-0.3 mg/kg/hr	• Bradycardia • Orthostatic hypotension • Anorexia, nausea, vomiting • Constipation • Urinary retention • Rash • Euphoria • Drowsiness, confusion • Dizziness • CNS depression • Respiratory depression	• Monitor HR, BP, RR and depth, urine output, patient evaluation of pain • Note contraindications: known hypersensitivity, hemorrhage, asthma, increased intracranial pressure • Use cautiously in liver disease, renal disease, head injury, respiratory depression, prostatic hypertrophy, addictive personality • Note that maximal respiratory depression occurs within 7 minutes after IV dose • Administer naloxone (Narcan) as indicated and prescribed for opiate overdosage
Nicardipine (Cardene)	**Calcium Channel Blocker** • Relaxes vascular smooth muscle, decreasing preload and afterload	• Hypertension • Angina pectoris	• PO: 20 mg tid initially; may be increased to 20-40 mg tid after 3 days if tolerated well • IV infusion: mix 25 mg in 240 ml (0.1 mg/ml) and infuse at 5 mg/hr (50 ml/hr); may be increased by 2.5 mg/hr (25 ml/hr) every 5 minutes until desired BP reduction is achieved • Do not mix in lactated Ringer's solution • Maximum 15 mg/hr	• Tachycardia • Hypotension • Nausea, vomiting, heartburn • Flushing • Headache • Chest pain • Heart failure • Hepatitis • Renal failure • Local irritation at injection site	• Monitor HR, BP • Note contraindications: known hypersensitivity, sick sinus syndrome, second- or third-degree AV block, systolic BP <90 mm Hg, severe aortic stenosis • Use caution in HF, hypotension, liver disease, renal insufficiency or failure, and in the elderly
Nifedipine (Procardia)	**Calcium Channel Blocker** • Relaxes vascular smooth muscle, decreasing preload and afterload • Relieves coronary artery spasm	• Coronary artery spasm • Angina pectoris • Mild HF • Hypertension • Raynaud's disease • Hypertrophic cardiomyopathy	• PO immediate release: 10-30 mg tid or qid; maximum 180 mg/24 hr • Not FDA approved for sublingual use and not recommended for sublingual use (causes precipitous drop in BP that may cause organ hypoperfusion) • PO sustained release: 30-120 mg/day	• Tachycardia • Dysrhythmias • Hypotension • Nausea, vomiting, heartburn • Diarrhea or constipation • Headache • Flushing • Fatigue • Dizziness • Rash • Pedal edema • Hypokalemia	• Monitor HR, BP, potassium • Note contraindications: known hypersensitivity, severe aortic stenosis • Use caution in HF, sick sinus syndrome, second- or third-degree AV block, systolic BP <90 mm Hg, liver disease, renal insufficiency or failure, and in the elderly

Continued

Drug	Classification/ Actions	Indications	Administration	Adverse Effects	Nursing Implications
Nitrates (nitroglycerin [Tridil], isosorbide dinitrate [Isordil])	**Nitrates** • Relax smooth muscle to reduce preload (PAOP) (and afterload [SVR] if >1 μg/kg/min) • Dilate coronary collateral circulation • Relieve coronary artery spasm	• Acute angina • Prophylactic use before activities that may cause angina • HF (preload reduction)	• Sublingual: 0.3-0.4 mg at 5-minute intervals to a maximum of three tablets or metered-dose sprays • PO (isosorbide): 5-40 mg every 6 hours • Transdermal: 1-4 inches every 8 hours • IV infusion: mix 50 mg in 250 ml (200 μg/ml); initial dose 5-10 μg/ min, increase by 5-10 μg/min every 5 minutes until desired results are achieved (e.g., control of chest pain, preload reduction) • Maximum: 400 μg/min • Administer in glass bottle and via non-PVC tubing	• Tachycardia or bradycardia • Hypotension or hypertension • Palpitations • Weakness • Apprehension • Flushing • Dizziness • Syncope • Headache • Methemoglobinemia with resultant reduction in Sao_2, Spo_2, and tissue oxygen delivery	• Monitor HR, BP, urine output • Monitor RAP, PA, PAOP, SVR, CI if hemodynamic monitoring if nitroglycerin is being administered IV and pulmonary artery catheter has been inserted • Note contraindications: known hypersensitivity, anemia, intracranial hypertension, cerebral hemorrhage, hypertrophic cardiomyopathy, right ventricular infarction • Use cautiously in hypotension • Decrease nitrate tolerance by scheduling oral nitrates with nitrate-free period at night and by removing transdermal nitrates at night • Administer ASA or acetaminophen for headache; usually dose-related • Teach patient to protect tablets from light and moisture and replace every 3 months • Teach patient to limit NTG to 3 tablets every 5 minutes and if no relief is obtained, to go to the ED • Teach patient to apply nitroglycerin paste to any relatively hairless area between the knees and shoulders and to rotate sites to prevent maceration • Note that patients receiving IV NTG and heparin IV concurrently require more heparin to achieve therapeutic aPTT; monitor aPTT closely with NTG dosage changes or discontinuance

Drug	Action	Indications	Administration	Adverse Effects	Nursing Considerations
Nitroprusside (Nipride)	**Vasodilator Antihypertensive** • Relaxes vascular smooth muscle, decreasing preload (PAOP) and afterload (SVR)	• Hypertensive crisis • HF (preload and afterload reduction) • Cardiogenic shock • BP control during and after vascular surgery	• IV infusion: mix 50 mg in 250 ml (200 µg/ml) and infuse at 0.5-10 µg/kg/min • Maximum: 10 µg/kg/min • Protect from light by wrapping aluminum foil around bag or bottle; it is not necessary to foil tubing, but avoid exposure of tubing to direct sunlight	• Nausea, vomiting, abdominal pain • Headache • Tinnitus • Dizziness • Diaphoresis • Apprehension • Hypotension • Tachycardia • Palpitations • Coronary artery steal, causing myocardial ischemia and chest pain • Intrapulmonary shunt, causing hypoxemia • Methemoglobinemia with resultant reduction in SaO_2, SpO_2, and tissue oxygen delivery	• Monitor HR, BP, urine output, neurologic status • Note contraindications: known hypersensitivity • Use cautiously in liver disease, renal disease, anemia, hypovolemia, hypothyroidism, older adults • Discard solution after 24 hours • Foil bottle to protect from light • Discard solution if dark brown, blue, green, or red • Monitor for thiocyanate toxicity • Thiocyanate levels should be determined daily if drug is used longer than 72 hours • Signs of thiocyanate toxicity: metabolic acidosis, confusion, hyperreflexia, seizures • Treatment includes amyl nitrate, sodium nitrate, and/or sodium thiosulfate • Simultaneous infusion with thiosulfate with NTP may prevent thiocyanate toxicity
Norepinephrine bitartrate (Levophed)	**Sympathomimetic** • Causes vasoconstriction, which increases afterload, SVR, BP	• Severe hypotension • Vasogenic forms of shock	• IV infusion: mix 4 mg in 250 ml (16 µg/ml) and infuse at 0.5-30 µg/min; titrate to BP response • Maximum: 30 µg/min • Administer through central venous catheter if possible; if administered peripherally, use a large vein • Do not administer with alkaline solutions	• Bradycardia • Ventricular dysrhythmias • Hypertension • Anxiety • Headache • Tremor • Dizziness • Chest pain • Metabolic (lactic) acidosis • Severe vasoconstriction may cause renal or mesenteric necrosis • Local necrosis with high dosages or if infusion infiltrates	• Monitor HR, BP, ECG, urine output, neurologic status • Note contraindications: known hypersensitivity, ventricular fibrillation, tachydysrhythmias, pheochromocytoma, narrow-angle glaucoma • Use cautiously in peripheral vascular disease, hyperthyroidism, CAD, hypertension, psychoneurosis, diabetes, patient receiving MAO inhibitors or tricyclic antidepressant, and in older adults • Note that this drug may cause a fluid shift from intravascular to interstitial space causing depletion of intravascular volume • Do not use discolored solution • Prevent extravasation because necrosis may occur; treat extravasation with phentolamine (Regitine)

Continued

Drug	Classification/ Actions	Indications	Administration	Adverse Effects	Nursing Implications
Octreotide acetate (Sandostatin)	**Growth hormone suppressant; Antidiarrheal** • Suppresses secretion of serotonin, gastroenteropancreatic peptides and growth hormones • Decreases splanchnic blood flow • Stimulates fluid and electrolyte absorption from GI tract and prolongs GI transit time	• Severe diarrhea associated with carcinoid tumors or vasoactive intestinal peptide tumors • Acromegaly • GI bleeding (investigational) • GI or pancreatic fistula (investigational) • After partial pancreatectomy (Whipple procedure) (investigational)	• SC: 50-150 µg bid or tid • IV injection (for GI bleeding): 50 µg followed by IV infusion • IV infusion (for GI bleeding): 50 µg/hr for 1-5 days	• Anorexia, nausea, vomiting • Abdominal pain • Diarrhea, constipation, steatorrhea • Abdominal bloating, flatulence • Increase in liver enzymes • Anxiety • Dizziness • Drowsiness • Heartburn • Hypoglycemia or hyperglycemia • Rectal spasm	• Monitor for GI complaints and/or bleeding and serum glucose • Note contraindication: known hypersensitivity • Note that this drug is tolerated better than vasopressin for GI bleeding, especially in patients with CAD • Do not administer if precipitation or discoloration occurs
Pancuronium (Pavulon)	**Neuromuscular Blocker (nondepolarizing)** • Blocks the transmission of nerve impulses at the skeletal neuromuscular junction • Causes paralysis of all striated muscle • Does not affect consciousness, cerebration, or relieve pain	• Adjunct to mechanical ventilation when control of spontaneous ventilation is required (e.g., PEEP, hyperventilation) • Facilitation of endotracheal intubation	• IV injection: 0.04-0.10 mg/kg initially followed by 0.01 mg/kg every 1 hour or as indicated by peripheral nerve stimulation *Other neuromuscular blockers* • Vecuronium bromide (Norcuron): mix 60 mg in 250 ml (240 µg/ml); loading dosage is 80-100 µg/kg followed by 0.8-1.2 µg/kg/min • Atracurium (Tracrium): mix 300 mg in 250 ml (1.2 mg/ml): loading dose is 0.4-0.5 mg/kg followed by 5-10 µg/kg/min • Mivacurium (Mivacron): mix 200 mg in 250 ml (0.8 mg/ml); loading dose is 0.15 mg/kg followed by 8-10 µg/kg/min	• Tachycardia or bradycardia • Hypertension or hypotension • Wheezing • Residual muscle weakness • Prolonged use may make weaning difficult due to muscle reconditioning	• Monitor HR, BP, serum electrolytes (especially potassium, magnesium), inspiratory effort, and nerve stimulation • Use this drug only with intubated patients • Note contraindications: known hypersensitivity • Use cautiously in CAD, renal disease, electrolyte imbalance, neuromuscular disease, pulmonary disease • Store in refrigerator • Inform patient that paralysis is temporary and always give analgesic and/or sedative concurrently • Provide eye care with artificial tears or Lacrilube to prevent corneal abrasion since the patient cannot blink • Evaluate dose by using peripheral nerve stimulation train-of-four; 1 to 2 twitches out of four indicates sufficient but not excessive dose; if no twitches out of four, decrease dosage; if 3 to 4 twitches, increase dosage

Drug	Classification/Action	Use	Dose	Side Effects	Nursing Considerations
Pentobarbital (Nembutal)	**Barbiturate** • Causes sedation • Decreases oxygen requirements when used to induce comatose state	For intracranial hypertension • Refractory intracranial hypertension • Status epilepticus	For intracranial hypertension • IV injection: 3 mg/kg IV slowly • IV infusion: mix 2 g in 500 ml (4 mg/ml); usual dose is 1-3 mg/kg/hr For status epilepticus • IV injection: 2-8 mg/kg IV slowly • IV infusion: mix 2 g in 500 ml (4 mg/ml); usual dose is 1-3 mg/kg • Therapeutic blood level: 25-40 mg/dl	• Bradycardia • Hypotension • Rash • Agranulocytosis, thrombocytopenia, anemia • Myocardial depression; may induce HF • Respiratory depression	• Monitor HR, BP, RR, neurologic status • Note that ICP monitoring is recommended because the most important indicator of neurologic status (level of consciousness) is eliminated by induced coma • Monitor for clinical indications of heart failure • Note contraindications: known hypersensitivity, respiratory depression, liver failure, renal failure • Use cautiously in anemia, liver disease, renal disease, hypertension, older adult
Phenylephrine (Neo-Synephrine)	**Sympathomimetic** • Causes vasoconstriction • Increases BP • Increases coronary artery perfusion pressure and coronary artery blood flow	• Vasogenic shock (e.g., septic, neurogenic, anaphylactic shock) • Postoperative CABG to increase CAPP and maintain graft patency	• IV infusion: mix 10 mg in 250 ml (40 μg/ml); usual dose is 20-60 μg/min; titrated to BP response	• Reflex bradycardia • Ventricular dysrhythmias • Hypertension • Nausea, vomiting • Paresthesia • Palpitations • Anxiety • Restlessness • Headache • Tremor • Chest pain	• Monitor HR, BP, ECG • Note contraindications: known hypersensitivity, ventricular fibrillation, tachydysrhythmias, pheochromocytoma, narrow-angle glaucoma • Use cautiously in older adults and those with hyperthyroidism, CAD, hypertension, psychoneurosis, diabetes mellitus, peripheral vascular disease • Prevent extravasation as necrosis may occur; treat extravasation with phentolamine (Regitine) • Treat reflex bradycardia with atropine • Discard if discolored or precipitate present
Phenytoin sodium (Dilantin)	**Anticonvulsant; Class IB Antidysrhythmic** • Thought to stabilize neurons • Decreases sodium influx during action potential of cardiac muscle	• Seizures • Digitalis-induced dysrhythmias (Note: although phenytoin has long been considered the drug of choice for digitalis-induced ventricular dysrhythmias, many physicians prefer to use lidocaine due to the hypotensive effects of IV phenytoin)	• PO: 300 mg daily • IV loading dose: 10-20 mg/kg at 50 mg/min • Do not mix with any other drugs or dextrose; flush tubing thoroughly with saline before and after administration • Therapeutic blood level: 10-18 μg/ml	• Hypotension if given too rapidly IV • Nausea, vomiting • Headache • Confusion • Nystagmus, diplopia • Dizziness, ataxia • Skin eruptions • Gingival hyperplasia • Slurred speech • Blood dyscrasias • Toxic hepatitis • Lymphadenopathy	• Monitor HR, BP, ECG, RR and depth, and response to therapy • Note contraindications: known hypersensitivity, psychosis, bradycardia, SA or AV block, sick sinus syndrome • Use cautiously in allergy, liver disease, renal disease • Note that fosphenytoin sodium (Cerebyx) may be used instead because it is less likely to cause hypotension and dysrhythmias

Continued

Drug	Classification/ Actions	Indications	Administration	Adverse Effects	Nursing Implications
Potassium chloride	**Electrolyte** • Corrects hypokalemia	• Hypokalemia	• IV infusion: 10 mEq/ 100 ml over 1 hour if given through a catheter in a peripheral vein; 10 mEq in 50 ml over 1 hour if given through a central venous catheter • Maximum: 20 mEq/hr with close monitoring of ECG and physical condition for serum potassium <2.5 mEq/L	• Ventricular dysrhythmias • AV block • Cardiac arrest • Hyperkalemia • Phlebitis • Burning/pain at injection site	• Monitor HR, BP, ECG • Note contraindications: hyperkalemia, renal failure, dehydration • Use cautiously in heart disease, acidosis, patient receiving potassium-sparing diuretics • Monitor for clinical indications of hyperkalemia: fatigue, irritability, muscle weakness, intestinal colic, diarrhea
Procainamide hydrochloride (Pronestyl)	**Class IA Antidysrhythmic** • Increases atrial refractoriness • Decreases automaticity, conductivity, contractility • Causes peripheral vasodilation	• Supraventricular dysrhythmias • Ventricular dysrhythmias	• PO 0.5-1 g every 4-6 hours • IM 250-500 mg every 4-6 hours • IV injection: 50-100 mg every 5 minutes • Stop injections and start maintenance infusion when suppression of dysrhythmia; widening of QRS by 50%; hypotension; or a total of 17 mg/kg occur • IV infusion: mix 2 g in 500 ml (4 mg/ml) and infuse at 1-4 mg/min • Therapeutic blood level 3-10 μg/ml	• Bradycardia • Hypotension • AV block • Dysrhythmias including torsades de pointes • Anorexia, nausea, vomiting, abdominal pain, diarrhea • Hepatic dysfunction • Bitter taste • Rash, urticaria • Fever • Mental depression • Hallucinations • Seizures • Bone marrow depression, thrombocytopenia • Worsening HF • Lupuslike syndrome	• Monitor HR, BP, ECG • ECG effects include increased PR interval, QRS width, and QT interval • Note contraindications: known hypersensitivity, myasthenia gravis, AV block • Use cautiously in renal disease, liver disease, HF, respiratory depression, patient receiving digitalis • Administer PO drug with food • Instruct patient to report fever, rash, muscle pain, bruising or bleeding, diarrhea, chest pain

Drug	Action/Classification	Use	Dosage	Side Effects	Nursing Considerations
Propafenone (Rythmol)	**Class IC Antidysrhythmic** • Blocks sodium influx during phase 0, which depresses the rate of depolarization • Does not change repolarization and action potential duration	• Life-threatening or refractory ventricular dysrhythmias	• PO: 150-300 mg tid; maximum 900 mg/day	• Proarrhythmia including PVCs, ventricular tachycardia, torsades de pointes, PACs, supraventricular tachycardia, bradycardia, SA block or arrest, AV block, bundle branch block • AV block • Nausea, vomiting, constipation • Heart failure • Dyspnea, bronchospasm • Dizziness • Diplopia • Paresthesia • Headache • Bitter or metallic taste • Leukopenia, agranulocytosis, thrombocytopenia, anemia • Bruising	• Monitor HR, BP, ECG • Report widening of QRS of greater than 25% • Monitor closely for clinical indications of heart failure • Note contraindications: heart failure, cardiogenic shock, SA, AV, bifascicular blocks or sick sinus syndrome without a pacemaker, myasthenia gravis, COPD, hypotension • Use cautiously in patients with renal or liver disease; dosage may be adjusted • Use cautiously if the patient is also receiving another negative inotropic agent (e.g., verapamil, procainamide, beta-blocker) • Use cautiously in patients receiving digitalis because this drug can increase plasma concentration • Use cautiously in patients receiving oral anticoagulants because propafenone can increase plasma concentration • Administer with food to diminish GI adverse effects • Correct electrolytes prior to therapy • Instruct patient to report recurrent or persistent infection
Propofol (Diprivan)	**Anesthetic Sedative-Hypnotic** • Provides conscious or unconscious sedation • Does not have analgesic properties	• Intraoperative anesthesia • Sedation of intubated, mechanically ventilated patients	• IV infusion: premixed in 10 mg/ml concentration, infuse 5-50 µg/kg/min • Maximum: 150 µg/kg/min • Use strict aseptic technique; discard tubing and unused solution at least every 12 hours	• Bradycardia • Hypotension • Decreased cardiac output • Nausea, vomiting • Headache • Twitching • Rash • Green urine • Respiratory depression • Reactions such as agitation, hyperactivity, combativeness may occur • Burning/pain at injection site • Infection	• Monitor HR, BP, ECG, sedation level • Note that this drug allows for faster weaning process and faster time to extubation than neuromuscular paralytics • Note contraindications: known hypersensitivity to propofol or lipid emulsion, hyperlipidemia and disorders of lipid metabolism, intracranial hypertension • Use cautiously in respiratory depression, dysrhythmias, pancreatitis, hypotension, hypovolemia, and in older adult • Correct hypovolemia before administration of propofol • Administer with analgesics if indicated • Wean by reducing the rate by 5-10 µg/kg/min every 10-15 minutes; stop when patient reaches baseline consciousness and orientation

Continued

Drug	Classification/ Actions	Indications	Administration	Adverse Effects	Nursing Implications
Propranolol (Inderal)	**Noncardioselective Beta-Blocker** **Class II Antidysrhythmic** • Decreases HR, contractility, automaticity, excitability, conductivity • Depresses sinus node automaticity • Increases AV nodal refractoriness and decreases conduction velocity • Decreases myocardial oxygen consumption	• Supraventricular and ventricular dysrhythmias • Hypertension • Angina • Pheochromocytoma • Hyperthyroid crisis • Myocardial infarction (primary prevention and secondary prevention of extension and reinfarction) • Hypertrophic cardiomyopathy	• PO: 10-80 mg tid or qid • IV injection: 0.1 mg/kg in 3 divided doses at rate not to exceed 1 mg/min • IV infusion: mix 20 mg in 250 ml (0.08 mg/ml); usual dose 3-8 mg/hr • Therapeutic blood level 0.04-0.90 μg/ml	• Bradycardia • AV block • Hypotension • Nausea, vomiting, diarrhea • Fatigue, lethargy • Rash • Syncope • HF • Bronchospasm, especially in patients with asthma • Mental depression • Hyperglycemia in type 2 DM • Asymptomatic hypoglycemia in type 1 DM • Impotence • Emotional lability • Insomnia • Agranulocytosis, thrombocytopenia	• Monitor HR, BP, ECG • Monitor for clinical indications of heart failure • Note contraindications: known hypersensitivity, sinus bradycardia, AV block greater than first degree, HF, shock, asthma, Raynaud's syndrome • Use cautiously in diabetes mellitus, renal disease, hyperthyroidism, COPD, liver disease, myasthenia gravis, peripheral vascular disease, hypotension • May potentiate the hypoglycemic effects of insulin and prevents sympathetic symptoms of hypoglycemia • Note that this drug limits cardiac reserve and exercise capacity since heart rate cannot increase • Note that this drug masks sympathetic clinical indications of shock since receptors are blocked
Quinidine sulfate	**Class IA Antidysrhythmic** • Decreases automaticity, excitability, conductivity, contractility • Increases AV nodal conduction	• Supraventricular dysrhythmias • Ventricular dysrhythmias	• PO, IM: 200-400 mg every 4-6 hours • Give PO dose with food • Therapeutic blood level 2-6 μg/ml	• Dysrhythmias including torsades de pointes • Hypotension • Anorexia, nausea, vomiting, diarrhea • Hepatotoxicity • Rash • Fever • Vertigo, lightheadedness • Headache • Tinnitus • Blurred vision • HF • Hemolytic anemia, thrombocytopenia, agranulocytosis	• Monitor HR, BP, ECG • Report widening of QRS greater than 25% or prolongation of QT interval to more than half of RR interval, hypotension • Note contraindications: known hypersensitivity, blood dyscrasia, AV block, myasthenia gravis • Use cautiously in renal disease, liver disease, HF, respiratory distress, potassium imbalance, patients on digitalis • May precipitate digitalis toxicity in patients receiving digitalis • Dose should be decreased in HF and liver disease • Instruct patient to report skin rash, fever, unusual bleeding, bruising, ringing in ears, or visual disturbances

Drug	Action	Indications	Dosage	Side Effects	Nursing Considerations
Ranitidine (Zantac)	**Histamine₂-Receptor Antagonist** • Decreases gastric acid secretion • Aids in prevention of stress ulcer	• Peptic ulcer disease • Prophylaxis for patients with high potential for stress ulcer • Hyperacidity	• PO: 150 mg twice daily with 300 at bedtime • IM: 50 mg every 6-8 hours • IV injection: 50 mg slowly every 6-8 hours or 50 mg in 100 ml over 15-20 minutes • IV infusion: mix 300 mg in 250 ml (1.2 mg/ml); usual dose 6.25-12.5 mg/hr	• Dizziness • Elevated liver enzymes, hepatotoxicity • Headache • Malaise	• Monitor HR, BP, liver enzymes, gastric pH • pH is maintained 3.5 or greater • Note contraindications: known hypersensitivity • Use cautiously in liver disease, renal disease
Recombinant plasminogen activator (r-PA) reteplase (Retavase)	**Thrombolytic (may also be referred to as *fibrinolytic*)** • Converts plasminogen to plasmin at fibrin surface • Causes clot-specific lysis	• Acute myocardial infarction (chest pain strongly suggestive of acute MI; ST segment of at least 1 mm in at least 2 leads)	• IV injection of 10 U over 2 minutes initially followed by 10 U over 2 minutes after 30 minutes • Heparin administered concurrently	• Severe, spontaneous bleeding including potential cerebral, retroperitoneal, GU, GI bleeding, surface bleeding • Reperfusion dysrhythmias	• Monitor aPTT, PT, thrombin time, neurologic status, and for signs of hemorrhage • Note contraindications: active bleeding; history of cerebral hemorrhage, intracranial neoplasm, AV malformation or aneurysm; recent (within 2 months) intracranial or intraspinal surgery or trauma; known bleeding disorder; severe uncontrolled hypertension; prolonged CPR • Use cautiously in recent (within 10 days) major surgery, GI, GU bleeding, or trauma; hypertension with SBP >180 mm/Hg or DBP >110 mm/Hg; high likelihood of left heart thrombus; acute pericarditis; significant liver dysfunction; pregnancy; retinopathy; septic thrombophlebitis; advanced age (>70-75 years); patients receiving oral anticoagulants; any condition in which bleeding constitutes a significant hazard or would be particularly difficult to manage because of its location • Identify indications of reperfusion in MI • Cessation of pain • ST segments descending back to baseline • Reperfusion dysrhythmias (ventricular ectopy including PVCs, VT or VF, accelerated idioventricular rhythm, junctional escape rhythms, bradycardia) • Early CK peak

Continued

Drug	Classification/Actions	Indications	Administration	Adverse Effects	Nursing Implications
					• Limit venipuncture and urinary catheterization as possible; use IV catheter with saline lock for blood sampling; avoid noncompressible IV sites • Avoid nasotracheal and nasogastric tubes if possible • Avoid automatic BP cuffs • Administer all drugs through existing IVs started before initiation of thrombolytic therapy or by mouth • Monitor oral secretions, sputum, vomitus, NG aspirate, stool, urine for blood • Bleeding precautions are maintained for 12-24 hours

Recombinant tissue plasminogen activator (rt-PA) alteplase (Activase)	**Thrombolytic (may also be referred to as fibrinolytic)**
	• Converts plasminogen to plasmin at fibrin surface
	• Causes clot-specific lysis
		• Acute myocardial infarction (chest pain strongly suggestive of acute MI; ST segment of at least 1 mm in at least 2 leads)
		• Massive pulmonary embolus (with RVF or refractory hypoxemia)
		• Thrombotic stroke
			For acute MI
			• IV injection: 15 mg followed by:
			• IV infusion: 0.75 mg/kg (not to exceed 50 mg) over next 30 minutes, followed by 0.5 mg/kg (not to exceed 35 mg) over the next 60 minutes
			• Heparin started within 1 hour of initial dose
			For acute pulmonary embolism
			• IV infusion: 100 mg at 50 mg/hr for 2 hours
			For thrombotic stroke
			• Total dose: 0.9 mg/kg with maximum dose of ≤90 mg
			• IV injection: 10% of this total dose over 1 minute followed by:
			• IV infusion: remaining 90% of this total dose administer over 60 minutes
				• Severe, spontaneous bleeding including potential cerebral, retroperitoneal, GU, GI bleeding, surface bleeding
				• Reperfusion dysrhythmias
					• Monitor aPTT, PT, thrombin time, neurologic status, and for signs of hemorrhage
					• Note contraindications: active bleeding; history of cerebral hemorrhage, intracranial neoplasm, AV malformation or aneurysm; recent (within 2 months) intracranial or intraspinal surgery or trauma; known bleeding disorder; severe uncontrolled hypertension; prolonged CPR
					• Use cautiously in recent (within 10 days) major surgery, GI, GU bleeding, or trauma; hypertension with SBP >180 mm Hg or DBP >110 mm/Hg; high likelihood of left heart thrombus; acute pericarditis; significant liver dysfunction; pregnancy; retinopathy; septic thrombophlebitis; advanced age (>70-75 years); patients receiving oral anticoagulants; any condition in which bleeding constitutes a significant hazard or would be particularly difficult to manage because of its location
					• Monitor for indications of reperfusion in MI
					  • Cessation of pain
					  • ST segments descending back to baseline

		• Reperfusion dysrhythmias (ventricular ectopy including PVCs, VT or VF, accelerated idioventricular rhythm, junctional escape rhythms, bradycardia) • Early CK peak • Note that signs of reperfusion are much more subtle in PE and thrombotic stroke • Limit venipuncture and urinary catheterization as possible; use IV catheter with saline lock for blood sampling; avoid noncompressible IV sites • Administer all drugs through existing IVs started before initiation of thrombolytic therapy or by mouth • Avoid nasotracheal and nasogastric tubes if possible • Avoid automatic BP cuffs • Monitor oral secretions, sputum, vomitus, NG aspirate, stool, urine for blood • Bleeding precautions are maintained for 12-24 hours
	• Anticoagulants and platelet aggregation inhibitors are not used for at least 24 hours • Reconstitution in sterile water only	
Sodium bicarbonate	**Metabolic Buffer** • Combines with free hydrogen acid to neutralize acid	• Metabolic acidosis with pH of 7.0 or less • Myoglobinuria, hemoglobinuria • Overdose of tricyclic antidepressants	• IV injection: 1 mEq/kg as initial dose; dose guided by arterial blood gases • Administer through a large peripheral vein or a central venous catheter • Do not administer with catecholamines (e.g., epinephrine, dopamine, isoproterenol, norepinephrine)	• Sodium and water retention • Metabolic alkalosis • Shift of oxyhemoglobin dissociation curve to the left making it more difficult for hemoglobin and oxygen to dissociate at the tissue level • Hypokalemia caused by shift back into the cell • Hypocalcemia caused by the change in the binding between calcium and albumin • Increased CO_2 production potentially causing worsening of respiratory acidosis	• Monitor ABGs, pH, respiratory rate, serum electrolytes • Note contraindications: hypertension, peptic ulcer, renal disease, hypocalcemia, hypokalemia • Use cautiously in HF, liver disease, toxemia, renal disease • Note that bicarbonate is given today only as absolutely necessary; treatment of metabolic acidosis should focus on treatment of cause (e.g., improve oxygenation and perfusion for lactic acidosis, insulin for diabetic ketoacidosis, dialysis for renal failure, etc.)

Continued

Drug	Classification/ Actions	Indications	Administration	Adverse Effects	Nursing Implications
Sotalol (Betapace)	**Class II and III Antidysrhythmic** • Depresses SA node automaticity • Increases refractory period of atrial and AV junctional tissue to slow conduction • Shortens action potential duration • Inhibits sympathetic activity • Blocks potassium movement during phase III • Increases action potential duration • Prolongs effective refractory period	• Life-threatening or refractory ventricular dysrhythmias	• PO: initial 80 mg bid followed by 160-320 mg/day divided into two to three doses	• Proarrhythmia including torsades de pointes, sinus bradycardia; second- or third-degree AV block • Heart failure • Hypotension • Dyspnea • Bronchospasm (especially in patients with history of asthma) • Headache	• Monitor HR, BP, ECG • Report prolongation of QT interval to more than half of RR interval or hypotension • Monitor serum glucose in patients with DM • Monitor closely for clinical indications of heart failure • Note contraindications: second- or third-degree AV block, SA block without pacemaker • Do not administer concurrently or within 4 hours of class IA antiarrhythmics or other class III antiarrhythmics; do not administer with other drugs that prolong the QT interval such as phenothiazines, tricyclic antidepressants • Correct electrolytes prior to therapy • Warn patient not to discontinue abruptly
Streptokinase (Streptase)	**Thrombolytic** • Activates plasminogen systemically and converts it to plasmin, which then degrades fibrin clots, fibrinogen, and other plasma proteins • Causes systemic lytic state	• Acute MI • Pulmonary embolism • Acute arterial thromboembolism	IV: mix 1.5 million U in 250 ml (6000 U/ml) • For acute MI usual loading dose 750,000 IV injection followed by 750,000 U IV infusion over next hour • For PE, arterial thromboembolism usual loading dose 250,000 over 30 minutes followed by 100,000 U/hr for up to 72 hours	• Allergic reaction (angioneurotic edema, pruritus, dyspnea, bronchospasm, dyspnea, hypotension, cyanosis, seizures, loss of consciousness) • Severe spontaneous bleeding • Cerebral, retroperitoneal, GU, GI, surface bleeding • Reperfusion dysrhythmias	• Monitor aPTT, PT, thrombin time, neurologic status, and for signs of hemorrhage • Note contraindications: patients who have had recent streptococcal infection or streptokinase within 6 months to 5 years • Note that indications in MI, contraindications, cautions, and signs of reperfusion after use for MI are as for tPA • Administer diphenhydramine (Benadryl) and hydrocortisone sodium succinate (Solu-Cortef) if chance of allergic reaction • Limit venipuncture and urinary catheterization as possible; use IV catheter with saline lock for blood sampling; avoid noncompressible IV sites • Administer all drugs through existing IVs started before initiation of thrombolytic therapy or by mouth • Avoid nasotracheal and nasogastric tubes if possible

Drug	Action/Use	Dosage	Side Effects	Nursing Considerations
				• Avoid automatic BP cuffs • Monitor oral secretions, sputum, vomitus, NG aspirate, stool, urine for blood • Maintain bleeding precautions for 48-72 hours due to fibrinogen depletion seen with streptokinase
Terbutaline sulfate (Brethine)	**Sympathomimetic Bronchodilator (Beta$_2$ Specific)** • Relaxes smooth muscle of bronchi	• PO: 2.5-5 mg/8 hr • Subcutaneous 0.25-0.5 mg/4 hr • Inhalation: 0.25-1 mg in 3 ml of normal saline	• Tachycardia • Palpitations • Nausea, vomiting • Anxiety • Tremor • Headache	• Monitor HR, BP, breath sounds • Note contraindications: known hypersensitivity, glaucoma, tachydysrhythmias; do not give with MAO inhibitors • Use cautiously in diabetes mellitus, hypertension, hyperthyroidism, cardiac disease, seizure disorder, prostatic hypertrophy • Do not administer with beta-blockers (they block effect)
Tirofiban HCl (Aggrastat)	**Platelet aggregation inhibitor (GP IIb/IIIa platelet receptor blocker)** • Inhibits platelet aggregation and platelet-mediated thrombosis	• Acute coronary syndrome with or without PCI	• Bleeding • Intracranial hemorrhage • Hematuria • Hematemesis • Bleeding at sheath site • Hypotension • Bradycardia • Pelvic pain	• IV infusion: premixed as 25 mg in 500 ml; usual dose is 0.4 μg/kg/min for 30 minutes and then continued at 0.1 μg/kg/min • Monitor PT, aPTT, or ACT, platelet count • Note contraindications: active internal bleeding, clinically significant bleeding in the GI or GU tract within the last 6 weeks, bleeding diathesis, history of CVA within the last two years or CVA with significant residual neurologic deficit, intracranial neoplasm, aneurysm, or AV malformation, severe uncontrolled hypertension, oral anticoagulants within 7 days unless prothrombin time is less than 1.2 × control, thrombocytopenia, presumed or documented history of vasculitis, major surgery or trauma within the last month, pericarditis, known hypersensitivity to tirofiban • Use cautiously in patients who weigh less than 75 kg, patients older than 65 years of age, patients with a history of GI disease, patients receiving thrombolytics, patients with thrombocytopenia • Administer with aspirin and heparin therapy as prescribed • Limit venipuncture and urinary catheterization as possible; use IV catheter with saline lock for blood sampling; avoid noncompressible IV sites • Monitor oral secretions, sputum, vomitus, NG aspirate, stool, urine for blood

Continued

Drug	Classification/ Actions	Indications	Administration	Adverse Effects	Nursing Implications
Tocainide (Tonocard)	**Class IB Antidys-rhythmic** • Blocks sodium influx during phase 0, which depresses the rate of depolarization • Shortens repolarization and action potential duration • Suppresses ventricular automaticity in ischemic tissue	• Ventricular dysrhythmias	• PO: initial dose of 600 mg; then 400 mg bid or tid; maximum 2400 mg/day	• Proarrhythmia including PVCs, ventricular tachycardia, torsades de pointes, PACs, supraventricular tachycardia, bradycardia, SA block or arrest, AV block, bundle branch block • Hypotension • Palpitations • Anorexia, nausea, vomiting, diarrhea, abdominal pain • Chest pain • Diaphoresis • Pulmonary fibrosis (dyspnea, cough, wheezing) • Mood changes • Headache • Dizziness • Paresthesias, tremors • Confusion • Diplopia, blurred vision • Seizures • Coma • Rash • Fever, chills • Thrombocytopenia, aplastic anemia, agranulocytosis	• Monitor HR, BP, ECG • Note contraindications: second- or third-degree block or sick sinus syndrome without pacemaker and patients with a history of allergic reactions to local amide type anesthetics • Use cautiously in older adults and patients with heart failure • Administer with meals to decrease GI adverse effects • Note that risk of toxicity is greater if patient is concurrently receiving cimetidine (Tagamet) or beta-blocker • Note that dosage is adjusted in heart failure or liver disease • Instruct patient to report dyspnea or cough (may indicate pulmonary fibrosis) or excessive bruising (may indicate thrombocytopenia) or frequent or unresponsive infection (may indicate agranulocytosis)
Vasopressin (Pitressin)	**Posterior Pituitary Hormone: Antidiuretic Hormone** • Reduces portal venous pressure through vasoconstriction • Increases water reabsorption in the renal tubule	• Upper GI hemorrhage • Diabetes insipidus	For GI hemorrhage • IV infusion: mix 100 U/100 ml (1 U/ml) and administer at 0.1-0.8 U/min (concurrent NTG is recommended with doses higher than 0.4 U/min) • Maximum: 0.9 U/min For DI • Aqueous vasopressin 5-10 U SC 2 to 3 times daily or 3 U/hr IV • Vasopressin in oil 5 U deep IM • Lypressin or DDAVP given by nasal spray	• Bradycardia • Hypertension • Fever • Water intoxication (SIADH), hyponatremia • Nausea, abdominal cramps • Tremor • Headache • Seizures • Coma • Constriction of cardiac arteries, resulting in chest pain and myocardial ischemia	• Monitor HR, BP, urine output, daily weight, serum sodium • Note contraindications: known hypersensitivity, nephritis • Use cautiously in coronary artery disease • Administer NTG as prescribed concurrently with IV vasopressin infusion to prevent potential complications related to cardiac ischemia • Prevent extravasation because necrosis may occur; treat extravasation with phentolamine (Regitine)

Drug	Classification/Action	Use	Dosage	Side Effects	Nursing Implications
Verapamil (Calan)	**Calcium Channel Blocker** **Class IV Antidysrhythmic** • Depresses rate of SA node • Increases refractoriness of AV node • Relaxes vascular smooth muscle decreasing SVR, BP	• Supraventricular dysrhythmias • Angina • Hypertension • Hypertrophic cardiomyopathy	• PO: 40-120 mg every 6 hours • IV injection: 0.075-0.15 mg/kg (5-10 mg); may be repeated in 15-30 minutes at 5-10 mg • Maximum: 20 mg • IV infusion: mix 50 mg in 250 ml (200 µg/ml); usual dose is 1-5 µg/kg/min • Therapeutic blood level 0.1-0.15 µg/ml	• Bradycardia • AV block • Hypotension • Nausea • Constipation or diarrhea • Elevated liver enzymes • Headache • Dizziness • Heart failure	• Monitor HR, BP, ECG, liver function studies, breath sounds, heart sounds • Note contraindications: known hypersensitivity, AV block, sick sinus syndrome, WPW, advanced HF, cardiogenic shock • Use cautiously in HF, hypotension, liver disease, renal disease, patients receiving digitalis or beta-blockers • Do not give concurrently with IV beta-blockers • Administer calcium (500 mg-1 g IV over 10 minutes) as prescribed prior to IV verapamil to prevent hypotension

Warfarin (Coumadin, Panwarfin)	**Anticoagulant**
	• Depresses synthesis of prothrombin by the liver
	• Prevents extension of clot and secondary thromboembolic complications
		• Deep vein thrombosis
		• Valvular heart disease
		• Atrial dysrhythmias
		• Postvalve replacement
			• PO: 2-10 mg daily depending on PT and international normalized ratio (INR)
			• INR 2.0-3.0
			  • MI
			  • DVT prophylaxis or treatment
			  • Pulmonary embolus
			  • Valvular heart disease
			  • Atrial fibrillation
			  • Tissue heart valve
			• INR 2.5-3.5
			  • Mechanical heart valve
				• Hemorrhage with excessive PT
				• Agranulocytosis, leukopenia
				• Hepatitis
				• Diarrhea
				• Fever
				• Rash
					• Monitor PT and for signs of hemorrhage
					• Note contraindications: known hypersensitivity, bleeding disorders, leukemia, peptic ulcer disease, liver disease, severe hypertension, endocarditis, acute nephritis, blood dyscrasias, eclampsia, suspected intracranial hemorrhage, open wounds, recent surgery, threatened abortion
					• Use cautiously in alcoholism, pregnancy, lactation, during menses, during use of any drainage tube, older adult, or in any patient in whom slight bleeding is dangerous
					• Ensure that vitamin K (AquaMephyton) is available
					• Avoid IM, arterial, or venous punctures if at all possible
					• Hold pressure for longer than usual if punctures necessary
					• Monitor oral secretions, sputum, vomitus, NG aspirate, stool, urine for blood
					• Do not discontinue suddenly
					• Teach patient to avoid trauma and increased amounts of vitamin K (green leafy vegetables), and how to monitor for bleeding
					• Teach the patient to report fever or rash; usually necessitates discontinuance

Bibliography and Selected References

Beyea S, Nicoll L: Back to basics: administering IM injections the right way, *AJN* 96 (1):34, 1996.

Bleck T: Thrombolysis for acute ischemic stroke: how, when—and why, *Journal of Critical Illness* 11 (10):645, 1996.

Bode C, et al.: Randomized comparison of coronary thrombolysis achieved with double-bolus reteplase (recombinant plasminogen activator) and front-loaded, accelerated alteplase (recombinant tissue plasminogen activator) in patients with acute myocardial infarction, *Circulation* 94 (5):891, 1996.

Brenner Z, Cannito M: Administering steroids successfully, *Nursing98* 28 (3):34, 1998.

Califf R et al: One-year results from the global utilization of streptokinase and TPA for occluded coronary arteries (GUSTO-I) trial, *Circulation* 94 (6):1233, 1996.

Chernow B, (Ed.): *The pharmacologic approach to the critically ill patient,* ed 3, Baltimore, 1994, Williams & Wilkins.

Covington H: Use of propofol for sedation in the ICU, *Critical Care Nurse* 18 (4):34, 1998.

Edwards J: Guarding against adverse drug events, *AJN* 97 (5):26, 1997.

Elder A: Adenosine: putting the brakes on SVT, *Nursing96* 26 (10):32aa, 1996.

Fette C, Enger E: Using amiodarone to tame cardiac arrhythmias, *Nursing96* 26 (3):32y, 1996.

Futterman L, Lemberg L: Amiodarone: a late comer, *Am J Crit Care* 6 (3):233, 1997.

Futterman L, Lemberg L: Low-molecular-weight heparin: an antithrombotic agent whose time has come, *Am J Crit Care* 8 (1):520, 1999.

Gahart B, Nazareno A: *1999 intravenous medications,* St Louis, 1999, Mosby.

Gregory S, Stockman L: Reducing the risks from postprocedure anticoagulation therapy, *Nursing97* 27 (8):32cc1, 1997.

Gysi J, Smull E: Speeding thrombolytic therapy, *Nursing97* 27 (5):32cc15, 1997.

Hadley S, Chang M, Rogers K: Effect of syringe size on bruising following subcutaneous heparin injection, *Am J Crit Care* 5 (4):271, 1996.

Halloran T, Pohlman A: Managing sedation in the critically ill patient, *Critical Care Nurse* August Supplement, 1995.

Harvey M: Managing agitation in critically ill patients, *Am J Crit Care* 5 (1):7, 1996.

Hock, N: Neuroprotective and thrombolytic agents: advances in stroke treatment, *J Neurosci Nurs* 30 (3):175, 1998.

Holcomb S: Understanding the ins and outs of diuretic therapy, *Nursing97* 27 (2):34, 1997.

Holcomb S: When beta-blockers aren't the drug of choice, *Nursing96* 26 (10):32dd, 1996.

Hutt N: Fosphenytoin for seizure control, *AJN* 99 (3):52, 1999.

Jerdee A: Heparin-associated thrombocytopenia: nursing implications, *Critical Care Nurse* 18 (6):38, 1998.

Kleinpell R et al: Use of peripheral nerve stimulators to monitor patients with neuromuscular blockade in the ICU, *Am J Crit Care* 5 (6):449, 1996.

Konick-McMahan J: Full speed ahead—with caution: pushing intravenous medications, *Nursing96* 26 (6):26, 1996.

Kost M: Conscious sedation—guarding your patient against complications, *Nursing99* 29 (4):34, 1999.

Kress J, et al: Sedating critically ill ventilated patients: a pharmacologic primer, *Journal of Critical Illness* 12 (5):287, 1997.

Lechner D: Sizing up your patients for heparin therapy, *Nursing98* 28 (8):36, 1998.

Lilley L, Guanci R: Neuromuscular blocking agents, *AJN* 97 (2):12, 1997.

Maljanian R, Quintiliani R: When once is enough—administering aminoglycosides effectively, *Nursing99* 29 (5):41, 1999.

Mayer D, Docktor W: Abciximab, a novel platelet-blocking drug: pharmacology and nursing implications, *Critical Care Nurse* 18 (2):29, 1998.

McCaffery M: Analgesics: mapping out pain relief, *Nursing96* 26 (1):41, 1996.

McCaffery M: How to make the most of nonopioid analgesics, *Nursing98* 28 (8):54, 1998.

McConnell E: Applying transdermal ointments, *Nursing98* 28 (10):30, 1998.

Pill M: Ibutilide: a new antiarrhythmic agent for the critical care environment, *Critical Care Nurse* 17 (3):19, 1997.

Seversen A, Baldwin L, DeLoughery T: International normalized ratio in anticoagulant therapy: understanding the issues, *Am J Crit Care* 6 (2):88, 1997.

Shawgo T, York N: Preoperative versus postoperative weights: Which one should be used for cardiac surgery patients' drug and hemodynamic calculations? *Critical Care Nurse* 19 (5):57, 1999.

Shirrell D, et al.: Understanding therapeutic drug monitoring, *AJN* 99 (1):42, 1999.

Sparks K: Are you up to date on weight-based heparin dosing? *AJN* 96 (4):33, 1996.

Strimike C, Wojcik J: Administering abciximab: a new drug for preventing coronary restenosis, *Nursing97* 27 (2):32aa, 1997.

Strimike C, Wojcik J: Stopping atrial fibrillation with ibutilide, *AJN* 98 (1):32, 1998.

Vitello J, et al.: Management of sedation: the nursing perspective, *Critical Care Nurse* August Supplement, 1996.

Wagner B, O'Hara D, Hammond J: Drugs for amnesia in the ICU, *Am J Crit Care* 6 (3):192, 1997.

Wait J, Karpel J: Managing acute respiratory failure in asthma: pharmacotherapy, *Journal of Critical Illness* 13 (7):440, 1998.

Wallace C: Nitroglycerin tolerance, *AJN* 98 (11):16CC, 1998.

Weissman C: Current strategies for providing short-term sedation in the ICU, *Journal of Critical Illness* 11 (4):225, 1996.

Woodin L: Resting easy—how to care for patients receiving IV conscious sedation, *Nursing96* 26 (6):33, 1996.

Index

Page numbers in *italic* indicate illustrations; page
numbers followed by *t* indicate tables.